Michael Reiners
7/30/97

Practical
Neurology

José Biller, MD

Professor and Chairman,
Department of Neurology,
Indiana University School of Medicine,
Chief, Neurology Services,
Department of Neurology,
Indiana University Medical Center, Indianapolis

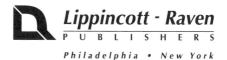

Lippincott - Raven
P U B L I S H E R S
Philadelphia • New York

Acquisitions Editor: Mark Placito
Manufacturing Manager: Dennis Teston
Production Manager: Bernie Richey
Production Editor: Julie Sullivan
Cover Designer: Karen Quigley
Indexer: AlphaByte, Inc.
Compositor: Compset, Inc.

Printed in the United States of America

9 8 7 6 5 4 3 2 1

Library of Congress Cataloging-in-Publication Data

Practical neurology / [edited by] José Biller.
     p.   cm.
   Includes bibliographical references and index.
   ISBN 0-316-09483-8
   1. Neurology.   I. Biller, José.
   [DNLM: 1. Nervous System Diseases—diagnosis.   2. Nervous System
Diseases—therapy.   3. Primary Health Care.   WL 141 P895 1997]
RC346.P685   1997
618.8—DC21
DNLM/DLC
For Library of Congress   97-4327
                                                              CIP

Contents

Contributing Authors

Harold P. Adams, Jr., MD

Professor, Department of Neurology, University of Iowa College of Medicine, Iowa City; Director, Division of Cerebrovascular Diseases, University of Iowa Hospitals and Clinics, Iowa City

John C. Andrefsky, MD

Assistant Director, Neuromedical/ Neurosurgical Intensive Care, The Cleveland Clinic Foundation, Cleveland

Martin J. Arron, MD

Assistant Professor of Medicine, Associate Division Chief, Division of General Internal Medicine, Northwestern University Medical School, Chicago; Associate Staff, Department of Medicine, Northwestern Memorial Hospital, Chicago

Birgitte H. Bendixen, MD, PhD

Assistant Professor, Department of Neurology, University of Iowa College of Medicine, Iowa City; Staff Physician, Division of Cerebrovascular Diseases, University of Iowa Hospitals and Clinics, Iowa City

José Biller, MD

Professor and Chairman, Department of Neurology, Indiana University School of Medicine, Indianapolis; Chief, Neurology Services, Department of Neurology, Indiana University Medical Center, Indianapolis

Randall L. Braddom, MD, MS

Professor and Chairman, Department of Physical Medicine and Rehabilitation, Indiana University School of Medicine, Indianapolis; Medical Director, Hook Rehabilitation Center Community Hospitals, Indianapolis

Allison Brashear, MD

Assistant Professor, Department of Neurology, Indiana University School of Medicine, Indianapolis; Staff Neurologist, Department of Neurology, Indiana University Medical Center, Indianapolis

Paul W. Brazis, MD

Consultant and Associate Professor, Department of Neurology and Ophthalmology, Mayo Clinic-Jacksonville, Jacksonville, Florida

Askiel Bruno, MD

Associate Professor, Department of Neurology, Indiana University School of Medicine, Indianapolis; Staff Neurologist, Department of Neurology, Indiana University Medical Center, Indianapolis

Bruce A. Cohen, MD
Associate Professor, Department of Neurology, Northwestern University Medical School, Chicago; Attending Physician, Department of Neurology, Northwestern Memorial Hospital, Chicago

James J. Corbett, MD
Professor of Neurology and Ophthalmology, Department of Neurology and Ophthalmology, University of Mississippi, Jackson; Chairman, Department of Neurology, University Medical Center, Jackson, Mississippi

James R. Couch, Jr., MD, PhD
Professor and Chairman, Department of Neurology, University of Oklahoma Health Sciences Center, Oklahoma City

Edward C. Daly, MD, PhD
Assistant Professor, Department of Neurology, Indiana University School of Medicine, Indianapolis; Staff Neurologist, Department of Neurology, Roudebush VA Medical Center, Indianapolis

Kathleen B. Digre, MD
Associate Professor, Department of Neurology and Ophthalmology, University of Utah Medical School, Salt Lake City; Director of Neuro-Ophthalmology, University of Utah Medical School, Salt Lake City

David W. Dunn, MD
Associate Professor, Departments of Neurology and Psychiatry, Indiana University School of Medicine, Indianapolis; Staff, Child Neurology and Psychology, Departments of Neurology and Psychiatry, Indiana University Medical Center, Indianapolis

André Durocher, MD, FRCP (C)
Staff Neurologist, Sciences Neurologiques, Hôpital Saint-Luc, Montreal, Quebec, Canada

Mark Eric Dyken, MD
Assistant Professor, Department of Neurology, University of Iowa College of Medicine, Iowa City; Director, Department of Neurology Sleep Disorders Center, University of Iowa Hospitals and Clinics, Iowa City

Rodger J. Elble, MD, PhD
Professor and Chairman, Department of Neurology, Southern Illinois University School of Medicine, Springfield; Director, Center for Alzheimer Disease and Related Disorders, Southern Illinois University School of Medicine, Springfield, Illinois

Martin R. Farlow, MD
Professor and Vice-Chairman for Research, Department of Neurology, Indiana University School of Medicine, Indianapolis; Staff Neurologist, Department of Neurology, Indiana University Medical Center, Indianapolis

Ann Ficco-D'Orazio, MS, CCC-SLP

Instructor, Department of Otorhinolaryngology, Division of Speech Pathology, University of Pennsylvania Medical School, Philadelphia; Supervisor of Speech Pathology, Department of Otorhinolaryngology, Division of Speech Pathology, University of Pennsylvania Medical Center, Philadelphia

Jeffrey I. Frank, MD

Director, Neuromedical/Neurosurgical Intensive Care, The Cleveland Clinic Foundation, Cleveland

Bhuwan P. Garg, MD

Professor, Department of Neurology, Indiana University School of Medicine, Indianapolis; Director, Section of Pediatric Neurology, Riley Hospital for Children, Indianapolis

Julius M. Goodman, MD

Chairman, Department of Neuroscience, Methodist Hospital of Indiana, Indianapolis; Clinical Professor, Section of Neurological Surgery, Indiana University School of Medicine, Indianapolis

Neill R. Graff-Radford, MB, BCh, MRCP (UK)

Professor, Department of Neurology, Mayo Medical School, Rochester, Minnesota; Chair, Department of Neurology, Mayo Clinic, Jacksonville, Florida

David Lee Gordon, MD

Associate Professor, Department of Neurology, University of Mississippi Medical Center Jackson; Director, Acute Stroke Unit, University Hospitals and Clinics, Jackson, Mississippi

Gregory Gruener, MD

Associate Professor of Clinical Neurology, Department of Neurology, Stritch School of Medicine, Maywood, Illinois; Attending Physician, Department of Neurology, Loyola University Medical Center, Maywood, Illinois

Timothy C. Hain, MD

Associate Professor, Departments of Neurology and Otolaryngology, Northwestern University Medical School, Chicago; Director, Vestibular Laboratory, Northwestern Memorial Hospital, Chicago

Aki Kawasaki, MD

Director of Research and Assistant Director of Neuro-Ophthalmology Clinic, Midwest Eye Institute, Indianapolis; Clinical Assistant Professor, Departments of Neurology and Ophthalmology, Indiana University School of Medicine, Indianapolis

John Collins Kincaid, MD

Associate Professor of Neurology, Indiana University School of Medicine, Indianapolis; Director of EMG Laboratories, Indiana University Hospitals, Indianapolis

Molly Kathleen King, MD

Assistant Professor, Department of Neurology, University of New Mexico School of Medicine, Albuquerque; Assistant Professor, Department of Neurology, Veterans Administration Medical Center, Albuquerque

Oldrich J. Kolar, MD

Professor, Department of Neurology, Indiana University School of Medicine, Indianapolis; Staff Physician, Department of Neurology, Indiana University Medical Center, Indianapolis

Marian P. LaMonte, MD, MSN

Assistant Professor, Department of Neurology, University of Maryland, Baltimore; Neurological Program Director, The Maryland Brain Attack Center, University of Maryland Hospital, Baltimore

Margaret A. Laycock, MD

Assistant Professor, Department of Neurology, Indiana University School of Medicine, Indianapolis; Staff, Department of Neurology, Indiana University Medical Center, Indianapolis

David Lefkowitz, MD

Associate Professor, Department of Neurology, Bowman Gray School of Medicine, Winston-Salem, North Carolina; Staff, Neurology Service, North Carolina Baptist Hospital, Winston-Salem, North Carolina

Bertrand C. Liang, MD

Assistant Professor, Department of Neurology, Medicine (Medical Oncology) and Pathology, University of Colorado, Denver; Neurologist, Neuro-Oncology Division, University of Colorado Cancer Center, Denver

Diane M. Liang, RN

Nurse, Department of Pediatrics, Aurora Pediatrics Associates, Aurora, Colorado

Jeri A. Logemann, PhD

Ralph and Jean Sundin Professor, Communication Sciences and Disorders, Department of Neurology and Otolaryngology, Northwestern University, Chicago; Associate Staff, Department of Neurology and Otolaryngology, Northwestern Memorial Hospital, Chicago

Betsy B. Love, MD

Assistant Professor, Department of Neurology, University of Iowa College of Medicine, Iowa City; Staff Physician, Division of Cerebrovascular Diseases and Clinical Outreach Program, University of Iowa Hospitals and Clinics, Iowa City

Kevin Edward Macadaeg, MD

Clinical Assistant Professor, Department of Anesthesiology, Indiana University School of Medicine, Indianapolis; Chronic Pain Specialist, Indiana Neurosurgical Associates, Indianapolis

Raúl N. Mandler, MD

Associate Professor, Department of Neurology, University of New Mexico Health Sciences Center, Albuquerque; Attending Neurologist and Electromyographer, and Director of Neuromuscular Program and MDA and ALS Clinics, Department of Neurology, University Hospitals of New Mexico, Albuquerque

Omkar N. Markand, MD

Professor, Department of Neurology, Indiana University School of Medicine, Indianapolis; Director, EEG/Epilepsy Section, Department of Neurology, Indiana University Medical Center, Indianapolis

Gary J. Martin, MD

Associate Professor of Medicine and Chief, Division of General Internal Medicine, Northwestern University Medical School, Chicago; Attending Physician, Department of Medicine, Northwestern Memorial Hospital, Chicago

Bette G. Maybury, MD

Clinical Assistant Professor, Department of Neurology, Indiana University School of Medicine, Indianapolis; Staff, Department of Neurology, Indiana University Medical Center, Indianapolis

Michael P. McQuillen, MD, MA

Professor of Neurology, Department of Neurology, University of Rochester School of Medicine and Dentistry, Rochester; Chief of Neurology, Department of Medicine, St. Mary's Hospital, Rochester, New York

Galen W. Mitchell, MD

Assistant Professor, Department of Neurology, University of Alabama College of Medicine, Birmingham, Alabama

Richard T. Miyamoto, MD

Arilla Apence DeVault Professor and Chairman, Department of Otolaryngology–Head and Neck Surgery, Indiana University School of Medicine, Indianapolis; Staff Physician, Department of Otolaryngology–Head and Neck Surgery, Indiana University Medical Center, Indianapolis

Catherine S. Mueller, RN, BNS

Neurology Outreach Nurse Coordinator, Joint Office of Clinical Outreach Services and Contracting for Patient Care, University of Iowa Hospitals and Clinics, Iowa City

Paul B. Nelson, MD

Professor and Chairman, Section of Neurological Surgery, Indiana University School of Medicine, Indianapolis; Chief of Neurosurgery, Indiana University Medical Center, Indianapolis

Robert M. Pascuzzi, MD	Professor and Vice Chairman, Department of Neurology, Indiana University School of Medicine, Indianapolis; Chief, Wishard Hospital Section, Department of Neurology, Wishard Memorial Hospital, Indianapolis
Hema Patel, MD	Clinical Assistant Professor, Department of Neurology, Section of Pediatric Neurology, Indiana University School of Medicine, Indianapolis; Child Neurologist, Department of Neurology, Section of Pediatric Neurology, Indiana University Medical Center, Indianapolis
Rahman Pourmand, MD	Associate Professor, Department of Neurology, Indiana University School of Medicine, Indianapolis; Staff Neurologist, Wishard Hospital Section, Department of Neurology, Wishard Memorial Hospital, Indianapolis
Eric Corey Raps, MD	William N. Kelley Associate Professor of Neurology, Department of Neurology, University of Pennsylvania School of Medicine, Philadelphia; Director, Division of Stroke and Neuro-Intensive Care, University of Pennsylvania Medical Center, Philadelphia
R. Venkata Reddy, MD	Associate Professor, Department of Neurology, Indiana University School of Medicine, Indianapolis; Consultant, Chronic Pain Management, Department of Neurology, Roudebush VA Medical Center, Indianapolis
Robert L. Rodnitzky, MD	Professor and Vice-Chairman, Department of Neurology, University of Iowa College of Medicine, Iowa City; Staff Neurologist, Department of Neurology, University of Iowa Hospitals and Clinics, Iowa City
Karen L. Roos, MD	Professor, Department of Neurology, Indiana University School of Medicine, Indianapolis; Staff Neurologist, Wishard Memorial Hospital, Indianapolis
Mark A. Ross, MD	Associate Professor, Department of Neurology, University of Iowa College of Medicine, Iowa City; Director, Neuromuscular Division and EMG Laboratory, Department of Neurology, University of Iowa Hospitals and Clinics, Iowa City
Jack M. Rozental, MD, PhD	Associate Professor, Department of Neurology, Northwestern University Medical School, Chicago; Chief, Neurology Service, VA Lakeside Medical Center, Chicago; Director, Medical Neuro-Oncology, Northwestern Memorial Hospital, Chicago

Frank A. Rubino, MD

Professor, Department of Neurology, Mayo Graduate School of Medicine, Rochester, Minnesota; Consultant, Department of Neurology, St. Luke's Hospital, Jacksonville, Florida

Vicenta Salanova, MD

Associate Professor of Neurology, Department of Neurology, Indiana University School of Medicine, Indianapolis; Staff Neurologist, Department of Neurology, Indiana University Medical Center, Indianapolis

Jeffrey L. Saver, MD

Assistant Professor, Department of Neurology, University of California School of Medicine, Los Angeles; Attending Physician, Neurobehavior Program, UCLA Medical Center, Los Angeles

Scott A. Shapiro, MD

Associate Professor of Neurosurgery, Section of Neurological Surgery, Indiana University School of Medicine, Indianapolis; Chief of Neurosurgery, Wishard Memorial Hospital, Indianapolis

Eric Siemers, MD

Clinical Associate Professor, Department of Neurology, Indiana University School of Medicine, Indianapolis; Director, Movement Disorder Clinic, Indiana University Medical Center, Indianapolis

Buckley terPenning, MD

Assistant Professor of Radiology/Nuclear Medicine, Department of Radiology, Uniformed Services University of the Health Sciences, Bethesda; Interventional Neuroradiologist, Department of Radiology, National Naval Medical Center, Bethesda, Maryland

Daniel Tranel, PhD

Professor, Department of Neurology, University of Iowa College of Medicine, Iowa City; Chief, Benton Neuropsychology Laboratory, University of Iowa Hospitals and Clinics, Iowa City

Bradley Todd Troost, MD

Professor and Chairman, Department of Neurology, The Bowman Gray School of Medicine, Winston-Salem; Chief, Neurology Service, North Carolina Baptist Hospitals, Winston-Salem, North Carolina

Ergun Y. Uc, MD

Associate, Department of Neurology, University of Iowa College of Medicine, Iowa City; Fellow, Movement Disorders, University of Iowa Hospitals and Clinics, Iowa City

Michael W. Varner, MD

Professor, Department of Obstetrics and Gynecology, University of Utah School of Medicine, Salt Lake City; Director, Maternal-Fetal Medicine, Department of Obstetrics and Gynecology, University of Utah School of Medicine, Salt Lake City

Melissa A. Waller, MS, CCC-A

Clinical Audiologist, Department of Otolaryngology, University of Texas Southwestern Medical Center, Dallas

Michael K. Wynne, PhD

Associate Professor, Department of Otolaryngology–Head and Neck Surgery, Indiana University School of Medicine, Indianapolis; Coordinator of Clinical Audiology, Department of Otolaryngology–Head and Neck Surgery, Indiana University Medical Center, Indianapolis

Thoru Yamada, MD

Professor, Department of Neurology, University of Iowa College of Medicine, Iowa City; Director, Division of Clinical Electrophysiology, University of Iowa Hospitals and Clinics, Iowa City

Robert D. Yee, MD

Professor and Chairman, Department of Ophthalmology, Indiana University School of Medicine, Indianapolis; Chief, Neuro-Ophthalmology Service, Indiana University Medical Center, Indianapolis

Phyllis C. Zee, MD, PhD

Associate Professor, Department of Neurology, Northwestern University, Chicago; Director, Sleep Disorders Center, Northwestern Memorial Hospital, Chicago

Preface

Neurology is often misrepresented as being esoteric and otherworldly. In surveys I conducted among various groups of graduating medical students, most respondents identified the study of neurology as an overwhelming and impractical one. Contributing to this perception is the widespread cliché that neurologists are therapeutic nihilists. To list neuronophobia as a result understates the problem. Certainly neurology draws on an intricate neurobiologic knowledge base. Inevitably, many young physicians become overwhelmed by the exponential increase in basic and applied information and give up on the subject.

With a high degree of specialization, the need for filtering relevant information becomes crucial. *Practical Neurology* has been written in an attempt to serve the neurology needs of primary care physicians, practicing neurologists, and residents in training. Because this book is unorthodox in its approach, it may help to clarify at the outset what it does and does not set out to accomplish. It is not meant to be a comprehensive neurology text. It is a book about relevant and practical neurology problems, written by practicing clinicians and educators. Indeed, the authors had no desire to amass a wealth of neurologic information, but rather to offer the broadest reliable information needed by the practicing physician caring for patients with neurologic disorders in a busy office practice.

The editing of this book has been challenging and instructive; I hope the book itself proves interesting and useful to those who read it. In addition, I hope that the body of information presented here serves to stimulate further study of the sound principles of neurologic diagnoses and management.

It remains only to thank my wife, Célika, and my children, Sofía, Gabriel, and Rebecca, for their encouragement and support, my colleagues and associates for the quality of their contributions, my students and residents for their relentless insistence on trying to answer all questions, and the editors at Little, Brown and Company and Lippincott–Raven for their support and advice.

José Biller, MD

Practical Neurology

Diagnosis

1

Approach to the Patient with Acute Confusional State (Delirium/Encephalopathy)

John C. Andrefsky
Jeffrey I. Frank

Delirium is a syndrome characterized by confusion accompanied by inattention, alteration of arousal, disorientation, and global cognitive impairment. All patients with delirium should be promptly evaluated because of the progressive and potentially lethal nature of many of the etiologies. Treatment of the underlying cause leads to resolution in most circumstances. In this chapter, the terms "delirium" and "confusion" will be used interchangeably.

I. **Etiology.** The common pathophysiology of all causes of delirium is the widespread dysfunction of both cortical and subcortical neurons leading to the characteristic global, nonfocal neurologic manifestations of most delirious patients. The spectrum of etiologies of delirium (Table 1-1) includes commonly encountered conditions (e.g., metabolic derangements) and rare conditions (e.g., acute intermittent porphyria), and many are reversible and carry excellent prognoses if treated in a timely manner. Following are the basic etiologic categories of delirium. Specific clinical features are outlined in subsequent sections and in Appendix A.

A. **Infections** represent one of the most common etiologies. Systemic infections should always be considered as potential causes of confusion, especially in elderly patients and those with prior brain damage who are particularly prone to encephalopathy resulting from systemic processes. Central nervous system (CNS) infections, although less commonly encountered than systemic infections, can cause severe brain damage if not recognized immediately and should be a primary consideration in postoperative neurosurgical and immunocompromised patients.

B. **Metabolic abnormalities** are common causes of delirium and often coexist with other precipitants of delirium such as sepsis and uremia. Often, the metabolic derangement must be extreme to cause confusion, and individual susceptibilities frequently dictate which patients will become symptomatic from a given metabolic abnormality.

C. **End-organ failure** presents with striking abnormalities on general physical examination and is usually readily recognized. Failure to provide prompt treatment of hypotension and hypoxia can result in severe brain damage.

D. **Endocrinopathies** present with abnormalities of multiple organ systems, usually of subacute onset, which must be specifically considered in recognizing the pattern of systemic involvement.

E. **Nutritional deficiencies** most often (in the United States) affect alcoholics, patients with systemic cancer, and those with malabsorption syndromes. If treated early, most of the neurologic sequelae can be prevented.

F. **Drug and alcohol intoxication and withdrawal** can be life-threatening and require prompt recognition and timely intervention and support.

G. **Medications** cause delirium in patients with impaired renal or liver function or metabolic interference from other drugs. Inquiry should be made about use of medications such as antipsychotics, tricyclic antidepressants, levodopa, antihistamines, digoxin, theophylline, corticosteroids, and anticholinergics, because these drugs can precipitate or aggravate delirium.

H. **Hemorrhage** in the CNS that causes delirium is usually associated with focal neurologic signs and represents an emergency frequently requiring neurosurgical intervention.

I. **CNS trauma** can cause concussion, brain contusion, and epidural and subdural hematomas (EDH and SDH), each potentially manifesting as a confused state with associated focal neurologic features. Confusion associated with traumatic hemorrhage can be immediate or delayed. The severity of the neurologic effects of brain contusions varies from transient loss of consciousness with minimal structural injury to progressive mental status deterioration with severe, life-threatening edema.

Table 1-1. Etiologies of delirium.

Infections

Non-central nervous system
  Sepsis
  Localized
Central nervous system
  Meningitis
    Bacterial
      Tuberculous
    Cryptococcal
    Syphilitic
    Toxoplasmosis
Tertiary syphilis
Encephalitis
  Herpes simplex
Progressive multifocal leukoencephalopathy
Human immunodeficiency virus
Abscess
  Brain
  Epidural
Subdural empyema
  Subacute spongiform encephalopathy
  Whipple's disease

Acute disseminated encephalomyelitis

Metabolic abnormalities

Electrolyte disorders
  Hyper-, hypo-osmolality
Central pontine myelinolysis
Hyper-, hyponatremia
Hypokalemia
Hypercalcemia
Hypophosphatemia
Hyper-, hypomagnesemia
Acid-base disorders
  Acidosis
  Alkalosis

End-organ failure

Hyperglycemia
  Diabetic ketoacidosis
  Hyperosmolar nonketotic hyperglycemia
Hypoglycemia
Hypercapnia
Hypoxia
Hypotension
Uremia
Hepatic encephalopathy
Reye's syndrome
Pancreatic encephalopathy
Acute intermittent porphyria

Endocrinopathy

Hyper-, hypothyroidism
Cushing's syndrome
Adrenal cortical insufficiency
Pituitary failure

Nutritional deficiencies

Wernicke's encephalopathy
Pellagra
Vitamin B_{12} deficiency

Intoxication

Acute alcohol intoxication
Alcohol withdrawal
Opioid intoxication
Cocaine intoxication
Amphetamine intoxication
Phencyclidine intoxication
Sedative-hypnotic intoxication
Sedative-hypnotic withdrawal
Barbiturate intoxication
Barbiturate withdrawal
Benzodiazepine intoxication
Benzodiazepine withdrawal
Lithium intoxication
Carbon monoxide poisoning

Medications

Hemorrhage

Intracranial hemorrhage
  Subarachnoid hemorrhage
    Aneurysm
    Arteriovenous malformation
    Disseminated intravascular coagulation

CNS trauma

Acute subdural hematoma
Subacute subdural hematoma
Epidural hematoma
Subarachnoid hemorrhage
Concussion
Contusion

Vascular

Transient ischemic attack
Cerebral infarction
Vasculitis
Venous occlusion

Tumors

Central nervous system
Paraneoplastic
  Limbic encephalitis

Seizures

Generalized
Partial
Postconvulsive

Hypertensive encephalopathy

Beclouded dementia

Postoperative delirium

J. Vascular etiologies usually present with focal neurologic signs. However, lesions localizing to particular areas of the posterior circulation and right hemisphere may present as confusional states with focal features discernible only by experienced neurologists. CNS vasculitis is often associated with headache and focal neurologic signs, as well as variable manifestations of systemic illness.

K. CNS tumors, malignant and benign, primary and metastatic, can cause prominent mental status changes including confusion, focal neurologic findings, headaches, and signs of increased intracranial pressure (ICP).

L. Seizures (absence and partial) and postconvulsive states (secondary to generalized tonic-clonic and partial seizures) are common causes of intermittent confusion.

M. Hypertensive encephalopathy requires prompt treatment in order to prevent end-organ damage and should be considered in patients presenting with extreme hypertension, mental status changes, and papilledema.

N. Beclouded dementia and postoperative delirium are encountered frequently by physicians practicing in a general medical setting. Demented patients are particularly sensitive to infections, metabolic abnormalities, and medications that may cause delirium. Patients become confused postoperatively secondary to metabolic aberrations, impaired gas exchange, infection, medication side effects, and the result of physiological derangements such as hypothermia and global hypoperfusion.

II. Clinical manifestations

A. Mental status. Examination of the delirious patient is challenging. Histories from encephalopathic patients must be interpreted with skepticism, underscoring the importance of seeking information from families and friends. The history and physical examination should be performed in a quiet room with few distractions or interruptions. Restraints should be avoided unless the safety of the patient or medical personnel is at risk. Much information regarding the mental status of the patient is obtained during the course of social interaction. Engage the patient in a friendly and polite manner. Note if the patient readily engages in greetings and conversation and follows a logical progression of thought. Frequent topic changes may signify confusion. Avoid frustrating questions that may sabotage patient cooperation for subsequent parts of the examination.

1. Attention. The hallmark of delirium is the inability to maintain selective attention to the environment and mental processes. Patients are easily distracted and often unable to engage in conversation or readily shift their attention from one task to another.

2. Orientation. Delirious patients are often disoriented to time and place with preserved orientation to person.

3. Arousal. Changes in the level of arousal are common, ranging from agitation with increased alertness to somnolence.

4. Memory. Because registration is dependent on the ability to focus attention, delirious patients are frequently unable to form new memories and do so only during lucid periods. Recall of recently learned material is usually impaired with preservation of remote memory.

5. Perception. Impairment of both qualitative and quantitative perception is common in the delirious patient. Hallucinations are usually either visual or auditory. Illusions and delusions are prominent.

6. Disordered thinking. Abnormalities of cognitive processing and problem solving are common.

7. Emotional disturbances. Marked emotional lability and inappropriate emotional responses occur frequently, but are not readily appreciated until the patient is engaged in conversation.

8. Language abnormalities. The inattention and distractibility of delirium challenge meaningful interactions and communication with others. Verbal output of delirious patients tends to be rambling and incoherent. Aphasia is often mistaken for confusion. Patients with focal disturbances of language (comprehension, repetition, expression, and naming) should be evaluated for focal processes.

9. Disturbances of the sleep-wake cycle are common. Patients may remain awake for most of the day and night with only brief naps or may reverse their normal sleep pattern. Many of the conditions that cause delirium also cause insomnia and the restless legs syndrome. Nocturnal exacerbation of confusion ("sundowning") in demented patients can be a source of frustration for caregivers.

B. Other neurologic findings

1. **Papilledema** is a sign of increased ICP or hypertensive encephalopathy. However, its absence does not rule out increased ICP, because the funduscopic changes evolve over hours to days.

2. **Pupil changes**

   a. Fixed and dilated pupils are observed with anticholinergic (e.g., atropine, scopolamine) intoxication.

   b. Enlarged but reactive pupils are present with increased sympathetic activity, intoxications with amphetamines and cocaine, and therapeutic use of epinephrine and norepinephrine as pressor agents.

   c. Midposition unreactive pupils can be caused by glutethimide overdose or focal midbrain dysfunction often from distortion by an expanding supratentorial mass.

   d. Use of opioids is associated with constricted pupils (<2 mm).

   e. The presence of a unilaterally dilated pupil with or without the other components of a cranial nerve III palsy is a sign of brainstem distortion. Until proven otherwise, this is a neurologic emergency requiring immediate diagnosis and treatment.

3. Abnormalities of **ocular motility** associated with confusion usually signal the presence of either increased ICP or brainstem distortion.

   a. An upgaze palsy suggests a lesion of the dorsal upper midbrain or distortion from hydrocephalus.

   b. Unilaterally impaired eye adduction (with pupillary dilatation) and diminished consciousness represent a nerve III palsy and constitute a neurologic emergency requiring immediate diagnosis and treatment until proven otherwise.

   c. Delirium with **quadriparesis** can occur as a result of central pontine myelinolysis (CPM), progressive multifocal leukoencephalopathy (PML), and acute disseminated encephalomyelitis (ADEM).

   d. Delirium with **paraparesis** can occur with cryptococcosis, vitamin B_{12} deficiency, and ADEM.

   e. Cushing's disease and hypokalemia can manifest as **proximal muscular weakness.**

4. **Abnormal limb movements** are often helpful in determining the etiology of delirium.

   a. **Myoclonus** is an asynchronous irregular twitching of single muscles, groups of muscles, or entire limbs, usually with proximal predominance, and it can be associated with metabolic abnormalities, hypoxic-ischemic injury, lithium intoxication, and CNS infections including tertiary syphilis and subacute spongiform encephalopathy (SSE).

   b. **Asterixis** is recurrent brief lapses of posture observed with arms raised and elbows and wrists extended, and it is a common manifestation of hepatic encephalopathy and uremia but can be associated with other metabolic encephalopathies.

   c. The **tremor** that is most frequently observed with delirium is coarse and irregular, most prominent in the fingers of the extended arms and absent at rest, and most commonly associated with hyperthyroidism, intoxications with sympathomimetics (amphetamine, cocaine, and phencyclidine), alcohol intoxication and withdrawal, and barbiturate and benzodiazepine withdrawal.

   d. **Gait ataxia** is prominent with intoxications, vitamin B_{12} deficiency, syphilis, and Wernicke's encephalopathy.

   e. **Seizures** can cause confusion and often signify a structural brain abnormality, metabolic abnormality, or intoxication or withdrawal state.

      (1) **Partial complex seizures** are the most common type of focal seizures that can cause confusion. Although rarely encountered, **epilepsia partialis continua (EPC)** is a focal motor epilepsy wherein clonic movements of the face, arm, and leg recur intermittently for long periods of time. This condition might go undiagnosed by the inexperienced clinician. The presence of EPC implies an irritative structural lesion involving cerebral cortex by any process that can cause focal cortical damage (e.g., stroke, encephalitis, or neoplasm).

(2) Generalized seizures can cause confusion or postconvulsive encephalopathy. **Absence seizures** represent generalized seizures that induce brief lapses of consciousness with prominent automatisms. Children that endure frequent interruptions in consciousness can be misdiagnosed with confusion or learning disabilities without recognition of the underlying seizure disorder.

III. Evaluation. The neurologic findings of delirious patients can be found in sec. **II.B.**

A. The **history** represents the most important part of the evaluation and often yields information that helps tailor an efficient investigation strategy, frequently with more rapid diagnosis and resolution of symptoms. Often family members and other observers must be the primary historians for delirious patients. Appendix A presents the characteristic clinical manifestations and laboratory and radiologic findings as a quick reference for specific etiologies of delirium.

1. **Headache.** Complaints of an acute headache in a confused patient can signify severe intracranial pathology such as subarachnoid hemorrhage (SAH) or intraparenchymal hemorrhage, whereas progressive headaches are more suggestive of a CNS neoplasm, infection, or hydrocephalus.
2. **Previous brain damage.** Patients with cerebral infarctions, progressive neurologic diseases, psychiatric illnesses, head trauma, and previous neurosurgical procedures are predisposed to delirium, often in association with other neurologic signs.
3. **Preexisting medical conditions** such as cardiac and lung disease represent risk factors for life-threatening conditions that cause delirium. Abnormal hepatic and renal function can cause impaired metabolism and excretion of medication.
4. **Drug history.** When evaluating a delirious patient, the clinician should always obtain a detailed substance abuse history. Inquiries about the specific substance abused, frequency of usage, and interval since last used are important.
5. **Exposure history.** Inquiries should be made about exposure to meningitis, human immunodeficiency virus (HIV), carbon monoxide, and other potential CNS toxins.
6. **Medications.** Addition of new medications or changes in dosage are frequently associated with confusion. Medications high in anticholinergic activity are particularly common culprits.

B. The general physical examination

1. **Abnormalities of the vital signs** often herald the presence of medical emergencies.
   a. **Hypotension** from dehydration, sepsis, cardiac arrhythmias, or congestive heart failure must be recognized and treated promptly to prevent further neurologic and other end-organ damage.
   b. **Tachycardia** can be a manifestation of infection, cardiac abnormality, hyperthyroidism, dehydration, withdrawal states, intoxication with sympathomimetic drugs, or sympathetic overactivity from delirium.
   c. **Hypoventilation** related to pneumonia or drug overdose can result in hypoxia or hypercapnia.
   d. **Increases in body temperature** are associated with infections, withdrawal states, and hyperthyroidism. Hypothermia is associated with sepsis and barbiturate overdose.
2. **Nuchal rigidity** is a sign of meningeal irritation, which frequently occurs with CNS infections and SAH. Meningitis, encephalitis, and SAH should be diagnostically pursued in the presence of nuchal rigidity or if clinical suspicion is high even in its absence.
3. In all cases of confusion, there should be a search for **evidence of head trauma** such as scalp laceration, depressed skull fracture, or hemotympanum. Signs of cerebrospinal fluid (CSF) leak are particularly important because they predispose patients to bacterial meningitis.
4. **Purulent drainage** from the nares or a **gray and immobile tympanic membrane** can represent sinusitis or otitis media, respectively. The nasal septum should also be examined for erosions secondary to cocaine use.
5. The **skin** should be examined for cyanosis, hirsutism, hyperpigmentation, and scaly dermatitis. The clinician should inspect the skin in all patients for the presence of track or "pop" marks which imply intravenous drug use.

6. **Examination of the heart** can reveal murmurs and irregular rhythms that predispose patients to cerebral circulatory compromise.

7. **Decreased or absent breath** sounds can be secondary to congestive heart failure or pneumonia with the resulting hypoxia potentially contributing to delirium.

8. Patients with **abdominal tenderness** should be evaluated for intra-abdominal infections. Neurosurgical patients with a ventriculoperitoneal shunt can manifest shunt infection as abdominal peritonitis.

9. Patients with delirium from hepatic failure can have **ascites, splenomegaly, spider telangiectasia, caput medusae, icteric sclera,** and **jaundice.**

C. **Ancillary tests**

1. **Serum electrolytes,** glucose, blood urea nitrogen, serum creatinine, complete blood count (CBC) (with differential), liver enzymes, prothrombin and partial thromboplastin times (PT and PTT), and an arterial blood gas (ABG) with arterial ammonia level will cover all of the metabolic abnormalities that need urgently to be identified.

2. **A drug screen** and a **blood alcohol level** should be included.

3. If all of the above laboratory tests are negative, the clinician should obtain an **HIV test,** a **fluorescent treponemal antibody-absorption (FTA-ABS) test, thyroid function tests,** and a **cortisol stimulation test.**

4. An **electrocardiogram** to rule out an arrhythmia and cardiac ischemia and a **chest x-ray** to rule out infections (e.g., pneumonia) that contribute to delirium or pulmonary processes that can compromise ventilation and oxygenation should be obtained.

D. **Lumbar puncture.** If meningitis or encephalitis is suspected, CSF analysis is mandatory. CSF examination is also indicated if a computerized axial tomography (CT) scan of the brain is negative in cases of suspected SAH. Routine CSF analysis consists of white blood cell (WBC) count with differential and red blood cell (RBC) count, glucose and total protein, and Gram stain and culture. Often, patients presenting with delirium need more than the basic CSF studies, and those used to evaluate specific entities that cause delirium are presented in Appendix A.

1. **Contraindications to lumbar puncture** include:

   a. A coagulopathy or platelet count less than $50,000 \text{ cm}^3$.

   b. Loss of cisternal spaces, evidence of brainstem distortion, an absent or distorted fourth ventricle, and any posterior fossa mass on CT scan.

   c. An abscess over the lumbar puncture site.

   d. Clinical suspicion of an intracranial mass lesion or increased ICP.

2. **The CSF WBC count** is considered abnormal when more than four WBCs of any type or one neutrophil are found. An increased WBC count is suggestive of CNS infection.

   a. Neutrophils predominate with bacterial infections of the CNS and early viral encephalitides (particularly enteroviruses).

   b. Lymphocytes predominate with tuberculous and cryptococcal meningitis, syphilitic infections, herpes simplex encephalitis, toxoplasmosis, and HIV.

3. **The presence of any RBCs** in the CSF is abnormal and requires explanation, traumatic tap being the most common cause.

   a. Two important pathologic processes that increase the RBC count are SAH and herpes simplex encephalitis. Cerebral infarctions, brain tumors (primary and metastatic), traumatic hematomas, and nontraumatic intracerebral hemorrhages inconsistently increase the CSF RBC.

   b. **Xanthochromia** is yellow color secondary to the presence of **oxyhemoglobin** and **bilirubin** from lysed RBCs in the supernatant of centrifuged CSF. Oxyhemoglobin reaches its peak level in about 36 hours and disappears after 7–10 days. Bilirubin appears in the CSF with SAH, reaches its maximum at about 48 hours, and disappears in 2–4 weeks.

4. A normal **CSF glucose** level is greater than 50% of the serum glucose level. Low CSF glucose is observed with CNS infections, SAH, hepatic failure, and hypoglycemia.

5. Increases in **CSF protein** accompany CNS infections, hemorrhages, and obstructions of CSF flow.

   a. Acute intermittent porphyria, hypothyroidism, and Wernicke's encephalopathy are associated with increased protein.

   b. Assuming a normal concentration of serum proteins, the CSF protein will increase by 1 mg/1000 RBCs. If a higher ratio is present, suspect the presence of a pathologic process.

6. **CSF Gram stains and cultures** should be obtained on all CSF specimens. In cases of suspected bacterial meningitis, latex agglutination testing provides rapid identification of some common bacterial antigens.

7. **Polymerase chain reactions (PCR)** can assist in identification of CNS infections resulting from organisms not readily grown on culture media (e.g., viruses). This test is performed infrequently, usually at tertiary care centers.

8. **India ink CSF staining** can be used for rapid determination of the presence of cryptococcus, but skepticism should be brought to a negative India ink study when clinical suspicion is high. Fungal cultures are more sensitive.

9. **CSF glutamine** is elevated in cases of hepatic encephalopathy, but in most cases of hepatic encephalopathy the diagnosis is self-evident without CSF examination. This test is rarely performed.

E. **Neuroimaging**
1. A **CT scan** can identify most causes of delirium that involve structural damage to the brain, including hemorrhages (intraparenchymal, epidural, subdural, and subarachnoid), tumors, infarctions, and edema.
   a. The CT scan may be normal in cases of early cerebral infarction, meningitis, or hemorrhages of low volume or in the severely anemic patient.
   b. IV contrast should be administered for cases of suspected brain abscess or tumors when the patient is medically and neurologically unstable and immediate neurosurgical intervention may be required. If the patient is stable, a magnetic resonance imaging (MRI) scan should be performed instead of a CT scan with contrast.
2. **MRI of the brain** is useful in evaluating delirious patients with suspected herpes simplex encephalitis, white matter processes (e.g., ADEM), a posterior fossa mass, multiple lesions (e.g., metastasis and septic emboli), or immunocompromise. The length of time necessary for completion of an MRI scan often precludes its use in the unstable and agitated patient.
3. **Magnetic resonance angiography (MRA) and venography (MRV) of the brain** are noninvasive diagnostic studies that can diagnose many conditions that affect the vasculature of the brain. Aneurysms, arteriovenous malformations (AVM), dissection of large vessels, cerebral venous sinus occlusion, and stenosis and occlusion of both intracranial and extracranial vessels can often be detected by MRA/MRV. Conventional angiography is more sensitive than MRA/MRV for the diagnosis of CNS vascular disease.
4. **Angiography** should be considered when aneurysm, arteriovenous malformation, venous occlusive disease, or CNS vasculitis is suspected and identification of the process will proximately affect therapeutic management decisions.

F. **Electroencephalography.**
The **electroencephalogram (EEG)** has a limited role in the evaluation of delirious patients.
1. Almost all patients with delirium will have an abnormal EEG with high-voltage delta or theta activity (slowing).
2. The EEG will help to diagnose complex partial status epilepticus and absence seizures and to identify abnormal brain activity that patients with seizures may manifest.
3. Specific EEG patterns such as triphasic waves (often observed with metabolic derangements) or high-voltage slowing with sharp waves on a flat background (often observed with SSE) can help corroborate some clinical diagnostic suspicions.

G. **Brain biopsy** is rarely indicated for the evaluation of delirium. It is necessary when histologic typing of CNS tumors will affect the management and outcome and in cases of suspected CNS vasculitis if the risks of empirical therapy outweigh the risks of the procedure. Encephalitis and SSE can be confirmed by means of brain biopsy.

IV. **Differential diagnosis.** Certain conditions can masquerade as delirium (Table 1-2), often requiring an experienced clinician to distinguish the actual process from delirium. Accurate diagnosis is imperative if the proper therapy is to be prescribed.

A. **Aphasia.** Language formulation disturbance (aphasia) can initially be misdiagnosed as confusion. Because other focal abnormalities (e.g., visual field defects, hemiparesis, and hemisensory loss) accompany aphasia more frequently than delirium, focal examination findings should drive a thorough "ruling out" of aphasia. Patients with "expressive" aphasia have normal language comprehension and

Table 1-2. Differential diagnosis of delirium.

Aphasia

Mania

Psychosis

Depression

Dementia

Transient global amnesia

sensorium but impaired spontaneous speech or mutism with writing difficulty paralleling the verbal expressive deficit. The expressively aphasic patient has a frustrated insight into the language problem. Differentiation of delirious patients from those with "receptive" aphasia can be difficult. Patients with "receptive" aphasia have severe comprehension problems but normal or only slightly impaired spontaneous speech, which is often nonsensical without any meaningful content. The receptively aphasic patient is unaware of the language problem and is frequently agitated, impairing interaction with others. However, attention is usually normal.

   B. **Psychiatric disorders** are usually characterized by prominent changes in several aspects of the mental status examination. Some examples include mania, depression, and schizophrenia. The manic patient has a consistently elevated mood, increased goal-directed activity, and a delusion of grandiosity. In contrast, the delirious patient has emotional lability and is unable to complete tasks.

   C. **Dementia.** Demented patients have memory impairment out of proportion to other aspects of the mental status examination. Focal neurologic findings such as aphasia, apraxia, and agnosia that are typically absent in the delirious patient may be present in the demented patient. Attention impairment usually occurs late in the course of dementia.

   D. **Transient global amnesia.** This syndrome usually occurs in middle-aged or elderly people and is an acute, self-limited episode of amnesia lasting for several hours. The memory deficit is for the present and recent past. The key features of delirium, such as inattention, disturbed language function, changes in the level of consciousness, and impaired cognitive abilities, are notably absent.

 V. **Diagnostic approach.** When evaluating the patient with delirium, a logical stepwise approach will enable the clinician to rapidly and accurately diagnose the underlying cause. The reader can refer to the algorithms included in this chapter (Figs. 1-1 to 1-4) as a practical guide to diagnosis.

   A. Upon presentation, consider causes, such as hypotension and hypoxia, that pose an immediate threat to life.

   B. If oxygenation and circulation are adequate, a neurologic examination searching for signs of increased ICP, intracranial hemorrhage, or CNS infection should be performed. If the examination is positive, an emergency CT scan of the brain should be performed.

   C. Upon arrival, admission tests should be performed to rule out a metabolic, cardiac, or toxic etiology.

   D. An EEG should be performed to rule out ictal activity, if seizures are suspected.

   E. A CT scan and EEG should be done if all laboratory work is negative.

   F. A lumbar puncture should be performed, assuming no contraindications (see sec. **III.D.**), if the CT scan and the EEG have not led to a diagnosis.

   G. An MRI scan should be performed, if the clinician suspects that a structural lesion exists despite a negative CT scan or if the patient is suspected of having encephalitis, a white matter process, multiple lesions, or a posterior fossa mass, or is immunocompromised.

   H. Figure 1-3 includes a list of entities to consider when all of the tests are nondiagnostic.

VI. **Criteria for diagnosis.** The diagnosis of delirium or acute confusion is given to any patient in whom the predominant abnormalities on mental status examination consist of inattention with a decline in general cognitive functioning. The *Diagnostic and Statistical Manual of Mental Disorders*, Fourth Edition (DSM-IV) lists the following criteria for the diagnosis of delirium resulting from a general medical condition.

   A. Disturbance of consciousness (i.e., reduced clarity of awareness of the environment) with reduced ability to focus, sustain, or shift attention.

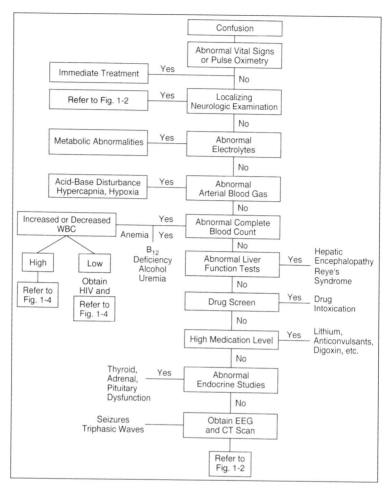

Figure 1-1. Algorithm for the initial work-up of a delirious patient. Conditions that require immediate diagnosis and treatment are included. (WBC = white blood cell count; HIV = human immunodeficiency virus; EEG = electroencephalogram; CT = computerized axial tomography).

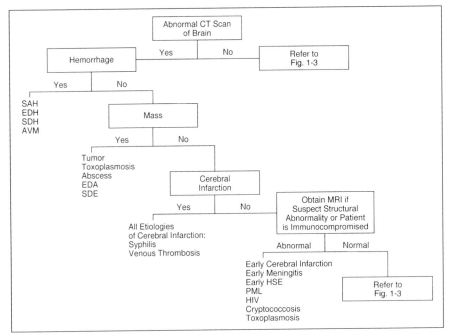

Figure 1-2. Algorithm for structural intracranial disease. (SAH = subarachnoid hemorrhage; EDH = epidural hematoma; SDH = subdural hematoma; AVM = arteriovenous malformation; EDA = epidural abscess; SDE = subdural empyema; MRI = magnetic resonance imaging; HSE = herpes simplex encephalitis; PML = progressive multifocal leukoencephalopathy).

   B. A change in cognition (such as memory deficit, disorientation, language disturbance) or the development of a perceptual disturbance that is not better accounted for by a preexisting, established, or evolving dementia.
   C. The disturbance develops over a short period of time (usually hours to days) and
   tends to fluctuate during the course of the day.
   D. There is evidence from the history, physical examination, or laboratory findings
   that the disturbance is caused by the direct physiological consequences of a general medical condition.*
VII. Referral. If the cause of delirium has been firmly established and the proper treatment initiated, no referral is necessary.
   A. A **neurologic consultation** should be obtained for a suspected primary CNS
   process, when diagnosis is unclear or when neurologic decline continues in spite
   of seemingly appropriate treatment for the underlying cause of delirium. Any focal neurologic abnormality indicates a condition that warrants the advice of a
   neurologist.
   B. Neurosurgical consultation is specifically indicated for assistance with management of intracranial mass lesions (e.g., neoplasm, hemorrhage, or edema) or
   for an invasive intracranial procedure (e.g., brain biopsy or ICP monitor placement).
   C. An **infectious disease consultation** is prudent when a CNS infection is suspected or for complex systemic infections such a those that occur in immunocompromised patients.
   D. Rheumatologic consultation can be helpful for assistance in diagnosis and
   management of collagen vascular diseases and patients with vasculitides.

*From the *Diagnostic and Statistical Manual of Mental Disorders*, 4th ed. Washington, DC,
American Psychiatric Association, 1994. Reprinted by permission.

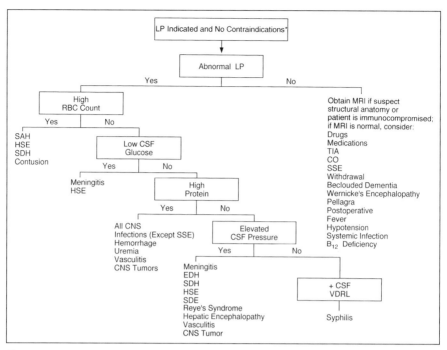

Figure 1-3. Algorithm for cerebrospinal fluid examination. (LP = lumbar puncture; RBC = red blood cell; CSF = cerebrospinal fluid; CNS = central nervous system; SSE = subacute spongiform encephalopathy; VDRL = venereal disease research laboratory test; TIA = transient ischemic attack; CO = carbon monoxide; * = contraindications for lumbar puncture).

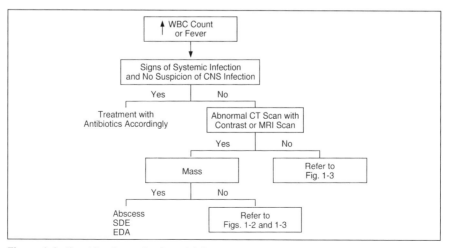

Figure 1-4. Algorithm for evaluation of delirious patients suspected of having infectious processes.

Recommended Readings

Aurelius E, et al. Rapid diagnosis of herpes simplex encephalitis by nested polymerase chain reaction assay of cerebrospinal fluid. *Lancet* 337:189–192, 1990.

Britton CB, Mills JR. Neurological complication in acquired immunodeficiency syndrome (AIDS). *Neurol Clin* 2:315–339, 1984.

Brown P, et al. Creutzfeld-Jakob disease: Clinical analysis of a consecutive series of 230 neuropathologically verified cases. *Ann Neurol* 20:597–602, 1986.

Busto U, et al. Withdrawal reaction after long-term therapeutic use of benzodiazepene. *N Engl J Med* 315:854–859, 1986.

Charness ME, et al. Ethanol and the nervous system. *N Engl J Med* 321:442–454, 1989.

Frey JL, Masferrer R. Postoperative encephalopathy. *Barrow Neurological Institute Quarterly* 6(4):30–34, 1990.

Greenlee JE. Progressive multifocal leukoencephalopathy. *Curr Clin Topics Infect Dis* 10:140–156, 1989.

Griggs RC, Satran R. Metabolic encephalopathy. In RN Rosenberg (ed.), *Comprehensive Neurology*. New York: Raven, 1991.

Horenstein S, et al. Infarction of the fusiform and calcarine regions: Agitated delirium and hemianopsia. *Trans Am Neurol Assoc* 92:85–89, 1967.

Lipowski ZJ. Delirium in the elderly patient. *N Engl J Med* 320:578–582, 1989.

Lockwood AH. Neurological complications of renal-disease. *Neurol Clin* 7:617–627, 1989.

Lowenstein DH, et al. Acute neurologic and psychiatric complications associated with cocaine abuse. *Am J Med* 83:841–846, 1987.

Mancall EL. Nutritional disorders of the nervous system. In MJ Aminoff (ed.), *Neurology and General Medicare*. New York: Churchill Livingstone, 1989.

Medina JL, et al. Agitated delirium caused by infarctions of the hippocampal formation and fusiform and lingual gyri. *Neurology* 24:1181–1183, 1974.

Medina JL, et al. Syndrome of agitated delirium and visual impairment: A manifestation of temporo-occipital infarction. *J Neurol Neurosurg Psychiatry* 40:861–864, 1977.

Mesulam MM, et al. Acute confusional states with right middle cerebral artery territory infarctions. *J Neurol Neurosurg Psychiatry* 29:84–89, 1976.

Mesulam MM, Geschwind N. Disordered state in the post-operative period. *Urol Clin North Am* 3:199–215, 1976.

Mullaly W, et al. Frequency of acute confusional states with lesions of the right hemisphere. *Ann Neurol* 12:113, 1982.

Pousada L, Leipzig RM. Rapid bedside assessment of postoperative confusion in older patients. *Geriatrics* 45(5):59–63, 1990.

Stern RH, et al. Osmotic demyelination syndrome following correction of hyponatremia. *N Engl J Med* 314:1535–1542, 1986.

Taylor D, Lewis S. Delirium. *J Neurol Neurosurg Psychiatry* 56(7):742–751, 1993.

Thompson TL, Thompson WL. Treating postoperative delirium. *Drug Ther* 13:30–31, 1983.

Tune LE, et al. Association of postoperative delirium with raised serum levels of anticholinergic drugs. *Lancet* 2:651–652, 1981.

Whitley RJ, et al. Herpes simplex encephalitis: Clinical assessment. *JAMA* 247:317–320, 1982.

2

Approach to the Patient with Dementia
Neill R. Graff-Radford

In the DSM-IV criteria, dementia is defined as a decline in memory and at least one other cognitive function (aphasia, apraxia, agnosia, or a decline in an executive function such as planning, organizing, sequencing, or abstracting). This decline should impair social or occupational functioning in comparison with prior functioning. The deficits should not occur exclusively during the course of delirium and should not be accounted for by another psychiatric condition such as depression or schizophrenia. Dementia is then further defined by a possible, probable, or definite etiologic diagnosis.

I. **Incidence and prevalence of dementia.** It is estimated that more than 4% of people over 65 years of age have dementia and about 50 to 75% of patients with dementia have Alzheimer's disease. It is also noteworthy that the incidence of Alzheimer's disease and vascular dementia (the second most common cause of dementia) is age related—i.e., the older the patient, the greater the chance of having one of these diseases. The prevalence of dementia is estimated to be 20% of people over the age of 85 years. These data should be analyzed in the context of the aging population. For example, in the United States, 50% of people are expected to live past the age of 75 years and 25% past the age of 85 years.

II. **Etiology.** Table 2-1 lists many of the etiologies of dementia. In a review by Clarfield of over 1000 patients in 11 studies for which follow-up data were available, the dementia was partially reversed in 8% of the cases and completely reversed in 3%. Metabolic disease was thought to be the cause in 16%, depression in 26%, and drugs in 28%.

III. **Criteria for diagnosis**
   A. Presented below are the **National Institute of Neurological and Communicative Disorders and Stroke** and the **Alzheimer's and Related Diseases Association (NINCDS-ARDA) criteria*** for the diagnosis of Alzheimer's disease, which is the most common cause of dementia.
      1. The criteria for the clinical diagnosis of **probable Alzheimer's disease** are as follows:
         a. Dementia established by clinical examination and documented by the Mini-Mental State Exam, Blessed Dementia Rating Scale, or some other similar examination, and confirmed by neuropsychological tests.
         b. Deficits in two or more areas of cognition.
         c. Progressive worsening of memory and other cognitive functions.
         d. No disturbance of consciousness.
         e. Onset between ages 40 and 90, most often after age 65.
         f. Absence of systemic disorders or other brain diseases that in and of themselves could account for the progressive deficits in memory and cognition.
      2. Supporting findings in the diagnosis of **probable Alzheimer's disease** include:
         a. Progressive deterioration of specific cognitive functions such as aphasia, apraxia, or agnosia.
         b. Impaired activities of daily living and altered patterns of behavior.
         c. Family history of similar disorders, particularly if confirmed neuropathologically.
         d. Laboratory results of:
            (1) Normal lumbar puncture as evaluated by standard techniques.

This work was supported by NIA grant AG08031-06S1 and the State of Florida Alzheimer's Disease Initiative.

*Reprinted with permission from *Neurology* 34:939–941, 1984.

Table 2-1. Etiologies of dementia.*

Degenerative	Psychiatric
Alzheimer's disease	*Depression*
Parkinson's disease	*Alcohol abuse*
Progressive supranuclear palsy	*Drug related*
Multiple system atrophy	*Personality disorder*
Huntington's disease	*Anxiety disorder*
Olivopontocerebellar degeneration	
Pick's disease	**Toxic/Metabolic**
Non-Pick frontal degeneration	B_{12} *deficiency*
Focal cortical degeneration	*Thyroid deficiency*
Diffuse cortical Lewy body disease	*System failure: liver, renal, cardiac, respiratory*
Corticobasilar degeneration	*Heavy metals*
	Toxins (e.g., glue sniffing)
Vascular	
Multiple infarction	**Traumatic**
Single stroke	*Subdural hematoma*
Binswanger's disease	*Closed head injury*
Vasculitis	*Open head injury*
Subarachnoid hemorrhage	Pugilistic brain injury
	Anoxic brain injury
Infectious	
Fungal meningitis	**Tumorous**
Syphilis	*Glioblastoma*
AIDS dementia	*Lymphoma*
Creutzfeldt-Jakob disease	*Metastatic tumor*
Post-herpes simplex encephalitis	
	Other
	Symptomatic hydrocephalus

*Causes in *italics* are at least partially reversible/treatable.

        (2) Normal pattern or nonspecific changes in EEG, such as increased slow-wave activity.

        (3) Evidence of cerebral atrophy on CT with progression documented by serial observation.

  3. Other clinical features consistent with the diagnosis of **probable Alzheimer's disease,** after exclusion of causes of dementia other than Alzheimer's disease, include:

    a. Plateaus in the course of progression of the illness.

    b. Associated symptoms of depression; insomnia; incontinence; delusions; illusions; hallucinations; catastrophic verbal, emotional, or physical outbursts; sexual disorders; and weight loss.

    c. Other neurologic abnormalities in some patients, especially those with more advanced disease and including motor signs such as increased muscle tone, myoclonus, or gait disorder.

    d. Seizures in advanced disease.

    e. CT normal for age.

  4. Features that make the diagnosis of **probable Alzheimer's disease** uncertain or unlikely include:

    a. Sudden, apoplectic onset.

    b. Focal neurologic findings such as hemiparesis, sensory loss, visual field deficits, and incoordination early in the course of the illness.

    c. Seizures or gait disturbance at the onset or early in the course of the illness.

  5. Clinical diagnosis of **possible Alzheimer's disease:**

a. May be made on the basis of the dementia syndrome, in the absence of other neurologic, psychiatric, or systemic disorders sufficient to cause dementia, and in the presence of variations in the onset, in the presentation, or in the clinical course.

b. May be made in the presence of a second systemic or brain disorder sufficient to produce dementia, which is not considered to be *the* cause of the dementia; and

c. Should be used in research studies when a single, gradually progressive severe cognitive deficit is identified in the absence of any other identifiable cause.

6. Criteria for diagnosis of **definite Alzheimer's disease** are the clinical criteria for probable Alzheimer's disease and histopathologic evidence obtained from a biopsy or autopsy.

7. Classification of Alzheimer's disease for research purposes should specify features that may differentiate subtypes of the disorder, such as: familial occurrence, onset before age 65, presence of trisomy 21, and coexistence of other relevant conditions such as Parkinson's disease.

B. Stroke. The diagnostic criteria proposed by the State of California Alzheimer's Disease Diagnostic and Treatment Centers (SCADDTC) for **ischemic vascular dementia (IVD)*** are as follows:

1. The criteria for **probable IVD** include all of the following:

a. Clinical characteristics of dementia.

b. Evidence of two or more ischemic strokes (history, neurologic examination, and imaging), or occurrence of a single stroke with clearly documented temporal relationship to the onset of dementia.

c. Evidence of at least one infarct outside the cerebellum (CT or MRI).

2. The criteria for **possible IVD** include clinical characteristics of dementia, and one or more of the following: a history or evidence of a single stroke (but not multiple strokes) without a clearly documented temporal relationship to the onset of dementia; or Binswanger's syndrome, which includes early-onset urinary incontinence not explained by peripheral cause, vascular risk factors, and extensive white matter changes on neuroimaging.

3. The criteria for **definite IVD** include:

a. Clinical evidence of dementia.

b. Pathological confirmation of multiple infarcts, some outside the cerebellum.

4. A diagnosis of **mixed dementia** should be made in the presence of one or more other system or brain disorders that are thought to be causally related to dementia.

It is important to realize that doctors using these criteria cannot be clinically certain of the cause of dementia in any single patient. The correlation of the clinical and autopsy diagnoses is about 85%. This discrepancy is the result of both imprecision of clinical diagnosis and evolution of pathological criteria.

IV. Evaluation

A. History. It is essential that the history be obtained not only from the patient but also from an independent informant—the spouse, for example. Often the informant may not want to speak openly in front of the patient, so you may wish to arrange a separate interview, perhaps while the patient is having another test or later by telephone.

1. Patient difficulties. Determine what difficulties the patient is having and what family members have noticed. Commonly a demented patient may not know that there is a memory difficulty or be able to give accurate details of the problem. Begin by asking the patient an open-ended question such as, "What problems are you having?" This often does not elicit the desired responses. Even if you ask specific questions such as, "Are you having difficulty with your memory?" you may not be told what the problems are. The best history usually is supplied by the informant—often the spouse. To obtain this you may have to speak to the informant separately, but in most instances you can say to the patient something like, "I am now going to ask your spouse some questions, and if your spouse makes any errors, feel free to make corrections." Then ask the informant, "What problems have the family noticed?" You may need to prompt

*Reprinted with permission from *Neurology* 42:473–480, 1992.

the informant with more specific questions, such as, "What can't the patient do now that he [she] could do before?" or "Does the patient sometimes ask the same question more than once in the same conversation?"

2. **Time course.** The time the family first noticed problems and the course the disease has taken over time are critical factors in the evaluation. A disease that is slowly progressive over time fits the profile of a degenerative disease such as Alzheimer's, whereas a disease that starts suddenly or follows a stepwise progression would be more in keeping with a vascular dementia.

3. **Functioning of the patient.** Determine how well the patient has been functioning at work and at home, including performance on basic activities of daily living. Ask what the patient does to keep busy. Does he or she read the newspaper, watch the news on television, keep the checkbook, do the shopping, prepare the meals, take part in a sport or hobby? Knowing this information helps you plan questions to ask during the mental status part of the examination.

4. **Issues of safety.** Ask if the patient drives. If so, has the patient ever become lost while driving or had any accidents, near-accidents, or traffic violations? If the patient prepares meals, has he or she ever left the stove on? Does the patient keep weapons, and if so, has this posed any danger to the patient or to others?

5. **Etiologically directed history.** Include a history of vascular disease and risk factors, head injury, toxic exposure, symptoms of infection or exposure to diseases such as tuberculosis, past psychiatric history such as depression, symptoms of depression (such as a change in weight, insomnia, crying, or anhedonia), medications, systemic illnesses, other past illnesses, and alcohol or tobacco use.

6. **Family history.** Ask what the patient's parents died from and at what ages. Ask specifically if there were memory problems in the later years. Then ask about the ages and health of the patient's siblings and children.

B. **Physical examination.** Give a **standardized short mental state test**—e.g., the Folstein Mini-Mental State Exam (Fig. 2-1). Test the patient's anterograde memory by asking about current events. Be sure that the patient has been exposed to this information. You may ask questions such as: Who is the president? What is his wife's name? Who was the last president? What is his wife's name? Which country did the United States and its allies fight in the Persian Gulf War? Asking such questions provides a very sensitive means of determining if the patient has a memory problem. Note any evidence of aphasia, apraxia, or agnosia.

Look for **cardiovascular risk factors** such as hypertension, arterial bruits, arrhythmias, and heart murmurs.

Complete a **full neurologic examination.** Pay special attention to focal deficits such as visual field cuts, pareses, sensory losses, and ataxia. Evaluate the patient for any extrapyramidal difficulties such as hypokinesia, increased muscle tone, a masklike face, and micrographia. Determine if the patient has any problem walking. This is often best undertaken in the hallway rather than in the examining room. Note the patient's step size, speed of walking, arm swing, and ability to turn. The palmomental reflex and snout reflex are not particularly helpful because they are commonly found in the normal elderly. The grasp reflex occurs late in the course of the disease.

C. **Laboratory studies**
1. **Recommended in all cases** are complete blood count, chemistry panel, sedimentation rate, thyroid function tests, vitamin B_{12} level, syphilis serology, computerized tomography or magnetic resonance imaging and neuropsychological evaluation.

2. **Recommended selectively** are electroencephalogram, lumbar puncture, chest x-ray, AIDS test, drug screen, single photon emission computerized tomography (SPECT) or positron emission tomography (PET) scan, and heavy metal screen.

3. An **electroencephalogram** may be useful in diagnosing Creutzfeldt-Jakob disease, distinguishing depression or delirium from dementia, evaluating for encephalitis, revealing seizures as causes of memory difficulties, and diagnosing nonconvulsive status epilepticus.

4. A **lumbar puncture** is recommended if the patient has cancer, infection is a possibility, hydrocephalus is seen on scan, the patient is under 55, the dementia is acute or subacute in onset, the patient is immunocompromised, or vasculitis or connective tissue disease is suspected.

Folstein Mini-Mental Status Examination

Patient's name _____   **Date test given** _____

Score 1 for each blank space

Please tell me the:

___ Year ___ Season ___ Date ___ Day ___ Month ___

___ State ___ County ___ City ___ Hospital ___ Floor ___

I am going to ask you to remember some words. First listen to me saying them, then say them back to me. (Score the number repeated on the first trial only). After patient learns all three, tell patient that he/she will be asked to remember these words later.

___ Orange ___ Airplane ___ Tobacco ___ (trials to learn all three items ___)

Subtract 7 from 100 and then subtract 7 from each answer, if patient misses twosubtractions, stop. If patient misses one but accurately subtracts 7 from the incorrect answer, score as correct (e.g., for 93, 87, 80, 73, 66 score 4).

___ 93 ___ 86 ___ 79 ___ 72 ___ 65 ___

If the patient can't do serial 7's, you can substitute: Spell the word WORLD backwards. Score 1 for each letter given in the correct order even if there is a missing letter (e.g., DLRW score 4) or a reversal of two letters (DLORW score 3).

___ D ___ L ___ O ___ R ___ W ___

What were the three words I asked you to remember earlier?

___ Orange ___ Airplane ___ Tobacco ___

Point to and ask the patient to name a

___ Pencil ___ Watch ___

Repeat the following phrase

___ No ifs, ands, or buts

___ **Read and obey   CLOSE YOUR EYES**

___ **Take this piece of paper with your right hand, ___ fold it in half, ___ and drop it on the desk ___ .**

___ **Copy the following drawing.**

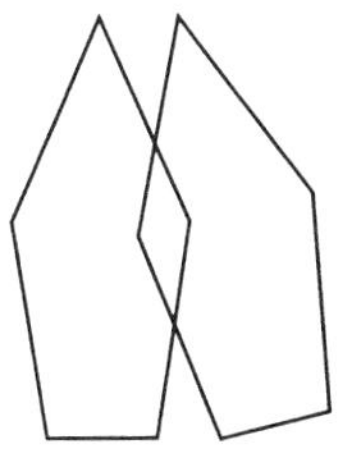

___ **Write a sentence.**

___ **Total**   (Cut-off scores of 21 for 8th grade or less, 23 for 12th grade, and 24 for college education, is abnormal.)

Figure 2-1. The Folstein Mini-Mental Status Examination. (Modified from Folstein MF. "Mini-mental state": A practical method for grading the cognitive state of patients for the clinician. *Journal of Psychiatric Research* 12:189–198, 1975.)

5. A **PET** or **SPECT scan** may be useful in distinguishing frontal dementia from Alzheimer's disease. In one blinded study in which PET imaging was used to evaluate demented and normal elderly patients, the sensitivity was only 38% and the specificity was 88%.

V. **Differential diagnosis.** Keep in mind the previously listed possible causes of dementia (see Table 2-1). The most important reversible causes include depression, medication, hydrocephalus, thyroid disease, vitamin B_{12} deficiency, fungal infection, neurosyphilis, subdural hematoma, and brain tumor. Alzheimer's disease is usually a slowly progressive dementia without focal neurologic deficits but with a prominent anterograde amnesia, followed by naming difficulties and visuospatial problems. Patients with cortical Lewy bodies with or without Alzheimer's disease have extrapyramidal deficits (without a resting tremor) and prominent psychiatric symptoms that include psychosis and depression. Vascular dementia (which constitutes 5 to 10% of cases) is characterized by a sudden onset, a stepwise progression, a history of stroke risk factors (previous stroke, transient ischemic attack, hypertension, atrial fibrillation, and coronary artery disease), focal signs, and imaging studies showing strokes. Mixed vascular dementia and Alzheimer's disease makes up about 10% of cases. When a patient exhibits a prominent change in behavior, perseverations, hyperphagia, poor insight, and, in the beginning, relative preservation of memory, suspect frontal dementia. Creutzfeldt-Jakob disease may present with a subacute course, myoclonus, visual changes, and ataxia. An EEG is often helpful in the diagnosis. Look for hydrocephalus if the patient has gait abnormality, memory loss, preserved naming, a large head (in about 10% of cases), and incontinence.

Recommended Readings

Alzheimer's Disease and Related Disorders Association (ADRDA), 919 North Michigan Avenue, #1000, Chicago, IL, 69611-1678, (800)272-3900.

Becker P, et al. The role of lumbar puncture in the evaluation of dementia: The Durham Veterans Administration/Duke University Study. *Journal of the American Geriatrics Society* 33:392–396, 1985.

Chui HC, et al. Criteria for the diagnosis of ischemic vascular dementia proposed by the State of California Alzheimer's Disease Diagnostic and Treatment Centers. *Neurology* 42:473–480, 1992.

Clarfield A. The reversible dementias: Do they reverse? *Ann Intern Med* 109:476–486, 1988.

Corey-Bloom J, et al. Diagnosis and evaluation of dementia. *Neurology* 45:211–218, 1995.

Diagnostic and Statistical Manual of Mental Disorders (4th ed.). Washington: American Psychiatric Association, 1994.

Folstein MF, Folstein SE, McHugh PR. "Mini-mental state": A practical method for grading the cognitive state of patients for the clinician. *Journal of Psychiatric Research* 12:189–198, 1975.

Graff-Radford NR, Godersky JC, Jones M. Variables predicting surgical outcome in symptomatic hydrocephalus in the elderly. *Neurology* 39:1601–1604, 1989.

Heston L. Morbid risk in first-degree relatives of persons with Alzheimer's disease. *Archives of General Psychiatry* 45:97–98, 1988.

Mortimer JA. The epidemiology of Alzheimer's disease: Beyond risk factors. In I Iqbal et al. (eds.), *Research Advances in Alzheimer's Disease and Associated Disorders*. New York: John Wiley and Sons, 1995.

McKhann G, et al. Clinical diagnosis of Alzheimer's disease: Report of the NINCDS-ADRDA Work Group under the auspices of the Department of Health and Human Services Task Force on Alzheimer's Disease. *Neurology* 34:939–944, 1984.

Morris JC, (ed.), *Handbook of Dementing Illnesses*. New York: Marcel Dekker, 1994.

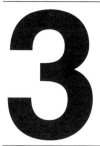

Approach to the Patient with Aphasia

Jeffrey L. Saver

Aphasia is a loss or impairment of language processing caused by brain damage. Language disorders are common manifestations of cerebral injury. Reflecting the centrality of language function in human endeavor, the aphasias are a major source of disability.

I. **Pathophysiology**

  A. **Cerebral dominance.** The left hemisphere is dominant for language in approximately 99% of right-handers and 60% of left-handers.

  B. **Neuroanatomy.** A specialized cortical-subcortical neural system surrounding the Sylvian fissure in the dominant hemisphere subserves language processing (Fig. 3-1). Circumscribed lesions in different components of this neurocognitive network produce distinctive syndromes of language impairment.

II. **Etiology**

  A. **Stroke.** Cerebrovascular disease is a frequent cause of aphasia. The perisylvian language zone is supplied by divisions of the middle cerebral artery, a branch of the internal carotid artery. The classic aphasic syndromes are most distinctly observed in ischemic stroke because vascular occlusions produce discrete, well-delineated brain lesions.

  B. **Other focal lesions.** Any focal lesion affecting the language cortices will also produce aphasia, including primary and metastatic neoplasms and abscesses. **Primary progressive aphasia** is an uncommon neurodegenerative syndrome characterized by slowly progressive, isolated language impairment in late life and focal atrophy of dominant frontotemporal cortices. Affected individuals frequently develop a generalized dementia after the first 2 years of illness. Among the causes of primary progressive aphasia are a focal variant of Alzheimer's disease, a focal variant of Pick's disease, and focal neuronal loss without specific histopathologic features.

  C. **Diffuse lesions.** Diseases producing widespread neuronal dysfunction will disrupt language processing along with other cognitive and noncognitive neural functions. **Traumatic head injury** and **Alzheimer's disease** are epidemiologically common causes of aphasic symptoms, although not of isolated aphasia.

III. **Clinical manifestations**

  A. **Nonfluency vs. fluency.** Fluency refers to the rate, quantity, and ease of speech production. In nonfluent speech, verbal output is meager (<50 words/min), phrase length shortened (one to four words per phrase), production effortful, articulation often poor, and the melodic contour (prosody) disturbed. Nonfluent speakers often preferentially employ substantive nouns and verbs, eliding small connecting grammatical/functor words ("telegraphic speech"). Conversely, in fluent speech, verbal output is generous (and may even be more abundant than customary), phrase length normal, production easy, articulation usually preserved, and the melodic contour intact.

    1. **Anatomic correlate.** Nonfluency indicates damage to the frontal language regions anterior to the fissure of Rolando. Fluency signals that these areas are intact.

  B. **Auditory comprehension impairment.** Impaired ability to understand spoken language ranges from complete mystification by simple one-word utterances to subtle failure to extract the full meanings of complex sentences. In informal conversation, aphasic patients often capitalize on clues from gestures, tone, and setting to supplement their understanding of the propositional content of a speaker's utterances. Examiners may underestimate the extent of auditory comprehension impairment if they fail to test formally a patient's comprehension deprived of nonverbal cues.

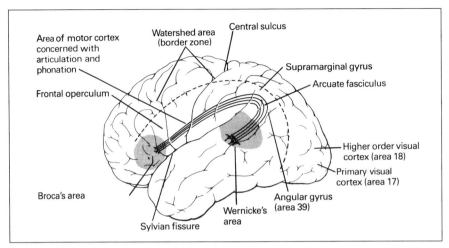

Figure 3-1. The neurocognitive network for language. The core perisylvian language cortices lie within the dashed line and include Broca's area in the inferior frontal gyrus, the supramarginal and angular gyri in the parietal lobe, the subjacent arcuate fasciculus white matter tract, and Wernicke's area in the superior temporal gyrus. Extrasylvian sites that produce transcortical aphasias are found in surrounding cortices (beyond dashed line). (Modified with permission from Mayeux R, Kandel ER. Disorders of language: The aphasias. In ER Kandel, JH Schwartz (eds), *Principles of Neural Science* (2nd ed). New York: Elsevier, 1985.

      1. Anatomic correlate. Comprehension impairment generally reflects damage to the temporoparietal language regions posterior to the fissure of Rolando. Preserved comprehension indicates that these areas are intact.*

   C. Repetition impairment. Repetition of spoken language is linguistically and anatomically a distinct language function. In most patients, repetition impairment parallels other deficits in spoken language. Occasionally, however, relatively isolated disordered repetition may be the dominant clinical feature (conduction aphasia). In other patients, repetition may be well-preserved despite severe deficits in spontaneous speech (transcortical aphasias). Rarely, such patients exhibit **echolalia,** a powerful, mandatory tendency to repeat all heard phrases.

      1. Anatomic correlate. Impaired repetition indicates damage within the core perisylvian language zone. Preserved repetition signals that these areas are intact.

   D. Paraphasic errors. Substitutions of incorrect words for intended words are paraphasias. Paraphasic errors are classified into three types.

      1. A **literal** or **phonemic paraphasia** occurs when only a part of the word is misspoken, as when "apple" becomes "tapple" or "apfle."

      2. A **verbal** or **global paraphasia** occurs when an entire incorrect word is substituted for the intended word, as when "apple" becomes "orange" or "bicycle." A **semantic paraphasia** arises when the substituted word is from the same semantic field as the target word ("orange" for "apple"). Fluent output contaminated by many verbal paraphasias is **jargon speech.**

      3. A **neologistic paraphasia** occurs when an entirely novel word not extant in the speaker's native lexicon is substituted for the intended word, as when "apple" becomes "brifun."

      4. Anatomic correlate. Paraphasic errors may occur with lesions anywhere within the language system and do not carry strong anatomic implications. To some extent, phonemic paraphasias are more common with lesions in the frontal language fields and global paraphasias more common with lesions in temporoparietal areas.

---

*Comprehension of grammar is an important exception to this rule. Agrammatism is associated with damage to inferior frontal language regions.

   E. **Word-finding difficulty (anomia).** Retrieval of target words from the lexicon
      is virtually always disturbed in aphasia. Patients may exhibit frequent hesita-
      tions in their spontaneous speech while they struggle with word-finding. **Cir-
      cumlocutions** transpire when patients "talk around" words they fail to re-
      trieve, providing lengthy definitions or descriptions to convey the meanings of
      words they are unable to access.
      1. **Anatomic correlate.** Word-finding difficulty occurs with lesions located
         throughout the language dominant hemisphere and possesses little localiz-
         ing value.
   F. **Reading and writing.** In most cases of aphasia, reading impairment (**alexia**)
      and writing impairment (**agraphia**) parallel oral language comprehension and
      production deficits. Occasionally, however, isolated reading impairment, writ-
      ing impairment, or both can occur in the setting of fully preserved oral lan-
      guage function.
      1. **Anatomic correlate.** The anatomy of reading and writing incorporates both
         the core perisylvian language zones and additional function-specific sites.
         Reading requires primary and higher-level visual processing in the occipital
         and inferior parietal lobes. Writing depends on visual stores in the inferior
         parietal lobe and graphomotor output regions in the frontal lobe.
IV. **Evaluation**
   A. **History.** Abrupt onset of language difficulty suggests a cerebrovascular lesion.
      Subacute onset may suggest tumor, abscess, or other more moderately progres-
      sive process. Slow onset suggests a degenerative disease, such as Alzheimer's
      or Pick's. Interviewing family members and other observers is crucial when the
      patient's language difficulty limits direct history-taking.
   B. **Physical examination**
      1. **Elementary neurologic signs.** A detailed elementary neurologic examina-
         tion allows identification of motor, sensory, or visual deficits that accom-
         pany the language disorder, aiding neuroanatomic localization. Important
         "neighborhood" signs are the presence or absence of hemiparesis, homony-
         mous hemianopia or quadrantanopia, and apraxia.
      2. **Mental status exam.** It is important to assess the patient's wakefulness and
         attentional function, lest language errors resulting from inattentiveness be
         wrongly ascribed to intrinsic linguistic dysfunction. Nonverbal tests to eval-
         uate memory, visuospatial, and executive functions should be utilized if se-
         vere language disturbance precludes routine verbal assessment.
      3. **Language exam.** A careful language exam is critical in the evaluation of
         aphasia, profiling the patient's impaired and preserved language abilities
         and allowing a syndromic, localizing diagnosis.
         a. **Spontaneous speech.** The patient's spontaneous verbal output, in
            the course of conversation and in response to general questions,
            should be judged for fluency versus nonfluency and presence or ab-
            sence of paraphasias. It is important to ask open-ended questions such
            as "Why are you in the hospital?" or "What do you do during a typical
            day at home?" because patients may mask major language derange-
            ments with yes-no answers and other brief replies to more structured
            interrogatories.
         b. **Repetition.** The patient is asked to repeat complex sentences. If diffi-
            culty is evidenced, simpler verbal sequences from single-syllable words
            to multisyllabic words and short phrases are given to determine the level
            of impairment. At least one sentence rich in grammatical/functor words,
            such as "No ifs, ands, or buts," should be employed to test for isolated or
            more pronounced difficulty in grammatic repetition, as may be seen in
            Broca's and other anterior aphasias.
         c. **Comprehension.** An initial judgment of auditory comprehension can be
            made in the course of obtaining the medical history and from sponta-
            neous conversation. Tests that require no or minimal verbal responses
            are essential to evaluation of auditory comprehension in individuals with
            severe disturbance of speech production and intubated patients.
            (1) **Commands.** One simple bedside test is verbally to instruct the pa-
               tient to carry out one-step and multistep commands, such as "Pick
               up a piece of paper, fold it in half, and place it on the table." Cau-
               tions to recall when interpreting results are: (1) apraxia and other
               motor deficits may cause impairment not related to comprehension

deficit, and (2) midline motor acts on command, such as closing/opening eyes and standing up, draw on distinct anatomic systems and may be preserved even in the setting of severe aphasic comprehension disturbance.

   (2) Yes/no responses. If the patient can reliably produce verbal or gestural yes/no responses, this output system may be used to assess auditory comprehension. Questions of graded difficulty should be employed for precise gauging of the degree of comprehension disturbance, using queries ranging from simple ("Is your name Smith?") to complex ("Do helicopters eat their young?").

   (3) Pointing. This simple motor response also permits precise mapping of comprehension impairment by means of questions of graded difficulty. The examiner should employ both simple pointing commands ("Point to the chair, nose, door") and more lexically and syntactically complex pointing commands ("Point to the source of illumination in this room").

   d. Naming. Difficulty with naming is almost invariable in all the aphasia syndromes. Consequently, naming tasks are sensitive, although not specific, means of testing for the presence or absence of aphasia.

   (1) Confrontation naming. The patient is asked to name objects, parts of objects, body parts, and colors pointed out by the examiner. Common, high-frequency words ("tie," "watch") and uncommon, low-frequency words ("knot" of the tie, "watchband") should be tested.

   (2) Word-List generation. Another type of naming test is to ask the patient to generate a list of items in a category (animals, cars) or words beginning with a given letter (F, A, S). Normal individuals produce 12 or more words per letter in 1 minute.

   e. Verbal automatisms. Patients with profound disruptions of speech production should be requested to produce (1) overlearned verbal sequences, including the numbers from 1 to 10 and the days of the week; (2) overlearned verbal material, such as the pledge of allegiance; and (3) singing, such as "Happy Birthday to You." These utterances draw on subcortical and nondominant hemisphere areas, and indicate residual capacities in impaired patients that may be capitalized on in rehabilitation.

   f. Reading. Patients should be asked to read sentences aloud. Written sentences that are commands ("Close your eyes") allow simultaneous testing of reading aloud and reading comprehension.

   g. Writing. In order of difficulty, patients may be asked to write single letters, words, and short sentences. Obtaining a signature is insufficient, because this overlearned sequence may be retained when all other graphomotor function is lost.

C. Laboratory studies

   1. Computed tomography (CT). A CT scan will delineate most focal structural lesions affecting the language regions of the brain. The CT scan may be normal in the first 24 hours following acute aphasia from new onset ischemic stroke.

   2. Magnetic resonance imaging (MRI). MRI is somewhat more sensitive than CT at detecting morphologic abnormalities, and is the preferred study if readily available. Imaging in the sagittal and coronal as well as axial planes allows precise mapping of lesions within known neural language regions.

V. Syndromic diagnosis. Distinctive features of a patient's language disturbance may be employed to assign a syndromic diagnosis that has localizing value (Table 3-1). Eight classical cortical aphasia syndromes are distinguished on the basis of fluency, comprehension, and repetition (Fig. 3-2). Approximately 60% of all aphasic patients exhibit one of these symptom clusters. Most of the remaining "atypical" aphasias will be found to harbor subcortical lesions. It is important to consider the time after onset when employing these syndromes for clinicoanatomic correlation. Soon after an acute insult, deafferentation, edema, and other mechanisms of diaschisis produce exaggerated clinical deficits. Later, neuroplasticity-mediated recovery of function reduces clinical deficits. The aphasia syndromes have maximal localizing value 3 weeks to 3 months after onset.

A. Perisylvian aphasias

   1. Broca's aphasia. Patients with Broca's aphasia exhibit (1) nonfluent,

Table 3-1. Clinical features of aphasia syndromes.

Syndrome	Language findings					Associated findings		
	Verbal output	Paraphasia	Comprehension	Repetition	Naming	Hemiparesis	Hemisensory loss	Visual field defect
Broca	Nonfluent	Rare-literal	Good	Poor	Poor	Common	Rare	Rare
Wernicke	Fluent	Frequent-mixed	Poor	Poor	Poor	Rare	Variable	Quadrantanopia (+/−)
Conduction	Fluent	Frequent-literal	Good	Poor	Poor	Rare	Common	Hemianopia (+/−)
Global	Nonfluent	Frequent-mixed	Poor	Poor	Poor	Common	Common	Hemianopia
Transcortical motor	Nonfluent	Rare	Good	Good	Poor	Occasional	Rare	Rare
Transcortical sensory	Fluent	Frequent-mixed	Poor	Good	Poor	Occasional	Common	Hemianopia
Mixed transcortical	Nonfluent	Rare	Poor	Good	Poor	Common	Common	Hemianopia (+/−)
Anomic	Fluent	Frequent	Good	Good	Poor	Rare	Rare	Rare
Striatocapsular	Nonfluent or Fluent	Frequent	Good	Good	Poor	Common	Variable	Rare
Thalamic	Fluent	Frequent	Poor	Good	Poor	Rare	Rare	Rare

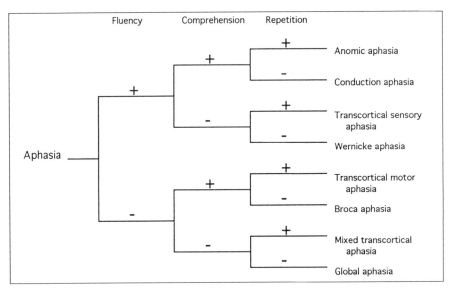

Figure 3-2. Algorithm for diagnosis of the eight classical cortical aphasias.

dysarthric, effortful speech; (2) similarly disordered repetition; and (3) relatively intact comprehension, with mild difficulty in understanding syntax and relational grammar. Their verbal output is often "telegraphic," containing substantive nouns and verbs but omitting small, connecting, functor words. Most patients exhibit a faciobrachial hemiparesis. Patients often exhibit frustration over their language deficits and are at elevated risk for depression.

    a. Lesions producing Broca's aphasia lie in the posterior portion of the inferior frontal gyrus (Broca's area) and extend to involve surrounding motor, premotor, and underlying white matter territories. Lesions restricted solely to Broca's area produce mild, transient aphasia and more persistent dysarthria.

    b. Broca's area is supplied by the superior division of the middle cerebral artery.

2. Wernicke's aphasia. Patients with Wernicke's aphasia evince fluent, effortless, well-articulated output, almost always contaminated with paraphasias and neologisms. Repetition demonstrates a parallel impairment, with fluent but paraphasic output. The leading feature of Wernicke's aphasia is a severe disturbance of auditory comprehension. Two types of behavioral responses to this comprehension deficit are observed. Most often in the acute phase, patients seem unaware of their inability to comprehend spoken language, calmly providing inappropriate and grossly paraphasic answers to observer inquiries. Less frequently, patients are irritable and paranoic, perhaps because of their inability to understand what others say. A superior homonymous quadrantanopia is frequently present. However, the absence of more dramatic motor or sensory deficits, and the fluid production of speech, may mislead medical personnel into believing that the patient is confused or psychotic rather than aphasic, and may delay diagnosis while metabolic or psychiatric disturbances are sought.

    a. The core of lesions engendering Wernicke's aphasia map to the posterior third of the superior temporal gyrus (Wernicke's area), an auditory association area. Lesion size may vary considerably, and damage often extends to the middle temporal gyrus and the inferior parietal lobe.

    b. Wernicke's area is supplied by the inferior division of the middle cerebral artery.

3. Global aphasia. The most profound form of aphasia, called global aphasia, is characterized by drastically nonfluent output, severe disruption of comprehension, and little repetitive ability. Spontaneous speech is often absent initially, or marked by production of a few stereotyped sounds. Patients neither read nor write. Hemiplegia is almost invariably present, and hemisensory loss and hemianopia are frequent.

 a. The typical insult involves the entire left perisylvian region, encompassing Broca's area in the inferior frontal lobe, Wernicke's area in the posterior temporal lobe, and all the interposed parietofrontal cortices. In rare cases, separate, discrete lesions of Broca's area and Wernicke's area produce global aphasia without hemiparesis.

 b. The perisylvian region lies within the territory of the middle cerebral artery, and internal carotid and middle cerebral artery occlusions are the most common causes of global aphasia.

4. Conduction aphasia. The hallmark of conduction aphasia is a disproportionate disruption of repetition. Comprehension of spoken language is relatively intact. Fluent spontaneous output is often marred by occasional hesitations and phonemic paraphasias, but is not as disturbed as repetition. Naming also tends to demonstrate mild paraphasic contamination. Motor and sensory disturbances are usually absent or mild.

 a. Two neural loci tend to give rise to conduction aphasia: (1) the supramarginal gyrus, sometimes with extension to the subinsular white matter, and (2) the primary auditory cortex, insula, and subjacent white matter. The arcuate fasciculus, a subcortical white matter tract connecting Wernicke's and Brodmann's areas, is often, but not invariably, involved.

 b. These regions are variably supplied by branches of the inferior or superior divisions of the middle cerebral artery.

B. Extrasylvian aphasias. The extrasylvian aphasic syndromes share the clinical characteristic of preserved repetition and the anatomic trait of sparing of the core perisylvian language zone. They occur less commonly than the perisylvian aphasias. Many arise from watershed infarcts, but they may also appear in conjunction with tumors, abscesses, hemorrhages, and other lesions.

1. Transcortical motor aphasia. Transcortical motor aphasia is characterized by discrepant spontaneous speech and repetition. Spontaneous output is severely disrupted, nonfluent, and halting. In contrast, the ability to repeat sentences verbatim is preserved, as is reading aloud. Comprehension is undisturbed. Naming may be mildly impaired.

 a. Transcortical motor aphasia results from damage at one of two foci: (1) prefrontal cortices and subjacent white matter anterior or superior to Broca's area, or (2) the supplementary motor area and cingulate gyrus. These lesions disconnect Broca's area from limbic areas and other sources of the drive to communicate.

 b. Lesions anterosuperior to Broca's area lie in the vascular border zone between the middle and anterior cerebral arteries. The supplementary motor area and cingulate gyrus regions are irrigated by the anterior cerebral artery.

2. Transcortical sensory aphasia. Patients with transcortical sensory aphasia exhibit severely disturbed comprehension of spoken language, but preserved repetition. Spontaneous speech is fluent, although often paraphasic. Echolalia—automatic repetition of overheard phrases—is common. Reading aloud may be fairly preserved whereas reading comprehension is quite poor. Motor deficits are generally absent, but hemisensory deficits are uncommon.

 a. Lesions may occur over a wide distribution posterior and superior to the posterior perisylvian region, including the middle temporal gyrus, the angular gyrus, and underlying white matter. These insults disconnect Wernicke's area from multiple posterior association cortices, preventing retroactivation by aural word forms of the widely distributed neural representations that convey their meanings.

 b. The lesions generally lie within the vascular watershed between the posterior and middle cerebral arteries.

3. Mixed transcortical aphasia. This rare and remarkable condition is analogous to global aphasia, except for preserved ability to repeat. Spontaneous speech is minimal or absent. Patients are unable to comprehend spoken language, name, read, or write. Repetition of spoken language, however, is preserved. Patients often are echolalic. Mild hemiparesis and hemisensory loss affecting proximal greater than distal extremities may be observed.

 a. Lesions are an additive combination of those producing transcortical motor and sensory aphasias. Insults anterosuperior to Broca's area and posterosuperior to Wernicke's area cut off the perisylvian language zone from access to other cortices. "Isolation of the speech area" is a synonym for mixed transcortical aphasia.

   b. The lesions fall in the crescentic vascular border zone among the anterior, middle, and posterior cerebral arteries.

4. Anomic aphasia. These patients exhibit difficulty retrieving verbal tags in spontaneous speech and confrontation naming. The remainder of language functions are relatively intact. Auditory comprehension, repetition, reading, and writing are normal. Spontaneous speech is preponderantly fluent, although interrupted by occasional hesitations for word-finding. In severe cases, output may be lengthy but empty, with recurrent circumlocutions.

   a. A wide variety of lesions, including nondominant hemisphere loci, may produce anomic aphasia. Particularly common sources are insults to (1) the dominant inferior parietal lobe and (2) the dominant anterior temporal cortices. The latter insults have been associated with category-specific naming deficits in which naming in different semantic categories (e.g., living versus nonliving entities) is differentially impaired.

   b. The angular gyrus and anterior temporal cortices are supplied by different branches of the inferior division of the middle cerebral artery.

C. Subcortical aphasia syndromes. Focal lesions confined to subcortical structures strongly interconnected with language cortices produce aphasia. The delineation of the subcortical aphasias is a rapidly evolving and still unsettled enterprise, but two major profiles can be discerned.

1. Striatocapsular aphasia. The language deficit in striatocapsular aphasia resembles that in anomic or transcortical motor aphasia. Patients may or may not be fluent but are almost invariably dysarthric. Mild to moderate anomia coexists with generally intact auditory comprehension, repetition, reading, and writing. Generation of complex syntactic sentences is impaired. Hemiparesis is common, hemisensory loss variable, and hemianopia infrequent. Lesions involve the dominant putamen, dorsolateral caudate, anterior limb of the internal capsule, and rostral periventricular white matter.

2. Thalamic aphasia. The language deficit in thalamic aphasia resembles that in transcortical sensory or mixed transcortical aphasia. Output may be nonfluent or relatively fluent, auditory comprehension is deficient, and repetition is preserved. Impairments of naming, reading comprehension, and writing are also present. A contralateral emotional facial paresis (diminished facial movement in expressing spontaneous emotions but preserved facial movements to command) and contralateral hypokinesia are often the only elementary neurologic deficits. Lesions are situated in the dominant anterolateral thalamus.

D. Additional classical syndromes. Strategically placed lesions may produce dissociated impairments of reading, writing, and oral language function. Three with well-characterized localizing properties will be reviewed.

1. Alexia without agraphia (pure alexia). Reading is severely impaired whereas spontaneous speech, repetition, and auditory comprehension are normal. Writing is preserved, but dramatically, after a delay, patients are unable to read phrases they themselves have written. Recognition of words spelled aloud and traced on the palm is normal. Only words presented visually pose difficulty. Patients frequently exhibit a slow, letter-by-letter reading strategy, painstakingly recognizing and stating aloud each letter in a word and then, from the spoken letters, string-determining the target word. A right homonymous hemianopia is common but not invariable. Disorders of color vision, including achromatopsia and color anomia, may be present.
The most common neuroanatomic substrate comprises simultaneous lesions of the left occipital lobe and the splenium of the corpus callosum, depriving the angular gyrus region critical for word recognition of visual input from either the left or right hemisphere. The smallest sufficient injury is a single lesion of the paraventricular white matter of the mesial occipitotemporal junction (the forceps major), interrupting interhemispheric and intrahemispheric visual tracts to the angular gyrus but sparing the corpus callosum and left occipital cortex.

2. Alexia with agraphia. Patients exhibit loss of literacy—inability to read or write—but relatively well-preserved oral language function. Speech is fluent, although anomia is often present, and auditory comprehension and repetition are intact. Hemisensory deficits are frequent, and hemiparesis and hemivisual disturbances are variable. A full-fledged Gerstmann's syndrome, including dyscalculia, dysgraphia, left-right confusion, and finger agnosia, may be present. The underlying lesion involves the dominant inferior parietal lobule (angular and supramarginal gyri).

3. **Pure word deafness.** Patients resemble Wernicke's aphasics. Comprehension and repetition of spoken language are impaired, whereas speech is fluent. Unlike in Wernicke's patients, however, paraphasias are rare and, more importantly, comprehension of written material is intact. Writing production is also normal. Although uncomprehending of word sounds, patients have intact hearing and generally are successful in identifying meaningful nonverbal sounds such as car horns or telephone rings.

Two types of lesions underlie pure word deafness, both disconnecting Wernicke's area from input from primary auditory cortices. Some patients harbor bilateral superior temporal lesions. A roughly equal number exhibit a single deep superior temporal lesion in the dominant hemisphere, blocking ipsilateral and crossing callosal auditory pathways.

E. **Aprosodia.** Meaning is conveyed not only through the propositional content of speech, but also through prosody—the melody, rhythm, timbre, and inflection of the speaker. Prosody is frequently disturbed in nonfluent aphasia. However, patients may have normal propositional language yet exhibit disturbances of the production, comprehension, or repetition of prosody. In general, the nondominant hemisphere plays a greater role in production and comprehension of emotional prosody than does the dominant hemisphere.

VI. **Differential diagnosis.** Acquired speech impairments may result from disruption of lower-order neural and muscular mechanisms for implementing sound production rather than disturbances of central processing of language. It is important to distinguish these nonaphasic speech impairments from genuine aphasia, because they differ in their localizing significance and spectrum of etiologic causes.

A. **Dysarthria.** Dysarthria is abnormal articulation of spoken language. At least five types of nonaphasic dysarthria may be distinguished. (1) **Paretic dysarthria** is caused by weakness of articulatory muscles. Soft, low-pitched, nasal voicing is characteristic. Causes include myopathies, neuromuscular junction disorders such as myasthenia gravis, and lower motor neuron disease. (2) In **spastic dysarthria,** speech is typically strained, slow, and monotonic. Bilateral upper motor neuron lesions compromising the corticobulbar tracts are the cause. (3) In **ataxic dysarthria,** jerky irregular speech rhythm and volume are noted, reflecting lesions to the cerebellum or its connections. Multiple sclerosis is a common cause. (4) **Extrapyramidal dysarthrias** include hypokinetic dysarthria, which is seen in parkinsonism, and choreic dysarthria, which is observed in Huntington's disease and other chorea syndromes. (5) In **aphemia (cortical dysarthria),** small lesions within Broca's area or the dominant frontal oral motor cortex produce dysarticulation without disturbing core language function.

Aphasic dysarthria—dysarticulation occurring as one manifestation of an aphasic language syndrome—is common with anterior aphasias such as Broca's syndrome. The nonaphasic dysarthrias may be distinguished from aphasic dysarthria by demonstrating preserved intrinsic language functions including naming, comprehension, and reading. Intact writing is most telling, showing normal productive language capacity when a nonoral output channel is employed.

B. **Mutism.** Aphasia—disordered language—can be securely diagnosed only on the basis of exemplars of disturbed output (or comprehension). Patients with acute onset aphasia, especially Broca's or global aphasia, are often unable to speak for the first few hours or days. However, a wide variety of other insults can produce total cessation of verbal output (Table 3-2). The full differential diagnosis of mutism includes (1) psychiatric etiologies (schizophrenia, depression, catatonia, and psychogenic illness); (2) abulia/akinetic mutism (bilateral prefrontal, diencephalic, and midbrain lesions); (3) acute dominant supplementary motor area lesions; (4) pseudobulbar palsy; (5) locked-in syndrome from bilateral ventral pontine or midbrain lesions; (6) acute bilateral cerebellar lesions; (7) lower motor neuron lesions; and (8) laryngeal disorders.

C. **Thought disorders.** When an intact language apparatus is placed in service of an underlying thought disorder, bizarre utterances arise that superficially re-

Table 3-2. Differential diagnosis of mutism.

Psychiatric disorders
  Schizophrenia
  Depression
  Catatonia
  Psychogenic

Aphasic syndromes (acute period)
  Global aphasia
  Broca's aphasia

Aphemia (acute period)

Dominant supplementary motor area lesion

Pseudobulbar palsy

Abulia

Akinetic mutism

Locked-in syndrome

Chronic vegetative state

Cerebellar lesions (bilateral)

Lower motor neuron lesions
  Guillain-Barré syndrome
Laryngeal disorders

semble the fluent aphasic output of patients with Wernicke's or conduction aphasia. Demographic features are helpful, recognizing that schizophrenia with psychotic speech of new onset tends to appear in individuals in their 20s and 30s whereas fluent aphasias cluster in older individuals with vascular risk factors. Several features of the utterances also distinguish thought-disordered from fluent aphasic speech. (1) Paraphasias are common in aphasia but rare in schizophrenia. (2) The neologisms of aphasics are frequent and changing, whereas those of schizophrenics are infrequent and consistent. (3) Open-ended questions tend to prompt briefer responses in aphasics than in schizophrenics. (4) Bizarre and delusional themes appear only in schizophrenic discourse.

VII. Course. Some degree of spontaneous recovery of language function is invariable after a static brain injury. An initial accelerated period of improved function occurs over the first few days or weeks after insult and is attributable to resolution of edema, ischemic penumbra, and other causes of dysfunction at a distance from the site of permanent injury. The second, slower phase of recovery reflects utilization of parallel circuits, retraining, and structural neural plasticity. The bulk of this functional recovery takes place in the first 3 months after injury, and some may continue up to 1 year, rarely longer. Among the aphasia syndromes, the greatest recovery compared with baseline tends to occur in Broca's and conduction aphasias. Anomic aphasia is a common end stage into which other aphasia subtypes tend to evolve.

Factors favoring greater spontaneous improvement, as well as response to speech therapy, are young age, left-handedness or ambidexterity, higher education, smaller lesion size, no or few nonlanguage cognitive defects, absence of emotional difficulties such as depression and neglect, and strong family support. Patients with traumatic aphasia tend to recover more fully than patients with ischemic lesions.

VIII. Referral

  A. Neurologist. Most patients with aphasia should undergo neurologic consultation. The neurology specialist will confirm the presence of aphasia, clarify the type, aid in etiologic diagnosis, and provide the patient and family with an informed prognosis.

    In selected cases, neurologists may consider pharmacotherapy of aphasia. Small case series have suggested that amphetamine and other norepinephrine agonists may increase neuroplasticity and facilitate recovery from aphasia when begun within 1 month of deficit onset. Dopamine agonists such as bromocriptine have been employed to improve output of speech in patients with speech initiation deficits, such as in transcortical motor aphasia. These non-FDA-approved uses of pharmacologic agents are the subject of active investigation.

B. Speech and language pathologist. All patients with aphasia should have an evaluation by a speech and language pathologist. The speech therapist will perform a formal diagnostic assessment, profiling the patient's language strengths and weaknesses with normed tests. A variety of standardized language assessment batteries, including the Boston Diagnostic Aphasia Examination, the Western Aphasia Battery, the Porch Index of Communicative Ability, and the Communication Abilities in Daily Living, may be drawn on to survey a patient's abilities. The therapist then employs the results to design and implement an individualized treatment program of aphasia therapy.

Although controversy regarding the effectiveness of aphasia therapy persists, the preponderance of evidence suggests that systematic language rehabilitation programs improve patient outcome. Treatment is tailored to each individual's pattern of linguistic and cognitive competencies and deficits, exploiting spared brain systems to reestablish, circumvent, or compensate for lost language capacities. A variety of deficit-specific programs are available to supplement general language stimulation. For nonfluency, treatments include (1) melodic intonation therapy, (2) sign language and other gestural communication training, and (3) communication boards. Syntax training may benefit agrammatism. Specific word-retrieval therapies have been developed for anomia and comprehension training programs for auditory comprehension deficits.

Speech therapy programs generally last for two to three months, in 30–60 minute sessions conducted two to five times per week. Self- and family-administered home exercises provide additional stimulation. Computer-based training is expanding in scope and sophistication.

C. Neuropsychologist. Patients who have major nonlinguistic cognitive deficits in addition to aphasia, and whose diagnosis is unclear, should undergo neuropsychological evaluation. Formal neuropsychological evaluation with tests that minimize language requirements allow a more detailed profiling of memory, visuospatial reasoning, executive function, praxis, and concept formation than can be obtained by bedside mental status examination. Findings may aid the physician in making a diagnosis by suggesting the pattern of neural system involvement and the speech pathologist in prescribing therapy by identifying the extent to which different extralinguistic capacities can support various compensatory strategies.

D. Patient support groups. The National Aphasia Association (P.O. Box 1887, Murray Hill Station, New York, NY 10156-0611, 1-800-922-4622) is an excellent resource for patients and their families. The American Heart Association and National Stroke Association also provide beneficial programs and information.

Recommended Readings

Alexander MP, et al. Distributed anatomy of transcortical sensory aphasia. *Arch Neurol* 46:885–892, 1989.

Alexander MP, et al. Broca's area aphasias: Aphasia after lesions involving the frontal operculum. *Neurology* 40:353–362, 1990.

Benson DF. Aphasia. In KM Heilman, E Valenstein (eds), *Clinical Neuropsychology* (3rd ed). New York: Oxford University Press, 1993. Pp 17–36.

Broca P. Remarks on the seat of the faculty of articulate speech, followed by the report of a case of aphemia (loss of speech). In DA Rottenberg, FH Hochberg (eds), *Neurologic Classics in Modern Translation*. New York: Hafner, 1977. Pp 136–149.

Cummings JL, et al. Mutism: Loss of neocortical and limbic vocalization. *J Nerv Ment Dis* 17:255–259, 1983.

Cummings JL, et al. Aphasia in dementia of the Alzheimer type. *Neurology* 35:394–397, 1985.

Damasio AR, et al. Category-related recognition defects as a clue to the neural substrates of knowledge. *Trends Neurosci* 13:95–98, 1990.

Damasio AR. Aphasia. *N Engl J Med* 326:531–539, 1992.

Damasio H. Neuroanatomical correlates of the aphasias. In M. Sarno (ed), *Acquired Aphasia* (2nd ed). New York: Academic, 1991. Pp 45–72.

Devinsky O. *100 Maxims in Behavioral Neurology*. London: Edward Arnold, 1992.

Geschwind N. Disconnexion syndromes in animals and man. *Brain* 88:237–294, 585–644, 1965.

Grodzinsky Y. The syntactic characterization of agrammatism. *Cognition* 16:99–120, 1984.

Kertesz A. Neurobiological aspects of recovery from aphasia in stroke. *International Rehabilitation Medicine* 6:122–127, 1984.

Mega MS, et al. Subcortical aphasia: The core profile of capsulostriatal infarction. *Neurology* 44:1824–1829, 1994.

Poeck K, et al. Outcome of intensive language treatment in aphasia. *J Speech Hearing Disord* 54:471–479, 1989.

Ross ED. The aprosodias: Functional-anatomic organization of the affective components of language in the right hemisphere. *Arch Neurol* 38:561–569, 1981.

Ross ED. Acute agitation and other behaviors associated with Wernicke aphasia and their possible neurological basis. *Neuropsychiat, Neuropsychol, Behav Neurol* 6:9–18, 1993.

Sabe L, et al. An open-label trial of bromocriptine in nonfluent aphasia. *Neurology* 42:1637–1638, 1992.

Schiff HB, et al. Aphemia: Clinical-anatomic correlation. *Arch Neurol* 40:720–727, 1983.

Starkstein SE, et al. Depression following cerebrovascular lesions. *Semin Neurol* 10:247–253, 1990.

Tranel D, et al. Global aphasia without hemiparesis. *Arch Neurol* 44:304–308, 1987.

Waler-Batson D, et al. Use of amphetamine in the treatment of aphasia. *Restorative Neurol Neurosci* 4:47–50, 1992.

Weintraub S, et al. Primary progressive aphasia. *Arch Neurol* 47:1329–1335, 1990.

Wertz RT, et al. Comparison of clinic, home, and deferred language treatment for aphasia. *Arch Neurol* 43:653–658, 1986.

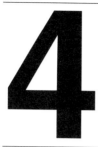

Approach to the Patient with Memory Impairment
Daniel Tranel

The term **amnesia** refers to conditions in which patients lose, partly or completely, the ability to learn new information or to retrieve information acquired previously. Amnesia (also referred to here as "memory impairment" or "memory dysfunction") is extremely common in neurologic diseases that affect the telencephalon or diencephalon, and is surely the most frequent complaint voiced by patients. In an outpatient setting, a substantial majority of patients manifest memory dysfunction, and varying degrees of amnesia are also common in inpatient populations. Amnesia, in fact, is a defining characteristic of some of the most frequently encountered neurologic diseases, including progressive dementia such as Alzheimer's disease. Complaints of memory impairment must be taken seriously, because such complaints frequently constitute one of the earliest manifestations of neurologic disease.

Accurate diagnosis and effective management of memory disorders are very important. A considerable clinical challenge is created, however, by the facts that (1) the most frequent neurologic diseases affect elderly persons and (2) a certain degree of decline in memory is associated with normal aging. Hence, it can be difficult to distinguish complaints of memory problems that are more or less normal manifestations of aging from complaints that signal the presence of neurologic disease. Memory complaints are also common in non-neurologic conditions, such as psychiatric disease, and this constitutes another reason for careful diagnosis. Such distinctions often require laboratory testing of the type that can be conducted by means of neuropsychological assessment procedures.

I. **Types of memory and memory systems in the brain.** There are several fundamental distinctions between different types of memory and the different neural systems to which different types of memory are related (see Table 4-1).
   A. **Anterograde and retrograde memory**
      1. **Anterograde memory** refers to the capacity to learn new information—i.e., to acquire new facts, skills, and other types of knowledge. Anterograde memory is closely dependent on neural structures in the mesial temporal lobe, especially the hippocampus and interconnected structures such as the amygdala, the entorhinal and perirhinal cortices, and other parts of the parahippocampal gyrus.
      2. **Retrograde memory** refers to the retrieval of information that was acquired previously—i.e., retrieval of facts, skills, and other knowledge learned in the recent or remote past. This type of memory is related to nonmesial sectors of the temporal lobe, including the polar region (Brodmann's area 38), the inferotemporal region (including Brodmann's areas 20, 21, and 36), and the occipitotemporal region (including Brodmann's area 37 and the ventral parts of areas 18 and 19). Autobiographical memory, a special form of retrograde memory that refers to knowledge about one's past, is linked primarily to the anterior part of the nonmesial temporal lobes.
   B. **Verbal and nonverbal memory.** Knowledge can be divided into that which exists in **verbal** form, such as words (written or spoken) and names, and that which exists in **nonverbal** form, such as faces, geographic routes, and complex musical patterns. This distinction is important, because memory systems in the two hemispheres of the human brain are specialized differently for verbal and nonverbal material (Table 4-2). Specifically, systems in the left hemisphere are dedicated primarily to verbal material, and systems in the right hemisphere are

Supported by NINDS Program Project Grant NS 19632.

33

Table 4-1. Subdivisions of memory.

Dichotomy	Characteristics
Retrograde	Retrieval of knowledge acquired previously, especially knowledge acquired prior to onset of brain injury
Anterograde	Learning of new knowledge, especially learning of knowledge after onset of brain injury
Verbal	Words, names, verbally coded facts; word-based material
Nonverbal	Faces, geographic routes, complex melodies; spatially based material
Declarative	Information that can be brought into consciousness; "declared"; held in the "mind's eye"
Nondeclarative	Performance-based; motor output; habits and conditioning; automatic tendencies
Short-term	Ephemeral (30–45 sec); limited capacity (7+/−2)
Long-term	Permanent; unlimited capacity

Table 4-2. Hemispheric specialization of memory systems.

Left	Right
Verbal	Nonverbal
Words	Patterns
Names	Faces
Stories	Geographic routes
Lyrics	Complex melodies
Sequential, feature-based	Holistic, gestalt-based
Lexical retrieval	Unique personal knowledge

dedicated primarily to nonverbal material. This arrangement parallels the general arrangement of the human brain, in which the left hemisphere is specialized for language, and the right hemisphere for visuospatial processing. This distinction applies to virtually all right-handed individuals, and to about two-thirds of left-handers (in the remaining minority of left-handers, the arrangement may be partially or completely reversed).

C. Declarative and nondeclarative memory

 1. **Declarative memory** (also known as **explicit memory**) refers to knowledge that can be "declared" and brought to mind for conscious inspection—e.g., facts, words, names, and individual faces that can be retrieved from memory, placed in the "mind's eye," and reported. Declarative memory is intimately linked to the functioning of the hippocampus and other mesial temporal lobe structures.

 2. **Nondeclarative memory** (also known as **implicit memory**) refers to various forms of memory that cannot be declared or brought into the mind's eye. Examples include sensorimotor skill learning, autonomic conditioning, and certain types of habits. Skating and skiing, for example, rely on motor skills that constitute forms of nondeclarative memory. Nondeclarative memory requires participation of the neostriatum, cerebellum, and sensorimotor cortices.

D. Short-term and long-term memory

 1. **Short-term memory.** This term is used to designate a time span of memory that covers from 0 to about 45 seconds, a brief period during which a limited amount of information can be held without rehearsal. Short-term memory (also known as **primary memory**) does not depend on the hippocampus or other temporal lobe memory systems, but is linked closely to cerebral mechanisms required for attention and concentration.

 2. **Long-term memory.** This term refers to a large expanse of time that covers everything beyond short-term memory—i.e., knowledge held for days, years, and even decades, in more or less permanent form. Long-term memory (also known as **secondary memory**) can be divided into **recent** (the past few weeks or months) and **remote** (years or decades ago). Unlike short-term

memory, the capacity of long-term memory is enormous, and information may be retained in long-term memory virtually indefinitely. The mesial temporal system, including the hippocampus, is required for acquisition of knowledge into long-term memory; other systems in the temporal lobe and elsewhere are required for retrieval of knowledge from long-term memory.

E. **Working memory** refers to a short time period during which the brain can hold several pieces of information in an active register and perform operations on them. Working memory is akin to short-term memory, but implies a somewhat longer duration (some several minutes) and more focus on the **operational** features of the mental process, rather than simply the acquisition of information. Working memory can be thought of as "on-line" processing and operating on knowledge that is being held in activated form. For example, consider the act of deciding to videotape a television program. One may consult a TV listing for the relevant information about channel, time, and so forth. One then programs the VCR, while holding in "working memory" the relevant information about the program, as well as bringing into mind knowledge that is required for operating the VCR.

II. **Clinical manifestations.** Several frequent neurologic conditions produce damage to memory-related neural systems, leading to various profiles and severities of amnesia (Table 4-3).

A. **Degenerative diseases**

1. **Cortical dementia**

a. **Alzheimer's disease.** The neuropathology of Alzheimer's disease (AD) is characterized by two principal features: the neurofibrillary tangle and the neuritic plaque. Early in the course of AD, the entorhinal cortex, which is a pivotal way station for input to and from the hippocampus, is disrupted by neurofibrillary tangles in cortical layers II and IV. The perforant pathway, which is the main route for entry into the hippocampal formation, is gradually and massively demyelinated. Eventually, the hippocampus is virtually deafferented from cortical inputs. AD also breaks down the efferent linkage of the hippocampus back to the cerebral cortex, through destruction of the subiculum and entorhinal cortex. The hallmark behavioral sign of this destruction is amnesia—specifically, an anterograde (learning) defect that covers declarative knowledge but largely spares nondeclarative learning and retrieval. Early in the course of the disease, retrograde memory is also relatively spared, but as pathology extends to nonmesial temporal sectors, a defect in the retrograde compartment (retrieval impairment) appears and gradually worsens.

b. **Pick's disease,** characterized by "Pick's bodies" (cells containing degraded protein material), is an uncommon form of cortical dementia that often shows a striking predilection for one lobe of the brain, producing a state of circumscribed lobar atrophy. The disease is often concentrated in the frontal lobes, in which case personality alterations, rather than amnesia, are the most prominent manifestations. However, the disease may affect one or the other temporal lobe, producing signs of a material-specific learning and retrieval disorder (verbal or nonverbal amnesia).

c. **Frontal lobe dementia** is another form of cortical dementia, involving

---

Table 4-3. Causes and conditions associated with amnesia.

Degenerative diseases (e.g., Alzheimer's, Pick's, Parkinson's)
Head injury
Cerebrovascular accident (e.g., infarction, ruptured aneurysm)
Toxic conditions (e.g., alcoholism)
Anoxia/ischemia
Herpes simplex encephalitis
Surgical ablation
Neoplasm
Normal pressure hydrocephalus
Transient global amnesia
Functional amnesia

focal atrophy of the frontal lobes, which causes personality changes and other signs of "executive" dysfunction. This condition is similar to Pick's disease, except that there is no predominance of Pick's bodies.

2. **Subcortical dementia**
   a. **Parkinson's disease.** With its pathology focused in subcortical structures, Parkinson's disease (PD) influences memory in a manner different from that of cortical dementias such as Alzheimer's and Pick's diseases. Disorders of nondeclarative memory (e.g., acquisition and retrieval of motor skills) are more prominent, and there may be minimal or no impairment in learning of declarative material. Also, PD patients often have more problems in **recall** of newly acquired knowledge than in **storage;** when cuing strategies are provided, the patients demonstrate normal levels of retention.
   b. **Huntington's disease.** Similar to Parkinson's disease, the pathology of Huntington's disease (HD) is concentrated in subcortical structures. The amnesia of HD patients also resembles that of PD patients, and in particular there is disproportionate involvement of nondeclarative memory. HD patients also tend to show disruption of **working memory** and have trouble holding information "on-line" and performing mental operations on it.
   c. **Progressive supranuclear palsy.** Progressive supranuclear palsy (PSP) is another primarily subcortical disease process that frequently produces problems with memory. In general, however, the amnesia of PSP is considerably less severe than that of Alzheimer's disease, and laboratory assessment often shows relatively mild defects in learning and retrieval, despite the patient's complaints of forgetfulness.
3. **Other degenerative conditions**
   a. **HIV/AIDS-related dementia.** HIV-positive persons and persons with AIDS frequently manifest varying degrees of memory impairment, with the severity being roughly proportional to the overall progression of the disease. Early in the course, memory defects may be the sole signs of cognitive dysfunction. The problems center on acquisition of new material, particularly material of the declarative type. Memory defects in this disease appear to be attributable mainly to defective attention, concentration, and overall efficiency of cognitive functioning, rather than to focal dysfunction of particular memory-related neural systems.
   b. **Multiple sclerosis.** Many patients with multiple sclerosis (MS) manifest varying degrees of amnesia, although the severity may wax and wane considerably in concert with other neurologic symptoms, and many MS patients show no memory defects at all during some periods of the disease process. When present, the memory impairment most commonly manifests as defective recall of newly learned information; encoding and working memory are normal or near-normal. Hence, MS patients benefit from cuing. Most often, the amnesia affects declarative material of both verbal and nonverbal types; defects in nondeclarative memory are rare.
B. **Head injury** is a frequent cause of amnesia, especially in young males, who sustain the vast majority of significant head injuries. There are several distinct types of amnesia associated with head injury.
   1. **Post-traumatic amnesia** (PTA) refers to the period of time following head trauma, during which patients fail to acquire new information in normal and continuous fashion, despite being conscious and "awake." During this time, the patient may appear alert and attentive, and may even deny memory problems, but it will become apparent later that the patient was not forming ongoing records of new experiences. Information is simply not encoded, and no amount of cuing will uncover memories that would normally have been acquired during this period. The **duration** of PTA is a reliable marker of the severity of head injury, and also constitutes one of the best predictors of outcome.
   2. **Retrograde amnesia.** Patients with head injuries often manifest retrograde amnesia—i.e., defective recall of experiences that occurred immediately prior to the injury. Information from the time period closest to the point of injury is most likely to be lost, and the further back in time one goes, the less the impairment. The extent of retrograde amnesia typically "shrinks" as the patient recovers, so that as time goes on, fewer and fewer retrograde memo-

ries will be missing. Patients may be left with only a small island of amnesia for the few minutes or hours immediately prior to the trauma.

3. **Learning defects (anterograde amnesia).** Moderate and severe head injuries often produce permanent damage to mesial temporal lobe structures such as the hippocampus, with resultant defects in learning (anterograde amnesia). The impairment is centered on declarative knowledge; nondeclarative learning is rarely affected. The defect may be unequal for verbal and nonverbal material, if there is asymmetry of the structural injury. Also, head injury patients tend to be exquisitely sensitive to distraction, fatigue, the effects of alcohol, and other influences that produce suboptimal learning performance.

C. Cerebrovascular disease

1. **Stroke** is a frequent cause of amnesia, and the nature and degree of memory disturbance are direct functions of which neural structures are damaged, and to what extent. Amnesia is most likely to result from infarctions that damage the mesial temporal region, the basal forebrain, or the medial diencephalon (especially the thalamus).

   a. **Mesial temporal lobe.** The parahippocampal gyrus and hippocampus proper can be damaged by infarcts in territories supplied by branches of the middle cerebral or posterior cerebral arteries. (Strokes in the region of the anterolateral temporal lobe are decidedly uncommon.) Infarctions of this type are almost always unilateral, and almost always produce incomplete damage to mesial temporal memory structures; hence, the profile is one of a partial material-specific (left–verbal; right–nonverbal) defect in anterograde memory for declarative knowledge.

   b. **Thalamus.** Damage to the thalamus can also produce amnesia. The most severe memory impairment results from infarcts that are bilateral and are situated in the anterior part of the thalamus in the interpeduncular profundus territory. Unilateral lesions caused by lacunar infarctions in anterior thalamic nuclei produce material-specific learning defects reminiscent of those observed with mesial temporal lobe lesions. Thalamic patients, however, tend to manifest both anterograde and retrograde defects. In the retrograde compartment, there is usually a **temporal gradient** to the defect—i.e., the further back in time one goes, the less the severity of the amnesia.

2. **Ruptured aneurysms.** Rupture of aneurysms located either in the anterior communicating artery or in the anterior cerebral artery almost invariably causes infarction in the region of the basal forebrain—a set of bilateral paramidline gray nuclei that includes the septal nuclei, the diagonal band of Broca, and the substantia innominata. The amnesia associated with basal forebrain damage has several distinctive features. Patients develop an inability to link correctly various aspects of memory episodes (i.e., "whens," "wheres," "whats," and "whys"). This problem affects both the anterograde and retrograde compartments. Confabulation is common in basal forebrain amnesias. Cuing markedly improves recall and recognition of both anterograde and retrograde material.

3. **Multi-infarct dementia** (MID; also known as **cerebrovascular dementia**) refers to conditions in which repeated infarctions produce widespread cognitive impairment, including amnesia. The term is used most commonly to denote multiple small strokes (lacunar strokes) in the arterioles that feed subcortical structures; hence, the usual picture is one of "subcortical" dementia. The memory impairment in MID generally affects encoding of new material (anterograde amnesia), and nondeclarative learning may also be defective. Retrograde memory tends to be spared.

D. Toxic conditions

1. **Alcoholism.** Chronic long-term alcohol abuse can produce permanent damage to certain diencephalic structures, particularly the mammillary bodies and dorsomedial thalamic nucleus, that has been linked to amnesic manifestations in these patients. This presentation is known as **alcoholic Korsakoff's syndrome** or **Wernicke-Korsakoff syndrome.** The amnesic profile in Korsakoff patients is characterized by (1) anterograde amnesia for both verbal and nonverbal material, with defects in both encoding and retrieval; (2) retrograde amnesia with a strong temporal gradient—i.e., progressively milder defects as one goes farther back in time; and (3) sparing of

nondeclarative memory. Confabulation is characteristic of Korsakoff patients, especially in the early days following detoxification.

2. **Other neurotoxins.** Amnesia can result from acute or chronic exposure to other neurotoxins, including metals (especially lead and mercury), solvents and fuels, and pesticides. The relationship between exposure to these substances and cognitive dysfunction is poorly understood, and conclusive scientific evidence for specific cause-and-effect relationships is virtually nonexistent. Nonetheless, there is little doubt that memory impairments do often result from excessive exposure to these neurotoxins. The amnesia tends to manifest as a deficiency in new learning (anterograde amnesia) that covers various types of material, including verbal, nonverbal, and nondeclarative. Defects of concentration, attention, and overall cognitive efficiency are frequent contributing factors, and in most cases the memory impairment occurs in the setting of more widespread cognitive dysfunction.

E. **Anoxia/ischemia.** Cerebral anoxia or global ischemia in the setting of cardiopulmonary arrest often leads to the selective destruction of cellular groups within the hippocampal formation. The extent of damage is linked fairly directly to the number of minutes of arrest. Brief periods of anoxia/ischemia may cause limited damage, and longer periods will produce greater destruction. With a critical length of deprivation, the damage will concentrate in the CA1 ammonic fields of the hippocampus, bilaterally, leading to a selective anterograde amnesia affecting declarative verbal and nonverbal material. The amnesia associated with anoxia/ischemia is quite reminiscent of the memory defect produced by early-stage Alzheimer's pathology.

F. **Herpes simplex encephalitis** (HSE) causes a severe necrotic process in cortical structures associated with the limbic system, some neocortical structures in the vicinity of the limbic system, and several subcortical limbic structures. The hippocampus, amygdala, and basal forebrain nuclei are frequent targets of HSE. Also, the parahippocampal gyrus—particularly the entorhinal cortex in its anterior sector and the polar limbic cortex (area 38)—are frequently damaged. Finally, HSE may also destroy neocortices of the anterolateral and anteroinferior regions of the temporal lobe (areas 20, 21, anterior 22, and parts of 36 and 37). The destruction is usually bilateral, although in recent years, with the advent of early diagnosis and treatment with acyclovir, circumscribed unilateral damage has been more common.

The profile of amnesia caused by HSE is dictated by the nature of neural destruction. Damage confined to the mesial temporal region (hippocampus, amygdala, and entorhinal cortex) will produce an anterograde declarative memory impairment. If both sides are involved, both verbal and nonverbal material will be affected. If the destruction is unilateral, a material-specific learning defect may appear—i.e., only verbal (left-sided damage) or nonverbal (right-sided damage) material will be covered by the amnesia.

When HSE-related pathology extends to nonmesial temporal structures in anterolateral and anteroinferior sectors, the amnesia will involve progressively greater portions of the retrograde compartment, and patients will not be able to retrieve memories from the past in addition to not being able to learn new information. The retrograde defect can be quite severe, if nonmesial temporal structures are extensively damaged. In the worst case, a patient may lose virtually all capacity to remember declarative information from the past. Such a defect, coupled with the anterograde impairment, constitutes **global amnesia.**

G. **Surgical ablation.** Surgical treatment of intractable epilepsy, especially temporal lobectomy, may result in memory impairment, depending on the nature of the resection. Even if the lobectomy spares most of the hippocampus proper, the resection usually involves other anterior regions of the mesial temporal lobe, including the amygdala and entorhinal cortex, resulting in mild but significant memory defects. In the most common presentation, the patient develops a material-specific learning defect following a temporal lobectomy. In addition to being material-specific (nonverbal if the resection is on the right; verbal if it is on the left), the amnesia will affect only declarative knowledge. However, mild retrograde amnesia may also result if there is sufficient involvement of the anterolateral and anteroinferior temporal sectors. Other factors being equal, patients whose seizures began at an early age (e.g., before age 5) are less affected by temporal lobectomies than are patients whose seizures began later (e.g., adolescence).

H. Neoplasm. Cerebral neoplasms can lead to amnesia, depending on their type and location. In fact, impaired memory is a common symptom of brain tumors, especially those centered in the region of the third ventricle (in or near the thalamus), or in the region of the ventral frontal lobes (in or near the basal forebrain). In addition, the most common treatments of high-grade malignant brain tumors, including resection and radiation, often produce memory defects. Radiation necrosis, for example, can damage the lateral portions of the temporal lobes, leading to a focal retrograde amnesia (in which new learning is spared).

I. Normal pressure hydrocephalus (NPH) is a partially reversible condition in which gait disturbance, incontinence, and dementia (especially memory impairment) comprise a hallmark triad of presenting features. Early in the course, memory impairment can be minimal, but most NPH patients go on to develop significant memory defects. The typical picture is one of anterograde amnesia for declarative material; however, significant problems with attention and concentration may exacerbate the amnesia and make the patient appear even more impaired than he or she actually is.

J. Transient global amnesia (TGA) is a short-lasting neurologic condition in which the patient develops a prominent impairment of memory in the setting of otherwise normal cognition and no other neurologic defect. The duration of TGA is typically in the range of about 6–7 hours, after which time the condition spontaneously remits and the patient returns to an entirely normal memory status. The cause of TGA is unknown, although psychological stress, vascular factors, and migraine have been proposed as potential etiologies. During the episode, the patient manifests a severe impairment of anterograde memory for verbal and nonverbal material. Retrograde memory is also impaired, although to a lesser degree. Following recovery, patients are unable to remember events that transpired during the TGA episode, and sometimes a short period of time immediately prior to the onset of TGA is also lost. Otherwise, there is no long-term consequence.

K. Functional amnesia. Amnesia can occur in the absence of any demonstrable brain injury, as a consequence of severe emotional trauma, hypnotic suggestion, or psychiatric illness. These presentations have been termed "functional" amnesias, to distinguish them from amnesias caused by "organic" factors, although at the molecular/cellular level the mechanisms may not be distinguishable. A common form is **functional retrograde amnesia,** in which the patient loses most or all memories of the past (including self-identity), usually following a severe emotional or psychological trauma. Curiously, anterograde memory may be entirely normal, and the patient may even demonstrate "relearning" of the past. Spontaneous recovery is frequent, although most patients will never be able to remember events that transpired during the episodes in which they were amnesic. Another interesting form is **posthypnotic amnesia,** which refers to the phenomenon whereby patients cannot remember events that transpired while they were under hypnosis (generally after being told by the hypnotist during the hypnosis that amnesia would ensue).

III. Evaluation

A. History

1. **Onset.** Through careful history-taking, the clinician should determine as precisely as possible the timing of the **onset** of the complaint. Memory defects that began years ago and have gradually worsened over time point to a degenerative disease, and Alzheimer's is the most likely candidate. Complaints of sudden onset of memory impairment in younger patients, in whom psychological factors (e.g., severe stress and depression) can be identified as being temporally related to the complaint, should raise the question of nonorganic etiologies.

2. **Course.** The history-taking should also document carefully the **course** of the problem. Progressive deterioration in memory signals a degenerative process. Memory defects following head injury or cerebral anoxia, by contrast, tend to improve gradually, and reports to the contrary raise the question of other factors (e.g., psychological illness).

3. **Nature.** The clinician should explore the **nature** of the problem. With what types of information, and in what situations, is the patient having trouble? Patients often produce vague, poorly specified complaints (e.g., "My memory is bad," "I can't remember things," or "I'm forgetful"), and it is important to request specific examples in order to form an idea as to the actual nature

of the problem. Also, patients tend to use the complaint of "memory impairment" to cover a wide range of mental status abnormalities, and, again, elicitation of examples is informative. Patients who complain that they "can't remember" may actually be suffering from circumscribed impairments in word-finding, proper name retrieval, or hearing or vision.

B. Bedside examination. Memory assessment is covered to some extent by virtually all bedside or screening mental status exams, including such measures as the Mini-Mental State Exam, the Blessed Dementia Rating Scale, and the Dementia Assessment Battery. If patients pass such exams, do not complain of memory impairment, and are not described by spouses or caretakers as having memory difficulties, it is safe to assume that memory is normal. If any of these conditions is not met, a more complete evaluation of memory is warranted. Referral for neuropsychological assessment provides the most direct access to such evaluation.

In bedside memory testing, there should be at least some coverage of the following aspects of memory and mental status.

1. **Learning.** Can the patient learn the examiner's name? three words? three objects?

2. **Working memory.** Backward spelling, serial subtraction, and the digit span backwards subtest from the Wechsler Adult Intelligence Scale-Revised are good probes of working memory.

3. **Delayed recall.** It is important to ask for retrieval of newly acquired knowledge after a delay—e.g., about 30 minutes. This may reveal a severe loss of information in a patient who performed perfectly in an immediate recall procedure.

4. **Retrograde memory.** The patient should be asked to retrieve knowledge from the past. This should be corroborated by a spouse or other "collateral," because patients with memory defects may otherwise confabulate and mislead the examiner.

5. **Orientation.** The patient should be asked for information about time, place, and personal facts. Defects in orientation are often early clues of memory impairment.

6. **Attention.** A significant impairment of attention will produce subsequent defects on most tests of memory. The diagnosis of amnesia, however, should be reserved for patients who have normal attention but still cannot perform normally on memory tests. Attentional impairment per se hallmarks other abnormalities, and not necessarily an amnesic condition.

C. Laboratory studies of memory are conducted in the context of neuropsychological assessment, which provides precise, standardized quantification of various memory capacities. Examples of some widely used procedures are as follows.

1. **Anterograde memory** is probed by most conventional neuropsychological tests of memory, including the Wechsler Memory Scale-Revised (WMS-R). The WMS-R and other such instruments assess **learning of declarative knowledge,** and it should not be assumed that all aspects of memory are normal simply because the patient passes these procedures. For example, these tests do not measure nondeclarative memory, and they rarely provide adequate investigation of the retrograde compartment. Nonetheless, the WMS-R and related procedures provide sensitive, standardized means of quantifying many aspects of memory.

   a. **Verbal.** In addition to several verbal memory procedures that comprise part of the WMS-R (e.g., paragraph recall and paired-associate learning), there are several well-standardized list-learning procedures in which the patient attempts to learn and remember a list of words. The Rey Auditory-Verbal Learning Test, for example, requires the patient to learn a list of 15 words. Five successive trials are administered, and then a delayed recall procedure is performed after about 30 minutes. The patient's learning capacity, learning curve, and degree of forgetting can be determined.

   b. **Nonverbal** memory tests typically involve the administration of various designs—e.g., geometric figures—that the patient must remember. The WMS-R includes one design-learning subtest. Another well-known test is the Benton Visual Retention Test, in which the patient is required to learn and reproduce various geometric figures. Face-learning procedures also provide good tests of nonverbal memory.

2. **Retrograde memory.** There are several standardized procedures for measuring retrograde memory, including the Remote Memory Battery, the Famous Events Test, and the Autobiographical Memory Questionnaire. These procedures probe recall and recognition of various historical facts, famous events and persons, and autobiographical knowledge. Corroboration of retrograde memory, particularly with regard to autobiographical information, is extremely important; otherwise, even mild confabulation can completely mislead the clinician into underestimating the severity of retrograde memory defects.

3. **Nondeclarative memory.** A standard procedure for measuring nondeclarative learning is the rotor pursuit task, which requires the patient to hold a stylus in one hand and attempt to maintain contact between the stylus and a small metal target while the target is rotating on a platter. Successive trials are administered, and then a delay trial, allowing measurement of acquisition and retention of the motor skill. Normally, patients show steady improvement on this task, which is retained after a delay period.

4. **Working memory.** The digit span backwards subtest from the Wechsler Adult Intelligence Scale-Revised provides a sensitive means of quantifying working memory. The Trail-Making Test, which requires the patient to execute a psychomotor response while tracking dual lines of information, is also a good probe of working memory. Another commonly used procedure is the Paced Auditory Serial Addition Test, in which the patient must add numbers in an unusual format under increasingly demanding time constraints.

5. **Long-term memory,** which depends not only on the ability to acquire new information but also on the consolidation and storage of that information and its retrieval at a later time, is the real crux of memory. In a practical sense, it is not very helpful to have normal short-term memory if one cannot transfer the information into a more permanent storage area. Hence, delayed recall and recognition procedures, which yield information about the status of long-term memory, are very important in memory assessment.

IV. **Differential diagnosis.** Different causes of amnesia have very different implications for diagnosis and management. There are several common differential diagnoses that are particularly challenging.

A. **Normal aging.** A seemingly minor but practically difficult challenge is to distinguish true memory impairment from the influences of normal aging. Aging produces certain declines in memory, which can be misinterpreted by patients and clinicians alike as signs of neurologic disease. Many elderly persons who complain of "forgetfulness" turn out to have peer-equivalent performances on all manner of standard memory tests, and the diagnosis of amnesia is not applicable. A considerable degree of "Alzheimer-phobia" has developed recently among elderly persons, as the devastating consequences and widespread nature of Alzheimer's disease have gained increasing attention in the popular media. Patients may be quick to interpret any episode of memory failure as a sign of Alzheimer's, or, alternatively, may adamantly deny memory dysfunction in the face of obvious real-world impairment. In both cases, careful quantification of the memory profile will aid in the differential diagnosis.

B. **Psychiatric disease.** Many psychiatric diseases produce some degree of memory impairment. Accurate diagnosis is critical, because memory defects resulting from psychiatric disease are generally reversible, unlike most of the amnesias that occur in the setting of neurologic disease.

1. **Pseudodementia.** A condition that produces memory impairment and other cognitive defects resembling "dementia," but which is not caused by neurologic disease, has been termed **pseudodementia.** Severe depression is the typical cause. Patients with pseudodementia often have memory impairments such as anterograde amnesia that are quite similar to those observed in the early stages of degenerative dementia. However, depressed patients will respond to treatment with antidepressant medications and psychotherapy; when the affective disorder lifts, memory returns to normal.

2. **Depression** is a very common cause of memory impairment, in all age groups. There are distinguishing features, however, that help differentiate amnesia as a result of depression from amnesia caused by neurologic disease. Depressed patients tend to have problems in concentration and attention, and they may manifest defects in working memory and other short-

term memory tasks. By contrast, long-term memory is less affected, and retrograde memory is normal. Apathetic, "don't know" responses are common in depressed patients, whereas neurologic patients more often give incorrect, off-target responses. Also, the history is often informative. In patients with depression, the clinician can usually find evidence of major stress, catastrophe, or other reasons for depression, and it is apparent that the onset of the memory complaints coincided with the onset of the affective disorder.

C. Medication side effects. Many medications commonly prescribed for elderly persons produce adverse side effects on cognitive functioning, including memory. It is important to know what medications a patient has been taking, and to account for the extent to which those medications may be causing memory impairment. The history often reveals that the onset of memory problems coincided with or soon followed the beginning of a particular medication. Also, memory defects caused by medication side effects tend to be rather variable—e.g., worse at certain times of the day. The main problem concerns attention, concentration, and overall cognitive efficiency; memory defects are secondary.

V. Diagnostic approach. The diagnostic approach to the patient with amnesia should include whatever procedures are necessary for establishing both the most likely **cause** and the precise **nature** of the memory impairment. The most commonly used procedures are as follows.

A. Neurologic examination should establish whether a memory complaint is present, the general degree of severity, and the history of the problem. It is not uncommon for patients with amnesia to underestimate or even deny the problem; hence, information from a spouse or caretaker is a critical part of the history. Careful mental status testing may provide sufficient characterization of the amnesia profile.

B. Neuroimaging procedures, including magnetic resonance imaging (MRI) and computed tomography (CT), are almost always helpful in diagnosing the cause of amnesia. Although MRI can be expensive, it is nearly always worth the cost.

C. Neuropsychological assessment provides detailed quantification of the nature and extent of memory impairment. Such testing should be considered for virtually all patients with amnesia, although there may be some instances in which the mental status testing portion of the neurologic examination provides sufficient information. The cost of neuropsychological testing varies considerably from one clinical center to another.

VI. Criteria for diagnosis. The diagnosis of amnesia is appropriate whenever there are memory defects that exceed those that would be expected given the patient's age and background. Some conditions, such as severe aphasia, make it difficult to assess memory in a meaningful fashion. Also, amnesia should not be diagnosed in patients with severe confusional states, where an attentional impairment, rather than memory dysfunction, is the principal manifestation. Otherwise, amnesia can present in isolation or coexist with virtually any other form of mental status impairment. It is customary to regard patients as **amnesic** if there is a significant discrepancy between the level of their intellectual function and one or more of their memory functions. There are many different subtypes of amnesia. Diagnosis of such subtypes usually requires fine-grained quantification such as that provided in the neuropsychological laboratory.

VII. Referral

A. Neuropsychologist. Neuropsychological testing is appropriate for virtually all patients with significant complaints or manifestations of amnesia. Several situations that occur commonly in clinical practice particularly call for such a referral.

1. **Precise characterization of memory capacities.** In a patient who has suffered brain injury, neuropsychological assessment provides detailed information regarding the strengths and weaknesses of the patient's memory, which is useful in planning for placement, rehabilitation, and return to work. In most instances, memory assessment should be performed as early in the recovery epoch as possible. This evaluation provides a baseline to which recovery can be compared. Follow-up assessments assist in monitoring recovery, determining the effects of therapy, and making long-range decisions regarding educational and vocational rehabilitation.

2. **Monitoring the status of patients who have undergone medical or surgical interventions.** Serial neuropsychological assessment of memory is used to track the courses of patients who are undergoing medical or surgical

treatment for neurologic disease. Typical examples include drug therapy for patients with Parkinson's disease or seizure disorders, and surgical intervention in patients with normal pressure hydrocephalus or brain tumors. Neuropsychological assessment provides a baseline memory profile with which changes can be compared and provides a sensitive means of monitoring changes in memory that occur in relationship to particular treatment regimens.

3. **Distinguishing "organic" from psychiatric disease.** Neuropsychological assessment can provide evidence crucial to the distinction between amnesic conditions that are primarily or exclusively "organic" and those that are primarily or exclusively "psychiatric." A common diagnostic dilemma faced by neurologists and psychiatrists is distinguishing between "true dementia" (e.g., cognitive impairment caused by Alzheimer's disease) and "pseudodementia" (e.g., cognitive impairment associated with depression).

4. **Medicolegal situations.** There has been a proliferation of cases in which "brain injury" and "memory impairment" are claimed as damages by plaintiffs who allegedly have sustained minor head injuries or have been exposed to toxic chemicals. In particular, there are many cases in which "hard" or "objective" signs of brain dysfunction (e.g., weakness, sensory loss, impaired balance) are absent, neuroimaging and EEG are normal, and the entire case rests on claims of cognitive deficiencies—particularly memory dysfunction. Neuropsychological assessment is crucial to the evaluation of such claims.

5. **Conditions in which known or suspected neurologic disease is not detected by standard neurodiagnostic procedures.** There are situations in which the findings of standard diagnostic procedures, including neurologic examination, neuroimaging, and EEG, are equivocal, even though the history indicates that brain disease and amnesia are likely. Examples include mild closed head injury, the early stages of degenerative demential syndromes (e.g., Alzheimer's disease and Pick's disease), and early HIV-related dementia. Neuropsychological assessment in such cases provides the most sensitive means of evaluating the patient's memory.

6. **Monitoring changes in cognitive function over time.** A situation that warrants special mention is the evolution of changes in memory over time. In the degenerative dementias in particular, equivocal findings in the initial diagnostic work-up are not uncommon. In such cases, follow-up neuropsychological evaluation can provide important confirming or disconfirming evidence regarding the status of the patient's memory.

B. **Rehabilitation.** Another common application of neuropsychological assessment is the case in which a patient undergoes cognitive rehabilitation for amnesia. Neuropsychological data collected at the initial assessment can help determine how to orient the rehabilitation effort. Subsequent examinations can be used to measure progress during the course of therapy.

Recommended Readings

Butters N, Stuss DT. Diencephalic amnesia. In F Boller, J Grafman (eds), *Handbook of Neuropsychology* (vol 3). Amsterdam: Elsevier, 1989. Pp 107–148.

Cohen NJ, Squire LR. Preserved learning and retention of pattern-analyzing skill in amnesia: Dissociation of knowing how and knowing that. *Science* 210:207–210, 1980.

Corkin S. Lasting consequences of bilateral medial temporal lobectomy: Clinical course and experimental findings in H.M. *Sem Neurol* 4(2):249–259, 1984.

Damasio AR. Time-locked multiregional retroactivation: A systems-level proposal for the neural substrates of recall and recognition. *Cognition* 33:25–62, 1989.

Damasio AR, Tranel D, Damasio H. Amnesia caused by herpes simplex encephalitis, infarctions in basal forebrain, Alzheimer's disease, and anoxia. In F Boller, J Grafman (eds), *Handbook of Neuropsychology* (vol 3). Amsterdam: Elsevier, 1989. Pp 149–166.

Damasio AR, et al. Amnesia following basal forebrain lesions. *Arch Neurol* 42:263–271, 1985.

Damasio AR, et al. Multimodal amnesic syndrome following bilateral temporal and basal forebrain damage. *Arch Neurol* 42:252–259, 1985.

Gabrieli JDE, et al. Intact acquisition and long-term retention of mirror-tracing skill in Alzheimer's disease and in global amnesia. *Behav Neurosci* 107:899–910, 1993.

Graff-Radford NR, et al. Diencephalic amnesia. In G Vallar et al. (eds), *Neuropsychological Disorders Associated with Subcortical Lesions*. New York: Oxford University, 1992. Pp 143–168.

Heindel WC, et al. Neuropsychological evidence for multiple implicit memory systems: A comparison of Alzheimer's, Huntington's and Parkinson's disease patients. *J Neurosci* 9:582–587, 1989.

Hyman BT, Kromer LJ, Van Hoesen GW. A direct demonstration of the perforant pathway terminal zone in Alzheimer's disease using the monoclonal antibody Alz-50. *Brain Res* 450:392–397, 1988.

Kapur N. Focal retrograde amnesia in neurological disease: A critical review. *Cortex* 29:217–234, 1993.

Kopelman MD. The neuropsychology of remote memory. In F Boller, J Grafman (eds), *Handbook of Neuropsychology* (vol 8). Amsterdam: Elsevier, 1993. Pp 215–238.

Lezak MD. *Neuropsychological Assessment* (3rd ed). New York: Oxford University, 1995.

Nahm FKD, et al. Cross-modal associations and the human amygdala. *Neuropsychologia* 31:727–744, 1993.

Poon L, ed. *Handbook of Memory Assessment of Older Adults*. Washington: American Psychological Association, 1987.

Squire LR. Memory and the hippocampus: A synthesis from findings with rats, monkeys, and humans. *Psych Rev* 99:195–231, 1992.

Thompson RF. The neurobiology of learning and memory. *Science* 233:941–947, 1986.

Tranel D. Neural substrates of memory. In VS Ramachandran (ed), *Encyclopedia of Human Behavior* (vol 3). New York: Academic, 1994. Pp 149–164.

Tranel D, Damasio AR. The covert learning of affective valence does not require structures in hippocampal system or amygdala. *J Cogn Neurosci* 5:79–88, 1993.

Tranel D, Damasio AR. Neurobiological foundations of human memory. In AD Baddeley, et al. (eds), *Handbook of Memory Disorders*. New York: Wiley, 1995. Pp 27–50.

Tranel D, et al. Sensorimotor skill learning in amnesia: Additional evidence for the neural basis of nondeclarative memory. *Learning Mem* 1:165–179, 1994.

Van Hoesen GW. The parahippocampal gyrus. *Trends Neurosci* 5:345–350, 1982.

Yanagihara T, Petersen RC (eds). *Memory Disorders: Research and Clinical Practice*. New York: Marcel Dekker, 1991.

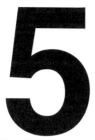

Approach to the Comatose Patient

Frank A. Rubino

Consciousness is the state of awareness of the self and the environment, and thus has two aspects: arousal and awareness. Awareness is the content of consciousness and is the sum of cognitive and affective mental functions such as learning, memory, self-awareness, and adaptive behavior. All of these functions are dependent on the functional integrity of cerebral cortical neurons and associated subcortical nuclei. Arousal is closely linked to wakefulness and is an independent autonomic-vegetative function maintained by deep brainstem and medial diencephalic structures. Awareness requires wakefulness, but mere arousal does not guarantee cognition. Unconsciousness implies global or total unawareness. **Coma** is a state of consciousness in which there is lack of both wakefulness and awareness; coma can be defined as unarousable unresponsiveness. Coma means advanced brain failure, and most causes of coma quickly and seriously threaten life or recovery of neurologic function. Thus, causes must be promptly identified and treated. Diagnosis and treatment have to proceed concurrently.

Coma tends to occur in conjunction with acute or subacute brain lesions. Altered or reduced consciousness implies either diffuse bilateral impairment of cerebral hemispherical function or failure of the brainstem ascending reticular activating system, or both. However, even functional impairment can later cause structural pathology, especially of the cortical neurons.

Diseases that produce coma fall into three categories:

1. Supratentorial lesions that also impair function of the opposite cerebral hemisphere or brainstem/diencephalic structures, or both.
2. Infratentorial lesions that directly impair the ascending reticular activating system.
3. Metabolic (systemic) disorders that diffusely impair the cerebral hemispherical functions and later brainstem/diencephalic structures. Supra- and infratentorial structural lesions usually produce focal neurologic signs as well as pupillary and ocular motility abnormalities, whereas systemic causes of coma usually present without focal neurologic signs or symmetric abnormalities (e.g., asterixis, myoclonus, or tremor).

I. Etiology (Table 5-1)

A. Supratentorial structural lesions
1. Unilateral cerebral hemisphere lesions cause focal neurologic signs but not coma.
2. Bilateral hemisphere lesions producing bilateral cerebral dysfunction can result in coma.
3. Unilateral lesions produce coma by secondarily encroaching on deep diencephalic structures so as to compress or damage physiological systems interacting with both hemispheres.
4. Typical lesions include cerebral infarction; primary and secondary neoplasm; subdural, epidural, and intracerebral hemorrhage; abscess; focal encephalitis (e.g., herpes simplex); granuloma; and venous sinus thrombosis.

B. Infratentorial structural lesions
1. Lesions directly damage the deeper activating systems of the upper brainstem, hypothalamus, and thalamus, which normally activate both cerebral hemispheres.
2. Typical lesions include brainstem infarction and hemorrhage, intra- and extra-axial neoplasms, abscess, and granuloma.
3. Importantly, one must consider lesions of the cerebellum that can secondarily compress the brainstem—especially infarction and hemorrhage.
   a. These lesions might require emergency neurosurgical decompression.
   b. These lesions may also cause acute obstructive hydrocephalus.

Table 5-1. Various etiologies of coma by approximate percentage.

Etiology	Percentage
Sedative drugs and toxins	40
Hypoxic-ischemic (cardiac arrest and anesthetic accidents)	25
Structural lesions	20
Other diffuse dysfunctions (metabolic disturbances, systemic infections, systemic organ failure, etc.)	15

C. **Primary neurologic diseases *not* producing mass effect or necessarily focal neurologic signs**
   1. Seizure disorders
      a. Postictal states
      b. Nonconvulsive status epilepticus
   2. Subarachnoid hemorrhage
   3. Diseases of the leptomeninges
      a. Infections: Meningitis and meningoencephalitis (viral, bacterial, or fungal)
      b. Neoplastic: Carcinomatosis and lymphomatosis of the leptomeninges
      c. Inflammatory: Sarcoidosis
D. **Diffuse diseases and systemic diseases (extracerebral causes)**
   1. These disorders widely depress or interrupt the functions of both the cerebral hemispheres and the brainstem.
   2. These disorders usually cause acute confusional states before causing stupor and coma.
   3. Causes:
      a. Anoxic ischemic conditions
      b. Toxins
      c. Metabolic disturbances
      d. Systemic infections
      e. Electrolyte imbalance
      f. Systemic organ failure of any type
      g. Hyperthermia-hypothermia
II. **Clinical manifestations**
   A. Between the extreme states of consciousness and coma are a variety of **altered states of consciousness.**
      1. Various confusing terms have been used in the literature.
      2. The following terms have been defined.
         a. **Drowsiness** is a state of apparent sleep from which the patient can be aroused, often only briefly by a verbal command.
         b. **Stupor** is a state in which the patient does not respond to verbal commands but does respond to some degree to painful or noxious stimuli.
         c. **Coma** is unarousable unresponsiveness.
         d. **Acute confusional state (delirium)** is a fluctuating state of impairment of both arousal and awareness and has been termed an attentional disorder.
   B. **The Glasgow Coma Scale** (Table 5-2)
      1. This scale may be a useful way to communicate the patient's clinical state to various medical personnel.
      2. Patients are considered to be in coma if they:
         a. Fail to open their eyes in response to verbal commands.
         b. Perform no better than weak flexion in response to pain.
         c. Utter only unrecognizable grunting in response to pain.
III. **Evaluation**
   A. **History**
      1. In general, coma is likely to present in one of the following three ways:
         a. As the predictable progression of an underlying illness
         b. As an unpredictable event in a patient with a previously known disease
         c. As a totally unexpected event
      2. Thus, the history obtained from witnesses reviews:
         a. The situation and the timing of the altered state of consciousness.
         b. Important previous medical and surgical illnesses.

Table 5-2. The Glasgow Coma Scale.

Circle the appropriate number and compute the total.

Eyes Open

Never	1
To pain	2
To verbal stimuli	3
Spontaneously	4

Best Verbal Response

No response	1
Incomprehensible sounds	2
Inappropriate words	3
Disoriented and converses	4
Oriented and converses	5

Best Motor Response

No response	1
Extension (decerebrate rigidity)	2
Flexion abnormal (decorticate rigidity)	3
Flexion withdrawal	4
Localizes pain	5
Obeys	6
Total	3–15

Adapted from Teasdale G, Jennett B. Assessment of coma and impaired consciousness. A practical scale. *Lancet* 2:81–84, 1974.

      c. Previous psychological and neurologic conditions.
      d. Medications, including over-the-counter drugs.
      e. Social history, including use of tobacco, alcohol, and "recreational drugs."
      f. History of immediate or recent trauma (even minor trauma).
      g. Family members' thoughts or theories (which at times may give valuable clues).
      h. Important information obtained from other witnesses, such as ambulance personnel and police.

B. Physical examination
  1. General physical examination. A rapid, thorough physical examination may provide clues to the cause of stupor and coma.
    a. Skin
      (1) Careful examination may reveal signs of trauma, especially about the head and neck.
      (2) There may be stigmata of liver disease, needle marks, and evidence of infection or embolic processes.
      (3) Anemia, jaundice, or cyanosis can be identified.
      (4) Exanthem may indicate a viral infection.
      (5) Petechial rash is an indication of meningococcal infection.
      (6) Hyperpigmentation suggests the possibility of Addison's disease.
      (7) Bullous lesions can be observed with barbiturate intoxication.
    b. Temperature
      (1) Fever usually indicates *infection* rarely a "central" cause.
      (2) Hypothermia may be due to exposure, intoxication with alcohol or barbiturates, peripheral circulatory failure, or, rarely, myxedema and Wernicke's encephalopathy.
    c. Breath
      (1) May give off the odor of alcohol.
      (2) May suggest hepatic disease (fetor hepaticus).
      (3) May give off the uriniferous smell of uremia.
      (4) May indicate ketoacidosis of diabetes.
    d. Blood pressure
      (1) Hypotension may indicate shock, septicemia, intoxication, myocardial infarction, or Addison's disease.

        (2) Hypertension is less helpful and may be the result or the cause of such lesions as cerebral hemorrhages and infarctions.

    e. Cardiovascular

        (1) An important arrhythmia may be detected.

        (2) Various valvular lesions may be detected.

    f. Abdomen

        (1) May reveal signs of trauma or rupture of viscera.

        (2) May exhibit hepatomegaly or splenomegaly.

2. Neurologic examination

    a. Rather than using vague and confusing terms, one should use everyday terms to describe the patient's responses to verbal, noxious, and painful stimuli.

        (1) For noxious stimuli, vigorously rub the sternum with the knuckles.

        (2) For painful stimuli, apply pressure with the fingers over the supra-orbital nerve area or press the base of the fingernails or toenails with the rounded surface of a pen or pencil.

        (3) Test pain with the gentle prick of a pin.

        (4) *Do not* use maneuvers that can potentially harm the patient, such as heavy pressure with a pin that draws blood or twisting the skin or nipples.

    b. Head and neck examination

        (1) It must be remembered that head and neck trauma are often associated with one another.

        (2) If no history is available, the neck must be immobilized until fracture dislocation of the cervical spine has been ruled out.

        (3) Then check the neck for signs of meningeal irritation.

        (4) Look for Kernig's sign, which is elicited by flexing the thigh of the recumbent patient to a right angle and then attempting to extend the leg at the knee; this is accompanied by pain, spasm of hamstring, and limitation of extension.

        (5) Look for Brudzinski's neck sign, in which passive flexion of the head on the chest is followed by flexion of both thighs and legs.

    c. State of consciousness

        (1) Describe the patient in everyday terms and also describe any spontaneous movements, either normal or abnormal, and the patient's response to various stimuli.

        (2) Such terms as semicoma, lethargy, and obtundation should be avoided.

        (3) The Glasgow Coma Scale may be used.

    d. Pupillary response

        (1) A patient cannot be in a coma resulting from a brainstem lesion without demonstrating impairment of pupillary function, ocular motility, or both.

        (2) The pupillary light reflex is very resistant to metabolic dysfunction.

        (3) The presence or absence of the light reflex is the single most important physical sign potentially distinguishing structural from metabolic coma.

        (4) A unilateral fixed dilated pupil suggests brain herniation (uncal herniation) or a posterior communicating artery aneurysm (in a conscious patient, a unilateral fixed dilated pupil is usually benign).

        (5) Midbrain lesions result in midposition pupils that do not react to light.

        (6) Pontine lesions can result in small, pinpoint pupils.

        (7) Most drug intoxications cause pupils to be small but sluggishly reactive.

        (8) Atropinic drugs can cause pupils to be large and unreactive.

        (9) Other agents that may cause pupils to be unreactive include barbiturates, succinylcholine, xylocaine, phenothiazines, methanol, and aminoglycoside antibiotics.

      (10) Hypothermia can fix the pupils.

      (11) Anoxia or ischemia, if severe, may lead to large, fixed pupils, which, if present beyond several minutes after an acute anoxic insult, carry a poor prognosis.

      (12) Examination of the optic fundi may reveal evidence of papilledema, hemorrhage, evidence of emboli, and subhyaloid hemorrhage (which is indicative of a subarachnoid hemorrhage).

e. Ocular motility

   (1) The pathway for ocular motility in the brainstem lies adjacent to the ascending reticular activating system in the PPRF (paramedian pontine reticular formation), making ocular motility an important clinical sign in stupor and coma.

   (2) Asymmetric ocular motility more often accompanies structural than metabolic causes of coma.

   (3) If the brainstem is intact, the eyelids are closed and the eyes, slightly divergent, drift slowly from side to side (roving eye movements).

   (4) Roving eye movements indicate that coma is a result of cerebral hemisphere dysfunction.

   (5) If ocular motility is severely impaired but the pupillary reflex is more or less still intact, the cause of the coma is metabolic and most likely attributable to abuse of drugs such as benzodiazepines, barbiturates, or alcohol.

   (6) Conjugate deviation of the eyes suggests the possibility of an ipsilateral cerebral hemispherical lesion or a contralateral brainstem lesion as the cause of the coma.

   (7) If there are no spontaneous eye movements, ocular motility can be tested by the oculocephalic reflex (doll's eye maneuver) and the oculovestibular reflex (caloric testing).

     (a) The oculocephalic reflex is tested by turning the patient's head from side to side; if the brainstem is intact, the eyes will move fully and conjugately to the opposite side.

     (b) The oculovestibular reflex provides a stronger stimulus and is tested after the head of the bed is elevated 30 degrees and an intact tympanic membrane is observed; 50 to 200 cc of ice water is instilled into the external auditory canal and after 5 minutes the opposite ear is tested.

       (i) The normal response in a conscious patient is the development of nystagmus with the fast component away from the site of stimulation.

       (ii) Nystagmus is not produced in response to the oculovestibular reflex in coma from any cause; thus the production of nystagmus indicates that the patient is conscious.

       (iii) A tonic conjugate full movement of the eyes toward the stimulated side indicates that the brainstem is intact and that the coma is a result of cerebral hemisphere dysfunction.

       (iv) A disconjugate response or no response indicates brainstem impairment.

       (v) Conjugate deviation of the eyes to one side as a result of a supratentorial lesion can usually be overcome by the oculovestibular reflex; conversely, conjugate deviation of the eyes to one side as a result of an infratentorial lesion *cannot* be overcome by the oculovestibular reflex.

       (vi) If a cerebral hemispherical lesion causes a conjugate deviation of the eyes, unless the patient is having a seizure, the eyes will "look toward the lesion," whereas with a brainstem lesion the eyes will "look away from the lesion."

       (vii) Drugs or conditions that can block the oculovestibular reflex include ototoxic drugs such as gentamicin; vestibulo-suppressant drugs such as barbiturates and other sedative drugs, phenytoin, and tricyclic antidepressants; neuromuscular blockers such as succinylcholine; and pre-existing vestibular disease.

f. Corneal reflex

   (1) The corneal reflex has a high threshold in comatose patients and is usually retained until coma is very deep.

(2) If there is a bilateral loss of the corneal reflex in a patient with light coma, one must consider drug-induced coma or a local anesthesia in both eyes.

(3) If there is a unilateral impairment of the corneal reflex, one might consider a focal neurologic lesion that causes decreased sensation on the ipsilateral side of impairment of eye closure from weakness on the ipsilateral side.

(4) Although unilateral impairment of the corneal reflex suggests a structural lesion, one cannot distinguish a cerebral hemispherical lesion from a brainstem lesion.

g. **Motor responses.** In eliciting motor responses, one looks for symmetric or asymmetric responses.

(1) An asymmetric response suggests a focal neurologic sign and thus a structural lesion in either the cerebral hemisphere or brainstem.

(2) Symmetric responses suggest a more diffuse process such as a metabolic encephalopathy.

(3) Paratonia (gegenhalten)

(a) This is a type of rigidity in which there is increased resistance in the opposite direction from which one passively moves a limb.

(b) This type of rigidity is very common in elderly patients with altered states of consciousness from any cause and is very prominent in the neck in all directions moved.

(c) In metabolic coma, paratonia is seen symmetrically in the limbs and neck.

(d) If there is paratonia of the limbs on one side and flaccidity of the limbs on the opposite side, this suggests a hemiparesis involving the flaccid limbs and thus indicates a structural lesion in the cerebral hemisphere or brainstem causing focal neurologic signs.

(4) Movement of the limbs

(a) The patient may move the limbs only on one side spontaneously or as a reaction to stimuli, suggesting a structural lesion in the cerebral hemisphere or brainstem.

(b) Rarely will metabolic coma be accompanied by hemiparesis.

(c) If the patient does not move the limbs spontaneously or in response to stimuli, one can lift the patient's arms from the bed and flex the patient's legs at the knees and release the limbs one at a time: in light coma, if the cause is a diffuse one, the limbs will fall slowly and symmetrically to the resting position; however, paretic limbs will fall like "dead weights" and thus a hemiparesis or monoparesis can be detected. Symmetric responses suggest a diffuse process; asymmetric responses suggest a focal, structural cause.

(5) Decorticate rigidity

(a) Characterized by adduction of the arm at the shoulder with flexion at the elbow and pronation and flexion at the wrist with the leg extended at the hip and knee.

(b) This usually indicates a structural lesion of the cerebral hemisphere or diencephalon with the decortication contralateral to the hemispherical lesion.

(6) Decerebrate rigidity

(a) The arm is extended, adducted, and internally rotated (hyperpronated), and the leg is extended.

(b) Supratentorial lesions causing downward herniation, upper brainstem structural lesions, and even severe metabolic disorders may give rise to decerebrate rigidity.

(7) Other movements

(a) Partial simple motor (focal motor) seizures usually result from focal cerebral hemisphere lesions, but are occasionally observed in metabolic comas such as nonketotic hyperosmolar coma.

(b) In general, asymmetric motor findings speak against metabolic encephalopathy.

        (c) Abnormal movements such as tremors, asterixis, myoclonus, and generalized tonic-clonic seizures are often observed in association with toxic-metabolic disorders; however, focal and multifocal motor seizures can accompany metabolic disorders such as nonketotic, hyperosmolar, and hyperglycemic states.

    h. Respiratory patterns

      (1) Abnormal respiratory patterns may be helpful in localizing the level of structural lesions in the central nervous system early in coma, but metabolic abnormalities may affect the respiratory centers of the brainstem and produce patterns resembling those observed in neurologic diseases.

      (2) A normal breathing pattern suggests that the brainstem is intact.

      (3) Cheyne-Stokes respiration also suggests that the brainstem is intact, and although this breathing pattern can have neurologic causes, it is usually observed in conjunction with metabolic disturbances.

      (4) Deep, rapid hyperventilation in a comatose patient suggests pneumonia or rectification of metabolic acidosis.

      (5) But central neurogenic hyperventilation may suggest a lesion in the midbrain or pons.

      (6) Apneustic breathing characterized by a deep inspiration followed by a pause suggests a lesion in the lower pons.

      (7) Cluster breathing characterized by clusters of breaths in an irregular sequence suggests a lesion in the low pons or high medulla.

      (8) Ataxic breathing characterized by an irregular pattern of breathing with inspiratory gasps of diverse amplitude and length and periods of apnea suggests a lesion of the respiratory center in the medulla.

      (9) Yawning and sneezing suggest that the brainstem is intact, but coughing, swallowing, or hiccuping can occur in patients with severe brainstem failure.

C. Laboratory studies

    1. Blood and urine screens for drugs and toxins

    2. CBC, urinalysis, blood chemistries, blood gases

    3. ECG

    4. Neuroimaging studies; CT or MRI scans

    5. Lumbar puncture

    6. EEG

IV. Differential diagnosis (Table 5-3)

A. Brain death

    1. Brain death is the permanent cessation of all brain functions.

    2. There is absence of function of both the cerebral cortex and the brainstem.

    3. Patients are *irreversibly* comatose and apneic, and have lost all brainstem reflexes and cranial nerve functions.

    4. Brain death is a *clinical diagnosis.*

B. Locked-in syndrome

    1. Consciousness and cognition are retained.

    2. Movement and communication are markedly impaired because of quadriplegia, inability to speak and swallow, and inability to move the eyes in a horizontal direction.

    3. This syndrome usually results from lesions of the corticospinal and corticobulbar pathways, frequently in the base of the pons.

Table 5-3. Differential diagnosis of coma.

Brain death
Locked-in syndrome
Persistent vegetative state
Frontal lobe disease
Nonconvulsive status epilepticus
Transient unresponsiveness in the elderly (idiopathic recurring stupor)
Psychiatric disorders (catatonia, depression)

   4. This syndrome has also been occasionally observed in patients with severe peripheral neuropathy (Guillain-Barré syndrome), with myasthenia gravis, and after the administration of neuromuscular blocking agents.
   5. The patient usually communicates by eye blinks or vertical eye movements.
   6. The syndrome has also been referred to as a de-efferented state.
C. **Persistent vegetative state**
   1. A state of wakefulness without detectable awareness.
   2. There is preservation of vital vegetative functions such as heart rate and rhythm, respiration, and maintenance of blood pressure.
   3. Patients remain unaware of self and environment.
   4. Patients have sleep-wake cycles, but no ascertainable cerebral cortical function.
   5. This state has been referred to as a de-afferented state.
   6. Patients are considered unconscious because, although they are wakeful, they lack awareness.
   7. Patients have extensive damage of the forebrain, especially the neocortex, with relative sparing of the brainstem.
   8. The most common acute causes are head trauma and hypoxic ischemic encephalopathy.
D. **Frontal lobe disease**
   1. Lesions are prefrontal and bilateral and include such disorders as hydrocephalus, subfrontal meningioma, bilateral frontal lobe tumors (primary or metastatic), intracerebral hemorrhages, cerebral trauma, and cerebral infarctions in the distribution of both anterior cerebral arteries.
   2. Patients are described as abulic.
      a. Patients exhibit long delays between a stimulus—noxious, painful, or verbal—and reaction.
      b. There is a slowness or "viscosity" that is applicable to verbal output and motor responsiveness.
E. **Nonconvulsive status epilepticus**
   1. Complex partial status epilepticus
      a. This is an important syndrome that is more common than suspected.
      b. This condition takes one of two forms:
         (1) A prolonged twilight state with partial responsiveness, impaired speech, and quasipurposeful automatisms.
         (2) A series of complex seizures with staring, total unresponsiveness, speech arrest, and stereotyped automatisms with a twilight state between seizures.
      c. There is often prolonged clouding of consciousness with cycling of ictal and postictal states.
   2. Absence status epilepticus
      a. Altered consciousness is often accompanied by mild clonic movements of the eyelids and hands with automatisms of the face and hands.
      b. There are bilateral synchronous spike-wave discharges on EEG.
      c. This is usually a disease of childhood.
      d. It can present in adults as an acute confusional state.
         (1) Usually no apparent cause.
         (2) Sometimes occurs in association with diffuse insults such as metrizamide myelography or electroconvulsive therapy.
         (3) Also reported after benzodiazepine withdrawal.
F. **Transient unresponsiveness in the elderly (idiopathic recurrent stupor)**
   1. This condition usually occurs in elderly people.
   2. There are one or more self-limited episodes of unresponsiveness unrelated to obvious structural, toxic, metabolic, convulsive, or psychiatric disorders.
   3. Flumazenil, a specific benzodiazepine receptor antagonist, may reverse the episodes.
G. **Psychiatric disorders**
   1. Pseudocoma (hysterical coma)
      a. This is a relatively rare syndrome and is a diagnosis of exclusion.
      b. Patient may hold eyes forcibly closed and resist eyelid opening or may keep eyes in a fixed stare interrupted by quick blinks.
      c. Pupils are of normal size, position and, reactivity (unless cycloplegic drugs have been used).
      d. Oculovestibular testing shows normal awake response.

   e. Patient may hyperventilate or breathe normally.
   f. EEG is normal.
   g. Harsh, painful stimuli are *inappropriate;* instead, one can stimulate the palpebral reflex or tickle the nose with a wisp of cotton.
  2. Severe vegetative depression
  3. Catatonia
   a. In the past, catatonia was considered to be a variety of schizophrenia.
   b. Catatonia can now occur as a conversion reaction or a dissociative state.
V. Diagnostic approach
 A. Screening the blood and urine for drugs and toxins can yield valuable information.
  1. Sedative drugs and alcohol overdoses are usually nonlethal and carry a good prognosis as long as circulation and respiration are supported.
  2. However, drugs often depress brainstem function and, if drug overdose is not suspected, the impairment of brainstem function might be misinterpreted as a poor prognostic sign.
 B. CBC, urinalysis, blood chemistries including electrolytes, and blood gases are all done to detect hepatic failure, renal failure, hyperglycemia, hypoglycemia, electrolyte disturbances, or acidosis.
 C. An ECG is important, of course, in detecting various cardiac arrhythmias.
 D. If a structural lesion is suspected in either of the cerebral hemispheres, the brainstem, or the cerebellum, neuroimaging needs to be done.
  1. A CT scan of the head without contrast is a good initial study because it can be done quickly and can identify acute intraparenchymal and subarachnoid hemorrhages better than the MRI scan.
  2. A plain CT scan of the head can detect most structural lesions causing stupor and coma, including subarachnoid hemorrhages as well as subdural and epidural hematomas.
  3. An MRI scan of the brain provides more information on lesions involving the temporal lobes, posterior fossa structures, and sellar and parasellar areas.
 E. A lumbar puncture with CSF analysis is necessary in suspected cases of meningitis or meningoencephalitis as well as other lesions involving the leptomeninges.
 F. Electroencephalography
  1. The major role of electroencephalography is in detecting nonconvulsive status epilepticus.
  2. It may also be helpful in detecting feigned or psychological coma, in which cases it will be normal.
  3. It can also detect postictal states and show diffuse abnormalities with metabolic and toxic causes of coma; certain drugs and toxins will also cause fast activity.
  4. The EEG, however, should not be used as a screening tool and is not needed in the emergency room unless nonconvulsive status epilepticus is suspected.
VI. Referral. Cases of coma should be referred to a neurologist or neurosurgeon if:
 A. There is structural cause in the cerebrum or brainstem.
 B. Seizures occur.
 C. The cause is obscure.
 D. Trauma is involved.
 E. There is involvement of the leptomeninges by a disease process (e.g., subarachnoid hemorrhage, meningoencephalitis, or neoplastic invasion).
 F. Brain death is suspected.
 G. Other states, such as locked-in syndrome or persistent vegetative state, are suspected.

Recommended Readings

Adams RD, Victor M. *Principles of Neurology* (5th ed). New York: McGraw-Hill, 1993.

Bates D. The management of medical coma. *J Neurol, Neurosurg Psych* 56:589–598, 1993.

Browning RG, et al. 50% Dextrose: Antidote or toxin? *Ann Emerg Med* 19:683–687, 1990.

Haimovic JC, Beresford HR. Transient unresponsiveness in the elderly. *Arch Neurol* 49:35–37, 1992.

O'Callahan W, Ranzi FP. Neurologic emergencies: Stupor and coma. In Stein, Chudnofsky (eds), *A Practical Approach to Emergency Medicine* (2nd ed). Boston: Little, Brown, 1994.

Plum F, Posner JB. *The Diagnosis of Stupor and Coma* (3rd ed). Philadelphia: Davis, 1980.

Samuels MA. The evaluation of comatose patients. *Hosp Practice* Mar 15, 1993:165–182.

Teasdale G, Jennett B. Assessment of coma and impaired consciousness. A practical scale. *Lancet* 2:81–84, 1974.

Tinuper P, et al. Idiopathic recurring stupor. *Neurology* 44:621–625, 1994.

Winkler E, et al. Use of flumazenil in the diagnosis and treatment of patients with coma of unknown etiology. *Critical Care Med* 21:538–542, 1993.

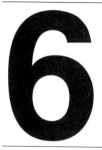

Approach to the Patient with Seizures

Vicenta Salanova

I. Introduction

  A. Seizures result from the paroxysmal, hypersynchronous, abnormal activity of neurons in the cerebral cortex. Seizures are common symptoms, and may be manifestations of toxic-metabolic abnormalities or of infections, may be secondary to a variety of disorders that affect neuronal function, or may be idiopathic with unknown cause.

    1. Nonrecurrent seizures: toxic-metabolic, hypoxia, etc.

    2. Recurrent seizures or epilepsy: inherited, acquired, or structural cortical lesions

  B. The **international classification of epileptic seizures** consists of two main categories: partial seizures and generalized seizures.

    1. Partial seizures (focal) result from localized epileptogenic lesions, except in children with benign focal epilepsy who have no structural lesions. Partial seizures are subdivided into:

      a. Simple partial seizures if there is preservation of consciousness.

      b. Complex partial seizures if there is impairment of consciousness. A partial seizure typically begins as a simple partial seizure consisting of an aura reflecting the site of seizure origin (or ictal spread to the symptomatogenic area), and then evolves into a complex partial seizure. Both simple and complex partial seizures may evolve into secondarily generalized seizures.

    2. Generalized seizures may be convulsive or nonconvulsive, and are subdivided into absence (typical and atypical absences), myoclonic, clonic, tonic, tonic-clonic, and atonic seizures.

  C. There is also an **international classification of epilepsy** and epilepsy syndromes. This classification takes into account the age of onset, possible etiologic factors, inheritance, neurologic examination, prognosis, and seizure type (partial or generalized).

    1. Localization-related epilepsies

      a. Idiopathic (benign childhood Rolandic and occipital epilepsy)

      b. Symptomatic, which are acquired and based mainly on the anatomic localization.

    2. Generalized epilepsies and syndromes

      a. Idiopathic, with age-related onset (benign neonatal familial convulsions, childhood and juvenile absence epilepsy, juvenile myoclonic epilepsy, epilepsy with grand mal seizures on awakening, etc.)

      b. Symptomatic (infantile spasms, Lennox-Gastaut syndrome, etc.). The international classification includes two other categories: epileptic syndromes with both focal and generalized seizures (acquired epileptic aphasia, etc.), and special syndromes (febrile convulsions, etc.). This chapter reviews the etiology, clinical manifestations, evaluation, and differential diagnoses of some of these types of seizures, with emphasis on those patients presenting with partial seizures.

II. Etiology

  A. Toxic-metabolic

    1. Systemic illness: hypoglycemia, nonketotic hyperglycemia, hypoxia, hypocalcemia (in patients with or without a history of hypoparathyroidism), hyponatremia (inappropriate antidiuretic hormone syndrome and water intoxication), hypomagnesemia, uremia and hepatic failure, sickle-cell anemia, thrombotic thrombocytopenic purpura, Whipple's disease

    2. **Drugs and toxins:** cocaine, amphetamines, phencyclidine, lidocaine, lead poisoning. Others may lower the seizure threshold and increase the risk of seizures usually in patients with other predisposing factors (tricyclics, theophylline, phenothiazine, penicillins).

    3. **Withdrawal syndromes:** alcohol, hypnotics

    4. **Pyridoxine deficiency**

B. **Acquired structural lesions**

    1. **Infections:** Brain abscess, meningitis, encephalitis (herpes simplex encephalitis, etc.), postinfectious encephalomyelitis, cysticercosis, opportunistic infections in AIDS, neurosyphilis

    2. **Vascular:** vasculitis (systemic lupus erythematosus, hypersensitivity, and infectious vasculitis), ischemic or hemorrhagic cerebrovascular disease, cerebral venous thrombosis, arteriovenous malformations (AVMs), cavernous angiomas

    3. **Trauma:** usually penetrating, subdural hematoma

    4. **Neoplasms** and other lesions: primary or metastatic tumors, hamartomas, cortical dysplasia

    5. **Mesial temporal sclerosis:** usually postfebrile convulsions

    6. **Others:** Alzheimer's disease, Creutzfeldt-Jakob disease, and, rarely, multiple sclerosis

C. **Familial**

    1. **Primary generalized epilepsies**

    2. **Benign focal epilepsies of childhood**

    3. **Febrile convulsions**

D. **Other genetic syndromes associated with seizures** (tuberous sclerosis, neurofibromatosis), disorders of amino acid, lipid, and protein metabolism (phenylketonuria, maple syrup urine disease, porphyria, etc.)

III. **Clinical manifestations**

A. **Metabolic-toxic and hypoxic insults.** Those patients with seizures attributable to metabolic or toxic causes exhibit generalized tonic-clonic seizures, but focal seizures and epilepsia partialis continua are observed in nonketotic hyperglycemia. Posthypoxic coma usually causes multifocal myoclonus; however, periodic lateralized epileptiform discharges (PLEDs) may be seen, at times associated with focal motor seizures.

B. **Meningitis and encephalitis** may cause either generalized or focal seizures with secondarily generalized seizures. Patients with herpes simplex encephalitis often present with complex partial seizures typical of those of temporal lobe origin. The electroencephalogram shows focal slowing in one or both temporal regions and periodic lateralized epileptiform discharges (PLEDs). Magnetic resonance imaging (MRI) shows hypodense lesions in one or both temporal lobes.

C. **Partial seizures** (functional-anatomic classification of the epilepsies). Clinical features and EEG findings indicate focal origin.

    1. **Temporal lobe seizures** are the most common partial seizures. In 30% of these patients, the seizures are refractory to medical treatment.

        a. **Signs and symptoms.** The neurologic examination is often normal. Most of these patients exhibit an epigastric aura (nausea, an epigastric rising sensation, or stomach upset). Other aurae consist of fear, complex visual or auditory hallucinations, déjà vu, and olfactory and gustatory sensations. The clinical manifestations are very stereotypic, and most patients have one seizure type. Most patients exhibit staring, unresponsiveness, oro-alimentary, and gestural automatisms. Some patients also have contralateral arm dystonic posturing. Ictal or postictal language difficulties also have lateralizing value. Ictal speech occurs in patients with seizures arising from the nondominant temporal lobe. Patients with seizures originating from the dominant temporal lobe may exhibit ictal and postictal dysphasia.

        b. **Etiologic factors and pathology.** Hippocampal sclerosis is the most common pathologic finding. There is a strong association between hippocampal sclerosis and prolonged complex febrile seizures in patients less than 5 years of age. There is usually a silent interval between the occurrence of febrile seizures and the onset of medial temporal lobe epilepsy, which often begins toward the end of the first decade of life or soon after.

    c. **EEG findings** include epileptiform discharges over the anterior temporal region, and often polymorphic slowing. Thirty to 40% of these patients have bitemporal independent interictal epileptiform discharges (usually with predominance on the side of ictal onset).

    d. **Imaging studies.** MRI volumetric studies usually show a smaller hippocampus and increased signal intensity on the T2 weighted images indicative of hippocampal sclerosis.

    e. **Secondarily generalized** tonic-clonic seizures and convulsive status epilepticus may occur; nonconvulsive complex partial status epilepticus is rare.

2. **Focal motor seizures.** These seizures originate in the vicinity of the rolandic motor cortex. Consciousness is preserved.

    a. **Signs and symptoms.** Examination may show a contralateral mild hemiparesis or hyperreflexia. Seizures commonly begin with focal contralateral twitching of the face or hand, and then spread to involve the remainder of the extremity. When seizures originate in the nondominant hemisphere, patients are usually able to speak during the seizures. When seizures originate in the dominant hemisphere, patients may exhibit ictal and postictal aphasia. Clonic eye movements, blinking, and conscious contraversion may also occur. Ictal focal motor manifestations, postictal hemiparesis, and postictal aphasia are contralateral to the side of seizure onset. Some patients may present with continuous focal motor activity (epilepsia partialis continua lasting weeks, months, or even years).

    b. **Imaging studies.** Focal structural lesions are common.

    c. **EEG findings** show focal slowing and focal epileptiform discharges over the frontal lobe; however, some of these patients have no epileptiform discharges on scalp recordings, or have bifrontal epileptiform abnormalities.

    d. These patients have to be distinguished from patients exhibiting benign rolandic epilepsy with centrotemporal spikes, which begins between the ages of 3 and 13 years. These children have normal neurologic examinations and imaging studies, nocturnal generalized seizures, and partial seizures with preservation of consciousness beginning in the face, at times with speech arrest. The EEG shows centrotemporal, high-amplitude, broad, sharp waves and slow discharges, with a horizontal dipole, occurring predominantly during sleep. The prognosis is excellent.

3. **Supplementary motor seizures** originate in the supplementary motor cortex, which is located in the mesial frontal lobe anterior to the primary motor leg area.

    a. **Signs and symptoms.** Examination is usually normal. Almost half of these patients exhibit a somatosensory aura consisting of tingling or numbness of the extremities, which may be contralateral or bilateral. These patients present with unilateral or bilateral tonic posturing of the extremities at onset, vocalization, speech arrest, and laughter. Other manifestations include fencing posture, thrashing, kicking, and pelvic movements. Responsiveness is preserved unless the seizure evolves into a secondarily generalized tonic-clonic seizure. Supplementary motor seizures are common during sleep and are of short duration without postictal confusion or amnesia.

    b. **Imaging studies.** Head MRI may show lesions in the supplementary motor area.

    c. **EEG findings** may show epileptiform discharges over the vertex, but some patients may have no interictal epileptiform discharges on scalp recordings. Ictal recordings are often nonlateralized and in a few patients may show no ictal EEG changes during scalp recordings.

4. **Complex partial seizures of frontal lobe origin**

    a. **Signs and symptoms.** Examination is usually normal. Patients may have a cephalic aura, followed by staring or looking ahead, unconscious contraversion, and complex motor automatisms such as bicycling, kicking, thrashing, running, and bouncing up and down. Vocalization and tonic posturing may occur toward the end of the seizure as manifestations of ictal spread to the supplementary motor area. Complex partial (nonconvulsive) status epilepticus, manifested by alteration of consciousness with automatic behavior often in a cyclical manner lasting hours to days, may also occur. Secondarily generalized tonic-clonic seizures and convulsive status epilepticus are believed to be more common in patients with frontal lobe seizures.

  b. Imaging studies. MRI may show lesions in the frontopolar, dorsolateral, orbitofrontal, and other frontal regions.

  c. EEG findings may show focal slowing and interictal epileptiform discharges over one frontal lobe, lateralized to one hemisphere, or bilateral frontal epileptiform abnormalities.

  5. Occipital lobe seizures are rare, but may be difficult to differentiate from seizures originating from the posterior temporal lobe.

  a. Signs and symptoms. Occipital manifestations are common. Patients may have visual field defects, visual aurae consisting of elementary visual hallucinations described as colored flashing lights, or ictal blindness. Other manifestations include contralateral eye deviation, a sensation of eye movement, nystagmoid eye movements, and blinking. Following the occipital manifestations, many patients have typical temporal lobe automatisms as well as focal motor seizure activity resulting from ictal spread to the temporal and frontal lobes. Because of these different spread patterns, many patients have more than one type of seizure. Almost two-thirds of patients have lateralizing clinical features, such as contralateral head deviation and visual field defects, contralateral to the epileptogenic zone.

  b. Imaging studies. Many patients have occipital lesions on CT and MRI ipsilateral to the epileptogenic zone.

  c. EEG findings may show focal slowing and epileptiform discharges over one occipital lobe. However, most often the EEG shows posterior temporal epileptiform discharges and, in some patients, bilateral posterior temporal-occipital epileptiform abnormalities.

  These patients have to be distinguished from patients with benign occipital epilepsy, who present in childhood and have similar symptoms but no occipital lesions. The age of onset ranges from 15 months to 17 years, and more than a third have family histories of epilepsy.

  6. Parietal lobe seizures are also uncommon.

  a. Signs and symptoms. The examination may show contralateral impaired two-point discrimination, but more often is normal. These patients present with somatosensory aurae described as contralateral tingling or numbness and painful and thermal sensations. Other aurae consist of disturbances of body image, a sensation of movement in one extremity, or a feeling that one extremity is absent. Vertiginous sensations and visual illusions can also occur, as well as aphasic aura. Some of these patients have seizures of multiple types as a result of ictal spread to the temporal and frontal lobes, and tonic posturing of extremities, focal motor clonic activity, head and eye deviations, and temporal lobe automatisms are commonly observed.

  b. Imaging studies. MRI may show focal lesions in the parietal lobe.

  c. EEG findings more often show lateralized epileptiform discharges to one hemisphere rather than localized discharges.

D. Primary (idiopathic) generalized epilepsies. The first clinical manifestations indicate involvement of both cerebral hemispheres. These epilepsies can be divided into convulsive and nonconvulsive.

  1. Childhood absence epilepsy begins between the ages of 4 and 8 years. The neurologic examination is normal.

  a. Signs and symptoms. There is a brief loss of consciousness usually lasting 10 seconds or less and almost always lasting less than 30 seconds. There is no aura or postictal confusion. Blinking, brief facial twitching, or other clonic component, decreased postural tone, and automatisms such as swallowing, lip smacking, and fumbling with clothes are common. Forty to 50% may also have tonic-clonic seizures.

  b. EEG findings show the typical generalized, bilaterally synchronous 3-Hz spike and wave epileptiform discharges. Hyperventilation for 3 to 5 minutes often provokes an absence seizure, with typical generalized, bifrontally dominant, regular, synchronous 3-Hz spike and wave complexes with abrupt onset and termination. In some patients the epileptiform discharges may be maximum over the posterior head regions.

   c. **Prognosis** is favorable, and in many patients the seizures remit in adolescence. The prognosis is less favorable if tonic-clonic seizures occur.

   d. **Absence status.** Rarely, patients may present with prolonged confusion, lasting hours or all day, associated with continuous 3-Hz spike-wave discharges.

2. **Juvenile absence epilepsy** is less common than childhood absence epilepsy. The clinical manifestations are similar, but seizures begin during puberty or later. The absences tend to occur on awakening and are not as frequent as those in the childhood form. Myoclonic seizures may also occur. The EEG may show generalized 3-Hz spike-wave discharges or higher-frequency (4–5-Hz) discharges. Prognosis is not as favorable as in the childhood form, and generalized tonic-clonic seizures are more frequent. Absence status is also more frequent than in the childhood form.

3. **Juvenile myoclonic epilepsy.** Age of onset is in the second decade. The neurologic examination is normal. The diagnosis is often missed because of failure to recognize the myoclonic jerks.

   a. **Signs and symptoms.** These patients have awakening myoclonic and generalized tonic-clonic seizures. Absence seizures occur in 15% of patients. During brief myoclonic jerks, consciousness is preserved. Myoclonic seizures may precede the onset of generalized tonic-clonic seizures by a few years, or they may have simultaneous onset. The generalized tonic-clonic seizures usually follow a series of myoclonic seizures. Seizures may be precipitated by sleep deprivation or alcohol intake.

   b. **EEG findings** show generalized polyspike and wave discharges in the majority of patients. Some patients are photosensitive, with photoparoxysmal responses. During the myoclonic jerks, the EEG shows abrupt onset of high-amplitude polyspike and wave complexes lasting from 2–10 seconds.

   c. **Prognosis.** Even though these patients have an excellent response to valproic acid, the electroclinical trait persists for life and most patients require lifelong treatment.

4. **Generalized tonic-clonic seizures.** The patient with primary generalized tonic-clonic seizures usually has a family history of epilepsy. Neurologic examination is normal. Age of onset is usually during puberty.

   a. **Signs and symptoms.** There is no aura. A few patients may have a prodrome (nervousness, irritability) hours before the seizure. The seizure begins with brief tonic flexion of the axial muscles and muscular contraction of the extremities, followed by a longer period of tonic extension of the axial muscles. The mouth is closed, and this may lead to tongue biting. Apnea may occur as a result of contraction of the respiratory muscles. The arms are semiflexed and the legs are extended. After the tonic phase, there is diffuse tremor, and then there is a clonic phase. Autonomic changes usually occur at the end of the tonic phase. Heart rate and blood pressure may more than double during the tonic phase. There is also increased bladder pressure.

   b. **Complications** during a prolonged tonic-clonic seizure may include tongue biting, dislocation of shoulders, vertebral compression fractures, aspiration pneumonia, and even sudden death. The mechanism of sudden death is unclear; several factors, such as apnea, pulmonary edema, and cardiac arrhythmias, may be involved.

   c. **EEG findings** show generalized 4–5-Hz spike-wave activity, or multiple spike-wave complexes. More irregular spike-wave discharges may also occur. The likelihood of recording the epileptiform discharges increases if the EEG is performed 1 to 5 days after a seizure. Some patients may have a photoparoxysmal response with bisynchronous, generalized irregular spike and spike-wave discharges. EEG ictal changes show generalized low-voltage fast activity (recruiting rhythm) followed by high-amplitude generalized polyspike or polyspike and wave discharges. During the clonic phase, there is high-amplitude polyspike or polyspike and wave discharges alternating with low-amplitude slowing. Postictally, there is low-amplitude slowing.

   d. **Generalized tonic-clonic status epilepticus** begins with recurrent brief tonic-clonic seizures without full recovery of consciousness, or with a prolonged generalized tonic-clonic seizure lasting 30 minutes.

E. Secondary (symptomatic) generalized epilepsy. These patients have multifocal cortical abnormalities, including infantile spasms (West's syndrome) and Lennox-Gastaut syndrome.

1. **West's syndrome.** The onset is usually between 3 and 6 months of age and always before 1 year. In some infants, there are no identifiable etiologic factors (cryptogenic subgroup). The symptomatic subgroup is more common and can result from trauma, infections, Down's syndrome, tuberous sclerosis, phenylketonuria, etc. These infants have frequent infantile spasms, developmental delay, and a characteristic EEG pattern (hypsarrhythmia).

2. **Lennox-Gastaut syndrome** is one of the most severe epileptic syndromes. These children usually exhibit developmental delay, neurologic deficits, and seizures of multiple types, which are often medically refractory (drop attacks, atypical absence, myoclonic, tonic, and tonic-clonic seizures). The EEG shows generalized slow (<2.5-Hz) spike and wave discharges.

   a. **Drop attacks** represent atonic seizures, and are characterized by sudden loss of tone, at times preceded by a generalized clonic jerk. There is head drop, and often the child collapses. The ictal EEG shows an electrodecremental response.

   b. **Atypical absences** usually last longer than typical absences and are commonly associated with motor findings and postictal confusion. They are more common during drowsiness and are not usually activated by hyperventilation. The EEG shows generalized slow spike-wave discharges and diffuse slowing of the background.

   c. **Absence status** is common. Patients present with prolonged absences (spike and wave stupor), blinking, and at times facial twitching, with continuous generalized spike and wave discharges.

   d. **Tonic seizures** are very common in Lennox-Gastaut syndrome. There is elevation of the arms in a semiflexed position with impairment of consciousness and autonomic changes.

IV. Evaluation

A. History

1. **Age of onset and frequency of seizures,** family history of epilepsy, psychosocial history, possible etiologic factors such as history of head trauma, difficult birth, febrile seizures, meningitis, or encephalitis. Precipitating factors include medical illnesses that may lead to metabolic abnormalities, and exposure to drugs or toxins.

2. **The presence and type of aura,** detailed description of the seizure by a family member, presence of automatisms, ictal speech, dystonic or tonic posturing, postictal language difficulties, Todd's paralysis, or the presence of myoclonus can help to distinguish focal from generalized seizures.

3. **Response to anticonvulsants,** and possible side effects.

B. Physical examination

1. **Detailed examination,** including the skin, for possible stigmata of neurocutaneous lesions associated with seizures such as neurofibromatosis, tuberous sclerosis, and Sturge-Weber syndrome. Cranial bruits may be present in patients with arteriovenous malformations, and cervical bruits in patients with seizures resulting from cerebrovascular disease.

2. **Limb asymmetries** suggestive of early life injuries. **Focal neurologic deficits,** such as subtle hemiparesis, hyperreflexia, decreased two-point discrimination, or visual field defects, may suggest the location of the epileptogenic lesion. Memory deficits can be elicited in some patients with bitemporal epilepsy.

C. Laboratory studies include CBC, ESR, VDRL, blood sugar, calcium, sodium, magnesium, liver and renal function tests, drug and toxicology screening if indicated by history or exam, and HIV testing for patients with risk factors.

D. CSF examination is performed if vasculitis or infection is suspected, or if serology is positive for syphilis.

E. EEG is essential to confirm the diagnosis of epilepsy and to characterize the seizure type, and usually shows focal slowing and epileptiform abnormalities in patients with partial seizures, or generalized epileptiform discharges in generalized seizures. Seizures are rarely recorded on routine EEGs, with the exception of absence seizures, which may be precipitated by hyperventilation. Metabolic encephalopathies associated with seizures usually show diffuse slowing or periodic patterns, such as triphasic waves, observed in patients with hepatic or renal failure.

1. **Activation procedures,** such as photic stimulation, hyperventilation, and sleep, are performed.
2. **Special electrodes.** Ear lobe, anterior temporal, or zygomatic electrodes are often used. Nasopharyngeal electrodes are traumatic and produce artifacts, and should not be used. Sphenoidal electrodes are reserved for those patients undergoing presurgical evaluation.
3. **Video EEG recordings.** In some patients with recurrent seizures and no interictal epileptiform discharges on serial EEGs, prolonged video EEG recording may be needed to confirm the diagnosis and to characterize the seizure type.

F. **Imaging studies.** When the history, neurologic examination, EEG findings, and seizure type are suggestive of partial seizures, the procedure of choice is a head MRI. Even though the head CT may be helpful, some patients with partial seizures have CT-negative lesions such as hamartomas, cortical dysplasia, low-grade gliomas, or cavernous angiomas.

V. **Differential diagnosis** includes many neurologic, psychiatric, and medical disorders. The most common are psychogenic seizures and syncopal episodes.

A. **Syncope** is defined as a brief episode of loss of consciousness as a result of transient decreases in cerebral blood flow. Episodes last a few seconds. Brief tonic-clonic movements and incontinence of urine and feces may occur (convulsive syncope). The EEG during the prodromal period (lightheadedness) shows diffuse high-amplitude slowing, and when tonic or clonic activity occurs the EEG is isoelectric.

B. **Psychogenic seizures** are suspected in patients with seizures precipitated by stress when others are present, no response to anticonvulsants, long duration up to 15 or 30 minutes or even hours, side-to-side head movements, pelvic thrusting, arrhythmic jerking, bilateral motor activity with preservation of consciousness, bizarre and aggressive behavior, and crying. There is no postictal confusion after generalized tonic-clonic jerking. However, some of these symptoms (bizarre complex automatisms, pelvic thrusting, bilateral motor activity, etc.) can occur in patients with complex partial seizures of frontal lobe origin and supplementary motor seizures.

C. **Panic attacks**

D. **Cerebrovascular:** transient global amnesia

E. **Basilar artery** migraine

F. **Sleep disorders:** narcolepsy

G. **Movement disorders:** myoclonus, choreoathetosis, familial paroxysmal dystonia

H. **Paroxysmal vertigo**

I. **Toxic-metabolic:** alcohol withdrawal, hypoglycemia

J. **Daydreaming episodes**

VI. **Diagnostic approach**

A. **History and examination** are central in order to determine the type of seizure (generalized or focal, psychogenic, related to syncope or metabolic causes, etc.), obtain descriptions of the aura (if present) and the seizure by a witness, identify subtle neurologic deficits, etc. It is helpful to ask a family member to mimic the seizure. After the initial evaluation, a presumptive etiologic diagnosis and a tentative seizure classification are often possible, and should determine the extent of the evaluation.

B. **Laboratory evaluation** should include serum electrolytes, baseline renal and hepatic function tests to rule out metabolic causes, drug screening, and other tests as indicated by history and examination.

C. If syncope is suspected, **EKG and Holter monitor** as indicated by history and examination. More extensive evaluation for cardiac causes of syncope may be needed.

D. **Sleep and awake EEG** with activation procedures (hyperventilation and photic stimulation) and special electrodes. Ambulatory EEG may be helpful in patients with suspected seizures or pseudoseizures or suspected convulsive syncopal episodes.

E. **Prolonged video EEG** may be needed to confirm the diagnosis, characterize the seizure type, and exclude psychogenic seizures. Patients with complex partial seizures of frontal lobe origin and supplementary motor seizures are often misdiagnosed as having psychogenic seizures, and ictal recordings are often needed.

F. Sleep studies (multiple sleep latency test and polysomnography) may be needed in some patients with suspected sleep disorders.

G. MRI should be performed in patients with partial seizures and secondary (symptomatic) generalized epilepsies.

VII. Referral. In patients with recurrent seizures, an initial neurologic consultation, including an EEG to clarify the seizure type, allows the proper choice of anticonvulsants. Whenever the diagnosis remains unclear after the initial evaluation or there is lack of response to anticonvulsants, the patient should be referred to a comprehensive epilepsy center. Evaluation at such centers includes prolonged video EEG recordings with sphenoidal electrodes.

A. Because the treatment and prognosis are based on the seizure type and epileptic syndrome, **ictal recordings** are invaluable and allow the proper choice of anticonvulsants.

B. Ictal recordings are the most effective way to diagnose psychogenic seizures, but patients with psychogenic seizures may also have epileptic seizures, and all the habitual seizure types should be recorded. To compound the problem, some patients with supplementary motor seizures and other simple partial seizures may exhibit no ictal EEG changes on scalp recordings, or the EEG may be obscured by muscle artifacts. Inpatient prolonged video EEG recordings with reduction of anticonvulsants may clarify the diagnosis by recording secondarily generalized seizures.

C. Identification of surgical candidates. Approximately 30% of patients with complex partial seizures of temporal lobe origin are refractory to medical treatment, and many benefit from surgery. Prolonged video EEG, MRI with volumetric studies, and tests of focal functional deficits (FDG-PET scans) are conducted at epilepsy centers to identify surgical candidates.

Recommended Readings

Aicardi J. *Epilepsy in Children.* In *International Review of Child Neurology Series.* New York: Raven, 1994.

Andermann F, Robb JP. Absence status: A reappraisal following review of 38 patients. *Epilepsia* 13:177–187, 1972.

Commission on Classification and Terminology of the International League Against Epilepsy. Proposal for classification of epilepsies and epileptic syndromes. *Epilepsia* 26:268–278, 1985.

Engel J. *Seizures and Epilepsy.* In *Contemporary Neurology Series.* Philadelphia: Davis, 1989.

French JA, et al. Characteristics of medial temporal lobe epilepsy: I. Results of history and physical examination. *Ann Neurol* 34:774–780, 1993.

Gloor P. Generalized epilepsy with spike and wave discharge: A reinterpretation of its electrographic and clinical manifestations. *Epilepsia* 20:571–588, 1979.

Gloor P, et al. The role of the limbic system in experiential phenomena of temporal lobe epilepsy. *Ann Neurol* 12:129–144, 1982.

Holmes G. *Diagnosis and Management of Seizures in Children* (vol 30). Philadelphia: Saunders, 1987.

Kanner AM, et al. Supplementary motor seizures mimicking pseudoseizures: Some clinical differences. *Neurology* 40:1404–1407, 1990.

Kotagal P, et al. Dystonic posturing in complex partial seizures of temporal lobe onset: A new lateralizing sign. *Neurology* 39:196–201, 1989.

Lüders H, Lesser R (eds). *Epilepsy: Electroclinical Syndromes.* London: Springer-Verlag, 1987.

Morris H, et al. Supplementary motor seizures: Clinical and electrographic findings. *Neurology* 38:1075, 1988.

Penfield W, Jasper H. *Epilepsy and the Functional Anatomy of the Human Brain.* Boston: Little, Brown, 1954.

Salanova V, Markand O, Worth R. Clinical characteristics and predictive factors in 98 patients with complex partial seizures treated with temporal resection. *Arch Neurol* 51:1008–1013, 1994.

Salanova V, et al. Occipital lobe epilepsy: Electroclinical manifestations, electrocorticography, cortical stimulation and outcome in 42 patients treated between 1930 and 1991. *Brain* 115:1655–1680, 1992.

Salanova V, et al. Frontal lobe seizures: Electroclinical syndromes. *Epilepsia* 36(1): 16–24, 1995.

Williamson PD, et al. Complex partial seizures of frontal lobe origin. *Ann Neurol* 18: 497–504, 1985.

Williamson PD, et al. Occipital lobe epilepsy: Clinical characteristics, seizure spread patterns and results of surgery. *Ann Neurol* 31:3–13, 1992.

Williamson PD, et al. Parietal lobe epilepsy: Diagnostic considerations and results of surgery. *Ann Neurol* 31:193–201, 1992.

Williamson PD, et al. Characteristics of medial temporal lobe epilepsy: II. Interictal and ictal scalp electroencephalography, neuropsychological testing, neuroimaging, surgical results and pathology. *Ann Neurol* 34:781–787, 1993.

Wyllie E, et al. The lateralizing significance of versive head and eye movements during epileptic seizures. *Neurology* 36:606–611, 1986.

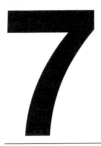

Approach to the Patient with Syncope

Gary J. Martin
Martin J. Arron

Syncope can be defined as a transient (less than 30 minutes) loss of consciousness accompanied by loss of postural control. Etiologies range from the relatively benign vasovagal syncope to life-threatening cardiac arrhythmias. This range is illustrated by several epidemiologic facts. Approximately one-third of healthy young adults have had at least one episode of loss of consciousness. For the majority of these individuals, it was a relatively benign event. On the other hand, 5% of sudden cardiac death victims have had a recent history of syncope. The potential prognostic significance of the syncopal event makes it necessary to evaluate each patient carefully.

I. Etiology

A. The major **mechanisms** of syncope include obstruction to cerebral blood flow, decreased cardiac output secondary to decreased heart rate or stroke volume, decreased peripheral vascular resistance, and insufficient blood constituents (oxygen and glucose). In the elderly, multiple mechanisms may contribute to the syncope. For example, postprandial fluid shifts may exacerbate mild preexisting orthostatic hypotension, sinus node dysfunction, and impaired autoregulation of cerebral blood flow.

B. Obstruction to **cerebral blood flow** is a rare cause of true syncope. Most carotid artery distribution (anterior circulation) transient ischemic attacks (TIAs) cause unilateral visual impairment, weakness, or loss of sensation. Posterior circulation (vertebral artery distribution) TIAs generally present with diplopia, vertigo, ataxia, or "drop attacks," but not loss of consciousness. Rarely, patients with TIAs may present with transient loss of consciousness, but isolated syncopal episodes without accompanying neurologic symptoms should not be ascribed to a TIA.

C. Generalized **hypotension** may cause inadequate cerebral perfusion. This is the main mechanism for most syncopal episodes. The hypotension may be cardiogenic, may result from rhythm disturbances such as bradycardia or tachyarrhythmia, which reduce cardiac output, or may be secondary to valvular dysfunction resulting in outflow obstruction, as observed in aortic stenosis or idiopathic hypertrophic subaortic stenosis (IHSS). Probably the most common mechanism of hypotension is loss of peripheral vascular tone. Vasovagal syncope is the most common disorder in this group. Drug toxicity and various disorders associated with orthostatic hypotension may also cause impaired peripheral vascular resistance.

D. Deficiencies in blood constituents, such as severe **hypoxemia** and **hypoglycemia,** are associated with true loss of consciousness. Profound hypoglycemia often causes longer episodes of impaired consciousness and may induce coma, as opposed to the brief, transient loss of consciousness characteristic of syncope.

E. Table 7-1 lists the common causes of syncope identified from a large number of prospective studies. Most common causes of syncope in patients presenting to emergency departments include vasovagal (vasodepressor) reactions, seizures, orthostatic hypotension, cardiac diseases such as dysrhythmia and outflow obstruction, situational syncope (postmicturition or post-tussive), and hypoglycemia. Rarer causes include transient ischemic attacks, migraine headaches, pulmonary embolism, and psychiatric disorders. Syncope of unknown origin is a legitimate diagnosis made after a careful history, physical examination, and selected laboratory tests have failed to elucidate a specific etiology. This diagnosis is clinically useful because it is associated with a distinct prognosis that is significantly better than that of patients who have identifiable car-

Table 7-1. Causes of syncope (1363 pooled patients).

Cause	Percentage	Cause	Percentage
Vasovagal	36%	Situational	4%
Idiopathic	24%	Psychogenic	3%
Cardiac	13%	Metabolic/drug	2%
Neurologic	11%	Miscellaneous	1–3%
Orthostatic	4%		

diac causes of syncope. Long-term follow-up studies have shown that the risk of sudden death in middle-aged and older patients with defined cardiac causes of syncope is as high as 24% during the first year after the syncopal event. Patients with a previous history of cardiac or neurologic disease also have a significantly increased long-term mortality. Patients with syncope of unknown cause have a relatively low incidence of sudden death (0–3%). Their risk is comparable to that of patients who, after further investigation, are diagnosed as having noncardiovascular causes of syncope.

II. **Clinical manifestations.** Table 7-2 lists associated signs and symptoms found in patients with syncope, grouped into two categories. The first few are fairly nonspecific symptoms associated with decreased cerebral perfusion regardless of the etiology. The second category of signs and symptoms are those that are somewhat more suggestive of specific etiologies.

III. **Evaluation**
  A. **History**
    1. Information about the **prodromal period** is most helpful diagnostically. A useful technique is to ask the patient to "walk through" the sequence of events occurring just prior to the loss of consciousness.
      a. A patient's activity and posture prior to the episode should be noted. A supine position suggests a cardiac dysrhythmia or seizure and makes a vasovagal reaction or syncope resulting from orthostatic hypotension very unlikely. Syncope during physical examination is a characteristic finding in aortic stenosis, whereas loss of consciousness after exercise indicates that idiopathic hypertrophic subaortic stenosis may be a causal factor. Loss of consciousness while urinating, coughing, or laughing is strongly suggestive of situational syncope. Episodes that follow the assumption of an upright posture, particularly if it occurs within 30 seconds to 2 minutes after standing, implies that orthostatic hypotension was the inciting cause. The nadir in blood pressure following a meal in the elderly occurs within 15–90 minutes. Syncope occurring within this time interval suggests a postprandial induction or exacerbation of orthostatic hypotension. Episodes that follow neck extension, flexion, or rotation implicate carotid sinus hypersensitivity, whereas those taking place during prolonged periods of standing are often the result of vasovagal reactions.
      b. Specific symptoms exhibited during the prodromal period are important predictors of the cause of the episode. The majority of symptoms are nonspecific and merely reflect the presence of cerebral hypoperfusion. Examples include lightheadedness, wooziness, nausea, a warm or flushed sensation, diaphoresis, paresthesias, and impaired visual acuity. Some of these symptoms are not unique to syncope and may also be felt just prior to a seizure. A classic but uncommon prodrome for a seizure disorder is a new smell or **olfactory hallucination.** Epigastric distress is observed with vasovagal syncope and inferior wall myocardial infarction. Although suggestive of pulmonary embolism, dyspnea can also be found in conjunction with hyperventilation and other psychiatric disorders associated with syncope. Facial pallor is very suggestive of decreased cerebral blood flow from any cause (orthostatic hypotension, vasovagal reactions, or arrhythmia) and helps rule out seizure. In the latter instance, facial cyanosis during the ictus epilepticus or postictal facial plethora is more typical.
      c. The perceived duration of the warning period provides clinically relevant information. Very brief intervals (<10 seconds) are characteristic

Table 7-2. Syncope: Associated signs and symptoms.

Nonspecific	Specific
Paresthesias	Aura
Diaphoresis	Palpitations
Dizziness	Vertigo and ataxia
Lightheadedness	Anginal or pleuritic chest pain
Blurred or fading vision	Diplopia
Auditory impairment	Olfactory hallucinations
Tinnitus	Dyspnea
Nausea	Epigastric discomfort

of cardiac causes, micturition syncope, orthostatic hypotension, and seizure disorders. On the other hand, vasovagal syncope typically has a more sustained warning period lasting 1 or 2 minutes. This can often be elicited with careful questioning.

    d. Focal neurologic symptoms may indicate a transient ischemic attack and can be present immediately before or after the loss of consciousness. Specific examples include vertigo, diplopia, ataxia, dysarthria, hemiparesis, and unilateral numbness. Posterior circulation TIAs usually present with a cluster of these symptoms.

    e. A variety of factors may trigger vasovagal syncope in predisposed individuals. Emotionally charged situations such as anger, fear, and seeing blood may induce vasodepressor activity. Pregnant patients as well as those suffering physical trauma, pain, fatigue, or sleep deprivation are at increased risk. Hot, enclosed, or crowded environments, particularly if the patient is standing for sustained periods of time, increase the likelihood of vasovagal syncope.

2. The events taking place during the syncopal period are of great importance in defining a specific etiology. A detailed history confirming the presence of a true transient episode of loss of consciousness and associated neuromuscular activity is extremely important to obtain.

    a. Given that patients are unconscious during most of this period, first-hand reports from witnesses are crucial. Clinicians should make sincere efforts to interview these individuals either in person or by telephone.

    b. Although prolonged episodes of cerebral anoxia (in excess of 10–15 seconds) may induce brief involuntary motor activity, the presence of more sustained episodes of alternating **tonic and clonic** muscle action is strongly suggestive of a seizure. The same is true for the presence of facial cyanosis, tongue biting, and excessive salivation.

    c. Brief episodes of unconsciousness are more typical of the majority of episodes of syncope resulting from cardiovascular causes. Hypoglycemia may induce episodes of more sustained durations. Seizures also tend to have more prolonged durations.

    d. Urinary incontinence is more frequently found in patients with seizure, although it may accompany syncope from any cause. Fecal incontinence is a finding that is more specific for seizures.

3. The events transpiring during the immediate postsyncopal period also provide important clues regarding the etiology of the loss of consciousness. Patients may be unable to recount specific details regarding this interval because they may have remained cognitively impaired during a significant portion of this time. It is important to seek out and interview individuals who may have witnessed the event.

    a. Prolonged durations of postictal confusion, **amnesia,** or lethargy implicate seizure or other primary CNS injury as the precipitating disorder.

    b. The presence of focal neurologic symptoms or signs points to an inciting neurologic event such as a seizure with residual functional deficit (Todd's paralysis) or ischemic injury.

    c. Facial **pallor** points to syncope, whereas facial **plethora** is more suggestive of seizure.

    d. Diffuse **muscle soreness** suggests seizure activity.

4. Past medical history

a. Comorbid disorders

(1) A variety of **cardiovascular disorders** are risk factors for syncope. Structural heart diseases such as coronary artery disease, congestive heart failure, hypertrophic obstructive cardiomyopathy, and valvular disorders predispose patients to syncope. Ventricular tachycardia, atrial fibrillation, and bradycardia are examples of dysrhythmias that may result in transient loss of consciousness. Chronic hypertension can induce left ventricular systolic and diastolic dysfunction, impair cerebrovascular autoregulation, and expose patients to hypotensive therapies.

(2) A variety of neurologic disorders predispose patients to syncope or seizure. Primary or metastatic neoplasia as well as scars from prior trauma, ischemic injury, or infection provide foci for seizures. Peripheral or autonomic neuropathy induced by diabetes mellitus, alcohol abuse, vitamin B_{12} deficiency, or other metabolic disorders can cause orthostatic hypotension. Preexisting cerebrovascular disease can make patients more susceptible to relatively minor reductions in cerebral perfusion. Various movement disorders such as Parkinson's disease are associated with a higher incidence of orthostatic hypotension and nonsyncopal falls.

(3) Anxiety disorders and depression are examples of psychiatric illnesses that have been linked to syncope.

b. A large number of medications can induce syncope. **Antihypertensive** drugs and **psychotropic** medications are the most risk prone. The former can impair cerebral perfusion by two primary mechanisms, either reducing cardiac output or lowering peripheral vascular resistance. Psychotropic medications can induce orthostatic hypotension and, in the case of the tricyclic antidepressants, predispose patients to a variety of cardiac rhythm disturbances.

c. A brief gynecologic history should be elicited to determine risk factors for pregnancy, particularly in ectopic locations. Gravid patients are at increased risk of syncope as a result of orthostatic hypotension and vasovagal reactions. Moreover, a ruptured ectopic pregnancy occasionally may present with syncope. The recent occurrence of sexual intercourse without the use of a contraceptive method, the presence of amenorrhea, and any symptoms of pregnancy should be elicited.

B. Physical examination

1. Accurate measurement of vital signs should be obtained. In order to detect accurately the presence of orthostatic hypotension, the supine blood pressure should be obtained after prolonged recumbency and the standing blood pressure measured after the patient has been erect for a minimum of 2 minutes. Blood pressure measurements in the sitting position do not accurately detect postural hypotension. Orthostatic hypotension has been arbitrarily defined as present if the systolic or diastolic arterial blood pressure falls 20 mm Hg or 10 mm Hg, respectively, after the patient goes from a supine to a standing posture.

2. A detailed cardiovascular examination should be performed. Palpation of the carotid arteries may reveal the pulsus tardus et parvus (delayed, low-volume carotid pulsation) associated with hemodynamically significant aortic stenosis or the pulsus bisferiens (equally intense, biphasic carotid pulsation) characteristic of idiopathic subaortic stenosis. The presence of a carotid bruit signifies a high likelihood of diffuse atherosclerotic vascular disease involving the cerebral, coronary, and peripheral vasculature. If continuous electrocardiographic monitoring is utilized and cardiac resuscitation equipment is readily available, carotid massage can be performed to detect the presence of carotid sinus supersensitivity. Cardiac examination should be performed to detect evidence of rhythm abnormalities, murmurs suggestive of significant valvular heart disease, or parasternal heaves or gallops characteristic of left ventricular dysfunction. Evidence of a subclavian steal syndrome, such as a supraclavicular bruit or a diminished upper extremity arterial pulsation, should be sought.

3. A screening **neurologic examination** should be pursued to detect postictal cognitive impairment, the presence of focal neurologic defects indicative of either an acute neurologic injury or a preexisting substrate for a seizure dis-

order, a peripheral neuropathy that would predispose to orthostatic hypotension, or a movement disorder that would cause nonsyncopal falls.
4. A digital rectal examination should be done to detect evidence of overt or occult gastrointestinal bleeding such as melena or hematochezia.

C. Laboratory studies

1. **Electrocardiography.** The resting **12-lead electrocardiogram** is the single most useful test for both prognosis and triage, despite the fact that it is diagnostic in only 5–10% of cases. It is uncommon for the etiologic rhythm disturbance to be detected on the tracing. However, research suggests that the presence of left axis deviation, left bundle branch block, or left ventricular hypertrophy points to an underlying cardiac cause. These are generally markers for the underlying substrate that can cause ventricular arrhythmias or bradyarrhythmias. Other less common electrocardiographic findings are helpful. Signs of acute right heart strain ($S_1Q_3T_3$ or right bundle branch block pattern) suggest a pulmonary embolism.

   More sophisticated forms of electrocardiographic monitoring are frequently helpful. **Ambulatory electrocardiography** is a moderately sensitive diagnostic tool. This test, however, has limited specificity, because certain rhythm disturbances such as brief pauses, premature atrial and ventricular contractions, as well as nonsustained ventricular tachycardia may be detected even when they are not responsible for the syncopal episode. If symptoms occur while the patient is monitored and no electrocardiographic abnormalities are detected, a rhythm disturbance is effectively excluded as an etiology. Continuous ambulatory monitoring in excess of 24 hours is usually unnecessary. Patient-activated loop recorders can be utilized for patients with recurrent but infrequent symptoms and a high pretest likelihood of a cardiac etiology. Exercise electrocardiography may be used in the uncommon instance when ischemically mediated rhythm disturbances are suspected. The roles of **signal averaged electrocardiography** (SAECG) and measurement of QT dispersion are less well defined. These two tests appear to be most useful in patients with moderate pretest probability of a causal cardiac dysrhythmia. In this instance, an abnormal test would prompt more sophisticated electrophysiologic testing. In patients for whom there is a reduced clinical suspicion, the positive predictive values are too low to be diagnostically useful.

2. **Serum chemistries.** The determination of serum electrolyte concentrations has limited utility. If evaluated within an hour of the syncopal event, some patients show a depressed **bicarbonate** level. This can be a clue to a seizure disorder because the **transient lactic acidosis** generated during a convulsion can cause a lowering of the serum bicarbonate concentration. This generally normalizes within an hour. Elevated **prolactin** levels have been reported in some patients hours after grand mal seizures. The same is true for creatine phosphokinase (CPK) levels, although increased serum concentrations may also be caused by injury during a syncopal episode. Serum **glucose** levels are most valuable at the time of the event, particularly in diabetic patients who have recently increased their insulin or oral hypoglycemic therapy or decreased their caloric intake.

3. **Complete blood counts.** The main component that is occasionally helpful is the **hemoglobin** level. It is most useful when acute or subacute blood loss or a severe anemia is suspected. In the former instance, clinically apparent bleeding is usually present.

4. **Arterial blood gas analysis.** Arterial **blood gases** can be useful in the occasional patient in whom pulmonary embolism is suspected by history, physical examination, or electrocardiography.

5. **Electrophysiologic studies (EPS).** This sophisticated assessment of the integrity of the cardiac conduction system is a reasonably accurate test. Its true sensitivity, specificity, and predictive values are unclear and often vary with the aggressiveness of the diagnostic protocol and the clinical suspicion of a dysrhythmia. It is most often abnormal in patients with known heart disease or those with significant abnormalities on routine electrocardiography. It should be pursued when there is a high clinical suspicion of life-threatening cardiac rhythm disturbances. It appears particularly useful in elderly individuals with organic heart disease, recurrent symptoms, and negative noninvasive evaluations.

6. **Tilt table testing.** The utility of both passive and active tilt table tests for the diagnosis of vasovagal syncope remains poorly defined. It is only a moderately sensitive and specific test. A positive test is reproducible only 70% of the time. Tilt table testing may also be used to gauge the effectiveness of therapy. The limited reproducibility of the test as well as the variable natural history of unexplained syncope reduce its utility in this latter role.

7. **Carotid sinus massage. Carotid sinus hypersensitivity,** a rare cause of syncope, can be detected by monitoring changes in blood pressure and heart rate following 5–40 seconds of unilateral carotid artery massage. Responses are characterized as cardioinhibitory if asystole lasting 3 seconds or more develops; vasodepressor if systolic arterial blood pressure falls 50 mm Hg or more without associated changes in heart rate or 30 mm Hg with associated syncope; and mixed when both cardioinhibitory and vasodepressor responses are present. Carotid sinus hypersensitivity occurs in a substantial minority of elderly patients, the vast majority of whom are asymptomatic. This diagnosis should be made only when the history is strongly suggestive and an abnormal response to carotid sinus massage is elicited.

8. **Radiographic testing.** Routine computed axial tomography (CT) and magnetic resonance imaging (MRI) of the head have low yields, but may be useful in patients who have sustained major head trauma, have newly diagnosed seizure disorders, or have focal deficits on the neurologic examination. Routine skull radiography, nuclear brain scans, and cerebral angiography are not useful screening tests for patients with syncope.

IV. **Differential diagnosis.** The differential diagnosis provided in Table 7-3 lists some clues for distinguishing seizure from syncope, as well as vasovagal syncope from cardiac syncope. This can be quite difficult in that patients frequently have unwitnessed events or witnesses are not available at the time of the physician's evaluation. It is also true that there is substantial overlap in the signs and symptoms typical of these disorders. For example, patients with decreased cerebral perfusion may have secondary brief (<10 seconds) seizure activity that can be mistaken for a primary seizure even by experienced observers. One of the main differentiating features is the prolonged duration of the postictal state following grand mal seizures. This may last 10–15 minutes as opposed to the relatively brief (<1 minute) confusional state that can follow syncope from cardiovascular causes.

V. **Diagnostic approach.** History and physical examination initially provide the etiology in one-half to more than two-thirds of diagnosed cases. Laboratory testing should be done selectively. A resting electrocardiogram should be obtained unless a benign, noncardiac cause of syncope is readily apparent. For patients in whom cardiac etiologies are suspected, up to 24 hours of ambulatory electrocardiographic monitoring is recommended. Loop recording devices are also quite useful in selected patients with recurrent but infrequent (every few weeks) symptoms. For those in whom significant arrhythmias have been detected or those with significant underlying heart disease and unexplained syncope (such as those with known myocardial infarction or left ventricular dysfunction), electrophysiologic studies (EPS) are often recommended. Signal averaged electrocardiography (SAECG) and QT dispersion may be helpful in patients with moderate suspicion of a cardiac arrhythmia. Those with abnormal results need EPS. In patients considered at high risk clinically, EPS should probably be done directly, because a negative SAECG would not be sufficiently reassuring.

Tilt table testing may be helpful for patients with unexplained syncope, particularly when a cardiac etiology is not suspected. However, therapy based on tilt table testing itself is not highly reliable. This is because the test-retest reliability of tilt testing is not high and because many patients improve over time without therapy (or with placebo). Its use should be reserved for patients with unexplained syncope who are older, have recurrent events, or have suffered significant injuries during their episodes. CT and MRI are of little value in most patients with syncope unless a true seizure disorder or a structural disease of the CNS is suspected.

VI. **Referral.** For patients in whom a seizure disorder is suspected, neurologic consultation is generally appropriate. For patients in whom a potentially life-threatening arrhythmia is strongly suspected or has been discovered, referral to a cardiologist, particularly one with advanced training in arrhythmias, would be helpful. Similarly, referral to a psychiatrist or psychologist may be indicated if the syncope is related to a psychiatric illness.

Table 7-3. Typical features of vasovagal syncope, cardiac syncope, and seizure.

	Vasovagal	Seizure	Cardiac
Onset	Subacute onset	Sudden onset or brief aura	Sudden onset Chest pain, dyspnea,
	Prodromal weakness, nausea, diaphoresis, or visual changes	Auditory hallucinations	palpitations, and other cardiac symptoms may be present
Typical milieu or precipitating factors	Fatigue Delayed meals Prolonged standing Crowded enclosed confines Pregnancy Pain or trauma Emotional situation	Spontaneous onset Triggered by flashing light or monotonous sensory simulation	Often spontaneous onset During or following exertion Known or suspected structural heart disease
Posture at time of onset	Standing or sitting	Standing, sitting, or supine	Standing, sitting, or supine
Appearance	Pallor Brief tonic-clonic motor activity possible Occasional urinary incontinence	Normal or cyanotic Stertorous respiration Stereotypic motor activity Transient loss of awareness Urinary and fecal incontinence common	Pallor Brief periods of tonic-clonic motor activity possible Urinary incontinence uncommon
Residual	Rapid recovery Reoccurence with resumption of upright posture possible	Delayed recovery Postictal cognitive impairment Todd's paralysis Todd's paralysis	Rapid or briefly delayed recovery If prolonged hypoxia, evidence of CNS injury present Symptoms of cardiac dysfunction

Recommended Readings

Benditt DB, et al. Cardiac pacing for the prevention of recurrent vasovagal syncope. *Ann Intern Med* 122:204–209, 1995.

Brignole M, et al. A controlled trial of acute and long-term medical therapy in tilt-induced neurally mediated syncope. *Am J Cardiol* 70:339–342, 1992.

Day SC, et al. Evaluation and outcome of emergency room patients with transient loss of consciousness. *Am J Med* 73:15–23, 1982.

Grubb BP, et al. Utility of upright tilt-table testing in the evaluation and management of syncope of unknown origin. *Am J Med* 90:6–10, 1991.

Hanlon JT, et al. Syncope and presyncope associated with probable adverse drug reactions. *Arch Intern Med* 150:2309–2312, 1990.

Kapoor W, Peterson J, Karpf M. A rapid identification of low-risk patients with syncope: Implications regarding hospitalization and cost. *Clin Res* 34:823A, 1986.

Kapoor W, et al. Predictors of sudden death in patients with syncope. *Clin Res* 33:255A, 1985.

Kapoor WN, et al. A prospective evaluation of syncope in patients presenting to the emergency department. *N Engl J Med* 309:197–204, 1983.

Kroenke MK. Orthostatic hypertension. *West J Med* 143:253–255, 1985.

Krol RB, et al. Electrophysiologic testing in patients with unexplained syncope: Clinical and noninvasive predictors of outcome. *J Am Coll Cardiol* 10:358–363, 1987.

Kuller L, Cooper M, Perper J. Epidemiology of sudden death. *Arch Intern Med* 129: 714–719, 1972.

Lipsitz LA, Wei JY, Rowe JW. Syncope in an elderly, institutionalized population: Prevalence, incidence, and associated risks. *Q J Med* 55:45–54, 1985.

Martin GJ, et al. Prospective evaluation of syncope in patients presenting to the emergency department. *Ann Emerg Med* 13:499–504, 1984.

Middlekauff HR, et al. Syncope in advanced heart failure: High risk of sudden death regardless of origin of syncope. *J Am Coll Cardiol* 21:110–116, 1993.

Murdoch BD. Loss of consciousness in healthy South African men: Incidence, causes and relationship to EEG abnormality. *S Afr Med J* 57:771–774, 1980.

Stumpf JL, Mitrzyk B. Management of orthostatic hypotension. *Am J Hosp Pharm* 51(1):648–660, 1994.

Thames MD, Alpert JS, Dalen JE. Syncope in patients with pulmonary embolism. *JAMA* 23:2509–2511, 1977.

Wayne HH. Syncope: Physiological considerations and an analysis of the clinical characteristics in 510 patients. *Am J Med* 30:418–438, 1961.

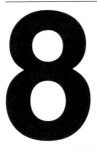

Approach to the Patient with Gait Disturbances and Recurrent Falls
Rodger J. Elble

Gait disturbances and **recurrent falls** are caused by many neurologic, visual, vestibular, and musculoskeletal illnesses. These illnesses are common in all age groups and are particularly common in older people. Impaired locomotion is a source of significant disability in roughly 15% of people over age 65, rivaling dementia as the leading form of neurologic impairment. Elderly Americans suffer approximately 250,000 hip fractures and 7000 deaths per year as a result of falls, and the estimated annual financial cost of this problem exceeds several billion dollars.

I. **Pathophysiology.** Successful locomotion requires the integrated control of posture and movement. Postural control is necessary for static and dynamic stability during stance and locomotion, respectively. Somatic, visual, and vestibular sensory information is used in complex feedback (reflex) pathways that enable the nervous system to respond to ever-changing environmental conditions. These sensory inputs are also combined with prior experience to adjust the pattern of stance or locomotion. This anticipatory or feedforward control of movement is critically important because reflex responses to the environment are too slow and inaccurate for normal locomotion. Altered sensorium and impaired cognition (i.e., memory, attention, motivation, visuospatial function, judgment, and insight) impede feedforward and voluntary modifications of stance and gait.

The basic locomotor rhythm emerges from spinal neuronal networks that interact directly with several brainstem nuclei and the cerebellum (Fig. 8-1). The midbrain locomotor region of the dorsolateral midbrain contains a heterogeneous group of neurons that connect with the basal ganglia and with raphe and reticular nuclei in the caudal pons and rostral medulla. The midbrain locomotor region and its connections play a critical role in the initiation of gait and in the control of posture. The cerebellum interacts with pontomedullary reticular nuclei, the red nucleus, and the vestibular nuclei in the control of posture and rhythmic limb motion. The cerebellum receives inputs from the spinal locomotor network, from peripheral somatosensory, vestibular, and visual pathways, and from the cerebral cortex by way of the pontine, olivary, and other brainstem nuclei. Consequently, the cerebellum is perfectly positioned in the feedback and feedforward control of posture and locomotion. The reticulospinal and vestibulospinal pathways in the ventral spinal cord are necessary for rudimentary control of the spinal networks, and corticospinal pathways are needed for flexible, adaptive control. The cerebral cortex has rich connections with the basal ganglia, thalamus, and cerebellum. Thus, the nervous system can modify posture and locomotion as dictated by environmental constraints, body mechanics, and personal desires.

II. **Etiology**

A. **Gait disturbances.** A disturbance of locomotion can occur at any level of the neuraxis. Gait disturbances are caused by any disease affecting the frontal and parietal lobes, basal ganglia, thalamus, brainstem motor nuclei, cerebellum, spinal cord, peripheral nerves, eyes, labyrinth, and musculoskeletal system. The etiologies of locomotor impairment are myriad. The list in Table 8-1 is not exhaustive, and multiple coexistent etiologies are common, particularly in older people. Neurologic disturbances commonly lead to secondary skeletal deformities, muscle deconditioning, and cardiopulmonary deconditioning, which cause further impairment of locomotion.

B. **Etiologies of recurrent falls.** Environmental hazards and errors in judgment are responsible for 35–50% of falls in some studies, but underlying neurologic, visual, or vestibular disease is present in most patients (see Table 8-1). Most

Supported by grant AG10837 from the National Institute on Aging.

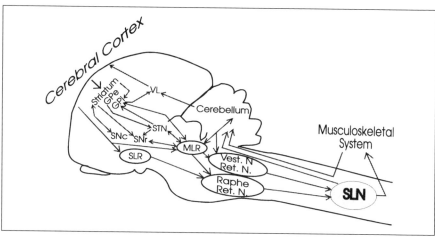

Figure 8-1. Schematic diagram of the principal neural pathways of locomotor control. GPe and GPi = globus pallidus externa and interna; VL = ventrolateral thalamus; SNc and SNr = substantia nigra pars compacta and reticulata; STN = subthalamus; SLR = subthalamic locomotor region; MLR = midbrain locomotor region; Vest. N. = lateral vestibular nucleus; Ret. N. = pontomedullary reticular nuclei; SLN = spinal locomotor network (central pattern generator).

Table 8-1. Etiologies of gait disturbances.

Vascular disease
  Stroke
  Binswanger's disease
  Collagen-vascular disease
Visual and vestibular disturbances
Degenerative movement disorders
  Basal ganglia (e.g., Parkinson's disease, progressive supranuclear palsy, Huntington's disease)
  Spinocerebellar degenerations (ataxias)
  Generalized dystonias (dystonia musculorum deformans, dopa-sensitive dystonia)
  Hereditary spastic paraparesis
  Amyotrophic lateral sclerosis
Cognitive disturbances
  Dementia (e.g., Alzheimer's disease, diffuse Lewy body disease, normal pressure hydrocephalus)
  Depression
  Acute confusional states
Metabolic and toxic disorders
  Vitamin B_{12} deficiency
  Thyroid disorders
  Ethanol
  Organic solvents
  Medications (neuroleptics, anticonvulsants, sedative-hypnotics, lithium, metoclopramide)
Skeletal disease
  Spinal and pelvic deformities
  Hip, knee, and ankle arthropathies
  Foot pathology (e.g., flatfoot, clubfoot)
Cervical spondylosis and other compressive myelopathies

Trauma
  Subacute and chronic subdural hematoma
  Post-traumatic positional vertigo
  Bilateral frontal lobe or brainstem contusions
  Spinal cord trauma and post-traumatic syringomyelia
Neoplasms
  Adults: frontal lobe (e.g., parasagittal), cerebellopontine angle, or spinal tumors
  Children: brainstem, cerebellar, and spinal tumors
  Carcinomatous meningitis, causing hydrocephalus
Multiple sclerosis, presenting as a spastic, hemiparetic, or ataxic gait
Infectious disease
  Creutzfeldt-Jakob disease, causing ataxic gait
  Chronic meningitis (e.g., cryptococcal), causing hydrocephalus
Neuromuscular (acquired and hereditary)
  Peripheral polyneuropathy
  Inflammatory myopathies
  Drug-induced myopathies
  Muscular dystrophies
  Congenital myopathies
  Muscular deconditioning
  Spinal muscular atrophies
Cerebral palsy
  Spastic diplegia
  Spastic quadriplegia

Table 8-1 *(continued)*

Spastic hemiparesis	Arnold-Chiari malformations
Choreoathetosis	Syringomyelia
Ataxia (rare)	Meningomyelocele
Congenital malformations	Aqueductal stenosis
Cerebellar dysgenesis	Acute cerebellar ataxia of childhood
Dandy-Walker syndrome	

older people who fall are impaired by previous stroke, Parkinson's disease, severe arthritis, orthostatic hypotension, dementia (confusion), poor vision, or vestibular disease. Medications are also a common contributing factor or primary etiology.

III. **Clinical manifestations.** The examination of gait is useful in neurologic diagnosis and functional assessment. However, most patterns of abnormal walking provide only rough indications of the site(s) of pathology (Table 8-2) and must always be interpreted in the context of other neurologic signs. The areas of the nervous system involved in locomotion are widely distributed and highly integrated (see Fig. 8-1), so lesions in one area can mimic damage to another. For example, damage to the frontal lobes, thalami, or cerebellum can produce similar ataxia of gait with poor balance and uncoordinated extremity motion.

A. **Features of normal walking.** Walking is a cyclical movement with two dimensions: time and length of stride. The gait cycle is defined as the time between successive heel-floor contacts with the same foot (Fig. 8-2). One gait cycle consists of two steps. From right heel-floor contact to left toe-off is a period of double-limb support, which lasts approximately 10% of the total gait cycle. This phase of the cycle is followed by the left swing phase, which is simultaneous with and equal to the right single-limb support phase. The time from left heel-floor contact to right toe-off comprises the second of two double-limb support phases in a gait cycle and is followed by the right swing phase and left single-limb support phase.

1. **Stride length (length of two successive steps) and cadence (steps per minute)** determine the velocity of walking (velocity = stride length × cadence ÷ 2). The magnitudes of arm swing, toe-floor clearance, and hip and knee rotations are proportional to stride length and velocity, whereas the

Table 8-2. Clinical manifestations and abbreviated differential diagnosis of gait disturbances.

Abnormal gait or sign	Related terms	Sites of pathology	Clinical conditions
Cautious gait	Senile gait	Any part of the central or peripheral nervous system involved in locomotion and higher cortical function	Mild neurologic and musculoskeletal disease Visual disturbances Vestibulopathy
Dysequilibrium	Frontal ataxia Thalamic ataxia Subcortical dysequilibrium Cerebellar ataxia Sensory ataxia	Frontal lobes Ventrolateral thalamus Brainstem motor nuclei Midline cerebellum and fastigial nucleus Multiple involvement of peripheral visual, vestibular, and somatosensory systems Spinal cord	Stroke Binswanger's disease NPH PSP MSA Hereditary ataxias and other SCDs Multiple sensory deficits Toxic-metabolic disorders

Table 8-2 *(continued)*

Abnormal gait or sign	Related terms	Sites of pathology	Clinical conditions
Dysrhythmic, uncoordinated movement of body segments	Cerebellar ataxia Reeling, lurching gait Ataxic gait	Cerebellum Brainstem motor nuclei Spinal cord	Hereditary ataxias and other SCDs PSP
Start hesitation	Gait ignition failure Gait apraxia Magnetic gait Frozen gait Akinetic gait Slipping clutch syndrome	Frontal lobes Basal ganglia Dorsolateral midbrain locomotor region	Binswanger's disease NPH Parkinson's disease PSP Frontal lobe (parasagittal) mass
Short, shuffling steps and en bloc turning, with or without festination	Parkinsonian gait Lower-half parkinsonism Marche à petits pas Gait apraxia Magnetic gait	Basal ganglia Frontal lobes	Parkinson's disease Binswanger's disease PSP MSA
Choreiform gait		Basal ganglia	Huntington's disease Sydenham's chorea Cerebral palsy
Dystonic gait		Basal ganglia	Torsion dystonia Dopa-sensitive dystonia Cerebral palsy
Hemiparetic gait	Hemiplegic gait Circumducting gait	Supraspinal pyramidal tract lesion	Stroke, tumor, abscess, trauma, demyelination, or other focal lesions
Spastic gait	Scissoring gait	Thoracic or cervical spinal cord damage	Myelopathy of any etiology affecting primarily the corticospinal tracts
Spastic diplegic gait	Crouch gait Scissoring gait	Bilateral perinatal frontal lobe damage	Cerebral palsy
Toe-walking		Tight heel cords Ankle contractures Bilateral pyramidal tract disease	Cerebral palsy Duchenne's muscular dystrophy Idiosyncratic
Waddling gait	Lordotic-waddling gait Myopathic gait	Weak hip girdle	Acquired and hereditary myopathies
Steppage gait	Bilateral foot drop	Bilateral weakness of muscles innervated by the peroneal nerves	Hereditary or acquired distal motor polyneuropathy Bilateral peroneal neuropathy
Antalgic gait	Hyperesthetic gait Limping gait	Foot, spine, pelvis, or lower extremity	Lumbar radiculopathy Skeletal pathology Foot deformities Tarsal tunnel syndrome Morton's neuroma

Table 8-2 *(continued)*

Abnormal gait or sign	Related terms	Sites of pathology	Clinical conditions
Ataxic gait	Tabetic gait Sensory ataxia Cerebellar ataxia Reeling, lurching gait	Dorsal spinal columns and spinocerebellar pathways Peripheral nerves Cerebellum Brainstem motor nuclei Spinal cord	Tabes dorsalis Pernicious anemia Hereditary ataxias and other SCDs PSP Alcoholic cerebellar degeneration Large-fiber sensory neuropathies Drug toxicity
Hysterical gait	Psychiatric astasia- abasia		Somatoform disorders Affective disorder with conversion reaction Factitious disorders, malingering

NPH = normal pressure hydrocephalus; PSP = progressive supranuclear palsy; MSA = multisystem atrophy; SCD = spinocerebellar degenerations.

percentage time in double-limb support increases with reductions in gait velocity.
2. **The total-body center of mass** oscillates vertically at a frequency equal to the cadence and horizontally at one-half the cadence. During a gait cycle, the two maxima in vertical oscillation occur at the middles of right and left single-limb support, and the two minima occur at the middles of the two phases of double-limb support. The left- and rightmost horizontal excursions of the center of gravity occur at the times of middle left and middle right single-limb support. These vertical and horizontal excursions of the center of mass are optimized in such a way that the center of mass (body) moves forward with the minimum amount of expended energy.
B. **Abnormal patterns of walking.** Descriptions of abnormal gaits have generated a fairly large and somewhat redundant terminology, which is summarized

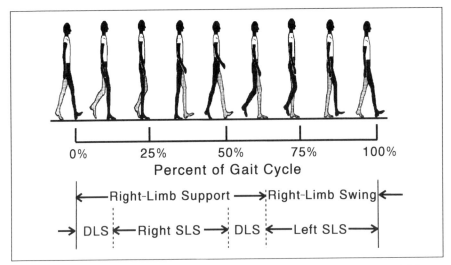

Figure 8-2. Phases of the normal gait cycle, expressed as percentages of total stride. DLS = double-limb support; SLS = single-limb support.

in Table 8-2. The characteristics of an abnormal gait are generally a mixture of primary abnormalities (i.e., direct effects of the underlying pathology), secondary musculoskeletal changes, and compensatory changes. All must be considered when deciphering a patient's gait.

1. **Cautious gait** is a slow, guarded, or restrained pattern of walking that resembles someone walking on a slippery surface or in a threatening environment. This pattern consists of stooped posture, reduced arm swing, increased time with both feet on the floor (double-limb support), loss of the normal heel-toe sequence of foot-floor contact during the stance phase, a slightly widened base, and reduced hip and knee rotations, all of which are commensurate with the patient's reduced stride and gait velocity. This gait is a nonspecific, largely compensatory response that is produced by most causes of impaired locomotion. The features of cautious gait frequently dominate the clinical picture of the patient with mild neurologic impairment, providing the clinician with few clues to the underlying pathology. **Senile gait** is a cautious gait in an older person.

2. **Dysequilibrium** is a disturbance of postural control and balance. Severe dysequilibrium produces a staggering, wide-based gait, particularly when the disturbance is acute. Mild or chronic dysequilibrium is often associated with a slow, cautious gait. Sudden or rapid movements (e.g., standing, turning, bending, and running) are avoided because they are most destabilizing. Dysequilibrium can result from damage at any level of the neuraxis (see Fig. 8-1). **Vestibular dysequilibrium** is associated with vertigo when the condition is acute. **Somatosensory dysequilibrium** is most evident when the eyes are closed.

3. **Dysrhythmic, uncoordinated limb movements** occur in patients with damage to the cerebellum or to those areas of the brainstem, ventrolateral thalamus, and frontal lobes with which the cerebellum is connected. Upper-limb movements are poorly coordinated with lower-extremity movements. Step length and width are often variable from stride to stride.

4. **Start hesitation** is a form of akinesia. Patients move their extremities relatively normally while they are seated or recumbent, but their feet appear to stick to the floor when they stand and attempt to walk. Gait typically is initiated, after a variable delay, with a few aborted, shuffling steps or is tricked into action by stepping over a self-imposed obstacle (e.g., the handle of an inverted cane) or by stepping onto a targeted spot on the floor. These tricks work best in patients with akinesia resulting from basal ganglia disease (e.g., Parkinson's disease and progressive supranuclear palsy). Environmental distractions and obstacles exacerbate start hesitation.

5. **Short, shuffling steps with en bloc turning** are common in patients with damage to the frontal lobes and basal ganglia. A greater reduction in arm swing than reduction in stride is characteristic of **Parkinson's disease.** Arm swing is increased relative to the reduced stride of **lower-half parkinsonism,** which is exhibited by patients with multiple small infarcts and subcortical white matter degeneration in the basal ganglia and frontal lobes. In **festination of gait,** the patient's forward lean increases as walking proceeds, and the steps become increasingly short and rapid. Festination is more common in idiopathic Parkinson's disease than in parkinsonism from other causes.

6. **Choreiform gait** consists of extremity movements and postural shifts that are interrupted by sudden, variable flinging or dancelike movements (chorea) of the extremities and torso. This gait appears bizarre and hazardous. Huntington's disease is the most common etiology. Suppression of chorea with haloperidol or other dopaminergic blockers frequently produces a disappointing improvement in gait, as a result of refractory concomitant disturbances in postural control.

7. **Dystonic gait** is a variable pattern of walking in which extremity movements and postural shifts are interrupted by tonic (sometimes phasic) co-contractions of antagonistic muscles in the limbs or trunk. The limbs, trunk, and neck may be contorted into bizarre postures that depend on the relative strengths of muscle contractions. Such dystonia may be focal or generalized and may emerge during a particular phase of the gait cycle (e.g., the swing phase). In addition to the conditions listed in Table 8-2, dystonia occasionally complicates the typical shuffling gait of Parkinson's disease.

8. **Hemiparetic gait** varies with the magnitude and distribution of weakness and spasticity. Reduced arm swing with flexor or dangling arm posture is observed in combination with a hyperextended lower extremity. Reduced hip and knee flexion and tonic ankle plantarflexion make foot-floor clearance during the swing phase of gait impossible, unless the patient leans away from the hemiparetic limb and swings the spastic lower extremity outward and forward (**circumduction**). The toes still scuff the floor, and the swing phase ends with the ball of the foot hitting the floor, instead of a normal heel strike. Patients with greater hip and knee mobility (and less spasticity) clear the floor during the swing phase with increased hip flexion.

9. **Spastic gait** varies with the magnitude and distribution of weakness and spasticity in the lower extremities and also varies with the degree of sensory loss. Movement of the upper extremities depends on the level of the pyramidal tract lesion. Upper-extremity movement may be increased relative to lower-extremity movement if the lesion is below the cervical cord. The upper extremities may dangle or exhibit flexor posturing in patients with high cervical or supraspinal lesions. Adduction or abduction of the upper extremities can occur. Relatively pure bilateral pyramidal tract dysfunction produces stiff, mechanical (i.e., deliberate), scissoring movements of the hyperextended lower extremities, which are tightly adducted. With less spasticity, the lower extremities move slowly and deliberately with little or no scissoring. Older people with mild to moderate cervical spondylosis and myelopathy frequently exhibit a nonspecific cautious pattern of walking.

10. **Spastic diplegic gait** is observed in some patients with cerebral palsy and is a result of perinatal bilateral corticospinal tract damage. The knees and hips are excessively flexed during the gait cycle, and the tightly adducted hips cause the lower extremities to move in a scissoring fashion. The upper extremities and speech (pseudobulbar palsy) are usually much less affected than the lower extremities, in contrast to the adult with bilateral hemiparesis and prominent pseudobulbar palsy. There is variable flexor posturing of the upper extremities and abduction of the arms.

11. **Gait disturbances resulting from neuromuscular weakness**
    a. **Waddling gait** is produced by muscle weakness in the hip girdle or, less commonly, by bilateral hip dislocations. Gait becomes increasingly wide-based and short-stepped. Increased lateral shoulder sway occurs during the stance phase in compensation for gluteus medius weakness. Increased arm abduction may also occur. Associated weakness in the paraspinal muscles produces exaggerated lumbar lordosis.
    b. **Steppage gait** is produced by distal symmetrical motor polyneuropathy or bilateral peroneal neuropathies. Weakness of ankle dorsiflexors interferes with foot-floor clearance during the swing phase of gait, so compensatory increases in hip and knee flexion are necessary to raise the foot higher. Steps are high and short. The foot commonly slaps the floor at the end of the swing phase. With polyneuropathy, there is often coexistent weakness of ankle plantar flexion, which limits propulsion of the body at the end of the support phase.

12. **Ataxic gait**
    a. **Cerebellar ataxia** occurs in patients with damage to the cerebellum or to those areas of the brainstem, ventrolateral thalamus, and frontal lobes that interact with the cerebellum. Gait is wide-based, erratic, and reeling. Upper- and lower-limb movements are uncoordinated. Abnormal postural sway during quiet stance is present with eyes open and closed. Damage to the midline cerebellum or fastigial nucleus produces a predominantly truncal disturbance, as in the rostral vermis degeneration of chronic alcoholism. Unilateral hemispheric lesions produce ipsilateral ataxia and falling toward the lesion.
    b. **Sensory disturbances** produce a variety of gait disturbances, depending on the magnitudes, locations, and chronicities of peripheral and central sensory dysfunction. Parietal and occipital sensory loss produces a cautious gait, and hemispatial neglect causes patients to veer toward the damaged parietal lobe. A cautious pattern of walking is also observed in patients with peripheral visual, vestibular, and somatosensory deficits, particularly when they are chronic. Deficits in two or three of these sen-

sory modalities produce marked postural instability, particularly in older people and in people with coexistent CNS disease.

c. **Sensory ataxia** is exhibited by patients with large-fiber sensory polyneuropathies or posterior spinal column disease, with or without spinocerebellar tract damage. Sensory ataxia consists of wide-based, irregular steps and postural dysequilibrium. Patients compensate for their loss of proprioception by watching their feet while walking. Postural sway is modest during quiet stance but increases markedly with eyes closed (Romberg's sign; loss of proprioception). Similarly, gait is more impaired in the dark. Sensory ataxia and steppage gait frequently coexist in patients with large-fiber sensorimotor polyneuropathy and in patients with degenerative diseases that affect both the spinal cord and peripheral nerves (e.g., tabes dorsalis, vitamin B_{12} deficiency, Friedreich's ataxia, and hereditary dysmyelinating diseases). Diseases affecting the dorsal and lateral columns of the spinal cord typically produce a gait with features of spasticity and sensory ataxia.

13. **Antalgic gait** occurs as a result of pain. Stance and gait are modified so as to reduce pain. Restricted (guarded) lower-extremity and pelvic rotations occur in locations dictated by the origin of pain. Limping is common.

14. **Hysterical gait.** Psychiatric gait disturbances are bizarre in appearance, and individual variation with time is typical. Patients frequently lean, lurch, and gyrate in a manner that requires good balance and coordination. Distracting the patient's attention tends to reduce these factitious abnormalities. For example, gait improves and stability increases when finger-to-nose testing is executed while the patient attempts to walk or stand. Gait may also improve when patients walk on their heels or toes. Tandem gait may initially seem impossible, but this task is frequently accomplished when attention is distracted with simultaneous performance of finger-to-nose testing or a difficult cognitive task (e.g., reciting the months of the year backwards), or both. Be careful when making this diagnosis. Dystonic gaits, choreatic gaits, and the gait disturbances produced by multiple lesions of multiple sclerosis can be so bizarre that an erroneous diagnosis of psychiatric disease is made.

IV. **Evaluation**

A. **History** is critical in determining a specific etiology and in identifying coexistent illnesses that might adversely affect the patient's performance (e.g., cardiopulmonary disease, arthritis, glaucoma, macular degeneration, and painful feet).

1. **Functional disability** is partly determined by taking a careful history. The frequency and circumstances of falls and the ability to perform various activities of daily living (dressing, bathing, climbing stairs, and getting in and out of bed and chairs) are important measures of disability.

2. **Associated symptoms** such as rest tremor (Parkinson's disease), oscillopsia and vertigo (vestibular or labyrinthine disease), urinary incontinence (frontal lobe lesions or hydrocephalus), dementia, numb clumsy hands (high cervical cord lesion causing loss of fine touch, vibration, and proprioception), speech and swallowing impairment (supraspinal pathology), and muscle wasting (peripheral neuromuscular disease) are helpful in making a diagnosis.

B. **Physical examination** is essential because abnormal patterns of gait often provide only rough indications of the locus of pathology (see Table 8-2). One must carefully search for more diagnostic or localizing neurologic signs (e.g., rest tremor and pyramidal tract signs) and general physical signs (cardiopulmonary disease, poor visual acuity, and musculoskeletal disease). The examination of gait and station is performed with the intent of localizing the lesion and establishing the degree of disability (Table 8-3). Bedside measurements of gait velocity, average step length, and cadence over a 40-ft walkway correlate well with all other valid measures of ambulatory ability.

C. **Laboratory studies** are useful mainly in corroborating the diagnosis derived from history and physical examination. A good argument can be made for performing a complete blood count and thyroid, renal, and liver function studies in all patients. Radiologic studies—such as x-rays of the hips, spine, and extremities; myelograms; and computed tomography (CT) or magnetic resonance imaging (MRI) scans of the head and spine—are performed as needed. Quantitative posturography and quantitative motion analysis with computerized pho-

Table 8-3. Performance-oriented examination of locomotion.

Static Posture
Curvature of spine
Head position
Pelvic tilt
Flexion of knees and hips
Stance base

Postural Control and Balance
Romberg's test
Nudge to the chest or back
Bending over
Reaching while standing

Walking
Sitting and rising from a chair
Initiation of gait
Coordination and amplitude of upper- and lower-limb movements
Step length, width, rhythmicity, and symmetry; gait velocity
Foot-floor clearance and contact
Walking path
Turning 180 degrees
Walking on heels and toes
Tandem walking

togrammetric methods do not have an established role in the evaluation of most patients. Eye movement recordings can be helpful in identifying subtle abnormalities and in distinguishing Parkinson's disease from other parkinsonian syndromes (e.g., progressive supranuclear palsy). Quantitative vestibular testing occasionally reveals vestibular dysfunction in patients with undiagnosed dysequilibrium.

V. **Differential diagnosis** is particularly difficult for those degenerative illnesses in older people that produce a roughly symmetrical gait disturbance with short, shuffling, hesitant steps (Table 8-4).

VI. **Diagnostic approach** is one of identifying the primary cause of gait impairment and all contributing illnesses. Many contributing illnesses are easily overlooked in patients with neurologic gait disturbances. Such illnesses include vitamin B_{12} deficiency, hypothyroidism, depression, foot pathologies (e.g., flat feet, painful feet, and clubfeet), muscle deconditioning, arthritic limbs, spinal deformities, cardiopulmonary disease, sleep apnea, orthostatic hypotension, visual impairment, benign positional vertigo, and medications (e.g., sedative-hypnotics, antipsychotics, and metoclopramide). These contributing illnesses are frequently more treatable than the primary neurologic condition.

VII. **Criteria for diagnosis** are well established for most illnesses (see Table 8-1). Many diagnoses are based largely or entirely on history and physical examination. The diagnosis of idiopathic normal pressure hydrocephalus (NPH) in older people is particularly difficult. The clinical triad of gait disturbance, urinary incontinence, and cognitive dysfunction is not specific and also occurs in patients with vascular dementias, chronic subdural hematomas, and degenerative dementias. In NPH, the cognitive dysfunction is a relatively mild and late-occurring component of the triad. Radiologic evidence of hydrocephalus is necessary but does not guarantee a beneficial response to ventriculoperitoneal cerebrospinal fluid (CSF) shunting. Improvement in gait after the removal of 30–40 ml of CSF by lumbar puncture supports the diagnosis but is not observed in all patients. Unfortunately, there is still no fully reliable method for predicting the response to CSF shunting. Improvement is achieved in roughly 50% of patients, sustained improvement in 30%, and complications in 20%. Patients with identifiable causes of hydrocephalus (e.g., aqueductal stenosis, Arnold-Chiari malformation, and prior meningitis or subarachnoid hemorrhage) are more likely to respond than those with idiopathic causes.

Table 8-4. Distinguishing the neurologic etiologies of symmetrical geriatric gait disturbances.

Other clinical and paraclinical features	Binswanger's disease	NPH	PD	PSP	Cervical spondylosis
Reduced arm swing			++	+	
Festination			+		
Rest tremor			++		
Numb, clumsy hands and a Romberg's sign					++
Stepwise progression	++				
Supranuclear gaze palsies				++	
Pyramidal tract signs in lower extremities	+				+
Speech impairment	+		+	+	
Extension of the neck and torso				++	
Urinary incontinence	+	+			+
Facial masking			++	+	
Prominent response to levodopa			++		
Definite improvement after LP (30–40 ml CSF removal)		++			
Spondylotic cervical spine and cord compression					+
Hydrocephalus (>5.5 cm across frontal horns)		+			
Subcortical white matter degeneration and microinfarcts	+				

NPH = normal pressure hydrocephalus; PSP = progressive supranuclear palsy; PD = Parkinson's disease; LP = lumbar puncture; CSF = cerebrospinal fluid; += suggestive; ++= very suggestive.

VIII. Referral
   A. Neurologic consultation is recommended whenever the primary physician is uncertain about or uncomfortable with the patient's diagnosis or treatment. A second opinion is advisable before shunting a patient with presumed NPH. Drug-resistant parkinsonism is fairly strong evidence against the diagnosis of idiopathic Parkinson's disease.
   B. Physical therapy and occupational therapy should be considered in most cases. An experienced occupational therapist, physical therapist, or visiting nurse can reduce falls and enhance mobility by performing a comprehensive safety evaluation of the patient's home. Handrails, raised toilet seats, adequate lighting, and rubber floormats are often helpful. Elimination of electrical cords, clutter, and throwrugs throughout the home and repair of uneven floors and cracked sidewalks are additional considerations. Shoes with slippery soles or high heels should be avoided. Properly prescribed walking aids are frequently useful.
   C. Orthopedic and rheumatologic referrals should be considered when skeletal and foot pathologies are impediments to ambulation.

Recommended Readings

Atchison PR, et al. The syndrome of gait ignition failure: A report of six cases. *Mov Disord* 8:285–292, 1993.

Baloh RW, Honrubia V. *Clinical Neurophysiology of the Vestibular System.* Philadelphia: Davis, 1990.

Ducroquet R, Ducroquet J, Ducroquet P. *Walking and Limping: A Study of Normal and Pathological Walking.* Philadelphia: Lippincott, 1968.

Elble RJ, Higgins C, Hughes L. The syndrome of senile gait. *J Neurol* 239:71–75, 1991.

Elble RJ, et al. The initiation of normal walking. *Mov Disord* 9:139–146, 1994.

Gage JR. *Gait Analysis in Cerebral Palsy.* New York: Cambridge University, 1991.

Garcia-Rill E. The basal ganglia and the locomotor regions. *Brain Res Reviews* 11:47–63, 1986.

Inglin B, Woollacott M. Age-related changes in anticipatory postural adjustments associated with arm movements. *J Gerontol* 43:M105–M113, 1988.

Inman VT, Ralston HJ, Todd F. *Human Walking.* Baltimore: Williams & Wilkins, 1981.

Lajoie Y, Teasdale N, Fleury M. Attentional demands for static and dynamic equilibrium. *Exp Brain Res* 97:139–144, 1993.

Mori S. Integration of posture and locomotion in acute decerebrate cats and in awake, freely moving cats. *Prog Neurobiol* 28:161–195, 1987.

Nutt JG, Marsden CD, Thompson PD. Human walking and higher-level gait disorders, particularly in the elderly. *Neurology* 43:268–279, 1993.

Riley DE, Fogt N, Leigh RJ. The syndrome of "pure akinesia" and its relationship to progressive supranuclear palsy. *Neurology* 44:1025–1029, 1994.

Smidt GL. *Clinics in Rehabilitation: Gait in Rehabilitation.* New York: Churchill Livingstone, 1990.

Sudarsky L. Geriatrics: Gait disorders in the elderly. *New Engl J Med* 322:1441–1446, 1990.

Sutherland DH. *Gait Disorders in Childhood and Adolescence.* Baltimore: Williams & Wilkins, 1984.

Thompson PD, Marsden CD. Gait disorder of subcortical arteriosclerotic encephalopathy: Binswanger's disease. *Mov Disord* 2:1–8, 1987.

Tinetti M. Performance-oriented assessment of mobility problems in elderly patients. *J Am Geriatr Soc* 34:119–126, 1986.

Vanneste JAL. Three decades of normal pressure hydrocephalus: Are we wiser now? *J Neurol Neurosurg Psychiatry* 57:1021–1025, 1994.

Yakovlev PI. Paraplegia in flexion of cerebral origin. *J Neuropath Exp Neurol* 13: 267–296, 1954.

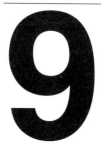

Approach to the Patient with Sleep Disorders

Mark Eric Dyken
Thoru Yamada

Sleep disorders are very common and may lead to, exacerbate, or result from various neurologic diseases. The foundation of an accurate clinical diagnosis is the history. Physicians often fail to ask the basic questions concerning sleep that can aid in diagnosing most sleep disorders.

I. General sleep

A. History. Because most patients with sleep disorders are not fully cognizant during the times when they are exhibiting their symptoms, the history should also be elicited from a bed partner, family member, or nursing staff member. In addition, a sleep diary, following the outline of the general sleep history, can be diagnostic, especially in cases of poor sleep hygiene or irregular sleep-wake schedules. Sleep disorders usually cause insomnia (difficulty initiating or maintaining sleep), excessive sleepiness, and abnormal behaviors and movements associated with sleep. The chronicity of symptoms and any precipitating, exacerbating, and alleviating factors should be assessed.

   1. Questions. What is the sleeping environment and what are the patient's habits associated with going to bed? When is bedtime (regular or irregular)? What is the sleep latency (the amount of time it takes the patient to fall asleep after "the head hits the pillow")? What is the quality of sleep? Is it restful or restless and, if restless, why? How many arousals occur per night and for what reasons? What is the patient's final awakening time? Is assistance in waking necessary? How does the patient feel on waking? How many hours of sleep does the patient estimate are necessary for refreshment? Does the subject suffer from excessive sleepiness or experience frank sleep attacks (while driving, waiting at stop lights, during conversation, during sex, or while eating)? Has this problem ever affected school or work performance or family life? Does the patient nap, and, if so, how often, how long, and how does the individual feel after the nap (refreshed, unchanged, worse)?

B. Exam. The patient examination is often normal, but in some disorders, such as obstructive sleep apnea, there are characteristic findings that may include obesity and a small oropharynx. Findings unique to specific disorders will be discussed in the appropriate sections to follow.

II. Diagnostic procedures

A. Polysomnography (PSG) is a combination of electroencephalography (EEG), electromyography (EMG), electro-oculography, a variety of other physiologic measures (heart rate, respiratory effort, airflow, etc.), and video monitoring. The PSG allows differentiation of five sleep stages (NREM stages 1 through 4 and REM sleep), which can be associated with specific disorders (Table 9-1).

B. Mean sleep latency testing (MSLT) allows detection of sleepiness that results from frequent arousals and microarousals associated with many sleep disorders. It is a cornerstone for the diagnosis of narcolepsy. The MSLT is a series of five 20-minute attempts at napping (during the patient's normal waking hours), which are separated by approximately 2-hour intervals. A mean sleep latency (the average time it takes the patient to fall asleep after the beginning of each individual nap period) of less than 5 minutes indicates pathologic sleepiness, a "diagnostic gray area" exists between 5 and 10 minutes, and a latency greater than 10 minutes is considered normal.

C. Other tests. A variety of medical and psychological disorders can produce insomnia and sleepiness. Routine laboratory studies may be needed to rule out anemia, hypoxemia, infection, and metabolic and endocrinologic abnormali-

Table 9-1. Classic PSG findings associated with specific sleep disorders.

Disorder	PSG
General insomnia	Increased sleep latency
	Frequent arousals
	Reduced sleep efficiency
Insomnia in endogenous depression	Reduced REM latency
	Increased rapid eye movements in the 1st REM period
SIRI	Apneas/hypopneas
	Obstructive
	Central
	Mixed
	Hypoventilation
	±Snoring
	±Cardiac arrhythmias
PLMD/RLS	PLMs often predominating in stage 2 NREM
RMD	HB, BR, LB from drowsiness/early NREM
RBD	Violent behavior from REM
	Elevated muscle tone in REM
	PLMs and nonperiodic movements in REM/NREM
NPD	Dystonia from REM/NREM
ST/SW	ST/SW from stage 3/4 NREM
CRD	
ASPS	Early BT, early AT
DSPS	Late BT, late AT
ISWP	Irregular sleep periods
Narcolepsy	Short SL/short RL
	MSLT with EDS, with REM on 2 or more naps
Epilepsy	Increase in interictal discharge
	±Clinical seizure
Cluster HA and PH	Headaches from REM
Fibromyositis	"Alpha-delta" sleep
	±PLMs

These are classic PSG findings that may not necessarily be captured during an isolated study or observed in every patient. MSLT may or may not show evidence of EDS.
PSG = polysomnogram; SIRI = sleep-induced respiratory impairment; PLMD = periodic limb movement disorder; RLS = restless legs syndrome; RMD = rhythmic movement disorder; HB = head banging; BR = body rocking; LB = leg banging; RBD = REM behavior disorder; PLMs = periodic limb movements; NPD = nocturnal paroxysmal dystonia; ST = sleep terrors; SW = sleepwalking; CRD = circadian rhythm disorder; ASPS = advanced sleep phase syndrome; DSPS = delayed sleep phase syndrome; ISWP = irregular sleep-wake pattern; BT = bedtime; AT = awakening time; SL = sleep latency; RL = REM latency; MSLT = mean sleep latency test; EDS = excessive daytime sleepiness; HA = headache; PH = paroxysmal hemicrania.

ties. A Minnesota Multiphasic Personality Inventory (MMPI), with an interview by a neuropsychologist or psychiatrist familiar with sleep disorders, may be helpful in cases where an affective disorder is suspected.

III. **Differential diagnosis.** Sleep disorders can result from, or be associated with, a multitude of environmental, medical, and psychophysiologic factors. Often they simply result from poor sleep hygiene practices, but on occasion they may exist without an obvious etiology (idiopathic insomnia) or as subjective complaints, with no objective evidence of a sleep disturbance (sleep state misperception or malingering).

IV. **Types of sleep disorders.** This discussion will use terminologies and outlines adapted from *The International Classification of Sleep Disorders* (ICSD): *Diagnostic and Coding Manual.*

  A. **Insomnia resulting from psychological concomitants.** Insomnia, the most common sleep problem, is only a symptom of many specific disorders. Difficulties with sleep are experienced by as much as 49% of the adult population in the United States, of which up to 75% result from specific problems with psychological associates, such as the intrinsic sleep disorder psychophysiologic insomnia, and from medical/psychiatric sleep disorders, which include depression, anxiety, and alcoholism.

1. **History.** Up to 15% of patients with sleep complaints have aspects of psychophysiologic insomnia. These patients have a tendency to respond to stress with somatized tension, which can occur in conjunction with learned sleep-preventing associations. Individuals generally are overconcerned with their insomnia and deny psychological concomitants. Paradoxically, their sleep problems become worse as they try harder to sleep, and improve when they do not try to sleep. Often they sleep much better in situations that differ from the routine sleep environment to which their somatized tension has been negatively conditioned, such as in the sleep laboratory.

   Because chronic insomnia can lead to depression, anxiety, and/or alcohol dependence, it is important to distinguish these secondary problems from primary disorders. In primary disorders, there is usually a history of major recurrent problems of mood, anxiety, or alcohol or drug abuse.

2. **PSG.** Insomnia in general is associated with an increased sleep latency and an increase in wakefulness after sleep onset, with a subsequent overall decrease in sleep efficiency. On occasion, a patient with psychophysiologic insomnia will report a much better night of sleep in the sleep laboratory setting than in the normal sleep environment. Patients with depression often have early onset of the first REM sleep period with an increased frequency of rapid eye movements, whereas patients with secondary depression generally have normal first REM period latencies of approximately 90 minutes. Chronic alcoholism can cause a reduction in slow wave sleep, which may improve only gradually after years of abstinence.

3. **MSLT.** If sleep disruption is significant, pathologic sleepiness can occur, although in patients with anxiety disorders there may be a normal or even increased sleep latency.

4. **Other tests.** Psychological testing with the MMPI and the Beck depression and anxiety inventories may show repression, denial, somatization, depression, or anxiety. In patients with histories of alcohol abuse, liver function tests may be of value.

B. **Sleep-induced respiratory impairments** are disorders that tend to occur more frequently in men and generally worsen with obesity and increasing age. Sleep-related breathing abnormalities are defined polysomnographically as apneas ("obstructive, central, or mixed"), "hypopneas," and hypoventilation.

   1. **General sleep-induced respiratory impairment assessment**

      a. **History.** Patients often complain of sleepiness and report short sleep latencies, restless or unrefreshing sleep, and extreme sleepiness or fatigue on awakening. Excessive sleepiness may be reported as memory loss, slow mentation, and amnestic periods associated with automatic behavior. Although insomnia often is not the major complaint, patients may report arousals associated with shortness of breath, choking, diaphoresis, palpitations, chest pains, and headaches. The bed partner and family members may complain of loud snoring, gasping respirations, and apneic episodes. Sleep-related breathing disorders have been associated with chronic systemic hypertension, pulmonary hypertension, congestive heart failure, and stroke.

      b. **PSG.** Respiratory events are often worse during REM sleep as a result of upper-airway hypotonia. Severity is determined by the number of abnormal respiratory events, the degree of oxygen desaturation associated with these events, and the patient's level of sleepiness determined with the MSLT.

      Apneas and hypopneas are associated with absent or markedly reduced airflow and oxygen desaturation. Apneas and hypopneas are further classified as obstructive, central, or mixed. Obstructions are associated with persistent respiratory effort, whereas during central events respiratory effort is absent. A mixed apnea has an initial central component, which is followed by an obstruction.

      Although there is considerable controversy concerning what constitutes polysomnographic significance in regard to sleep-induced respiratory impairment, the following standards are often used to rate disorder severity, using the apnea/hypopnea (A/H) index (the average number of abnormal respiratory events per hour) and the lowest value of oxygen saturation ($SatO_2$) during an event. An A/H index of 0–10 is considered relatively insignificant, 10–20 mild, 20–50 moderate, and greater than 50 severe. An $SatO_2$ of 90% or greater is considered normal, 80 to less than 90% mildly significant, 70–80% moderately severe, and less than 70% (or any event that appears to induce a significant cardiac arrhythmia) severe.

c. **MSLT.** The MSLT should be performed 1½ to 3 hours after the completion of the PSG. An MSLT should not be performed as an isolated test without the PSG. Disrupted sleep continuity associated with any sleep disorder can produce significant sleepiness, which can be life-threatening in many situations, such as when driving.

d. **Other tests.** In general, an ABG and a CBC with differential, liver, renal, and thyroid function tests screen for many concomitant medical disorders that may induce or exacerbate sleep-induced respiratory abnormalities and sleepiness.

2. **Obstructive sleep apnea (OSA) syndrome** is often seen in middle-aged, overweight men who snore and report excessive sleepiness. Women are less commonly affected. This disorder is associated with adenotonsillar hypertrophy, acromegaly, myxedema, micrognathia, kyphoscoliosis, hypertension, and pulmonary, cardiac, or neurologic disease.

a. **History.** The bed partner often reports heroic snoring, which may be exacerbated by fatigue, alcohol, weight gain, and supine sleeping position. Snoring severity may force the individual to sleep alone and may persist even when sitting up. OSA and snoring are associated with a compromised oropharynx.

b. **Exam.** The blood pressure, body mass index (BMI), and neck circumference should be documented. Oro- and nasopharyngeal patency should be assessed with a search for enlarged tonsils or adenoids, nasal-septal deviation, enlarged turbinates, temporomandibular joint abnormalities, retro- or micrognathia, large tongue, or general fatty infiltration of soft tissues in the upper airways.

c. **PSG.** During obstructive apneic events, profound surges in blood pressure and tachybradyarrhythmias can occur. Mixed apneas and hypopneas are frequently observed and in general have the same significance as classic obstructive apneas. Central apneas may also be appreciated, and in such cases the diagnosis is dependent on which phenomena (obstructions or central events) are most prevalent.

d. **Differential diagnosis.** Loud snoring may exist as a problem independent of OSA, and has been associated with the "upper airway resistance syndrome," where partial airway obstruction may lead to frequent nocturnal arousals and hypersomnolence. One should also consider primary disorders of excessive sleepiness such as narcolepsy.

e. **Other tests.** Because OSA has been associated with multiple medical problems, an interdisciplinary approach, with appropriate referrals, is often necessary. Cephalometric evaluations of the upper airway, pulmonary function tests, and extensive cardiovascular/cerebrovascular assessments may be appropriate.

3. **Central sleep apnea (CSA) syndrome.** Injury to brainstem medullary respiratory centers ("Ondine's curse") and congestive heart failure (CHF), with or without a Cheyne-Stokes respiratory pattern, can be associated with central sleep apnea. In most cases, a specific anatomic lesion cannot be discerned.

a. **History and exam.** Patients often present with sleep maintenance ("middle") insomnia. One should carefully assess for brainstem injury and CHF.

b. **PSG.** Care must be taken not to overinterpret physiologic central apneas, which normally occur with sleep stage transitions and during the phasic eye movements of REM sleep. These phenomena are not associated with significant oxygen desaturations.

c. **Differential diagnosis.** Metabolic disorders, such as renal failure, may be associated with a Cheyne-Stokes respiratory pattern. Alcohol and other CNS depressants can cause or exacerbate CSA.

d. **Other tests.** A magnetic resonance imaging (MRI) study of the brain and brainstem, chest radiogram, EKG, cardiac enzyme studies, and drug screens may be helpful.

4. **Hypoventilation syndrome.** Acquired hypoventilation can be caused by obesity ("pickwickian syndrome") and diseases affecting the lungs and res-

piratory musculature. In the absence of a primary cause, this disorder is believed to be the result of intrinsic dysfunction of medullary respiratory centers, and is referred to as the central alveolar hypoventilation syndrome.

- **a. History.** Idiopathic hypoventilation appears in early adulthood and causes insomnia and sleepiness. Other forms of hypoventilation can occur at any age in association with brainstem and cervical spine injury, anterior horn cell disease, poliomyelitis, dysautonomias, muscular dystrophies, and diseases affecting the thorax and diaphragm.
- **b. Exam.** The BMI test, oral and nasopharynx tests, and signs of cardiac and cerebrovascular disease should be addressed.
- **c. PSG.** Hypoventilation appears as prolonged periods of reduced respiratory effort associated with sustained reductions in oxygen saturation. Hypoventilatory episodes may on occasion be difficult to differentiate from central apneas.
- **d. Other tests.** Generally, pulmonary function tests are normal, but there may be reduced respiratory responses to hypoxemia and hypercarbia during wakefulness or sleep. In cases of secondary hypoventilation, an MRI of the brain and brainstem, and EMG and nerve conduction velocity (NCV) studies, may be helpful.

C. Movement disorders
  1. **Periodic limb movement disorder (PLMD) and restless legs syndrome (RLS).** PLMD and RLS often occur concomitantly. Periodic limb movements, often inappropriately referred to as "nocturnal myoclonus," are sleep-related movements, affecting primarily the lower extremities, which can lead to insomnia and daytime sleepiness. Patients with RLS complain of dysesthesias and an uncontrollable need to move the legs that occurs on lying down to sleep or after sitting for prolonged periods. Although frequently observed in otherwise normal middle-aged and elderly adults, PLMD and RLS are associated with pregnancy, iron deficiency anemia, uremia, tricyclic antidepressant use or drug withdrawal, and a variety of CNS disorders. PLMD can be familial and has no gender predominance.
  - **a. History.** It is essential that the bed partner be questioned, because the patient may be unaware of these movements. These movements increase with age and generally are not appreciated in patients under 30 years of age. With RLS, patients classically report minutes to hours of lower-extremity discomfort that is associated with rest, substantially improves with leg movement, and returns with rest.
  - **b. Exam.** The physical and neurologic examinations are usually normal.
  - **c. PSG.** Periodic limb movements appear as elevated EMG activity from the tibialis anterior muscle, which persists for 0.5–5.0 seconds and coincides with episodes of repetitive, stereotypic extension of the large toe with ankle, knee, and hip flexion. Consecutive movements, with inter-movement intervals of 4–90 seconds, arise primarily from stage 2, NREM sleep. The number of periodic limb movements per hour (the PLM index) is used to quantify severity: five or more movements per hour but less than 25 is considered mild; 25 or more but less than 50 is moderate; and 50 or more is severe. When PLMs are followed by an arousal, a PLM-arousal index of five or more movements per hour is significant, and more than 25 is considered severe.
  - **d. Differential diagnosis.** Nonperiodic myoclonic movements associated with epilepsy and many neurodegenerative disorders should be considered. RLS-like complaints may be associated with muscle overuse syndromes, nocturnal leg cramps, peripheral neuropathic dysesthesias, and rheumatologic pain disorders.
  - **e. Other tests.** Routine laboratory analyses should include a CBC, iron and folate studies, a serum glucose, and renal function tests. Drug screens, a rheumatoid factor, and possibly a pregnancy test may be considered. If a neurologic lesion is suspected, an MRI of the brain and brainstem, or EMGs and NCVs, may be helpful.
  2. **Rhythmic movement disorder (RMD).** RMDs are parasomnias that primarily affect children. These are sleep-related, stereotypic, repetitive movements of the head, neck, or large muscle groups, often associated with rhythmic vocalizations, that include head banging (jactatio capitis nocturna), body rocking, and leg banging.

   a. History. Rhythmic body movements often begin in normal children between 8 and 18 months of age, and rarely lead to injury. These movements generally resolve by 5 years, although persistence may be associated with stress, stimulus deprivation, or CNS lesions. Head banging is more common in boys. Both head banging and body rocking may occur in families. Family members generally complain of the noise, and sometimes violent nature, associated with these behaviors. Repeated, rhythmic striking of the head generally occurs in the supine position, whereas body rocking is associated with anteroposterior whole-body movements and can occur in many positions.
   b. PSG. Because RMDs may not occur nightly, several consecutive study nights, using infrared-video analysis, are often scheduled. Rhythmic movements generally occur with a frequency of 0.5–2 Hz during drowsiness and light sleep and may last from 15 minutes to 4 hours.
   c. Differential diagnosis. Seizures, night terrors, sleepwalking, and self-abusive and other psychogenic behaviors should be considered.
   d. Other tests. A baseline EEG (awake and sleeping) should be considered to rule out seizure. If the disorder is persistent, neuropsychiatric assessment may be appropriate.
3. **REM sleep behavior disorder (RBD).** This disorder is associated with violent behaviors during sleep that reflect dream enactment. Events begin during REM ("dreaming" or "paralyzed") sleep and are followed, after arousal, by reports of dream imagery that are compatible with the actions observed during the spell.
   a. History. This disorder generally appears, although not exclusively, in elderly men, often with neurologic disease, with histories of potentially harmful sleep-related body movements associated with dreaming. Patients frequently report sleep-related injuries, which include bruises, lacerations, dislocations, fractures, and subdural hemorrhages.
   b. PSG. Because major episodes may occur only once every 2–3 weeks, several consecutive study nights may be scheduled. During REM sleep, the muscle tone is generally elevated and a variety of nonviolent movements, such as PLMs, can occur in REM and NREM sleep. Behaviors, appearing as dream enactment, may be appreciated during REM sleep.
   c. Differential diagnosis. Violent behaviors associated with dreams have been reported in association with the post-traumatic stress disorder and sleep apnea, whereas elevated muscle tone in REM sleep may be observed with narcolepsy, drug use, and neurodegenerative diseases. Excessive movements during sleep have been associated with some psychiatric disorders (dissociative states and nocturnal panic attacks).
   d. Other tests. RBD appears to result from dysfunction of the brainstem generators responsible for the atonia that is normally associated with REM sleep. This permits movement (dream enactment) during REM sleep, a state otherwise associated with essential paralysis. Although anatomic injury may not be appreciated with imaging studies, an MRI of the brain/brainstem may be helpful in some cases. MSLT, drug screening, and/or neurocognitive and psychiatric testing may be considered for specific patients.
4. **Nocturnal paroxysmal dystonia (NPD).** NPD exists within a spectrum of disorders that includes paroxysmal arousals and episodic nocturnal wanderings. The clinical characteristics, interictal EEG findings, and response to anticonvulsants suggest that NPD may actually be a complex-partial seizure disorder originating from the fronto-orbital or mesial-temporal area, but much controversy continues to surround the true nature of this phenomena, because the EEG is generally normal during a typical spell.
   a. History. NPD has an onset that ranges from infancy to late middle age and shows no gender preference. It is generally not considered a familial disorder. Episodes may persist for more than 20 years and have been associated with reports of daytime and nocturnal seizures. "Short-lasting" spells of NPD generally last 1 minute and can occur up to 20 times nightly. The spells begin during sleep with several seconds of stereotypic dystonic, choreoathetotic, or opisthotonic posturing of the head, trunk, and extremities, which is often followed by semipurposeful, repetitive, violent movements. Patients may appear awake, although not necessar-

ily fully conscious. After the spell the patient is coherent and often goes back to sleep immediately. The episodes may be associated with partial amnesia, are not linked with dreamlike imagery, and are not associated with tongue biting or bowel and bladder incontinence.

b. Exam. The physical and neurologic examinations are generally normal.

c. PSG. Onsets of spells have been reported during stage 2 NREM sleep (occasionally following K-complexes, which are phenomena often associated with arousal), in stage 3 and 4 NREM sleep, and during transitions to REM sleep. The event persists during apparent arousal with a normal waking EEG pattern (although electroencephalographic evidence of epileptiform activity followed by generalized tonic-clonic activity has been reported).

d. MSLT. Because frequent NPD can cause significant sleep interruption, daytime sleepiness may be documented.

e. Differential diagnosis. NPD may mimic sleep terrors, nightmares, somnambulism, RMD, or RBD, and at times may suggest a conversion disorder or malingering. Atypical reports include a long-lasting form of NPD, which is associated with 2–50 minutes of dystonic or dyskinetic (choreoathetoid, ballistic) movements (one individual with this form of NPD developed familial Huntington's disease 20 years after disease onset) and patients with characteristic movements precipitated during wakefulness.

f. Other tests. Brain imaging studies and interictal EEGs are generally normal, although on occasion the interictal, sleep-deprived EEG may show focal slowing, paroxysmal bursts of theta activity, and generalized and focal epileptic discharges from the temporal lobes. Positron emission tomography (PET) scans have demonstrated frontal and temporal hypometabolism.

5. **Sleep terrors (pavor nocturnus in children, pavor incubus in adults) and sleepwalking (somnambulism).** These phenomena are closely related parasomnias that can occur in a familial pattern, are observed primarily in children, and begin in slow wave (stage 3 and 4 NREM) sleep. These spells are associated with a general lack of responsiveness to the environment, with automatic actions, confusion, disorientation, and occasional injuries. After these events, from which the patient is generally unarousable, there is usually amnesia without dream recall. These disorders generally resolve by puberty, but when diagnosed in adults they may be associated with psychopathology.

a. History. Sleep terrors tend to occur more often in boys, with an onset between 4 and 12 years and resolution by puberty. During the spell, the patient often appears glassy-eyed and frightened, with tachycardia, tachypnea, diaphoresis, and inconsolable screaming and crying that may last from a few seconds to 20 minutes. Sleepwalking generally occurs at 4–8 years of age, often after sleep terrors have resolved. Patients ambulate in a confused manner and are subject to injury.

b. Exam. The physical and neurologic exams are generally normal. Assess for evidence of infection, fever, or drug use, any of which can exacerbate these parasomnias.

c. PSG. Because these spells may not occur nightly, several consecutive nights of video-PSG should be considered. Classically, an event follows a sudden arousal from stage 3 and 4 NREM sleep, in the first third of the night. Partial arousals from stage 3 and 4 sleep are not uncommon. Often a spell cannot be captured and the diagnosis is based primarily on the history.

d. MSLT. One may be able to document sleepiness, because sleep deprivation can precipitate or exacerbate these disorders.

e. Differential diagnosis. The differential diagnosis includes nightmares, seizures, RMD, RBD, psychogenic disorders, and malingering. Confusional arousals (arousals from sleep not associated with fear, walking, or hallucinations) must also be considered.

f. Other tests. When the disorder is persistent, is associated with injury, or affects an adult, an MMPI and neuropsychological assessment may be important. A baseline EEG (awake and asleep) may be necessary to evaluate for seizures.

D. Circadian rhythm disorders (disorders of the timing of the sleep-wake pattern). These disorders occur when there are incongruencies between the sleep-wake schedule demanded by society and the intrinsic sleep-wake pattern of the patient (determined in large part by the circadian pacemaker—the suprachiasmatic nuclei of the anterior hypothalamus). When not extrinsic or self-imposed ("jet lag" or shift work), these problems are believed to result from abnormal intrinsic physiologic responses to environmental time cues ("Zeitgebers") such as sunlight (which exerts its effects through retinal-hypothalamic pathways). Subsequently the patient's state of sleepiness or arousal is out of synchrony with that of the general population, resulting in alternating complaints of sleepiness and insomnia when the patient tries to follow a normal schedule.

1. **History.** In many cases, the diagnosis can be made using a sleep log. By accurately documenting, for a period of 1–2 months, all bedtimes, final awakening times, and all nap times, a sleep log can help differentiate a circadian rhythm disorder from poor sleep hygiene. The log should be filled out during a vacation or "free" time so as to avoid societal constraints that prevent the patient from following his or her intrinsic sleep-wake pattern.

2. **PSG.** The PSG should corroborate the sleep log reports.

3. **MSLT.** In general, if patients are allowed to follow their intrinsic sleep-wake rhythm, there should be no evidence of sleepiness during normal waking hours.

4. **Differential diagnosis.** Poor sleep hygiene, drug use, affective problems, and a variety of disorders that may be distinguished using PSG and MSLT must be considered.

5. **Other tests.** Some sleep disorders centers can monitor hormonal rhythms (such as those of cortisol and melatonin) and 24-hour body temperature fluctuations, which can lose normal circadian fluctuations and amplitudes in circadian sleep pathologies. Referral to such centers may be necessary.

6. **Other syndromes**
   a. **Advanced sleep-phase syndrome.** When free to follow their desired sleep-wake schedules, these individuals go to sleep very early in relation to the setting of the sun, arise very early in relation to sunrise, and do not complain of excessive sleepiness during their "normal" waking hours. This tendency increases with age, and is generally addressed only if it significantly impairs the quality of the patient's work, social, or family life.
      (1) **Sleep log.** The sleep log reveals a consistently early bedtime and early final awakening time with normal sleep continuity and total sleep time. Patients do not report excessive sleepiness unless they attempt to follow societal schedules.
      (2) **PSG/MSLT.** In the ICSD it is suggested that the patient history can be confirmed by performing consecutive sleep studies. All PSGs should show early evening sleep onsets, with normal sleep latencies and sleep architectures, and early morning final awakenings. MSLT should not reveal excessive sleepiness.
   b. **Delayed sleep-phase syndrome.** This disorder is observed primarily in adolescents. Patients complain of chronically late bedtimes with late final awakening times.
      (1) **Sleep log.** The sleep log confirms that the patient's complaints are associated with normal sleep continuity and normal total sleep times. These patients do not complain of sleepiness unless they attempt to follow the normal societal sleep-wake schedule.
      (2) **PSG.** When the patient is allowed to follow his or her "normal" sleep pattern, the PSG reveals a very late sleep onset and a late final awakening. The sleep latency is usually greater than 30 minutes (this subsequently leads to a relatively low sleep efficiency). Sleep continuity and architecture are otherwise normal.
   c. **Non-24-hour sleep-wake syndrome (hypernyctohemeral syndrome).** These patients have an inability to synchronize ("entrain") the physiologic desire for a sleep-wake schedule that is greater than 24 hours with a normal 24-hour day. Subsequently these patients continually "phase delay," and on a day-to-day basis show a progressive 1–2-hour delay of their bedtimes and final awakening times. When they attempt to

keep regular sleep-wake schedules (with fixed bedtimes and final awakening times), they experience recurrent periods without sleep complaints (when their intrinsic schedules match society's), which are then followed by the gradual onset of periods associated with sleep onset insomnia, difficulty waking in the morning, and daytime sleepiness (when their intrinsic schedules are out of synchrony with society's).

    (1) History. Often these patients are blind (from a variety of etiologies, including tumors of the optic chiasm). The disorder has been reported in association with mental retardation and schizophrenia, and only rarely in the normal population.

    (2) Sleep log. The sleep log reveals a day-to-day delay in bedtimes and final awakening times.

    (3) Other tests. Imaging studies of the brain may be considered, because this disorder has been associated with suprasellar lesions.

  d. Irregular sleep-wake pattern. In this disorder there is no definitive sleep-wake rhythm. Subsequently, patients suffer from intermittent nocturnal insomnia and variable periods of daytime sleepiness, which generally result in three or more irregularly timed naps during a 24-hour period. The total sleep time during a 24-hour period is normal, but the timing of sleep is not predictable.

    (1) History/exam. This disorder is common in patients with significant congenital, developmental, and degenerative brain disorders.

    (2) PSG. A prolonged, continuous PSG for 24–72 hours shows irregular periods of sleep that vary from day to day. In patients with significant brain injury, the presence of diffuse, slow wave activity with a loss of normal sleep architecture is not unusual.

    (3) Other tests. Imaging studies of the brain should be considered.

E. Sleep disorders associated with the central nervous system

  1. Narcolepsy is generally considered a disorder of excessive sleepiness. Although some investigators believe a history of pathologic sleepiness and cataplexy is sufficient for diagnosis, narcolepsy may involve the classic full clinical tetrad of excessive sleepiness, cataplexy, sleep paralysis, and hypnagogic hallucinations.

    a. History. The onset generally begins during puberty or young adulthood, with symptoms of excessive sleepiness and sleep attacks. Sleep attacks may occur while driving, during active conversation, or while eating. Brief 10–20-minute naps may refresh the patient for hours. Once the sleepiness complaints stabilize, they generally do not progress, whereas the other symptoms associated with narcolepsy may come and go. Cataplexy, often precipitated by strong emotion, involves attacks that range from brief sensations of weakness to essential paralysis. The spells are transient and do not produce cognitive impairment. Hypnagogic (at sleep onset) and hypnopompic (on awakening) hallucinations are generally frightening visual, auditory, or movement perceptions that essentially represent dreaming while awake. Sleep paralysis occurs during the transition from sleep to waking (or waking to sleep). The patient may experience brief paralysis (seconds to minutes) with the inability to speak. Other symptoms of narcolepsy can include insomnia, poor memory, depression, and automatic behaviors.

    b. PSG. Normally, REM sleep begins approximately 90 minutes after sleep onset. The REM latency in narcoleptics may be less than 20 minutes. In addition, a short sleep latency and a reduced sleep efficiency may be appreciated.

    c. MSLT should show evidence of excessive sleepiness with two or more REM onset sleep periods, although a variety of factors, including a noisy testing environment (hospitals in general), can produce false-negative results. For a 2-week period prior to the sleep studies, the patient should keep a diary, documenting good sleep hygiene and the avoidance of centrally active drugs. Both sleep deprivation and drug withdrawal can be associated with REM rebound, which may mimic narcolepsy electrophysiologically.

    d. Genetic testing. The major histocompatibility complex (MHC) contains genetic markers for narcolepsy, the strongest being human leukocyte antigen (HLA) DR2. The presence of such markers correlates strongly with narcolepsy, but these markers have been associated with false-positive and false-negative results.

e. Differential diagnosis. Many sleep disorders can disrupt sleep continuity and produce sleepiness and an MSLT suggesting narcolepsy. A thorough sleep history and an accurate sleep log, along with PSG and MSLT, generally prevent misdiagnosis in such cases. In addition, cataplectic-like events can occur in conjunction with sleep drunkenness, complex partial seizures, fugue states, and transient global amnesia.

Idiopathic (CNS) hypersomnolence can be differentiated from narcolepsy by means of history and sleep studies. This is a lifelong disorder, beginning during adolescence or young adulthood, that is associated with continual sleepiness without cataplexy. Naps are long and unrefreshing, and drowsiness generally precedes sleep attacks. PSG reveals a normal sleep, whereas MSLT confirms sleepiness. However, REM onset sleep is not recorded by MSLT.

The history usually distinguishes narcolepsy from disorders of recurrent hypersomnolence such as the Kleine-Levin syndrome, which primarily affects adolescent boys. These patients suffer two to 12 sleep attacks per year, lasting hours to days, that have been associated with hyperphagia and sexual inappropriateness.

2. Sleep-related epilepsy. In epileptics, focal interictal discharges and secondarily generalized tonic-clonic seizures during NREM sleep are not unusual. Sudden death during sleep is rarely observed, but it has occurred in association with poor seizure control and nontherapeutic anticonvulsant levels. Seizure disorders associated with sleep (although not necessarily occurring exclusively in sleep) include juvenile myoclonic epilepsy (with seizures often occurring shortly after awakening), electrical status epilepticus of sleep (primarily an EEG phenomenon that occurs during sleep and that is otherwise not associated with clinical seizures), and the Landau-Kleffner syndrome (an acquired epileptic aphasia associated with mental deterioration).

a. Diagnosis. Nocturnal seizures often can be diagnosed using the history and the baseline waking-sleeping EEG. If necessary, several consecutive nights of extended PSG/EEG monitoring may be helpful.

b. Differential diagnosis. Other sleep disorders associated with sleep-related movements, such as OSA, PLMD, RMD, RBD, and NPD, should be considered.

3. Sleep-related pain

a. Headaches. Sleep studies often can lead to the diagnosis of, and assist in differentiating, primary sleep-related headaches (associated with specific sleep stages) and secondary sleep-related headaches that occur as a result of intrinsic sleep pathologies such as OSA and epilepsy. Headaches that can be exacerbated by lying down or by sleep include those associated with cerebral edema, intracranial hypertension, and obstructive hydrocephalus, and often present with a "crescendo time profile" (generally over a period lasting up to 3 months). The most frequent type of morning headache is associated with the "hangover" that results from alcohol use and whose differential diagnosis includes headaches associated with systemic hypertension, depression, sinus inflammation, and sleep apnea. Postictal headaches associated with seizures may occur anytime throughout sleep, whereas headaches reported to occur just before sleep onset may represent the "exploding-head syndrome" (a disorder associated with a sudden sensation of an explosion going off in the head).

(1) Cluster headaches. Patients usually also experience daytime headaches (from one every other day to eight per day), although as much as 75% of the headaches may occur during REM sleep.

(a) History. These headaches afflict men far more frequently than they do women, and tend to occur during periodic "clusters" lasting from 7 days to 1 year (generally 2 weeks to 3 months) and separated by at least 14 pain-free days. Patients wake with severe, unilateral eye and facial pain, often associated with tearing, conjunctival vasodilation, rhinorrhea, nausea, vomiting, and occasionally a Horner's syndrome. Episodes may last 15 to 180 minutes and can occur several times per night.

(b) PSG. Typical headaches, associated with arousals from REM sleep, may be captured during extended PSG monitoring.

(2) Paroxysmal hemicrania ("REM sleep-locked headache"). These headaches occur primarily in adult women and, like cluster headaches, are unilateral and associated with REM sleep, but they generally are briefer and occur more frequently than cluster headaches. These headaches can last from 2 to 45 minutes (usually 5 to 20 minutes) and occur day or night during waking or sleep, as many as 30 times during a 24-hour period. Therapeutically they respond with an absolute effectiveness to indomethacin.

b. Fibrositis syndrome (fibromyalgia, fibromyositis) is a chronic disorder of diffuse musculoskeletal pain, which is often worse at night and can lead to insomnia and sleepiness.

(1) History. This disorder, when it first appears, generally affects young adults, women more than men, often following a febrile illness. Symptomatically these individuals report diffuse myalgias and arthralgias, which may be exacerbated by climatologic changes and minimal trauma. The chronicity of the disorder can lead to psychological concomitants.

(2) Exam. Diffuse tenderness, most prominent in the neck and shoulder musculature, can be appreciated with deep palpation. Specific areas to assess include the medial borders of the trapezius and scapula, the sternal border of the pectoralis major and the second costochondral junction, the cervical and lumbar erector spinae and intervertebral ligaments, the middle aspect and upper outer quadrant of the gluteus maximus, the anterior superior iliac spine, the lateral portions of the elbows, and the medial aspects of the knees.

(3) PSG may show "alpha-delta" sleep patterns, in which alpha EEG activity (the normal 8–12-Hz occipital activity observed in waking patients when their eyes are closed) appears in the slow waves of stage 3 and 4 NREM, or "delta," sleep. Occasionally, periodic limb movements may be appreciated.

(4) Differential diagnosis includes myopathies, polymyalgia rheumatica, arthritis, chronic fatigue syndrome, and primary affective disorders.

(5) Other tests. Laboratory tests for inflammation, infection, and rheumatologic disorders, and radiographic studies, should be normal. Associated affective disorders may require neuropsychological evaluations.

4. Dysfunction of specific neurologic systems. In general, injury and trauma to the CNS can lead to sleep-related problems through diffuse effects that often involve the hypothalamus and brainstem.

a. Large hemispheric strokes are associated with sleepiness and insomnia, which may be attributable to an inversion of the sleep-wake rhythm. The loss of sleep spindles and normal stage 2 NREM sleep architecture are associated with a poor prognosis.

b. Diencephalic lesions involving the anterior hypothalamus, and injuries to the preoptic area and the amygdala, as reported in conjunction with some encephalitides, can result in insomnia. Lesions of the posterior hypothalamus can cause hypersomnia. Symptomatic narcolepsy/cataplexy can occur in association with several diseases involving the hypothalamic–upper brainstem area and the third ventricle, including craniopharyngiomas, gliomas, sarcoidosis, colloid cysts, pituitary adenomas, and mesencephalic gliomas.

c. Brainstem lesions involving the mesencephalon and the rostral-central tegmentum (as in the "top of the basilar syndrome") can produce sleepiness (possibly as a result of reticular activating system injury), gaze palsies, hallucinations, and unreactive, dilated pupils. Pontine lesions, often with involvement of the median raphe, resulting from vascular (medial tegmental pontine stroke), inflammatory (poliomyelitis), and degenerative (spinocerebellar degeneration) diseases, can produce indeterminate sleep patterns, with a paucity of normal sleep architecture, and insomnia. RBD has been reported with dorsopontomesencephalic lacunar infarctions. Damage to tegmentoreticular tracts are hypothesized to produce disconnection of peri–locus caeruleus centers (generators of muscular atonia) from the medullary inhibitory center of Magoun and Rhines.

Bulbar poliomyelitis, lower brainstem stroke, spinal (high cervical) surgery, syringobulbia, encephalitides, striatonigral degeneration, Creutzfeldt-Jakob disease, and olivopontocerebellar degeneration are associated with CSA. Apneas can present as "Ondine's curse," where no spontaneous respirations occur during sleep, necessitating continuous ventilatory support. The Arnold-Chiari malformation can be associated with central and obstructive respiratory phenomena. Associated cranial nerve dysfunction may reduce the oropharyngeal opening as a result of jaw and tongue instability, phrenic nerve dysfunction, and atrophy of accessory respiratory muscles.

d. **Degenerative disorders,** including Parkinson's disease, the Shy-Drager syndrome, progressive supranuclear palsy, olivopontocerebellar and spinocerebellar degeneration, fatal familial insomnia, Huntington's chorea, dyssynergia cerebellaris myoclonica of Ramsay Hunt, and many dementias, have been associated with a variety of sleep disorders including insomnia, indeterminate sleep, daytime sleepiness, nocturnal myoclonus, sleep apnea, and RBD. In some cases, sleep disorders may be related to psychological concomitants or medications. Dopaminergic agents may improve sleep disturbances in some patients, but in others may have an alerting effect, enhancing hallucinations and exacerbating nightmares.

e. **Myopathies** may predispose patients to sleep-related respiratory disorders by reducing tidal volumes during REM sleep. Myasthenia gravis can lead to mixed, obstructive, and central apneas in REM sleep. Myotonic dystrophy (possibly attributable to dorsomedial thalamic dysfunction) has been associated with hypersomnia, although craniofacial characteristics and impaired upper-airway and inspiratory muscle function may contribute to OSA, CSA, sleep-related alveolar hypoventilation, and sleepiness.

f. **Acquired autonomic neuropathies,** such as those associated with diabetes, may lead to irregular breathing patterns, a decrease in tidal volume in NREM sleep, and hypoventilation and apneas in REM sleep.

V. **When to refer to a sleep disorders center.** Sleep disorders are very common, and general practitioners see many patients with sleep-related complaints. Accurate clinical diagnoses can often be made if a full sleep history is routinely incorporated into the general examination. On occasion, successful treatment of many sleep problems can be achieved by correcting poor sleep hygiene practices and/or addressing the primary social, psychological, and medical concomitants when they exist. When sleep problems persist, significantly impair the patient's quality of life, or require formal sleep studies for diagnosis or therapy (as in narcolepsy and sleep apnea), referral to a reputable sleep disorders center should be considered.

Recommended Readings

General

Carskadon MA, et al. Guidelines for the multiple sleep latency test (MSLT): A standard measure of sleepiness. *Sleep* 9:519–524, 1986.

Culebras A. The neurology of sleep. *Neurology* 42(suppl 6), 1992.

Kryger MH, Roth T, Dement WC. *Principles and Practice of Sleep Medicine* (2nd ed). Philadelphia: Saunders, 1994.

Rechtschaffen A, Kales A. A manual of standardized terminology, techniques and scoring system for sleep stages of human subjects. *Natl Inst Health* 204, 1986.

Thorpy MJ and the Diagnostic Classification Steering Committee. *The International Classification of Sleep Disorders: Diagnostic and Coding Manual.* Rochester, MN: American Sleep Disorders Association, 1990. Pp 38–43.

Insomnia Resulting from Psychological Concomitants

Hauri PJ. Consulting about insomnia: A method and some preliminary data. *Sleep* 16(4):344–350, 1993.

Morin CM. *Insomnia: Psychological Assessment and Management.* New York: Guilford, 1993.

Sleep-Induced Respiratory Impairments

Deveraux MW, Keane JR, Davis RL. Automatic respiratory failure associated with infarction of the medulla: Report of two cases with pathologic study of one. *Arch Neurol* 29:46–52, 1973.

Dyken ME, Somers VK, Yamada T. Stroke, sleep apnea and autonomic instability. In K Togawa, et al. (eds), *Sleep Apnea and Rhonchopathy.* Basel: Karger, 1993. Pp 166–168.

Hung J, et al. Association of sleep apnoea with myocardial infarction in men. *Lancet* 336:261–264, 1990.

Kales A, et al. Sleep apnoea in a hypertensive population. *Lancet* 2:1005–1008, 1984.

Young T, et al. The occurrence of sleep-disordered breathing among middle-aged adults. *N Engl J Med* 328:1230–1235, 1993.

Movement Disorders

Culebras A, Moore JT. Magnetic resonance findings in REM sleep behavior disorder. *Neurology* 39:1519–1523, 1989.

Dyken ME, Rodnitzky R. Periodic, aperiodic and rhythmic motor disorders of sleep. In A. Culebras (ed), The neurology of sleep. *Neurology* 42(6):68–74, 1992.

Dyken ME, et al. Violent sleep related behavior leading to subdural hemorrhage: Polysomnographically documented REM sleep behavior disorder with split-screen electroencephalographic-video analysis. *Arch Neurol* 52:318–321, 1995.

Keefauver SP, Guilleminault C. Sleep terrors and sleepwalking. In MH Kryger, T Roth, WC Dement (eds), *Principles and Practice of Sleep Medicine* (2nd ed). Philadelphia: Saunders, 1994. Pp 567–573.

Lugaresi E, Cirignotta F. Hypnogenic paroxysmal dystonia: Epileptic seizure or a new syndrome? *Sleep* 4(2):129–138, 1981.

Mahowald MW, Schenck CH. REM sleep behavior disorder. In MH Kryger, T Roth, WC Dement (eds), *Principles and Practice of Sleep Medicine* (2nd ed). Philadelphia: Saunders, 1994. Pp 574–588.

Salva MAQ, Guilleminault C. Olivopontocerebellar degeneration, abnormal sleep, and REM sleep without atonia. *Neurology* 36:576–577, 1986.

Schenck CH, et al. A polysomnographic and clinical report on sleep-related injury in 100 adult patients. *Am J Psychiatry* 146(9):1166–1172, 1989.

Circadian Rhythm Disorders

Campbell SS, et al. Exposure to light in healthy elderly subjects and Alzheimer's patients. *Physiol and Behavior* 42:141–144, 1988.

Rosenthal NE, et al. Phase-shifting effects of bright morning light as treatment for delayed sleep phase syndrome. *Sleep* 13(4):354–361, 1990.

Sleep Disorders Associated with the Central Nervous System

Dyken ME, et al. Narcolepsy: Unequivocal diagnosis after split-screen, video-polysomnographic analysis of a prolonged cataplectic attack. *Neurology* 44:760–761, 1994.

Moscovitch A, Partinen M, Guilleminault C. The positive diagnosis of narcolepsy and narcolepsy's borderland. *Neurology* 43:55–60, 1993.

Mouret J. Differences in sleep in patients with Parkinson's disease. *Electroencephalogr Clin Neurophysiol* 38:653–657, 1975.

Niedermeyer E. Epileptic seizure disorders. In E Niedermeyer, F Lopes da Silva (eds), *Electro-Encephalography: Basic Principles, Clinical Applications and Related Fields* (2nd ed). Urban and Schwarzenberg, 1987. Pp 405–510.

Olesen J and Headache Classification Committee of the International Headache Society. Classification and diagnostic criteria for headache disorders, cranial neuralgias, and facial pain. *Cephalgia* 8:1–96, 1988.

Plum F, Posner JB. *The Diagnosis of Stupor and Coma* (3rd ed). Philadelphia: Davis Company, 1980.

Yasuhara A, et al. Epilepsy with continuous spike-waves during slow sleep and its treatment. *Epilepsia* 32:59–62, 1991.

10

Approach to the Patient with Visual Loss

James J. Corbett

When **visual loss** is a patient's primary complaint, symptoms vary depending on whether one or both eyes are affected; whether the visual loss is abrupt in onset, gradual in onset, or suddenly discovered long after its onset; whether the visual loss is complete or partial; and, finally, whether the visual loss is manifested as visual hallucinations or illusions. The probable causes of visual loss are narrowed down to a very few possibilities on the basis of the patient's symptoms, the patient's age and sex, and the presumed anatomic location of the lesion (Table 10-1).

Patients with primary visual complaints usually seek the attention of an ophthalmologist or optometrist. Referral to a neurologist commonly occurs with a CT or MRI already in hand. If the problem appears to be a tumor, the patient more often will be referred directly to a neurosurgeon. The pattern of referral and the tests done before referral further reduce the number of probable diagnostic options.

The visual pathway consists of elements easily examined directly at the bedside, such as the pupils, the retina, and the optic disk, and those that are indirectly examined using subjective tests, such as the more posterior elements of the optic nerve, chiasm, optic tract, lateral geniculate, geniculocalcarine tract, and visual cortex. Damage to visual association cortices, parietal and inferior temporal, will produce symptoms with preservation of visual acuity and sometimes normal visual fields.

I. **Bedside or office clinical examination of the visual system**
   A. **Visual acuity.** Although it is best to examine visual acuity using a distance chart, the neurologist almost always examines visual acuity using a near card. This should be done with a hand-held Snellen chart or a Jaeger print card. If a near card is being used, be sure that patients are using their reading glasses. Push patients to give you the very best acuity possible. Do not rush them. Do not start with the largest type; rather, ask patients to read the 20/25 line and then the 20/20 line. If this fails, gradually work your way up. Three fingers held up are the equivalent of the big E on the distance acuity chart, and a patient who can count fingers at 20 feet has 20/200 acuity. Thus, counting fingers at 5 feet would be equivalent to 20/800 acuity. Visual acuity should be normal in a pure homonymous hemianopia or pure bitemporal hemianopia. Acquired visual acuity deficits that are not attributable to refractive error imply a central scotoma.
   B. **Confrontation visual fields** should be done at a distance of 1 m from the patient. Have the patient cover one eye with the palm of the hand and look at your nose. Present your fingers (one, two, or five) rapidly in each quadrant. Slowness to respond in one quadrant or hemifield may be the earliest sign of a homonymous visual field defect. After rapid finger counting, present your hands, palms forward, first in the two upper quadrants and then in the two lower quadrants. Ask the patient to compare the palms for brightness and clarity. Finally, place one finger on your nose and one at a distance of ½ m from your nose, in the nasal, temporal, superior, and inferior fields, and ask which of the two fingers is brightest and clearest. This tests for a central scotoma. Holding one of your hands above and one below the horizontal meridian and having the patient compare the two for brightness and clarity helps identify the altitudinal defects that accompany retinal and disk diseases.
   C. **Color vision testing.** A book of Ishihara's color plates can be used one eye at a time to test color acuity. Although these plates were designed for testing red-green color blindness, this test can be used as a rough indicator of color acuity, which is a macular function. Test one eye at a time, and use this test especially when looking for evidence of optic nerve damage.

Table 10-1. Etiology of visual loss by anatomical location.

Retina[a]	Optic disk[b]	Optic nerve[c]	Chiasm/tract[d]	Retrochiasmal[e]
Detachment	Ischemic optic	Demyelination	Tumor	Tumor
Ischemia	neuropathy	Tumor	Pituitary	Glioma
(embolic)	Arteritic	Meningioma	Glioma	Meningioma
Infections	Nonarteritic	Glioma	Cranio-	Metastasis
CMV	Optic neuritis	Sarcoid	pharyn-	Stroke
Histoplas-	(papillitis)	Mucocele	gioma	Demyelination
mosis	Papilledema	Pituitary	Mucocele	Alzheimer's
Toxoplas-	Glaucoma	tumor	(sphenoid)	disease
mosis	Pits/colobomas	Cranio-	Meningioma	Creutzfeldt-
Toxic	Tumors	pharyn-	Rathke's cleft	Jakob disease
Phenothia-	Sarcoid	gioma	cyst	(Heidenhain)
zine	Degenerative	Rathke's cleft	Aneurysm	
Ethambutol	Carcinoma-	cyst	Trauma	
Degenerative	associated	Aneurysm	Demyelination	
Aging	optic	Thyroid	Vascular	
macular	neuropathy	ophthalmop-	Toxic	
degenera-		athy		
tion		Inflammation		
Retinitis		Trauma		
pigmentosa		(indirect		
Carcinoma-		traumatic		
associated		optic		
retinopathy		neuropathy)		

[a]Appearance of fundus or disk and mode of presentation are key. Visual fields helpful.
[b]Appearance of fundus or disk and mode of presentation are key. Visual fields helpful.
[c]Optic nerve function, appearance of disk, proptosis, and appearance of disk and retinal nerve fiber layer are key. Visual fields helpful.
[d]Visual function—acuity, fields, fundus exam, and visual complaints—are key.
[e]Associated general neurologic findings, visual fields, and CT or MRI findings are key.

   D. **Pupil tests.** The single most useful objective bedside test of visual function is the pupillary light response test. When there is damage to the ganglion cells or their axons in one eye, optic disk, or optic nerve, there will be a less vigorous (less complete) response to a light shone in that eye than to a light shone in the unaffected or normal eye. Damage to both eyes will show a defect in the eye with the greatest amount of visual field loss. There is no describable entity such as bilateral afferent pupil defect. Swinging the light from eye to eye will elicit a brisker reaction (a more complete response) to light in the unaffected eye and a less brisk reaction or dilation of the pupil in the affected eye. This is the relative afferent pupillary defect (RAPD). If one eye is blind, the reaction to light will be gone completely—this is an amaurotic pupil. For the details of the examination of the pupil for RAPD, refer to Chap. 11.
   E. **Ophthalmoscopy.** The fundus examination is, of course, key in establishing the appearance of the optic disk—pallor, swelling, or anomalous appearance—and the appearance of the retina and macula. In chronically choked optic disks, the venous drainage is frequently diverted into collaterals known as optociliary collateral vessels, which drain the venous blood out through the vortex veins into the orbit rather than into the cavernous sinus.
   F. **Visual evoked potentials.** This test tends to be overused, but it can be valuable for two types of patients: (1) the patient with a past history suggestive of optic neuritis and exhibiting minimal or no residual signs, who frequently has an abnormally prolonged latency; and (2) the patient who is functionally blind, provided the patient is attentive. Uncooperative subjects with functional visual loss can focus past the visual evoked potential (VEP) screen, defocus or look around the screen, and alter VEP latencies (implicit times). Thus, a normal latency in this setting is useful, but an abnormal latency may be a red herring.
   G. **Formal visual field testing** consists of three types of tests.
      1. The **tangent screen exam** is carried out on a flat black screen located 1 m from the patient. It is especially helpful in that it allows the examiner to

back the patient up to 2 or 3 m and use the tangent screen to look for tunnel vision or to magnify small central visual defects. This type of visual field is useful only for the inner 20 to 30 degrees of vision. This is the most common type of formal field testing done in a neurologist's office, but today it is uncommon to see a neurologist who actually carries out such studies.

   2. **Kinetic perimetry** is carried out on a Goldmann perimeter using suprathreshold kinetic targets and is done in an ophthalmologist's office. This form of perimetry is being supplanted by the static or Humphrey perimeter (see item 3).

   3. The **static (Humphrey) perimeter** tests threshold static targets. This test is also done in an ophthalmologist's office.

II. Acute transient monocular visual loss (TMVL)

   A. Clinical features. Acute TMVL is relatively common and comes in a host of different forms (Table 10-2). First, before concluding that the patient has had a monocular event, explore the possibility that the "monocular" event was really binocular—i.e., a homonymous hemianopia. Patients with homonymous visual defects complain that half of objects are gone or that they cannot see well to one side. They may insist that when they close one eye and then the other, the visual loss is only unilateral, but frequently they are simply seeing what they think they should be seeing. Also, monocular visual loss is occasionally reported as being sudden in onset when in reality it was suddenly and unexpectedly discovered when the normal eye was covered and the patient could not see well out of the affected eye. The most common important cause of true monocular visual loss is artery-to-artery or cardiac-to-artery embolism, but there are *many* causes of transient or permanent acute visual loss (see Table 10-2).

   B. Approach to TMVL

   1. Be sure historically that the spells are in one eye and not homonymous.

   2. Look for evidence of optic disk anomaly, swelling, or residues of retinal embolism (hemorrhages, soft exudates, embolic plugs of cholesterol, platelets, fibrin, or calcium).

   3. Look for RAPD, visual field loss, and loss of visual acuity.

   4. Look for proptosis (sign of intraorbital mass lesion) causing intermittent amaurosis as a result of vascular compression by eye movement.

   5. Auscultate the heart and carotid arteries for murmurs and bruits.

   6. Laboratory studies should include:

   a. CBC, including platelets

   b. Sedimentation rate

   c. C-reactive protein

   d. In young patients under age 40, strongly consider evaluation for hypercoagulable states:

   (1) Protein C

   (2) Protein S

   (3) Antithrombin III

   (4) PT and PTT

   (5) Lupus anticoagulant

   (6) Anticardiolipin antibodies

   (7) Fibrinogen

   7. Perform transthoracic and transesophageal echocardiograms, looking especially at the aortic arch and at the atrial septum for evidence of patent foramen ovale, atrial septal defect, atrial septal aneurysm (>1.0 cm), and atrial myxoma.

   8. Perform carotid doppler and transcranial doppler.

   9. Consider cerebral angiography.

   It should be remembered that emboli from the carotid arteries are only one cause of TMVL and that there may be more than one convincing potential cause of TMVL. It is always valuable to refer the patient with visual loss as a primary problem for examination by an ophthalmologist, who can measure intraocular pressure, perform a dilated indirect ophthalmoscopic examination, perform formal visual fields, and obtain fundus photos. Most patients seen by neurologists have already been seen by an ophthalmologist or optometrist if the primary complaint is visual.

III. Subacute monocular visual loss may occur in two age groups: 15 to 45, where it is usually painful, especially with eye movement; and over 50, where it is usually stepwise and painless.

   A. Clinical syndromes

   1. **Optic neuritis** occurs in younger patients with monocular painful visual

Table 10-2. Sources of transient monocular visual loss (TMVL).

Intraocular
Recurrent hyphema (intraocular lens haptics)
Glaucoma*
Papilledema*
Disk drusen*
Congenital cavitary disk anomalies*
Anterior ischemic optic neuropathy
  Arteritic
  Nonarteritic
Choroidal insufficiency (ocular ischemia)

Intraorbital (intermittent vascular compression)
Hemangioma
Osteoma
Meningioma

Intracranial
Arteriovenous malformations
Brain tumors

Embolic to retina (central or branch retinal artery occlusion)
Intracranial aneurysm
Cardiac
  Valvular debris:
    Subacute bacterial endocarditis
    Rheumatic valvular disease
    Bicuspid aortic valve
    Mitral valve prolapse
  Clot
    Atrial fibrillation
    Ventricular subendocardial ischemia
    Akinetic segment
    Ventricular aneurysm
    Right-to-left shunt
      Patent foramen ovale
      Atrial septal defect
      Atrial septal aneurysm
    Atrial myxoma
Aortic atherosclerosis
Carotid disease
  Dissection
  Atherosclerosis
  Fibromuscular dysplasia
Fat embolism
  Pancreatitis
  Fractures

Hematologic
Polycythemia
Sickle cell disease
Thrombocytosis

Hypotension

Demyelinating disease
Uhthoff's phenomenon

Vasospasm
Hypertensive crises, especially in paraplegic or quadriplegic patients
Migraine

*These causes of TMVL usually last seconds and are known as transient visual obscurations, or TVOs. They are frequently binocular as well as monocular.

loss. Visual loss may follow the pain by a matter of days. Pain is worse with eye movement. The visual loss is characterized as a "skim, scum, blur, fog, or haze" or may be described as if there were a cloud in front of the eye. Vision may be characterized as dim, dark, or bright.

Colors are dim, washed out, or gone entirely, and low-contrast images are lost. One-third of patients have swollen optic disks. Occasionally, patients complain of photopsias (spots and sparkles) with loud noise. Visual acuity may range from 20/20 to no light perception, but 20/50 to 20/200 is the rule. The visual field loss is monocular and usually central and/or altitudinal. Prognosis for visual return is excellent within weeks.

2. **Anterior Ischemic Optic Neuropathy (AION).** The older patient with monocular subacute, occasionally stepwise visual loss that is painless is suffering from ischemia to the optic disk known as **anterior ischemic optic neuropathy (AION).** This condition has two forms.

   a. **Nonarteritic AION (NAION).** The nonarteritic form of AION is believed to be in large part related to ischemia predisposed by an anatomically small scleral canal through which all of the axons of the optic nerve pass on their way to the chiasm and beyond. This small scleral canal causes the disk to be small, tightly packed, and a set-up for an ischemic cascade that may be abrupt and cataclysmic or gradual and stepwise. NAION is painless and usually produces inferior altitudinal, inferior nasal quadrantic, or central scotomatous visual field defects. In 40% of patients the second eye is affected within 2 years.

   b. **Arteritic AION.** The major difference between NAION and the arteritic form of AION is age. Arteritic AION is attributable to giant cell arteritis and is usually a disease of the elderly. The added features with suspected giant cell arteritis include headache, and superimposed antecedent brief amaurotic attacks resulting from choroidal ischemia especially affecting the optic disk. Other symptoms include tenderness of scalp, jaw claudication, aching pains in the shoulders and hips, weight loss, fever, and night sweats. Arteritic AION causes sudden severe visual loss and is a diagnostic emergency. Visual acuity is 20/200 or less, and the visual field shows an altitudinal defect with a large central scotoma. There is a relative afferent pupillary defect (RAPD), or in some cases an amaurotic (blind and unreactive) pupil. In addition to erythrocyte sedimentation rate and C-reactive protein tests, a temporal artery biopsy should be performed. As with NAION, the disk is swollen, but it is usually very pallid with a few small splinter hemorrhages. Prognosis for visual return is poor. Risk of second eye involvement, if left untreated, is very high.

   c. **Leber's optic neuropathy** is a syndrome of painless monocular visual loss over days, characteristically observed in men in the teens to 20s (male-female ratio of 8:1). It is a disorder of mitochondrial DNA. The second eye is involved weeks to months after the first eye. The disk is slightly swollen and exhibits tortuous small telangiectasia vessels. After a few weeks, the nerve fiber layer becomes atrophic. This occurs first between the 7 and 11 o'clock positions in the right eye and between the 1 and 5 o'clock positions in the left eye. Later, both disks become diffusely pale. Visual loss ranges from acuity of 20/80 to 20/800 and central scotomas that may extend (break out) into the periphery of the visual field. The diagnosis is confirmed by examination of mitochondrial DNA appropriate mutations.

B. **Approach to permanent or long-lasting monocular visual loss**

   1. Try to determine historically the pace of visual loss. Was it suddenly discovered by accident? Was there gradual and progressive visual dysfunction in that eye, or did the visual loss occur abruptly and the vision remain poor?
   2. Look for evidence of optic disk swelling or pallor and for evidence of embolic material in the retina.
   3. Look for RAPD, do confrontation visual fields, and document visual acuity.
   4. Decide whether or not this visual loss appears to have resulted from vascular embolic disease, in which case proceed as if the patient has TMVL—i.e., look for an embolic source.
   5. If the visual loss appears to be attributable to optic neuritis (pain on eye movement, and subacute visual loss over a few days), proceed to do MRI and lumbar puncture tests.

6. If it appears that the visual loss was actually more gradual in onset or has been present longer than recognized and there is evidence of optic disk pallor, do CT and MRI scans, looking for a compressive lesion from orbital apex to optic chiasm.

IV. **The syndrome of chronic progressive monocular visual loss** is characteristic of optic nerve compression. Visual acuity may well be normal early, but patients will notice that something is not quite right. They will complain of blurs or smudges and may repeatedly clean their glasses or have their refractions checked, resulting in one of the "handful of glasses" syndromes (Table 10-3). Visual loss is usually painless. If the optic nerve is being compressed by a mass in the orbit, there may be proptosis, limitation of ocular motility, and chemosis. If the optic nerve compression is in the optic canal or is intracranial, proptosis will occur only late.

Severe loss of visual acuity may occur rapidly, and visual field testing reveals a central scotoma that may "break out" (extend) into the periphery. Color vision is defective, and there is an RAPD (Marcus Gunn pupil) in the affected eye. Optic disk swelling, pallor and atrophy, or a mixture of pallor and swelling is common. Optociliary collateral shunt vessels appear on the disk and are evidence of chronic optic nerve compression occurring at the level of the disk with chronic papilledema, of end-stage glaucoma, or, most importantly, of retrobulbar strangulation of the optic nerve by meningioma, glioma, or sarcoidosis.

VEP in the early stages of optic nerve compression with normal or near-normal acuity reveals a prolonged latency. After visual acuity has dropped, latency becomes strikingly prolonged and the amplitude drops. Consultation with an ophthalmologist is appropriate to rule out other treatable ocular causes of visual loss and to obtain formal visual fields, and, when appropriate, photos of the optic disks.

V. **Binocular visual loss that is abrupt in onset** (Table 10-4) is rarely caused by bilateral optic disk disease such as ischemic optic neuropathy or optic neuritis. However, when this occurs the typical patient announces that the vision in both eyes has acutely or subacutely been lost and, on examination, one optic disk is pale and atrophic and the other is swollen. This **"Foster Kennedy syndrome"** is classically attributed to a frontal tumor causing monocular visual loss and optic atrophy in one eye and papilledema in the other eye. However, the most common cause of this ophthalmoscopic combination of atrophy/pallor and disk swelling is the **pseudo–Foster Kennedy syndrome** of bilateral sequential anterior ischemic optic neuropathy in a patient who failed to notice visual loss in the first eye. The loss of vision in the only properly seeing eye suddenly plunges the patient into unexpected bilateral visual loss.

Transient visual obscuration (TVO) observed in patients with papilledema, drusen of the disk, and other conditions (see Table 10-2) will cause transient bouts of binocular dimming or blindness precipitated by Valsalva's maneuvers or postural changes. Examination of the fundus should identify any of the congenitally anomalous or swollen disks.

Longer-lasting binocular visual disturbances of rather rapid onset occasionally afflict migraineurs who have basilar migraine. This is a historical diagnosis, and lab examination is helpful only in ruling out other conditions.

Binocular visual loss abrupt in onset occurs on rare occasions following radiographic procedures. The use of metrizamide for myelography or for intracranial positive contrast studies may occasionally result in bilateral blindness from a toxic-metabolic cause (cortical hypoglycemia). Posterior fossa angiography and coronary angiography are also occasionally attended by what appears to be a toxic reaction to contrast associated with vasospasm.

VI. **Binocular visual loss as a result of chiasmal damage** is observed in the pure form, in which there is no damage to optic nerves or optic tracts.

Table 10-3. "Handful of glasses" syndromes.

Early optic nerve compression
Bitemporal hemianopia with hemifield slide
Alexia without agraphia
Bilateral small occipital tip lesions
Eye-movement-induced myopia with convergence-retraction nystagmus

Table 10-4. Causes of bilateral visual loss (excluding occipital lobe).

Ocular causes
Anomalous disks*
Papilledema*
Disk drusen*
Pseudo–Foster Kennedy syndrome (bilateral anterior ischemic optic neuropathy)
Toxic
   Nutritional (tobacco-alcohol amblyopia)
   Medications: ethambutol, chloramphenicol, plaquenil, thioridazine
   Leber's optic neuropathy

Intracranial causes
Chiasmal
Tumor (craniopharyngioma, Rathke's cleft cyst, pituitary tumor, meningioma, and other rarer
   tumors)
Aneurysm
Sphenoid mucocele
Trauma (chiasmal tear)
Pituitary apoplexy
Demyelination
Vascular (dolichoectatic anterior cerebral artery)

Combined chiasmal and optic nerve disease caused by any of the above will result in
   combinations of bitemporal and central visual loss.

Optic tract
Tumor—same as chiasm
Demyelination
Trauma

*These causes result in transient visual obscurations, which may be bilateral.

A. Clinical features

1. **Bitemporal visual loss.** If the lesion is coming from below (typically a pituitary adenoma), the visual loss is superior bitemporal. If the compression is from above (typically an aneurysm of the anterior cerebral artery or a craniopharyngioma), the visual field defect is inferior bitemporal. Complete, macula-splitting, bitemporal defects are usually attributable to tumors or traumatic chiasmal tears.

   The visual complaints of patients with bitemporal visual loss are *not* losses of peripheral vision but rather symptoms caused by instability of the two nasal visual fields abutting the midline. These symptoms consist of intermittent and brief doubling of objects, loss of objects, and strange visual effects as a result of vertical sliding of the two hemifields, causing the right halves of images to slip vertically in relation to the left halves. These symptoms are known collectively as the "hemifield slide phenomena" and are another cause of the "handful of glasses" syndrome (see Table 10-3). Because patients with visual symptoms see eye doctors first, and rarely articulate the nature of the visual dysfunction adequately, they are commonly provided with new refractions.

2. **Junctional syndrome.** If the chiasmal compression is far anterior, one optic nerve may be compressed at the junction with the chiasm. This produces symptomatic optic nerve compression (see sec. **IV**) and asymptomatic superior temporal quadrantic visual loss in the other eye. This is caused by damage to a loop of fibers from the inferior nasal part of the contralateral eye that loops into the optic nerve at its junction with the chiasm (Wilbrand's knee). Thus a visual field combination of central loss in one eye and a superior temporal defect in the other eye is known as a **junctional syndrome.**

3. **Pituitary apoplexy.** Abrupt onset of unilateral or bilateral visual loss, usually with ocular motility disturbances resulting from pareses of cranial nerves III, IV, and VI and associated with headache, agitation, fever, stiff neck, and blood in the CSF, occurs with hemorrhage into a pituitary tumor either spontaneously or from emboli following carotid endarterectomy or

cardiac surgery. Diagnosis must be suspected and will be confirmed with MRI or CT scan, but patient agitation frequently makes these studies less than optimal for interpretation. Although pituitary apoplexy rarely causes purely visual loss, and usually involves some ocular motility disturbance, it should be high on the list of causes of sudden onset of bilateral visual loss.

4. **Combination of central and bitemporal visual loss.** Both optic nerves may be gradually compressed by large lesions that also compress the chiasm. This causes both central visual loss and a bitemporal visual field defect. Unless the bitemporal field loss is complete, it is rare for the amount of field loss to be the same in both eyes. Thus the eye with the greatest visual field loss will have an RAPD.

B. **Clinical approach to binocular visual loss that is subacute or chronic**

1. Look for symptoms in the patient's history that are consistent with hemifield slide and determine which eye seemed to be more affected.
2. Do confrontation visual fields to look for bitemporal and central visual field losses. Do visual acuity testing to look for evidence of optic nerve disease. Perform ophthalmoscopy to look for evidence of optic disk swelling or pallor.
3. Perform a CT or MRI scan to look especially at the suprasellar space, the pituitary fossa, and the sphenoid sinus.
4. Fundus findings in chiasmal compression depend on the nature of the lesion and whether or not there is an associated increase in intracranial pressure. Papilledema is rarely observed with pituitary adenomas unless the tumor has caused hydrocephalus, and even then optic atrophy may preclude disk swelling. For reasons that are not clear, disk swelling is fairly common in patients with craniopharyngiomas, as is severe optic atrophy.

VII. **Bilateral visual loss resulting from homonymous hemianopia** can be caused by lesions in the optic tract, geniculate nucleus, geniculocalcarine tract, or occipital cortex.

A. **Localization of lesions.** If the hemianopia is complete and splits fixation and there are no other symptoms or signs, the lesion is in either the optic tract or the occipital cortex. Lesions between the optic tract and visual cortex rarely produce complete hemianopia without creating other problems such as hemiparesis, hemisensory loss, aphasia, or neglect. Most hemianopias are incomplete, and their location, density, and congruity (superimposability of one field on the other) help to tell where in the neuraxis the lesion is located. With CT and MRI, however, these lesions are rarely a mystery, and homonymous and visual field defects caused by tumors, strokes, and arteriovenous malformations (AVMs) are easily accounted for with these techniques. Occipital lobe damage produces pure visual loss if damage is confined to the calcarine cortex. Total loss of calcarine cortex on one side produces a complete homonymous hemianopia, which is rare. More commonly, the macular area is "spared" to some extent because so much of the visual cortex subserves the inner 20 degrees of vision. Conversely, small infarcts in the cortex that represents the inner 20 degrees of the visual field may cause small but very disturbing visual field loss that may not be discovered on Goldmann or Humphrey perimetry and is best identified using a tangent screen. These patients complain bitterly of visual loss that cannot be corrected with glasses (see Table 10-3) and frequently go from one eye doctor to another without having the occipital lobe damage discovered.

B. **Migraine auras.** Far and away the most common cause of repeated homonymous visual loss is the visual aura (a visual hallucination) of migraine. This is frequently mistaken for visual loss in one eye. The characteristic features of this visual event are movement and "buildup" of the visual loss usually beginning in the center and moving over minutes to the periphery of the visual field. The hallucinations consist of zigzag lines—silvery, colored, bright white, and black—that pulsate, turn, swirl, or glimmer. Although most patients characterize this as a "circle" or "horseshoe" shape to one side, some patients describe a visual image that is central in both eyes "as if a flashbulb just went off" or an arc of shimmering, flashing zigzags in both the right and left fields "like a rainbow." The next most common description is a "heat wave" sensation or the image of water running down a window. These visual events usually last from 5 to 45 minutes and are followed by a headache. The headache is usually unilateral but may be generalized and need not be severe or long-lasting. Some patients have only the visual aura and no headache—the so-called acephalgic migraine.

C. **Visual seizures.** Metastatic brain tumors, primary gliomas, and AVMs may cause primary visual seizures with no secondary generalization. These seizures produce sparkles, flashes, and colors, but, unlike migraine, there is no characteristic "buildup" and progression of the visual event from center to periphery. CT and MRI scans rapidly identify these conditions, and EEG shows epileptiform activity.

   D. Degenerative diseases. The common causes of homonymous hemianopsia either are benign and leave no trace (migraine) or produce lesions in the brain that can be detected by CT or MRI (stroke or tumor). Creutzfeldt-Jakob disease may present with homonymous hemianopia (the so-called Heidenhain variety), and focal Alzheimer's disease may also present with homonymous hemianopia. Neither of these conditions shows any specific CT or MRI findings. Progressive multifocal leukoencephalopathy, a condition much more common in immune-compromised patients, often presents with dense homonymous hemianopia and large demyelinating plaques detected by MRI in the white matter, which characteristically spares the U-fibers and the cortex.

VIII. Syndromes of visual disturbances resulting from higher cognitive dysfunction, although sometimes caused by tumors, primary or metastatic, are mostly attributable to strokes and are particularly common after cardiac surgical procedures. They frequently go unrecognized.

   A. Alexia without agraphia. This syndrome is caused by damage to the connections between the primary visual cortices and the angular gyrus resulting either from a lesion in the left splenial outflow and the connections of the left occipital lobe to the angular gyrus or from a combination of a left occipital infarct and a callosal splenium lesion. Patients frequently appear with a history of many visits to eye doctors for new glasses because of their inability to read.

   B. Balint's syndrome, which is caused by bilateral damage to the watershed between the middle and posterior cerebral circulation, consists of visual disorientation, spasm of fixation (apraxia of gaze), optic ataxia or ataxia of visually guided hand movements, and simultanagnosia (loss of panoramic vision). Patients do not deny their visual troubles but usually suffer in silence unable to verbalize satisfactorily what is wrong. They are not agitated and are not aphasic or demented.

   C. Bilateral inferior temporal lobe syndrome. Damage to the inferior temporal lobe bilaterally in the region of area V4 of the fusiform gyrus causes one or both of the following syndromes: **prosopagnosia** (the inability to recognize faces) and **central achromatopsia** (central color vision loss).

      1. Prosopagnosia presents with either sudden bilateral visual disturbance or a previously damaged inferior temporal lobe (which may or may not have been recognized) and then a second lesion in the other inferior temporal lobe. Occasionally, patients have only one lesion, usually in the left hemisphere. They complain of being unable to recognize faces, but they also have trouble picking out their own cars from other cars and their own dogs from other dogs. In short, although they can identify classes of objects, they have trouble singling out specific items from the general class or group without other clues. Distinguishing features of a person's voice or the way a person walks become the cues to identifying people. These patients commonly complain that colors are washed out and that whites (linens, snow) look dirty or brownish. They may have homonymous superior quadrantic visual field disturbances or may have no visual field loss.

      2. Central achromatopsia. Patients with central achromatopsia may also have prosopagnosia or a unilateral defect in color vision known as central hemiachromatopsia. Color loss may be profound or it may consist simply of the desaturation and dirtying of color complained of by patients with prosopagnosia.

   D. Anton's syndrome consists of visual loss produced by bilateral damage to the occipital and parietal lobes and the denial of blindness. Patients confabulate elaborately in response to questions about their visual environments.

   E. Approach to patients with homonymous visual field defects:
      1. Obtain best corrected visual acuity.
      2. Confrontation visual fields will tell you the completeness and the location of the visual field defect.
      3. Fundus examination will confirm that no significant disease of the retina or disk is responsible for the visual loss.
      4. Perform a CT scan or preferably an MRI scan.

    5. Refer the patient to an ophthalmologist for visual fields.
    6. Perform neuropsychological evaluation of patients with higher cortical defects.

IX. Functional visual loss. Patients with functional visual loss can claim either total or partial loss in one or both eyes. Whatever the motivation or underlying problem, it is possible to uncover functional monocular visual loss simply by looking for a relative afferent pupillary defect (RAPD). In the absence of an RAPD, severe (or even moderate), neurologically significant visual loss does not occur. Patients with functional binocular blindness can be uncovered in one of two ways. Use of an optokinetic target (tape or drum) is usually sufficient, but some patients are able to "look through" these targets. A foolproof method that can be used to test for one "blind" eye or bilateral "blindness" is the use of a mirror held in front of the patient's face and tilted up, down, and from side to side. This maneuver produces an irresistible sensation of environmental movement, and the patient's eyes move in an orienting response. Such eye movement proves that the patient can see at least partially.

The most difficult problem is that of the patient who presents with moderate functional visual loss that is equal in both eyes (e.g., 20/50 OU). An RAPD is of no help, and the acuity is too good to make the mirror or optokinetic target (OKN) useful. In this setting and in the setting of other functional visual loss, a referral to an ophthalmologist to ensure that there is no underlying serious ocular pathology is in order. Remember that it is possible for patients to alter the VEP latency and wave form voluntarily, and thus an abnormal VEP is not helpful. A normal VEP *is* helpful, however. Accurate color identification suggests that the central vision is better than the patient claims. Before pronouncing a patient's visual loss functional, be sure to use a pinhole to "refract" or to send the patient for an ophthalmological refraction.

  A. Approach to the patient with functional visual loss:
    1. Document every visual test performed and the patient's response. This includes how the patient entered the examining room, found the chair and sat down, and regarded the examiner, and how vigorously the testing was resisted.
    2. The greater the resistance and complaints about the test, the more likely it is that the patient is a deliberate malingerer, whereas the more naive functional patient will gladly go along with the exam regardless of the obvious contradictions in performance behavior.
    3. Confrontation of the patient with accusations of malingering is fruitless and counterproductive. Gentle suggestion that vision is "better than the patient thinks it is" and that the patient's vision is likely to improve will reassure almost all but the hard-core malingerer.
    4. Radiographic or electrophysiologic studies should be done and interpreted for the patient to ensure that no nagging doubts remain. The patient should be told that no disease of the central or peripheral nervous system has been identified.
    5. Do not give drops or pills or refer the patient to a psychiatrist. Prescriptions for medication give double messages (i.e., "nothing is wrong, but take this medication"), and psychiatric referrals for functional problems do not produce useful results. Simple reassurance is the key.

  B. General rules for referral of patients who complain of visual loss:
    1. If the patient has seen several eye-care specialists (optometrists or ophthalmologists) and continues to complain of visual loss, consider the syndromes in Table 10-5.
    2. Imaging studies should be done with the visual pathways in mind. If the visual loss is monocular, look at the orbit and intracranial optic nerve. If the visual loss is bitemporal, look at chiasm and perichiasmal structures.
    3. Enlist an ophthalmologist for visual examination if the patient has not yet seen one. Ask for visual fields to be done and for an interpretation of the findings. If the optic disk looks abnormal or the fundus appears abnormal, have photographs taken. As physicians, we get chest x-rays for lung disease, and we should obtain fundus photos for eye disease. Remember that the ophthalmologist will be able to put corneal, lenticular, and visible vitreous and retinal diseases into perspective in regard to visual loss.
    4. If a tumor or stroke is causing visual loss, referral to a neurologist is appropriate. If the problem is pituitary apoplexy, refer immediately and emergently to a neurosurgeon.

Table 10-5. Syndromes of transient visual loss.

Name	Synonyms	Duration	Pain	Characteristics
Amaurosis fugax	Transient monocular visual loss, transient monocular blindness	Seconds to hours, usually less than 5 minutes	Rare	Complete, altitudinal, or quadrantic loss; spots or constriction
Transient visual obscuration	Transient obnubilation	Seconds	No	Gray-, black-, or white-out of vision
Uhthoff's phenomenon	None—usually in an eye that has had optic neuritis	Minutes to 1 hour	No	Precipitated by heat or exercise
Migraine aura	Fortification specters or spectra, teichopsias	Five to 45 minutes	Usually following the visual symptoms, but occasionally painless (so-called acephalgic migraine)	Zigzags, flashes, lights, sparkles, heat wave, or water-on-window sensation

Recommended Readings

Aldrich MS, et al. Cortical blindness: Etiology, diagnosis and prognosis. *Ann Neurol* 21:149–158, 1987.

Barton JJS, Corbett JJ. Neuro-ophthalmologic vascular emergencies in the elderly. *Clin Geriat Med* 7:525–548, 1991.

Bernstein EF (ed). *Amaurosis Fugax.* New York: Springer-Verlag, 1987.

Brown G, Tasman W. *Congenital Anomalies of the Optic Disc.* New York: Grune & Stratton, 1983.

Bruno A, et al. Transient monocular visual loss patterns and underlying vascular abnormalities: A prospective study of 100 consecutive patients. *Stroke* 21:34–39, 1990.

Carr RE, Siegel IM. *Electrodiagnostic Testing of the Visual System: A Clinical Guide.* Philadelphia: Davis, 1990.

Damasio A, et al. Central achromatopsia: Behavioral, anatomic and physiologic aspects. *Neurology* 30:1064–1071, 1980.

Frisén L. The neurology of visual acuity. *Brain* 103:639–670, 1980.

Grant M. *Toxicology of the Eye* (3rd ed). Springfield, IL: Thomas, 1986.

Hughes B. Indirect injury to the optic nerves and chiasm. *Bull Johns Hopkins Hosp* 111:98–126, 1963.

Hupp SL. Syndromes of the optic chiasm. In RJ Tusa, SA Newman (eds), *Neuro-Ophthalmological Disorders: Diagnostic Workup and Management.* New York: Marcel Dekker, 1995. Pp 65–75.

Hupp SL, et al. Visual disturbances of migraine. *Surv Ophthalmol* 33:221–236, 1989.

Kathol RG, et al. Functional visual loss: Follow up of 42 cases. *Arch Ophthalmol* 101:729–735, 1983.

Lessell S. Indirect optic nerve trauma. *Arch Ophthalmol* 107:382–386, 1989.

Rizzo M. The role of striate cortex: Evidence from human brain lesion studies. In A Peters, K Rockland (eds), *Cerebral Cortex* (vol 10). New York: Plenum, 1994. Pp 504–540.

Rizzo M, Nawrat M. Human visual cortex and its disorders. *Curr Opin Ophthalmol* 4:30–37, 1993.

Thompson HS. Functional visual loss. *Am J Ophthalmol* 100:209–213, 1985.

Thompson HS, Corbett JJ. Swinging flashlight test. *Neurology* 39:154–156, 1989.

Trobe JD, et al. Confrontation visual field techniques in the detection of anterior visual pathway lesions. *Ann Neurol* 10:28–34, 1981.

Wray SH. Amaurosis fugax. In RJ Tusa, SA Newman (eds), *Neuro-Ophthalmological Disorders: Diagnostic Workup and Management.* New York: Marcel Dekker, 1995. Pp 3–26.

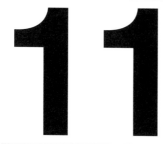

Approach to the Patient with Abnormal Pupils

Aki Kawasaki

The pupillomotor pathway is composed of an afferent limb (the input signals stimulating the pupillomotor centers) and an efferent limb (the output signals that actually direct pupillary movement). A lesion in one afferent limb diminishes the amplitude of the pupil reaction in both eyes (direct and consensual responses) when that side is stimulated, in comparison with the amplitude of the pupil reaction elicited by stimulating the intact side. Pupil sizes are equal as long as the output signals are equal. Therefore, unequal pupil size is evidence of an output (efferent) defect on one side.

Proper equipment for pupillary examination includes a millimeter ruler, a bright hand-held light source (a nonhalogen penlight is not bright enough), a darkened room, 4% or 10% cocaine HCl eyedrops, and 1% pilocarpine eyedrops. Be sure to ask the patient if any ophthalmic medications have been used in the past 24 hours.

I. **Pupillary examination.** *Objective:* To recognize abnormal pupils and then distinguish between afferent versus efferent pupillary defects.

   A. **Pupil size.** Average pupil diameter is greatest (7.0–7.5 mm) during the teenage years, then gradually decreases with increasing age. Have the patient fixate on a distant target and note each pupil diameter in light and in darkness. Size asymmetry of 0.4 mm or more is clinically visible. If any inequality exists, carefully measure each pupil diameter under the following three conditions.

   1. **In darkness.** Turn off the room lights and hold the handlight at the level of the patient's chin. Illuminate the patient's face from below, just enough to view (and measure) the pupils.

   2. **In light.** Turn on all room lights, including the handlight, then view (and measure) the pupils.

   3. **To near response.** Turn room light to mid-level. Ask the patient to slowly follow your finger towards his or her nose. Watch the patient's eyes converge and pupils constrict. Do this two or three times to maximize the patient's effort.

      a. Normal pupils are sometimes slightly unequal in size, but seldom by more than 1.0 mm, and the difference may increase a bit in darkness. (See sec. **III.B.1,** Physiologic anisocori.)

      b. Significant anisocoria usually indicates an efferent pupillomotor problem (see sec. **III,** Efferent pupillary defect).

      c. A subtle Horner's syndrome can be missed because there may be very little anisocoria under regular room lighting conditions. Remember to view pupils in light *and* in darkness. (See sec. **IV.A.1,** Horner's syndrome.)

   B. **Pupillary light reaction**

   1. **Direct response.** Have the patient fixate on a distant target in a dark room. Shine a bright focal light directly onto one pupil for 3 seconds and note the amplitude and velocity of constriction of the illuminated pupil. Do this to each pupil two or three times for a mental "average."

   2. **Consensual response.** Sometimes it may be important to view the consensual response, even though it is difficult to do so because the consensual pupil remains in darkness during light stimulation of the other side. If one pupil consistently has lesser direct *and* consensual light reactions, it has an efferent defect and there is probably an anisocoria. Repeat, if necessary, the procedure for measuring pupil diameter presented in sec. **I.A.**

      a. Noting that a pupil is "sluggish" to direct light stimulation alone does not differentiate between afferent and efferent pupillary defects. (See also sec. **I.C.**)

      b. Remember that an *afferent* pupillary defect does *not* produce an anisocoria.

109

C. **Alternating light test.** This is the standard clinical technique for identifying an asymmetry of input between the two eyes. This asymmetry is referred to as a relative afferent pupillary defect (RAPD), formerly called "Marcus Gunn pupil." Have the patient fixate a distant target in a dark room. Shine a bright focal light directly onto one pupil for 3 seconds, then quickly swing the light onto the other pupil for 3 seconds, and repeat this for four or five alternations. Watch only the directly illuminated pupil. The normal response is a matching pupillary constriction followed by equal redilation in both eyes.

   1. **Large RAPD.** In this eye, the pupil fails to constrict or may simply dilate when the light falls on it.

   2. **Small-to-moderate RAPD.** In this eye, the pupil may exhibit an initial constriction to direct light, but it will be less vigorous than the constriction exhibited by the contralateral pupil when stimulated. It may also "escape"— i.e., redilate—sooner after the initial constriction.

      a. Neutral density filters can be used to "titrate" the pupil responses to a balance point and quantitate the RAPD.

      b. An underlying large anisocoria adds another dimension to pupillary light testing. The larger pupil lets in more light than the smaller pupil, and this resultant asymmetry of pupillomotor input can produce a small RAPD in the eye with the smaller pupil.

      c. If only one pupil is working properly, compare its direct light response to its consensual light response. The reactions should be equal if the afferent functions of both eyes are intact.

      d. Younger patients may exhibit a wide range of physiologic pupillary unrest (known as hippus), which can be mistaken for early pupillary escape—i.e., a small RAPD.

II. **Afferent pupillary defect.** A relative afferent pupillary defect (RAPD) is a sensitive indicator of unilateral or asymmetric injury to the afferent pupillary pathway. If an RAPD is found, it needs to be investigated. In general, the size of the RAPD correlates with the asymmetry of visual field loss and the resultant asymmetry of pupillomotor input. It also tends to vary with the location of the lesion within the afferent pathway (Fig. 11-1).

A. **Retina**

   1. Large unilateral retinal lesions produce a clear RAPD (e.g., retinal detachment or central retinal artery occlusion). Acuity might be good if the macula is spared. A careful dilated funduscopic examination is usually diagnostic, and so an ophthalmology consultation is important.

   2. Cataracts and corneal opacities are not causes of afferent pupillary defects.

B. **Optic nerve.** Damage to the optic nerve almost always produces an RAPD. Visual acuity loss may be mild or severe, but a visual field abnormality can almost invariably be detected by formal perimetry testing. The optic disk may appear normal or acutely swollen but will later develop pallor. Examples of optic nerve disorders include optic neuritis, ischemic optic neuropathy, hereditary optic neuropathy, compressive lesions, toxins, trauma, and cellular infiltration. (See Chap. 10, Approach to the Patient with Visual Loss.)

   1. The largest afferent defects occur in association with unilateral optic nerve disorders.

   2. "Resolved" optic neuritis may result in optic disk pallor and RAPD despite recovery to normal visual acuity and normal visual field.

   3. The extent of damage in bilateral optic nerve disorders is rarely perfectly symmetrical. Therefore, an RAPD will be found on the side with greater damage. Look carefully.

C. **Optic chiasm**

   1. Compressive lesions of the optic chiasm can produce asymmetric visual loss and, therefore, an RAPD. Commonly, a junctional scotoma is found.

   2. Symmetric bitemporal hemianopsia is not associated with an RAPD, because injury to the visual and pupillary pathways is symmetric.

D. **Optic tract.** Slightly more nerve fibers decussate at the chiasm than do not. A pure optic tract lesion will produce a small RAPD in the *contralateral* eye. Thus, a complete homonymous hemianopsia with an afferent defect in the eye with the temporal field loss should raise the possibility of a tract lesion as the cause of visual loss.

E. **Pretectal nucleus**

   1. The pretectal nucleus in the dorsal midbrain is the final synapse site of

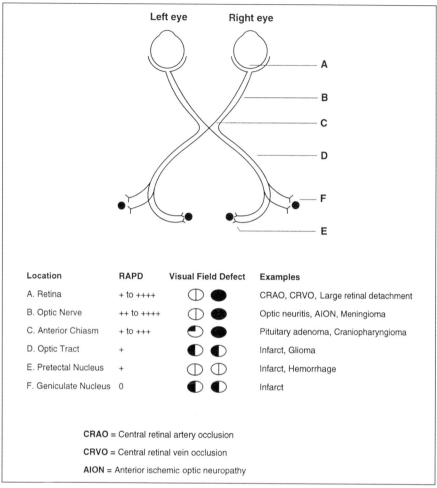

Figure 11-1. Localization of lesions causing visual field defects.

pupillary fibers coming from the optic tract via brachium of the superior colliculus. Visual fibers, however, have separated off to go on to the lateral geniculate nucleus. Therefore, a dorsal midbrain lesion can produce a small contralateral RAPD and *no* visual loss.

2. Afferent pupillary defects from optic tract or midbrain injury are usually small and are fairly rare.

III. **Efferent pupillary defect.** Unequal pupil size in the awake, alert patient who casually presents to an outpatient clinic is virtually never the result of a compressed oculomotor nerve from impending tentorial herniation. This section is designed for the evaluation of anisocoria in the noncomatose patient (Fig. 11-2).

A. **Structural iris damage: "ophthalmologic" anisocoria.** The iris contains two muscles that modulate pupil size and shape: the circular sphincter and the radial dilator. Therefore, structural iris defects can distort pupil size, shape, and both light and near reactions even though the neural afferent and efferent pathways are intact. If iris mechanics are suspect, refer the patient to an ophthalmologist, because this might avoid unnecessary ancillary tests.

1. **History.** Inquire about any previous ocular infection, inflammation, trauma, or surgical procedures. Consult the patient's primary ophthalmologist.

2. **Examination.** Some iris defects—e.g., iris coloboma and iridectomy—are visually apparent, whereas others—e.g., synechiae (adhesions) and small

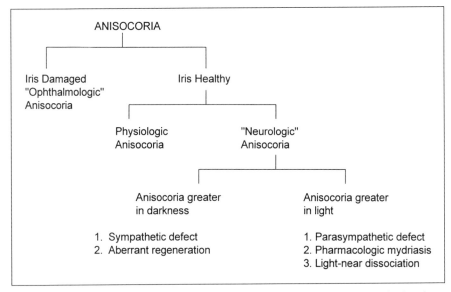

Figure 11-2. Differential diagnosis of anisocoria. Sometimes it is difficult to say whether the anisocoria gets worse in dark or light. In this circumstance, a detailed history and other examination findings may provide clues.

sphincter tears—require slit-lamp biomicroscopy. Marked irregularity of the pupillary margin, unusual distortions of pupillary shape, and differences in iris color are clues that iris damage may be present. A dusting of iris pigment may be observed in a ring on the lens of a patient who has had a blow to the eye.

B. Structurally intact iris. If the iris appears healthy, the next important decision is whether or not the anisocoria is physiologic.

   1. Physiologic anisocoria

      a. This disorder has been called benign or essential anisocoria but is now known as simple central anisocoria.

      b. Incidence. Approximately 20% of the normal population have pupillary inequalities of 0.4 mm or more in dim lighting.

      c. Clinical characteristics

         (1) Anisocoria is less than 1.0 mm in diameter.

         (2) Anisocoria is slightly increased in darkness.

         (3) Anisocoria can vary in amplitude (even within a few minutes).

         (4) Anisocoria can even "reverse" sides—i.e., the larger pupil can be on one side at first but on the other side later.

         (5) Pupillary constriction to light and near stimulation is normal in both eyes.

         (6) Pupillary dilation to darkness is normal.

      d. Work-up: none. Physiologic anisocoria may occasionally be confused with Horner's pupil, because both conditions cause an increase in anisocoria in darkness. Look for other clinical evidence of oculosympathetic damage (see sec. **IV.A.1,** Horner's syndrome).

   2. "Neurologic" anisocoria. Because our discussion of neurologic anisocoria is lengthy, it is ascribed a major heading of its own and presented as sec. **IV,** below. Section **IV** assumes that the iris is healthy and that physiologic anisocoria has been ruled out, and the guidelines that it presents are not applicable to bilateral or mixed sympathetic or parasympathetic pupil defects.

IV. Neurologic anisocoria. (Read sec. **III** first.) Two iris muscles regulate pupil size. The sphincter (pupilloconstrictor) is innervated by the parasympathetic system and the dilator (pupillodilator) is innervated by the sympathetic system. Determine whether anisocoria is greater in darkness (dilation problem in the eye with the smaller pupil) or in light (constriction problem in the eye with the larger pupil).

A. Anisocoria greater in darkness
  1. Horner's syndrome (oculosympathetic defect)
    a. Clinical characteristics
      (1) Ptosis. There is upper lid ptosis and "upside-down" lower lid ptosis (elevation of the lower lid). Together, they create the impression of enophthalmos but do not constitute a true enophthalmos. The upper-lid ptosis of Horner's syndrome is generally mild. Especially in older patients, it can be inapparent if the opposite eyelid is dehisced or droopy from age-related skin changes.
      (2) Smaller pupil. The anisocoria is usually not marked but is more apparent in darkness. Remember that the relative miosis stems from a failure to dilate, not a failure of pupilloconstriction.
      (3) Dilation lag. When the lights are first turned off, a normal pupil dilates promptly but the smaller Horner's pupil initially dilates more slowly—i.e., "lags." Illuminate the patient's face from below with a flashlight. Turn the room lights off and watch the anisocoria slowly change. The anisocoria will be barely visible in bright light, then maximally visible at 5 seconds of darkness, and then smaller again after 15–20 seconds of darkness as the Horner's pupil finally dilates. (Drowsiness causes miosis and obscures dilation lag. Arouse the patient before testing for dilation lag.)
      (4) Ipsilateral facial anhidrosis. This finding is not present with postganglionic sympathetic lesions (see sec. **IV.A.1.c**).
      (5) Heterochromia iridis (different iris color) accompanies congenital Horner's syndrome.
    b. Pharmacologic testing: cocaine test. Cocaine inhibits presynaptic reuptake of released norepinephrine at the postganglionic neuromuscular synapse. When the entire oculosympathetic pathway is intact, cocaine normally dilates the pupils. (Inform the patient that the urine will test positive for cocaine for the next 48–72 hours.)
      (1) Do not touch the corneas or use eyedrops prior to the cocaine test—i.e., do not check corneal reflexes or intraocular pressures. Contact lenses should not be worn 24 hours prior to the test.
      (2) Place 2 drops (1 minute apart) of 4% to 10% cocaine HCl ophthalmic solution in each eye. Wait 40–60 minutes.
      (3) The normal pupil will dilate. A Horner's pupil will fail to dilate. Postcocaine anisocoria of 1.0 mm or greater is considered diagnostic.
    c. Anatomy of the oculosympathetic pathway
      (1) The central oculosympathetic neuron originates in the posterolateral hypothalamus and descends in the lateral brainstem to the spinal cord.
      (2) The preganglionic neuron originates in the lateral horn of the spinal cord at C_8-T_2, "the ciliospinal center of Budge-Waller." Its fibers skirt across the apex of the lung and under the subclavian artery before ascending in the anterior neck.
      (3) The postganglionic neuron originates in the superior cervical ganglion, and its pupillary fibers are intimately associated with the internal carotid artery through the neck, base of the skull, and cavernous sinus. (The vasomotor sympathetic fibers travel separately with the external carotid artery.) In the orbit, the oculosympathetic fibers are carried in the long ciliary nerves.
    d. Etiology of Horner's syndrome. In general, a central Horner's syndrome is stroke-related. Preganglionic lesions may be neoplastic and postganglionic lesions are mostly benign. (See Table 11-1 for more details.)
    e. Work-up of Horner's syndrome
      (1) Clinical localization
        (a) A central Horner's syndrome is usually accompanied by other symptoms or signs of brainstem dysfunction (e.g., Wallenberg syndrome). There is also anhidrosis throughout the ipsilateral face, neck, and body.
        (b) Preganglionic Horner's syndrome causes ipsilateral anhidrosis of the face only. Weakness and wasting of the ipsilateral hand muscles suggest injury to the C_8-T_2 spinal rootlets or brachial

Table 11-1. Causes of injury to the oculosympathetic pathway (Horner's syndrome).

Central	Preganglionic	Postganglionic
Hypothalamus	Cervicothoracic cord/spinal	Superior cervical ganglion
Infarct	roots	Iatrogenic (surgical
Tumor	Trauma	removal, tonsillectomy)
Brainstem	Intramedullary or	Trauma
Ischemia	paravertebral tumor	Internal carotid artery
Hemorrhage	Syrinx	Dissection
Tumor	AVM	Trauma
Demyelination (MS)	Spondylosis	Thrombosis
Cervical cord	Epidural anesthesia	Tumor
Trauma	Lower brachial plexus	Migraine/cluster headache
Tumor	Birth trauma	Base of skull/carotid canal
Syrinx	Acquired trauma	Tumor (e.g., nasopharyn-
AVM	Pulmonary apex/under sub-	geal CA, lymphoma)
	clavian artery	Trauma
	Vascular anomalies	Middle ear
	(e.g., subclavian	Tumor (e.g., cholestea-
	aneurysm, aortic tortu-	toma)
	osity)	Infection
	Pancoast, apical lung	Cavernous sinus
	tumor	Tumor (meningioma, pitu-
	Cervical rib	itary adenoma)
	Iatrogenic (e.g., chest	Inflammation (Tolosa-Hunt
	tube)	syndrome)
	Infection (e.g., apical TB)	Cavernous carotid
	Anterior neck	aneurysm
	Iatrogenic (thyroid sur-	Thrombosis
	gery, neck dissection,	Fistula
	catheters)	
	Trauma	
	Tumor (lymphoma, breast	
	metastases)	

Of all outpatient cases of Horner's syndrome, 3–13% have a central etiology. Of all outpatient cases of Horner's syndrome, 41% have a preganglionic etiology, and of these, 50% are neoplastic. Many cases of benign postganglionic Horner's syndrome are associated with pain. Every infant or child with congenital Horner's syndrome requires evaluation for mediastinal neuroblastoma.
MS = multiple sclerosis; AVM = arteriovenous malformation; TB = tuberculosis; CA = carcinoma.

plexus. If there is also pain in the supraclavicular fossa, an apical lung tumor may be suspected. Inquire about any past surgery or trauma to the neck or chest—e.g., central catheters, thyroidectomy, or history of physical assault/choking.

(c) A Horner's syndrome in a patient with vascular headaches is usually postganglionic in origin. There is no clinically appreciable facial anhidrosis. Sudden pain in the jaw, ear, throat, or peritonsillar area is characteristic of carotid dissection. A painful postganglionic Horner's syndrome with ipsilateral trigeminal dysfunction (dysesthesia, numbness) is called Raeder's paratrigeminal syndrome and has been associated with a variety of lesions in the parasellar/cavernous sinus region.

(2) Pharmacologic localization: 1% hydroxyamphetamine. Hydroxyamphetamine testing distinguishes a central or preganglionic Horner's syndrome from a postganglionic Horner's syndrome. Hydroxyamphetamine releases stored catecholamines from the postganglionic fiber terminal if the postganglionic fiber is intact. Therefore, the pupil of the eye with a postganglionic oculosympathetic defect fails to dilate to hydroxyamphetamine. Referral to neuro-ophthalmology may be necessary because hydroxyamphetamine is not readily available.

(a) **Central or preganglionic Horner's syndrome.** If no brain-stem symptoms or signs exist, scan the neck and chest (CT or MRI). If these scans are negative, do a cranial MRI. If brainstem signs are present, cranial MRI is indicated first.

(b) **Postganglionic Horner's syndrome** requires a head and neck MRI. Angiography may be considered if carotid dissection is a diagnostic differential. Cluster headaches may cause a postganglionic Horner's pupil in up to 22% of cases. If the history is typical and other neurologic deficits are absent, no radiologic studies are necessary.

2. **Aberrant regeneration**
   a. **Pathophysiology.** When a structural lesion compresses or transects the oculomotor (third) nerve, the fibers innervating the extraocular muscles may sprout misguided collaterals that aberrantly innervate the iris sphincter.
   b. **Clinical characteristics**
      (1) **Simultaneous unilateral pupilloconstriction** accompanies adduction, supraduction, or infraduction of the globe.
      (2) **Miosis.** The aberrantly innervated pupil is typically smaller than the normal pupil, and, because it does not dilate well, the anisocoria is more apparent in darkness.
      (3) **Reversed anisocoria.** Although aberrantly innervated, the original parasympathetic innervation to the iris sphincter has been disrupted by the structural lesion, damaging the oculomotor nerve. Therefore, that pupil has a smaller amplitude of constriction to light and it may appear to be the *larger* pupil under bright lights.
   c. **Other lesions**
      (1) Primary ischemic injury to the oculomotor nerve essentially never causes aberrant regeneration.
      (2) A tonic pupil may also seem to have "reverse" anisocoria, where it is the larger pupil in light and the smaller pupil in dark. This is also a result of aberrant regeneration. (See sec. **IV.B.2,** Tonic pupil.)
3. **Physiologic anisocoria.** (See sec. **III.B.**)

B. **Anisocoria greater in bright light**
   1. **Oculomotor (third) nerve palsy**
      a. **Clinical characteristics**
         (1) **Ptosis.** Upper-lid ptosis is usually present but can be absent, slight, or complete. Lower-lid ptosis is not present.
         (2) **Larger pupil.** Anisocoria is more apparent under bright lighting. The pupil is rarely "blown"—i.e., completely nonreactive—in the *noncomatose* patient with an acute third nerve palsy.
         (3) **Ophthalmoplegia.** The patient complains of diplopia resulting from limitation of adduction, supraduction, and infraduction.
      b. **Anatomy of the oculoparasympathetic pathway**
         (1) **The oculomotor nerve.** The preganglionic neuron originates in the Edinger-Westphal subnuclei in the dorsal midbrain. Its fibers exit at the interpeduncular fossa and then enter the cavernous sinus. At the anterior cavernous sinus/superior orbital fissure, the oculomotor nerve divides into a superior division innervating the levator palpebrae and superior rectus muscles and an inferior division that contains fibers for accommodation and pupilloconstriction as well as innervation of the inferior rectus, medial rectus, and inferior oblique muscles.
         (2) **The short ciliary nerves.** The postganglionic neuron originates in the ciliary ganglion of the orbit. The ciliary ganglion is located mesial to the lateral rectus, approximately 1 cm behind the globe. Its fibers are the short ciliary nerves that serve both accommodation and pupilloconstriction.
      c. **Etiology of an oculomotor nerve palsy.** See Table 11-2. (For further details, refer to Chap. 12, Approach to the Patient with Diplopia.)
      d. **Work-up.** Any painful oculomotor nerve palsy with pupillary involvement warrants *emergent* angiographic consideration to look for an expanding or ruptured posterior communicating artery aneurysm. Remem-

Table 11-2. Etiology of oculomotor nerve palsy.

Preganglionic (oculomotor nerve)	Postganglionic: "tonic pupil" (ciliary ganglion or short ciliary nerve)
Brainstem (midbrain)—"fascicular"	Intraorbital
Ischemia	Viral ganglionitis
Hemorrhage	Trauma
Tumor	Ocular surgery
AVM	Tumor
Interpeduncular fossa/subarachnoid space	Systemic peripheral neuropathy
Basal aneurysm	Hereditary (e.g., Charcot-Marie-Tooth
Basal infections	disease, Riley-Day syndrome)
(granulomatous meningitis, fungal	Acquired (diabetes, alcohol, toxins,
meningitis)	amyloid, vasculitis)
Intraneural ischemia—"vasculopathic"	Idiopathic ("Adie's") tonic pupil
(e.g., diabetes, hypertension)	
Cavernous sinus/superior orbital fissure	
Tumor (e.g., meningioma, pituitary	
adenoma)	
Inflammation (Tolosa-Hunt syndrome)	
Cavernous carotid aneurysm	
Thrombosis	
Fistula	

Brainstem "fascicular" oculomotor nerve palsies occasionally occur as isolated findings but are more commonly associated with other neurologic deficits (i.e., Weber's, Benedikt's, Claude's, and Nothnagel's syndromes). Vasculopathic oculomotor nerve palsies tend to spare the pupil. Compressive lesions typically involve the pupil.
AVM = arteriovenous malformation.

ber that early compression by aneurysm can cause a partial oculomotor palsy and no initial pupil dysfunction.

2. Tonic pupil (Adie's pupil). The site of injury for a tonic pupil is the ciliary ganglion cell bodies or their postganglionic parasympathetic fibers carried in the short ciliary nerves.

  a. Symptoms include anisocoria, photophobia, and blurred near vision.

  b. Clinical characteristics

    (1) Larger pupil. A fresh tonic pupil is very large but gets smaller over several months.

    (2) Poor light reaction. Pupillary constriction to light stimulation is minimal and segmental when present but may be completely absent.

    (3) Light-near dissociation. Pupillary constriction to near stimulation is delayed in onset and slow in velocity. The pupil remains tonically constricted; thus, it is called "tonic." The amplitude of the near reaction exceeds the amplitude of the light constriction, which is why there is light-near dissociation.

    (4) Pupillary redilation after near constriction is slow owing to the tonic constriction. Thus, it also has "tonic" redilation.

    (5) Accommodation paresis. Acutely, accommodation is lost but may gradually improve.

    (6) Segmental palsy of the iris sphincter requires a slit lamp. On near effort, the innervated areas of sphincter will draw up like a pulled purse string, but the denervated areas will flatten out. A tonic pupil is the larger pupil in light because it reacts to light poorly, but because it also dilates tonically, it may be the smaller pupil in darkness. (See sec. **IV.A.2,** Aberrant regeneration.)

  c. Pharmacologic testing: 0.1% pilocarpine

    (1) Dilute regular strength 1% pilocarpine to a 1:10 weak strength ophthalmic solution (0.1%).

    (2) Place 2 drops (1 minute apart) in each eye. Wait 25–30 minutes.

(3) Weak (0.1%) pilocarpine generally does not affect the normal pupil sphincter but induces constriction of the suspected tonic pupil because of cholinergic denervation supersensitivity of the sphincter. (The diagnostic utility of weak pilocarpine testing assumes that there is one tonic pupil and one normal pupil for comparison.)

d. Pathophysiology

(1) Acute denervation. An injury to the ciliary ganglion or short ciliary nerves denervates the ciliary muscle and its sphincter; thus, accommodation and pupilloconstriction are acutely abolished.

(2) Aberrant reinnervation. Neurons originally destined for the ciliary muscle for accommodation regrow and correctly reinnervate the ciliary muscle but in addition sprout collaterals to aberrantly reinnervate the iris sphincter. Accommodation improves and tonic pupilloconstriction accompanies accommodation (near effort).

e. Etiology. See Table 11-2. The most common tonic pupil is idiopathic and unilateral, typically affects women between the ages of 20 and 40 years, and may be associated with generalized hyporeflexia (Adie's syndrome) and/or segmental anhidrosis (Ross' syndrome).

f. An isolated tonic pupil does not require any imaging studies.

3. Pharmacologic mydriasis

a. Mydriatic ophthalmic agents include atropine, scopolamine, homatropine, cyclopentolate, tropicamide, Neo-Synephrine, phenylephrine, cocaine, and hydroxyamphetamine.

b. The pupil is maximally dilated and nonresponsive to light or near stimulation.

c. Other ocular or neurologic findings are absent. There is no history of recent ocular trauma.

d. Instillation of regular strength 1% pilocarpine fails to produce *any* constriction in a pharmacologically dilated pupil. A pupil dilated as a result of a parasympathetic defect (third nerve palsy or tonic pupil) will promptly constrict to regular strength 1% pilocarpine.

4. Light-near dissociation (LND). Typically, the amplitude of pupilloconstriction to a light stimulus is greater than to a near stimulus. Never test the near response with a bright light, because the two stimuli summate and create the false impression of LND. Light-near dissociation occurs under the following two circumstances.

a. The light response limb of the reflex is defective (reduced), but the near response is spared (normal). This circumstance arises with any isolated lesion to the afferent pupillary pathway. It is said that the most common cause of LND is an optic neuropathy.

b. The light response *and* the near response are defective, but only the near response is restored—i.e., aberrant regeneration. The classic example is the tonic (Adie's) pupil.

c. Specific examples of LND

(1) Midbrain LND (sylvian aqueduct syndrome, dorsal midbrain syndrome). Both pupils are typically midsize with light-near dissociation. Associated motility dysfunctions include bilateral lid retraction, supranuclear vertical gaze palsy, and convergence-retraction nystagmus.

(2) Argyll Robertson pupils. Both pupils are typically small in size and irregular in shape with an impaired light response, brisk near response, and poor dilation in darkness. Visual function is intact. Originally, these pupils were described as a sign of central nervous system syphilis.

(3) Bilateral LND. Bilateral old Adie's pupils and diffuse peripheral neuropathy such as diabetes may also cause bilaterally small pupils that have light-near dissociation. Any bilateral light-near dissociation warrants syphilis serologies.

V. Referral. Any diagnostic dilemma regarding the afferent or efferent pathways should be referred to a neuro-ophthalmologist.

Recommended Readings

Corbett JJ, Thompson HS. Pupillary function and dysfunction. In AK Asbury, GM McKhann, WI McDonald (eds), *Diseases of the Nervous System: Clinical Neurobiology.* Philadelphia: Saunders, 1992.

Cox TA, Thompson HS, Corbett JJ. Relative afferent pupillary defects in optic neuritis. *Am J Ophthalmol* 92:685–690, 1981.

Cremer SA, et al. Hydroxyamphetamine mydriasis in Horner's syndrome. *Am J Ophthalmol* 110:71–76, 1990.

Czarnecki JSC, Thompson HS. The iris sphincter in aberrant regeneration of the third nerve. *Arch Ophthalmol* 96:1606–1610, 1978.

Digre KB, et al. Selective MR imaging approach for evaluation of patients with Horner's syndrome. *AJNR* 13:223–227, 1992.

Grimson BS, Thompson HS. Horner's syndrome: Overall view of 120 cases. In HS Thompson (ed), *Topics in Neuro-Ophthalmology.* Baltimore: Williams & Wilkins, 1979.

Kardon RH, et al. Critical evaluation of the cocaine test in the diagnosis of Horner's syndrome. *Arch Ophthalmol* 108:384–387, 1990.

Lam BL, Thompson HS, Corbett JJ. The prevalence of simple anisocoria. *Am J Ophthalmol* 104:69–73, 1987.

Loewenfeld IE. The Argyll Robertson pupil, 1869–1969. A critical survey of the literature. *Surv Ophthalmol* 14:199–299, 1969.

Loewenfeld IE. "Simple, central" anisocoria: A common condition, seldom recognized. *Trans Am Acad Ophthalmol Otolaryngol* 83:832–839, 1977.

Loewenfeld IE, Thompson HS. The tonic pupil: A re-evaluation. *Am J Ophthalmol* 63:46–87, 1967.

Loewenfeld IE, Thompson HS. Mechanism of tonic pupil. *Ann Neurol* 10(3):275–276, 1981.

Maloney WF, Younge BR, Moyer NJ. Evaluation of the causes and accuracy of pharmacologic localization in Horner's syndrome. *Am J Ophthalmol* 90:394–402, 1980.

Miller NR. Disorders of pupillary function, accommodation and lacrimation. In BD Tansill (ed), *Walsh and Hoyt's Clinical Neuro-Ophthalmology.* Baltimore: Williams & Wilkins, 1985.

Thompson HS. The pupil. In WM Hart Jr. (ed), *Adler's Physiology of the Eye: Clinical Application* (9th ed). St. Louis: Mosby-Year Book, 1992.

Thompson HS, Corbett JJ. Swinging flashlight test (letter). *Neurology* 39:154–156, 1989.

Thompson HS, Corbett JJ, Cox TA. How to measure the relative afferent pupillary defect. *Surv Ophthalmol* 26:39–42, 1981.

Thompson HS, Kardon RH. Pretectal pupillary defects (editorial comment). *J Clin Neuro-ophthalmol* 11(3):173–174, 1991.

Thompson HS, Kardon RH. Clinical importance of pupillary inequality. Focal points: clinical modules for ophthalmologists. *Amer Acad Ophthalmol* 10(10):1–12, 1992.

Thompson HS, Newsome DA, Loewenfeld IE. The fixed dilated pupil. Sudden iridoplegia or mydriatic drops? A simple diagnostic test. *Arch Ophthalmol* 86:21–27, 1971.

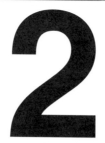

Approach to the Patient with Diplopia
Robert D. Yee

Misalignment of the eyes causes **binocular diplopia.** Both images are equally clear, and covering either eye abolishes the double vision. Abnormalities of the ocular media (e.g., cornea and lens) create **monocular diplopia** (see below). When the patient covers the normal eye, the double vision persists. However, diplopia disappears when the abnormal eye is occluded. Disorders of the extraocular muscles, orbit, cranial nerves, and brainstem cause binocular diplopia. The physical examination reveals the location of the abnormality, and the history usually indicates its etiology. The work-up and management of diplopia usually are not urgent and allow time for observation, except when the etiology might be an intracranial aneurysm. An aneurysm can cause sudden pain, diplopia, and a third nerve palsy with dilated pupil and abnormal pupillary reactions. Because of the risk of severe morbidity and mortality with rupture of the aneurysm, magnetic resonance imaging, magnetic resonance angiography, and perhaps cerebral angiography should be ordered immediately. Phycomycosis of the orbit, cavernous sinus thrombosis, pituitary apoplexy, and ischemia of the extraocular muscles cause sudden diplopia and ophthalmoplegia and must be evaluated immediately.

I. Etiology and clinical manifestations
  A. Extraocular muscles. Table 12-1 describes the patterns of eye findings that establish the anatomic locations of lesions causing ophthalmoplegia. Table 12-2 lists the common and/or potentially serious causes of diplopia arranged according to anatomic location. Diseases that affect the extraocular muscles (EOMs) directly (ocular myopathies) include myasthenia gravis, chronic progressive external ophthalmoplegia, muscular dystrophies, myositis, and Graves' ophthalmopathy. Ocular myopathies usually do not limit extraocular movements in patterns suggesting cranial nerve palsies. However, when they do, the presence of ptosis (drooping of the upper eyelid), weakness of the orbicularis oculi muscles (inability to keep the eyelids shut), and retraction/edema of the eyelids can indicate that a myopathy exists.

    1. Patients with **myasthenia gravis** usually have ptosis and a history of variable diplopia throughout the day (worse in the evening) and from day to day. Asymmetric ptosis and weakness of the eyelid closure (orbicularis oculi) are usually present. EOM weakness is also asymmetric and produces a pattern that may mimic a cranial nerve palsy or internuclear ophthalmoplegia (limitation of adduction). Pupillary reactions are always normal. Voluntary eye movements (saccades) made by affected muscles can have normally high velocities.

    2. Chronic progressive external ophthalmoplegia (CPEO) is a mitochondrial disorder that presents as a progressive, bilateral ptosis over years. Patients with CPEO usually do not complain of diplopia because ptosis occludes one eye, the characteristically symmetric EOM weakness does not cause misalignment of the eyes, or one eye's image is suppressed by the brain. As in myasthenia gravis, the orbicularis oculi are weak. Because weakness is usually symmetric among each eye's EOMs and between the two eyes, CPEO usually does not mimic a cranial nerve palsy. However, as in myasthenia gravis, the medial rectus muscles are often most affected and a pattern of pseudointernuclear ophthalmoplegia results. Saccades are very slow. CPEO and atypical retinitis pigmentosa comprise the **Kearns-Sayre syndrome.** Cardiac conduction defects can develop in this syndrome. **Oculopharyngeal dystrophy** and **myotonic dystrophy** are autosomal dominant muscular dystrophies that cause ophthalmoplegia.

    3. Myositis is a form of idiopathic inflammatory pseudotumor of the orbit in

Table 12-1. Patterns at anatomic locations.

Extraocular muscles
Individual muscles (usually not cranial nerve pattern)
Pseudocranial nerve palsy
Pseudo-internuclear ophthalmoplegia
Ptosis
Facial muscle paresis

Orbit
Individual muscles
Cranial nerve palsies
Proptosis
Periocular edema and inflammation
Visual loss (orbital apex syndrome)
Infraorbital nerve sensory loss

Cranial nerve palsy
Third nerve palsy
  Exotropia and hypotropia
  Limited adduction (medial rectus), supraduction
    (superior rectus), infraduction (inferior
    rectus), supraduction in adduction (inferior
    oblique)
  Pupillary dilation, diminished constriction to
    light and near reflex
  Decreased accommodation (ciliary muscles)
Fourth nerve palsy
  Hypertropia and excyclotorsion
  Deviation increases in contralateral horizontal
    gaze, downgaze, and head tilt to ipsilateral
    shoulder
  Limited infraduction in adduction
Sixth nerve palsy
  Esotropia
  Limited abduction

Cavernous sinus/superior orbital fissure
Single nerve palsy or multiple nerve palsies
Complete or partial pupil-sparing third nerve palsy
Horner's syndrome (sixth nerve palsy)
Facial sensory loss (1st and 2nd divisions of fifth nerve)
Decreased orbital venous return (dilated retinal veins)

Brainstem
Oculomotor nucleus
  Ipsilateral third nerve palsy
  Bilateral limited supraduction
  Bilateral ptosis
Trochlear nucleus
  Contralateral fourth nerve palsy
Abducens nucleus
  Ipsilateral horizontal gaze palsy
Fascicles
Internuclear ophthalmoplegia
  Ipsilateral limited adduction
  Slow saccades by ipsilateral medial rectus
  Abducting nystagmus in contralateral gaze
Skew deviation

Table 12-2. Location and causes of ophthalmoplegia.

Extraocular muscles
Myasthenia gravis
Chronic progressive external ophthalmoplegia
Muscular dystrophies (oculopharyngeal dystrophy, myotonic dystrophy)
Myositis (idiopathic inflammatory pseudotumor of orbit)
Graves' ophthalmopathy
Metastatic tumors, lymphomas
Botulism

Orbit
Idiopathic inflammatory pseudotumor of orbit
Primary neoplasms
Metastatic neoplasms
Vascular malformations
Paranasal sinus mucoceles
Orbital cellulitis (bacterial infections, phycomycosis)
Orbital wall fractures

Cranial nerves
Microvascular occlusion (diabetes mellitus, hypertension, arteriosclerosis, migraine)
Intracranial aneurysms
Trauma
Inflammation
Infection (Gradenigo's syndrome, meningitis, herpes zoster)
Neoplasms (parasellar, meninges, clivus)
Transtentorial herniation
Increased intracranial pressure
Subarachnoid hemorrhage
Congenital

Cavernous sinus/superior orbital fissure
Tumors (meningioma, hemangioma, pituitary neoplasms, parasellar tumors, metastatic
   tumors)
Intracavernous aneurysm
Cavernous sinus thrombosis
Carotid-cavernous fistulas
Tolosa-Hunt syndrome
Herpes zoster

Brainstem
Demyelination (multiple sclerosis, postviral)
Ischemia
Hemorrhage
Trauma
Infection (encephalitis, AIDS)
Tumors
Vascular malformation
Congenital hypoplasia

which the EOMs are infiltrated by chronic inflammatory cells. Impaired contraction of muscle fibers and restriction limit eye movements. Severe pain accompanies the gradual or sudden onset of diplopia. The conjunctiva and lids might be injected and edematous.

4. In **Graves' ophthalmopathy,** lymphocytes, plasma cells, and edema distend the EOMs, causing restriction. Supraduction and abduction are typically impaired. Lid retraction, periocular edema, conjunctival injection, and proptosis often occur in both eyes. The ophthalmopathy usually follows a period of hyperthyroidism. However, some patients with Graves' disease show ophthalmopathy before developing hyperthyroidism or have normal thyroid function tests (euthyroid Graves' disease).

5. On rare occasions, **metastatic tumors** and **lymphomas** infiltrate the EOMs, and occasionally **giant cell arteritis** causes ischemia of the EOMs.

Acute **botulism** causes dilated, areflexic pupils and ophthalmoplegia by blocking transmission at cholinergic synapses.

B. Orbit. Masses in the orbit displace the globe, mechanically interfere with the EOMs, and cause cranial nerve palsies. **Mass lesions** include orbital inflammatory pseudotumor, lymphoma, primary tumors (cavernous hemangioma, rhabdomyosarcoma, and lacrimal gland neoplasms), metastatic tumors (adenocarcinomas, leukemia, and neuroblastoma), vascular lesions (venous varix and arteriovenous malformation), and lesions of the paranasal sinuses. Most orbital disorders produce **proptosis.**

1. The rapidity of onset and progression depend on the behavior of the mass lesions. For example, cavernous hemangiomas cause a gradual, painless, forward displacement of the eye over many years. Diplopia develops late in the clinical course. A **venous varix** presents as intermittent proptosis and diplopia precipitated by a Valsalva's maneuver. **Mucoceles** of the frontal and ethmoid sinuses gradually displace the eye downward and laterally, but may cause sudden pain and diplopia with infection (pyomucocele).

2. Inflammation, infection, and neoplasms at the **orbital apex** impair eye movements (nerve palsies or mechanical restriction) and damage the optic nerve. **Phycomycosis** in patients with metabolic acidosis (e.g., diabetic ketoacidosis) extends from the nasopharynx, oropharynx, and paranasal sinuses into the orbit and causes a fulminant orbital apex syndrome.

3. A blow to the face might cause an **orbital wall fracture.** In blowout fractures of the orbital floor, entrapment of the inferior rectus muscle and other tissues in the fracture restricts supraduction. Damage to the infraorbital nerve causes numbness below the eye. The medial rectus muscle can be caught in a medial wall fracture, producing limitation of abduction.

C. Cranial nerves. Microvascular occlusion, aneurysms, tumors, trauma, inflammations, infection, and increased intracranial pressure cause acquired cranial nerve palsies.

1. The pattern of a **third nerve palsy** includes ptosis, pupillary dilation, decreased pupil reactions to light and in the near reflex, and limitation of adduction (medial rectus), supraduction (superior rectus and inferior oblique), and infraduction (inferior oblique). The affected eye is deviated laterally (exotropia) and downward (hypotropia).

2. A **fourth nerve palsy** causes limitation of infraduction while the eye is adducted (superior oblique). The affected eye is deviated upward (hypertropia) and the 12 o'clock position of the cornea is rotated laterally relative to the visual axis (excyclotorsion). The patient complains of vertical and torsional diplopia.

3. The pattern of a **sixth nerve palsy** includes impaired abduction (lateral rectus) and nasal deviation of the eye (esotropia).

4. The most common etiology in older adults is microvascular occlusion causing ischemia of the peripheral cranial nerves. The common associated systemic diseases are **diabetes mellitus, hypertension, arteriosclerosis,** and **migraine.** Diplopia occurs suddenly and is often accompanied by retrobulbar pain. In third nerve palsies, pupillary size and reactions are normal or nearly normal (pupil sparing). Spontaneous improvement occurs in a few weeks, and complete resolution occurs in almost all patients within 6 months.

5. **Intracranial aneurysms** create third and sixth nerve palsies. The onset can be abrupt or gradual, and moderate or severe pain often exists. In third nerve palsies, the pupil is dilated and the pupillary contractions to light and near are diminished. Pain may accompany cranial nerve palsies caused by **tumors** (sellar and parasellar neoplasms). Diplopia usually begins slowly and gradually increases.

6. **Head trauma** produces sudden diplopia and is the most frequent etiology of fourth nerve palsies.

7. **Aberrant regeneration** after a traumatic third nerve palsy results in pupillary miosis and/or lid elevation on attempted adduction or infraduction, or adduction on attempted up or down gaze. Oculomotor synkinesis occurs a few months after trauma or compression by aneurysms or tumors. The upper eyelid elevates or the pupil constricts, or both, when the eye adducts or infraducts. Regenerated axons that originally innervated the medial rectus or inferior rectus muscles reach the eyelid levator muscle or the iris sphincter muscle. If aberrant regeneration is found without a history of acute ocu-

lomotor paralysis, a slowly growing, parasellar neoplasm—e.g., meningioma of the cavernous sinus—should be suspected.

8. **Inflammatory disorders**—e.g., sarcoidosis or postviral encephalitis—can produce cranial nerve palsies. The diplopia and pain respond quickly to systemic corticosteroids.

9. **Increased intracranial pressure** creates bilateral papilledema and unilateral or bilateral sixth nerve palsies. Fourth nerve palsies occur occasionally, and third nerve palsies rarely.

10. Inflammatory, infectious, and neoplastic disorders of the **meninges** and head **trauma** with shearing forces can damage single or multiple cranial nerves. Severe mastoiditis causes a sixth nerve palsy associated with ipsilateral facial pain and facial palsy.

11. The **Guillain-Barré syndrome** and its variant, the **Miller-Fisher syndrome** (ophthalmoplegia, ataxia, and areflexia), can cause cranial nerve palsies.

12. **Transtentorial herniation** can compress the third nerve, initially producing pupillary dilation and later causing EOM paresis as it progresses.

13. **Congenital cranial nerve palsies** are less common than acquired palsies. Patients with congenital third nerve palsies usually have miotic pupils with abnormal reflexes. The miosis results from aberrant regeneration. Congenital sixth nerve palsies are usually associated with other neurologic or systemic malformations—e.g., **Möbius' syndrome** (bilateral sixth and seventh nerve palsies). In **Duane's retraction syndrome,** a sixth nerve palsy is associated with narrowing of the ipsilateral palpebral fissure and retraction of the paretic eye backward into the orbit when the paretic eye adducts.

D. **Cavernous sinus.** Because nerves in the cavernous sinus continue into the adjacent superior orbital fissure, syndromes of both structures are similar. Lesions in the cavernous sinus—e.g., **tumors, aneurysms,** and **carotid-cavernous fistulas**—produce single or multiple cranial nerve palsies.

1. Granulomatous inflammation at the superior orbital fissure or in the cavernous sinus in the **Tolosa-Hunt syndrome** also causes multiple cranial nerve palsies and severe pain. The pain and diplopia improve with systemic corticosteroids. However, ophthalmoplegia caused by aneurysms and tumors can produce the same findings that also respond to corticosteroids.

2. The third, fourth, sixth, and fifth nerves (sensory divisions 1 and 2) and the postganglionic sympathetic axons to the eye traverse the cavernous sinus. Sensory loss in the face and **Horner's syndrome** (sympathetic axons travel with sixth nerve in posterior part of cavernous sinus) might accompany diplopia.

3. In third nerve palsies, the pupils are totally or partially spared and are normal in size or only slightly dilated. Simultaneous damage to postganglionic, sympathetic axons to the iris dilator muscle prevents greater pupillary dilation. Lesions of the cavernous sinus often cause dilation of the retinal veins by obstructing venous flow from the eye and orbit into the cavernous sinus.

4. **Meningiomas** are the most common primary tumors in adults. **Pituitary tumors** can extend into an adjacent cavernous sinus. Hemorrhagic infarction of a pituitary adenoma produces severe pain, obtundation, bilateral cranial nerve palsies, and bilateral blindness (pituitary apoplexy).

5. **Cavernous sinus thrombosis** from bacterial infection extending from the orbit (orbital cellulitis) into the cavernous sinus causes unilateral or bilateral cranial nerve palsies, severe pain, and dilation of retinal veins, and is also a medical emergency.

6. **Intracavernous carotid aneurysms** cause cranial nerve palsies, often with pain. The risk of rupture is less than that with other intracranial aneurysms because the intracavernous aneurysm is supported by the surrounding venous sinus.

7. **Traumatic and spontaneous carotid cavernous fistulas** cause unilateral or bilateral cranial nerve palsies, periocular edema, and dilation (arterialization) of conjunctival veins arranged radially around the corneas.

E. **Brainstem.** Brainstem lesions cause diplopia from nuclear and fascicular cranial nerve palsies, internuclear ophthalmoplegia, and skew deviation. Common etiologies are **demyelination** (multiple sclerosis and postviral) and **ischemia** (hypertension, diabetes mellitus, arteriosclerosis, and vasculitis).

1. Unilateral lesions of the **oculomotor nucleus** cause ipsilateral paresis of the EOMs innervated by the third nerve, bilateral ptosis, and bilateral supe-

rior rectus paresis. The ipsilateral superior rectus subnucleus projects to the contralateral superior rectus. The crossing fibers from the contralateral subnucleus to the ipsilateral superior rectus are interrupted by the nuclear lesion. Patients have bilateral ptosis because the levator superioris palpebrae subnucleus that innervates both lid levators is located in the midline.

2. The **trochlear nucleus** innervates the contralateral superior oblique muscle. Head trauma and hydrocephalus can produce bilateral fourth nerve palsies by damaging the fascicles decussating in the anterior medullary velum.

3. Lesions of the **abducens nucleus** cause an ipsilateral horizontal gaze palsy. The nucleus contains motor neurons of the ipsilateral lateral rectus and interneurons that decussate and project through the contralateral medial longitudinal fasciculus (MLF) to the contralateral medial rectus subnucleus.

4. **Fascicular lesions** or **nuclear lesions** of each cranial nerve usually damage adjacent structures in the brainstem. The syndromes that result include Nothnagel's syndrome (third nerve palsy and contralateral cerebellar ataxia), Benedikt's syndrome (third nerve palsy and contralateral tremor), Weber's syndrome (third nerve palsy and contralateral hemiparesis), Foville's syndrome (ipsilateral horizontal gaze palsy or sixth nerve palsy, facial palsy, facial analgesia, loss of taste, Horner's syndrome, deafness, and contralateral hemiplegia), Raymond's syndrome (sixth nerve palsy and contralateral hemiplegia), and the Millard-Gubler syndrome (ipsilateral sixth nerve palsy, facial palsy, and contralateral hemiplegia).

5. Damage to the MLF produces **internuclear ophthalmoplegia** (INO). INO is characterized by paresis of the ipsilateral medial rectus, slowing of saccades generated by the medial rectus, overshooting of abducting saccades (contralateral lateral rectus), and dissociated nystagmus in contralateral gaze (nystagmus in abducting eye larger than in adducting eye). Patients complain of diplopia in contralateral gaze. In addition, upbeat nystagmus and skew deviation are often present. Demyelination is the most common cause of bilateral INO; ischemia is the most common etiology of unilateral INO.

6. **Skew deviation** is a vertical misalignment of the eyes that is not a result of a third or fourth nerve palsy. It is usually caused by lesions of the brainstem or cerebellum.

II. Evaluation

A. History. The type of onset (gradual or sudden); the presence, type, and location of pain; and the progression over time (increasing, decreasing, stable, or variable) should be questioned. The history should establish the direction of the diplopia (vertical, horizontal, oblique, or torsional) and whether or not closure of either eye abolishes diplopia (binocular diplopia vs. monocular diplopia). Other ocular symptoms (ptosis, pupillary dilation, visual loss, periocular edema, injection, ptosis, and proptosis), neurologic symptoms, and the existence of systemic diseases are important.

B. Physical examination. The general physical examination and neurologic examination should look for a compensatory head position (face turn in third and sixth nerve palsies and head tilt in fourth nerve palsy), facial palsy, and sensory loss in the face (fifth cranial nerve). The ocular examination measures visual acuity and confrontation visual fields, and seeks signs of ptosis or retraction of

Table 12-3. Eye tests for ophthalmoplegia.

Monocular occlusion (monocular vs. binocular diplopia)
Cover test for tropia (primary gaze, eccentric gaze)
Alternate cover test for phoria
Hirschberg corneal reflex test for tropia
Ductions
Oculocephalic maneuver
Saccades
Eyelid position and movement
Pupil size and reflexes
Proptosis and periocular signs
Facial sensation

the eyelids, periocular inflammation, proptosis, and anisocoria. Table 12-3 lists the eye tests that evaluate ophthalmoplegias.

1. Covering each eye differentiates **monocular diplopia** from **binocular diplopia** (see below).
2. The **cover test** detects a tropia, which is a misalignment of the eyes when both eyes are opened and binocular vision is possible. While the patient fixates a small target straight ahead, cover one eye with an occluder and watch the other eye. If that eye makes a refixation movement, it was not aligned on the target. If the eye moves nasally, it was misaligned temporally and the patient has an exotropia. Refixation temporally signifies an esotropia, downward movement indicates a hypertropia, and upward movement reveals a hypotropia. If the eye does not refixate, remove the occluder and pause momentarily to allow binocular vision to be reestablished. Then cover the second eye and look for refixation of the first eye.
   a. Third nerve palsies produce exotropia and hypotropia of the paretic eye. Sixth nerve palsies cause an esotropia of the affected eye. Fourth nerve palsies create a hypertropia and excyclotorsion of the paretic eye.
   b. Tropias are commonly caused by **nonparalytic strabismus** beginning in childhood. The image from the deviated eye is suppressed, and there is no diplopia. Patients do not have an ophthalmoplegia, and there is no limitation of eye movements. The cover test can be repeated in eccentric horizontal and vertical gazes. In nonparalytic strabismus, the amount of tropia does not change.
   c. In paralytic strabismus, the tropia increases when the eyes gaze in the direction of action of the paretic muscle in which the muscle is maximally active, and decreases in the opposite direction of gaze in which the paretic muscle is relaxed.
   d. Patients often have a habitual face turn that moves the eyes away from the field of action of the paretic muscle and minimizes the tropia and diplopia. For example, a patient with a right sixth nerve palsy turns the face to the right, placing the eyes in left gaze. The right sixth nerve palsy produces an esotropia of the right eye in center gaze. The esotropia increases in right gaze and decreases in left gaze. Patients with fourth nerve palsies often tilt their heads toward the shoulder opposite the side of the paretic superior oblique muscle to decrease the hypertropia and cyclotorsional diplopia.
   e. The **Park's three-step test** detects the pattern of a fourth nerve palsy.
      (1) In center gaze, the hypertropic eye is the paretic eye. For example, a right fourth nerve palsy produces a right hypertropia.
      (2) The hypertropia increases when the patient looks to the opposite side. For example, the right hypertropia is greater looking to the left than to the right.
      (3) The hypertropia increases when the patient tilts the head to the same side. For example, the right hypertropia is larger when the head tilts toward the right shoulder than when it tilts toward the left shoulder.
3. If the cover test reveals no tropia, test for a phoria with the **alternate cover test.** A phoria is misalignment of the eyes when binocular vision is absent. While the patient looks at the target straight ahead, cover one eye with the occluder and then move the occluder quickly to cover the other eye so that there is no opportunity for binocular vision to be established. Move the occluder alternately between the eyes. If the eyes make refixation movements when they are uncovered, they were misaligned when occluded. Nasal movements identify an exophoria (each eye was deviated temporally under cover), temporal movements an esophoria, and vertical refixation movements a hyperphoria. Phorias do not cause diplopia because the eyes are aligned when both eyes are opened simultaneously. However, under certain conditions—e.g., fatigue or generalized CNS depression—phorias can "break down" and become tropias, causing diplopia.
4. When a patient cannot fixate a small target (poor vision or cooperation), the **Hirschberg corneal reflex test** can detect a tropia. Position a penlight in front of the eyes so that the bright corneal reflex is centered in the pupil of one eye. If the reflex in the other eye is also in the center of the pupil, the eyes are aligned. If it is displaced temporally, the eye is deviated nasally (es-

otropia). Nasal displacement signifies an exotropia, upward displacement a hypotropia, and a downward deviation a hypertropia.

5. The **ductions** (ranges of motion) of the EOMs should be tested. While the first eye is occluded, the second eye follows the examiner's target—e.g., pen point held in front of the patient. The examiner moves the target horizontally and vertically into the primary fields of action of the EOMs. The maximum range of motion from center gaze is normally 45–50 degrees. The examiner should try to estimate the range of motion—e.g., one-third of the maximum is 15 degrees, one-half is 30 degrees, and full movement is 45 degrees. This measurement reflects the severity of EOM palsy. The examiner covers the second eye and measures the first eye's ductions. Ductions should be tested with monocular viewing, because binocular viewing can give a false impression of limited ductions when a nonparalytic strabismus is present. For example, if a patient has a nonparalytic left esotropia and fixates the target with the right eye, in left gaze the left eye will not be fully abducted, giving the impression that weakness of the left lateral rectus muscle exists.

6. The **oculocephalic maneuver** (doll's eye test) evaluates ductions when the patient is unconscious. The examiner rapidly thrusts the patient's head horizontally and vertically. The vestibulo-ocular reflex rotates the eyes in the opposite direction. This maneuver can also identify a supranuclear gaze palsy in an alert patient. For example, patients with Parinaud's syndrome and a supranuclear palsy of up gaze cannot voluntarily look up, but thrusting of the head down rotates the eyes upward. Forced closure of the eyelids normally causes the eyes to supraduct (Bell's phenomenon). A patient with a supranuclear palsy of upgaze might still show a normal Bell's phenomenon.

7. **Saccades** are rapid, conjugate, voluntary eye movements between objects. The examiner holds small targets (e.g., the fingertips) 30 degrees to the patient's right and 30 degrees to the left, or 30 degrees up and 30 degrees down, and verbally commands the patient to look back and forth between the targets. Normal saccades have high velocities (up to 800 degrees per second) and are accurate.

   a. Most ophthalmoplegias—e.g., cranial nerve palsies, internuclear ophthalmoplegia, and CPEO—cause slowing of saccades. When the paretic eye makes a saccade into the field of action of the weak muscle, the examiner detects that that eye reaches the target *after* the normal eye. The examiner can watch one eye and notice that the paretic eye has slow saccades into the field of the weak muscle and normal saccades into the opposite field. Slowing of saccades is a more sensitive sign of most ophthalmoplegias than limitation of duction.

   b. Many patients with myasthenia gravis can make small saccades with normal velocities despite very limited ductions. Saccades in restrictive orbitopathies—e.g., Graves' ophthalmopathy and orbital blowout fracture—can have normal velocities until they are made into the field of restriction.

8. The examiner should measure **lid position.** The margins of the upper eyelids usually intersect the edges of the corneas at the 10 and 2 o'clock positions. A higher position might signify pathologic lid retraction in Graves' ophthalmopathy or Parinaud's syndrome. A lower position might indicate ptosis.

   a. When asymmetric lid positions are present, the difference should be measured with a ruler. The examiner measures the actions of the lid levators, levator palpebrae superioris, by measuring the excursion of the upper eyelid margin from extreme downgaze to extreme upgaze. The normal excursion is about 15 mm. In ptosis due to paresis of the lid levator, the excursion is decreased.

   b. Myasthenia gravis causes fatigue of the lid levator. The examiner uses fingers of one hand to press against the eyebrows to prevent brow lift, and holds a target above the patient for 30 sec. As the patient maintains upward gaze, the examiner watches for a gradual descent of the upper lids. Myasthenia gravis can cause Cogan's lid twitch sign. The patient looks from downgaze to center gaze. The upper eyelid momentarily overshoots the normal lid position.

9. The examiner observes **pupillary size** and **reflexes.** The patient fixates a small distant target in a well-lit room. A difference in pupillary diameter between the eyes (anisocoria) of 1 mm can be normal.

   a. If the examiner finds a small anisocoria (1–2 mm), the upper lid is 1–2 mm lower in the miotic eye, and the lower lid in the same eye is 1 mm higher, a Horner's syndrome might be present. The examiner should measure the pupillary diameters in a dark room. In Horner's syndrome, the anisocoria increases in the dark. Administration of topical cocaine can confirm the presence of a Horner's syndrome. Topical hydroxyamphetamine can identify damage to the third-order neuron in the sympathetic pathway to the iris dilator muscle.

   b. In third nerve palsies, parasympathetic innervation to the iris sphincter muscle can be interrupted or spared (pupil sparing). If it is interrupted, the pupil is dilated, and pupillary constrictions to direct stimulation by light and in the near reflex (focusing on a near target) are decreased or absent. While the patient fixates a distant target, the examiner shines a bright penlight beam into each eye and compares the speeds and amplitudes of the pupillary constrictions of the two eyes. If the parasympathetic innervation is partially interrupted (partial pupil sparing), the pupil is slightly dilated and its reactions are decreased, but still present.

10. The examiner looks for **proptosis** and **periocular signs.**

   a. Narrow palpebral fissures (openings between upper and lower lids) give the appearance of enophthalmos (recession of the eye into the orbit), and wide palpebral fissures make the eye look proptotic (bulging out of the orbit). To confirm the presence of enophthalmos or exophthalmos, the examiner stands behind the patient, looks over the patient's brows, and compares the positions of the two corneas relative to themselves and to the superior orbital rims.

   b. A mass in the orbit increases resistance in the orbit. The examiner gently pushes against the closed eyelids and judges the resistance to retrodisplacement of each eye. The orbit with a mass lesion causing proptosis seems stiffer.

   c. The examiner also should look for lid edema and conjunctival injection.

   d. Perception of light touch and pin prick in the three sensory divisions of the trigeminal nerve should be tested.

C. Laboratory studies. The probable localizations and etiologies of ophthalmoplegia dictate which laboratory tests should be ordered.

1. Blood tests

   a. The work-up of myopathies and orbital disorders includes antiacetylcholine (anti-ACh) receptor antibody titers and antistriated muscle antibody titers for myasthenia gravis, and T-3, T-4, and thyroid-stimulating hormone (TSH) levels for Graves' ophthalmopathy. If myasthenia gravis affects only or primarily the extraocular muscles (ocular myasthenia gravis), anti-ACh receptor titers are elevated in only about 50% of patients. There is no direct correlation between thyroid hormone levels and the activity of Graves' ophthalmopathy. However, abnormal hormone levels indicate abnormal thyroid function, which can corroborate the ocular diagnosis, and hormone testing is important for the patient's general health.

   b. The work-up of an isolated cranial nerve palsy should include tests for diabetes mellitus and vasculitis. Because a cranial nerve palsy can be the initial sign of type II diabetes, a fasting blood sugar, a 2-hour postprandial blood sugar, and a serum hemoglobin A_{1c} level should be ordered. A CBC, an antinuclear antibody titer, an anti-DNA titer, and a Westergren sedimentation rate can identify vasculitides, such as systemic lupus erythematosus and giant cell arteritis. The work-up of brainstem lesions includes the tests for vasculitis. If ischemia is a possible cause in a young adult, the lupus anticoagulant syndrome might be considered and antiphospholipid antibody titers measured.

2. Cerebrospinal fluid. A lumbar puncture (LP) should evaluate the CSF in cranial nerve palsies if the examiner suspects that increased intracranial pressure causes a cranial nerve palsy or that inflammatory, infectious, or neoplastic diseases produce cranial nerve palsies or brainstem disorders. The opening pressure must be recorded, and a CT or MRI scan should be obtained before the LP if increased intracranial pressure is suspected.

3. CT and MRI scans. Neuroradiologic tests are indicated in some myopathies, orbital disorders, cranial nerve palsies, and brainstem disorders.

CT scanning is usually satisfactory in studying disorders of the EOMs and orbits. The examiner should request direct coronal and axial views of the orbits and paranasal sinuses with intravenous contrast administration. Patients with obvious Graves' ophthalmopathy do not need CT scans unless visual loss from optic nerve compression occurs. MRI scans are usually better than CT scans in imaging the orbital apex, superior orbital fissure, cavernous sinus, sella, and sphenoid bone. The examiner should request coronal and axial views with and without injection of gadolinium and with fat-suppression techniques for the orbit. MRI scans of the posterior fossa should be used to evaluate brainstem disorders.

   4. Other tests
      a. If myasthenia gravis is a likely etiology for diplopia and ophthalmoplegia, the examiner should perform an antiacetylcholinesterase test. **Edrophonium (Tensilon)** should be used for adults and older children, and **neostigmine (Prostigmin)** is used for young children and other patients whose ability to cooperate is limited. The examiner must measure the ptosis, tropia, and/or limitation of ductions before and after drug administration. For the edrophonium test, a short intravenous line (e.g., butterfly) is placed in a hand or arm vein and is kept opened and flushed with a 10- or 20-ml syringe of saline. In adults, 0.4 mg of atropine (1 ml of a 0.4 mg/ml solution) is given to block some of the systemic side effects of edrophonium. Saline flushes the IV line after each drug injection. The examiner injects small amounts of edrophonium (10 mg/ml) with a 1-ml tuberculin syringe. Aliquots of 1, 3, 3, and 3 mg are given serially to reduce systemic side effects. After each aliquot, the examiner measures the eye findings over the next 2 minutes. If a definite improvement occurs, the next aliquot is not injected. Alternatively, the examiner injects 0.04 mg/kg of neostigmine intramuscularly (up to the adult dose of 1.5 mg) and measures the eye signs 30 minutes later. Whereas the effects of edrophonium persist for only several minutes, those of neostigmine can last up to 1 hour.
      b. Patients with CPEO should have an **EKG** to detect a cardiac myopathy (conduction defect) caused by the mitochondrial cytopathy.
III. Differential diagnosis. The disorders described above produce misalignment of the eyes and **binocular diplopia.** Covering either eye abolishes the diplopia. In **monocular diplopia,** the eyes are not misaligned. One eye usually has an abnormality of the ocular media and produces multiple images. When the abnormal eye is covered, the diplopia disappears. Covering the abnormal eye does not abolish the diplopia. Uncorrected refractive errors—e.g., astigmatism, irregularities of the corneal surface, corneal opacities, and cataracts—are the most common etiologies of monocular diplopia. When the subject views with the abnormal eye, one image is usually clear and the second image is blurred (ghost image). Refraction or viewing through a pinhole usually abolishes monocular diplopia. In rare cases, lesions in the parieto-occipital cortex cause monocular diplopia.
IV. Referral. If a patient complains persistently of diplopia, a tropia is detected, or a limitation of ductions is found, the patient should be referred to a neurologist, ophthalmologist, or neuro-ophthalmologist. These specialists can confirm the findings, suggest the differential diagnosis, recommend laboratory tests, and help treat the patient. Treatment could include temporary patching of one eye, eyeglasses with prisms, or EOM surgery. Most cases of diplopia and ophthalmoplegia do not require urgent referral. However, when patients are likely to have diseases that can quickly cause severe morbidity or mortality, the referral, work-up, and treatment must proceed rapidly. The subsections that follow describe the initial management of patients with cranial nerve palsies (intracranial aneurysms), orbital apex syndrome (phycomycosis), cavernous sinus thrombosis (bacterial orbital cellulitis), pituitary apoplexy (pituitary adenoma), and ischemic myopathy (giant cell arteritis) as examples of why urgent referrals might be needed.
   A. Cranial nerve palsy
      1. Compression by an aneurysm at the junction of the posterior communicating artery and internal carotid artery is an infrequent, but important, cause of third nerve palsy because of the risk of spontaneous rupture and high risk of severe morbidity and mortality if a rupture occurs. Aneurysms of the posterior inferior cerebellar artery, basilar artery, and intracavernous carotid artery less frequently cause sixth nerve palsy. Intracavernous aneurysms are

less likely to rupture because the venous structures and dura of the cavernous sinus surround them. Aneurysms rarely produce fourth nerve palsy.

2. Ischemia of the subarachnoid or intracavernous portions of the cranial nerves is the most common etiology of isolated cranial nerve palsies in adults (microvascular cranial nerve palsies). Patients usually have histories of diabetes mellitus, hypertension, arteriosclerosis, or migraine. Obstruction of small blood vessels supplying the peripheral nerve produces sudden diplopia and ophthalmoplegia that are often accompanied by pain behind the affected eye. Improvement in the diplopia and ophthalmoplegia occurs within the following 4 to 6 weeks, and recovery is complete within 6 months in the large majority of patients.

3. **Microvascular third nerve palsy** usually spares pupillary reactions. If the extraocular muscles innervated by the third nerve are severely affected, but pupillary size and reactions to light and near are normal **(pupil-sparing third nerve palsy),** the most likely etiology is ischemia and an aneurysm is unlikely. After doing the initial examination and obtaining the screening laboratory tests mentioned above, the examiner reevaluates the patient in 2 weeks if diabetes mellitus, hypertension, arteriosclerosis, or migraine is present. If there is no history of these systemic diseases, the patient should return in 1 week to be examined for signs of pupillary involvement or progression of paresis. The paretic eye can be patched to avoid diplopia. In microvascular cranial nerve palsies, signs of improvement should be observed within 4–6 weeks after the onset. The examiner must measure the tropia, ductions, and lid findings at the initial examination so that improvement can be detected in follow-up visits.

4. If the pupil becomes affected, EOM paresis increases, improvement does not occur within 4–6 weeks, or full recovery does not occur within 6 months, an MRI scan of the orbits, sella, and posterior fossa with and without gadolinium, as well as MR angiography and an LP, should be ordered to seek other etiologies.

5. If the extraocular muscles are severely paretic, the pupil is mildly dilated, and pupillary reactions are slightly decreased **(partial pupil-sparing third nerve palsy),** a microvascular third nerve palsy is probably present and aneurysmal compression is still unlikely. The patient can be followed as described above. Compression of the third nerve in the cavernous sinus—e.g., by a meningioma of the cavernous sinus—often produces this type of third nerve palsy, but in this case the palsy usually does not show spontaneous improvement.

6. If the pupil is widely dilated and pupillary reactions are absent **(non-pupil-sparing third nerve palsy),** a microvascular cause is unlikely. Compression by an aneurysm or tumor, inflammation, or infiltration is often the etiology. Occasionally, diabetes mellitus causes a non-pupil-sparing third nerve palsy, but aneurysmal compression is the most common cause. The examiner should request an MRI study of the orbits, sella, and posterior fossa, with and without gadolinium, and an MR angiography of the intracranial arteries immediately. The MRA can detect intracranial aneurysms with diameters of 5 mm or greater. The most common site of an aneurysm causing a third nerve palsy is the junction of the posterior communicating artery and the internal carotid artery. However, MRA cannot exclude smaller aneurysms. Although small aneurysms are less likely to rupture than larger ones, the cerebral angiogram is still the gold standard test and should be ordered if the MRA is normal. The examiner should perform an LP if the neuroimaging studies are normal.

7. Pupil sparing when the third nerve EOMs are only mildly paretic or when some third nerve EOMs are not affected is not as reassuring that there is a microvascular etiology as pupil sparing with severe EOM paresis. Compressive lesions in the subarachnoid space and cavernous sinus, including aneurysms and tumors, can produce pupil-sparing third nerve palsies. However, the EOM paresis is usually partial. In this instance, both MRI and MRA should be ordered. If they are normal, the patient is reevaluated in 1 month.

8. Patients with multiple cranial nerve palsies should have MR scans with and without gadolinium to seek lesions at the orbital apex, superior orbital fissure, cavernous sinus, sella, meninges, and brainstem.

B. Phycomycosis of the orbit. The phycomycetes—e.g., mucor—cause opportunistic infections of the oronasopharynx and paranasal sinuses in patients with metabolic acidosis. Diabetic ketoacidosis is a frequent predisposing disorder. The infection rapidly spreads to the orbits, producing a painful orbital apex syndrome with ophthalmoplegia and loss of vision. The examiner should look for black, necrotic lesions of the mouth and nose; immediately obtain a CT scan of the orbits and paranasal sinuses; and request consultations to treat the acidosis, begin antimicrobial medications, and obtain biopsies. Prompt reversal of acidosis, intravenous administration of amphotericin B, lavage of infected tissues with amphotericin B, and excision of necrotic tissue can achieve recovery without extensive debridement of infected tissues.

C. Cavernous sinus thrombosis. Bacterial infection of the cavernous sinus causes abrupt, painful, bilateral cranial nerve palsies. Multiple cranial nerves to both eyes are affected because the cavernous sinuses are connected. The retinal veins are dilated because venous return from the orbits into the cavernous sinuses is obstructed. Cavernous sinus thrombosis usually occurs after an orbital cellulitis has been present. Orbital cellulitis usually follows trauma to the eyelids or orbits, and is rarely caused by hematogenous spread of bacteria. The examiner should immediately order CT scans of the orbits, paranasal sinuses, and cavernous sinuses, and request consultations for drainage of an abscess, culturing of infected tissues, and institution of systemic antibiotics.

D. Pituitary apoplexy. Hemorrhagic infarction of a pituitary tumor causes sudden, severe pain, bilateral ophthalmoplegia, binocular loss of vision, and prostration from pituitary insufficiency. Cranial nerves in both cavernous sinuses and both intracranial optic nerves are damaged. The retinal blood vessels are dilated. The examiner should immediately begin treatment for pituitary insufficiency and obtain an MRI or CT scan of the sella and cavernous sinuses. Urgent transsphenoidal decompression of the sella may salvage vision and cranial nerve function.

E. Ischemic myopathy and cranial nerve palsy from giant cell arteritis. Giant cell arteritis (temporal arteritis) produces characteristic systemic symptoms in the elderly. These symptoms include headache, enlarged and tender temporal arteries, scalp tenderness, jaw claudication, myalgias of limb muscles, fatigue, weight loss, and fever. Infarction of the short posterior ciliary arteries that supply the optic disks causes sudden, severe visual loss and pale swelling of the optic disk of one eye (anterior ischemic optic neuropathy). Giant cell arteritis rarely produces sudden ophthalmoplegia and diplopia by obstructing ophthalmic artery branches to the EOMs or ischemia of the cranial nerves. If a patient with sudden ophthalmoplegia has systemic symptoms suggestive of giant cell arteritis, the examiner should immediately obtain a Westergren sedimentation rate and C-reactive protein level. The sedimentation rate normally increases with age. Dividing a male's age (in years) by 2 approximates the upper limit of the normal sedimentation rate (mm/hr) for that patient. In females, the patient's age plus 10 is divided by 2. Giant cell arteritis and other systemic inflammatory disorders also increase C-reactive protein level. If the sedimentation rate and C-reactive protein level are abnormally high, the patient should begin taking 100 mg of prednisone q.d. immediately, and a temporal artery biopsy should be performed in the next several days. The examiner obtains the laboratory tests and begins treatment immediately to avoid permanent visual loss from anterior ischemic optic neuropathy (infarction of the optic disk from occlusion of branches of the posterior ciliary arteries).

Recommended Readings

Biller J, et al. Oculomotor nuclear complex infarction: Clinical and radiological correlation. *Arch Neurol* 41:985, 1984.

De Keizer RJW. Spontaneous carotid-cavernous fistulas. *Neuro-ophthalmology* 2:35, 1981.

DiNubile MJ. Septic thrombosis of the cavernous sinuses. *Arch Neurol* 45:567, 1988.

Feldon SE, Weiner JM. Clinical significance of extraocular muscle volumes in Graves' ophthalmopathy: A quantitative computed tomographic study. *Arch Ophthalmol* 100:1266, 1982.

Forteza G, Burgeno M. Rhinocerebral mucormycosis: Presentation of two cases and review of the literature. *J Craniomaxillofac Surg* 16(2):80, 1988.

Gerbitz KD, et al. Mitochondrial myopathies: Divergences of genetic deletions, biochemical defects and the clinical syndromes. *J Neurol* 237:5, 1990.

Goldberg RT. Ocular muscle paresis and cranial arteritis: An unusual case. *Ann Ophthalmol* 15:240, 1983.

Harley RD. Paralytic strabismus in children: Etiologic incidence and management of third, fourth, and sixth nerve palsies. *Ophthalmology* 86:24, 1980.

Hirst LW, Miller NR, Johnson RT. Monocular polyopia. *Arch Neurol* 40:756, 1983.

Hunt WE, Brighton RP. The Tolosa-Hunt syndrome: A problem in differential diagnosis. *Acta Neurochir Suppl (Wien)* 42:248, 1988.

Kline LB. The Tolosa-Hunt syndrome. *Surv Ophthalmol* 27:79, 1982.

Kushner BJ. Errors in the three-step test in the diagnosis of vertical strabismus. *Ophthalmology* 96:447, 1989.

Leigh RJ, Zee DS. *The Neurology of Eye Movements* (2nd ed). Philadelphia: Davis, 1991.

McKhann GM. Guillain-Barré syndrome: Clinical and therapeutic observations. *Ann Neurol* 27(suppl):S13, 1990.

Meienberg O, Buttner-Ennerver JA, Kraus-Ruppert R. Unilateral paralysis of conjugate gaze due to lesion of the abducens nucleus. *Neuro-ophthalmology* 2:47, 1981.

Meienberg O, Ryffel E. Supranuclear eye movement disorders in Fisher's syndrome of ophthalmoplegia, ataxia, and areflexia. *Arch Neurol* 40:402, 1983.

Miller NR. *Walsh and Hoyt's Clinical Neuro-Ophthalmology* (4th ed, vol 2). Baltimore: Williams & Wilkins, 1994.

Newman NJ. Third-, fourth-, and sixth-nerve lesions and the cavernous sinus. Chapter 194 in DM Albert, FA Jacobiec (eds), *Principles and Practice of Ophthalmology. Clinical Practice* (vol 4). Philadelphia: Saunders, 1994.

Palestine AG, Younge BR, Piepgras DG. Visual prognosis in carotid-cavernous fistula. *Arch Ophthalmol* 99:1600, 1981.

Richards BW, Jones FR, Younge BR. Causes and prognosis in 4,278 cases of paralysis of the oculomotor, trochlear, and abducens cranial nerves. *Am J Ophthalmol* 113:489, 1992.

Sibony PA, Lessell S, Gittinger JW. Acquired oculomotor synkinesis. *Review Surv Ophthalmol* 28:382, 1984.

Soliven BC. Sero-negative myasthenia gravis. *Neurology* 38:514, 1988.

Soni SR. Aneurysms of the posterior communicating artery and oculomotor paresis. *J Neurol Neurosurg Psychiatry* 37:475, 1974.

Striph GG, Burde RM. Abducens nerve palsy and Horner's syndrome revisited. *J Clin Neuro-Ophthalmol* 8:13, 1988.

Terranova W, Palumbo JN, Breman JG. Ocular findings in botulism type B. *JAMA* 241:475, 1979.

Trobe JD. Isolated pupil-sparing third nerve palsy. *Ophthalmology* 92:58, 1985.

Trobe JD, Glaser JS, Post JD. Meningiomas and aneurysms of the cavernous sinus: Neuro-ophthalmologic features. *Arch Ophthalmol* 96:457, 1978.

Wakai S, et al. Pituitary apoplexy: Its incidence and clinical significance. *J Neurosurg* 55:187, 1981.

Yee RD, et al. Rapid eye movements in myasthenia gravis. II: Electro-oculographic analysis. *Arch Ophthalmol* 94:1465, 1976.

Yee RD, et al. Saccadic eye movements in myasthenia gravis. *Ophthalmology* 94:219, 1987.

Younge BR, Sutula F. Analysis of trochlear nerve palsies: Diagnosis, etiology, and treatment. *Mayo Clin Proc* 52:11, 1977.

13

Approach to the Patient with Facial Numbness

Betsy B. Love
Catherine S. Mueller

I. Introduction
  A. Definition of facial numbness. Isolated facial numbness is often descriptive of impairment of sensation of the face as a result of dysfunction of the trigeminal system or central trigeminal pathways. Patients may complain of unilateral or bilateral facial numbness, paresthesias (a spontaneous abnormal sensation), or dysesthesias (an unpleasant abnormal sensation produced by normal stimuli). There may be associated symptoms of altered sensation of the mucous membranes of the nose, mouth, gums, palate, or teeth. Facial numbness may be a part of a syndrome involving other cranial nerves, in addition to the trigeminal nerve. Trigeminal nerve dysfunction associated with pain is discussed in Chap. 14.
  B. Types. The types of facial numbness that are covered in this chapter include conditions that may present with isolated facial numbness, including lesions of the trigeminal nerve branches (e.g., trauma, tumor, connective tissue diseases, etc.), the gasserian ganglion or root (infection, tumors, nontumorous masses, etc.), and the central trigeminal pathways (stroke, tumor, vascular anomalies, etc.). Facial numbness is an uncommon, but not rare, condition. A patient with a complaint of facial numbness may present to a dentist, primary physician, neurologist, or otolaryngologist. The typical clinical scenario is a gradual onset of numbness in one or more regions of the face, usually unilaterally. Because the presence of facial numbness may indicate a serious underlying condition, each patient with this symptom requires a thorough evaluation.
  C. Facial numbness as a symptom of a life-threatening disorder. Facial numbness may represent not only a serious underlying condition that needs to be evaluated expeditiously but in some rare instances a medical condition that needs to be dealt with emergently. Facial numbness is rarely the presenting sign of an internal carotid artery dissection, carotid aneurysm, intracranial hemorrhage, or intracranial or nasopharyngeal tumor. However, in most instances, there are associated features that may point to one of these serious etiologies. If there are features suggestive of a carotid artery dissection or intracranial aneurysm, an emergent brain CT and a cerebral arteriogram are warranted. An MRI scan of the head with contrast is indicated if there is suspicion of an intracranial tumor. A brain CT without contrast is indicated if an intracranial hemorrhage is a concern. An otolaryngology consultation should be obtained if symptoms suggest a nasopharyngeal tumor.
II. Etiology. A brief review of the trigeminal pathways is necessary for an understanding of the location of dysfunction with facial numbness.
  A. Neuroanatomy of the trigeminal nerve
    1. The trigeminal (V) nerve is a mixed sensory and motor nerve.
      a. The sensory portion of the nerve is the largest portion, transmitting sensation from areas of the face, oral cavity, and nasal passages.
      b. There are three divisions of the sensory portion of the nerve (Fig. 13-1):
        (1) Ophthalmic (V1). The ophthalmic division provides cutaneous supply to the forehead and anterior scalp to approximately the vertex, parts of the nose and the upper eyelid, and the upper half of the cornea. Branches of this division to the facial structures are the nasociliary, infratrochlear, supratrochlear, lacrimal, and supraorbital nerves.
        (2) Maxillary (V2). The maxillary division provides cutaneous supply to portions of the nose, upper lip, cheek, lower half of the cornea, upper gums and teeth, palate, and nasal mucosa. Branches of this

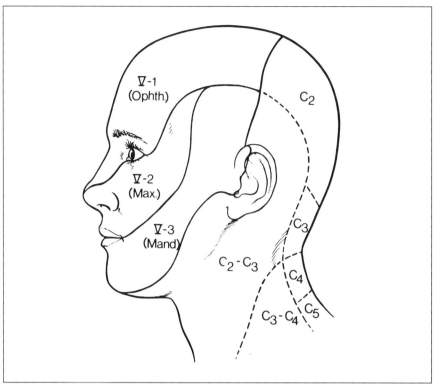

Figure 13-1. Regions of the face supplied by the three sensory divisions of the trigeminal nerve (V1, V2, V3). (From Sears ES, Franklin GM. Diseases of the cranial nerves. In RN Rosenberg (ed), *Neurology.* New York: Grune & Stratton, 1980, with permission.)

divalion are the zygomaticofacial, zygomaticotemporal, and infraorbital nerves.

(3) **Mandibular (V3).** The mandibular division provides cutaneous supply to the lower lip, chin, portions of the jaw, ear, and mouth, lower gums and teeth, and the anterior two-thirds of the tongue. Branches of this division are the auriculotemporal, buccal, and mental nerves. The combined nerve trunk of the mandibular division and the motor portion gives rise to the inferior alveolar nerves and the lingual nerves.

c. The motor portion of the trigeminal nerve is a smaller division that travels with V3. It provides motor function to the muscles of mastication and the tensor tympani. This portion will not be discussed further. However, it is important to examine the patient for dysfunction of the motor portion of the nerve.

2. The three sensory divisions (V1, V2, and V3) enter the cranial cavity through the superior orbital fissure, foramen rotundum, and foramen ovale, respectively, to unite in the gasserian or semilunar ganglion, which lies at the apex of the petrous bones.

3. Second-order sensory neurons enter the pons at the sensory root.

B. **Localization of the lesion with facial numbness** (Table 13-1). Facial numbness is usually unilateral and may be partial or total. Bilateral numbness may be associated with brainstem involvement, leptomeningeal disease, or systemic diseases, or it may be idiopathic. There are some generalizations that help localize the lesion.

1. Lesions of the divisions of V have distinct areas of sensory loss (see Fig. 13-1).

Table 13-1. Types of numbness associated with lesions in different areas of the trigeminal sensory system.

Location of lesion	Areas of facial sensory loss
Ophthalmic (V1) division	Forehead, scalp, nose (except inferolateral), upper eyelid, upper half of cornea
Maxillary (V2) division	Lateral nose, upper lip, cheek, lower half of cornea, upper gums, palate, mucosa of lower nasal cavity
Mandibular (V3) division	Lower lip, lower jaw, chin, tympanic membrane, auditory meatus, upper ear, floor of mouth, lower gums and teeth, anterior two-thirds of tongue
Proximal to gasserian ganglion	Entire face and all structures listed above
Brainstem	Onionskin sensory loss

    2. Lesions proximal to the gasserian ganglion cause cutaneous numbness of the entire face and the anterior scalp (Fig. 13-2).

    3. Lesions of the brainstem may produce an onionskin distribution of sensory loss (Fig. 13-3).

    4. Lesions of V typically spare the angle of the jaw, which is supplied by C2 and C3 (see Fig. 13-1).

  C. Causes of facial numbness (Table 13-2). There are many causes of facial numbness. The different causes will be discussed according to the known or presumed site of involvement of the trigeminal pathway.

    1. Lesions peripheral to the gasserian ganglion (V1, V2, and V3)

      a. Trauma. Injury to the peripheral branches of the trigeminal nerve may occur with head or facial trauma, dental trauma or surgery, or any surgery of the face (e.g., ENT or dermatologic surgery).

        (1) Head or facial injury. The most frequently affected nerves are the superficial branches, including the supraorbital (branch of V1), supratrochlear (branch of V1), and infraorbital (branch of V2) nerves. The sensory loss is temporally related to the injury. Nerve regeneration may be accompanied by facial pain. The supraorbital branch may be damaged by blunt injury or as a result of a fracture of the upper margin of the orbit. The infraorbital nerve may be injured with closed head injuries or maxillary fractures. The entire ophthalmic division (V1) may be damaged in fractures through the foramen ovale. Transverse basilar skull fractures may injure the gasserian ganglion, resulting in anesthesia of the entire face and weakness of the masticatory muscles.

        (2) Dental trauma. Facial numbness may occur after tooth extraction. The lingual nerve may be damaged, usually resulting in transient anesthesia. Also, direct nerve injury may occur as a result of needle trauma during dental anesthesia. Chronic denture use may cause pressure on the mental nerve, resulting in chin numbness.

        (3) Facial surgery. Any surgical procedure involving the face may lead to trigeminal nerve injury.

      b. Infection

        (1) Leprosy. Worldwide, lepromatous leprosy is the most common cause of facial numbness. There can be facial hypalgesia and resultant inadvertent mutilation of the face.

        (2) Herpes zoster. Although the herpes zoster virus resides in the gasserian ganglion, evidence of active infection usually involves a division of the trigeminal nerve. The most commonly affected division is the ophthalmic division.

      c. Systemic diseases

        (1) Sickle cell anemia. Numbness of the chin and lower lip resulting from a mental neuropathy has been described with a sickle cell crisis.

        (2) Diabetes. Facial numbness has been reported with diabetes and may accompany other sensory neuropathies.

        (3) Diffuse connective tissue disease. The presence of facial numb-

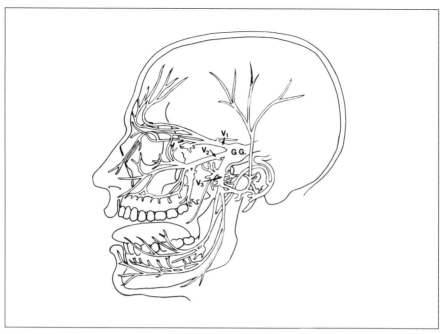

Figure 13-2. Relationship of the divisions of the trigeminal nerve and the gasserian ganglion (GG).

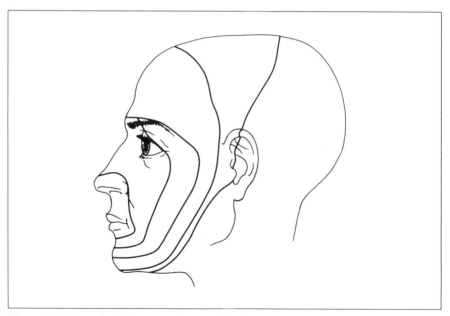

Figure 13-3. The onionskin sensory loss resulting from brainstem lesions.

Table 13-2. Causes of facial numbness.

Lesions Peripheral to the Gasserian Ganglion
Trauma (accidental, dental, surgical)
Infection (leprosy, herpes zoster)
Systemic diseases (sickle cell anemia, diabetes, diffuse connective tissue disease)
Tumor
Inflammatory
Drugs or toxins (stilbamidine, cocaine, others)
Idiopathic trigeminal sensory neuropathy

Lesions of the Gasserian Ganglion Root
Infections (syphilis, tuberculosis, herpes zoster)
Tumor
Nontumorous mass lesions (aneurysm, hydrocephalus)
Sarcoidosis
Arachnoiditis
Amyloid
Drug (trichloroethylene)

Lesions of the Central Trigeminal Pathways
Stroke
Tumor
Syringobulbia
Demyelinating disease
Vascular anomalies

Denotes presumed site of pathology.
(Modified from Hagen et al. with permission)

ness with a connective tissue disorder is rare. It has been associated with scleroderma, Sjögren's syndrome, mixed connective tissue disease, systemic lupus erythematosus, rheumatoid arthritis, and dermatomyositis.

   d. **Tumors.** Regional spread of tumors along the trigeminal nerve can occur. Disease (most commonly lung and breast) metastasizing to the lower jaw may affect the inferior alveolar or mental nerves, causing numbness of the chin and lower lip. Cheek or malar numbness has been described with local spread of tumors along V2 or with leptomeningeal involvement with tumors. Nasopharyngeal tumors (squamous cell carcinoma is most common) arise most frequently in the roof of the pharynx. They may encroach on the trigeminal nerve, producing facial numbness. Associated features may include excessive lacrimation, facial pain, proptosis, hearing loss, and Horner's syndrome.

   e. **Inflammatory lesions.** Paranasal sinusitis may affect some branches of the trigeminal nerve.

   f. **Drugs and toxins**
      (1) **Stilbamidine** is an agent that has been used to treat leishmaniasis and multiple myeloma. Unilateral or bilateral facial numbness and anesthesia have been reported after treatment.
      (2) **Cocaine** abuse by the nasal route is a cause of facial numbness in the territory of the maxillary division (V2). Usually there is associated traumatic and ischemic necrosis of the nasal mucosa.
      (3) **Other drugs.** Many drugs can cause facial paresthesias. Circumoral paresthesias have been reported with labetalol, and a mandibular neuropathy has been reported with allopurinol.

   g. **Vascular disorders.** Rarely, a carotid artery dissection may produce facial numbness.

   h. **Idiopathic trigeminal sensory neuropathy.** This diagnosis is one of exclusion, after serious etiologies have been ruled out. This is discussed further in sec. **III** (Clinical manifestations).

2. **Lesions of the gasserian ganglion or root**

   a. **Infections** of the gasserian ganglion may occur with syphilis, tuberculosis, and herpes zoster.

  b. **Tumors.** Various tumors may affect the gasserian ganglion or root. Tumors that arise in the ganglion (ganglioneuroma or gangliocytoma) tend to have early, associated pain. In contrast, those tumors that arise primarily in the root (neurinoma or neurofibroma) tend to have predominant sensory loss without pain. Tumors that may compress or invade the ganglion or root include acoustic neuromas, meningiomas, schwannomas, metastasis, cholesteatomas, pituitary adenomas, chordomas, and nasopharyngeal carcinomas.
  c. **Nontumorous mass lesions (aneurysm, hydrocephalus)**
  d. **Sarcoidosis**
  e. **Arachnoiditis**
  f. **Amyloid.** Rarely, the gasserian ganglion or root may be the solitary site of amyloid deposits.
  g. **Drug: Trichloroethylene** is an industrial solvent that has been associated with facial numbness.
3. **Lesions of the central trigeminal pathways**
  a. **Stroke.** An infarction in the lateral tegmentum of the medulla (Wallenberg's syndrome) may produce ipsilateral facial numbness, along with other cranial nerve deficits and long tract signs. Rarely, a lateral pontine hemorrhage may cause isolated facial numbness, perhaps as a result of involvement of the main sensory nucleus of the trigeminal nerve.
  b. **Tumors.** Tumors of the pons or medulla may affect the sensory nucleus of V, but there are usually other signs, including long tract and cranial nerve findings.
  c. **Syringobulbia.** This central cavitation of the medulla or pons may be associated with facial numbness.
  d. **Demyelinating disease.** Facial numbness is the initial symptom in 2–3% of patients with multiple sclerosis.
  e. **Vascular anomalies.** Very rarely, isolated facial numbness results from a posterior fossa aneurysm or other vascular malformation.
III. **Clinical manifestations**
  A. **Trigeminal sensory neuropathy.** The literature is rather unclear in its definition of trigeminal sensory neuropathy (TSN). TSN has been used to describe different populations of patients with facial numbness. Blau et al. (1969) described a population of patients with TSN who had self-limited facial paresthesias that in half of the cases resolved in several months. There were no associated neurologic deficits. On neurologic examination, the corneal response was intact and the only finding was a subjective decrease in light touch and pinprick over the involved trigeminal distribution. Only 10% of these patients had identifiable causes of TSN, and 10% went on to develop trigeminal neuralgia.
  In contrast to this population, with a seemingly benign course, Horowitz (1974) found that 88% of a population with facial numbness had an identifiable, usually serious condition. This population almost always had other neurologic deficits (cranial nerve or ataxia). It may be concluded that these two studies involved quite different populations.
  TSN is best defined as a general term for facial numbness of which there are many different causes, as previously discussed. Any area of the face may be involved. Idiopathic TSN is used to describe patients with a purely sensory impairment in a territory of the trigeminal nerve (usually V2 or V3) on one or both sides of the face, of unknown etiology. It may be associated with pain, paresthesias, or dysfunction of taste. Because the data currently available do not allow one to distinguish consistently between facial numbness that is benign and facial numbness that is attributable to a serious condition, idiopathic TSN remains a diagnosis of exclusion after an appropriate, thorough evaluation. Available data do indicate that the presence of associated neurologic signs and deficits usually points to a more ominous process.
  B. **Numb chin and numb cheek syndromes**
  1. **Numb chin syndrome.** Isolated chin numbness is not a common syndrome of facial numbness. However, the numb chin syndrome is rarely caused by benign lesions and often is a symptom of involvement of the mental or inferior alveolar nerves (branches of V3) by systemic cancer. Any tumor metastasizing to the jaw may produce this syndrome, but breast, lung, and lymphoreticular malignancies are observed most commonly. Leptomeningeal

involvement with malignancies, such as lymphoma, is a less common cause. Most patients already have a known diagnosis of cancer. However, a mental neuropathy may be the initial symptom of a malignancy or it may herald tumor recurrence or progression.

The clinical presentation involves ipsilateral numbness or anesthesia of the skin and mucosa of the lower lip and chin, extending to the midline. There is usually no associated pain, but there may be lip swelling and ulcerations from biting of the numb lip.

The evaluation of patients with numb chin syndrome should include x-rays of the mandible, with particular attention to the mental foramen, x-rays of the basal skull, an MRI scan of the brain with contrast, and if there is concern of leptomeningeal infiltration, CSF analysis.

Although a numb chin is a seemingly benign complaint, it should be thoroughly evaluated because of its clinical importance as a possible sign of malignancy.

2. **Numb cheek syndrome.** Numbness over the malar region may have implications that are similar to those of the numb chin syndrome. Squamous or basal cell carcinomas of the face may spread along the trigeminal nerve. Such tumors may also spread from regional nerves to the skull base and into the intracranial space. Numbness of the anterior gums and teeth suggests a more peripheral lesion, whereas both anterior and posterior gum and teeth involvement suggests leptomeningeal disease.

IV. **Evaluation**
  A. **History.** It is important to obtain as much detailed information as possible about the patient's facial numbness. The points that should be addressed include the following.
    1. **Site(s) of numbness,** including whether unilateral or bilateral.
    2. **Duration of numbness**
    3. **Quality of numbness**
    4. **Associated features** (pain, altered taste, and nasal, dental, and cerebrovascular symptoms)
    5. **History of trauma** (accidental, dental, or surgical)
    6. **History of malignancy**
    7. **Medications used currently and in the past**
  B. **Physical examination**
    1. **General physical examination.** A thorough, *complete* examination is necessary to evaluate for a potential cause of the facial numbness. Particular attention needs to be paid to evaluating for an underlying malignancy (including a nasopharyngeal tumor), a dental etiology, or an underlying rheumatologic condition. Although many different areas need to be assessed, the following areas are especially important.
      a. **Head and neck.** Inspection of the nose, mouth, and teeth, and palpation for adenopathy, are important.
      b. **Vascular disorders.** Bilateral blood pressures should be checked to evaluate for vascular disease. Auscultation for carotid or vertebral bruits should be performed. If there is suspicion of an intracranial aneurysm, listen for cranial bruits.
      c. **Breast**
      d. **Pulmonary**
      e. **Lymphatic**
      f. **Rheumatologic**
      g. **Skin**
    2. **Neurologic examination.** A thorough neurologic examination is necessary. It is particularly important to evaluate all of the functions of the trigeminal nerve and to evaluate for evidence of dysfunction of other cranial nerves.
      a. **Clinical evaluation of the trigeminal nerve**
        (1) **Sensory evaluation.** Touch, pain, and temperature are tested in the distribution of the three divisions. Each division is tested individually and is compared with the opposite side. The sensation in the nasal and oral mucosa, the anterior two-thirds of the tongue, and the anterior portion of the ear (tragus and anterior helix) should be assessed.
        (2) **Motor evaluation.** The motor functions of the trigeminal nerve are assessed by testing the muscles of mastication. By having a patient

clench the jaw, the strength of the masseters and temporalis can be tested bilaterally. Weakness is evidenced by absent or reduced contraction of the muscles on the side of the lesion. Test the lateral pterygoids by having the patient move the jaw from side to side against the resistance of your hand. The jaw will deviate toward the paralyzed side on opening the mouth because of contraction of the intact contralateral lateral pterygoid muscle. It cannot be deviated to the opposite, nonparalyzed side. Finally, the patient should be asked to protrude the jaw. Any evidence of atrophy or fasciculation is noted.

    (3) Reflex evaluation

        (a) Corneal reflex. This reflex is performed by touching a wisp of a sterile cotton-tipped applicator to the edge of the cornea (not the sclera) bilaterally. The afferent portion of the reflex is carried by V1 (upper cornea) and V2 (lower cornea), and the efferent portion is carried by cranial nerve VII, both ipsilaterally and contralaterally. Lesions of the trigeminal nerve may cause a diminished or absent response both ipsilaterally and contralaterally.

        (b) Orbicularis oculi reflex (blink reflex). This reflex is performed by tapping the glabella or supraorbital ridge. This illicits an early ipsilateral blink followed by bilateral blinking.

        (c) Sternutatory reflex. This reflex is performed by checking light touch sensation of the lateral nasal mucosa with a cotton-tipped applicator. The appropriate response is immediate withdrawal from the irritating stimulus. This reflex may be diminished or absent in lesions of the maxillary division (V2).

        (d) Masseter reflex or jaw jerk. This reflex is performed by tapping the slightly opened lower jaw. Lesions of the trigeminal nerve may result in a hypoactive ipsilateral jerk, whereas bilateral supranuclear lesions may result in a hyperactive response.

  b. The remainder of the neurologic examination

    (1) Speech. Dysarthria may be present with profound facial, tongue, or oral sensory deficits.

    (2) Cranial nerves. Careful attention should be paid to associated abnormalities of cranial nerves, especially II, III, IV, VI, VII, and VIII.

    (3) Motor and deep tendon reflexes

    (4) Sensory loss. It is important to evaluate for evidence of other regions of sensory loss, especially a generalized sensory neuropathy.

    (5) Coordination. Coordination may be impaired by a process such as a tumor in the cerebellopontine angle.

    (6) Gait and station

C. Laboratory studies

  1. Biochemical tests include CBC with differential, a complete chemistry profile including liver function tests and glucose, and a sedimentation rate. In certain situations, a Venereal Disease Research Laboratory (VDRL) test, antinuclear antibody (ANA) determination, rheumatoid factor (RF), extractable nuclear antigen antibodies, or an angiotensin-converting enzyme (ACE) level may be necessary. A skin scraping or biopsy is necessary when leprosy is a consideration.

  2. A **purified protein derivative (PPD) test** should be done if there is suspicion of tuberculosis.

  3. A **chest roentgenogram** should be obtained to evaluate for a pulmonary malignancy or tuberculosis.

  4. Skull and/or sinus roentgenogram. A mandible x-ray is indicated if there is a numb chin.

  5. A **lumbar puncture** is essential if there is suspicion of an infection or a leptomeningeal malignancy.

  6. A **blink reflex** may be elicited electrophysiologically by electrical stimulation of the supraorbital nerve. It may be helpful in detecting subtle central or peripheral lesions of the trigeminal nerve.

  7. Brain imaging. All patients with facial numbness should undergo brain imaging by magnetic resonance imaging (MRI) of the brain. MRI is more sensitive than computed tomography (CT) as a detector of lesions of the trigeminal nerve, and of posterior fossa abnormalities such as acoustic neuroma.

Suspicion of an acoustic neuroma may necessitate special cuts through the acoustic canals with administration of contrast. Suspicion of an intracranial tumor may necessitate administration of contrast. CT with and without contrast may be indicated if MRI is not available or if there are contraindications for MRI.

V. Differential diagnosis. Specific locations of lesion causing facial numbness are detailed in Table 13-1.

    A. Tumor
    B. Infection
    C. Trauma
    D. Connective tissue diseases
    E. Drug or toxin
    F. Nontumor mass lesions
    G. Vascular disorders
    H. Demyelinating disorders
    I. Other systemic or rare diseases
    J. Idiopathic disorders

VI. Diagnostic approach

    A. The first step is to define clinically whether the deficit involves a division or divisions of the trigeminal nerve, the gasserian ganglion or root, or the central trigeminal pathways. Involvement of other cranial nerves or stigmata of associated diseases may help to limit the number of diagnostic possibilities.

    B. Appropriate tests are ordered depending on the results of the examination. Unless there is an obvious history of trauma, the following tests should be obtained: CBC with differential, chemistry profile, sedimentation rate, chest roentgenogram, and brain MRI. In selected individuals, other tests are indicated, such as Venereal Disease Research Laboratory (VDRL), ANA, extractable nuclear antigen antibodies, ACE, PPD, blink reflex, lumbar puncture, skull roentgenogram, sinus roentgenogram, and brain CT. The tests that may be indicated, and their relative costs, are listed in Table 13-3.

VII. Referral. Because there is such a wide range of possible underlying diseases that can cause facial numbness, it is often necessary to employ a teamwork approach to this problem. A neurologist, who should be most familiar with the localization of lesions of the trigeminal nerve, should be consulted initially. It is often necessary to consult an otolaryngologist to evaluate for the presence of a nasopharyngeal tumor, an acoustic neuroma, or sinusitis. A dentist or an oral surgeon may be needed to assist in ruling out a dental cause of facial numbness. In selected instances, a rheumatologist may be required if there is evidence of an associated connective tissue disease.

Table 13-3. Tests used in the evaluation of facial numbness and their relative costs.

Test	Cost*
CBC with differential	$
Chemistry profile	$
Sedimentation rate	$
VDRL	$
ANA	$
RF	$
Extractable nuclear antigen antibodies	$$
ACE	$
PPD	$
Chest roentgenogram	$$
Skull roentgenogram	$$
Sinus roentgenogram	$$
Lumbar puncture	$$
Blink reflex	$$
Brain CT	$$$
Brain MRI	$$$$

*$ = relatively inexpensive; $$ = moderately expensive; $$$ = expensive; $$$$ = very expensive.

Recommended Readings

Ashworth B, Tait GBW. Trigeminal neuropathy in connective tissue disease. *Neurology* 21:609, 1971.

Blau JN, et al. Trigeminal sensory neuropathy. *N Engl J Med* 281:873, 1969.

Brazis PW, Masdeu JC, Biller J. The localization of lesions affecting cranial nerve V. *Localization in Clinical Neurology* (3rd ed). Boston: Little, Brown, 1996.

Bruyn RPM, Boogerd W. The numb chin. *Clin Neurol Neurosurg* 93:187, 1991.

Burt RK, et al. Mental neuropathy (numb chin syndrome): A harbinger of tumor progression or relapse. *Cancer* 70:877, 1992.

Francis KR, et al. Facial numbness and dysesthesias: New features of carotid artery dissection. *Arch Neurol* 44:345, 1987.

Gibbin KP, Griffith IP. Idiopathic sensory trigeminal neuropathy. *J Laryngol Otol* 92:915, 1978.

Goldstein NP, et al. Trigeminal neuropathy and neuritis: A study of etiology with emphasis on dental causes. *JAMA* 184:458, 1963.

Goor C, Ongerboer De Visser BW. Jaw and blink reflexes in trigeminal nerve lesions: An electrodiagnostic study. *Neurology* 26:95, 1976.

Greenberg HS, et al. Metastasis to the base of the skull: Clinical findings in 43 patients. *Neurology* 31:530, 1981.

Hagen NA, et al. Trigeminal sensory neuropathy associated with connective tissue disease. *Neurology* 40:891, 1990.

Holtzman RNN, et al. Lateral pontine tegmental hemorrhage presenting as isolated trigeminal sensory neuropathy. *Neurology* 37:704, 1987.

Horowitz SH. Isolated facial numbness: Clinical significance and relation to trigeminal neuropathy. *Ann Intern Med* 80:49, 1974.

Kuntzer T, et al. Herald facial numbness. *Eur Neurol* 32:297, 1992.

Lecky BRF, et al. Trigeminal sensory neuropathy: A study of 22 cases. *Brain* 110:1463, 1987.

Massey EW, et al. Mental neuropathy from systemic cancer. *Neurology* 31:1277, 1981.

Searles RP, et al. Isolated trigeminal sensory neuropathy: Early manifestation of mixed connective tissue disease. *Neurology* 28:1286, 1978.

Sears ES, Franklin GM. Diseases of the cranial nerves. In RN Rosenberg (ed), *Neurology*. New York: Grune & Stratton, 1980.

Thrush DC, Small M. How benign a symptom is facial numbness? *Lancet* 2:851, 1970.

14

Approach to the Patient with Facial Pain

Julius M. Goodman

A careful work-up usually reveals the source of most **facial pain,** but there are some patients with severe facial pain problems who have normal physical examinations and diagnostic tests. It is important for the primary care physician to realize that some of these patients may have pain of neurologic or psychological origin. Sometimes such pain is erroneously attributed to disorders of the paranasal sinuses, teeth, or jaw, leading to a series of therapeutic misadventures by surgical and dental specialists with interest in facial pain. This chapter reviews an approach to patients with **trigeminal** and **glossopharyngeal neuralgia, cluster headache,** and **herpetic** and **postherpetic neuralgia.** Other related neurologic conditions and causes of facial pain are mentioned. Some patients with chronic facial pain of unknown etiology may have the **atypical facial pain** syndrome, which is thought to be of psychological origin. Long-term management and guidance of these distraught patients may become the responsibilities of the primary care physician.

  I. **Trigeminal neuralgia (TN)** (tic douloureux or tic) is the most common paroxysmal pain disorder of the face and one of the most painful afflictions known.
  A. **Etiology.** The exact mechanism for TN has not been definitely established. Some cases have been associated with structural lesions (symptomatic), but in most patients imaging studies fail to reveal a cause (idiopathic).
    1. **Symptomatic.** Approximately 1–2% of patients with TN have a posterior fossa lesion in the area of the ipsilateral trigeminal nerve: tumor (epidermoid, acoustic schwannoma, or meningioma), vascular malformation, or anomaly or tumor of the skull. At times, there is a mass on the side opposite the pain or even in the supratentorial area, and in such cases it has been postulated that secondary distortion of the brainstem is responsible.
    2. **Idiopathic.** Most patients with TN have no discernible lesions. Some neurosurgeons feel that the majority, but not all, may have compression of the fifth nerve root near its exit from the brainstem by a normal or ectatic artery or a vein. It has been postulated that vascular pulsations cause an area of demyelination on the trigeminal root with resulting ephaptic (nonsynaptic) transmission or "short circuit" from thickly myelinated sensory fibers to thinly myelinated pain fibers.
  B. **Symptoms.** Most patients with TN are more than 50 years old. Women are affected somewhat more frequently than men. TN is characterized by intermittent paroxysms of severe, brief (seconds), lancinating, "shocklike" pain. Patients often use phrases such as "a bolt of lightning" or "an electric shock" when describing the pain. TN pain may occur spontaneously or be brought on by talking, eating, brushing the teeth, washing, or lightly touching the face. Some patients refuse to go outdoors, fearing that a breeze will precipitate pain. Most patients have a **trigger zone,** which is a localized area of skin or mucous membrane that is highly sensitive. When this area is touched lightly, a paroxysm of pain can be "triggered." The first attack of TN may be so spectacular that the patient can usually describe it vividly, even after many years. Often the patient initially consults a dentist and undergoes tooth extractions or root canals to no avail.
  Tic pain usually involves a single trigeminal division or two adjacent divisions simultaneously, but rarely all three; the first (ophthalmic) division is least involved. The pain never crosses the midline. In 4% of patients, symptoms may become bilateral, but simultaneous bilateral pain is extremely rare. Patients with multiple sclerosis are more prone to eventual bilateral involvement.

Spontaneous remissions of TN pain, lasting months to years, are not uncommon, especially at the onset. After many years, TN pain may change to a more constant discomfort with fewer lancinating pains, thus making the diagnosis more difficult. When seeing a patient at this stage for the first time, it is helpful to ask the patient to describe the pain initially experienced at the onset of the disorder.

C. **Signs.** The neurologic exam for TN is characteristically normal and the diagnosis must be suspected from the history. Actually, the patient may refuse to give a history for fear of setting off pain. Watching a patient experience a startle reaction to a spontaneous TN pain while talking is almost diagnostic. Also, light touching of a trigger area, if the patient allows it, may result in a very brief sudden startle or jump, during which the patient may draw a hand up toward the face. If this typical quick jerk can be described or mimicked by a member of the patient's family, the diagnosis of TN can be clinched. **The presence of objective or subjective sensory loss, facial weakness, decreased hearing, or ataxia should raise suspicion of a mass lesion.** Signs and symptoms of multiple sclerosis should also be sought.

D. **Diagnosis.** There is no laboratory test for TN. The key to diagnosis is an accurate history. A dramatic response to carbamazepine is reassuring, because this medication rarely relieves facial pain from other causes. Imaging studies to rule out a structural lesion are not essential in the elderly patient with a normal neurologic exam, but an MRI scan before embarking on surgical treatment is advisable. MRI scanning should also be considered for most patients below age 60 and for all those with abnormal neurologic exams or in whom multiple sclerosis is suspected. MRI with and without contrast enhancement is preferred over CT because of its superiority in visualizing intra- and extra-axial lesions of the posterior fossa. Angiography is not indicated to rule out microvascular compression of the trigeminal nerve, even if microvascular decompression is contemplated. Small-vessel compression cannot be detected on angiography, and ectatic displacement of the basilar and vertebral arteries is evident on good-quality MRI scans. Electrophysiologic studies are not helpful.

II. **Glossopharyngeal neuralgia (GN)** is characterized by paroxysmal lancinating pain similar to TN pain but centered around the tonsil and ear. Pain may be triggered by swallowing, yawning, or food contact on the pharynx. GN is quite rare in comparison with TN. **It is more often associated with neoplasms involving the skull base.** Again, the diagnosis is made by history. All of these patients should undergo ear, nose, and throat consultation to look for occult neoplasms. Anesthetizing the pharynx with topical anesthesia may temporarily halt lancinating pain triggered by touch or swallowing and may be of some diagnostic help. An occasional GN patient has episodes of bradycardia or apnea secondary to increased reflex sensitivity in the distribution of the ninth and tenth cranial nerves.

III. **Herpes zoster virus neuralgia** has no relationship to TN in regard to etiology, symptoms, or management. The thoracic dermatomes are most commonly involved with herpes zoster (HZ), but in 10–20% of patients the ophthalmic division (V1) of the trigeminal nerve is affected, resulting in facial pain. Zoster infection results from reactivation of latent varicella-zoster virus in the gasserian (trigeminal) sensory ganglion, usually in elderly patients with declining immune systems and in association with diseases involving compromised immunity. Two pain syndromes are associated with HZ involving the face: acute **herpes zoster ophthalmicus,** which includes the preeruptive phase, the skin lesion discomfort, and persistent pain for one month; and chronic **postherpetic neuralgia,** which is a central pain syndrome that occurs in some patients after the acute phase.

A. **Herpes zoster ophthalmicus (HZO)** in the preeruptive phase may be difficult to diagnose and can be confused with other types of facial neuralgias and cranial arteritis until the characteristic ulcerative rash appears. There may be burning or lancinating pain in the V1 distribution associated with nausea, malaise, and mild fever. The skin lesions usually appear within 4 days of onset, but sometimes can be delayed for many days. Rarely, there may be pain without skin lesions, and if the diagnosis is suspected, it can be confirmed by rising HZ virus antibody titers. Any portion of the globe can also be involved with HZ, leading to ocular pain and visual loss.

B. **Postherpetic neuralgia (PHN)** involving the face, usually the ophthalmic division, is a central type of pain and is not caused by stimulation of pain nerve endings by damaged tissue as in the acute infection. PHN is more common following acute HZ of the face than of the thoracic area. Patients with severe pain in the acute phase and those over 80 are more prone to develop PHN. The disorder is very incapacitating to the suffering patient and extremely frustrating for the physician attempting to treat it.

1. **Symptoms** of PHN begin approximately 4 weeks after the cutaneous phase has subsided at the site of the herpetic eruption (shingles). Most PHN patients describe their pain as "burning" or "ice burning." The pain is different from the pain of shingles and is not considered a continuation of that pain. Patients with PHN may have tactile allodynia—i.e., pain caused by a nonnoxious stimulus. Hair brushing or wind may set off this pain, but it should not be confused with the electric-shock-like pain of TN, which can be set off with similar stimuli. Sometimes patients put a moist cloth over the skin for some relief. They can usually sleep without being awakened by pain, but emotional stress may aggravate symptoms, as in other kinds of central pain.

2. **Signs.** Residual skin scarring of HZO may be evident. Careful sensory testing in the involved areas may reveal deficits in response to light touch, pinprick, hot and cold, and two-point discrimination.

IV. **Cluster headache** (migrainous neuralgia) is a paroxysmal, recurring disorder of unknown etiology that is characterized by episodes of intense, strictly unilateral facial pain lasting about 30 minutes to 2 hours. The pain tends to occur once or several times daily over a period of weeks to months, followed by spontaneous remissions lasting months to years.

A. **Symptoms.** Periocular pain is characteristic, but the cheek and forehead may be involved. The pain is as excruciating as in TN but is of longer duration. Occasionally it may be lancinating, but the existence of a trigger area is rare. The pain frequently awakens the patient from sleep, which is uncommon with TN. There are no auras, and nausea and vomiting are not usual. Unlike migraine, (1) the disorder is more common in men, (2) onset in childhood is unusual, and (3) a family history of migraine is rare.

B. **Signs.** Neurologic examination is normal except for an occasional partial Horner's syndrome manifested by slight ptosis and miosis during episodes of pain. Horner's syndrome associated with any other type of facial pain is ominous and deserves a detailed search for a structural lesion. During an attack there may be flushing of the face, conjunctival injection, and ipsilateral nasal stuffiness.

C. **Variants**

1. **Cluster-tic syndrome.** A rare patient with cluster headache may also have symptoms of trigeminal neuralgia. The pain is always on the same side, is in the same division, and can be provoked by the same stimuli, suggesting that this is a separate entity and not the coexistence of the two disorders. The success rate of medical or surgical therapy is not well established.

2. **Cluster-migraine.** Migraine headaches occur in 1–3% of patients with cluster headaches, and vice versa.

3. **Chronic paroxysmal hemicrania.** In this condition, the pain is similar to cluster headache but shorter in duration with more frequent episodes. It occurs much more commonly in women than in men and responds rapidly and specifically to indomethacin.

4. **Post-trauma cluster headaches.** Occasionally, clusterlike headaches have occurred after facial trauma. The mechanism is not known, and these headaches are more resistant to abortive and prophylactic treatments.

V. **Atypical facial pain** is a term used to describe facial pain for which no organic cause can be found and which does not meet the criteria for the facial pain syndromes described above.

A. **Signs and symptoms.** The typical patient is a middle-aged woman with continuous deep facial pain that is poorly localized and not in the anatomical distribution of one of the trigeminal branches. Initially the pain is unilateral, but in one-third of cases bilateral symptoms may eventually occur. The patient may have difficulty describing the pain, but terms such as "pulling," "aching," "tearing," and "drawing" are frequently used. The intensity of the pain may fluctuate, but discomfort is always present. Activities and weather may aggravate the pain, but not to the extent observed in TN. These patients are often prone to exaggeration and may claim that the pain is ruining their lives, but they may not look very sick. Mood swings, irritability, and insomnia are common symptoms. Patients may carry lists of medications that have failed to alleviate their suffering or to which they are allergic. Typically, the patient has already seen numerous specialists and may have undergone numerous negative diagnostic studies, unsuccessful anesthetic blocks, and failed surgical procedures. Those suffering with atypical facial pain may be looking forward to additional operations, hoping that eventually someone will find the cause of and a cure for their discomfort.

   B. Etiology. About half the patients with atypical facial pain attribute the onset to trauma or a dental procedure. Most authorities believe that the disorder is primarily psychological.

VI. Other causes of facial pain that deserve comment are as follows.

   A. Paranasal sinus disease. Acute sinusitis is usually clinically evident, and chronic sinusitis is rarely a cause of facial pain. However, isolated sphenoid sinusitis may be an obscure cause of headache and pain referred to the face. Remember that thickened mucous membranes are often evident on routine imaging studies in asymptomatic patients.

   B. Temporomandibular joint (TMJ) disorders are frequently diagnosed in patients with chronic facial pain. The diagnosis should be considered when there is pain on jaw movement, restriction of mouth opening, localized trauma, and abnormal imaging studies. However, the diagnosis of TMJ is controversial and difficult. It is important for the primary care physician to keep this in mind when monitoring the evaluation and treatment of patients.

   1. Many patients have dental malocclusion but no TMJ symptoms.

   2. Many asymptomatic individuals have abnormal TMJ imaging studies and arthrograms, including arthritis and TMJ meniscus disorders.

   3. Symptoms decrease with age, which would be unusual if degenerative disease of the TMJ were the cause of pain.

   4. Joint tenderness and EMG abnormalities occur with equal frequency in patients labeled with TMJ disorders and in controls.

   Multiple opinions and prolonged conservative treatment should be considered before a patient is advised to proceed with a TMJ procedure.

   C. Toothache is an easily diagnosed cause of acute facial pain, but sometimes bad teeth may coexist with a neurologic disorder such as trigeminal neuralgia that may not be appreciated by the patient or the dentist. Moreover, some dentists believe that small cavities in the jaw, apparently occurring after tooth extraction but not visible on radiographs, can cause chronic oral pain. If the pain is relieved with a block, curettage of the mandible is usually recommended. However, these procedures may not be successful in relieving chronic facial pain.

   D. Temporal arteritis may present in an elderly individual with pain in the distribution of the external carotid artery. Discomfort from chewing, tenderness and thickening over the branches of the superficial temporal arteries, and occasional redness or ulceration of the skin of the forehead may be present. The sedimentation rate is almost always elevated.

   E. Cranial nerve disorders may present with pain before neurologic examination makes the cranial nerve involvement obvious.

   1. Optic neuritis or retrobulbar neuritis may present with retro-orbital pain that precedes visual loss by hours or days. An early abnormal afferent pupillary reflex should be sought.

   2. Ischemia or infarction of the oculomotor or other cranial nerves may present simultaneously with pain that may overshadow the neurologic deficit, such as in early diabetic oculomotor palsy.

   F. Ocular pain

   1. Acute glaucoma as a cause of pain in the eye and adjacent face is usually obvious by virtue of clouding of the cornea and other changes in the globe. However, subacute glaucoma may present with eye pain and physical findings that may not be readily evident to an inexperienced examiner.

   2. Refractive errors and squint should not ordinarily be diagnosed as causes of unexplained facial pain.

   G. Thalamic pain, a manifestation of a central pain syndrome, may develop after a thalamic infarction and may occasionally be limited to the face. The patient suffers pain and dysesthesias of the opposite face. There is usually some sensory loss, but this finding may be difficult to elicit. A good-quality MRI scan may show a thalamic infarct.

   H. Anesthesia dolorosa, another form of central pain, may occur as a complication of any of the surgical procedures for trigeminal neuralgia. A constant and very unpleasant feeling is noted in an area of skin or mucous membrane with profound sensory loss following an ablative operation.

    1. Symptoms usually begin weeks to months after the procedure. The patient describes the unpleasant sensation as burning or stinging. A feeling of crawling and itching sometimes occurs around the mouth or eye. There may be an irrepressible urge to scratch the anesthetic area with resulting erosion or abrasion of skin. Night pain causing insomnia is common.

    2. Management by medication or operation is very difficult.

  I. Cancer may be a very indolent cause of facial pain. Even though the patient may have seen numerous physicians, each new consultant as well as the patient's own physician must periodically repeat a complete history and examination and review previous imaging studies. If the patient's symptoms change or fail to respond to treatment, further imaging studies should be considered. **The presence of a subjective or objective sensory deficit in the trigeminal distribution, hearing loss, serous otitis, chronic nasal obstruction, enlarged cervical lymph nodes, weakness or atrophy of the muscles of mastication, cranial nerve palsy, diplopia, proptosis, lid edema, subjective or objective bruits, and Horner's syndrome should raise the possibility of a serious structural lesion.**

VII. Referral

  A. When a **structural lesion** is noted or a **neoplasm** is suspected (see sec. **VI.I**), referral should be made to the appropriate specialist for an evaluation.

  B. Trigeminal neuralgia should be evaluated by a neurologist or neurosurgeon if the diagnosis is in doubt, if there are abnormal neurologic signs, symptoms, or imaging studies, or if there is failure to respond, relapse, or inability to tolerate carbamazepine. If a surgical procedure is contemplated, the primary physician should be aware of the various available percutaneous and open operations, because certain centers and surgeons may be biased toward particular procedures. Dental operations, including extractions and root canals, do not relieve TN pain, and alcohol blocks by dentists should ordinarily be avoided.

  C. Glossopharyngeal neuralgia is rare and difficult to diagnose. A neurologist or neurosurgeon should be involved. Because of the high incidence of malignancy associated with this condition, an otolaryngologist should also be consulted.

  D. Cluster headache and its variants should be referred to a neurologist if there is doubt about the diagnosis or failure to respond to the usual medications.

  E. Herpes zoster ophthalmicus and **postherpetic neuralgia** involving the face do not ordinarily require neurologic referral once the diagnosis has been established. Many specialists have experience with these disorders, including ophthalmologists, dermatologists, oncologists, and infectious disease physicians. The primary care physician, however, should monitor the patient. As a "last resort" treatment for postherpetic neuralgia, a sympathetic or overzealous surgeon may recommend an ablative procedure used for trigeminal neuralgia. These interventions should be avoided, because they do not relieve postherpetic pain and may make the patient worse.

  F. Atypical facial pain is notoriously difficult to treat. A neurologist or a neurosurgeon with an interest in facial pain may be helpful in establishing the diagnosis and suggesting medication. The advice of other consultants, such as otolaryngologists, ophthalmologists, and oral surgeons, may be needed to exclude occult disorders that could cause facial pain. However, the generalist should screen and protect the patient against futile nerve blocks and dental or surgical operations done on the "hope" that they might relieve the patient's pain. Surgical procedures, often advised by some out-of-town consultant as acts of desperation, are fraught with hazard, because they often aggravate an already bad situation. Referral to a psychotherapist who lacks special interest and expertise with atypical facial pain is usually another bad experience for the patient. Support and a compassionate relationship between the patient and the primary physician is important.

Recommended Readings

Adams CBT. Microvascular compression: An alternative view and hypothesis. *J Neurosurg* 70(1):1–12, 1989.

Ferrante L, et al. Glossopharyngeal neuralgia with cardiac syncope. *Neurosurgery* 36(1):58–63, 1995.

Janetta PJ. Trigeminal neuralgia: Treatment by microvascular decompression. In RH Wilkins, SS Rengachary (eds), *Neurosurgery*. New York: McGraw-Hill, 1996. Pp 3961–3968.

Lichtor T, Mullen JF. A 10 year follow-up review of percutaneous microcompression of the trigeminal ganglion. *J Neurosurg* 72:49–54, 1990.

Metheetrairut C, Brown MB. Glossopharyngeal neuralgia and syncope secondary to neck malignancy. *J Otolaryng* 22(1):18–20, 1993.

Nugent GR. Trigeminal neuralgia: Treatment by percutaneous electrocoagulation. In RH Wilkins, SS Rengachary (eds), *Neurosurgery*. New York: McGraw-Hill, 1996. Pp 3945–3951.

Pellock JM, Willmore LJ. A rational guide to routine blood level monitoring in patients receiving antiepileptic drugs. *Neurology* 41:961–964, 1991.

Resnick DK, Jannetta PJ. Microvascular decompression for glossopharyngeal neuralgia. *Neurosurgery* 36(1):64–69, 1995.

Rovit R, Murali R, Jannetta P (eds). *Trigeminal Neuralgia*. Baltimore: Williams & Wilkins, 1990.

Solomon S, Lipton RB. Facial pain. *Neurolog Clinics* 8(4):913–928, 1992.

Taha JM, Tew JM, Buncher CR. A prospective 15-year follow up of 154 consecutive patients with trigeminal neuralgia treated by percutaneous stereotactic radiofrequency thermal rhizotomy. *J Neurosurg* 83(6):989–993, 1995.

Watson CPN (ed). *Herpes Zoster and Postherpetic Neuralgia*. Berlin: Elsevier, 1993.

15

Approach to the Patient with Facial Weakness

Askiel Bruno
Molly Kathleen King

Facial weakness is a common neurologic problem that can be caused by a large number of diverse disorders. The diagnosis needs to be established rapidly in order to minimize the neurologic damage and prevent recurrence. A systematic approach to lesion localization and differential diagnosis optimizes patient management.

I. **Etiology.** Table 15-1 summarizes the causes of facial weakness. The innervation of the facial muscles starts in the precentral gyrus of the cerebral motor cortex. The region controlling the facial muscles is located most laterally and inferiorly near the sylvian fissure. Above this region is the cortical region for hand movement, then the region for arm movement, and finally, on the medial surface, in the interhemispheric fissure, the region for leg movement. Blood flow to the lateral portion of the cerebral motor cortex controlling face and arm movement is supplied by the middle cerebral artery. Blood flow to the medial portion of the cerebral motor cortex controlling leg movement is supplied by the anterior cerebral artery. From the motor cortex, the axons pass through the centrum semiovale and converge in the internal capsule. Within the internal capsule the motor fibers to the face are located at the genu, the fibers to the arm are located posteriorly to the facial fibers, and the fibers to the leg are posterior to the arm fibers. The motor fibers continue down through the cerebral peduncles in the midbrain, where the facial fibers are most medial, the arm fibers are lateral to them, and the leg fibers are most lateral. The motor fibers then continue down to the lower pons, where they innervate part of the ipsilateral facial nucleus and also cross to innervate the contralateral facial nucleus. From the facial nucleus, the fibers travel through the pons, the subarachnoid space, the temporal bone, the parotid gland, and the subcutaneous facial region to the muscles of facial expression. The differential diagnosis of facial weakness depends on which segment of this pathway is affected.

II. **Clinical manifestations.** In patients with facial weakness, the appearance of the face at rest changes and the weakness becomes obvious during testing. It is important to determine whether the facial weakness is caused by an upper or a lower motor neuron lesion. This distinction can be easily made on examination (Fig. 15-1 and sec. **III.B**). Drooping of one side of the face with flattening of the nasolabial fold is observed at rest. With lower motor neuron type weakness, flattening of the forehead wrinkles and palpebral fissure widening may also be apparent. The eye may be red and dry as a result of impaired blinking or decreased lacrimation. Speech is usually slurred.

Taste may be impaired if the facial nerve is lesioned proximal to the chorda tympani nerve branch, within the temporal bone, which carries taste sensation from the ipsilateral anterior two-thirds of the tongue. Sounds may be exaggerated (hyperacusis) if the facial nerve is lesioned proximal to the stapedius nerve branch in the temporal bone, which supplies the ipsilateral stapedius muscle to dampen loud sounds.

III. **Evaluation**

A. **History.** The most useful facts to be obtained from the medical history are the rate of onset of the weakness, whether there are any other neurologic symptoms, and what preexisting medical problems might possibly be causing the facial weakness. Sudden or rapid onset (within hours) of nontraumatic facial weakness suggests a vascular etiology such as stroke or peripheral ischemic neuropathy if the weakness is unilateral, and Guillain-Barré syndrome if the weakness is bilateral. Facial weakness progressing over days or weeks is most likely idiopathic (Bell's palsy) or the result of an infection or a tumor.

The status of eye closure on the affected side and the presence or absence of

Table 15-1. Causes of facial weakness.

Upper Motor Neuron Causes
Stroke: 85% ischemic, 15% hemorrhagic
Brain tumor: metastatic or primary, hemispheric or brainstem
Brain abscess

Lower Motor Neuron Causes
Bell's palsy
Guillain-Barré syndrome (may be HIV associated)
Direct facial nerve infections: herpes viruses
Vasculitis
Sarcoidosis, Behçet's syndrome, polyarteritis nodosa, Sjögren's syndrome, syphilis
Meningitis: common bacteria (pneumococcus, meningococcus, *Haemophilus influenzae*),
    Mycobacterium tuberculosis, Lyme borreliosis, syphilis, fungi
Meningeal carcinomatosis
Temporal bone fracture
Temporal bone tumors: metastatic, invasive meningioma
Middle ear infections: common organisms, *Pseudomonas aeruginosa*
Middle ear tumors
Parotid gland tumors or infections
Facial lacerations

Disorders Affecting the Neuromuscular Junction
Myasthenia gravis
Botulism

Disorders Affecting the Facial Muscles
Muscular dystrophies
Myopathies

---

other neurologic symptoms help localize the lesion. Inability to close the eye suggests a motor neuron lesion, and preservation of eye closure suggests an upper motor neuron (cerebral) lesion. Presence of CNS symptoms such as hemiparesis, hemisensory loss, or hemineglect, in addition to facial weakness, suggests a brain lesion. Presence of lower motor neuron symptoms, such as sensory disturbances in distal lower extremities or muscle atrophy, suggests a neuropathy.

Certain medical conditions predispose to facial weakness. Increasing age, tobacco smoking, diabetes mellitus, and hypertension increase the risk of ischemic stroke as well as ischemic peripheral neuropathy. Ear and parotid gland infections increase the risk of facial nerve damage. Head trauma with basal skull fracture may cause facial nerve compression or laceration within the temporal bone. Malignancies predispose to metastatic facial nerve infiltration and carcinomatous meningitis.

B. **Physical examination** confirms the suspicions from clinical history and uncovers additional useful findings. Upper motor neuron facial weakness can be distinguished from lower motor neuron weakness rapidly and reliably by examination (see Fig. 15-1). Upper motor neuron facial weakness is caused by contralateral brain lesions above the level of the facial nucleus (lower pons). Only the lower facial muscles are affected. The appearance of the forehead and the width of the palpebral fissure are normal. Eyebrow elevation, forehead wrinkling, and eye closure are intact. The nasolabial fold is flattened, the corner of the mouth is lowered, and smiling and grinning are impaired. Speech is usually slurred, and when the cheeks are puffed with air, the air escapes between the lips on the weak side. The corneal reflex is intact because the lesion is above this reflex arc. Emotional facial movements, such as smiling, are usually intact despite weakness of voluntary facial movements.

The reason that the upper facial muscles are spared by upper motor neuron lesions is that the portion of the facial nerve nucleus that controls the upper facial muscles receives bilateral cerebral innervation. Therefore, a unilateral cerebral lesion impairs only the lower facial muscles. The reason that emotional facial movements are intact when voluntary facial movements are not is that facial innervation for voluntary movements comes from the pyramidal motor cortex

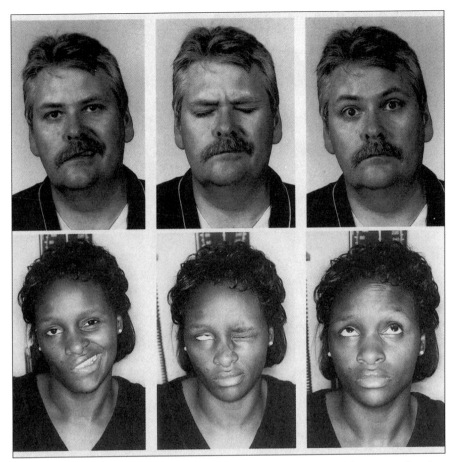

Figure 15-1. Right facial weakness resulting from left cerebral infarction (upper panel) and from Bell's palsy (lower panel). At rest, there was no obvious facial weakness in either patient (not shown). Voluntary smiling produces obvious facial asymmetry with a similar appearance of the facial weakness in both patients (images at left). Eye closure (middle images) and eyebrow elevation (images at right) are impaired only in the patient with lower motor neuron facial weakness. The upward eye deviation observed during eye closure (lower middle image) is the normal Bell's phenomenon.

whereas facial innervation for emotional facial expressions comes from extrapyramidal cerebral regions. In patients with upper motor neuron weakness of voluntary facial movements, emotional movements are usually intact.

Lower motor neuron facial weakness is caused by lesions affecting the facial nerve nucleus, its fibers within the lower pons, or the peripheral portion of the facial nerve. The facial nucleus and nerve contain all the nerve fibers that innervate the ipsilateral facial muscles. Therefore, a lesion in the facial nucleus or nerve impairs all the ipsilateral facial muscles. In addition to the lower facial weakness, the forehead creases are flattened, the palpebral fissure is widened, and the patient is unable to raise the eyebrow, wrinkle the forehead, or close the eye tightly. Emotional movements are also impaired. The corneal reflex is impaired because the lesion affects the efferent part of this reflex arc. The distinction between upper and lower motor neuron facial weakness made on examination is very reliable if made during acute weakness. However, after a partial recovery has occurred, lower motor neuron facial weakness may occasionally resemble upper motor neuron weakness.

The remainder of the neurologic examination is important as a means of looking for other focal deficits that will help localize the lesion or lesions and suggest the best differential diagnosis. Multiple cranial neuropathies suggest basilar meningitis or vasculitis. Hemiparesis on the same side as the facial weakness suggests a hemispheric brain lesion contralateral to the weakness. Hemisensory loss on the side opposite the lower motor neuron facial weakness, or gaze palsy on the same side as the facial weakness, suggests a pontine lesion on the side of the facial weakness (see sec. **V.B.4**).

Examination of the ear is very important. Infections and tumors in the tympanic cavity can be detected with an otoscope and can account for facial nerve damage. The facial nerve passes near the tympanic cavity in the temporal bone. Vesicles on the external ear suggest herpetic facial neuropathy (Ramsay Hunt syndrome). Parotitis and parotid tumors also can cause peripheral facial palsy.

C. **Laboratory studies**
   1. **Magnetic resonance imaging (MRI)** is indicated when a brain lesion is suspected. Overall, it is a more sensitive brain imaging test than CT, specially in the posterior fossa, where CT is limited by bone artifacts.
   2. **Computed tomography (CT)** is superior to MRI in demonstrating basal skull fractures. When an acute stroke is suspected, CT is preferred as the initial neuroimaging study in order to differentiate hemorrhage from ischemia.
   3. **Lumbar puncture (LP)** should be done when there is an indication of possible meningitis or vasculitis, such as fever, headache, nuchal rigidity, or systemic signs of vasculitis.
   4. **Electrodiagnostic studies** such as electroneurography are used to prognosticate recovery, but are not needed to make the diagnosis.

IV. **Differential diagnosis**
   A. **Guillain-Barré syndrome** is a serious acute neurologic disorder involving multiple peripheral nerves. Sometimes facial weakness is the predominant presenting finding. In that situation, the facial weakness is bilateral. Weakness in other muscles and loss of tendon reflexes are always part of this syndrome. The most dreaded acute complications are respiratory insufficiency resulting from neurogenic respiratory muscle weakness and autonomic instability resulting from autonomic neuropathy. Prompt diagnosis is essential for optimal management.
   B. **Acute stroke** can present with predominantly facial weakness. Usually there are other deficits, such as hemiparesis or hemisensory loss. Upper motor neuron facial weakness develops suddenly or over minutes to a few hours.
   C. **Meningitis** is manifested by headache, fever, and nuchal rigidity. The infection or inflammation can damage the facial nerve as it passes through the subarachnoid space and the meninges to enter the temporal bone. Infectious (bacterial or fungal) meningitis needs to be distinguished, by cerebrospinal fluid (CSF) analysis, from carcinomatous meningitis caused by metastatic infiltration of the meninges.
   D. **Otitis media** is manifested by ear pain and inflammation in the tympanic cavity. Because the facial nerve passes very close to the tympanic cavity, it can become damaged by otitis media.
   E. **Brain tumor or abscess.** Cerebral hemispheric tumor or abscess can present with upper motor neuron facial weakness as the predominant finding. Infiltrating pontine tumors, such as glioma or lymphoma, or a cerebellopontine angle tumor, can present with lower motor neuron facial weakness as the predominant finding. The weakness progresses over days to months, and often there is headache or fever.
   F. **Bell's palsy** is diagnosed when there is peripheral facial nerve palsy (lower motor neuron facial weakness) without other neurologic deficits and without an apparent cause. Serologic and pathologic evidence suggests that a large proportion of apparently idiopathic facial neuropathies may be caused by neuronitis resulting from one of the herpes viruses. In a patient with vascular risk factors, ischemic facial neuropathy is a likely etiology.

V. **Diagnostic approach.** First determine if the facial weakness is of the upper or lower motor neuron type (see Fig. 15-1). Second, determine the rate of onset of facial weakness and if there are other associated symptoms. Third, determine if there are other neurologic deficits and if they represent a central or a peripheral lesion. Fourth, localize the problem to a single lesion if possible, or to multiple lesions. Fifth, generate a differential diagnosis list based on the lesion localization and rate of onset of the facial weakness (Fig. 15-2). Sixth, obtain the diagnostic

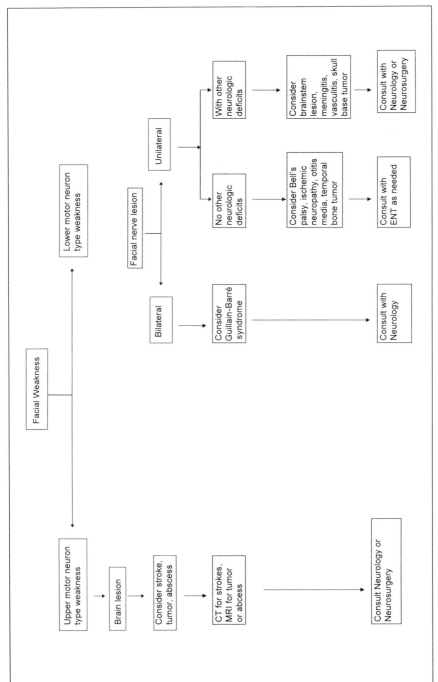

Figure 15-2. Diagnostic algorithm for evaluation of patients with facial weakness.

tests needed to confirm or exclude the serious or treatable conditions in the differential diagnosis list.

A. Upper motor neuron facial weakness indicates a brain lesion. Sudden onset of weakness suggests a stroke, and weakness progressing over days or weeks suggests a brain tumor or an abscess. If an acute stroke is suspected, cranial computed tomography (CT) should be done without contrast. This test easily and reliably distinguishes ischemic from hemorrhagic stroke. If another brain pathology is suspected, MRI should be done, usually with contrast, to distinguish among the various possible causes.

B. Lower motor neuron facial weakness indicates involvement of the facial nerve.

1. **Isolated unilateral lower motor neuron facial weakness,** without other neurologic deficits, is most likely idiopathic (Bell's palsy) or ischemic and the result of small vessel disease. If the patient has no vascular risks, such as hypertension, smoking, diabetes mellitus, or advanced age, the most likely diagnosis is Bell's palsy. If the patient has vascular risks, the diagnosis of ischemic facial neuropathy is likely.

2. **Bilateral facial weakness.** Rapid onset of bilateral facial weakness should alert the physician to the possibility of Guillain-Barré syndrome, sarcoidosis, or other vasculitis causing multiple cranial neuropathies (see Table 15-1). With Guillain-Barré syndrome, there is progressive weakness over hours to days, other muscles usually are weak, including the respiratory muscles and extremities, and the muscle stretch reflexes are always absent or depressed.

   Slow-onset or long-standing bilateral facial weakness should alert the physician to the possibility of muscular dystrophy, such as facioscapulohumeral muscular dystrophy, of myasthenia gravis, or of congenital hypoplasia of the facial nuclei (Möbius' syndrome). In muscular dystrophy and in myasthenia gravis, other muscles are always involved. In facioscapulohumeral muscular dystrophy, there is bilateral proximal upper extremity weakness. In myasthenia gravis, there is usually weakness in the ocular muscles, neck muscles, pharynx, or proximal limbs, and the weakness is intermittent throughout the day. In Möbius' syndrome, there also may be hypoplasia of the abducens (cranial nerve VI) nucleus and other brainstem nuclei.

3. **Multiple cranial nerve deficits.** If multiple cranial nerve deficits are associated with facial weakness, infectious and carcinomatous basilar meningitis, vasculitis, and basilar skull tumor should be considered. Any of these problems is likely to cause headache, fever, nuchal rigidity, and elevated erythrocyte sedimentation rate (ESR). However, these findings are nonspecific. Presence of extracranial malignancy suggests possible carcinomatous meningitis. Presence of collagen vascular disease suggests possible vasculitis. MRI should be done to rule out a basal skull tumor. If a lesion is detected, gadolinium-enhanced MRI should be obtained to determine the enhancement pattern. A tumor excision or a biopsy usually is needed for definitive diagnosis. If the MRI is negative, a lumbar puncture should be done to look for meningitis. The spinal fluid should be stained and inspected for bacteria, fungi, and malignant cells. It should also be cultured for bacteria and fungi. Bacterial stains and cultures should always include mycobacteria. The CSF protein, glucose, and cell count abnormalities are important indicators of disease, but they cannot reliably differentiate among the various disorders in question.

4. **Brainstem lesions.** The facial nerve and nucleus can be involved by lesions within the pons. Because of the proximity of other structures in the pons to the facial nucleus and nerve, additional neurologic deficits help establish the correct diagnosis. The facial nerve fibers wrap around the abducens nucleus (cranial nerve VI), located dorsally to the facial nucleus. A lesion in the abducens nucleus produces lateral gaze palsy on the side of the lesion. The spinal trigeminal nucleus and tract are lateral to the facial nucleus. A lesion in the trigeminal tract or nucleus produces pain and temperature sensory loss on the same side of the face. The trigeminothalamic and spinothalamic tracts are located ventrally to the facial nucleus. A lesion in the trigeminothalamic tract produces pain and temperature sensory loss on the other side of the face, and a lesion in the spinothalamic tract produces pain and temperature sensory loss on the other side of the body below the neck. Cere-

bellar fibers from above and from below travel to the cerebellum through the pons, and a lesion involving these fibers produces dysmetria of the arm or leg, or both, on the same side. Large pontine lesions may involve the ventrally located corticospinal tract and cause hemiparesis on the other side of the body. The so-called "crossed signs"—cranial nerve deficit contralateral to hemiparesis or hemisensory loss—can be explained by a single lesion only in the brainstem.

VI. Referral

A. None. When the history and physical examination are consistent with Bell's palsy or ischemic facial neuropathy, referral may not be necessary. Slow spontaneous improvement is expected.

B. Neurologist. Consultation with a neurologist is indicated when there is suspicion of acute stroke, Guillain-Barré syndrome, meningitis, or vasculitis.

C. Ear, Nose, and Throat. An ENT specialist should be consulted when unusual otitis media or tumor in the tympanic cavity or parotid gland is suspected.

D. Neurosurgeon. A neurosurgeon should be consulted when a tumor or abscess is demonstrated.

Recommended Readings

Adour KK. Diagnosis and management of facial paralysis. *N Engl J Med* 307:348–351, 1982.

Bateman DE. Facial palsy. *Br J Hosp Med* 47:430–431, 1992.

Brazis PW, Masdeu JC, Biller J. The localization of lesions affecting cranial nerve VII. *Localization in Clinical Neurology* (3rd ed). Boston: Little, Brown, 1996.

Engstrom M, et al. Facial nerve enhancement in Bell's palsy demonstrated by different gadolinium-enhanced magnetic resonance imaging techniques. *Arch Otolaryngol Head Neck Surg* 119:221–225, 1993.

Finestone AJ, Byers K. Acute facial paralysis: Is it a stroke or something else? *Geriatrics* 49:50–52, 1994.

Furuta Y, et al. Latent herpes simplex virus type 1 in human geniculate ganglia. *Acta Neuropathol* 84:39–44, 1992.

Keane JR. Bilateral seventh nerve palsy: Analysis of 43 cases and review of the literature. *Neurology* 44:1198–1202, 1994.

Morgan M, Nathwani D. Facial palsy and infections: The unfolding story. *Clin Infect Dis* 14:263–271, 1992.

Murr AH, Benecke JE Jr. Association of facial paralysis with HIV positivity. *Am J Otolaryngol* 12:450–451, 1991.

Olsen KD. Facial nerve paralysis: General evaluation, Bell's palsy. *Postgrad Med* 75:219–225, 1984.

Olsen KD. Facial nerve paralysis: All that palsies is not Bell's. *Postgrad Med* 76:95–105, 1984.

Walling AD. Bell's palsy in pregnancy and the puerperium. *J Fam Pract* 36:559–563, 1993.

16

Approach to the Patient with Dizziness and Vertigo
Timothy C. Hain

Dizziness and **vertigo** are common symptoms: about 2.5% of all primary care visits are for dizziness and about 1% are for vertigo. Dizziness and vertigo have diverse etiologies. For this reason, a broadly based approach to the dizzy patient is necessary, at times requiring serious and life-threatening medical problems such as cardiac arrhythmia to be distinguished from the more common inner ear disease and dizziness from unlocalizable sources.

I. **Etiology.** Vertigo can be categorized into four types: otologic, central, medical, and unlocalized (Table 16-1). The largest category, unlocalized vertigo, includes roughly 50% of patients with vertigo.

A. **Otologic vertigo** is caused by dysfunction of the inner ear. It accounts for about one-third of all patients with vertigo. Table 16-1 lists entities that account for about 95% of all cases of otologic vertigo.

1. **Benign paroxysmal positional vertigo (BPPV)** is the most common single type of otologic vertigo, accounting for roughly 50% of all cases. BPPV presents with brief vertigo provoked by changes in the orientation of the head to gravity. BPPV is caused by loose debris within the posterior canal of the inner ear.

2. **Vestibular neuritis** presents with vertigo, nausea, ataxia, and nystagmus. It is attributed to a viral infection of the vestibular nerve. **Labyrinthitis** presents with the same symptom complex, combined with tinnitus and/or hearing loss. Vestibular neuritis and labyrinthitis together account for about 15% of all otologic vertigo cases.

3. **Ménière's disease** presents with intermittent vertigo accompanied by hearing complaints (see the so-called "hydrops" symptom complex in sec. **IV.A.3**). It is attributed to dilation and periodic rupture of the endolymphatic compartment of the inner ear. Ménière's disease accounts for about 15% of otologic vertigo cases.

4. **Bilateral vestibular paresis** presents with oscillopsia and ataxia, usually caused by loss of vestibular hair cells. The typical history comprises treatment for several weeks with an intravenous or intraperitoneal ototoxic antibiotic (of which gentamicin is the most commonly encountered). Bilateral vestibular loss is uncommon.

5. **Perilymph fistula (PLF)** presents with the pressure sensitivity or hydrops symptom complexes (see sec. **IV** for details), or as ataxia provoked by activity. In PLF, a rupture has occurred between the fluid-filled inner ear and the air-filled middle ear. Barotrauma, such as from scuba diving, is the common mechanism. PLF is very uncommon.

6. **Tumors compressing the eighth nerve** present with asymmetric hearing combined with mild ataxia. Eighth nerve tumors are very uncommon in the vertiginous population (but are more common in the unilaterally hearing impaired).

B. **Central vertigo** is caused by dysfunction of central structures that process sensory input from the inner ear. Central vertigo accounts for 2–23% of vertigo diagnoses, depending on the specialty setting in which patients are seen. In a majority of cases, central vertigo is caused by vascular disorders such as stroke, transient ischemic attack, and vertebrobasilar migraine. Table 16-1 lists entities accounting for only about 60% of central vertigo diagnoses, the remainder being made up of individual unusual conditions (e.g., spinocerebellar degeneration).

1. **Stroke** and **transient ischemic attack (TIA)** involving the brainstem or

Table 16-1. Etiologies of vertigo.

Otologic Vertigo
BPPV
Vestibular neuritis and labyrinthitis
Ménière's disease
Bilateral vestibular paresis or loss
Perilymph fistula
Tumors compressing the eighth nerve

Central Vertigo
Stroke and transient ischemic attack
Vertebrobasilar migraine
Seizures
Multiple sclerosis
Arnold-Chiari malformation

Medical Vertigo
Postural hypotension
Arrythmia
Hypoglycemia and diabetes
Medication effect
Viral syndrome

Unlocalized Vertigo Syndromes
Unknown
Anxiety and panic
Post-traumatic vertigo
Hyperventilation
Malingering

cerebellum causes about one-third of all central dizziness cases. Pure vertigo can occasionally be the only symptom preceding a posterior fossa stroke, and there are no reliable means of distinguishing a TIA affecting the vestibular nucleus from another process affecting the vestibular nerve or end organ.

2. **Vertebrobasilar migraine** ordinarily presents with vertigo and headache, but it can also present as isolated vertigo. Migraine causes about 15% of central vertigo cases. Migraine is particularly common in women in their thirties.

3. **Seizures** present with vertigo combined with motor symptoms or confusion, or more frequently as quick spins. About 5% of central vertigo cases are caused by seizures.

4. **Multiple sclerosis (MS)** combines vertigo with other central signs, such as cerebellar dysfunction. MS is an uncommon source of vertigo, although many patients suspect it as a cause of symptoms. MRI assists in the diagnosis. About 2% of central vertigo cases are caused by MS.

5. The **Arnold-Chiari malformation** is a hindbrain malformation wherein the cerebellar tonsils herniate 5 mm or more below the foramen magnum. These patients complain of vertigo, ataxia, and posterior headaches, and often have downbeat nystagmus. Like perilymph fistula, symptoms may be precipitated by straining or coughing. MRI of the posterior fossa establishes the diagnosis. About 1% of the cases of central vertigo are caused by the Arnold-Chiari malformation.

C. **Medical vertigo** is caused by altered blood pressure, decreased blood sugar, and/or metabolic derangements associated with medication or systemic infection. Medical vertigo is largely encountered in the emergency room, where it accounts for about 33% of all cases of dizziness. Medical vertigo is unusual in subspecialty settings (2–5%). Table 16-1 lists nearly all causes of dizziness reported in studies of vertigo as it presents to emergency rooms.

1. **Postural hypotension** presents as giddiness, lightheadedness, or syncope. Dizziness occurs only while the patient is upright.

2. **Cardiac arrythmia** presents with syncope or drop-attacks. Like those of postural hypotension, symptoms are characteristically present only when patients are upright.

3. **Hypoglycemia** and **metabolic derangements associated with diabetes** present with giddiness or lightheadedness. Together they account for about 5% of the cases of dizziness in general medical settings.

4. **Medication effect** or **substance abuse** usually presents with giddiness or lightheadedness, but also can present with true vertigo. These diagnoses account for about 16% of the dizzy patients seen in the emergency setting, but are rare outside the emergency room. Medications commonly encountered include antihypertensive agents, especially alpha-1 adrenergic blockers such as terazosin (Hytrin), calcium channel blockers with strong vasodilating effects such as nifedipine (Procardia), and sedatives. Certain common benzodiazepines, such as Xanax, cause dizziness as part of the withdrawal syndrome. Vestibular suppressant medications, such as meclizine (Antivert) and scopolamine (Transderm-Scōp), can cause dizziness through direct effects on central vestibular pathways.

5. **Viral syndromes** not involving the ear are the reported cause of dizziness in 4–40% of all cases seen in the emergency room setting. Such syndromes might include, for example, gastroenteritis and influenza-like illnesses.

D. **Unlocalized vertigo** patients include those whose symptoms are attributed to psychiatric disorders, those whose symptoms are attributed to events without further definition (such as head trauma), and those with vertigo and dizziness of unknown origin. Common variants of unlocalized vertigo include psychogenic vertigo, hyperventilation syndrome, post-traumatic vertigo, and nonspecific dizziness. About 50% of all patients with dizziness or vertigo fall into this category.

1. **Unknown.** Diagnostic procedures are insensitive, and in dizziness evaluations it is usual to have a significant population of patients without any detectable abnormalities on careful clinical examination and thorough testing. Unfortunately, some authors wrongly define psychogenic vertigo as the complaints of patients falling into this category. About 75% of the unlocalized vertigo category consists of patients in whom there are no abnormalities on examination and testing.

2. **Anxiety and panic.** These patients complain of dizziness, ataxia, and autonomic symptoms. This is a common presentation. It is often difficult to determine whether or not anxiety is the cause or a reaction.

3. **Post-traumatic vertigo** patients complain of vertigo following head injuries but present no findings on examination or vestibular testing. Post-traumatic vertigo is common.

4. **Hyperventilation syndrome.** These patients have vertigo resulting from hyperventilation, without other findings. Most authors report that hyperventilation syndrome is uncommon.

5. **Multisensory disequilibrium of the elderly.** Most elderly people have age-related multisensory impairment. Like the diagnosis of psychogenic vertigo, this diagnosis is often used in situations where examination is otherwise normal.

6. **Malingering.** Because vertigo can be intermittent and disabling, and frequently follows head injury, vertigo may be claimed in an attempt to obtain compensation. Malingering is common only among patients who are being compensated for illness.

II. **Clinical manifestations**

A. **Primary symptoms.** The primary symptoms listed in Table 16-2 are mainly the result of a disturbed sensorium.

1. **Vertigo** denotes a sensation of rotation—either of the person or of the world. Vertigo can be horizontal, vertical, or rotatory (about the front-back axis). It is also described as visual "blurring" or "jumping." Horizontal vertigo is the most common type, usually resulting from dysfunction of the inner ear. Vertical vertigo is rarer. When transient, it is usually caused by BPPV. When constant, it is usually of central origin and accompanied by downbeat or upbeat nystagmus. Rotatory vertigo is the least frequent. When transient, rotatory vertigo is usually caused by BPPV. When chronic, it is always central and is usually accompanied by rotatory nystagmus.

2. **Impulsion** denotes a sensation of translation, usually described as brief sensations of being pushed or tilted. Variants include rocking, floating, and perceived changes in the directions of up and down. Impulsion indicates dysfunction of the otolithic apparatus of the inner ear or central processing of otolithic signals.

Table 16-2. Symptoms in patients with dizziness and vertigo.

Primary Symptoms
Vertigo
Impulsion and rocking
Oscillopsia
Ataxia
Hearing symptoms

Secondary Symptoms
Nausea, emesis, diarrhea
Pallor, bradycardia
Fatigue
Headache
Visual sensitivity

Nonspecific Symptoms
Giddiness
Lightheadedness

3. **Oscillopsia** is an illusory movement of the world evoked by head movement. Patients with bilateral vestibular loss are unable to see when their heads are in motion because of oscillopsia. Patients with unilateral vestibular loss often complain that "the world doesn't keep up" when they rapidly move their heads laterally to the side of the bad ear.

4. **Ataxia,** unsteadiness of gait, is nearly universal in patients with otologic or central vertigo, and is variably observed in patients with medical and unlocalized vertigo.

5. **Hearing symptoms.** Vertigo is often accompanied by tinnitus, hearing reduction or distortion, and aural fullness.

B. **Secondary symptoms** include nausea, autonomic symptoms, fatigue, headache, and visual sensitivity. These symptoms accompany vertigo in varying amounts according to individual susceptibility. Although most secondary symptoms are self-explanatory, **visual sensitivity,** also known as the "grocery store syndrome," is not encountered frequently in other contexts. Patients complain of dizziness related to the types of patterned visual stimulation that occur when one views grocery store aisles, drives past picket fences or through bridges, or views large screen movies. The grocery store syndrome is a nonspecific common late symptom in patients with vertigo, and presumably reflects a visual-vestibular mismatch.

C. **Giddiness and lightheadedness.** These terms have no precise meanings in common usage. They are rarely used by patients with documented inner ear dysfunction but are frequently used by patients with vertigo related to medical problems (e.g., postural hypotension or hypoglycemia).

III. **Evaluation**

A. **History.** Because of the numerous potential causes of vertigo cutting across four subspecialty areas, the history must either be all-encompassing or follow a heuristic technique whereby questions are dynamically selected as the interview progresses. Here we outline the all-encompassing approach.

1. **Definition.** Does the patient complain of vertigo (spinning), a secondary symptom (such as nausea), a nonspecific symptom (giddiness or lightheadedness), or something entirely different (e.g., confusion)?

2. **Timing.** Are symptoms constant or episodic? If episodic, how long do they last?

3. **Triggering or exacerbating factors** are listed in Table 16-3. All patients should be queried regarding these factors, either by going through them one by one, or by using an interview heuristic whereby one attempts to rule in or rule out a symptom complex (see sec. **IV**).

4. **Otologic history.** Ask about hearing loss, tinnitus, and fullness. Positives indicate an audiogram. Ask about the type of tinnitus—"roaring" tinnitus suggests Ménière's disease.

5. **Medication history.** Numerous medications can induce vertigo, including ototoxins (especially gentamicin), anticonvulsants, antihypertensives, and

Table 16-3. Triggering or exacerbating factors.

Changes in position of the head or body
Standing up
Rapid head movements
Walking in a dark room
Loud noises
Coughing, blowing the nose, sneezing, straining, or laughing
Underwater diving, elevators, airplane travel
Exercise
Later times in the day
Shopping malls, narrow or wide-open spaces, grocery stores, escalators
    (visual sensitivity complex)
Foods, not eating, salt, monosodium glutamate
Alcohol
Menstrual periods
Boat or car travel
Anxiety or stress

---

sedatives. All current medications, as well as previous exposure to ototoxins, should be considered as sources of vertigo.

6. **Family history.** Has anyone in the immediate family had similar symptoms? Is there a family history of migraine, seizures, Ménière's disease, or early-onset hearing loss?

7. **Review of systems** should explore psychiatric problems (anxiety, depression, and panic), vascular risk factors, cancer, autoimmune disease, neurologic problems (migraine, stroke, TIA, seizures, and MS), otologic surgery, and general medical history (especially thyroid dysfunction, diabetes, and syphilis).

8. **Previous studies** relevant to dizziness (see sec. **III.C**) should be reviewed.

B. **Physical examination.** The physical examination of the vertiginous patient is outlined in Table 16-4. It is ordered in such a way that procedures may be added on the basis of previous results. Because a full examination may be quite lengthy, it is most practical to expand or contract the examination dynamically. As an exception to the following procedure, if there is a history of positional vertigo, it is best to go immediately to the Dix-Hallpike test (see sec. **III.B.5.b**).

1. **General examination.** Blood pressure and pulse are taken with the patient standing. Arrythmia is noted, if present. If the standing blood pressure is low (110/70 or lower), check blood pressure with the patient lying flat. The heart and the carotid and subclavian arteries are auscultated. In patients with potential syncope, who are less than 70 years of age, 10 seconds of carotid sinus massage may be undertaken. This is done with the patient in the sitting position, first on one side and then on the other, to see if symptoms are reproduced.

2. **Balance** is assessed via observation of gait (apraxic, antalgic, ataxic, bizarre, normal, or parkinsonian) and the eyes-closed tandem Romberg test. The tandem Romberg test is extremely useful. Low normal performance consists of the ability to stand heel-to-toe, with eyes closed, for 6 seconds. Young adults should be able to perform this test for 30 seconds, but performance declines with age.

It is helpful to develop a judgment of how much ataxia is appropriate for a given degree of ear injury. Patients with **bilateral vestibular loss** are moderately ataxic—they make heavy use of vision and are unsteady when their eyes are closed (with a narrow base). No patient with bilateral loss can stand in the eyes-closed tandem Romberg test for 6 seconds. Patients with an additional superimposed position sense deficit are unsteady with eyes open (with a narrow base). Patients with **chronic unilateral vestibular loss** show very little ataxia, and they are usually normal on the eyes-closed tandem Romberg test. The need to gauge ataxia does not come up in patients with recent unilateral vestibular imbalance, because these patients

Table 16-4. Examination procedures for dizziness and vertigo.

Procedures in *italics* are always performed; procedures not in italics are performed only for certain symptom complexes.

Procedures	Triggers for additions
General Examination	
Orthostasis	
Arrythmia	
Carotid sinus hyperreactivity	Syncope
Balance Assessment	
Observe gait	
Eyes-closed tandem Romberg test	
Pulsion and retropulsion	Parkinsonian gait
Otologic Examination	
Hearing	
Tympanic membranes	
Neurologic Examination	
Cranial nerves	
Long tract signs	
Cerebellar	
Position sense testing	Fails Romberg test
Nystagmus Assessment	
Spontaneous nystagmus	
Dix-Hallpike positional test	
Head-shake test	Negative exam so far
Fistula test	Pressure sensitivity
Hyperventilation	Negative exam so far
VOR Gain Assessment	
Dynamic illegible "E" test	Fails Romberg test
Ophthalmoscope test	Fails "E" test

have prominent nystagmus. Patients with **cerebellar disorders,** such as alcoholic cerebellar degeneration, have greater ataxia than is appropriate for their degree of nystagmus or vestibular paresis. Patients who are **malingering** also typically emphasize imbalance, which is the disabling aspect of their symptoms.

In head injury or where there is other reason to suspect a CNS origin of imbalance, also test basal ganglia function (pulsion/retropulsion tests).

3. **Otologic examination.** A brief screening test is adequate for hearing. The examiner's thumb and first fingers are rubbed together at arm's length from one of the patient's ears. Persons with normal hearing can perceive this sound at an arm's length. If the sound is not perceived, the source is brought in closer and closer until it is heard, and the distance is recorded. This simple test identifies high-tone hearing loss—for example, most elderly are able to hear at about 6 inches on either side. The tympanic membranes should be inspected for wax, perforation, otitis, discoloration, and mass lesions. Wax should always be removed before more sophisticated diagnostic procedures are performed.

4. **Neurologic examination.** An abbreviated neurologic examination is adequate. The cranial nerve examination includes ophthalmoscopy, extraocular movements (range, saccadic accuracy and velocity, and pursuit), and facial movement. It usually is convenient to check the vestibuloocular reflex (VOR) and nystagmus with the ophthalmoscope at this point (see secs. **III.B.5.a** and **III.B.6.b**). The motor examination includes tests for reflexes, Babinski signs, and gross assessment of power. The cerebellar examination includes finger-to-nose testing and rapid alternating movement testing. Sensory examination of position sense is done when ataxia is present.

5. **Nystagmus** (involuntary movement of the eyes) indicates an inner ear, brain, or ocular muscle disorder.

  a. **Spontaneous nystagmus** is best assessed using Frenzel's goggles, which are illuminated, magnifying goggles worn by the patient. The goggles are placed on the patient and the eyes are observed for spontaneous nystagmus for 10 seconds. The typical nystagmus produced by inner ear dysfunction is a primary position "jerk" nystagmus—the eyes slowly deviate off center and then there is a rapid "jerk," which brings them back to the center position. Most nystagmus of other patterns (e.g., sinusoidal, gaze-evoked, and saccadic) is of central origin.

   If Frenzel's goggles are not available, similar information about nystagmus can be obtained from the ophthalmoscopic exam. One simply monitors movement of the back of the eye. As the back of the eye moves oppositely to the front of the eye, for horizontal and vertical movement, one must remember to invert the direction of the nystagmus when making notes. Fixation can be removed by covering the opposite eye. Nystagmus deriving from the inner ear is increased by removal of fixation.

  b. **Dix-Hallpike positional test** (Fig. 16-1). The Frenzel goggles are temporarily removed, and the patient is repositioned on the examination table so that, on lying flat, the head extends over the end of the table. If Frenzel's goggles are available, they are replaced on the patient, but ordi-

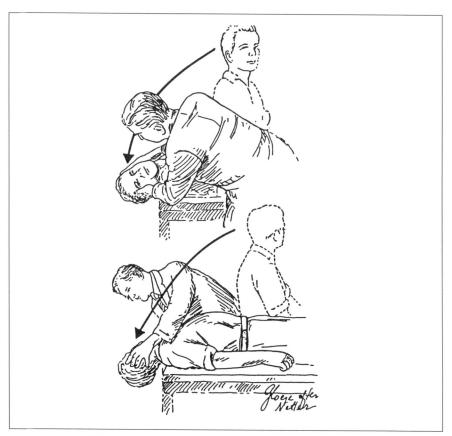

Figure 16-1. Dix-Hallpike positional test. To precipitate the characteristic nystagmus of benign paroxysmal positional vertigo (BPPV), the patient is rapidly brought into a head position that makes the posterior canal vertical and also brings it through a large angular displacement. (From Bahloh RW, Honrubia V. *Clinical Neurophysiology of the Vestibular System* (2nd ed). Philadelphia: Davis, 1990. P 124)

narily one can get by without them. The patient is then moved rapidly to the head-hanging position. If no dizziness or nystagmus is appreciated after 20 seconds, the patient is sat back up. The head is then repositioned to 45 degrees right, and the patient is brought down to the head-right supine position. After another 20 seconds, the patient is sat up again, and the procedure is repeated to the left (head-left position). One hopes to see a burst of nystagmus provoked by either the head-right or the head-left position. The nystagmus of classic BPPV beats upward and also has a rotatory component, such that the top part of the eye beats toward the down ear. The nystagmus typically has a latency of 2–5 seconds, lasts 5–60 seconds, and is followed by a downbeat nystagmus when the patient is sat up. There is also a lateral-canal variant of BPPV in which the eyes beat horizontally, toward the down ear.

    c. Head-shake nystagmus. If there is no spontaneous nystagmus or positional nystagmus and if Frenzel's goggles are available, the head-shake test may be performed. The patient's eyes are closed and the head is moved in the horizontal plane, back and forth, for 20 cycles. One aims for a 45-degree excursion of the head to either side and a frequency of 2 cycles per second. A nystagmus lasting 5 seconds or more is an indication of an organic disorder of the ear or central nervous system, and supports further investigation.

    d. The **fistula test** is performed if there is a pressure sensitivity symptom complex on history (see sec. **IV**). Three or four pulses of pressure are delivered to each external ear canal in turn while the patient watches an eye chart. A positive test consists of dizziness or apparent movement of the eye chart correlated with pressure.

    e. The **hyperventilation test** is performed if so far the examination has been entirely normal. The patient takes 30 deep, hard breaths. Immediately after hyperventilation, the eyes are inspected for nystagmus with the Frenzel's goggles and the patient is asked if the procedure has reproduced the symptoms. A positive test without nystagmus suggests the diagnosis of hyperventilation syndrome. Nystagmus induced by hyperventilation suggests a tumor of the eighth nerve or MS.

  6. Assessment of VOR gain. These maneuvers are aimed at documenting bilateral vestibular loss. They need not be done unless the patient has failed the eyes-closed tandem Romberg test.

    a. The dynamic illegible "E" test. Using an eye chart at a distance of at least 10 ft, visual acuity is recorded with the head still. Then the examiner gently moves the patient's head horizontally at roughly 1 Hz, ±30 degrees, and visual acuity is again recorded. Normal subjects drop from zero to two lines of acuity with head movement. Patients with partial to complete bilateral loss of vestibular function drop from three to seven lines of acuity. Patients with complete bilateral loss usually drop seven lines of acuity.

    b. The **ophthalmoscope test** is done when the illegible "E" test is positive, to obtain objective corroboration. The examiner focuses on the optic disk and then gently moves the head as described above. If the disk moves with the head, this confirms that the VOR gain is abnormal. This test is less sensitive than the illegible "E" test.

C. Laboratory studies. Table 16-5 enumerates laboratory procedures commonly used for evaluation of patients with vertigo and dizziness, with indications. For efficiency and cost containment, procedures should be selected according to specific symptom complexes and be done sequentially. Algorithms are discussed in secs. **IV** and **V**.

  1. Audiologic testing is not needed for every dizzy patient but may be appropriate when there are hearing complaints. Audiometry is the most generally applicable technique and is recommended even for patients who have no hearing abnormalities, if the diagnosis is uncertain.

    a. Audiogram. The audiogram measures hearing. Abnormalities suggest otologic vertigo. Audiograms often include a battery of procedures including tympanometry and acoustic reflex testing. In situations where cost containment is important, the two latter procedures may be omitted.

    b. The **brainstem auditory evoked response (BAER)** test assesses the auditory nerve and brainstem pathways. Because BAERs are of little use

Table 16-5. Laboratory procedures for dizziness and vertigo.

Test	Indication
Audiologic Tests	
Audiogram	Vertigo, hearing symptoms
BAER	Asymmetric hearing loss
ECOG	Secondary test for Ménière's disease and PLF
MLR	
Otoacoustic emissions	
Vestibular Tests	
ENG	Vertigo
Rotatory chair test	Bilateral loss, secondary to confirm ENG
Fistula test	Pressure sensitivity
Posturography	Malingering
Blood Tests	
FTA-ABS	Vertigo with hearing symptoms
Glycohemoglobin	Hydrops symptom complex
ANA	Hydrops symptom complex
TSH	Hydrops symptom complex
Radiologic Tests	
MRI of head	Central vertigo, abnormal BAER
MRA, vertebrobasilar	TIA
CT scan of temporal bone	PLF, mastoiditis, congenital abnormality, significant head trauma
Other Tests	
EEG	Quick spins, head trauma
Ambulatory event monitoring (Holter monitoring)	Cardiogenic syncope
Tilt table test	

for patients who have no high-frequency hearing, audiometry is recommended prior to BAER testing. Abnormal BAERs should trigger an MRI of the posterior fossa (T1 with contrast). For cost efficiency, BAER need not be obtained if an MRI is planned.

    c. **Electrocochleography (ECOG)** is a variant of the BAER test in which needle electrodes are used. Like BAER, ECOG also requires reasonable high-frequency hearing. An abnormal ECOG is suggestive of Ménière's disease.

    d. **Miscellaneous tests.** The MLR or middle latency response is a central variant of the BAER test. Otoacoustic emissions measure sounds generated by the ear itself. At the present writing, neither of these recently developed tests has found a place in the usual diagnostic process.

2. **Vestibular testing** is not needed for every dizzy patient. The primary study—the electronystagmography (ENG) test—is helpful when there is no clear diagnosis after history and examination.

    a. **Electronystagmography (ENG)** is a battery of procedures that can identify vestibular asymmetry (such as that caused by vestibular neuritis) and document spontaneous or positional nystagmus (such as that caused by BPPV). ENG is an intrinsically inaccurate test, and an abnormal result that doesn't fit the clinical picture should be confirmed by rotatory chair testing.

    b. **Rotatory chair testing** measures vestibular function of both inner ears together. Rotatory testing is highly sensitive and specific for bilateral loss of vestibular function. In unilateral loss, it is sensitive but nonspecific. Also, it does not identify the side of the lesion.

    c. **Fistula testing** involves recording of nystagmus induced by pressure in the external ear canal. Its sensitivity to perilymph fistula is only 50%.

    d. **Posturography** is an instrumented Romberg test. Except to document malingering, posturography has no diagnostic value.

3. **Blood tests** are triggered by specific symptom complexes (see sec. **IV**), and there is no "routine" set obtained for every dizzy patient. In particular, chemistry panels, CBCs, glucose tolerance tests, and allergy tests need not be routinely ordered.
4. **Radiologic investigations.** Skull films, cervical spine films, CT scans of the head, and CT scans of the sinuses are *not* recommended routinely in the evaluation of vertigo.
   a. **MRI scan of the head** evaluates the structural integrity of the brainstem, cerebellum, periventricular white matter, and eighth nerve complexes. The T1 MRI with contrast is the most useful variant. MRI is not routinely needed to evaluate vertigo without accompanying neurologic findings. Although MRI may show enhancement of the vestibular nerve in vestibular neuritis, it seems unreasonable to use this expensive test to document the existence of a self-limited condition.
   b. **CT scan of the temporal bone** provides higher resolution of ear structures than MRI and also is better for evaluating lesions involving bone.
5. **Other tests**
   a. **Electroencephalography (EEG)** is used to diagnose seizures. Because EEGs are insensitive procedures, several may be required.
   b. **Ambulatory event monitoring,** or Holter monitoring, is used to detect arrythmia or sinus arrest.
   c. **Tilt table testing** is sometimes advocated for diagnosis of syncope. However, because of a present lack of data establishing a link between tilt table test abnormalities and successful treatment outcomes, the appropriate role of the tilt table test in the evaluation of dizzy patients is presently unclear.

IV. **Differential diagnosis.** We will now discuss symptom complexes, their differential diagnosis, and algorithms used to narrow down the differential. This approach can be time-consuming, and is intended for use by an examiner who has about an hour to make an evaluation. Table 16-6 enumerates five specific symptom complexes. When a patient does not fit into a complex in Table 16-6, one may fall back to grouping patients by duration of symptoms only, as in Table 16-7.
   A. **Approach based on specific symptom complexes**
      1. **Bed spins and positional syndromes.** Patients complain of a brief burst of rotatory vertigo when getting into or out of bed, or on rolling over from

Table 16-6. Specific symptom complexes.

Positional Vertigo (Bed Spins)
BPPV (95%)
Central vertigo
Vestibular neuritis
Postural hypotension

Headaches and Vertigo
Vertebrobasilar migraine
Post-traumatic vertigo
Arnold-Chiari malformation
Unlocalized vertigo

Hydrops Symptom Complex (Fluctuating Hearing, Vertigo, Tinnitus, Fullness)
Ménière's disease
Perilymph fistula
Post-traumatic hydrops
Syphilis

Pressure Sensitivity Symptom Complex
Perilymph fistula
Ménière's disease
Arnold-Chiari malformation
Stapes malformation

Medicolegal Situations
Malingering and disability evaluations

Table 16-7. Typical duration of selected conditions causing dizziness.

1–3 Seconds (Quick Spins)
Epilepsy
Vestibular nerve irritation
Ménière's disease variants
BPPV variants

Less than 1 Minute
BPPV
Arrythmia
Ménière's disease variants

Minutes to Hours
TIA
Ménière's disease
Panic attacks, situational anxiety, hyperventilation
Orthostasis

Hours to Days
Ménière's disease
Vertebrobasilar migraine

Two Weeks or More
Vestibular neuritis and labyrinthitis
Central vertigo with structural lesion
Anxiety
Malingering
Bilateral vestibular paresis or loss
Multisensory disequilibrium of the elderly
Drug intoxications

one side to the other. This symptom strongly suggests the diagnosis of benign paroxysmal positional vertigo (BPPV).

a. **BPPV.** If a typical nystagmus is observed on Dix-Hallpike positional testing, no other diagnoses need be considered. Because roughly 95% of all positional nystagmus is caused by BPPV, even in cases in which an atypical positional nystagmus is observed, it is usually most efficient to try one of the currently available treatments before considering other diagnoses. MRI of the head is indicated when an atypical BPPV is refractory to treatment.

b. **Central disorders.** Strong positional nystagmus may also accompany brainstem and cerebellar disorders (for example, medulloblastoma and the Arnold-Chiari malformation). MRI is indicated when positional nystagmus is combined with an abnormal neurologic examination or when an atypical BPPV is refractory to treatment.

c. **Vestibular neuritis.** A weak horizontal positional nystagmus may be found in peripheral vestibulopathies. ENG and audiogram are indicated.

d. **Postural hypotension** also presents with dizziness on getting out of bed, but never occurs in bed. It is diagnosed by a symptomatic decrease in blood pressure or increase in pulse rate between the supine and standing positions. A drop of 20 mm of mercury is significant.

2. **Headaches and vertigo**

a. **Migraine.** One large group of patients are women in their thirties with perimenstrual exacerbations. Food triggers, motion sickness, and positive family history are frequent associations. Empirical trials of antimigraine medication (verapamil) may be the only way to make this diagnosis.

b. **Post-traumatic vertigo.** Audiometry, ENG, CT scan of the head, and EEG are indicated.

c. **Arnold-Chiari malformation.** The headache is posterior, and there is downbeat nystagmus and ataxia. Diagnosis is done by sagittal T1-MRI.

d. **Unlocalized vertigo.** Audiometry and ENG are indicated for the vertigo component. The headache component (tension, migraine, sinus, etc.) is considered separately.

3. **Hydrops.** Patients complain of spells of vertigo, roaring tinnitus, and transient hearing loss, preceded by aural fullness. Audiometry should be obtained in all patients, as well as fluorescent treponemal antibody absorption (FTA), sedimentation rate, and thyroid-stimulating hormone (TSH) blood tests.

   a. **Ménière's disease.** The usual duration of vertigo is 2 hours, but it can vary from seconds to weeks. Audiometry is crucial to document the fluctuating low-tone sensorineural hearing loss (Fig. 16-2). The diagnosis of Ménière's disease is highly probable when a typical history is obtained, and when fluctuating hearing is documented. ECOG testing may be performed in difficult cases, in an attempt to "rule in" the diagnosis. About 10% of all cases of bilateral Ménière's disease are autoimmune. Thyroid disease is frequent in patients with Ménière's disease.

   b. **Perilymph fistula (PLF).** Occasionally, fistula presents with hydrops rather than the pressure sensitivity symptom complex (see sec. **IV.A.4**). The only clue may be a history of barotrauma. Fistula testing is indicated.

   c. **Post-traumatic hydrops** is a variant of the Ménière's disease symptom complex that appears after a significant blow to the ear, with presumed bleeding into the inner ear.

   d. **Syphilis.** Hearing loss is bilateral. Diagnosis is by FTA-ABS.

4. **Pressure sensitivity.** Patients complain of dizziness or ataxia evoked by nose blowing, high-speed elevators, cleaning of the ear with a cotton swab, straining as at stool, after the landing of an airplane, or after diving. In addition to pressure sensitivity, patients with fistula may report vertigo induced by loud noises (Tullio's phenomenon) and by exercise. Patients are often extremely motion-intolerant and visually sensitive. Audiometry and the fistula test are indicated.

   a. **Perilymph fistula** is the main source of pressure sensitivity. Most patients have a history of barotrauma. Audiometry and the fistula test are indicated. The ECOG may be used as a secondary test if audiometry and the fistula test fail to establish the side of injury.

   b. **Ménière's disease.** Mild pressure sensitivity occurs in about one-third of patients with Ménière's disease. See the hydrops symptom complex description (sec. **IV.A.3**) for a differential diagnosis.

   c. **Arnold-Chiari malformation.** Vertigo is correlated with straining but not with pressure in the external ear canal. The downbeat nystagmus and abnormal MRI found in the Arnold-Chiari malformation also separate it from the other entities.

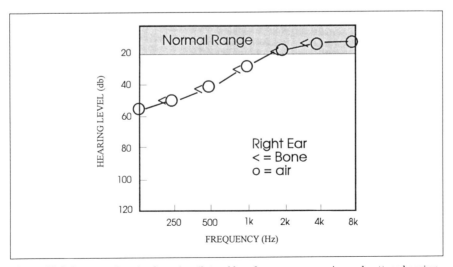

Figure 16-2. Low-tone hearing loss. A unilateral low-frequency sensorineural pattern hearing loss is often observed in early Ménière's disease.

d. Stapes malformation. Remarkable pressure sensitivity with torsional movement of the eye occurs in patients with congenital malformations of the stapes footplate and also in patients in whom stapes prostheses (for otosclerosis) of excessive length have been inserted. A CT scan of the temporal bone is indicated in this situation, if there has been no stapes surgery.

5. **Medicolegal situations.** The possibility of malingering often comes up in disability evaluations, worker's compensation cases, and legal situations where patients may potentially be compensated for being vertiginous. These patients usually present no objective evidence on physical examination or testing. Often they may resist examination, by closing their eyes at inappropriate times or refusing to perform key positional maneuvers. Their complaints often cannot be resolved into one of the symptom complexes discussed above. Objective testing (audiometry, ENG, or an MRI scan of the head) is nearly always appropriate. In addition, posturography may be helpful. This test can trick the malingering patient by presenting a series of protocols that gradually become more and more difficult. The malingerer who is trying to fail the posturography test will frequently perform equally poorly on the easy and difficult subtests, producing a nonphysiologic pattern.

B. **Approach based on timing only.** These categories, as documented in Table 16-7, are less useful for diagnosis than those based on symptom complexes, but can be used when patients don't fall into any category. As such, they form a clinical "fall back" strategy.

1. **Quick spins** are brief spells (1–3 seconds) of true vertigo, unaccompanied by secondary symptoms. EEG and BAER should be obtained. A trial of carbamazepine may be helpful.

   a. **Epilepsy.** Spells are often very frequent (20 per day), and there is often a history of head injury. Cognitive impairment is frequent.

   b. **Microvascular compression syndrome.** Frequent spells are also possible. There may also be hearing symptoms such as a "sizzling" tinnitus. The BAER may be abnormal. Magnetic resonance angiography (MRA) occasionally documents a vertebral or basilar artery compressing the brainstem. If the EEG is normal, a good response to carbamazepine suggests the diagnosis.

   c. **Ménière's disease variants.** Frequency of spells is daily at most. Hearing is often affected. For diagnosis, see hydrops symptom complex (sec. **IV.A.3**).

   d. **BPPV variants.** Spells are of no more than daily frequency. Presumably, otoconial debris is caught on a canal wall and suddenly slips down. Diagnosis is done by the Dix-Hallpike maneuver. It may take several visits to get a positive result.

2. **Less than 1 minute.** These are mainly postural syndromes.

   a. **Classic BPPV.** If there is positional vertigo, this diagnosis is easy. However, poor "historians" may omit to mention that they have adopted sleeping strategies (e.g., two pillows) by which bed spins are avoided. BPPV can also be triggered by unusual head positions such as looking up at the "top shelf." Diagnosis is done by the Dix-Hallpike maneuver.

   b. **Cardiac arrythmia.** The clue is usually that vertigo spells occur *only* while standing, and that lightheadedness is a more prominent symptom than spinning. Ambulatory event monitoring is the best method of documenting this problem. Holter monitoring may be used in contexts where event monitoring is not available.

   c. **Ménière's disease variants.** See sec. **IV.B.1.c**.

3. **Minutes to hours**

   a. **TIA.** Spells of pure vertigo lasting roughly 30 minutes, of abrupt onset and offset, in a patient with significant vascular risk factors are diagnosed as TIA until proven otherwise. MRA of the vertebrobasilar circulation is the single most useful test.

   b. **Ménière's disease.** The typical Ménière's attack lasts 2 hours. If there are hearing symptoms, see the hydrops symptom complex (sec. **IV.A.3**). If not, be cautious about proposing this diagnosis. Sometimes the term "vestibular Ménière's disease" is used to denote episodic vertigo, having the typical timing of classic Ménière's disease but without any ear symptomatology. It is presently unclear whether this entity exists, and there is no method of confirming this diagnosis.

c. **Panic attacks, situational anxiety,** and **hyperventilation** may produce symptoms of this duration (minutes to hours). These patients ordinarily are not symptomatic during examination. A detailed history is the most useful diagnostic test. If hyperventilation reproduces symptoms in patients without other findings, the diagnosis is hyperventilation syndrome. If hyperventilation also induces nystagmus, MRI is indicated.

d. **Cardiac arrythmia and orthostasis**

4. **Hours to days**

a. **Ménière's disease**

b. **Vertebrobasilar migraine.** Migraine is so common in the general population that even unusual variants, such as manifestation solely as a vertiginous aura, are common. Diagnosis is suggested by age (twenties and thirties), sex (usually female), positive family history, and attacks provoked by the usual migraine triggers.

5. **Two weeks or more**

a. **Vestibular neuritis.** Diagnosis is made by combining a long duration with spontaneous nystagmus or an abnormal ENG test. The ENG may document nystagmus or a significant vestibular paresis (a conservative criterion is a paresis of 40% or more). After 2 months of vertigo, central vertigo becomes more likely and an MRI is indicated. For **labyrinthitis** the diagnosis is made by combining the vestibular neuritis pattern with hearing symptoms. Audiometry, serum FTA, sedimentation rate, and fasting glucose are indicated.

b. **Central vertigo with a fixed structural CNS lesion.** This diagnosis should be considered when there are neurologic symptoms or signs accompanying vertigo. Central vertigo may last indefinitely. For example, the combination of a peripheral vestibular loss with a cerebellar lesion may occur after acoustic neuroma surgery. MRI is the most effective method of diagnosis.

c. **Anxiety.** With this duration of symptoms (2 weeks or more), patients may be complaining of vertigo in your office. If a patient is presently complaining of vertigo, but no spontaneous nystagmus is evident under Frenzel's goggles, one may reasonably conclude that the vertigo is probably functional in origin. Patients with anxiety typically report that nearly every trigger factor in Table 16-4 exacerbates their symptoms. Interestingly, whereas most patients with inner ear problems report that stress makes their symptoms worse, patients with anxiety frequently are sensitive about this diagnosis and perversely claim that everything *except* stress triggers vertigo. A positive response to a trial of a benzodiazepine such as lorazepam supports this diagnosis but does not establish it, because many organic vestibular disorders also respond well to these medications.

d. **Malingering.** Malingerers persist in reporting symptoms as long as necessary to accomplish their purpose of obtaining favorable court settlements or disability rulings. Posturography may be helpful.

e. **Bilateral vestibular paresis or loss.** These patients universally fail the dynamic illegible "E" test and the eyes-closed tandem Romberg test. Their ataxia is worse in the dark. On audiometry, usually only high-frequency hearing is affected. Rotary chair testing is the best way to confirm this diagnostic impression.

f. **Multisensory disequilibrium of the elderly** is essentially an unlocalized vertigo in an elderly patient. If the diagnosis is accurate, this is usually a permanent condition.

g. **Drug intoxications.** Diagnosis depends on withdrawal of medications.

V. **Diagnostic approach**

A. Perform history and examination as outlined in secs. **II** and **III**.

B. Approximately 20–40% of patients are diagnosed immediately on examination.

1. BPPV patients on Dix-Hallpike maneuver (15–20% of vertigo population)

2. Orthostatic hypotension, arrythmia, and carotid sinus hypersensitivity (2–5%)

3. Bilateral vestibular paresis or loss on dynamic illegible "E" test (5%)

4. Fistula on fistula test (0–5%)

       5. Acute vestibular neuritis via spontaneous nystagmus (2–5%)

  C. For the remaining patients, proceed as follows.

       1. If patient fits into a symptom complex category, follow procedures presented in sec. **IV.A.**

       2. If patient does not fit into a symptom complex, follow procedures outlined in sec. **IV.B.**

         a. If symptoms are intermittent, follow procedures in sec. **IV.B.1–3.**

         b. Otherwise, if symptoms are constant, proceed as follows.

            (1) If duration has been less than 2 weeks, treat symptomatically or simply reassure and have patient return if symptoms persist beyond 2 weeks.

            (2) If duration has been more than 2 weeks, follow the procedures outlined in sec. **IV.B.**

VI. Referrals

  A. Otology

       1. Cerumen disimpaction and microscope exam. Ear wax can be safely removed with the examining microscope, a standard piece of otologic equipment.

       2. Progressive or acute hearing loss has potential medicolegal ramifications, and otologic consultation should be obtained.

       3. A **perforated tympanic membrane** or **mass** in the canal or behind the tympanic membrane may require referral for closure of the perforation or surgical management of the tumor.

       4. Mastoiditis or chronic otitis media. These patients are commonly managed with a mixture of surgery, cleaning, antibiotics, and antiseptics that requires otologic supervision.

       5. Surgical management of acoustic neuroma, Ménière's disease, fistula, and cholesteatoma

  B. Internal medicine

       1. Cardiac or blood pressure problems

       2. Management of diabetes or thyroid dysfunction

  C. Psychiatry

       1. Undiagnosed patients (after thorough evaluation)

       2. Patients with anxiety or panic

       3. Patients who may be malingering

Recommended Readings

Brandt T. *Vertigo. Its Multisensory Syndromes.* London: Springer-Verlag, 1991.

Drachman D, Hart CW. An approach to the dizzy patient. *Neurology* 22:323–334, 1972.

Fisher CM. Vertigo in cerebrovascular disease. *Arch Otolaryngol* 85:85–90, 1967.

Herr RD, Zun L, Mathews JJ. A directed approach to the dizzy patient. *Annals Emerg Med* 18:664–672, 1989.

Kroenke K, et al. Causes of persistent dizziness. *Ann Int Med* 117:898–904, 1992.

Kroenke K, et al. Psychiatric disorders and functional impairment in patients with persistent dizziness. *J Gen Int Med* 8:530–535, 1993.

Macrae D. The neurologic aspects of vertigo. Analysis of 400 cases. *California Med* 92:255–259, 1960.

Madlon-Kay DJ. Evaluation and outcome of the dizzy patient. *J Family Practice* 21:109–113, 1985.

Nedzelski JM, Barber HO, McIlmoyl L. Diagnoses in a dizziness unit. *J Otolaryngol* 15:101–104, 1986.

Sloane PD. Dizziness in primary care. Results from the national ambulatory medical care survey. *J Family Practice* 29:33–38, 1989.

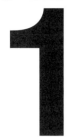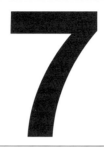

Approach to the Patient with Hearing Loss

Richard T. Miyamoto
Michael K. Wynne

Hearing loss is the most prevalent physical ailment in the United States, affecting approximately 1 in 10 individuals. It produces significant communication problems and may be the presenting symptom of serious underlying medical disorders. A detailed medical and audiologic evaluation is required to establish a specific etiology and management plan.

I. **Etiology.** There are various and complex causes of hearing loss. In many cases, particularly in children, the etiology of the hearing loss may remain unknown or idiopathic even after an extensive medical and audiologic work-up. Despite the diversity of patients and presenting symptoms, the etiology of hearing loss can be classified as either hereditary or adventitious, although there is no clear distinction between the two (e.g., certain populations have a genetic disposition that causes greater susceptibility to noise-induced hearing loss). In addition, the onset of the hearing loss serves as a useful indicator when describing the etiology of the hearing loss. The hearing loss is considered congenital when caused prior to birth, perinatal when occurring during the birthing process, and postnatal when the onset occurs after birth. Finally, nonorganic hearing losses are not uncommon and can be found in young children or in patients with previously confirmed organic hearing loss.

II. **Anatomy and physiology of the auditory system.** The auditory system is divided into four anatomic regions: (1) the external ear, (2) the middle ear, (3) the inner ear, and (4) the central auditory pathway.

A. **External ear.** The external ear, consisting of the pinna and the external auditory canal, collects and directs sound to the tympanic membrane. Because of its physical dimensions, it provides a significant resonance boost between 2000 and 5000 Hz, a frequency range that contributes to the perception of speech.

B. **Middle ear.** The middle ear consists of the tympanic membrane, three ossicles (malleus, incus, and stapes), two middle ear muscles (tensor tympani and stapedius), and the ligaments that suspend the ossicles in the middle ear cavity. The middle ear structures transmit acoustic energy from the external environment to the inner ear and serve as a mechanical transformer recovering energy that would otherwise be lost as sound is transmitted from a gaseous medium (air) to a liquid medium (endolymph).

Two middle ear mechanisms restore most, but not all, of the sound pressure lost in the energy transfer. Most of the mechanical gain results from a concentration of the energy collected by the relatively large tympanic membrane on the small oval window. The areal ratio between the tympanic membrane and the oval window recovers approximately 23 dB of the 30 dB lost. An additional 2 or 3 dB is gained as a result of a lever action that occurs because the handle of the malleus is slightly longer than the long process of the incus.

C. **Inner ear.** The inner ear is divided into the vestibular portion, which consists of three semicircular canals as well as the utricle and saccule, and the auditory portion, which consists of the cochlea. The semicircular canals provide information regarding angular acceleration, and the utricle and saccule provide information regarding gravitational or linear acceleration. The vestibular system, coupled with the visual and proprioceptive systems, functions as the body's balance mechanism. The cochlea is the end organ of hearing. The cochlea is a fluid-filled cavity that is divided by the cochlear partition into three cavities: the scala vestibuli, the scala media, and the scala tympani. With stapes displacement, a traveling wave moves up the cochlear partition, displacing the basilar membrane. This displacement results in a shearing action of the stereocilia at the top of the one set of inner hair cells and the three sets of outer hair cells. The inner hair cells are considered sensory cells and the outer hair cells are considered motor cells. When the stereocilia of the inner hair cell are sheared toward the cell's basal body (the human cochlear hair cell does not have a kinocilium but, rather, a basal body located at the base of the "U" or "W" pattern of the stereocilia), the inner hair cell depolarizes and discharges neurotransmitters at its base and into the synaptic space with the afferent eighth nerve fibers. Because of the stiffness and mass characteristics of the cochlear partition, the traveling wave envelope reaches its peak at a given location along the cochlear partition and then the displacement is heavily damped. This location corresponds to a specific frequency region that is equivalent to the frequency of the auditory stimulus. Thus, the inner ear acts like a low-pass filter with high-frequency sounds encoded at the basal region of the cochlea and low-frequency sounds encoded at the apical region of the cochlea. This tonotopic arrangement is then maintained throughout the central auditory system.

   D. Central auditory system. The central auditory system consists of the auditory portion of the eighth cranial nerve, the cochlear nucleus, the intermediate stria or trapezoid body, the superior olivary complex, the lateral lemniscus, the inferior colliculus, the medial geniculate body of the thalamus, and finally the auditory cortex. The level of neural complexity rises exponentially with each higher-order neuron or central auditory nucleus.

III. Medical evaluation of the auditory system is accomplished by obtaining a detailed history, a physical examination, and audiologic studies. In selected cases, radiologic imaging is indicated.

   A. History. The otologic history includes inquiry into symptoms of ear disease, including hearing loss, ear pain (otalgia), discharge from the ear (otorrhea), tinnitus and other head noises, and vertigo or dizziness. If any of these symptoms is present, a detailed characterization is performed. The clinical significance of hearing loss is related to its time and acuity of onset, its severity, and its tendency to fluctuate or progress. The deleterious effects of hearing loss are particularly great when its onset occurs prior to the development of spoken language (prelingually).

   B. Physical examination. The otologic examination begins with inspection of the pinna and palpation of periauricular structures including periauricular and parotid lymph nodes. Otoscopic examinations of the external ear canal and the tympanic membranes are performed to identify abnormalities of these structures. Pneumatic otoscopy is helpful in assessing tympanic membrane mobility and is particularly useful in identifying subtle middle ear effusions. A complete head and neck examination is performed, including a cranial nerve screen and cerebellar testing.

   1. Tuning fork tests remain an important part of the otologic functional examination for hearing acuity. They are particularly useful in the differentiation between conductive and sensorineural hearing losses. The most useful tuning forks are those with vibrating frequencies of 512 and 1024 Hz.

   The two most commonly used tuning fork tests are Weber's test and Rinne's test. To perform **Weber's test,** the stem of the tuning fork is placed on the midline plane of the skull and the patient is asked to identify the location of the auditory percept within the head. The signal lateralizes to the ear with a conductive hearing loss, provided that there is normal hearing in the opposite ear. This occurs because the ambient room noise in the usual testing situation tends to mask the normal ear, but the poorer ear with a conductive loss does not hear such noise and better hears bone-conducted sound. If a sensorineural loss is present in one ear and the opposite ear is normal, the fork is heard louder in the better ear. **Rinne's test** is performed by alternately placing a ringing tuning fork opposite one external auditory meatus and firmly on the adjacent mastoid bone. The loudness of the tuning fork in these two locations is compared. The normal ear hears a tuning fork about twice as long by air conduction as by bone conduction. A conductive hearing loss reverses this ratio, and sound is heard longer by bone conduction than by air conduction. Patients with sensorineural hearing loss hear better by air conduction than by bone conduction, although hearing sensitivity by both air and bone conduction is reduced.

IV. Hearing. The audiologic evaluation characterizes the type, severity, and configuration of a hearing loss. Loss of hearing can be either partial or total. It can affect the low, middle, or high frequencies and any combination thereof. The acuity of onset and the tendency to fluctuate or progress in severity influence the negative impact of hearing loss.

A. Range of hearing. Although the human ear is sensitive to frequencies from 20 to 20,000 Hz, the frequency range of 300–3000 Hz is the most important for the understanding of speech. During an audiologic evaluation, pure tone thresholds are routinely obtained for frequencies at octave intervals of 250–8000 Hz. This approximates a range from middle C (262 Hz) to one octave above the highest note on a piano (4165 Hz). The range of sound pressure to which the human ear responds is immense. An infinitesimal movement of the hair cells produces a just-audible sound, and yet a trillionfold increase is still tolerable. The large range of numbers required to describe audible sound pressure is best represented by a logarithmic ratio comparing a sound with a standard reference sound. This ratio is called the decibel (dB). The decibel is defined in relation to the physical reference of sound, or sound pressure level (SPL); to the average threshold of normal hearing for young adults, or hearing level (HL); or to a patient's own threshold for the sound stimulus, or sensation level (SL).

Speech sounds vary in their acoustic characteristics. Vowels tend to have most of their energy in the low to middle frequencies and are produced at intensities higher than those of consonants. Thus, vowels carry the power of speech. In contrast, consonants tend to contain higher-frequency information and have lower power. Much of the actual understanding of speech is dependent on the correct perception of the consonants. Consequently, speech may not be audible for patients with significant hearing losses across the entire frequency range. However, in patients with significant hearing losses in the higher frequencies, speech may be heard but not understood.

B. Audiogram. A graphic representation of pure tone responses is provided by the audiogram presented in Figure 17-1. Frequency (pitch) is represented on the horizontal axis and intensity (loudness) on the vertical axis. The 0 dB HL line represents the average threshold level for a group of normal-hearing young adults with no history of otologic disease or noise exposure. Conversational speech at a distance of 1 m has an intensity level of approximately 50–60 dB HL. Most individuals with normal hearing or sensorineural hearing losses would find speech uncomfortably loud at about 80–90 dB HL.

V. Hearing loss is broadly classified into two types: conductive and sensorineural. Each type has a wide variety of pathologic causes. Table 17-1 presents a summary of the diagnostic and audiologic findings associated with various types of hearing loss.

A. Conductive hearing loss occurs when sound cannot efficiently reach the cochlea. The blockage may be the result of abnormalities of the ear canal, the tympanic membrane, or the middle ear ossicles, including the footplate of the stapes. Hearing loss caused by obstruction of the external auditory canal may result from impacted cerumen, foreign bodies in the canal, or swelling of the canal during an infection. Cerumen impaction is the most common cause of conductive hearing loss. Cerumen is normally secreted by glands in the outer one-third of the ear canal to protect the ear canal skin from moisture. It is normally carried to the outside by the canal skin as it migrates from the tympanic membrane to the external auditory meatus. Another cause is congenital atresia of the external auditory canal, in which the canal fails to develop.

Conductive hearing loss may result from damage to the tympanic membrane or middle ear as a result of trauma or infection. Tympanic membrane perforations or ossicular discontinuities are surgically correctable. Otitis media with effusion is the most common cause of conductive hearing loss in children. This condition may be associated with adenoid hypertrophy. The middle ear effusion may require treatment with a myringotomy and tube placement. Otosclerosis is the most common cause of conductive hearing loss in people 15–50 years of age. Otosclerotic bone progressively fixes the stapes in the oval window. This condition can be successfully treated by stapedectomy.

B. Sensorineural hearing loss results from lesions central to the footplate of the stapes, involving the cochlea or cochlear division of the eighth cranial nerve. When the lesion is located within the cochlea, the hearing loss is considered to be sensory (end organ), whereas when the lesion is located within the neural pathways, the hearing loss is neural or retrocochlear. In sensorineural hearing losses, both air- and bone-conduction thresholds are outside the normal range of hearing sensitivity.

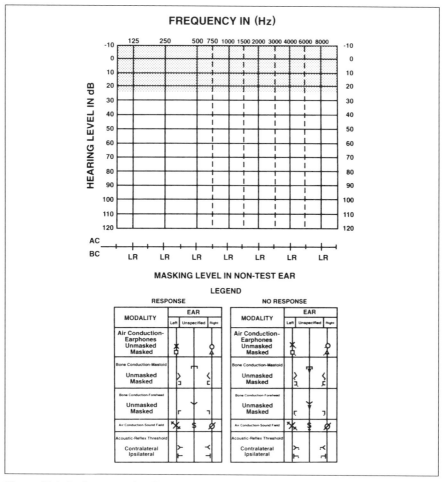

Figure 17-1. Audiogram and audiometric symbols.

Sensorineural hearing loss may be hereditary, and at least 100 genetic syndromes that involve hearing loss have been identified. It has been estimated that 50% of childhood sensorineural hearing loss is caused by genetic factors (Northern and Downs). Genetic forms of hearing loss may be congenital or delayed in onset, unilateral or bilateral, and progressive or nonprogressive. Several viruses, including cytomegaloviruses, rubella, and herpes simplex, have been implicated as etiologic agents for congenital and acquired hearing loss. Congenital syphilis and bacterial meningitis are contemporary causes of deafness in spite of greatly improved treatment modalities. Other common etiologies of sensorineural hearing loss are noise exposure, metabolic and systemic changes in the auditory system, ototoxic medications, aging (presbycusis), and head trauma. In patients with unilateral progressive sensorineural hearing loss, acoustic neuroma must be suspected. Bilateral acoustic neuromas are the hallmark of neurofibromatosis II and must be suspected in patients with positive family histories (autosomal dominant inheritance).

C. **Mixed hearing loss** exists when both conductive and sensorineural hearing losses occur in the same ear. The lesions are additive, resulting in significant air-to-bone gaps with the bone-conduction thresholds falling outside the normal range of hearing sensitivity.

D. **Central auditory processing disorder.** In addition to the classical types of hearing loss discussed above, some patients present with central auditory processing disorders. They fail to perceive and use acoustic information because

Table 17-1. Summary of the types of hearing loss with general diagnostic and audiologic patterns.

Type of lesion	Characteristics	Tuning fork	Speech audiometry	Tympanogram	Acoustic reflexes	Recruitment/adaptation
Conductive	Unilateral or bilateral hearing loss Rising or flat audiometric configuration Bone-conduction thresholds—normal Maximum conductive loss cannot exceed 60–70 dB HL. Paracusis Willisii: "I hear better in a noisy place." If speech is presented at a sufficient intensity, discrimination is excellent. No loudness tolerance difficulties Often can be treated medically Can be transient or fluctuating Examples: cerumen impaction, otitis media, otosclerosis, tympanic membrane (TM) perforation	Weber: to ear with greatest conductive loss Rinne: negative, bone is better than air Bing: no occlusion effect	SRT: consistent with pure tone average Discrimination: excellent Normal dynamic range	Jerger Type B: fluid in middle ear space Jerger Type C: retracted TM Jerger Type A or A_S: otosclerosis or ossicular fixation Jerger Type A_D: tympanosclerosis or ossicular discontinuity	Absent	None seen
Sensorineural	Unilateral or bilateral hearing loss ranging from mild to profound in severity Flat or falling audiometric configuration—may have notch if noise induced or rising in Ménière's disease No air-to-bone gap, bone-conduction thresholds are poorer than normal limits Speech discrimination is variable, depending on severity, configuration, and etiology of hearing loss.	Weber: to ear with best cochlear reserve Rinne: positive, air is better than bone Bing: occlusion effect	SRT: consistent with pure tone average Discrimination: excellent to minimal Reduced dynamic range	Jerger Type A: normal TM compliance at normal pressure	Present but may vary as a function of the severity of the hearing loss	Partial or complete recruitment; no adaptation

Type						
(Sensorineural, continued)	Abnormal growth of loudness and reduced dynamic range Otoacoustic emissions are generally absent. BSER has normal latencies for high-intensity clicks—recruitment. Tinnitus is common, ranging from high-pitched ringing to low-frequency roar to unusual head noises. Some patients experience vertigo. Occasionally can be treated medically Can be assisted with hearing aids, cochlear implants, assistive listening devices, and speech reading Examples: presbycusis, NIHL, Ménière's disease, ototoxicity, congenital loss					
Mixed	Combination of the two types of hearing loss described above Significant air-to-bone gaps with bone-conduction thresholds poorer than normal Conductive component may respond to medical treatment but will still require amplification or other aural rehabilitation strategies.	Weber: to ear with greatest conductive loss Rinne: negative, bone is better than air Bing: no occlusion effect	SRT: consistent with pure tone average Discrimination: excellent to minimal Dynamic range may be reduced	Jerger Type B: fluid in middle ear space Jerger Type C: retracted TM Jerger Type A or A_S: otosclerosis or ossicular fixation Jerger Type A_D: tympanosclerosis or ossicular discontinuity	Absent	None seen because of the overriding conductive component

Table 17-1 (*continued*)

Type of lesion	Characteristics	Tuning fork	Speech audiometry	Tympanogram	Acoustic reflexes	Recruitment/adaptation
Neural	Usually a unilateral or asymmetric hearing loss, ranging from normal hearing to profound loss Characterized by asymmetric configuration No air-to-bone gaps Speech discrimination is generally poorer in the affected ear. Abnormal adaptation Otoacoustic emissions may be present or absent. BSER shows prolonged latencies between waves I and V or between ears. Vertigo and tinnitus are common. Is often treated surgically, trying to preserve hearing when possible	Weber: to ear with best cochlear reserve Rinne: positive, air is better than bone Bing: occlusion effect	SRT: consistent with or poorer than pure tone average Discrimination: poor to minimal in affected ear Reduced dynamic range	Jerger Type A: normal TM compliance at normal pressure	Elevated or absent; abnormally rapid decay	Can have partial or complete recruitment; abnormal adaptation is common.
Central or central auditory processing disorder	Example: acoustic neuroma Audiogram is generally normal, but could have any other type of hearing loss. Characterized by difficulties processing speech in the presence of noise Often diagnosed by abnormally poor scores on specialized speech tests Otoacoustic emissions are usually normal but may have unusual contralateral suppression characteristics. BSER is normal, but middle and late evoked potentials and event-related potentials may be abnormal. Generally poor academic and reading performance	Normal	SRT: consistent with pure tone average Discrimination: excellent in quiet, reduced in noise or if signal is distorted Normal dynamic range	Jerger Type A: normal TM compliance at normal pressure	Generally present at normal levels	None seen

the central auditory system is incapable of appropriately processing the signals transduced by the cochlea. Patients with central auditory processing disorders can be taught compensation strategies to improve their ability to comprehend speech. In addition, many adults with sensorineural hearing loss may have concomitant central auditory processing disorders confounding the evaluation and management of the sensorineural hearing loss.

E. Degree of hearing loss. Although a hearing handicap can be quantified as a percentage of normal hearing for medicolegal purposes (Table 17-2), the degree of hearing loss cannot be completely defined as a percentage because the effects of the loss are dependent on its type, severity, and configuration. Table 17-3 presents the ranges and effects of the various degrees of hearing loss, particularly as those degrees affect educational outcomes for children. Table 17-4 presents some of the common hearing loss configurations.

VI. Audiologic evaluation

A. Screening for hearing loss. Because hearing is critical for speech and oral language development in children, the early identification of hearing loss is a primary concern for health care professionals and educators. The recent *Joint Committee on Infant Hearing 1994 Position Statement* endorses the concept of universal hearing screening of infants and recommends that this screening be conducted before 3 months of age. The position paper identifies indicators associated with sensorineural and conductive hearing loss that can be used to identify infants who should receive hearing screening (Table 17-5).

B. Pure tone threshold audiometry. The thresholds obtained during pure tone threshold audiometry are the faintest intensity levels at which pure tone stimuli can be detected by patients. Thresholds are generally obtained for air-conduction stimuli presented through earphones or in a sound field and for bone-conduction stimuli presented by means of a vibrator placed on the mastoid or forehead.

For adults and compliant older children, pure tone testing simply requires behavioral responses to pure tone stimulation. For infants above 5 months of age, visual reinforcement audiometry (VRA) can be used to obtain thresholds as well as to obtain information about other auditory functions. In VRA testing, infants are reinforced by illuminated, animated toys when they demonstrate a head-turn response away from the midline and toward the reinforcer. VRA is a very successful means of measuring the hearing status of older infants and young toddlers. Play audiometry is typically used to assess the hearing status of preschool children. In this technique, play activities are used as operant reinforcers for a child's response to auditory signals. If an older infant or a child fails to condition using visual reinforcement audiometry or play audiometry, electrophysiologic testing may be required.

C. Speech audiometry. Speech signals can be used to assess hearing sensitivity as well as processing capabilities of the auditory system. Speech must first be audible to be understood. However, even when speech is audible, various physiologic and environmental factors can reduce the intelligibility of the speech signal so that the patient can have difficulties understanding the speech in spite of hearing it. Two different types of tests are used to measure these two different parameters: (1) speech threshold tests and (2) speech recognition or discrimination tests.

1. Speech threshold tests. In testing for hearing sensitivity, a speech recognition threshold (SRT) or a speech awareness threshold (SAT) is obtained for

---

Table 17-2. Calculation of hearing handicap as a percentage.

1. Obtain air-conduction thresholds in dB HL for both ears.
2. Calculate the average of the thresholds obtained for 500, 1000, 2000, and 3000 Hz for each ear.
3. If the average exceeds 25 dB (low fence), subtract 25 and multiply the remainder by 0.015 up to a maximum of 1.0 (100%), which is reached at a little less than 92 dB (high fence). This score represents percent monaural impairment.
4. If the percent monaural impairment is the same for both ears, that figure expresses the percent handicap. If the percent monaural impairment is not the same for both ears, multiply the smaller percentage (better ear) by 5, add the product to the larger percentage (poorer ear), and divide the sum by 6 to arrive at the total hearing handicap.

Table 17-3. Degrees and possible effects of hearing loss.

Range of hearing loss	Severity	Possible effects	Possible educational needs
−10–15 dB HL	Normal	None	None
16–25 dB HL	Slight	The child may have difficulties hearing faint speech, especially in difficult listening situations. The child may be unaware of subtle conversational cues, which could cause inappropriate behavior. The child may become fatigued by the increased listening effort.	The child will benefit from preferential seating and possibly from routine medical and/or audiologic monitoring. The child may benefit from mild gain hearing assistance technologies. The child may require speech-language services.
26–40 dB HL	Mild	At 30 dB, a child can miss 25–40% of the speech signal. In difficult listening environments, up to 50% of the primary speech signal may be missed. The child may not attend to speech and becomes easily fatigued by the increased listening effort.	The child will benefit from amplification and hearing assistance technologies. The child may need additional educational services to address any deficits in speech-language skills and academic performance. Teacher in-service is strongly recommended.
41–55 dB HL	Moderate	The child likely understands conversational speech only when it is clear and distinct, at close proximity, and in a favorable listening situation. The hearing loss is likely to have some effect on the child's speech and language skills and academic performance.	Amplification and hearing assistance technology are essential in the classroom. The child will likely benefit from additional educational services to address any deficits in speech-language skills and academic performance. Teacher in-service is strongly recommended.
56–70 dB HL	Moderate to severe	Without amplification, conversational speech is very difficult to hear. The child will have some delayed or disordered speech and language skills. Needing constantly to wear hearing aids, the child is perceived as a special learner.	Full-time amplification is required, and hearing assistance technologies are essential in the classroom. The child will likely require additional educational services to address any deficits in speech-language skills and academic performance. Teacher in-service is necessary.
71–90 dB HL	Severe	Without amplification, speech must be very loud if it is to be heard. Even when aided, the child may have significant difficulties hearing and understanding speech. The child will have some delayed or disordered speech and language skills. Needing constantly to wear hearing aids, the child is perceived as a special learner.	In addition to the communication and educational needs listed above, the child may require the use of a sign language system as part of the overall communication program.

Table 17-3 (*continued*)

Range of hearing loss	Severity	Possible effects	Possible educational needs
>90 dB HL	Profound	Even with conventional hearing aids, speech is very difficult to understand. In many cases, the child may be only aware of the sound and not appropriately perceive it. The child will likely rely on visual cues to communicate effectively.	In addition to the communication needs described above, the child may require cochlear implants or tactile aids to perceive the acoustic cues of speech. Some families may choose a bilingual, bicultural approach to language development.

each ear individually or for both ears in the sound field. The SRT is obtained at the lowest intensity level at which the patient can repeat the spondee words (two-syllable words with equal stress on each syllable) 50% of the time. The SAT is the lowest intensity level at which the patient gives any consistent behavioral response to the presentation of speech stimuli. Both the SRT and the SAT are used to provide valid estimates of hearing sensitivity and to verify the accuracy and reliability of the pure tone thresholds when they are available. The SRT and the pure tone average of the thresholds obtained at 500, 1000, and 2000 Hz should be within ± 7 dB of one another. If a discrepancy exists, the examiner should doubt the validity or accuracy of the patient's thresholds.

2. **Speech recognition or discrimination tests.** Word recognition or speech discrimination testing determines how well a patient can "understand" speech when the stimuli are above threshold. Speech recognition or discrimination scores are dependent on the type, severity, and configuration of the hearing loss as well as the type of ear pathology. In addition, the scores are dependent on several stimulus and response characteristics. Finally, the patient's attending and cognitive skills can influence the results, particularly when one is working with children or the elderly. Although several pathologies can result in markedly reduced speech recognition or discrimination scores, a rollover phenomenon in which the scores first rise and then dramatically fall with increasing presentation levels is characteristic of retrocochlear lesions. For patients who demonstrate excellent word recognition scores at or near their thresholds for speech, the results often have nonor-

Table 17-4. Configurations (slopes) of hearing loss audiograms.

Configuration	Slope characteristics
Flat	Approximately equal hearing loss at all frequencies, <15 dB variation across frequencies
Gradually sloping	Progressively greater hearing loss at higher frequencies at a slope of 5–10 dB per octave
Sloping	Progressively greater hearing loss at higher frequencies at a slope of 15–20 dB per octave
Precipitously sloping	Progressively greater hearing loss at higher frequencies at a slope of >20 dB per octave
Rising	Progressively better hearing at higher frequencies
Notch	A precipitously sloping hearing loss reaching a peak with some precipitous rise to better hearing in the higher frequencies above the center frequency. At least a 15-dB drop and recovery must occur within two octaves before the hearing loss is considered to have a notch.
"Cookie bite"	Greater loss in the middle frequencies with at least 20-dB better hearing in the lower and higher frequencies

Table 17-5. Indicators associated with sensorineural and/or conductive hearing loss from the Joint Committee on Infant Hearing 1994 Position Statement.

For use with neonates (birth to 28 days) when universal screening is not available:
  Family history of hereditary childhood sensorineural hearing loss
  In utero infections, such as cytomegalovirus, rubella, syphilis, herpes, and toxoplasmosis
  Craniofacial anomalies, including morphologic abnormalities of the pinna and ear canal
  Birth weight less than 1500 g (3.3 lb)
  Hyperbilirubinemia at serum levels requiring exchange transfusion
  Ototoxic medications including but not limited to the aminoglycosides used in multiple
    courses or in combination with loop diuretics
  Bacterial meningitis
  Severe depression at birth with Apgar scores of 0–4 at 1 minute or 0–6 at 5 minutes
  Prolonged mechanical ventilation lasting 5 days or longer (e.g., persistent pulmonary
    hypertension)
  Stigmata or other findings associated with a syndrome or a conductive hearing loss, or both
For use with infants (29 days to 2 years) when certain health conditions develop that require
    rescreening:
  Parent/caregiver concern regarding hearing, speech, language, or developmental delay
  Bacterial meningitis and other infections associated with sensorineural hearing loss
  Head trauma associated with loss of consciousness or skull fracture
  Stigmata or other findings associated with a syndrome known to include a sensorineural or
    conductive hearing loss, or both
  Ototoxic medications including but not limited to chemotherapeutic agents or
    aminoglycosides used in multiple courses or in combination with loop diuretics
  Recurrent or persistent otitis media with effusion for at least 3 months
For use with infants (29 days to 3 years) who require periodic monitoring of hearing
    (indicators associated with delayed-onset sensorineural hearing loss):
  Family history of hereditary childhood hearing loss
  In utero infections, such as cytomegalovirus, rubella, syphilis, herpes, and toxoplasmosis
  Neurofibromatosis type II and neurodegenerative disorders
  Persistent pulmonary hypertension in the newborn period
For use with infants (29 days to 3 years) who require periodic monitoring of hearing
    (indicators associated with conductive hearing loss):
  Recurrent or persistent otitis media with effusion
  Anatomic deformities and other disorders that affect eustachian tube function
  Neurodegenerative disorders

ganic components. Children and adults with central auditory processing disorders show markedly reduced scores when the speech signals are altered in their frequency content or when the speech is presented against background noise but at a favorable message-to-competition ratio (MCR).

VII. **Physiologic measures of audition.** Whenever possible, behavioral measures of hearing should be used to assess the status of the auditory system, because such measures provide more specific descriptions of which auditory stimuli can elicit responses in a patient and how that patient perceives and responds to those stimuli. Owing to many variables that can affect the validity and reliability of these measures, particularly in testing of infants and young children, physiologic techniques can be used to assess the integrity of the auditory system and, in some instances, provide excellent estimates of hearing sensitivity.

  A. **Immittance audiometry** consists of measuring the impedance of the tympanic membrane for the transmission of a tone or the amount of sound reflected back from the tympanic membrane.

  1. **Tympanometry** is sensitive to middle ear pathologies affecting the tympanic membrane, middle ear space, and ossicular chain. It is particularly useful in documenting the presence of middle ear effusions, ossicular discontinuities, and ossicular fixations. However, it lacks specificity for infants younger than 6 months of age because of the high compliance of their external ear canal walls. Figure 17-2 illustrates typical test results obtained during tympanometry.

  2. **Acoustic reflex.** When an ear with normal hearing is exposed to an intense auditory signal, the stapedius muscle contracts and then changes the orien-

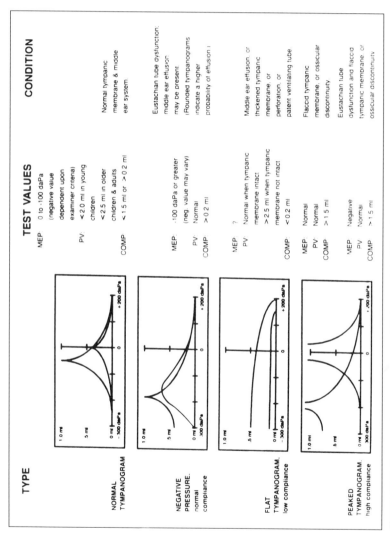

Figure 17-2. Common tympanograms and their associated disorders.

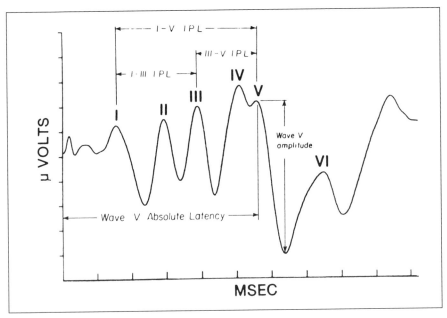

Figure 17-3. A normal BSER obtained from a young adult.

tation of the stapes footplate to the oval window, creating additional impedance to the flow of energy to the inner ear. This acoustic reflex occurs bilaterally regardless of which ear is stimulated, if the system is functioning normally. The presence or absence of the reflex as well as the intensity levels at
which the reflex is obtained provide information useful in identifying lesions
within the auditory system up to the level of the superior olivary complex. In
cases of eighth nerve lesions, the decay of the acoustic reflex occurs rapidly,
indicating an abnormal adaptation of the neural response.

B. **Brainstem evoked response (BSER) audiometry** consists of measuring the
electrical potentials generated by the neurons within the eighth cranial nerve
and lower auditory brainstem in response to rapid-onset, short-duration
acoustic signals such as the click stimulus. Because these signals are low level
and are often buried in noise, signal averaging techniques are used to record
the electrical response of the auditory system. An example of the normal BSER
results obtained from an adult patient is presented in Figure 17-3. The response
is judged by the presence of positive wavelets occurring within a certain latency range. The latencies, amplitudes, and morphologies of the responses are
dependent on the patient's age, the stimulus characteristics, and the recording
parameters. Individuals with normal peripheral ear and lower auditory brainstem system integrity will demonstrate a response to clicks at intensities as low
as 15 dBnHL (dB "normalized" hearing level). Under most stimulus conditions,
the response is sensitive to the hearing status between 2000 and 4000 Hz. Although different methods of evoked potential testing can estimate hearing sensitivity outside this frequency range, such testing is more difficult and the results are less reliable.

The test parameters and interpretation criteria for BSER audiometry are dependent on the nature of the questions asked by the clinicians. Because the amplitude measures are highly variable and more susceptible to artifacts, clinicians typically use latency measures to assess the integrity of the system. When
screening for hearing loss, the clinician examines the waveform for the presence of distinctive peaks, particularly wave V, as the intensity of the stimulus
changes and compares any measurable latency with the normative values available for the type of patient being tested. When used for differential diagnosis of
retrocochlear pathology, a prolonged latency difference between waves I and V
becomes the most sensitive indicator of this pathology, although other pro-

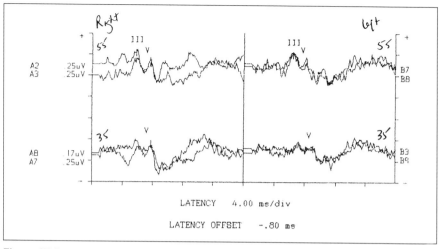

Figure 17-4. A normal series of BSERs obtained from an infant (when screened for hearing loss).

longed values for interpeak latencies and interaural latency differences can be diagnostic. Absolute latency values tend to be the least diagnostic for retro-cochlear lesions. Knowledge of the hearing sensitivity between 2000 and 4000 Hz in each ear is critical for the appropriate interpretation of BSER results during differential diagnosis.

BSER can be obtained without intentional responses from patients, and frequency is used to assess the integrity of the auditory system in populations such as infants. Although the click-evoked BSER can appear as early as the twenty-fifth week of gestation and is typically present at the twenty-seventh week of gestation, there are developmental changes in the response until about 2 years of age. The decrease in the absolute latencies of the response is the most salient change during this maturational period. Therefore, interpretation of the BSER to identify hearing loss depends on age-appropriate norms. Still, if wave V of the BSER is present in a test ear at 35 dBnHL, it is likely that the infant has normal hearing sensitivity between 2000 and 4000 Hz in the test ear. An example of normal results from a BSER screening of an infant is presented in Figure 17-4. It must be pointed out that clinicians must resist the urge to "peak pick" when judging a BSER waveform with either poor morphology or low-amplitude wavelets.

C. **Otoacoustic emissions.** Otoacoustic emission testing is a relatively new means of detecting hearing loss. The cochlea generate a low-intensity acoustic echo in response to an auditory stimulus in individuals with normal hearing. Hearing losses resulting from cochlear and/or middle ear pathologies can be readily identified using otoacoustic emissions; however, these measurements generally fail to define the severity of the hearing loss. There are two classes of otoacoustic emissions: spontaneous otoacoustic emissions (SOAEs) and evoked otoacoustic emissions. Evoked otoacoustic emissions can be further divided, according to the type of stimulus used during measurement, into stimulus frequency emissions (SFEs), transient evoked otoacoustic emissions (TEOAEs), and distortion product otoacoustic emissions (DPOAEs). TEOAEs and DPOAEs tend to be preferred for clinical measurements because of the equipment difficulties encountered in trying to obtain SFEs. Figure 17-5 illustrates a TEOAE from a school-age child whose hearing was evaluated as a baseline measure of auditory sensitivity prior to the administration of ototoxic medication and radiation to treat an intracranial tumor. Recent studies have suggested that otoacoustic emissions may be a very effective means of identifying hearing loss in infants and young children.

VIII. **Management and referral lists.** When any hearing loss is suspected or identified, the patient should be referred for otologic examination and audiologic evaluation to determine the appropriate means of treatment. The following organizations can

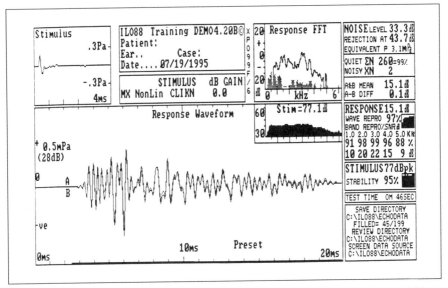

Figure 17-5. A normal transient evoked otoacoustic emission (TEOAE) from a young child.

assist readers in locating patient education materials and appropriate otologic and audiologic service providers in their geographic areas.

American Academy of Otolaryngology—Head and Neck Surgery
1 Prince St.
Alexandria, VA 22314
(703) 836-4444

American Academy of Audiology
1735 N. Lynn St., Suite 950
Arlington, VA 22209-2022
(800) 222-2336

Recommended Readings

Allen JB, Neely ST. Micromechanical models of the cochlea. *Physics Today* 45(7):40–47, 1992.

American Speech-Language-Hearing Association. Joint Committee on Infant Hearing 1994 Position Statement. *Asha* 36:38–41, 1994.

American Speech-Language-Hearing Association. Report on audiologic screening. *Amer J Aud* 4(2):24–40, 1995.

Anderson KL. Hearing conservation in the public school revisited. *Sem Hear* 12:340–363, 1991.

Bess FH, Humes LE. *Audiology: The Fundamentals* (2nd ed). Baltimore: Williams & Wilkins, 1994.

Diefendorf AO, et al. Pediatric assessment: TIPS (testing-interpreting-promoting-securing) for early amplification. In FH Bess, JS Gravel, AM Tharp (eds), *Amplification for Children with Auditory Deficits*. Nashville: Bill Wilkerson Center, in press.

Ginsberg IA, White TP. Otologic disorders and examination. In J Katz (ed), *Handbook of Clinical Audiology* (4th ed). Baltimore: Williams & Wilkins, 1994.

Hall JW III, et al. Audiologic assessment and management of central auditory processing disorder (CAPD). *Sem Hear* 14:254–263, 1993.

Jerger J, et al. Effects of age and gender on dichotic sentence identification. *Ear Hear* 15:274–286, 1994.

Kemp DT, Ryan S. The use of transient evoked otoacoustic emissions in neonatal hearing screening. *Sem Hear* 14:30–44, 1993.

Miyamoto RT, et al. The role of cochlear implants in deaf children. *Scand Audiol Supple* 30:121–126, 1988.

Miyamoto RT, et al. Comparison of sensory aids in deaf children. *Ann Oto Rhino Laryngo* 98(Suppl 142):2–7, 1989.

Møller MB. Audiological evaluation. *J Clin Neurophysiol* 11(3):309–318, 1994.

Northern JL, Downs MP. *Hearing in Children* (4th ed). Baltimore: Williams & Wilkins, 1991.

Northern JL, Roush J. Diagnostic audiology. In GM English (ed), *Otolaryngology.* Philadelphia: Lippincott, 1994.

Norton SJ. Application of transient evoked otoacoustic emissions to pediatric populations. *Ear Hear* 14:64–73, 1993.

Nozza RJ, et al. Towards the validation of aural acoustic immittance measures for diagnosis of middle ear effusion in children. *Ear Hear* 13:442–453, 1992.

Pender DJ. *Practical Otology.* Philadelphia: Lippincott, 1992.

Pickles JO. *An Introduction to the Physiology of Hearing* (2nd ed). New York: Academic, 1988.

Picton TW. Clinical usefulness of auditory evoked potentials: A critical evaluation. *J Sp Lang Path Aud* 15:3–29, 1991.

Ruenes R. *Otologic Radiology with Clinical Correlations.* New York: Macmillan, 1986.

Sataloff RT, Sataloff J. *Hearing Loss* (3rd ed). New York: Marcel-Dekker, Inc., 1993.

Schuknecht HF. *Pathology of the Ear* (2nd ed). Philadelphia: Lea & Febiger, 1993.

Widen JE. Adding objectivity to infant behavioral audiometry. *Ear Hear* 14:49–57, 1993.

Yost WA. *Fundamentals of Hearing: An Introduction* (3rd ed). San Diego: Academic, 1994.

18

Approach to the Patient with Dysphagia
Jeri A. Logemann

I. **Dysphagia: difficulty in swallowing.** Oropharyngeal swallowing problems are common in patients with degenerative neurologic diseases such as motor neuron disease, including amyotrophic lateral sclerosis and postpolio syndrome, myasthenia gravis, multiple sclerosis, and Parkinson's disease, and may be the first symptom of the disease. Dysphagia is also common after sudden-onset neurologic damage such as stroke, head injury, or spinal cord injury. It is critical to identify the presence of a swallowing problem early, define the exact nature of the physiologic or anatomic problem, and institute appropriate compensatory or therapy procedures to prevent costly medical complications (see sec. **I.B.4**).

A. **Symptoms of oropharyngeal dysphagia**
   1. Coughing at meals
   2. Struggling to eat
   3. Taking longer to eat
   4. Chronic excessive secretions, including tracheal secretions, chronic bronchitis, and asthma
   5. Weight loss of unexplained origin
   6. Pneumonia, especially recurrent
   7. Gurgly voice quality, especially during or after meals
   8. Recurrent fevers or increased secretions 1 to 1½ hours after meals
   9. Elimination of some consistencies of foods from the diet
   10. Difficulty managing own saliva
   11. Patient complaint of difficulty swallowing

B. **Effects of dysphagia on health and the healthcare system**
   1. **Aspiration pneumonia.** A significant positive correlation has been found between the aspiration observed during a modified barium swallow test and the development of pneumonia within the next 6 months.
   2. **Malnutrition**
   3. **Dehydration**
   4. **Increased costs of healthcare,** including hospitalization for aspiration pneumonia and other costly medical complications, nonoral feeding, and nursing care, if dysphagia is not managed properly.

C. **Prevention: the reason for evaluation and treatment of oropharyngeal dysphagia.** In patients with neurologic damage or disease, dysphagia cannot be prevented, but the expensive medical complications that result from swallowing disorders *can* be prevented by means of appropriate assessment and treatment.
   1. **Prevention of expensive medical complications.** Aspiration pneumonia alone is a significant cost to the healthcare system. In the Midwest, an average hospital stay for aspiration pneumonia costs $18,000 to $20,000 in 1995 dollars.
   2. **Facilitation of the patient's return to safe and efficient oral intake.** Nonoral feeding requires greater nursing care and often specially prepared feedings, both of which are more costly than oral feeding.

II. **Normal swallowing.** At all ages, normal swallowing is safe and efficient, moving food and liquid from the mouth, through the pharynx and into the cervical esophagus in 2 seconds or less, and through the esophagus in an additional 8–20 seconds.

A. **Swallowing stages**
   1. **Oral preparatory stage (variable duration).** The oral preparatory stage includes chewing and other oral manipulations that reduce food to a consistency appropriate for swallowing and provide taste and pleasure of eating.

This stage does not depend on good dentition. Included in this stage are lip closure; circular, rotary action of the tongue; normal facial tone; and rotary jaw action. Circular tongue action and fine motor control of the tongue are most important, because tongue action controls food in the mouth.

2. **Oral stage (approximately 1 second).** The tongue is responsible for propelling food through the oral cavity and for providing sensory input that contributes to triggering of the pharyngeal stage.

3. **Pharyngeal triggering (½ second or less).** Pharyngeal triggering involves sensory input from the oral cavity to the cortex and brainstem that is recognized as a swallow stimulus in the nucleus tractus solitarius (NTS) in the brainstem. This sensory information is passed to the nucleus ambiguous (NA), which triggers the pharyngeal motor response.

4. **Pharyngeal stage (less than 1 second).** The pharyngeal stage involves closure of the airway to prevent entry of food into the airway (aspiration), opening of the upper esophageal sphincter (UES) to allow food to pass into the esophagus, and application of pressure to the bolus by the tongue and pharyngeal walls to clear food efficiently into the esophagus.

5. **Esophageal stage (8 to 20 seconds).** The esophageal stage involves sequential contraction of the esophageal muscle fibers from top to bottom, propelling the bolus ahead of the contractile wave into the stomach. It also involves relaxation of the lower esophageal sphincter to allow the bolus to pass into the stomach.

B. **Neuromuscular components of the normal swallow**

1. **Lip closure** is maintained from the time food is placed in the mouth until the pharyngeal swallow is completed. If lip closure cannot be maintained, the nasal airway may not be patent.

2. **Lingual control.** Oral tongue action is required in oral preparation, because the tongue controls the food in the mouth during chewing. The tongue also forms the food into a ball or bolus in preparation for the swallow, subdividing the food in the mouth if necessary, to ensure the bolus of appropriate size for swallowing. The oral portion of the tongue then propels the food through the oral cavity and into the pharynx.

3. **Rotary, lateral jaw motion.** Jaw action crushes the food, which is placed on the biting surface of the teeth by the tongue.

4. **Velar or soft palate elevation and closure of the velopharyngeal port.** Velopharyngeal closure prevents food from entering the nasal cavity.

5. **Tongue base posterior motion** generates pharyngeal pressure on the bolus, as does sequential contraction down the pharyngeal wall.

6. **Airway closure** prevents aspiration. Airway closure begins at the true vocal folds, proceeds to the level of the airway entrance—i.e., the false vocal folds, the arytenoids, and the base of the epiglottis, and ends as the epiglottis is folded over the airway. The most critical level of airway closure is at the entrance—i.e., the arytenoid cartilage and the base of the epiglottis and false vocal folds. This level of closure prevents food from entering the airway.

7. **Opening of the upper esophageal sphincter (UES)** involves a complex set of actions, including (1) relaxation of the cricopharyngeal muscular portion of the valve that does not open the sphincter; (2) laryngeal upward and forward motion, which opens the sphincter by carrying the anterior wall of the sphincter, the cricoid cartilage, away from the pharyngeal wall; and (3) arrival of the bolus under pressure, which increases the width of the opening of the upper sphincter.

8. **Esophageal peristalsis** begins when the tail of the bolus enters the esophagus and follows the bolus through the esophagus.

C. **Systematic changes in oropharyngeal swallow with changes in volume and viscosity of the incoming food and voluntary control.** Not all swallows are alike. Normal oropharyngeal swallow physiology changes systematically as the volume and viscosity of the food being swallowed increase. A great deal of voluntary control can also be exerted over the oropharyngeal swallow. These systematic changes help to explain why patients have more difficulty with one type of food than another. The swallows are, in fact, different for different foods.

1. **As bolus volume increases,** the durations of the oral and pharyngeal stages of the swallow increase. The duration of airway closure and cricopharyngeal opening increase systematically.

    2. Increasing viscosity of food increases the width of the cricopharyngeal opening.

    3. Volitional control also changes the characteristics of the oropharyngeal swallow.

       a. Breath-holding can extend the duration of airway closure at the vocal folds or at the entrance to the airway. This is often done in anticipation of swallowing a large volume of liquid, as from a cup.

       b. Volitional control can open the UES and prolong the duration of UES opening.

       c. Volitional control can extend the duration and extent of laryngeal elevation.

       d. Increasing effort during the swallow increases oropharyngeal pressures.

D. Effects of normal aging

    1. Oral transit time slows by ½ to 1 second with increasing age, probably because older adults hold the bolus on the anterior floor of the mouth and must pick it up with the tongue to begin the swallow.

    2. There is a slightly slower shift from the oral to the pharyngeal stage in individuals over age 60, probably because of slower neural processing.

    3. After age 80, the range of motion of pharyngeal structures is reduced—i.e., there is less muscle reserve and less flexibility in the swallow.

    4. Over age 60, the esophageal peristalsis becomes less efficient.

    5. Healthy elderly individuals do not aspirate more often than young people. Elderly patients (over age 80) who become generally weak and sick demonstrate a weak swallow, which can cause aspiration because of reduced muscular reserve.

E. Efficiency and safety

    1. Normal swallows are efficient, quickly moving food through the mouth and pharynx and into the esophagus (in less than 2 seconds).

    2. Aspiration occurs only occasionally—usually when the mechanism is stressed or when eating and talking occur simultaneously in a social situation.

    3. Efficiency and safety do not change significantly with age.

III. Swallowing disorders can occur in any stage of swallow and may involve one or more of the neuromuscular actions or sensory inputs described above as involved in the swallow.

A. Swallowing disorders can be **anatomic** or **physiologic** in nature.

B. Effective treatment requires identification of the specific anatomic or physiologic abnormalities in each patient's swallow, such as reduced laryngeal elevation, poor airway closure, reduced tongue base movement, etc.

C. Aspiration and **oral or pharyngeal residue** are *symptoms* of swallowing disorders rather than disorders. These symptoms disappear when the patient's swallowing physiology returns to normal.

IV. Definitive assessment of the oropharyngeal swallow: the modified barium swallow

A. The **modified barium swallow (MBS)** is performed by a speech-language pathologist or radiologist. This radiographic (videofluorographic) test examines the anatomy and physiology of the oral and pharyngeal stages of swallowing. These stages must be examined separately from the esophagus, which is anatomically and physiologically distinct from the oral cavity and pharynx and requires a different technique for assessment (a **barium swallow**). An MBS assessment examines the ability of the pharynx to manage small to large volumes and thin to thick viscosities of food. An esophageal assessment requires presentation of a large bolus to distend the esophagus, which as a collapsed muscular tube cannot be examined adequately unless distended.

    1. Purpose. The purpose of the MBS is to:

       a. Define oral and pharyngeal swallow physiology in relation to the patient's swallow symptoms.

       b. Define swallow physiology symptomatic of neurologic disease.

       c. Examine the effectiveness of management strategies designed to assist patients in continuing to eat safely by mouth or beginning to eat safely by mouth.

       d. Define a treatment plan to rehabilitate oropharyngeal swallow physiology and eliminate symptoms of dysphagia, including aspiration, thereby preventing the development of aspiration pneumonia.

2. Procedure. The procedure for the MBS is designed to minimize the risk of aspiration by presenting calibrated amounts of liquid, pudding, and masticated material as tolerated by the patient.

   a. The patient is seated upright initially and examined in the lateral plane to determine the speed, efficiency, and safety (aspiration) of the swallow.

   b. Liquids are given in 1-ml, 3-ml, 5-ml, 10-ml, and cup-drinking amounts (two swallows each) to observe the "dose response" of the pharynx and to define the optimal volume for each patient.

   c. If and when the patient aspirates or has a highly inefficient swallow, various treatment strategies are provided and their effects observed radiographically, including:

   (1) Posture changes

   (2) Increased sensory input

   (3) Therapy procedures (require normal cognition)

   (4) Increased bolus viscosity

   d. Pudding (1–2 ml) and a small bite of cookie are given (two swallows each), as tolerated by the patient.

   e. The patient is turned and examined in the A-P plane to define the symmetry of the swallow.

   f. The report contains descriptions of the oral and pharyngeal anatomy and swallow physiology causing the patient's dysphagia symptoms, identification of the types and amounts of foods safely swallowed, whether or not partial or full nonoral feeding is necessary, and the effectiveness and need for compensatory strategies or swallow therapy.

3. Reevaluation. To ensure patient safety, the patient's oropharyngeal swallow may need to be reevaluated when the patient appears ready to move to oral intake.

B. Barium swallow. The barium swallow examines the esophageal stage of swallowing, particularly esophageal anatomy and any anatomic abnormalities such as stricture, tumors, etc. Because this assessment requires the patient to swallow larger volumes of liquid, it should be completed after an oropharyngeal assessment—i.e., the modified barium swallow—to be sure the patient can tolerate these larger volumes.

1. The barium swallow assesses esophageal anatomy and peristaltic action.

2. The barium swallow misses reflux disease 60 to 80% of the time.

V. Screening tests for oropharyngeal dysphagia are not definitive and tend to overidentify patients at risk for swallowing disorders in the pharyngeal stage of swallowing.

A. A **bedside or clinical exam** is usually performed by a speech-language pathologist. A bedside or clinical, noninstrumental assessment of swallowing cannot reliably define swallow physiology or dysphagia symptoms such as aspiration. The exam includes:

1. A complete history of the swallowing problem.

2. A complete oromotor test of lip, jaw, tongue, and laryngeal function.

3. Observation of trial swallows of small amounts of food.

B. The 3-oz water test involves giving the patient 3 oz of water to swallow continuously.

1. If the patient coughs or has difficulty, referral for a modified barium swallow should be made.

2. The 3-oz water test can be dangerous if the patient aspirates a large amount of liquid.

3. This test does not identify the patient's swallow physiology, and so treatment cannot be planned.

VI. Referrals for further testing

A. CT or MRI for lesion localization. A small lesion causing dysphagia may not be detected by these procedures.

B. Other instrumental assessments of the oropharyngeal swallow, such as endoscopy, are more limited in their views of the swallow. None of these procedures is as useful as a modified barium swallow.

1. Endoscopy, which is usually performed by an otolaryngologist or a speech-language pathologist, examines the pharynx from above, both before and after, but not during, a swallow.

2. Ultrasound visualizes the oral stages of the swallow, but cannot image the pharynx. It is usually performed by a speech-language pathologist.

C. **Neurologic evaluation.** Some patients with swallowing complaints and no known diagnosis need in-depth neurologic testing before an accurate diagnosis can be made.

D. **Gastroenterology consultation** may be needed during diagnosis of esophageal aspects of the patient's swallowing disorder.

E. **Otolaryngology consultation** may be helpful if voice changes are present.

F. **Speech-language pathology consultation** may be helpful in defining the voice, speech, and swallowing disorders indicating neurologic disease.

VII. **Swallowing problems in patients with known neurologic damage or disease**

A. **Progressive neurologic disease.** Dysphagia is frequently observed in progressive neurologic disease at some point in the patient's deterioration, and many neurologic diseases can first present with swallowing difficulties.

1. **Parkinson's disease**

   a. **Onset.** The swallowing problem may come early or late in the progression of the disease.

   b. The patient may **aspirate silently**—i.e., no cough.

   c. **Symptoms of swallowing disorders**

   (1) The patient may slow down while eating, because of a characteristic (pathognomonic) rocking, rolling tongue motion.

   (2) The patient may swallow two or three times for each bite of food because the swallow is not efficient and leaves residue in the pharynx.

   (3) There are increased chest secretions and "bronchitis" with chronic cough, which are actually signs of chronic aspiration.

   (4) There is a gurgly voice quality because of residual food remaining at the top of the airway.

   d. **Referrals**

   (1) Modified barium swallow (MBS)

   (2) Swallowing therapy as indicated by MBS

   e. **Progression** is slow. The condition may worsen very slowly over 10 years, 20 years, or more.

   f. **Parkinson medications** may improve the swallowing disorder.

   g. **Swallow therapy.** Patients respond moderately well to swallow therapy.

2. **Amyotrophic lateral sclerosis**

   a. A swallowing or speech disorder may be the first symptom. It usually affects the oral stage of the swallow first, reducing tongue strength and fine control so that chewing is increasingly difficult.

   b. **Symptoms of swallowing disorders**

   (1) **Diet change.** The patient eliminates foods that require chewing and thicker foods that require more muscle effort to swallow.

   (2) **Weight loss**

   (3) **Coughing** occurs, usually during swallowing of liquids, which are not well controlled by the tongue and splash into the pharynx and the open airway.

   (4) There may be **slight aspiration.**

   c. **Referrals.** Modified barium swallows are indicated at regular intervals (3–4 months) in patients with brainstem involvement to define optimum eating strategies. Direct exercise fatigues muscles.

   d. **Progression**

   (1) Progression is often rapid in predominantly brainstem-involved patients. The patient may be advised to stop eating and accept gastrostomy within 1½–2 years of diagnosis because of chronic aspiration.

   (2) Progression is very slow in patients with predominantly spinal involvement. It may be 10 to 15 years before dysphagia is severe enough to cause weight loss or chronic aspiration.

3. **Postpolio syndrome**

   a. **Onset.** Dysphagia may begin as patients reach their forties or fifties—particularly patients with histories of bulbar polio.

   b. The patient may have **reduced awareness** of the swallowing problem.

   c. **Symptoms of swallowing disorders**

   (1) **Feeling of food left in the throat**—particularly thicker, heavier foods, which require increased muscle activity to swallow

   (2) **Fatigue** as meal progresses

   d. Referrals. An MBS is indicated to define optimum eating strategies. Often the problem is unilateral weakness of the pharynx, and head rotation toward the damaged side of the pharynx during eating facilitates clearance of food. Direct exercise fatigues the mechanism.
   e. Progression is slow, worsening over a period of years.
4. Myasthenia gravis
   a. A swallowing or speech disorder may be the first symptom.
   b. Symptoms of swallowing disorders
      (1) Fatigue in selected muscles of the mouth or pharynx as eating progresses.
      (2) Increasing nasality, hoarseness, and imprecision in speech sounds as patient continues to talk.
   c. Referrals. An MBS is indicated to define the involved musculature and the extent of fatigue.
   d. Progression. Symptoms worsen slowly. Medication may significantly improve swallowing.
5. Multiple sclerosis
   a. A swallowing problem may be the first symptom, but is more likely to occur as the disease progresses. The patient is often unaware of the swallowing problem.
   b. A wide range of swallowing disorders may occur as various parts of the nervous system become affected.
   c. Symptoms of swallowing disorders
      (1) Difficulty swallowing liquids, with coughing, because of pharyngeal swallow delay.
      (2) Complaints of food "stuck in the throat" because of reduced strength of tongue base and pharyngeal wall movement.
   d. Swallowing therapy. Patients respond well.
   e. Referrals
      (1) Modified barium swallow (MBS)
      (2) Swallowing therapy, if indicated by MBS
B. Sudden-onset neurologic disorders. Strokes, head injuries, and spinal cord injuries may cause dysphagia that has potential for recovery with appropriate management. The focus of management should be early radiographic assessment (MBS) with swallowing therapy to prevent medical complications. The more medical problems and complications the patient sustains, the longer the recovery time.
1. Stroke. Single or multiple strokes can cause swallowing problems.
   a. A **single infarct** in the cortex, subcortical region, or brainstem can cause swallowing problems that are worst within the first week after the stroke. By 3 weeks after the stroke, patients usually are functional swallowers unless they are taking medications that affect swallowing or have additional medical complications that slow swallowing recovery.
   b. Brainstem stroke patients are at greatest risk for dysphagia. Some brainstem stroke patients, particularly those with lateral medullary syndrome, need intensive swallowing therapy.
   c. Multistroke patients often exhibit more severe swallowing problems and require more rehabilitation, but usually do recover to full oral intake.
   d. Referrals
      (1) Modified barium swallow. An MBS is performed when the patient is alert and awake (3–4 days poststroke) to determine the need for nonoral feeding and swallowing therapy. The study is repeated at 3 weeks poststroke to determine progress and discontinue nonoral feeding if it is no longer needed.
      (2) Swallowing therapy, if indicated by MBS
2. Head injury. Approximately one-third of the patients with head injuries exhibit swallowing problems. Dysphagia may result from the neurologic injury, from other injuries of the head or neck (such as laryngeal fractures), or from acute care procedures, such as long-term intubation. Usually, neuromuscular damage is present in both the oral and pharyngeal phases of swallowing.
   a. Referrals
      (1) Modified barium swallow
      (2) Swallowing therapy, if indicated by MBS

b. Most patients regain oral intake with therapy. Some patients with severe head injuries require maintenance therapy from caregivers to maintain safe and adequate oral intake.

3. Cervical spinal cord injury. Patients with cervical spinal cord injuries who undergo anterior spinal fusions are at greatest risk for dysphagia. The pharyngeal swallow is usually impaired.

  a. Referrals
    (1) Modified barium swallow
    (2) Swallowing therapy
  b. Swallowing problems occur most often in the pharyngeal phase of the swallow.
  c. With swallowing therapy, most patients recover. The duration of recovery depends on the extent of physical damage and the number of medical complications sustained.

VIII. Patients with complaints of swallowing disorders but no medical diagnosis

  A. Most often these patients have neurologic disease, have had a stroke, or have a brain tumor. Rarely does the dysphagia indicate a head or neck cancer.

  B. Testing

    1. History. A complete medical and swallowing history should be taken, including:

      a. Pattern of difficulty
        (1) Fatigue at the end of the meal, which could indicate myasthenia gravis
        (2) Foods that the patient finds difficult to swallow
        (3) Gradual or sudden onset. Gradual onset usually indicates neurologic disease. Sudden onset may indicate a stroke.
      b. Family history of any swallowing problem

    2. Symptoms. Asking patients to describe their symptoms is helpful.
      a. Food remains in the mouth, which indicates an oral stage problem.
      b. Food hesitates at the top of the neck, which may indicate difficulty in triggering the pharyngeal stage.
      c. Food remains in the throat, which may indicate pharyngeal stage problems.
      d. A feeling of pressure at the base of the neck or that food remains at the base of the neck usually indicates an esophageal stage problem.
      e. A feeling of pressure in the chest or that food is caught in the chest usually indicates esophageal stage problems.

    3. Other motor signs
      a. Gait changes
      b. Tremor in the tongue, jaw, pharynx, or larynx. Tremor at rest may indicate Parkinson's disease.
      c. Speech or voice changes. Many patients with neurologic diseases may exhibit speech or voice changes *and* swallowing problems.

IX. Summary. Early MBS assessment by a speech-language pathologist can reduce the medical complications from dysphagia and thereby reduce the costs to the healthcare system. One hospitalization for aspiration pneumonia can cost as much as MBSs and follow-up swallowing therapy for three to five patients for 3 months. Careful and aggressive management of dysphagia can save the healthcare system significant amounts in hospitalization and other medical costs.

Recommended Readings

DePippo KL, Holas MA, Reding MJ. Validation of the 3 oz water swallow test for aspiration following stroke. *Arch Neurol* 49:1259–1261, 1992.

Dodds WJ, Logemann JA, Stewart ET. Radiological assessment of abnormal oral and pharyngeal phases of swallowing. *AJR* 154:965–974, 1990.

Ergun GA, Miskovitz PF. Aging and the esophagus: Common pathologic conditions and their effect upon swallowing in the geriatric population. *Dysphagia* 7:58–63, 1992.

Horner J, et al. Aspiration following stroke: Clinical correlates and outcomes. *Neurology* 38:1359–1362, 1988.

Jacob P, et al. Upper esophageal sphincter opening and modulation during swallowing. *Gastroenterology* 97:1469–1478, 1989.

Kahrilas PJ, et al. Pharyngeal clearance during swallow: A combined manometric and videofluoroscopic study. *Gastroenterology* 103:128–136, 1992.

Kasprisin AT, Clumeck A, Nino-Murcia M. The efficacy of rehabilitative management of dysphagia. *Dysphagia* 4:48–52, 1989.

Langmore SE, Schatz K, Olsen N. Fiber optic endoscopic examination of swallowing safety: A new procedure. *Dysphagia* 2(4):216–219, 1988.

Lazarus C, Logemann JA. Swallowing disorders in closed head trauma patients. *Arch Phys Med Rehabil* 68:79–87, 1987.

Lazarus CL, et al. Effects of bolus volume, viscosity and repeated swallows in normals and stroke patients. *Arch Phys Med Rehabil* 74:1066–1070, 1993.

Logemann J, et al. The benefit of head rotation on pharyngoesophageal dysphagia. *Arch Phys Med Rehabil* 70(10):767–771, 1989.

Logemann JA. *Evaluation and Treatment of Swallowing Disorders.* Austin, TX: Pro-Ed, 1983.

Logemann JA (ed). Swallowing disorders and rehabilitation. *J Head Trauma Rehabil* 4(4), 1989.

Logemann JA. Head and neck diseases in the elderly: Effects of aging on the swallowing mechanism. *Otolaryngol Clin North Am* 23(6):1045–1056, 1990.

Logemann JA. The dysphagia diagnostic procedure as a treatment efficacy trial. *Clin Common Dis* 3(4):1–10, 1993.

Logemann JA. A Manual for Videofluoroscopic Evaluation of Swallowing (2nd ed). Austin, TX: Pro-Ed, 1993.

Logemann JA, Kahrilas PJ. Relearning to swallow post CVA: Application of maneuvers and indirect biofeedback: A case study. *Neurology* 40:1136–1138, 1990.

Logemann JA, et al. Closure mechanisms of the laryngeal vestibule during swallowing. *Am J Physiol* 262:G338–344, 1992.

Martin BJ, et al. The association of swallowing dysfunction and aspiration pneumonia. *Dysphagia* 9:1–6, 1994.

Rasley A, et al. Prevention of barium aspiration during videofluoroscopic swallowing studies: Value of change in posture. *AJR,* 160, 1005–1009, 1993.

Robbins J, Levine R. Swallowing after unilateral stroke of the cerebral cortex: Preliminary experience. *Dysphagia* 3:11–17, 1988.

Robbins J, Logemann J, Kirschner H. Swallowing and speech production in Parkinson's disease. *Ann Neurol* 19:283–287, 1986.

Robbins JA, et al. Oropharyngeal swallowing in normal adults of different ages. *Gastroenterology* 103:823–829, 1992.

Schmidt J, et al. Videofluoroscopic evidence of aspiration predicts pneumonia and death but no dehydration following stroke. *Dysphagia* 9:7–11, 1994.

Splaingard M, et al. Aspiration in rehabilitation patients: Videofluoroscopy vs. bedside clinical assessment. *Arch Phys Med Rehabil* 69:637–640, 1988.

Tracy JF, et al. Preliminary observations on the effects of age on oropharyngeal deglutition. *Dysphagia* 4:90–94, 1989.

Veis SL, Logemann JA. Swallowing disorders in persons with cerebrovascular accident. *Arch Phys Med Rehabil* 65:372–375, 1985.

19

Approach to the Patient with Dysarthria

Marian P. LaMonte
Eric Corey Raps
Ann Ficco-D'Orazio

Communication disorders are common in neurologic practice and are the result of congenital, developmental, and acquired abnormalities. **Dysarthria** is a collective name for a group of motor speech disorders that result from focal, multifocal, or diffuse damage to the central or peripheral nervous system, or both. The dysarthrias are classified using descriptive categories that have been correlated previously with specific lesion sites and neuropathologies (Table 19-1). Production of speech occurs through the interaction of five systems: (1) respiration, (2) phonation, (3) resonance, (4) articulation, and (5) prosody. Examination of each system facilitates not only the diagnosis of a specific type of dysarthria, but also the neuroanatomic localization and, ultimately, the appropriate therapeutic intervention.

I. **Etiology.** Neurologic conditions that produce dysarthria are both numerous and diverse. Furthermore, dysarthric symptoms may remain stable, improve, or progress, depending on the etiology. Most patients who present with dysarthria have preceding significant neurologic symptoms or accompanying neurologic signs that assist in diagnosis of the dysarthria type. Lesions along the neuroaxis that produce motor dysfunction of any of the five speech systems produce a type of dysarthric speech. The lesions may be unilateral or bilateral and localize to cortex, subcortex, brainstem, cranial nerves, or upper cervical nerves. There are several possible classification schemes for etiology (Table 19-2). In Table 19-3 we present disease processes by time of onset.

II. **Clinical manifestations** of particular types of dysarthria are the result of nervous system damage to particular speech system components, and the effects present as patterns of dysfunctional speech. Table 19-4 presents a classification of dysarthria, clinical manifestations of speech abnormalities identified by examination, location of pathology, and typical neurologic causes. The dysfunctional patterns are classified descriptively. An understanding of the normal speech system components, followed by identification of specific system abnormalities and their common causes, will clarify the resulting clinical manifestations.

A. **Normal speech systems**

1. **Respiration**
   a. Anatomic components include the lungs, chest wall, diaphragm, and abdominal muscles.
   b. Physiologically, respiration provides the air source and subglottal pressure necessary to force a constant column of air through the larynx and vocal folds.
   c. Respiration is dependent on intact connections from medullary centers to respiratory muscles.

2. **Phonation**
   a. The anatomic unit is the larynx.
   b. Physiologic changes in vocal fold length, thickness, opposition, and vibratory pattern, as well as changes in the relationships between cartilage and muscle, bring about vocalization.
   c. Each individual has a unique fundamental frequency as a controlled stream of air passes through the vocal folds. Pitch is a function of fundamental frequency changes produced by elevation and depression of the larynx. Laryngeal movement results in position and tension changes of the true vocal folds.

The authors acknowledge Dr. Jeffrey Metter's outstanding contribution to the understanding of dysarthria by basing this chapter on his diagnostic approach.

Table 19-1. Classification of dysarthrias.

Central Types
Spastic: bilateral upper motor neuron disorders
Hyper/hypokinetic: extrapyramidal disorders
Ataxic: cerebellar disorders

Peripheral Types
Flaccid dysarthrias: individual nerve disorder or diffuse neuromuscular disorder

Mixed Types
Spastic-flaccid: amyotrophic lateral sclerosis
Spastic-hypokinetic-ataxic: Wilson's disease
Other mixed type: multiple sclerosis

Adapted from Darby JK (ed). *Speech and Language Evaluation in Neurology.* Englewood Cliffs, NJ: Prentice-Hall, 1985.

3. **Resonance**
   a. The anatomic units are the oropharynx and the nasopharynx, but contributions are made by all the components of the respiratory outflow tract.
   b. Physiologically, the supraglottic space provides a chamber in which various harmonics of the fundamental frequency are resonated to create more complex sounds.
   c. Specific consonants rely on specific intact functions. Examples are as follows:

Unit/Function	Production	Consonants
Nasopharynx	Nasal resonance	/m/ as in "met"; /n/ as in "no"
Soft palate closure	Stop consonants	/p/ as in "put"; /b/ as in "bed"; /k/ as in "key"

4. **Articulation**
   a. Anatomic components include the lips, teeth, cheeks, tongue, and soft palate.
   b. Manipulation of the size and shape of the oral cavity, in conjunction with the positions of the lips, teeth, and tongue, produces phonemes—distinctive units of speech sound.
   c. Production of vowels and consonants is accomplished by means of lingual positioning plus relative opening of the vocal tract. Vowel sounds are created with the vocal tract remaining in an open position; consonants are formed by a range of vocal tract constriction. Sonorant consonants require a relatively open tract (e.g., /m/ as in "mad"; /l/ as in "live"), and obstruent consonants require a degree of closure (e.g., /g/ as in "got"; /s/ as in "soup").

5. **Prosody**

Table 19-2. Classification schemes for the dysarthrias.

Category	Examples
Age at onset	Congenital or acquired
General cause	Vascular, neoplastic, traumatic, infectious, etc.
Disease processes	Multiple sclerosis, myasthenia gravis, parkinsonism, etc.
Neuroanatomic area involved	Cerebral, cerebellar, brainstem, etc.
Cranial nerves involved	V, VII, IX, X, XI, XII
Speech processes involved	Respiration, phonation, resonance, articulation, prosody
Speech valves involved	Respiratory, laryngeal, pharyngeal, velar, lingual, dental, labial
Speech events involved	Neural, muscular, structural, aerodynamic, acoustic, perceptual

Adapted from Johns DF (ed). *Clinical Management of Neurogenic Communication Disorders* (2nd ed). Boston: Little, Brown, 1985.

Table 19-3. Etiologies of dysarthria.

Congenital/developmental	Acquired
Cerebral palsy	Acute
	Drugs
	Trauma
	Toxins
	Vascular
	Encephalitis
Muscular dystrophy	Subacute
	Inflammation/infection
	Expanding mass lesion
	Metabolic derangement
Agenesis of the lower cranial nerves	Progressive/chronic
	Multiple sclerosis
	Basal ganglia degenerative diseases
	Parkinson's disease
	Huntington's disease
	Dementias
	Motor neuron disease (amyotrophic lateral sclerosis)
Hearing disorders	
Basal ganglia degenerations	
Wilson's disease	
Hallervorden-Spatz disease	
Cerebellar degenerations	
Hereditary ataxias	
Inborn errors of metabolism	

    a. Neurologic control of the speech system that produces prosody is diverse, with brain control and programming of speech organized as for other movements.

    b. Integration of the functions of the premotor and motor cortex, the pyramidal and extrapyramidal systems, the cerebellum, afferent sensory nerves, and peripheral nerves results in control of the sequencing, timing, and rate of speech production.

    c. By alterations in pitch, stress, and rhythm, different meanings and emphases are conveyed.

  B. Abnormalities in speech systems

    1. Abnormalities in respiration result from hypofunction or hyperfunction.

      a. Hypofunction is associated with decreased vital capacity, expiratory volumes, and expiratory force.

        (1) Diseases include obstructive and restrictive pulmonary diseases; chest wall restriction (i.e., kyphoscoliosis); nerve (mononeuropathy or polyneuropathy), neuromuscular junction, and muscle diseases; and intrathoracic and intra-abdominal masses.

        (2) The results are quick fall-offs in pitch and loudness, loss of strength of voiceless consonants (e.g., /p/ as in "put"), shortened speech phrasing, and interruption by frequent wheezing and inspiratory stridor.

      b. Hyperfunction is related to upper motor neuron dysfunction, both pyramidal and extrapyramidal.

        (1) Constant hyperfunction is associated with spasticity and results from asynchrony between respiratory muscles. This condition is observed in pseudobulbar palsy and cerebral palsy and is characterized by choppy and explosive speech.

        (2) Intermittent hyperfunction accompanies the hyperkinetic movement disorders of chorea and dystonia, wherein sudden changes in muscle tone result in abrupt stops and breaks in inspiration and expiration, leading to unwanted pauses and changes in pitch and loudness. These individuals speak in short phrases because of frequent changes in voice.

    2. Abnormalities in phonation. Abnormalities that produce faulty approxi-

Table 19-4. Mayo Clinic classification of dysarthria.

Dysarthria type	Neurologic condition(s)	Location of pathology	Most distinctive speech deviations
Flaccid	Bulbar palsy	Lower motor neuron	Marked hypernasality, often with nasal air emission; continuous breathiness; audible inspiration
Spastic	Pseudobulbar palsy	Upper motor neuron	Very imprecise articulation; slow rate; low pitch; harsh strained/strangled voice
Ataxic	Cerebellar ataxia	Cerebellum	Excess stress and mono-stress; phoneme and interval prolongation; dysrhythmia of speech and syllable repetition; slow rate; some excess loudness variation
Hypokinetic	Parkinsonism	Extrapyramidal system	Monopitch, monoloudness, reduced overall loudness; variable rate; short rushes of speech; some inappropriate silences
Hyperkinetic 1. Quick	Chorea	Extrapyramidal system	Highly variable pattern of imprecise articulation; episodes of hypernasality; sudden variations in loudness
	Myoclonus		Rhythmic hypernasality; rhythmic phonatory interruption
	Gilles de la Tourette's syndrome		Sudden ticlike grunts, barks, coprolalia
2. Slow	Athetosis	Extrapyramidal system	Distinctive deviations unreported
	Dyskinesias		Distinctive deviations unreported
	Dystonia		Prolongations of phonemes, intervals; unsteady rate, loudness
Mixed	Amyotrophic lateral sclerosis	Multiple motor systems	Grossly defective articulation; extremely slow, laborious rate; marked hypernasality; severe harshness, strained/strangled voice; nearly complete disruption of prosody
	Multiple sclerosis		Impaired control of loudness; harshness
	Wilson's disease		Reduced stress; monopitch; monoloudness; similar to hypokinetic dysarthria except no short rushes of speech

Adapted from Johns DF (ed). *Clinical Management of Neurogenic Communicative Disorders* (2nd ed). Boston: Little, Brown, 1985.

mation of vocal folds (nerve, muscle, or joint injuries), or variation in vocal mass (tumors, nodules, inflammation, or edema), result in three types of abnormal phonatory patterns, as follows.

    a. Hypofunction results from impaired adduction of the vocal folds, as occurs with nerve injuries and mass lesions. There is excessive escape of air through a patent glottis, leading to loss of clear tonal musical sound. Instead, a breathy quality is heard. This condition can result from laryngeal nerve injury, tumor, surgical procedure, or recent extubation.

    b. Hyperfunction is the result of overadduction of the vocal folds and results in increased pitch and evidence of a strained or strangled quality resulting from the greater effort to create a voice. This condition accompanies pseudobulbar palsy, dystonias, and cerebellar disease.

    c. Mixed phonation combines pathologic elements of both hypofunction and hyperfunction and imparts both a breathy and a harsh or hoarse character to the voice. Mixed phonation occurs in association with structural lesions of the vocal folds, such as tumors, polyps, and inflammation.

3. Abnormalities in resonance. Defects in the shape of the vocal tract above the level of the larynx result in two types of resonance changes: variations in nasality, which are discussed below; and variations in articulation, which are discussed in sec. **II.B.4.**

    a. Hypernasality is associated with velopharyngeal incompetence, or weakness of the soft palate. There is an excess escape of air through the nasal cavity and into the nose during speaking.

    b. Hyponasality results from obstruction within the velopharyngeal opening or within the nostrils. Acoustic energy is dissipated through the mouth during speaking.

        (1) For example, the nasal consonants /m/ as in "met" and /n/ as in "net" resemble their non-nasal counterparts /b/ as in "bet" and /d/ as in "debt."

        (2) Vowel sounds are also altered in hyponasal speech, producing an overall dull or muffled speech.

4. Abnormalities in articulation. The presence of a general articulatory abnormality alone does not distinguish the type of dysarthria. Articulation disorders are either generalized or specific.

    a. Generalized articulation disorders involve articulatory problems affecting all or most phonemes and occur with either CNS or systemic disease.

    b. Specific articulatory disorders involve problems affecting specific groups of phonemes and are associated with local structural pathology or damage to one or more nerves.

    c. Errors

        (1) The types of errors that occur during articulation include omissions, distortions, substitutions, and additions of phonemes.

        (2) Dysarticulations may be secondary to faulty lip, tongue, dental, or oral cavity manipulation (e.g., common lisps), and when dysarticulation is the only abnormality, it is not considered a dysarthria, but a developmental dysarticulation disorder.

5. Abnormalities in prosody are common to all dysarthrias. There are three types of prosodic errors: (1) hyperprosody, (2) hypoprosody, and (3) dysprosody. Both hyperprosodic and hypoprosodic errors tend to be constant in the nature of the dysfunction, whereas dysprosody exhibits errors that vary from moment to moment.

    a. Hyperprosody consists of exaggerated variations in stress, as observed in Broca's aphasia, or in pitch and stress, as in the mania of bipolar disorder.

    b. Hypoprosody is evidenced by decreased stressing or lack of stressing, reduced loudness, monopitch, and lack of rhythm. It is observed in dysarthrias associated with parkinsonism and with right hemispheric lesions.

    c. Dysprosody, which involves errors in pitch, rhythm, or stress, is observed in cerebellar dysarthrias.

III. Evaluation
    A. History

1. **Onset.** When did the patient or family first notice the change in speech? Were there preexisting developmental dysarticulation problems?
2. **Tempo.** Did the speech change come on suddenly or gradually, and has it improved, stabilized, or progressed since it was first noticed? Has it fluctuated in severity? Have there been normal periods of speech among periods of abnormality?
3. Coexisting neurologic symptoms, especially those related to the upper or lower motor system of the brain or to the cranial or cervical nerves
4. Previous neurologic diagnoses and previous treatment
5. Medication history and nonprescription drug use
B. **Physical examination**
   1. There are three steps in the physical examination.

      Step 1. Obtain adequate samples of both spontaneous and tested speech.
      Step 2. Interpret the speech samples by focusing on each system and determining whether it is normal or abnormal, and, if it is abnormal, the nature of the abnormality. Include a physical examination of the oral cavity, the oropharynx, the nasopharynx, and chest wall movement.
      Step 3. Categorize the pattern of abnormalities noted in the previous steps, and compare it with known patterns resulting in clinical diagnoses of dysarthria (see Table 19-4).

   2. **Specific system testing**
      a. **Respiration.** Have the patient sustain a constant vowel sound /a/ for as long as possible. Normal vital capacity allows a duration of 20–25 seconds. Note pitch fall-off, loudness, length of speech phrasing, choppiness, or explosiveness during attentive listening. Test fatiguability by having the patient count numbers during one breath.
      b. **Phonation.** Have the patient phonate a constant vowel syllable /ah/ as clearly and for as long as possible. Other phonemes, such as /ee/, place greater stress on the vocal folds, and the examiner should listen for variations in quality, duration, pitch, steadiness, and loudness. To assess true vocal fold efficiency, compare the times that the patient can sustain the /s/ and /z/ phonemes. Normal function makes it possible to sustain phonation of these two consonants for equal lengths of time. If /z/ is sustained for a significantly shorter period, inefficient use of the true vocal folds is indicated. Have the patient give a crisp cough to see if the abnormality clears. Refer the patient to an otolaryngologist for laryngoscopic visualization if abnormalities are noted.
      c. **Resonance** is evaluated by having the patient selectively pronounce words that emphasize nasal and plosive phonemes. Watch the soft palate at rest and during the phonation of /ah/. Have the patient sustain phonation as long as possible. Watch for fatigue. Another measure of nasality is taken by having the patient sustain /ah/ while the examiner occludes the nares. Feel for vibration, which indicates diminished palatal function/ closure. Note periodic movements of the palate, which may accompany palatal myoclonus. Use a nasopharyngeal mirror to examine the nasopharynx indirectly.
      d. **Articulation.** During attentive listening, note whether the abnormality is general (mispronunciation of all or most phonemes) or specific (mispronunciation of only certain phonemes). By having the patient pronounce a series of diphthongs, the examiner can assess which structures are involved in dysarticulation—e.g., lips, tongue, soft palate, or a combination thereof. Have the patient pronounce each of the following diphthongs repeatedly: "puh," "tuh," and "kuh." "Puh" is specific for bilabial function, "tuh" is specific for lingual-alveolar function, and "kuh" is specific for lingual-palatal function. Then have the patient rapidly alternate among all the diphthongs to bring out dysdiadochokinesia and errors in prosody. Alternatively, an expression that has more contextual meaning may be used to assess dysarticulation, such as "buttercup" or "pattycake." Inspection and palpation of intraoral structures is performed to search for abnormal coloration, clefts, malocclusion, missing teeth, and masses.
      e. **Prosody.** In careful listening to spontaneous speech, note rate, timing, spacing, valving, melody, and emphasis. Have the patient imitate varied

stress and intonation patterns using a common phrase such as "How are you?"

f. Test hearing by recognition of words whispered into each ear, or with a tuning fork.

C. Laboratory studies

1. **Brain or cervical neuroimaging** is indicated in acute or subacute instances, and in cases of progressive or chronic disorders when treatable illness is possible.

2. **Electromyography** is used to diagnose specific peripheral nerve injury or focal dystonia, polyneuropathy, myopathy, bulbar palsy, motor neuron disease, or myasthenia gravis.

3. **Other blood testing** is specific to the diagnostic possibilities producing the dysarthria.

IV. **Differential diagnosis.** As with the classification of the dysarthrias, differential diagnosis can be approached in several different ways. If a general neurologic diagnosis and neuroanatomic localization are arrived at prior to speech testing, a relatively accurate diagnosis of the type of dysarthria can be made using attentive listening during conversation with the patient. Alternatively, if the neurologic diagnosis or neuroanatomic localization is elusive, careful application of the steps used to characterize the type of dysarthria may narrow the diagnostic search. Table 19-4 summarizes the dysarthria type, neuroanatomic localization, differential diagnoses for dysarthria type, and the most prominent features on testing. Adherence to the method of testing is necessary because certain diagnoses can be made by specific testing of each of the five systems involved in speech production: respiration, phonation, resonance, articulation, and prosody.

A. **Respiration.** The differential diagnosis for respiration problems falls mainly into two categories: primary pulmonary diseases and neurologic diseases. Patients with pulmonary diseases show diminished breath support, phrase length, and voice quality, but other parameters are most often normal. Primary neurologic disorders characterized by respiration system abnormalities include injury or dysfunction of the intercostal nerves, phrenic nerve, sympathetic plexus, spinal cord, brainstem, or vagus nerve; myopathic processes; and neuromuscular junction disorders. Diseases include:

1. **Myopathic disorders**
   a. Acute myopathy syndrome
   b. Hypokalemic periodic paralysis
   c. Periodic paralysis

2. **Neuromuscular junction disorders**
   a. Persistent neuromuscular blockade
   b. Myasthenia gravis
   c. Hypermagnesemia

3. **Peripheral nerve disorders**
   a. Critical illness polyneuropathy
   b. Guillain-Barré syndrome
   c. Acute intermittent porphyria
   d. Phrenic and intercostal nerve lesions from trauma or tumor infiltration
   e. Intoxications

4. Multiradiculopathy from carcinoma, lymphoma, or degenerative cervical spine disease

5. Anterior horn cell disease

6. Spinal cord disorder

B. **Phonation** is dependent on the integrity of the vagus nerve and specifically its branches.

1. The recurrent laryngeal nerve innervates the true vocal folds.
   a. Lesions. A unilateral lesion produces vocal fold paralysis in the paramedian position. The result is a flaccid dysphonia, which is characterized by breathiness, lowered pitch, and possibly diplophonia (a stereophonic-type sound caused by unequal frequencies of vibration of the two vocal folds). There may be special difficulty with vowels. Rarely, unilateral lesions of the vagus or recurrent laryngeal nerves can result in a normal voice, because the normal vocal fold may adduct across the midline to approximate the weaker vocal fold. Bilateral lesions produce vocal folds in the paramedian position with severe compromise of the airways, and

speech may be dysphonic or aphonic. There may be a tense or tight quality to the voice, which may result in monostress and monopitch.

    b. **Common causes** include accidental injury during open heart surgery, especially to the left recurrent laryngeal nerve as it passes around the aorta; trauma as from gunshot or knife wounds; tumor infiltration; and laryngitis.

2. The superior laryngeal nerve innervates the cricothyroid muscle. Bilateral damage results in loss of pitch control. The voice is hoarse and deep, and fatigues quickly.

3. An intramedullary or extramedullary lesion at the brainstem level affecting the main trunk of the vagus nerve produces a unilateral or bilateral true vocal fold paralysis in the abducted position, causing considerable glottic air escape and a severely breathy voice quality combined with hypernasality (see sec. **IV.C.1,** below).

4. Adductor palsy is usually psychogenic, and loss of speech is out of proportion to involvement.

5. Paradoxical vocal cord motion occurs when the inspiratory phase is out of synchrony with vocal fold abduction. Speech and biofeedback therapy are important interventions.

C. Resonance. Normal resonance depends on the integrity of the oropharynx, nasopharynx, nares, and mouth cavities.

1. The pharyngeal nerve branch of the vagus innervates the soft palate. Lesions produce unilateral or bilateral weakness of the soft palate and incompetence of the velopharyngeal seal during speech and swallowing. Speech is hypernasal owing to escape of air through the nares. The problem is more prominent if the head is tipped forward, because the soft palate collapses onto the posterior oropharynx.

2. Lesion of the trigeminal nerve or its mandibular branch produces flaccidity of the floor of the mouth because of loss of innervation of the mylohyoid and anterior digastric muscles.

3. Obstruction along the nasal passage by a mass, by inflammation, or by edema results in excess escape of air through the mouth, giving the speech a hyponasal quality.

D. Articulation. Disordered articulation results from dysfunction of cranial nerves VII and XII (predominantly XII), but also, although less commonly, the trigeminal nerve that serves to open and close the jaw. Normal function of the muscles of facial expression and tongue are required for production of accurate phonemes. Acquired dysfunction is traditionally differentiated from childhood developmental dysarticulation (developmental articulatory dyspraxia), which is the imprecise imitation, movement, or coordination of the elements of speech production in children with otherwise normal mentation and muscle tone.

1. The facial nerve provides innervation for motor manipulation of the mouth and lips. Paralysis produces problems with bilabial (e.g., /b/ as in baby) and labiodental (e.g., /f/ as in father) phonemes.

    Common causes of facial nerve lesions include idiopathic (Bell's palsy), tumor within the temporal bone, Ramsay Hunt syndrome, mass lesions such as acoustic neuromas, aneurysm, Lyme disease, sarcoidosis, Guillain-Barré syndrome, trauma, and both supranuclear and pontine lesions.

2. The hypoglossal nerve provides innervation for tongue manipulation, and lesions result in lingual dysarticulations. Two types of lingual dysarticulations occur commonly. The first is the lisp, a distortion of sibilant phonemes (e.g., "thoup" for "soup" or "thebra" for "zebra"). The second is lalling, a distortion of phonemes produced by the tongue tip (e.g., "wime" for "rhyme" and "yime" for "lime").

    Common causes of hypoglossal nerve lesions include motor neuron disease; posterior fossa and basilar skull masses; retropharyngeal, retrostyloid, and neck masses; infections; trauma; and radiation therapy exposure.

3. Dental malocclusion, dental absence, and structural deformity of the tongue can also bring about dysarticulation.

E. Prosody. Dysprosody or aprosody, as mentioned above, may be the result of a lesion anywhere along the motor speech neuroaxis, but is most prominently associated with brain hemispheric disease.

V. Diagnostic approach

      A. Perform the three-step physical examination outlined in sec. **III.B.**

      B. Initiate a therapeutic plan based on system dysfunction and dysarthria type.

VI. Referral

      A. Otolaryngology consultation may be necessary for evaluation of the larynx and pharynx, especially if hypernasality is of recent onset, to rule out structural lesion and hearing problems. If a patient has been extubated for longer than 7 days and vocal quality remains impaired or not improving, referral may be indicated for nasopharyngeal laryngoscopy.

      B. Speech pathology consultation is necessary to aid in diagnosis of speech and swallowing and to provide and administer a therapeutic plan.

Recommended Readings

Adams RD, Victor M. Affection for speech and language. In RD Adams, M Victor (eds), *Principles of Neurology* (5th ed). New York: McGraw-Hill, 1993.

Barry WR (ed). *Clinical Dysarthria*. San Diego: College Hill, 1983.

Bladle AJ (ed). Language and motor speech. *Clinical Examinations in Neurology* (6th ed). St. Louis: Mayo Foundation, 1991.

Brazis PW, Masdeu JC, Biller J. The localization of lesions affecting cranial nerve XII. *Localization in Clinical Neurology* (3rd ed). Boston: Little, Brown, 1996.

Brookshire RH. *An Introduction to Neurogenic Communication Disorders* (4th ed). Philadelphia: Mosby, 1992.

Chapey R (ed). *Language Intervention Strategies in Adult Aphasia* (2nd ed). Baltimore: Williams & Wilkins, 1986.

Costello J. *Speech Disorders in Adults*. San Diego: College Hill, 1985.

Critchley EMR. *Language and Speech Disorders: A Neurophysiological Approach*. Hillsdale, NJ: CNS Clinical Neuroscience, 1987.

Darby JK (ed). *Speech and Language Evaluation in Neurology: Adult Disorders*. Boston: Grune & Stratton, 1985.

Duus P. *Topical Diagnosis in Neurology* (2nd ed). New York: Thieme, 1989.

Eldridge M. *A History of the Treatment of Speech Disorders*. London: Livingstone, 1968.

Groher ME. *Dysphagia: Diagnosis and Management* (2nd ed). Boston: Butterworth-Heinemann, 1992.

Hartman DE, Abbs JH. Dysarthria associated with focal unilateral upper motor neuron lesion. *Eur J Disord Commun* 27(3):187–196, 1992.

Hird K, Krisner K. Dysprosody following acquired neurogenic impairment. *Brain and Language* 45(1):46–60, 1993.

Ichikawa K, Kageyama Y. Clinical anatomic study of pure dysarthria. *Stroke* 22:809–812, 1991.

Johns DF. *Clinical Management of Neurogenic Communicative Disorders* (2nd ed). Boston: College Hill, 1985.

Johnson JA, Pring PR. Speech therapy in Parkinson disease: A review on further data. *Disord Commun* 25(2):183–194, 1990.

Lass NJ, et al. *Handbook of Speech, Language Pathology, and Audiology*. Philadelphia: BC Decker, 1988.

Love RJ, Webb WG. *Neurology for the Speech-Language Pathologist* (2nd ed). Boston: Butterworth-Heinemann, 1992.

Matas M. Psychogenic voice disorders: Literature review and case report. *Can J Psychiatry* 36(5):363–365, 1991.

Metter J. *Speech Disorders: Clinical Evaluation and Diagnosis*. Dana Point, CA: PMA, 1985.

Moore CA, Yorkston KM, Beukelman DR (eds). *Dysarthria and Apraxia of Speech: Prospective on Management*. Baltimore: PH Brooks, 1991.

Nation JE, Aram DM. *Diagnosis of Speech and Language Disorders* (2nd ed). San Diego: College Hill, 1984.

Singh S, Lynch J. *Diagnostic Procedures in Hearing, Language, and Speech*. Baltimore: University Park, 1978.

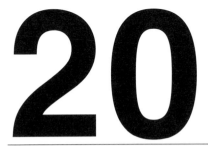

20

Approach to the Patient with Acute Headache
David Lee Gordon

Acute headache is one of the most common reasons for visits to emergency rooms. **Primary headache**—e.g., migraine and cluster—is a condition in which headache is a primary manifestation and no underlying disease process is present. **Secondary headache** is a condition in which headache is a secondary manifestation of an underlying disease process. The majority of patients with acute headache have primary headache, particularly migraine. Performing an expensive battery of tests on all patients with acute headache is neither cost-effective nor appropriate. However, failure to perform diagnostic tests on certain patients with acute headache results in failure to detect life-threatening, yet treatable, causes. The challenge to the clinician in the emergency setting is not to be lulled to sleep by the frequent migraine attacks and to remain vigilant for the other causes of acute headache. Migraine is so common that many patients with secondary headaches have past histories of migraine, making diagnosis in the acute setting quite difficult. Certain clues on history and examination should lead to the performance of a diagnostic evaluation in search of the cause of secondary headache. The primary goals of the clinician managing a patient with acute headache are threefold: (1) diagnose the cause of headache, (2) provide emergency therapy, and (3) provide the patient with a means of long-term care. These same goals apply for patients with primary or secondary headaches; primary headaches are chronic conditions manifested by multiple acute attacks, and secondary headaches generally result from diseases requiring both urgent and prolonged care. This chapter deals with the diagnosis of acute headache. The diagnosis of chronic headache and the therapies for conditions that cause headache are dealt with elsewhere in this text.

I. **Pathophysiology.** Headache description alone cannot reliably predict whether a headache is primary or secondary—e.g., hemicranial throbbing pain is not always a feature of migraine and may be a feature of intracranial disease. This suggests that primary and secondary headaches share common pathophysiologic mechanisms. Although the current understanding of the etiology of head pain is not complete, a plausible explanation of headache pathophysiology, emphasizing the common final pathway of primary and secondary headaches, is depicted in Figure 20-1. The schema provides an explanation for the "migrainous" characteristics of some secondary headaches. Older theories regarding the vascular origin of migraine and the muscle-contraction etiology of tension headache are not likely to be true.

II. **History**
   A. **Previous history of headaches** is perhaps the most important historical information needed to determine whether a diagnostic evaluation is necessary. A history of similar headaches for many years suggests a primary headache disorder. If, on the other hand, the current headache is the *first* headache of the patient's life, if it is the *worst* headache that the patient has had, if it is *different* in character from past headaches, or if the pain is *persistent* despite the use of measures that have relieved previous headaches, a secondary headache is much more likely. In addition, if the patient has suffered similar headaches for only a few months, weeks, or days, the possibility of secondary headache increases and further investigation is warranted. Although it is common for the character of primary headache disorders to change throughout one's lifetime, if the current headache differs from previous headaches, the clinician is obligated to investigate.
   B. **Age of onset** of primary headache disorders is generally childhood to young adulthood. Onset at an age greater than 50 years is particularly suspicious for secondary headache.

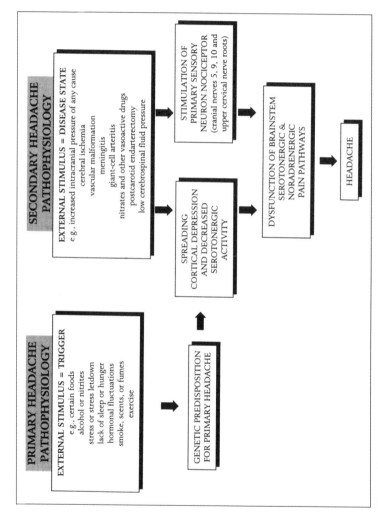

Figure 20-1. Plausible schema for headache pathophysiology, depicting the common final pathway of primary and secondary headaches.

C. **Activity at onset** of headache may suggest the cause of headache. Although migraine can be precipitated or exacerbated by Valsalva's maneuver, changes in position, or head trauma, the presence of any of these features on history should raise the suspicion of secondary headache. **Valsalva's maneuver,** which occurs with lifting, straining, or squatting, may precipitate aneurysmal rupture and resultant subarachnoid hemorrhage. Headache during coitus may occur as a result of aneurysmal rupture or as a result of coital migraine; the first time a person experiences coital headache, he or she should undergo a complete evaluation to rule out aneurysmal subarachnoid hemorrhage. **Changes in position** exacerbate several types of headaches. Headaches that are worse in the supine position suggest sinusitis, cerebral venous thrombosis, or an intracranial mass. Headaches that improve in the supine position and worsen on sitting or standing are characteristic of low-pressure headaches. Headaches that occur only in a particular head position may be attributable to a mobile intracranial tumor that intermittently obstructs the ventricles (and thereby increases intracranial pressure), such as a third ventricle colloid cyst. Although **head trauma** may serve as a "trigger" for migraine, subdural hematoma must be ruled out before this diagnosis is possible. **Exercise** may precipitate a migraine headache.

D. **Headache characteristics** are most helpful in determining whether the current headache is different from previous headaches. Certain characteristics are suggestive of, but not pathognomonic for, certain causes of headache.

   1. **Severity** of pain is important in that any patient who complains of "the worst headache of my life" deserves an urgent and complete evaluation, with subarachnoid hemorrhage highest in the differential diagnosis. Both primary headaches and secondary headaches, however, can present with either very severe or very mild pain.

   2. **Temporal onset** of pain is more discriminating. The sudden onset of a headache suggests a sudden increase in intracranial pressure such as occurs with subarachnoid hemorrhage. Mass lesions such as tumors, abscesses, and subacute or chronic subdural hematomas usually present gradually over days to months. Gradual onset of headache over minutes to hours is consistent with migraine. The headache of giant cell arteritis tends to be subacute to chronic in presentation.

   3. **Duration** of primary headaches is variable, although they typically last for hours to days. Headaches that persist for longer periods of time despite treatment are worrisome for underlying cranial pathology.

   4. **Location** of headache and radiation of pain are nonspecific. Many posterior lesions cause frontal headaches. Both primary and secondary headaches may be unilateral or bilateral. The pain of both migraine headaches and secondary headaches may radiate.

   5. **Quality** of headache is nondiscriminating. Despite the traditional teaching that migraines must be pounding or throbbing, they are just as often presurelike, squeezing, sharp, stabbing, or dull. Cluster headaches are typically described as boring, sharp, or lancinating, but so might the headaches associated with other pathologies.

   6. **Associated symptoms** of the headache may offer important clues to its cause.

      a. **Nausea** and **vomiting** are common features of migraine, but their presence in a person with new or sudden headache is worrisome for either increased intracranial pressure or a posterior fossa lesion.

      b. **Photophobia** and **phonophobia** may be associated with either a migraine or a meningeal process such as subarachnoid hemorrhage or meningitis.

      c. **Neck stiffness** is typical of a meningeal process.

      d. **Changes in consciousness** are rare in patients with primary headache; such changes should alert the clinician to more serious causes of headache.

      e. **Focal neurologic symptoms** (e.g., aphasia, visual symptoms, vertigo, ataxia, hemiparesis, or hemisensory deficit) may occur suddenly in association with headache in patients with stroke, seizure, subdural hematoma, and migraine. In this case, migraine is a diagnosis of exclusion and the clinician is obligated to investigate for underlying disease. Transient ischemic attacks (TIAs) typically last 5–20 minutes.

Symptoms of stroke and subdural hematoma persist. The Todd's paralysis of partial seizures and the aura of migraine often last for hours. The focal symptoms of ischemia and hemorrhage are typically static, whereas the focal symptoms of migraine typically travel over minutes to hours—e.g., numbness that begins in the fingertips and progresses to involve the entire arm and perhaps the ipsilateral face or leg. Partial seizures may result in symptoms that travel over seconds. Binocular visual symptoms may be migrainous or the result of occipital pathology. A headache in a person more than 50 years old with monocular blurred vision and a swollen optic disk suggests the anterior ischemic optic neuropathy of giant cell arteritis. Certain visual symptoms are classic for migraine, such as scintillating scotomata (blind areas surrounded by sparkling zig-zag lines), photopsia (unformed flashes of color), and fortification spectra (slowly enlarging, sparkling, serrated arcs).

f. Fever, diaphoresis, chills, or **rigors** are worrisome for infection. Fever of any cause or a generalized infection may cause headache, but if headache, neck stiffness, and decreased consciousness are prominent symptoms, meningitis is highest in the differential diagnosis.

E. Family history of headache is important, yet extremely difficult to obtain in the emergency setting of an acute headache. Patients may be distracted by their pain and nausea and may have cognitive dysfunction as a feature of the headache (whether primary or secondary). Even if the patient is coherent or an accompanying relative is available, it is common for the patient not to be aware of a family history of headaches. Migraines tend to be most prominent in early adulthood, when children are too young to realize the parent has headaches and the patient no longer lives under the same roof with parents or siblings. In addition, rationalizations of relatives regarding the cause of their headaches (e.g., "sinus" or "tension") are usually believed by the patient, making it difficult to obtain a family history of "migraine."

III. Physical examination may reveal signs of a disease that causes secondary headache. A detailed neurologic examination is particularly important; any subtle abnormality should be enough to indicate a diagnostic evaluation.

A. General examination

1. Vital signs. Fever suggests infectious cause of headache. Arterial hypertension in a patient with headache is common and is not necessarily causative. Hypertension occurs as a result of migraine attacks, cerebral ischemia, and intracranial hemorrhage. In certain cases, especially when it comes on abruptly and reaches extreme levels, hypertension may be a primary cause of headache.

2. General appearance. Cachexia may be present in patients with chronic diseases such as cancer, AIDS, tuberculosis, and sarcoidosis. Headache resulting from tumor, abscess, granuloma, or meningitis may be the presenting symptom in such patients.

3. Head. Evidence of cranial trauma includes face and scalp abrasions and contusions and the signs of skull fracture: depressed section of skull, Battle's sign (postauricular ecchymosis that occurs with basilar skull fracture), raccoon sign (periorbital ecchymosis), hemotympanum, and cerebrospinal fluid rhinorrhea. Skull tenderness to palpation may occur as a result of subdural hematoma. Poor dentition or dental abscess may result in intracranial abscess. Tenderness to palpation over the mastoid process, frontal sinus, or maxillary sinus may suggest infection of these structures. Migraine, however, frequently results in external carotid territory vasodilatation with resultant sinus "fullness," "pressure," and tenderness. The presence of purulent discharge from the sinuses is more helpful in diagnosing sinusitis. Otoscopic examination may reveal ear infection as well as hemotympanum. Temporal tenderness or diminished temporal artery pulses in a person aged 50 or more are consistent with giant cell (temporal) arteritis. Auscultation of the skull may reveal cranial bruits that occur as a result of arteriovenous malformation.

4. Neck. Meningeal signs include nuchal rigidity (neck stiffness in the anteroposterior direction), Kernig's sign (inability to extend the knee after passive hip flexion in the supine position), and Brudzinzki's sign (involuntary hip flexion after passive flexion of the neck in the supine position) and imply the presence of meningitis or subarachnoid hemorrhage. Evidence of neck trauma includes pain on lateral neck movement and neck immobility.

5. **Skin.** Examination may reveal bruising suggestive of a bleeding diathesis, splinter hemorrhages of the distal digits suggesting cardioembolism, or lesions suggestive of a neurocutaneous disorder such as neurofibromatosis, tuberous sclerosis, or cutaneous angiomatosis. These conditions are associated with intracranial lesions that may cause headache. Melanoma suggests the possibility of cerebral metastasis as a cause of headache. Lesions of Kaposi's sarcoma are consistent with acquired immunodeficiency syndrome (AIDS), which is associated with several intracranial diseases that cause headache.

6. **Lymph nodes.** Lymphadenopathy occurs in patients with cancer, AIDS, chronic infections, and chronic inflammatory diseases. The possible presence of any of these conditions should stimulate evaluation for cause of secondary headache.

B. **Neurologic examination** is normal in patients with primary headache. A change in consciousness or focal deficit raises the possibility of secondary headache. The funduscopic examination may reveal papilledema (swollen disk with normal visual acuity) in patients with increased intracranial pressure, anterior ischemic optic neuropathy (swollen disk with decreased visual acuity and/or relative afferent pupillary defect) in patients with giant cell arteritis, or preretinal hemorrhages in patients with intracranial hemorrhage. Headache in association with either a partial third nerve palsy or a complete but pupil-sparing third nerve palsy is worrisome for a posterior communicating artery aneurysm. Patients with these findings warrant urgent four-vessel cerebral arteriography. The combination of proptosis, oculomotor findings, and headache suggests disease in the orbit, superior orbital fissure, or cavernous sinus; evaluation should be urgent. Acute glaucoma can present with headache, especially periorbitally. An injected conjunctiva and a hard globe are consistent with this diagnosis. Horner's syndrome (miosis, subtle upper- and lower-lid ptosis, and anhydrosis) may occur in isolation, ipsilateral to a carotid dissection.

IV. **Laboratory studies** are necessary for any patient suspected of having secondary headache. There are no laboratories that identify patients with primary headache.

A. **Blood evaluation**

1. **Complete blood count (CBC).** Leukocytosis is consistent with infection, and marked leukocytosis is found in leukemia, which can cause headache associated with carcinomatous meningitis or cerebral venous occlusion. Leukopenia accompanies AIDS. Anemia may occur in patients with cancer or giant cell arteritis; it may also be associated with a low-flow state that precipitates cerebral venous thrombosis. Essential thrombocythemia is a hypercoagulable state that can cause arterial or venous occlusions in the brain, and resultant headache.

2. **Chemistries.** Renal failure may be associated with headache. Both renal function and liver enzyme abnormalities have implications regarding past drug use and options for future medical management. In general, however, abnormalities in serum chemistries may provide clues of a generalized, underlying disease process that can cause headache.

3. **Erythrocyte sedimentation rate (ESR)** and **C-reactive protein (CRP)** are the initial tests to perform if giant cell arteritis is suspected. Moderate elevations in ESR (up to 50 mm/hr) are common in healthy elderly patients. Both ESR and CRP are nonspecific; elevations may be present in patients with infection, inflammatory disease, or cancer. Still, marked elevations of ESR or any elevation of CRP in a patient with new-onset headache over age 50 should prompt the administration of high-dose steroids and a temporal artery biopsy.

4. **Increased prothrombin time (PT)** and **partial thromboplastin time (PTT)** may provide evidence of a bleeding diathesis that results in intracranial hemorrhage and headache.

5. **Thyroid function tests.** Thyroid disease may result in headache by serving as a trigger in a migraine patient, or may cause headache by other mechanisms.

6. **Hypercoagulable profile** is indicated in any patient with suspected cerebral venous thrombosis and in any patient younger than 50 with suspected TIA (new-onset headache with transient neurologic deficit). In addition to CBC, PT, and PTT, the minimal evaluation should include fibrinogen, protein

C, protein S (total and free), antithrombin III, lupus anticoagulant, and anti-cardiolipin antibodies (IgG and IgM). If the platelet count is abnormal, platelet function studies should be performed.

7. **Arterial blood gas.** Hypoxia can cause headache; arterial blood gas should be performed if clinically indicated.

8. **Drug screen.** Sympathomimetic drugs such as cocaine and amphetamines may be associated with intracranial hemorrhage or cerebral ischemia and resultant headache. Salicylate toxicity may result in diffuse cerebral edema with headache worsening. The use of excessive analgesics, whether over-the-counter or narcotic, can cause chronic analgesic rebound headache and interfere with acute headache management.

B. **Urine evaluation** may reveal nephrotic syndrome (which can be associated with a hypercoagulable state and resultant cerebral venous thrombosis), infection (organisms and white blood cells), evidence of peripheral embolization (red blood cell casts), or use of illicit or analgesic drugs.

C. **X-rays.** Chest x-rays may reveal hilar adenopathy or pulmonary lesions that provide clues regarding the identity of intracranial lesions that cause headache. Cervical spine x-rays may reveal evidence of neck trauma.

D. **Computed tomography (CT)** is the preferred initial cerebral imaging study because of its sensitivity in detecting acute blood. A noncontrast scan is mandatory, because both contrast and acute blood are white (hyperdense) on CT. If only a contrast scan is obtained, there may be confusion about whether a lesion is a hemorrhage or an enhancing mass. With time, blood becomes increasingly dark on CT. Consequently, a subacute (2–14-day) subdural hematoma is isodense with parenchyma on CT and may be difficult to detect. MRI is better at detecting subacute blood. The odds of detecting subarachnoid hemorrhage on CT decreases with time from onset of symptoms; within a few days, a large percentage of CTs are negative. Even in the acute phase, at least 5% of patients with subarachnoid hemorrhage will have normal CTs. In any patient with suspected subarachnoid hemorrhage, if CT is negative, the clinician is obligated to perform lumbar puncture. Once a noncontrast CT is obtained, if a mass lesion is suspected, a contrast scan should be obtained. Mass lesions such as tumors and abscesses disrupt the blood/brain barrier and cause seepage of dye around or in the lesion. A mass lesion may be isodense with parenchyma on noncontrast CT and therefore difficult to detect. A contrast scan greatly increases the chance of detecting such a lesion. Patients with known allergic reactions to the iodine-based dye should be pretreated with steroids. CT contrast is nephrotoxic and should not be used for patients with renal failure.

E. **Magnetic resonance imaging (MRI)** is a secondary cerebral imaging procedure for acute headache because of its inability to detect acute blood. It is better than CT, however, in the detection of subacute blood and is especially useful in patients with suspected subacute subdural hematoma. MRI is also superior to CT and even to angiography in the detection of vascular malformations. Any patient with suspected unruptured arteriovenous malformation as a cause of headache should undergo MRI. MRI is superior to CT in detection of parenchymal lesions and visualization of the posterior fossa and inferior temporal lobes. Unlike CT, MRI provides information regarding blood flow in cerebral vessels. MRI is the procedure of choice for patients with suspected cerebral venous thrombosis; it detects both parenchymal and venous abnormalities and is diagnostic in cerebral venous thrombosis approximately 75% of the time. MRI contrast (i.e., gadolinium) is not iodine based, is not nephrotoxic, and generally does not cause allergic reactions.

F. **Magnetic resonance angiography (MRA)** is indicated for patients with suspected cerebral venous thrombosis who do not undergo conventional angiography. MRA offers a noninvasive way of evaluating the cerebral vessels; contrast is not necessary. MRA, however, uses very complex technology and can mislead the clinician if not performed and interpreted properly. MRA uses gradient-recall echo technology; vessels with abnormal flow are not visualized, slow flow may mimic occlusion, and subacute thrombus may mimic normal flow. Selective MR venography (MRV) may be obtained by saturating arterial inflow. Images should be acquired perpendicular to flow in order to avoid in-plane flow artifacts. Two-dimensional time-of-flight images are preferred for venography, although additional phase-contrast images may be necessary for clarification.

G. Lumbar puncture (LP)

1. **Indications.** LP for cerebrospinal fluid (CSF) analysis is indicated if acute or chronic meningitis, subarachnoid hemorrhage, pseudotumor cerebri, or low-CSF-pressure headache is suspected.

2. **Timing in relation to CT.** It is preferable to perform CT before LP. If the CT shows a significant mass effect, such as shift across the midline, obliterated basilar cisterns, or a compressed fourth ventricle, LP should be avoided in order to avoid precipitation of uncal or central herniation of brain tissue through the foramen magnum. If CT shows subarachnoid hemorrhage, LP is not necessary. If meningitis is suspected and CT is to be delayed for more than a few minutes, antibiotics should be started on the way to the CT, and LP should be performed after normal CT. If the CT is to be delayed for hours and meningitis is highly suspected, it is necessary to perform LP and treat with appropriate antibiotics without CT. Prognosis in patients with meningitis is heavily influenced by promptness of treatment.

3. **CSF analysis.** Opening pressure is most important in patients with suspected pseudotumor cerebri (generally >250 mm Hg) or low-CSF-pressure headache. If subarachnoid hemorrhage is suspected, one should obtain cell counts in the first and last tubes of CSF and also test for xanthochromia. Knowing that the number of red blood cells did not change significantly between the two tubes helps to confirm the diagnosis and avoids the common dilemma of determining whether or not a bloody tap is "traumatic." Xanthochromia is the yellowish color of CSF supernatant that results from either the presence of hemoglobin breakdown products or a very high protein concentration. If the patient presents days after a subarachnoid hemorrhage, there may be no red blood cells in the CSF, but xanthochromia resulting from hemoglobin breakdown persists for up to 2 weeks. Cultures for bacteria, fungus, and tuberculosis should be sent for analysis. Polymerase chain reaction (PCR) is a sensitive means of detecting the presence of infection. VDRL and cryptococcal antigen tests should be done as well. If cancer is suspected, at least 10 cc of fluid should be sent for cytologic analysis.

H. Cerebral angiography should be performed urgently for any patient with subarachnoid hemorrhage on CT or LP. A four-vessel arteriogram is mandatory, because predictions of aneurysm location based on CT are not always accurate, and many patients have multiple aneurysms. Delayed venous phase films are the gold standard for the evaluation of cerebral venous thrombosis, which can also cause subarachnoid bleeding.

I. Electroencephalography (EEG) is indicated if seizures are suspect. Headaches often occur in association with seizures. Partial seizures can result in transient neurologic deficits and can be difficult to distinguish from migraine with aura and TIA.

V. Differential diagnosis

A. Primary headache

1. **Migraine**

   a. **Definition.** Migraine is a genetic condition in which the patient has a predisposition to suffer episodic headache, gastrointestinal dysfunction, or neurologic dysfunction. Contrary to popular belief, severe headache need not be a feature of migraine. The International Headache Society definition of migraine is quite specific for the purpose of research, but is probably too limiting in clinical practice. Migraine is inherited in an autosomal-dominant fashion and generally is not life-threatening—i.e., it is inherited in the same way brown eyes are inherited. It stands to reason that approximately two-thirds of all people suffer from migraine. There is convincing evidence that **tension-type headache** is a form of migraine, rather than a separate entity.

   b. **Triggers.** A migraine attack occurs as a result of an external stimulus or trigger affecting a person with the genetic predisposition to migraine. Examples of triggers include hormonal change, stress, stress letdown, certain foods, alcohol, smoke, certain scents, fumes, exercise, fatigue, lack of sleep, hunger, and head trauma. Women suffer more migraine attacks than men because they are more frequently exposed to triggers (estrogen-level fluctuations during menstruation, pregnancy, oral contraceptives, and menopause), but they are not more likely than men to have the genetic predisposition.

c. Phases. There are four main phases of migraine: prodrome, aura, headache, and postdrome. Not all phases need be present in any one migraine attack.

(1) The **prodrome** occurs hours to days before the headache and consists of mood changes (irritability or depression) or food cravings. Although chocolate is often thought to be a migraine trigger, more frequently a craving for chocolate is part of the migraine prodrome.

(2) The **aura** may be visual, sensory, motor, or reflective of brainstem (e.g., vertigo or diplopia) or cerebral cortex (e.g., aphasia) involvement. The symptoms are typically traveling in nature—e.g., moving or pulsating spots in the vision, or numbness that starts in part of one extremity and travels over several minutes to hours to involve the entire extremity or other extremities. The traveling nature of the symptoms reflects the spreading wave of cortical depression that occurs during migraine. The visual symptoms may be of any shape (spots, circles, or wavy or zig-zag lines), may be of any color (clear, silver, black, white, or brightly colored), may be hemianopic or present throughout the visual field, and typically move (traveling across vision, floating, pulsating, or heat-wave sensation). An aura may be the only symptom of a migraine attack (aura without headache—acephalgic migraine); may occur before, during, or after the headache (headache with aura—classic migraine); or may not be present at all (headache without aura—common migraine).

(3) The **headache** quality is not as helpful in diagnosis as is generally believed. Although the headache may be severe, throbbing, and hemicranial, it need not have any of these characteristics. Migraine headaches are frequently mild, squeezing, or dull in nature, or bilateral. The onset of headache is typically gradual over minutes to hours, and the duration is typically several hours to a few days. The headache may be associated with nausea, vomiting, photophobia, phonophobia, or difficulty in concentrating.

(4) The **postdrome** is marked by malaise for several hours after the headache. Mood changes, impaired concentration, and scalp or muscle tenderness may also be present. Sleep often helps migraine attacks, and the patient tends to crave rest in a dark, quiet room.

d. Difficulties in diagnosis. The diagnosis of migraine is a purely historical diagnosis. Influenced by folklore and advertising for over-the-counter medications, patients tend to believe that their recurrent headaches are attributable to "sinus," "tension," or "regular headache." Consequently, obtaining a past history of "migraine" is often difficult. It may be beneficial to educate the patient regarding migraine prior to obtaining a history. If there is any doubt in the clinician's mind regarding the diagnosis of migraine, a diagnostic evaluation is necessary to rule out other causes of headache.

2. Cluster headache is much less common than migraine. It occurs primarily in men and is manifested by severe, stabbing, periorbital pain with associated ipsilateral tearing, injected conjunctiva, nasal congestion, and rhinorrhea. Alcohol often precipitates attacks. The attacks occur most frequently at night, last 30 minutes to 3 hours, and may occur several times per day. Unlike migraine patients, cluster patients prefer to pace and keep active during attacks. The term "cluster" refers to the seasonal occurrence of multiple episodes over weeks to months with intermittent periods of remission. There are both episodic and chronic forms.

B. Secondary headache

1. Subarachnoid hemorrhage (SAH) is the most important consideration in patients with a "first-or-worst headache," and yet it is frequently missed: 25% of patients with SAH are initially treated for other conditions. The majority of patients with SAH have headache as their initial symptom. The headache is unilateral in 30% of patients, and neurologic examination may be normal. Many patients (estimates range from 20–95%) have milder "sentinel" headaches that precede the cataclysmic event. The clinician should consider the sentinel headache of SAH in patients with mild, yet different, headaches. CT is usually diagnostic, but if SAH is suspected clinically and CT is normal,

LP is mandatory. One should examine the CSF as described in sec. **IV.G.** Once SAH has been diagnosed by CT or LP, urgent four-vessel angiography is required to identify aneurysms amenable to surgical clipping.

2. **Meningitis,** particularly bacterial and viral meningitis, often presents as acute headache. Fever, neck stiffness, confusion, decreased consciousness, and cranial neuropathies may also be present. Bacterial meningitis is fatal if not treated. If bacterial meningitis is suspected, CSF analysis is mandatory. If CT is available within minutes, CT should be performed before LP to rule out mass effect. Section **IV.G** describes steps to take if CT is not immediately available. Broad-spectrum antibiotics should be started either just before or immediately after LP; the antibiotics can be adjusted once culture results are known. Aseptic meningitis and the chronic meningitides may also present as acute, persistent headache. Cranial neuropathies are more common and neck stiffness is less common in the chronic meningitides. Conditions associated with chronic meningitis include syphilis, fungal infection (especially cryptococcus), tuberculosis, sarcoidosis, Lyme disease, cancer, and lymphoma. Any AIDS patient with headache and normal contrast brain CT should be given an LP to search for cryptococcal meningitis. In patients with suspected carcinomatous or lymphomatous meningitis, multiple LPs for cytologic analysis of CSF may be necessary before the diagnosis is confirmed.

3. **Subdural hematoma** occurs as a result of the tearing of bridging veins. When acute, it presents as a rapidly progressive neurologic deficit, but headache may be the only symptom of subacute or chronic subdural hematoma. Although subdural hematoma is typically caused by closed head trauma, in many cases a history of trauma is absent, especially in older patients. CT is usually diagnostic, but subacute blood (2 days to 2 weeks) is isodense with brain parenchyma on CT, making it difficult to detect. MRI, although inferior to CT in the detection of acute blood, is superior in the detection of subacute blood. **Epidural hematoma,** resulting from a ruptured meningeal artery and usually associated with skull fracture, usually presents with rapidly progressive neurologic deficit and decreased consciousness, rather than headache; the classic sequence of events is head trauma, brief loss of consciousness, lucid interval, and then rapid progression to coma.

4. **Intracerebral hemorrhage** presents with focal neurologic findings and usually a change in consciousness or cognition. Estimates of headache incidence with intracerebral hemorrhage vary depending on the size and location of the hemorrhage. Among patients who are able to communicate, headache is more common with larger hemorrhages and those in the cerebellum and cortex (i.e., lobar hemorrhages). The classic description of cerebellar hemorrhage is acute-onset posterior headache with nausea, vomiting, and inability to stand. CT is diagnostic, and emergency surgery may be lifesaving.

5. **Ischemic stroke** and **transient ischemic attack (TIA)** are always present with a focal neurologic deficit. Headache occurs in 15–20% of patients with acute cerebral ischemia. The presence of headache with acute cerebral ischemia suggests at least temporary large-artery-territory ischemia, even if only a subcortical, "lacunar" infarct is detected on CT or MRI (not all small-artery "occlusions" result from small-artery "disease"). Despite traditional teaching, it is unclear whether headaches are more common in association with cardioembolic rather than atherothromboembolic stroke. CT is often normal in the first 24–48 hours of ischemic stroke. Stroke should be the first consideration for a patient with acute-onset focal neurologic deficit with headache. Patients with acute-onset focal brain or brainstem dysfunction, headache, and a CT that is normal or demonstrates focal hypodensity should be given a thorough evaluation for cause of ischemic stroke or TIA; the evaluation should include assessment of cerebral arteries and heart for embolic source and, in certain circumstances, assessment of the aorta and blood (i.e., hypercoagulable or vasculitic profile).

6. **Cervicocephalic arterial dissection** may not be associated with trauma. When trauma is the cause, symptoms may be delayed for several minutes to hours. Headache, facial pain, or neck pain may be the only symptom. Carotid dissection usually results in ipsilateral, steady, nonthrobbing headache and ipsilateral Horner's syndrome. Throat pain and focal cerebral ischemia are also prominent. Vertebrobasilar dissection results in occipital headache or

neck pain and may be associated with neck manipulation or whiplash injury. Definitive diagnosis of arterial dissection requires cerebral angiography.

7. **Giant cell arteritis** is almost exclusively a disease of people more than 50 years of age, and is much more prevalent among those over 60. It should be considered in any person over 50 with a persistent or new headache. The term "temporal arteritis" is misleading, because this condition often affects the short posterior ciliary arteries of the eye and external carotid artery branches other than the temporal artery; it may also affect cerebral and coronary arteries. Possible associated symptoms include visual loss (arteritic anterior ischemic optic neuropathy), temporal tenderness, weight loss, malaise, fever, chills, polymyalgia rheumatica (pain without tenderness in the shoulders, neck, and hips), and jaw claudication. Anemia, leukocytosis, and elevated liver enzymes may be present. CRP elevation is more sensitive and more specific than ESR elevation. Definitive diagnosis is made by temporal artery biopsy. Steroids should be started as soon as serologic results are known; the treatment does not affect biopsy results for weeks to months. Because of the frequent presence of "skip lesions," long segments of artery should be taken and bilateral biopsies may be necessary.

8. **Cerebral venous thrombosis** is probably more common than it was previously thought to be and often goes unrecognized; it is a condition that occurs as a consequence of a predisposing disease. Diffuse headache resulting from increased intracranial pressure may be the only symptom. Other common symptoms include seizure, focal neurologic deficit, and change in consciousness. Predisposing conditions fall into one of three categories: hypercoagulable states, low-flow states, and vessel-wall abnormalities. Primary hypercoagulable states include deficiencies in the naturally occurring anticoagulants, lupus anticoagulant, and anticardiolipin antibodies (see sec. **IV.A.6**). A personal or family history of past clotting episodes (deep-vein thrombosis, pulmonary embolism, stroke, myocardial infarction, or multiple miscarriages) suggests a primary hypercoagulable state. Secondary hypercoagulable states include those associated with late pregnancy, the puerperium, and cancer. Low-flow states include dehydration, anemia, congestive heart failure, sickle cell disease, and compression of cerebral sinus by tumor. Vessel-wall abnormalities can occur as a result of trauma, infection, cancer, or inflammatory process. Because the cerebral sinuses lie in the midline, lesions are often bilateral and parasagittal. Venous edema, infarct, or hemorrhage can occur; edema and infarct cannot be distinguished on cerebral imaging. CT is often suggestive but not diagnostic. MRI is diagnostic 75% of the time, but MRV and conventional cerebral angiography (with delayed venous films) are the definitive studies for diagnosis. Cerebral venous thrombosis should be considered for any patient with a "pseudotumor" syndrome (especially men and thin women; see sec. **V.B.9,** below); for any patient with headache and history consistent with hypercoagulable state; and for any patient with headache and bilateral "infarcts" or hemorrhages on cerebral imaging.

9. **Idiopathic intracranial hypertension (IIH, pseudotumor cerebri)** is primarily a condition of young obese women. Diagnosis is made by the clinical presentation of headache and papilledema, normal cerebral imaging, and elevated opening CSF pressure (>250 mm Hg) on LP. Brain tumor and cerebral venous thrombosis in particular must be ruled out. Recent reports suggest that papilledema need not be present for diagnosis. The serious sequela of IIH is blindness caused by chronic papilledema. Several drugs can cause intracranial hypertension, mimicking the idiopathic condition; these drugs include tetracycline, aminoglycosides, and vitamin A. The syndrome of intracranial hypertension in a patient taking oral contraceptives should stimulate investigation for cerebral venous thrombosis, because oral contraceptives may exacerbate or cause a hypercoagulable state.

10. **Unruptured arteriovenous malformation (AVM)** may result in migraine-like headaches. If an apparent migraineur always has hemicranial headaches on the same side, and there is no known family history of migraine (realizing the pitfalls of family headache history), one should rule out an unruptured AVM with MRI. It is likely that ischemia or rapid changes in cerebral blood flow incite spreading cortical depression and a migraine-like attack.

11. **Postcarotid endarterectomy** headaches occur in approximately 40% of

patients undergoing the procedure. The headache usually develops several hours to days following the endarterectomy, occurs ipsilateral to the side of the operation, and resembles a migraine. Patients with histories of migraine may suffer typical attacks. The presence of associated focal neurologic symptoms is concerning to patient and physician alike, but usually the headache lasts only a few hours and the neurologic symptoms resolve without sequelae. Nausea is often present. As is the case with AVMs, the rapid change in cerebral blood flow may incite spreading cortical depression and migraine-like phenomena. Seizures and intracerebral hemorrhages may occur after endarterectomy as well, and should be included in the differential diagnosis.

12. **Bell's palsy**—i.e., idiopathic mononeuropathy of cranial nerve VII—is often associated with retroauricular pain. Pain may be the first symptom and may be severe enough to be the patient's chief complaint, rather than the ipsilateral facial weakness involving the forehead, eye closure, and lips.

13. **Cerebral tumors and abscesses** usually present similarly with gradually progressive headache over weeks to months. They may be associated with gradually progressive neurologic deficits as well. Both primary brain tumors and metastatic lesions may present acutely if associated with hemorrhage or seizure. Abscesses generally do not hemorrhage, but they frequently cause seizures and may be associated with fever and other signs of sepsis. Any patient with a known history of cancer and new headache should be evaluated for cerebral metastasis. Colloid cysts may present with positional headaches, as noted above.

14. **Dental abscesses** usually present with oral or jaw pain first, but if untreated may result in more diffuse headache.

15. **Sinusitis** is a much less common cause of acute headache than is generally imagined. A sensation of nasal congestion is common in migraine as a result of external-carotid-territory vasodilatation; this can even result in a clear nasal drainage or mild nosebleed. Surgery for sinusitis should not be undertaken to treat the headache alone, because in most patients the headache associated with sinus congestion is a result of migraine. The diagnosis of sinusitis is more likely if the headache is associated with fever, purulent nasal discharge, cranial sinuses that are exquisitely tender to palpation, and increased densities in the sinuses on CT.

16. **Trigeminal neuralgia** is usually described as a sharp or burning pain, rather than an ache, and most commonly occurs unilaterally in the maxillary distribution of the trigeminal nerve—i.e., over the cheek. It may occur sporadically or may represent a symptom of multiple sclerosis (see Chap. 40).

17. **Low-CSF-pressure headache** may occur when the CSF pressure is abnormally low, such as occurs after LP (i.e., post-LP headache) or after nerve-root-sleeve trauma and subsequent CSF leak. Symptoms typically resolve in the supine position and recur when the patient is upright.

18. **Acute glaucoma** often presents with periorbital headache. Pupillary changes, conjunctival injection, lens clouding, and a hard ocular globe to palpation are typical. Elevated intraocular pressure confirms the diagnosis.

19. **Arterial hypertension** most often occurs as a result of, rather than as a cause of, headache; migraine and stroke both cause the arterial blood pressure to rise. In circumstances wherein the blood pressure rises markedly and acutely, however, the hypertension may cause headache; causes of acute hypertension and headache include pheochromocytoma and drugs such as cocaine, amphetamines, phenylpropanolamine, and monoamine oxidase inhibitors. Patients are often confused, and papilledema may be present.

VI. **Diagnostic approach.** The diagnosis of primary headache conditions is based on a supportive detailed history and a normal neurologic examination. If the clinician has any suspicion at all that the patient may be suffering a secondary headache, a series of diagnostic tests is indicated to determine the cause of headache. Many of the conditions that cause secondary headache are fatal or disabling if left untreated. Fortunately, in many cases the conditions are treatable. Figure 20-2 depicts a diagnostic algorithm for patients with suspected acute secondary headache. If a patient has any one of the clinical features suggestive of secondary headache, the diagnostic evaluation should be undertaken, beginning with laboratory tests and noncontrast CT.

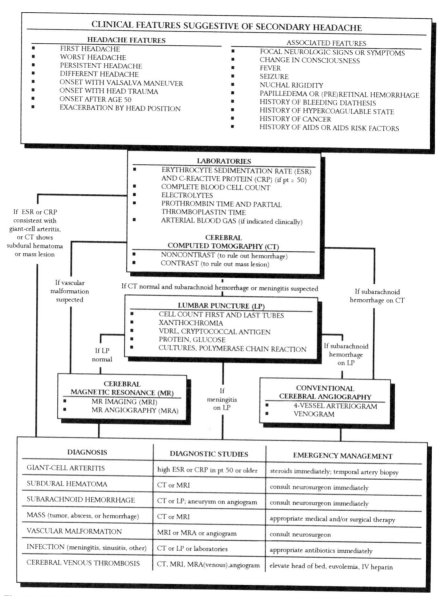

Figure 20-2. Diagnostic algorithm for patients with suspected acute secondary headache.

VII. Referral

A. Primary headache. Migraine, cluster, "tension-type," and analgesic rebound headaches are chronic conditions that present acutely. The proper treatment of primary headache conditions requires long-term care. Once the acute care clinician diagnoses primary headache and offers emergency treatment, she or he is obligated to counsel the patient regarding the importance of long-term care and to refer the patient to a neurologist or generalist for definitive treatment. Patient education leads to improved patient care and lower healthcare costs by not spending emergency room resources on recurrent headache patients.

B. Secondary headache. After initial diagnosis and emergency management, the definitive treatment of patients with secondary headache usually requires admission to a hospital and referral to a specialist. A neurosurgeon should be intimately involved in all aspects of the care of patients with subarachnoid hemorrhage, subdural hematoma, or epidural hematoma. Patients with intracranial masses require immediate referral to a neurologist and often a neurosurgeon as well. If the mass turns out to be a tumor, referral to a neuro-oncologist may be necessary. If the mass is an abscess, referral to a specialist in infectious diseases is appropriate. Most patients with sinusitis and headache are best cared for by a generalist or infectious disease expert; if surgery is deemed necessary, referral to an otolaryngologist is appropriate, because surgery may be necessary. Patients with suspected giant cell arteritis should be treated with high-dose steroids by the acute care clinician and then referred immediately to both a medical physician for chronic steroid administration (usually a neurologist or rheumatologist) and a surgical physician for temporal artery biopsy (usually an ophthalmologist or neurosurgeon); one should not wait for the biopsy before beginning steroids. Patients with cerebral venous thrombosis require immediate referral to a neurologist or primary care physician for anticoagulation and hypercoagulable evaluation.

Recommended Readings

Gordon DL. Cerebral venous thrombosis. In J Biller, KD Mathews, BB Love (eds), *Stroke in Children and Young Adults.* Boston: Butterworth-Heinemann, 1994.

Koudstaal P, van Gijn J, Kappelle J. Headache in transient or permanent cerebral ischemia. *Stroke* 22:754–759, 1991.

Mathew NT. Cluster headache. *Neurology* 42(suppl 2):22–31, 1992.

Moskowitz MA. Basic mechanisms in vascular headache. *Neurol Clin* 8:801–815, 1990.

Olesen J, Tfelt-Hansen P, Welch KMA (eds). *The Headaches.* New York: Raven, 1993.

Rapoport AM, Silberstein SD. Emergency treatment of headache. *Neurology* 42(suppl 2):43–44, 1992.

Raskin NH. *Headache* (2nd ed). New York: Churchill Livingstone, 1988.

Saper JR, et al. *Handbook of Headache Management.* Baltimore: Williams & Wilkins, 1993.

Silberstein SD. Advances in understanding the pathophysiology of headache. *Neurology* 42(suppl 2):6–10, 1992.

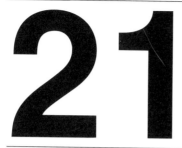

Approach to the Patient with Chronic and Recurrent Headache

David Lefkowitz

Most **chronic and recurrent headaches** represent a benign recurrent headache syndrome. Migraine, tension-type headache, cluster headache, and chronic daily headache represent the overwhelming majority of headaches encountered in primary care. The primary goal of the evaluation of headache patients should be the accurate distinction of benign headache syndromes from serious organic pathologies.

I. Etiology and clinical manifestations. The classification of headache was revised in 1988 by the International Headache Society (IHS). The new classification scheme is a phenomenologic one, based on symptoms and signs. The characteristics of the various forms of primary benign recurrent headache are summarized in Table 21-1.

   A. Migraine is no longer referred to as migraine headache of the vascular type, reflecting growing evidence that it is a neurogenic disorder and that observed vascular changes are secondary to other, underlying mechanisms.

   1. The following clinical characteristics of migraine are outlined in the IHS classification system.

   a. The duration of headache is 4–72 hours.

   b. The quality of headache fulfills at least two of the following criteria: unilaterality, pulsatility, moderate to severe intensity, and aggravation by routine physical activity.

   c. There is at least one of the following associated features: nausea, vomiting, photophobia, and phonophobia.

   d. Migraine, like other benign headache syndromes, is a diagnosis of exclusion without evidence of organic disease.

   e. A history of stereotypy is sought. There should be at least five such episodes if there is no aura, or at least two if an aura is present.

   2. Migraine may be associated with **focal neurologic symptoms and signs.** A distinction is made between migraine with aura, in which neurologic features are present (formerly classical migraine), and migraine without aura (formerly common migraine). A spreading wave of cortical depolarization analogous to Leão's spreading depression may be an important mechanism in migraine with aura.

   a. By definition, the aura should meet at least three of the following criteria.

   (1) It consists of one or more fully reversible symptoms of focal cerebral and/or brainstem dysfunction.

   (2) One aura symptom develops gradually over more than 4 minutes, or two or more symptoms occur in succession.

   (3) No aura symptom lasts more than 60 minutes, or proportionately longer if there is more than one.

   (4) Headache follows within 1 hour of the aura, or the onset of the aura precedes, or occurs simultaneously with, the headache. An aura need not begin before the headache.

   b. Typical migraine auras consist of homonymous visual disturbance, unilateral paresthesias or numbness, unilateral weakness, aphasia, or unclassifiable speech disturbance. Sensory auras typically have a cheiro-oral distribution, and there may be a "march" from one body part to another.

   c. Migraine with prolonged aura (formerly referred to as complicated migraine) may be diagnosed if at least one aura symptom persists for more than 1 hour but less than 7 days and neuroimaging studies remain normal.

Table 21-1. Characteristics of benign recurrent headache disorders.

	Migraine	Tension-type headache	Cluster headache	Chronic daily headache
Age of onset	10–30 years	Any age	Middle age	3rd–4th decade
Gender	F >M	F >M	M >F	F >M
Duration	4–72 hours	30 minutes to 7 days	15–180 minutes	Constant or nearly constant
Frequency	Variable	Occasional to daily	At least daily for weeks to months	Daily or constant
Time of day	Any time	Later in day	Nocturnal awakening	Constant
Quality	Pulsatile	Dull, aching, bandlike	Severe, boring	Variable
Location	Retro-orbital, temporal, hemicranial, or holocephalic	Bilateral, temporal, or occipitonuchal	Unilateral, retro-orbital	Variable
Associated symptoms	Nausea/vomiting, photo/phonophobia, with or without neurologic accompaniments	Other symptoms are rare, association with stress in episodic form	Ipsilateral autonomic symptoms	Migraine history, psychopathology, analgesic overuse common

    d. Migrainous infarction is classified as a complication of migraine. It occurs when symptoms of the aura do not completely resolve within 7 days and there is evidence of infarction on imaging studies.

    e. Migraine aura without headache (previously referred to as migraine equivalents) occurs when the aura is not followed by a headache.

    f. Migraine is often associated with specific triggers, including ingestion of tyramine-containing foods, use of alcohol, changes in sleep patterns, and emotional stress. There is also a relationship with hormonal factors. Migraine is more common in females than in males, but the gender predilection does not occur until after the age of menarche. In most women, migraine is more frequent or severe at or around the time of menses, and the headaches often improve after menopause.

B. Tension-type headache was previously diagnosed as tension headache, but the terminology has been changed in the IHS system because it is now widely believed that muscle tension is not the underlying etiology of this type of headache.

    1. Clinical characteristics of tension-type headache include the following features.

        a. Headache duration is 30 minutes to 7 days.

        b. Pain conforms to at least two of the following: pressing or tightening in quality, nonpulsatile, mild to moderately intense, bilateral, and not aggravated by routine physical activity.

        c. There should be no nausea or vomiting, although anorexia is permissible. There may be photophobia or phonophobia, but not both simultaneously.

        d. There is no evidence of organic disease.

    2. There may or may not be tenderness or increased electromyographic activity in the pericranial muscles.

    3. Tension-type headache is episodic when there are fewer than 15 headache days per month or 180 days per year for at least 6 months and chronic when headache frequency exceeds these limits. There should be a history of 10 similar headaches for a diagnosis of episodic tension-type headache.

C. Cluster headache is less common than migraine but is quite characteristic and can be readily diagnosed from the history and physical examination.

    1. A diagnosis can be made using IHS criteria when there have been five or more attacks with the following features.

    a. Severe unilateral supraorbital or temporal pain lasting 15–180 minutes. The pain is usually described as boring in quality.

    b. Patients invariably have at least one of the following ipsilateral autonomic signs: conjunctival injection, eyelid edema, lacrimation, nasal congestion or rhinorrhea, forehead and facial sweating, miosis, or ptosis (oculosympathetic paresis).

    c. Attacks occur from once every other day to as many as eight times daily. There is a tendency for attacks to occur at the same time each day or to awaken the patient from sleep, usually in the early morning when the patient is entering rapid eye movement (REM) sleep.

  2. The typical episodic pattern, which gives this entity its name, consists of periods of headache lasting 1 week to 1 year separated by remissions of at least 2 weeks. When recurrent headaches persist for at least 1 year without interruption or remissions last less than 2 weeks, the disorder is referred to as chronic cluster headache.

  3. Variants of cluster headache

    a. Chronic paroxysmal hemicrania is now classified as a variant of cluster headache. This is an unusual disorder affecting primarily women with multiple, brief, unilateral clusterlike headaches occurring daily and absolute indomethacin responsiveness.

    b. Raeder's paratrigeminal neuralgia. Raeder originally described five patients with a parasellar syndrome of neuralgic pain in the trigeminal distribution, oculosympathetic paresis, and dysfunction of the trigeminal and multiple other cranial nerves. The term "Raeder's syndrome" has come to be applied to a very different syndrome of non-neuralgic head pain and oculosympathetic paresis without other cranial nerve palsies. This latter syndrome usually represents a variant of cluster headache.

    c. Cluster headache variant. This is an entity consisting of multiple daily atypical cluster headaches, a constant background vascular headache, multiple sharp jabs, and response to indomethacin.

    d. Lower-half headache refers to several arcane syndromes, referred to variously as Sluder's neuralgia, sphenopalatine neuralgia, vidian neuralgia, and greater superficial petrosal neuralgia, and manifested by face pain and ipsilateral nasal congestion or rhinorrhea. These syndromes probably represent cases of cluster headache.

D. Other considerations regarding classification of recurrent headaches

  1. Benign recurrent headache. It is theorized that the benign headache syndromes are different manifestations of a single entity sharing a common abnormality of serotoninergic mechanisms with migraine and tension-type headache occupying opposite ends of a spectrum.

  2. Differentiating migraine from episodic tension-type headache. In some individuals it may be difficult to distinguish migraine without aura from episodic tension-type headache, because both may be bilateral, nonthrobbing, moderately severe, and associated with anorexia, photophobia, or phonophobia without violating IHS criteria. Both types of headaches may occur in the same patient. IHS criteria no longer recognize the existence of combined or mixed headaches having properties of both migraine and tension-type headache.

  3. Chronic daily headache

    a. There are some limitations in the way IHS criteria handle chronic daily headache. Most cases are classified as chronic tension-type headache, although the majority probably are transformed migraine. Many patients with chronic tension-type headache also have acute exacerbations of headache fulfilling IHS criteria for migraine.

    b. Rebound headache. Rebound or withdrawal headache related to overuse of narcotics, butalbital-containing analgesics, or ergotamine is frequently a factor in chronic daily headache. In these patients, there is a rhythmic cycle of headache and medication use. The patient awakens with early morning headache resulting from medication withdrawal, and the headache is relieved only by the next dose of medication. Patients may begin to use analgesics in anticipation of pain. Other symptoms of medication withdrawal, including irritability, asthenia, and insomnia, may also occur.

II. Differential diagnosis

A. **Tumor.** Head pain in patients with brain tumor is thought to arise from traction or pressure on pain-sensitive intracranial structures or by production of increased intracranial pressure. There is nothing pathognomonic about headache in patients with brain tumor, but there are some general rules.

1. In most cases, headache is described as dull, aching, or pressurelike and resembles tension-type headache in quality. The headache is intermittent and moderate to severe in most patients. Worsening with bending or Valsalva's maneuver is not unusual. "Tumoral headache" mimicking migraine is rare.

2. The typical history of severe headache associated with exacerbation in the morning and nausea or vomiting is relatively uncommon, accounting for only 17% of patients in one series. Other kinds of headaches that should raise the physician's suspicion of tumor, such as postural, cough, or exertional headache, are likewise rare.

3. If the headache is unilateral, the pain is usually on the side of the lesion. When the headache is bilateral, it is usually a result of the presence of increased intracranial pressure or either midline or bilateral tumor.

4. Supratentorial tumors generally produce frontal or bifrontal, relatively mild headache.

5. The headache of infratentorial tumors is generally localized to the occiput.

6. Increased intracranial pressure produces severe headache in the frontal area, vertex, or neck with associated nausea and vomiting.

7. Involvement of the dura or skull may produce localized pain.

B. **Cerebrovascular disease.** Headache, nausea, and vomiting are more commonly associated with intracranial hemorrhage than with strokes of other subtypes. In some patients, recurrent subarachnoid hemorrhage may mimic migraine. There is controversy about how often unruptured aneurysms cause recurrent headache. Headache occurs in 30–40% of patients with cerebral infarction and in 25–40% of those with transient ischemia. It is usually nonthrobbing, ipsilateral to the infarct, and self-limited. In patients with chronic or recurrent headache, the following diagnoses should be considered.

1. **Dissection.** An ipsilateral throbbing or steady headache, with or without neck or jaw pain, frequently accompanies carotid dissections. When these symptoms occur in the setting of a fixed or reversible neurologic deficit, one should consider dissection in the differential diagnosis. Oculosympathetic paresis, visual scintillations, and dysgeusia are also clues to this diagnosis. Dissections may be difficult to recognize when they occur without a previous history of trauma or follow relatively trivial injuries.

2. **Atherosclerotic TIA or infarction versus late-life migraine.** When headache recurs in association with focal neurologic deficit, it may be challenging to distinguish between migrainous accompaniments and atherosclerotic cerebrovascular disease, especially in elderly patients. There need not be a history of preexisting migraine, and headache does not have to be a prominent feature of the individual episodes. Fisher described this entity in detail in 1980. He suggested the following as criteria for late-life migraine accompaniments.

   a. Scintillations or other typical visual displays are common manifestations, and they may expand or "build up" after onset.

   b. There may be a sensory "march" from one body part to another or spreading to the opposite side of the body, which is unusual with other causes of cerebrovascular disease.

   c. One accompaniment may progress to another without delay.

   d. Episodes may be stereotyped, which should be less common in embolism.

   e. Headache is frequently associated with the episode.

   f. The attacks occur in characteristic midlife flurries with a benign course.

   g. Other causes of focal deficit, including atherosclerosis, should be excluded.

C. **Headaches resulting from disorders of intracranial pressure**

1. **Pseudotumor cerebri (benign intracranial hypertension, or BIH).** The primary features of this disorder are headache and visual disturbance (enlargement of the blind spot, visual obscurations, and progressive visual loss) resulting from elevated intracranial pressure. There may also be tinnitus, dizziness, and nausea. BIH is most commonly encountered in obese young women. There is frequently a history of menstrual irregularities. Physical

findings are limited to papilledema and nonlocalizing abducens nerve palsies. Papilledema may be unilateral, asymmetric, or even absent in pseudotumor cerebri. The cerebrospinal fluid (CSF) is acellular with elevated pressure, and the protein content may be low. Imaging may reveal slit-like ventricles or an empty sella, but no mass lesion. Some cases are idiopathic, whereas others may be symptomatic of a disorder such as vitamin A intoxication, steroid withdrawal, hypoparathyroidism, systemic lupus erythematosus, or side effects of nalidixic acid. In some patients with BIH, imaging studies may reveal signs of thrombosis of the superior sagittal or lateral sinuses. When sinovenous occlusion occurs in the setting of ear infection, it has been referred to by the misnomer "otitic hydrocephalus."

2. **Obstructive hydrocephalus.** Headache is not typically a symptom of communicating hydrocephalus, but it is a common symptom of obstructive hydrocephalus. The headache is usually occipital and may be associated with neck pain or stiffness, vomiting, or visual abnormalities. The headache may be present on awakening and more severe in the morning. Obstructive hydrocephalus resulting from intraventricular tumors may cause positional headache and may produce life-threatening increases in intracranial pressure.

3. **Intracranial hypotension.** Postspinal headache may occasionally become protracted or complicate the evaluation of patients with chronic or recurrent headaches resulting from other causes. A history of postural headache worsened or initiated by assumption of the upright position, often with accompanying nausea or dizziness, and relieved by lying down is typical. When there is a history of a preceding lumbar puncture, the diagnosis is obvious. Youth, female gender, lower body mass index (BMI), and larger-diameter LP needles are associated with a higher risk of post-LP headache, but the duration of recumbency after the procedure is not. In some cases, CSF hypotension may occur without a history of diagnostic LP as a result of CSF leakage following head trauma, Valsalva's maneuver, or nerve-root avulsion.

D. **Pheochromocytoma.** Approximately 10% of patients with pheochromocytoma present with headache. The headache is usually bifrontal, severe, and throbbing. It may be exacerbated by coughing, bending, straining, or lying flat. The headache is associated with paroxysmal hypertension caused by release of catecholamines from the tumor.

E. **Inflammatory disorders**

1. **Giant cell arteritis** is rare before age 50. Giant cell or temporal arteritis may present with constitutional symptoms, headache, joint complaints, or jaw claudication. Headache is the most common presenting symptom; it is often, but not always, localized to the temple and is sharp, throbbing, or boring in quality. Blindness from ischemic optic neuropathy is the most feared complication. Diplopia may also occur as a result of ischemia of oculomotor nerves and extraocular muscles. Physical findings include a tender, nodular, nonpulsatile, thickened superficial temporal artery. The Westergren erythrocyte sedimentation rate is elevated in approximately 85% of patients. Other common laboratory abnormalities include elevated C-reactive protein, thrombocytosis, and anemia. Definitive diagnosis rests on the use of superficial temporal artery biopsy, but the biopsy may be negative because of patchy involvement (skip lesions).

2. **Systemic lupus erythematosus (SLE).** Migrainous headaches, often associated with focal neurologic auras, are frequently encountered in patients with systemic lupus. Visual scintillations have been reported anecdotally as the presenting symptom of lupus.

    a. Evidence suggests that the headaches are related to the lupus and not merely coincidental. In a case-controlled prospective study of patients with SLE, there was a higher incidence of migraine, a higher percentage of migraine with aura, and later age of onset of migraine than in controls. There was also a tendency for headaches to parallel the activity of the lupus and sometimes to respond to steroids or immunosuppressive therapy.

    b. There is no proven association of antiphospholipid antibodies with migraine in SLE patients or with neurologic deficits in migraine patients who do not have lupus.

F. **Post-traumatic headache**

1. **Postconcussion syndrome** is a distinct clinical entity following relatively minor head injuries that is manifested by recurrent headache, memory disturbances, irritability, difficulty in concentrating, dizziness, and depressive symptoms. There is still controversy surrounding the etiology of this syndrome and whether it results from "compensation neurosis" or organic brain damage. Symptoms are usually self-limited and resolve within 6 months in most patients. Chronic subdural hematoma should be excluded.

2. **Occipital neuralgia.** The occipital nerve may be traumatized directly or compressed by spasm of the trapezius or semispinalis capitis muscle. There is usually a lancinating, neuralgic component to the pain and a Tinel's sign when the nerve is percussed by the examiner.

3. **Post-traumatic migraine and tension-type headaches.** In some patients, head trauma may precipitate headaches identical in quality to migraine or tension-type headache. Post-traumatic cluster headache has also been reported, although rarely. In some patients, headache is associated with scarring at the site of a scalp laceration and is relieved by infiltration of a local anesthetic.

4. **Post-traumatic dysautonomic cephalalgia.** Vijayan and Dreyfus described this syndrome in 1975. Throbbing headaches associated with nausea, photophobia, and signs of ipsilateral sympathetic overactivity such as sweating and mydriasis occur as delayed sequelae of penetrating neck injuries that damage the sympathetic fibers in the carotid sheath. This disorder should not be confused with cluster headache, which it superficially resembles.

G. **Temporomandibular joint (TMJ) dysfunction** is believed to be a myofascial syndrome related to dental malocclusion or bruxism. It may cause recurrent preauricular or temporal pain radiating into the neck. The pain is typically aggravated by chewing and is frequently worse in the morning. Physical findings include lateral jaw deviation and crepitus of the joint on opening the mouth and tenderness or spasm of the masticatory muscles.

H. **Trigeminal neuralgia** is usually included in the differential diagnosis of headache, particularly of cluster headache, although typical trigeminal neuralgia is rarely confused with other entities. Onset is usually later in life except when it occurs as a manifestation of multiple sclerosis. The IHS defines trigeminal neuralgia as follows.

1. Paroxysmal attacks of facial or frontal pain lasting a few seconds to less than 1 minute

2. The attacks have at least four of the following characteristics.
   a. Distribution along one or more divisions of the trigeminal nerve
   b. Sudden, intense, sharp, superficial, stabbing or burning quality
   c. Severe intensity
   d. Precipitation by stimulation of trigger areas or by daily activities such as eating, talking, washing the face, or cleaning the teeth
   e. The patient is asymptomatic between the paroxysms

3. Absence of neurologic deficit

4. Attacks are stereotyped.

5. Most cases result from microvascular compression of the trigeminal nerve, but trigeminal neuralgia may also be secondary to cerebellopontine angle tumors or vascular abnormalities.

III. **Evaluation**

A. **History.** In most cases, the history is the most important factor in the accurate diagnosis of headache. It is usually helpful to ask the patient to describe a typical headache, beginning with its onset. It is important to remember that as many as 30–40% of headache patients have more than one headache type. Because the head does not exist in isolation, disorders of other organ systems may cause or modify headache. Therefore, the physician must inquire about general symptoms and signs of CNS dysfunction and conduct a detailed review of the medical history. The headache history should specifically include questions regarding the following areas.

1. **Age of onset.** Onset of most benign headache syndromes occurs early in life, usually between childhood and the third decade, although tension-type headache may begin at any time. Late onset may suggest a more serious condition.

2. **Site and radiation of headache.** The location of headache may help in de-

termining its etiology. Migraine is frequently unilateral, alternates sides, and involves the temple or retro-orbital area. Tension-type headache is usually bilateral, frontal, or occipital, and radiates into the neck and shoulders. Brief attacks of strictly unilateral orbital pain suggest cluster headache or chronic paroxysmal hemicrania. Dental, ocular, and sinus disorders often produce frontal pain. The site of headache may be of localizing value in patients with mass lesions, as discussed above (see sec. **II.A**).

3. **Temporal pattern.** Headache syndromes may have characteristic patterns of headache duration and frequency. In general, longer-lasting headaches tend to be benign, particularly when headache is constant over more than several months without change in character or development of new signs. Headache resulting from meningitis may be constant, but not usually over a prolonged duration. Benign headache syndromes typically produce episodic headache. For instance, migraine usually lasts several hours and occurs several times a month. Cluster headache has a characteristic periodicity. Acute tension-type headache is usually brief and associated with emotional stress, but in its chronic form, tension-type headache becomes more frequent, prolonged, or constant and loses its association with psychosocial stressors. The mode of onset may also be helpful. Does the headache begin gradually or start suddenly? Sudden headache onset is of greater concern because it may indicate intraparenchymal or subarachnoid hemorrhage. In some patients, sudden onset of an intense headache referred to as thunderclap headache simulates subarachnoid hemorrhage but actually represents a benign syndrome that may be a variant of migraine. Day and Raskin have reported a patient with recurrent thunderclap headache who proved to have an unruptured internal carotid artery aneurysm. The headaches ceased after surgical correction of the aneurysm. It was hypothesized that stretching of the aneurysm wall had accounted for the headache.

4. **Quality and severity of pain** are often very difficult for patients to verbalize. There is a tendency for the headache patient to describe the severity rather than the quality of pain. It may be necessary for the interviewer to provide the patient with some pain characteristics from which to choose. Migraine and headache associated with fever are usually throbbing and pulsatile, for instance. Tension-type headache is usually described as dull and nagging, tight and constricting, or bandlike. Tumor and meningitis typically produce a steady, aching pain. Severity of pain can be ranked on a scale of 1–10. Another indicator of severity is whether or not headache interferes with routine activity such as work or school attendance.

5. **Modifying factors**
   a. **Prodromal and associated symptoms.** Symptoms that precede or coincide with headache onset may be valuable clues to the nature of the underlying headache. The patient with migraine may have mood or behavioral changes for several days before the headache. Visual scintillations and fortification spectra are typical migraine prodromes, but visual symptoms may also be associated with carotid dissections and occipital arteriovenous malformations. Ipsilateral autonomic features are almost always present in cluster headache.
   b. **Precipitating factors.** The provoking factors may suggest the diagnosis, as in the lancinating pain of trigeminal neuralgia precipitated by cutaneous stimulation or the onset of migraine headache following ingestion of certain foods or alcohol or in response to stress, glare, hypoglycemia, or sleep deprivation. Bruxism may be associated with the headache of temporomandibular joint dysfunction. Identification of precipitants may also provide information that will be helpful in treatment.
   c. **Sleep onset.** Migraine, hypertension, and cluster headache may awaken patients from sleep. Tension-type headache does so only rarely.
   d. **Relieving or exacerbating factors.** Patients with migraine, for instance, typically state that their pain is aggravated by movement, bending, straining, and coughing and is relieved by lying flat, by avoiding bright light, and sometimes by pressure over the superficial temporal artery or after vomiting.

6. **Family history.** About 20–60% of patients with migraine report having at least one similarly affected family member. However, 6% of men and 18% of

women report migraine, and thus it is not unusual for there to be a migraine history even for patients presenting with other types of headaches.

B. Physical examination. Vital signs should be checked for fever and hypertension. In addition to a thorough general and neurologic examination, certain areas require special attention.

1. **Inspection, palpation, and percussion of the skull** should be performed to check for signs of trauma, including areas of localized tenderness or scarring. There may be tenderness at the site of a skull neoplasm. Percussion over the site of a tumor or subdural hematoma may also produce pain. In children, head circumference should always be measured.

2. **Assessment of the ears, tympanic membranes, and mastoids.** Examination of the ears may reveal evidence of otitis or mastoiditis.

3. **Evaluation of the temporomandibular joints.** The temporomandibular joint and masticatory muscles may be tender to palpation, or there may be an audible or palpable "click" when the patient opens and closes the mouth. This can be felt externally or with the examiner's fingers in the external auditory canals. The jaw should also be observed for lateral deviation when the mouth is opened. When temporomandibular joint dysfunction results from muscle spasm, the joint is tender to direct palpation but not to palpation through the ear canal.

4. **Palpation of glandular and lymphatic tissues.** Examination of the soft tissues of the neck may reveal evidence of infection or malignancy of the head and neck, sarcoidosis, or Behçet's syndrome.

5. **Inspection of the teeth and oropharynx.** In some patients, headache may be referred from dental disease, although headache rarely occurs without concomitant tooth pain. Percussion of the teeth and examination for evidence of caries or periodontal disease may suggest a dental origin. Percussion of the maxillary teeth may also hint at maxillary sinusitis, which can arise from dental root infection.

6. **Assessment of the nose and paranasal sinuses.** The nasal mucosa should be examined for polyps, septal deviation, and secretions. The maxillary and frontal sinuses may be palpated or percussed for tenderness. The ethmoid and sphenoid sinuses are not adequately evaluated by bedside techniques. The sinuses can also be transilluminated with a flashlight in a darkened room.

7. **Assessment of the eyes.** Ocular causes of headache are uncommon. Patients frequently attribute chronic headache to eye strain or refractive errors and often consult an ophthalmologist or optometrist before seeking a neurologic opinion, but eye strain and refractive errors rarely prove to be responsible. (Acute glaucoma may sometimes present primarily with head pain.) Nevertheless, examination of the eyes may provide valuable information on the nervous system, such as the presence of papilledema or abducens palsy resulting from increased intracranial pressure, optic disk pallor from a compressive lesion, or ischemic optic neuropathy associated with giant cell arteritis.

8. **Assessment of the extracranial vasculature** is especially important in cases of suspected giant cell or temporal arteritis, in which the superficial temporal artery may be tender, nodular, and nonpulsatile. Bruits may result from arterial stenosis or increased venous outflow in patients with arteriovenous malformations. Increased collateral flow may be a source of headache when there is extracranial vascular disease. In patients with migraine, compression of the superficial temporal artery may temporarily relieve the headache.

9. **Palpation of the scalp and neck musculature and neck mobility.** Tenderness of the pericranial muscles and limited or painful range of motion of the neck may suggest tension-type headache or spinal pathology. Spinal disease may cause headache referred to the frontal area. Resistance to passive anteroposterior neck movement, and Kernig's and Brudzinski's signs, are indications of CNS infection or subarachnoid bleeding.

10. **A low hairline** may be a clue to cervicocranial junction abnormalities such as an Arnold-Chiari malformation, basilar impression, or invagination.

IV. Indications of structural disease. Acute recurrent headache is usually migraine. Chronic nonprogressive headache usually represents analgesic overuse, benign intracranial hypertension, or chronic tension-type headache. Features that suggest structural disorders are as follows:

A. **Altered consciousness or behavior.** Although loss of consciousness during headache may result from vasovagal syncope or as a manifestation of basilar migraine, in most cases it is a sign of increased intracranial pressure, seizure activity, or ischemia. Sudden headache with altered consciousness may represent subarachnoid hemorrhage. Changes in cognitive function may also accompany destructive lesions.

B. **Neurologic deficit developing simultaneously or following the onset of headache.** In general, the neurologic symptoms associated with migraine arise prior to the onset of headache, although this is not necessary by definition. For the other benign headache disorders except cluster headache, nonspecific subjective neurologic symptoms occur more often than objective signs of neurologic dysfunction. When a neurologic deficit develops at or after onset of headache, differential considerations include tumor, stroke, and abscess.

C. **Headache associated with fever or meningeal signs** should suggest infections such as encephalitis, meningitis, subdural empyema, or abscess. Recurrent meningitis may occur in patients with anatomic defects, after splenectomy, or when there is immune compromise. Noninfectious causes of recurrent meningitis include craniopharyngiomas, dermoid cysts, sarcoidosis, Behçet's syndrome, and the Vogt-Koyanagi-Harada syndrome. Recurrent aseptic meningitis associated with large mononuclear endothelial cells is referred to as Mollaret's meningitis. Tuberculous and fungal meningitides are likely to present chronically. Subarachnoid hemorrhage may also produce meningismus and low-grade fever. Fever and headache may also accompany sinusitis or dental abscess, but the physician should keep in mind the possibility of intracranial complications of extracranial infections of the head and neck.

D. **Headache occurring exclusively on one side over time.** Side-locked headache has traditionally been described as a warning sign of structural disease—particularly vascular abnormalities. In reality, many benign headache syndromes, such as migraine, cluster, and atypical facial pain, may consistently affect one side of the head.

E. **Onset after age 50.** Benign headache syndromes generally begin early in life.

F. **Change in character or response to treatment of preexisting headache.** There is no reason why a patient with chronic recurrent headache cannot develop a second disorder. Therefore, the clinician should carefully approach the patient in whom a change in the pattern or quality of long-standing headaches occurs or in whom a progressive increase in frequency or severity of headache occurs over several months, particularly when presenting with sudden onset of the "worst headache of [his/her] life."

G. **Vomiting preceding headache by days to weeks.** Vomiting, with or without preceding nausea, may be a sign of increased intracranial pressure resulting from tumor, hydrocephalus, or chronic infection.

H. **Headache associated with paroxysmal hypertension.** In addition to headache, pheochromocytomas cause tachycardia, tremor, nausea, or diaphoresis. In a small minority of patients, the tumor is located in the bladder and symptoms follow urination.

I. **Associated endocrine changes.** The association of subacute or chronic headache with signs of secondary hypothyroidism, galactorrhea, hypo- or hypercortisolism, or other evidence of pituitary dysfunction raises suspicions of a sellar lesion such as a pituitary adenoma. Hypopituitarism may also occur with craniopharyngiomas.

J. **Headache precipitated by rapid changes in head position or head movement.** Rapid changes in head position may produce pain when there is an intracranial mass. Intraventricular lesions such as colloid cysts of the third ventricle may cause obstructive hydrocephalus with a change in posture.

K. **Headache initiated by Valsalva's maneuver or associated with exercise or sexual activity.** Although migraine is often exacerbated by Valsalva's maneuver, the onset of headache with Valsalva's maneuver may have more ominous significance. About 10% of patients with exertional or cough headache have an underlying structural abnormality—usually a craniocervical junction abnormality. Other abnormalities associated with exertional headache include posterior fossa subdural hematoma, abscess, or tumor and pituitary tumor. These patients should always have MRI scans. Some patients with exertional headache have a benign disorder that is usually considered a form of migraine. The headaches are often self-limited and respond to indomethacin. Coital headache is usually bilateral, throbbing, and intense. It is more common in men than in women and usually occurs just prior to orgasm. The major differential diagnosis is subarachnoid hemorrhage, especially after the first episode.

L. Headache not conforming to known functional headache patterns

V. Laboratory studies. In many patients a diagnosis can be made on clinical grounds alone and treatment can be initiated without any further testing. Headache is rarely the sole symptom of serious nervous system disorders. Patients with any of the historical factors discussed in the preceding section or with fever, focal signs, changes in cognition or consciousness, or stiff neck on examination should be evaluated more extensively.

A. Blood work. Occasionally, routine blood work may provide evidence of infection, anemia, or electrolyte or hormonal abnormalities that are related to headache. Erythrocyte sedimentation rate (ESR) should be checked in all elderly patients with headache due to the possibility of giant cell arteritis. When the ESR is not elevated, other acute phase reactants such as C-reactive protein, haptoglobin, or the platelet count may be increased.

B. Imaging

1. Uninfused CT is the procedure of choice for diagnosis of intracranial hemorrhage. Sagittal MRI is superior for diagnosis of Arnold-Chiari malformations. MRI is also preferable to CT for imaging of dural sinus or vein occlusions. Neither CT nor MRI, including magnetic resonance angiography (MRA), is adequate for excluding aneurysms; conventional angiography is still necessary.

2. Imaging studies in patients presenting with headache are of limited value unless there is something unusual in the history or abnormal on examination. In a prospective consecutive series of 350 patients studied with CT for headache, 2% had clinically significant abnormalities, including metastatic tumor, epidural abscess, chronic subdural hematoma, and hydrocephalus. Another 7% of the patients had clinically insignificant CT abnormalities. Of those patients with abnormal examinations, 10% had clinically significant CT abnormalities compared with 11% if there was either an unusual history or an abnormal examination and none if both the history and the physical were normal.

3. In patients with histories consistent with migraine, the yield of imaging studies is exceptionally low. Frishberg reviewed retrospective and prospective CT or MRI studies of patients with headaches and normal examinations and found that of 897 patients with histories compatible with migraine, only 0.4% had abnormal imaging studies. Of 1825 patients whose headaches were nonmigrainous, 2.4% had positive scans. Frishberg concluded that for patients with histories of migraine, imaging studies were unnecessary unless there was a history of a seizure, a change in headache pattern, or a focal neurologic sign. For patients with "nonspecific" headaches, the role of imaging was not clear.

C. Lumbar puncture (LP) has a role in the diagnosis of headache syndromes.

1. **Exclusion of subarachnoid hemorrhage.** CT is very sensitive to the presence of subarachnoid blood but still misses about 5–10% of acute subarachnoid hemorrhages. In these patients, the presence of CSF blood or xanthochromia may be diagnostic.

2. **Diagnosis of CNS infection.** In patients with suspected encephalitis or meningitis, LP may indicate the presence of CSF pleocytosis. Patients should have an imaging procedure prior to undergoing LP except when bacterial meningitis is strongly suspected, in which case LP should be done immediately to prevent a potentially life-threatening delay in institution of antibiotic therapy.

3. **Confirmation of elevated CSF pressure in BIH.** For the patient with chronic headache and signs of increased intracranial pressure, such as papilledema or small ventricles, especially in young obese women, benign intracranial hypertension should always be included in the differential diagnosis. When imaging studies exclude a mass lesion, LP should be performed to confirm an elevation of CSF pressure.

4. **Cisternal taps.** Cisternal puncture may increase the likelihood of diagnosing fungal or tuberculous meningitis, which may primarily affect basal meninges.

D. Biopsy of pathologic material is indicated under certain circumstances.

1. **Diagnosis of giant cell arteritis.** Temporal artery biopsy is helpful in diagnosing cranial arteritis. A specimen of adequate length is imperative because of the tendency of this disorder to affect the temporal artery at irregular intervals. The incidence of positive biopsy results falls rather dramatically after even short trials of steroids, but the risk of blindness in the untreated patient is sufficient to warrant initiation of steroids as soon as the diagnosis of cranial arteritis is contemplated. In addition, the biopsy is a relatively benign procedure. Therefore, moving to biopsy rapidly is recommended. If temporal artery biopsy is negative and there is still a high degree of suspicion, the clinician should consider a biopsy of the contralateral superficial temporal artery. If the biopsy is positive, it should also be recalled that other arteritides—particularly polyarteritis nodosa—may involve the temporal artery.
2. **Meningeal biopsy.** In patients with chronic meningitis, meningeal biopsy may help establish diagnoses such as granulomatous angiitis, sarcoidosis, or meningeal carcinomatosis.

Recommended Readings

Allison MC, Gallagher PJ. Temporal artery biopsy and corticosteroid treatment. *Ann Rheum Diseases* 43(3):416–417, 1984.

Day JW, Raskin NH. Thunderclap headache: Symptom of unruptured cerebral aneurysm. *Lancet* II:1247–1248, 1986.

Fisher CM. Late-life migraine accompaniments as a cause of unexplained transient ischemic attacks. *Can J Neurol Sci* 7(1):9–17, 1980.

Forsyth PA, Posner JB. Headaches in patients with brain tumors: A study of 111 patients. *Neurology* 43(9):1678–1683, 1993.

Frishberg BM. The utility of neuroimaging in the evaluation of headache in patients with normal neurologic examinations. *Neurology* 44(7):1191–1197, 1994.

Gorelick PB, et al. Headache in acute cerebrovascular disease. *Neurology* 36(11): 1445–1450, 1986.

Guralnick W, Kaban LB, Merrill RG. Temporomandibular joint afflictions. *N Engl J Med* 299(3):123–129, 1978.

Headache Classification Committee of the International Headache Society. Classification and diagnostic criteria for headache disorders, cranial neuralgias and facial pain. *Cephalalgia* 8(suppl. 7):1–96, 1988.

Kovanen J, Sulkava R. Duration of postural headache after lumbar puncture: Effect of needle size. *Headache* 26(5):224–226, 1986.

Kuntz KM, et al. Post-lumbar puncture headaches: Experience in 501 consecutive procedures. *Neurology* 42(10):1884–1887, 1992.

Leone M, et al. Clinical considerations on side locked unilaterality in long-lasting primary headaches. *Headache* 33(7):381–384, 1993.

Marcelis J, Silberstein SD. Idiopathic intracranial hypertension without papilledema. *Arch Neurol* 48(4):392–399, 1991.

Markus HS, Hopkinson N. Migraine and headache in systemic lupus erythematosus and their relationship with antibodies against phospholipids. *J Neurol* 239(1):39–42, 1992.

Medina JL, Diamond S. Cluster headache variant: Spectrum of a new headache syndrome. *Arch Neurol* 38(11):705–709, 1981.

Mitchell C, Osborn RE, Grosskreutz SR. Computed tomography in the headache patient: Is routine evaluation really necessary? *Headache* 33(2):82–86, 1993.

Porter M, Jankovic J. Benign coital cephalgia: Differential diagnosis and treatment. *Arch Neurol* 38(11):710–712, 1981.

Raeder JG. "Paratrigeminal" paralysis of oculo-pupillary sympathetic. *Brain* 47:149–158, 1924.

Rando TA, Fishman RA. Spontaneous intracranial hypotension: Report of two cases and review of the literature. *Neurology* 42(3):481–487, 1992.

Silberstein SD, et al. Classification of daily and near-daily headaches: Proposed revision to the IHS criteria. *Headache* 34(1):1–7, 1994.

Vijayan N, Dreyfus PM. Posttraumatic cephalalgia. *Arch Neurol* 32:649–652, 1975.

Wong RL, Korn JH. Temporal arteritis without an elevated erythrocyte sedimentation rate. *Am J Med* 80(5):959–964, 1986.

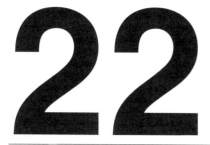

Approach to the Patient with Neck Pain, with and without Associated Arm Pain

Scott A. Shapiro

I. Traumatic neck pain without arm pain

A. Introduction. Trauma to the neck secondary to a motor vehicle accident, work-related injury, or athletic injury is a common cause of musculoskeletal neck pain. In the vast majority of patients, post-traumatic neck pain is a self-limited problem that is not serious.

B. Etiology. Straining of anterior/posterior cervical muscles and tendons is the mechanism of pain for most post-traumatic neck pain syndromes. The most common cause in clinical practice is vehicular accidents with hyperextension/flexion to the neck (whiplash). Altercations, athletic injuries (especially football), and lifting/tugging work injuries also occur.

C. Evaluation

1. History and physical examination. The primary complaints are post-traumatic neck pain and neck stiffness. The paracervical muscles are tender with limitation of motion, spinous process point tenderness may be present, and there may be some associated interscapular pain and headache. Complaints of patchy arm numbness are occasionally reported, but the neurologic exam in the upper extremities is normal for the vast majority of patients.

2. Radiographs

a. Plain x-rays rule out most fractures and ligamentous instability. In the under-40 age group, the most common finding is loss of the lordotic curve from muscle spasm. In the over-40 age group, x-rays often show degenerative changes such as narrowed disk spaces and osteophyte (bone spur) formation. The accident is not the cause of these roentgenographic changes, but certainly these changes can predispose the patient to more pain than a normal spine.

b. CT scan/MRI scan. In the modern era, any clinical or radiographic evidence for acute fracture, subluxation (instability), or spinal cord injury requires a thorough evaluation including plain films with five cervical views (anteroposterior, lateral, right and left obliques, and open-mouth odontoid), a CT scan, consultation with a spine specialist, and, more often than not, an MRI scan.

D. Referral

1. First 2–3 weeks (medicate and wait)

a. Soft collar. The post-traumatic neck pain usually subsides on its own over a week or two. A narrow soft cervical collar can be helpful in taking the weight of the head off the neck and transferring it to the shoulders. The collar should not be so wide that it forces the patient into hyperextension, which is uncomfortable.

b. Medication. Over-the-counter nonsteroidal anti-inflammatory medication (ibuprofen with or without acetaminophen) is the ideal analgesic. Other analgesics, such as propoxyphene, codeine, and codeine analogs, are acceptable, but no schedule 3 narcotics, such as oxycodone, demerol, and morphine, should be used. Muscle relaxants such as methocarbamol (Robaxin) 500 mg PO q6–8h, cyclobenzaprine (Flexeril) 10 mg PO tid, and chlorzoxazone (Parafon forte) 500 mg PO q6–8h can help. Do not use benzodiazepines, because of the abuse potential. In the patient whose stomach is sensitive to nonsteroidal medication, an evening dose of an H-2 receptor blocker, such as cimetidine 300–600 mg PO every hour, can help prevent gastritis.

     c. Time off from work. Desk-bound workers with mild to moderate neck pain can work, and most ambitious people are able to function. Heavy laborers may benefit from light duty or 1–2 weeks off work. Beware of patients who exhibit symptom magnification and functional overlay for purposes of secondary gain (worker's compensation and litigation). They have the tendency to abuse time off work. In these scenarios, early referral to a physical medicine and rehabilitation specialist who can scientifically assess for malingering may be helpful.

  2. Weeks 3–6 if pain is still present

     a. Physical therapy. If the neck pain does not subside after 2 weeks, physical therapy—heat, ultrasound, massage, and transcutaneous electrical nerve stimulation (TENS)—is reasonable.

     b. Pain clinic. Trigger-point injections of anesthetic/steroid can be helpful but are probably best scheduled after evaluation by a spine specialist.

  3. After 6–8 weeks. When neck pain persists after 6–8 weeks despite rest and therapy, and the pain remains severe enough to interfere with work or recreation, the next diagnostic test should be a cervical MRI scan to evaluate the cervical disks. Usually the study is normal or shows mild cervical disk dehydration with disk bulging. Neck pain from cervical disk dehydration can best be treated by cervical traction. Minor cervical disk bulging, presenting with chronic pain with a normal neurologic exam, is rarely sufficient indication for surgery. At this point it is best to get the opinion of a neurosurgeon.

II. Nontraumatic neck pain of arthritic origin

  A. Introduction. Neck pain from degenerative arthritis of the neck is of epidemic proportion (60–80%) in the elderly population.

  B. Etiology. Degenerative arthritis of the cervical spine occasionally manifests itself as early as the third decade of life but is much more common with increasing age. Disk dehydration and disk space narrowing with osteophyte formation is a process that occurs naturally with age. Facet arthritis also occurs. Small nerve fibers innervating the disk and facet can be involved, leading to neck pain. Dural impingement by osteophytes can also produce neck pain—especially with extension or lateral gaze.

  C. Evaluation

    1. History and physical examination. Nontraumatic neck pain in the over-40 age group is most often secondary to cervical degenerative arthritis. The pain is gradual in onset and initially intermittent and then becomes more constant. There can be associated occipital headache and interscapular pain. Motion, especially extension or lateral gaze, can aggravate the pain.

    2. Radiographs. X-rays show narrowing of disk spaces with bone spur formation. At least 70% of the population over the age of 65 have significant changes in degenerative arthritis. Regardless of how bad the x-rays look, if the patient is neurologically normal, MRI or surgery is not absolutely indicated.

  D. Referral

    1. Medication. Over-the-counter nonsteroidal anti-inflammatory medication (ibuprofen with or without acetaminophen) is the ideal analgesic. Other analgesics, such as propoxyphene, codeine, and codeine analogs, are acceptable, but no schedule 3 narcotics should be used. Muscle relaxants such as methocarbamol 500 mg PO q6–8h, cyclobenzaprine 10 mg PO tid, and chlorzoxazone 500 mg PO q6–8h can help. Do not use benzodiazepines, because of the abuse potential. In the patient whose stomach is sensitive to nonsteroidal medication, an evening dose of an H-2 receptor blocker, such as cimetidine 300–600 mg PO every hour, can help prevent gastritis.

    2. Physical therapy. Heat, ultrasound, massage, and TENS therapy can help.

    3. Pain clinic. Trigger-point injections can help.

    4. Alternative therapies. Although chiropractors can help many people, we cannot advocate manipulation of the neck when obvious bone spurs exist. Neurologic catastrophes and lawsuits have occurred in such cases. Patients can seek chiropractic care at their own risk.

    5. Spine specialist. In the majority of patients with neck pain and no arm pain, surgery is not indicated. The removal of large osteophytes ventral to the spinal cord can improve severe neck pain and occipital headache and actually improve range of motion. Only an experienced spinal surgeon should make this decision, on the basis of a CT scan or MRI scan and repetitive physical exams over a period of time.

III. Neck pain with arm pain (radiculopathy) from soft cervical disk bulges/herniations

A. Etiology. In the under-50 age group, the most common cause of this condition is a single-level soft cervical disk. The concept of a soft cervical disk means either an eccentric disk bulge or a free-fragment herniation compressing a root. A disk consists of an inner water-laden mucoid nuclear material and an outer fibrous annulus. The annulus can fissure, allowing the nucleus either to bulge or to herniate out. There is no osteophyte involved in the compression. The posterior longitudinal ligament extends beneath the entire spinal cord, protecting the cord from disk herniation, and so a disk herniation primarily projects laterally into the foramen, compressing the nerve only. In rare cases, sufficient force, such as in trauma, can lead to a large disk herniation, causing an acute myelopathy.

B. Anatomy. A disk is named by the bordering vertebral bodies. Thus, the disk between vertebral bodies C5 and C6 is named the C5-C6 disk. The nerve root whose number corresponds to that of a given vertebral body exits above that body's pedicle. Thus a C5-C6 disk compresses the C6 nerve root.

C. Evaluation

1. History. In the classic story, there is intermittent neck pain and then severe neck pain and arm pain develop. Rarely is this condition traumatic in origin. The pain radiates down the shoulder and into the arm. There are some dermatomal patterns of radiation that can help discern the level of herniation. Patients may complain of various combinations of suboccipital headache, interscapular pain, numbness, tingling, and weakness. The pain often awakens the patient from sleep.

2. Physical examination

a. Neck examination. There is posterior tenderness, especially tenderness at the process near the level of involvement and paracervical tenderness. Painful limitation of motion with extension and lateral gaze to the side of the arm pain is classic.

b. Arm examination

(1) C5 radiculopathy (C4-C5 disk herniation) presents with pain and numbness radiating to the shoulder along with a weak deltoid muscle (shoulder abduction). Simultaneous testing of both deltoid muscles by compression on the outstretched upper arms detects minor weakness. There is no true reflex to test.

(2) C6 radiculopathy (C5-C6 disk herniation). C5–C6 disk herniation is the second most common cervical disk herniation. Pain and numbness radiate across the top of the neck and along the biceps to the lateral aspect of the forearm and dorsal thumb and index finger. Numbness is usually more distal. A weak biceps, a reduced biceps reflex, and weak wrist extension are observed.

(3) C7 radiculopathy (C6-C7 disk herniation). This is the most common disk herniation. Pain radiates across the top of the neck, across the triceps, and down the posterolateral forearm to the middle finger. Numbness again is more distal. A weak triceps and a reduced triceps reflex are observed.

(4) C8 radiculopathy (C7-T1 disk herniation) is very uncommon. Pain and numbness radiate across the neck and down the arm to the small finger and ring finger. Wrist flexion and the intrinsic muscles of the hand are weak.

3. Radiographic evaluation

a. Plain x-rays provide very little help. They may show slight narrowing of the disk space involved and loss of lordosis.

b. MRI scan without contrast is the study of choice for demonstrating a soft cervical disk herniation (Fig. 22-1).

4. Electromyogram (EMG) and nerve conduction velocity (NCV) studies. An EMG for a single-level disk herniation with a radiculopathy is not absolutely necessary. An EMG can help when other disorders, such as amyotrophic lateral sclerosis, carpal tunnel syndrome, and brachial plexopathy, need to be ruled out.

D. Referral

1. Physical therapy. After diagnosis by MRI, a patient with a motor strength rating of 4/5 or more (Table 22-1) can be referred for cervical traction, heat,

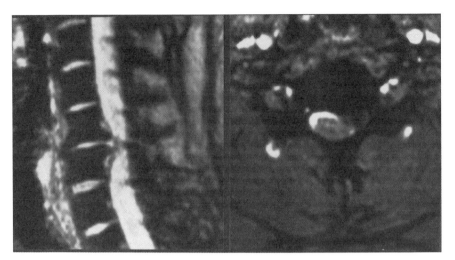

Figure 22-1. *Left:* Sagittal MRI scan shows a large C5-C6 disk herniation. *Right:* Axial MRI demonstrates a large eccentric cervical disk herniation compressing the spinal cord and nerve root.

ultrasound, massage, and a soft collar. Initially, cervical traction should be done by a physical therapist. Inform the therapist that if traction is tolerated, the patient is to be instructed in home cervical traction at 10 lb for ½ hour every night. Approximately 60–80% of soft disk herniations improve to the point of resolution of the radiculopathy with traction alone within 4–6 weeks. Not every patient can tolerate traction.

2. **Medication.** A trial of 4-mg self-weaning methylprednisolone (Medrol) dose pack can be used early in the treatment prior to nonsteroidals with some success. Over-the-counter nonsteroidal anti-inflammatory medication (ibuprofen with or without acetaminophen) is the ideal analgesic. Other analgesics, such as propoxyphene, codeine, and codeine analogs, are acceptable, but no schedule 3 narcotics should be used. Muscle relaxants such as methocarbamol 500 mg PO q6–8h, cyclobenzaprine 10 mg PO tid, and chlorzoxazone 500 mg PO q6–8h can help. Do not use benzodiazepines, because of the abuse potential. In the patient whose stomach is sensitive to nonsteroidal medication, an evening dose of an H-2 receptor blocker, such as cimetidine 300–600 mg PO every hour, can help prevent gastritis.

3. **Time off from work.** Desk-type workers with mild to moderate neck/arm pain can work, and most ambitious people are able to function. Heavy laborers may benefit from light duty or 1–4 weeks off work. Beware of patients who exhibit symptom magnification and functional overlay for purposes of secondary gain (worker's compensation and litigation). They have the tendency to abuse time off work. In these scenarios, early referral to a physical medicine and rehabilitation specialist who can scientifically assess for malingering may be helpful.

4. **Spine specialist.** In any patient with 3/5 strength or worse, immediate referral to a spine surgeon is indicated. The longer a root is compressed with severe weakness, the less likely strength will return to normal. If the strength remains 4/5 or better but pain persists after 3–6 weeks of traction, referral to a spine surgeon is also indicated. A well-trained spine surgeon should achieve improvement of arm pain and weakness in 90–95% of soft cervical disk herniations.

IV. **Neck pain with arm pain from bone spurs (hard disk, cervical spondylosis)**
   A. **Introduction.** The combination of neck pain and arm pain in cervical spondylosis is also of epidemic proportions in the elderly population.
   B. **Etiology.** Disk dehydration and narrowing lead to bone spur formation at the margins of the vertebral body. The spurs can project into the foramen or canal, compressing the nerve root or the spinal cord, or both. In addition, facet arthritis

Table 22-1. Medical Research Council motor strength classification.

Grade	Description
0	No movement
1	Flicker of movement
2	Able to move but not against gravity
3	Able to move against gravity but offers no resistance
4	Offers resistance but able to overcome or easy fatigue
5	Normal

with resultant hypertrophy and ligamentous hypertrophy also narrow the spinal canal and neural foramens. With progressive age, more than one disk space is usually involved. The center of the process usually extends from C4 to C7.

C. Evaluation

1. **History.** This condition occurs primarily in patients older than soft cervical disk herniation patients, although the two groups overlap. About 90% of patients have gradual onset of neck pain with progression to neck and arm pain. The pain radiates down the shoulder and into the arm. There are some dermatomal patterns of radiation that can help discern the level of root compression. Various complaints of suboccipital headache, interscapular pain, numbness, tingling, and weakness may also be present. The pain often wakes the patient up from sleep. About 10% of patients have asymptomatic degenerative arthritis, and then symptoms of neck pain and arm pain are often precipitated by hyperextension/flexion injuries from trauma (motor vehicle accidents). A large percentage have multiple disk spaces involved, making it more difficult to determine which level or levels caused the radiculopathy.

2. **Physical examination**

   a. **Neck examination.** There is posterior tenderness, especially tenderness at the spinous process near the level of involvement and paracervical tenderness. Painful limitation of motion with extension and lateral gaze to the side of the arm pain is classic.

   b. **Arm examination** (see Table 22-1)

      (1) **C5 radiculopathy (C4-C5 disk degeneration)** presents with pain and numbness radiating to the shoulder along with a weak deltoid muscle (shoulder abduction). Simultaneous testing of both deltoid muscles by compression on the outstretched upper arms detects minor weakness. There is no true reflex to test.

      (2) **C6 radiculopathy (C5-C6 disk degeneration).** The C5-C6 level is the second most common level for disk disease with spurring. Pain and numbness radiate across the top of the neck and along the biceps to the lateral aspect of the forearm and dorsal thumb and index finger. Numbness is usually more distal. A weak biceps, a reduced biceps reflex, and weak wrist extension are observed.

      (3) **C7 radiculopathy (C6-C7 disk degeneration).** The C6-C7 level is the most common level for disk space involvement. Pain radiates across the top of the neck, across the triceps, and then down the posterolateral forearm to the middle finger. Numbness is again more distal. A weak triceps and a reduced triceps reflex are observed.

      (4) **C8 radiculopathy (C7-T1 disk degeneration)** is very uncommon. Pain and numbness radiate across the neck and down the arm to the small finger and ring finger. Wrist flexion and the intrinsic muscles of the hand (especially those for finger extension) are weak.

   c. **Leg examination** (Table 22-2). Gait is usually normal even in the face of significant radiographic evidence of spinal cord compression. Occasionally, myelopathy is present. Early on, the gait is normal in the face of increased muscle stretch reflexes and a Babinski sign. With more severe and prolonged compression, one can observe spastic gait with bowel and bladder problems. In the most severe cases, the patient requires a cane or a walker. Rarely is the condition allowed to progress to wheelchair dependency.

Table 22-2. Nurick classification.

Grade	Description
1	Signs of spinal cord disease but normal gait
2	Slight gait abnormality not preventing full-time employment
3	Gait abnormality severe enough to prevent employment or housework. Still able to ambulate independently.
4	Requires a walker or someone else's help to ambulate
5	Wheelchair bound

   3. Radiographs
      a. Plain x-rays show disk space narrowing with osteophyte (bone spur) formation. Oblique films can exhibit neuroforaminal narrowing.
      b. MRI scan (Fig. 22-2). MRI is excellent for demonstrating nerve-root compression and cord compression from bone spurs. It does not provide as much detail about bone anatomy as the CT scan.
      c. CT scan (Fig. 22-3). CT shows better bone detail than MRI but is not as good at showing the neural structures. The two studies together are ideal for this group of patients, but this is obviously not cost-effective, and so MRI is the first choice.
   4. Electromyogram (EMG) and nerve conduction velocity (NCV) studies. The EMG can be helpful in discerning which roots are most involved in patients with multilevel spondylosis.
 D. Referral
   1. Medication. Initially, over-the-counter or prescription nonsteroidal anti-inflammatory medication with or without acetaminophen is ideal. An evening dose of an H-2 receptor blocker such as cimetidine can prevent the gastritis associated with nonsteroidals. Analgesics such as propoxyphene, codeine,

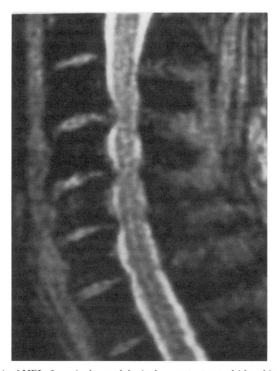

Figure 22-2. Sagittal MRI of cervical spondylosis demonstrates multi-level involvement.

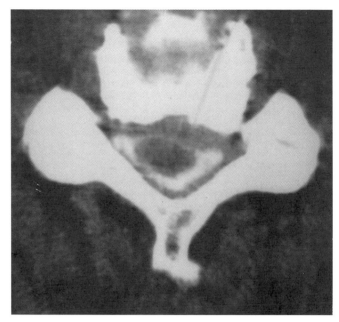

Figure 22-3. Axial CT scan of cervical spondylosis with canal and foraminal stenosis in a patient with cervical spondylotic radiculomyelopathy.

and codeine analogs are acceptable. Occasionally, muscle relaxants such as methocarbamol can help. Again, schedule 3 narcotics and benzodiazepines are ill-advised because of the chronic nature of the disorder. However, abuse of these medications is less likely in the elderly, and thus one may be more willing to prescribe them for elderly patients.

2. **Soft cervical collar**
3. **Physical therapy.** Heat, ultrasound, massage, traction, and TENS can reduce the symptoms. Approximately 20% of the radiculopathies (arm pain/strength) can be successfully improved with medicine and therapy alone for many years. The majority of patients have some pain with persistent mild weakness (if any weakness is present). Rarely does myelopathy develop in this group of patients.
4. **Spine specialist.** Surgery for cervical spondylotic radiculopathy is almost always elective. Results of surgery are much better for single-level disease than for multi-level disease—especially for neck pain. Arm motor strength rating of 3/5 or worse and any evidence of myelopathy are indications for immediate referral to a spine surgeon. The anterior approach is superior to the posterior approach if bone spurs project under the entire spinal cord. Surgery helps the radiculopathy in 90–95% of both single-level disease and multilevel disease patients, but neck pain improves in only 70–75% of multilevel disease patients. Complete relief of radicular pain occurs in approximately 60–80% of the cases. There is no age cutoff for surgery as long as the patient is in reasonable medical condition. The elderly tolerate surgery very well with minimal morbidity. If a myelopathy is present with gait abnormality and an aggressive decompression is performed, an improvement of one grade on the Nurick scale (see Table 22-2) can be expected in 70–80% of patients. Duration of symptoms is very important for patients with gait problems. Thus, early referral is indicated.

V. **Neck pain with and without arm pain as a result of metastatic cancer of the cervical spine**
   A. **Introduction.** As patients live longer with various malignancies, the number of patients who present with spine metastases also increases. The tumors that most commonly involve the spine are lung tumors, breast tumors, prostate tumors, lymphomas, and multiple myelomas. As many as 20% of these tumors will

develop symptomatic spinal involvement. In approximately 10% of patients, metastatic spinal involvement will be the mode of presentation with no known primary tumor.

B. Evaluation

    1. History and physical examination. Both primary and metastatic tumors of the spine initially present with pain that is often worse at night. The pain continues to worsen over a very short period, and then neurologic symptoms such as radiculopathy and myelopathy develop fairly quickly. It is best to make the diagnosis when neurologic symptoms are minimal.

    2. Radiographs

        a. Plain x-rays can show destruction of the vertebral bodies and pedicles. Pathologic compression fractures and lytic pedicles are very common. The sensitivity of plain x-rays is approximately 60%.

        b. Bone scans are very sensitive—approaching 100%—in showing spine metastases, including asymptomatic areas with no destruction.

        c. MRI scans are ideal for delineating canal involvement, cord compression, and surgical feasibility.

C. Referral

    1. Radiation therapy. Diffuse disease involving large amounts of the spine is treated primarily with steroids and radiation therapy. Radiation is usually reserved for the symptomatic areas only. Dexamethasone 2–20 mg PO q6h can be quite helpful in improving pain and neurologic symptoms.

    2. Surgery. Early referral to a spine surgeon is warranted following diagnosis regardless of the neurologic exam. If surgery is indicated, it is often best to perform it prior to radiation therapy, because this reduces the wound complication rate. In the face of a cervical myelopathy resulting from diffuse canal involvement and cord compression, a laminectomy can be performed. Patients with lung cancer do very poorly, and it is hard to justify surgery scientifically for metastatic lung cancer. Other tumors do better, but a good rule is that 30–50% of all tumors are improved by laminectomy, with a 10% mortality rate. Isolated vertebral body disease can be resected from an anterior approach—especially in breast cancer, prostate cancer, lymphoma, and renal cell cancer—with excellent long-term results.

VI. Miscellaneous neck pain with and without arm pain

A. Rheumatoid arthritis

    1. Etiology. Rheumatoid arthritis can affect the C1-C2 articulation, leading to erosion of the odontoid process and transverse atlantal ligament, which in turn leads to C1-C2 instability and cord compression from the developing panus.

    2. Evaluation

        a. History and physical examination. Severe neck pain is usually followed by arm pain and a progressive myelopathy.

        b. Radiographs. Plain x-rays and MRI scans are best for showing erosion of the odontoid process with subsequent instability.

    3. Referral and therapy. Place the patient in a soft collar and refer immediately to a spine surgeon. Posterior C1-C2 fusion with transarticular screws is ideal for this problem. Occasionally, an anterior transoral odontoidectomy is required. These treatments are not without risk and must be individualized.

B. Diskitis/osteomyelitis

    1. Introduction. Bacterial diskitis/osteomyelitis is extremely uncommon in the cervical spine, and fever may not be present.

    2. Evaluation

        a. History and physical. There may be a prior history of skin infection, urinary tract infection, or pulmonary infection. Iatrogenic diskitis/osteomyelitis complicating cervical spine surgery is known to occur. Perhaps the most common cause in urban settings is a history of IV drug abuse. Progressive neck pain with a rapidly progressive myelopathy is the usual presentation.

        b. Radiographs. Plain x-rays show disk space collapse with erosion of the bordering vertebral bodies. MRI shows epidural spinal cord compression from kyphosis or epidural abscess.

    3. Referral. The patient should be immediately referred to either a spine specialist or an infectious disease specialist. An immediate radiology-directed needle biopsy/culture or open biopsy/culture, and administration of intravenous bactericidal antibiotics for at least 6 weeks, are indicated. Surgical debridement and decompression are performed for severe kyphosis and neurologic problems.

Recommended Readings

Adams R, Victor M (eds). *Principles of Neurology.* New York: McGraw-Hill, 1993.

Bracken M, et al. Methylprednisolone or naloxone treatment after acute spinal cord injury: 1 year follow up data. Results of the Second National Acute Spinal Cord Injury Study. *J Neurosurg* 76:23–31, 1992.

DePalma A, et al. The natural history of severe cervical disc degeneration. *Acta Orthop Scand* 43:392–396, 1972.

Kricun M (ed). *Imaging Modalities in Spinal Disorders.* Philadelphia: Saunders, 1988.

Lunsford L, et al. Anterior surgery for cervical disc disease. Part 1: Treatment of lateral cervical disc herniation in 253 cases. *J Neurosurg* 53:1–11, 1980.

Modic M, Masaryk T, Ross J (eds). *Magnetic Resonance Imaging of the Spine.* Chicago: Year Book, 1989.

Pellicci P, et al. A prospective study of the progression of rheumatoid arthritis of the cervical spine. *J Bone Joint Surg* 63-A:342–350, 1981.

Rothman R, Simeone F (eds). *The Spine* (vols 1 and 2). Philadelphia: Saunders, 1992.

Shapiro S, et al. Cervical spondylosis with radiculopathy and no myelopathy. Proceedings of 9th Annual Meeting of the Joint Section on Disorders of the Spine and Peripheral Nerves, 1993. P 77.

Shapiro S, et al. Cervical spondylosis with myelopathy. Proceedings of the 9th Annual Meeting of the Joint Section on Disorders of the Spine and Peripheral Nerves, 1993. P 160.

Wilkins R, Rengachary S (eds). *Neurosurgery* (vols 1–3). New York: McGraw-Hill, 1985.

Wong D, Fornasier V, Mac Nab I. Spinal metastases: The obvious, the occult and the imposters. *Spine* 15:1–4, 1990.

23

Approach to the Patient with Low Back Pain and Lumbosacral Radiculopathy

Paul B. Nelson

I. Introduction
  A. **Acute low back pain.** Back pain is extremely common. Most adults can re-member at least one episode of back pain sometime in their lives. Approxi-mately 50% of working adults have back pain at least 1 day per year. Back pain has become one of the most expensive healthcare problems and has become a leading cause of disability under the age of 45. The estimated cost of medical care for patients with low back pain is greater than 8 billion dollars.
  B. **Lumbar disk disease with sciatica.** Patients with back and leg pain (sciatica) most likely have nerve-root compression secondary to a ruptured lumbar disk. Although ruptured disk is occasionally observed in the pediatric and geriatric age groups, it generally occurs in the third to fifth decades of life. Approxi-mately 90% of the ruptured lumbar disks occur between L4-L5 and L5-S1; 5% oc-cur at L3-L4. The incidence of disk rupture is the same in males and in females.
  C. **Lumbar spinal stenosis** is any type of narrowing of the spinal canal, lateral recess, or intervertebral foramina secondary to congenital causes, disk degen-eration, bony hypertrophy, ligamentous hypertrophy, or spondylolisthesis. Be-cause the disease is caused primarily by degenerative change, it seldom occurs before the fifth decade of life. The mean age of patients undergoing operative procedures for lumbar stenosis is the sixth decade, although it sometimes oc-curs in the seventh and eighth decades. Lumbar stenosis is most commonly ob-served at L4-L5 and L3-L4.
II. Etiology
  A. **Acute low back pain.** Only about half of the patients with low back pain have associated injuries. With the disorder being so common and so often unassoci-ated with injury, back pain must be considered a normal part of aging. Degener-ative changes in the spine begin by the end of the second decade of life and are extremely common by the fifth decade.
     A small percentage of patients have structural abnormalities that account for their low back pain. Spondylolisthesis, which is a forward slipping of one verte-bral body over another, is caused by defects in the pars interarticularis (spondy-lolysis) in the younger age group and by degenerative changes in the older age group. Lumbar scoliosis, which is a lateral deformity of the spine, is usually caused by degenerative disease. Primary or metastatic bone tumors or infec-tions of the disk or epidural space are much less common causes of back pain.
  B. **Lumbar disk disease with sciatica.** A lumbar disk acts as an articulation be-tween the vertebrae and as a cushion. It is composed of a cartilaginous end plate and an outer annulus that surrounds the nucleus. Degenerative changes begin in the disk by the late twenties and are common by the fourth decade. Al-terations in the lumbar disk from age alone and major or minor trauma may cause an intervertebral disk to rupture. The disk most commonly ruptures in a posterolateral direction. Disk extrusions and some protrusions may cause neural, nerve-root, or (most frequently) cauda equina compression.
  C. **Lumbar spinal stenosis.** With the exception of the patient born with short pedicles, spinal stenosis develops secondary to degenerative changes and many years of repetitive trauma. With age, the disk loses its water content and stops functioning as a cushion. There is increased stress on the bony vertebrae, the ligaments, and the facets. There is increased mobility of the vertebral bod-ies, ballooning of the disk, and hypertrophy of the ligaments. All of these changes may cause narrowing of the lumbar canal. Absolute spinal stenosis is

defined as a midsagittal diameter of less than or equal to 10 mm. A normal lumbar canal is 15–25 mm in diameter.

III. **Clinical manifestations and evaluation**
   A. **History**
      1. **Acute low back pain.** The history must determine if there is an associated injury. It must also determine if there are any "red flags" that would suggest more serious causes of the back disorder (Table 23-1). Symptoms and histories that should alert the physician that there may be a disorder more serious than regular mechanical low back pain include night pain, fever, severe back spasms, leg pain, leg weakness, leg numbness, bladder or bowel dysfunction, major trauma, minor trauma in an orthopedic patient, weight loss, lethargy, back pain in a child, history of previous bacterial infection, history of carcinoma, history of IV drug use, and a worker's compensation or legal claim.
      2. **Lumbar disk disease with sciatica.** The patient with sciatica usually has a history of back pain for several days before the development of leg pain. In L4-L5 and L5-S1 disk disease, the back pain may actually improve somewhat as the patient goes on to develop a burning discomfort in the buttocks and unilateral pain in the posterolateral aspects of both the upper and lower leg. There may also be numbness or tingling in a portion of the foot or toes. The less common L3-L4 disk disease may cause pain in the groin and anterior aspects of the thigh and upper leg. Occasionally the history is one of severe sciatic pain from the onset. Bilateral leg pain and bladder or bowel dysfunction suggest a large midline disk extrusion.
      3. **Lumbar spinal stenosis.** In spinal stenosis, the history is more important than the examination. Typically, the patient complains of back and leg discomfort, numbness, or heaviness with standing or walking. Symptoms improve with rest or forward bending. The leg symptoms are usually asymmetrical. Occasionally, the patient may have true sciatica.
   B. **Physical examination**
      1. **Acute low back pain.** Examination of the patient with acute low back pain should begin with inspection and palpation of the low back. Paravertebral muscle spasms may be present. In most cases of mechanical back pain, straight leg raise testing causes back pain only. Straight leg raise testing that causes back and leg pain and a neurologic exam that reveals neurologic deficits in the lower extremities suggest a root or cauda equina compression. The neurologic examination should include walking on the heels and toes, squatting, and individual testing of the foot and toe dorsiflexors, the quadriceps, and the iliopsoas muscles. The general exam should include palpation of the abdomen, to rule out an abdominal aortic aneurysm, and a rectal examination.
      2. **Lumbar disk disease with sciatica.** The patient walks in a slow, deliberate fashion with a slight forward tilt of the trunk. Paravertebral muscle tightness may cause decreased range of motion of the back, and asymmetrical muscle tightness may cause an associated scoliosis. The patient prefers to stand or

Table 23-1. "Red flags" that suggest serious causes of low back pain.

Symptoms/histories	Possible diagnosis
Night pain	Tumor
Fever, history of recent bacterial infection or IV drug use, severe back spasms	Diskitis and epidural abscess
Leg pain	Nerve-root compression
Bilateral lower extremity weakness/numbness, bladder or bowel dysfunction	Cauda equina or conus compression
Major trauma	Fracture/dislocation
Minor trauma in an osteoporotic patient	Compression fracture
History of carcinoma	Metastatic disease
Systemic symptoms such as fever, weight loss	Multiple myeloma
Back pain in a child	Tumor, tethered cord
Worker's compensation or legal claim	Secondary gain

lie rather than sit. The best position is usually lying on the unaffected side with the affected leg slightly bent at the knee and hip. The pain is frequently worsened by Valsalva's maneuvers.

Straight leg raise testing is important in the diagnosis of lumbar disk disease. The patient is in a supine position with the knee extended and the ankle plantar flexed. The examiner raises the leg slowly. Normally, the leg can be raised to 90 degrees without discomfort or with slight tightness in the hamstring. When the nerve root is compressed by a ruptured disk, the straight leg raise is limited and causes back and leg pain. It is worsened with dorsiflexion of the foot. In most cases, the straight leg raise test is positive only on the side of the disk rupture. If lifting the asymptomatic leg causes pain in the symptomatic leg, one must consider a disk rupture in the axilla of the nerve root.

Motor testing is directed to the nerve roots most commonly affected. L5 nerve-root compression may result in foot and great toe dorsiflexion weakness (tibialis anterior and extensor hallucis longus). When the compression is severe, the patient may exhibit a foot drop. S1 nerve-root compression may cause plantar flexion weakness. This is difficult to detect at the bedside and is best tested by having the patient do toe raises one leg at a time. L4 weakness may cause quadriceps weakness. The patient may have the sensation that the leg is giving way. Disease of the L3-L4 disk causes a decrease in the knee reflex, and disease of the L5-S1 disk causes a decrease in the ankle reflex.

Sensory loss resulting from a disk rupture seldom occurs in a dermatomal pattern. Rupture of the L5-S1 disk may cause relative hypalgesia in the lateral aspect of the foot and little toe. Rupture of the L4-L5 disk may cause relative hypalgesia in the dorsum of the foot and great toe. Rupture of the L3-L4 disk may cause sensory loss in the anterior thigh and shin.

3. **Lumbar spinal stenosis.** The neurologic examination of the lower extremities may be relatively unremarkable at rest. Occasionally, one may find evidence of mild nerve-root dysfunction such as L5 numbness and weakness.

IV. Differential diagnosis
A. Acute low back pain with and without sciatica
1. Lumbosacral sprain
2. Degenerative arthritis
3. Fracture
4. Metastatic disease
5. Primary bone tumor
6. Diskitis
7. Epidural abscess
8. Ankylosing spondylitis
9. Paget's disease
10. Tethered spinal cord
11. Spondylolisthesis
12. Conversion reaction

B. Lumbar spinal stenosis
1. **Peripheral vascular disease.** Arterial vascular insufficiency may also cause leg discomfort during walking, but is relieved by simply stopping rather than bending forward or sitting.
2. **Degenerative hip disease** may also cause limitation of standing and walking. The pain usually comes on with any type of weight bearing. Examination reveals a decreased range of motion of the hip, and hip rotation may exacerbate the discomfort. The pain associated with degenerative hip disease is most likely to be located in the proximal hip, thigh, and knee.

V. Diagnostic approach
A. Acute low back pain.
In the absence of red flags that suggest a more serious disorder, most testing should be delayed for 4 weeks. If the patient fails to respond to conservative treatment in 4 weeks, however, the following studies may be considered.
1. Lumbosacral spine x-rays
2. Magnetic resonance imaging (MRI)
3. A CT scan should be done if an MRI is not available or if the patient is claustrophobic. The CT scan should include L3-L4, L4-L5, and L5-S1.
4. Lumbosacral myelography and postmyelography CT are seldom needed unless it is impossible to obtain an MRI.

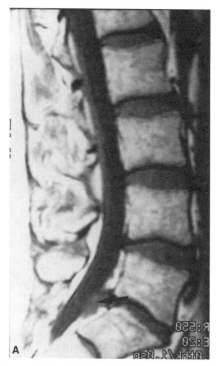
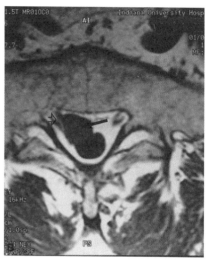

Figure 23-1. (A) T1-weighted sagittal MRI showing a lumbar disk extrusion at L5-S1 that has gone down the lumbosacral canal (closed arrow). (B) T2-weighted axial MRI showing a large extruded L5-S1 disk fragment (solid arrow) that is compressing the right S1 nerve root (open arrow).

  5. Laboratory tests include a CBC and differential, and ESR.
  6. A bone scan can be done, especially if there is a previous history of carcinoma.
B. Lumbar disk disease with sciatica. Few tests are needed in the first 4 weeks if the signs and symptoms are mild to moderate. Severe sciatica, and sciatica associated with significant neurologic deficits with significant weakness of bladder and bowel movements, should be evaluated earlier.

The presence of a disk rupture on an imaging study does not necessarily imply nerve-root dysfunction. About 75% of asymptomatic adult patients have disk bulges or protrusions. Most severe sciatica is associated with disk extrusion.
  1. Plain lumbosacral spine x-rays
  2. MRI is the procedure of choice for evaluating a lumbar disk rupture. An L5-S1 disk extrusion causing severe right S1 nerve-root compression is shown in Figure 23-1.
  3. A CT may be used for a patient who is unable to tolerate an MRI.
  4. Myelography and postmyelography CT scanning may occasionally be used if the MRI and CT scans are nondiagnostic.
  5. Electromyogram (EMG) and nerve conduction velocity (NCV) studies may be helpful if the signs and symptoms do not correlate well with the MRI or CT scan and if one suspects a peripheral nerve problem.
C. Lumbar spinal stenosis. Unless the symptoms are severe, testing may not be done in the early stages of spinal stenosis. The patient who seeks medical treatment for spinal stenosis usually has a walking tolerance of less than one to two blocks and a standing tolerance of less than or equal to 20 minutes.
  1. Plain lumbosacral spine x-rays are indicated to assess the degree of degenerative change and bone density. Flexion/extension lateral views are needed to detect degenerative spondylolisthesis (Fig. 23-2). Degenerative spondylolisthesis is frequently associated with spinal stenosis.

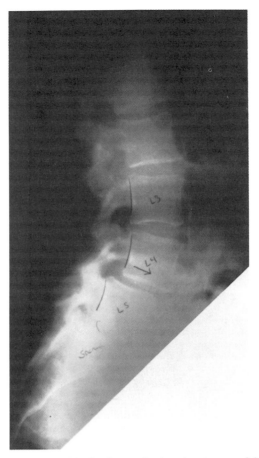

Figure 23-2. Lateral plain x-ray of the lumbosacral spine, showing spondylolisthesis of L4 on L5.

2. **MRI** is the best test for evaluating the number of levels involved and the severity of the spinal stenosis. An MRI showing severe stenosis at L4-L5 is shown in Figure 23-3.
3. **CT** may be used if MRI is not available, but CT does not show the complete lumbar spine and has poorer resolution.
4. A **bone scan** should be done if there is a history of malignancy.
5. **X-rays** of the hip are needed if there is decreased range of motion of the hip or pain with rotation of the hip.
6. **Laboratory values.** CBC and differential, sedimentation rate, and possibly serum and urine protein electrophoresis should be obtained if there are systemic symptoms. A prostatic specific antigen (PSA) should be obtained in a male patient more than 50 years of age.
7. **Arterial Doppler ultrasonography** should be obtained in a patient with diminished or absent peripheral pulses.

VI. **Treatment**

A. **Acute low back pain.** Approximately 90% of patients with acute low back pain will recover within 1 month. Treatment is as follows.
   1. Restrict patient activities as tolerated.
   2. Acetaminophen
   3. Nonsteroidal anti-inflammatory drugs (NSAIDs) (ASA, ibuprofen)
   4. Opioids can be given, but for no longer than 2 weeks.
   5. Short course of steroids (3–5 days)

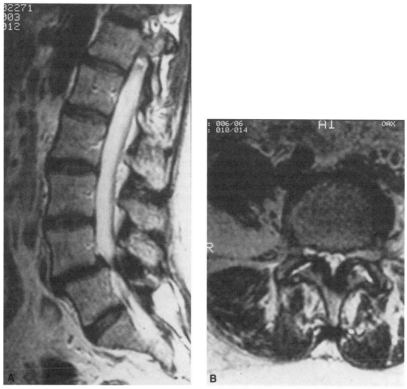

Figure 23-3. (A) T2-weighted sagittal MRI showing segmental stenosis at L4-L5. (B) Axial T2-weighted MRI showing severe stenosis at L4-L5. There is marked facet and ligamentous hypertrophy.

6. Muscle relaxants
7. Heat
8. Limit lifting to 20 lb for moderate to severe back pain. Activity restrictions at work should seldom be extended beyond 3 months.

B. **Lumbar disk disease with sciatica.** The initial treatment for sciatica is similar to treatment for acute low back pain. At least one-half of the patients with sciatica improve within 1 month.
1. Two to 4 days of rest with gradual return to normal activities
2. Acetaminophen
3. NSAIDs (ASA and ibuprofen)
4. Short course of opioids (no more than 2 weeks)
5. Short course of steroids (3–5 days)
6. Muscle relaxants
7. Heat
8. Limit lifting to 20 lb. Try to keep work-related activity restrictions to no more than 3 months.
9. Epidural steroids may be considered if initial conservative therapy is not successful.

C. **Lumbar spinal stenosis**
1. **Conservative therapy** requires that patients be taught to live within the limits of their walking and standing tolerances. They must realize that they should get off their feet, if possible, when they become symptomatic. The patient with severe limitation to walking may benefit from the use of a handicap license plate. Patients with degenerative spondylolisthesis may benefit from lumbosacral supports. Flexion exercises should also be considered.
2. **Surgical treatment** should be considered only if the patient is medically

stable and can no longer live with his or her degree of spinal claudication. True sciatica that does not respond to conservative therapy may also be considered for surgery. The surgical procedures that can be considered include lumbar laminectomy, lateral recess decompression, and spinal fusion. Seldom is surgery for spinal stenosis necessary in the first 3 months of symptoms and, in most cases, the patient will be symptomatic for 12–18 months.

VII. Surgical referral
  A. Severe and disabling sciatica
  B. Significant neurologic deficits such as foot drop or bladder and bowel disturbance
  C. Poor response to at least 4 weeks of conservative therapy
  D. Other "red flags" (see Table 23-1)

Recommended Readings

Clinical Practice Guidelines, Acute Low Back Problems in Adults: Assessment and Treatment. US Department of Health and Human Services. AHCPR, Publication #95-0643, December, 1994.

Frymoyer JW. *The Adult Spine: Principles and Practice.* New York: Raven, 1991.

Jansen MC, et al. Magnetic resonance imaging of the lumbar spine in people without back pain. *N Engl J Med* 331:69–73, 1994.

Malmivaara A. The treatment of low back pain—bed rest, exercise, or ordinary activity? *N Engl J Med* 332:351–355, 1995.

Mixter WJ, Barr JS. Rupture of the intervertebral disc with involvement of the spinal canal. *N Engl J Med* 211:210–215, 1934.

Rockman RH, Simeone FA. *The Spine.* Philadelphia: Saunders, 1992.

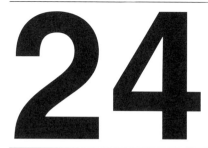

Approach to the Patient with Upper Extremity Pain and Paresthesias and Entrapment Neuropathies

Mark A. Ross

Upper extremity (UE) pain and paresthesias are extremely common complaints. Disorders producing these symptoms are usually not life-threatening, but prompt evaluation is necessary because these disorders can cause significant impairments that often are reversible. Musculoskeletal (MSK) disorders are common causes of UE pain without neurologic manifestations. Peripheral nervous system (PNS) disorders causing these symptoms are cervical radiculopathy (see Chap. 22), brachial plexopathy, and peripheral nerve injuries (mononeuropathies). Symptoms vary depending on the specific etiology and its severity, and often include motor abnormalities—e.g., weakness and atrophy. Sensory and motor symptoms can be collectively called "sensorimotor" symptoms. The locations of symptoms and signs generally reflect PNS anatomy, and hence knowledge of PNS anatomy is fundamental for diagnosis. Electrodiagnostic studies (EDS) are critically important for diagnostic accuracy, because symptoms and physical findings of PNS disorders overlap considerably. Determination of the specific cause is possible by integrating clinical history, physical findings, and results of diagnostic studies.

I. **Differential diagnosis and etiology of UE pain.** See Table 24-1.
II. **Evaluation**
   A. **History**
      1. **Description of symptoms.** The examiner should consider not only the affected UE, but also the unaffected UE and legs, to address the possibility of a generalized process.
         a. **Sensory symptoms**
            (1) **Pain.** Descriptions of pain are never pathognomonic of specific disorders. Tingling or radiating pain suggests a peripheral nerve, plexus, or root disorder, whereas dull, aching, nonradiating pain is typical of MSK disorders. Exceptions to this generalization occur frequently. Acute onset of excruciating pain in the shoulder or arm is common with idiopathic brachial plexopathy. Pain radiating from the neck to the arm or hand is suggestive of radiculopathy (Chap. 22). The location of pain may suggest the root involved—e.g., lateral arm (C5), lateral forearm or thumb (C6), middle finger (C7), or medial aspect of hand and forearm (C8). Pain localized to the shoulder may result from MSK disorders such as bicipital tendinitis, rotator cuff injury, and adhesive capsulitis, or from PNS disorders such as C5 radiculopathy, brachial plexopathy, and entrapment of the suprascapular or dorsal scapular nerves. Pain radiation to sites distant from the causative pathology may give misleading localization—e.g., carpal tunnel syndrome rarely manifests as forearm or shoulder pain. Forearm pain may occur with C6 radiculopathy, plexopathy, or entrapment of nerves in the forearm. Pain involving specific digits can help narrow diagnostic considerations. Involvement of the thumb, index finger, or middle finger, or some combination thereof, suggests a median mononeuropathy, a disorder of the upper or middle component of the brachial plexus, or a C6 or C7 radiculopathy. Pain involving the ring and little fingers suggests an ulnar mononeuropathy, a lower plexus disorder, or C8-T1 radiculopathy. Digital pain may also result from local MSK disorders—e.g., arthritis. Bizarre descriptions of pain are typical of psychological or functional disorders.
            (2) **Paresthesias and sensory loss.** Paresthesias are spontaneous sensations originating from nerve fibers, which patients may describe as

Table 24-1. Differential diagnosis and etiology of upper extremity pain.

Disorder	Common etiologies
PNS Disorders	
Radiculopathy	Root compression (disk, bone), trauma
Brachial plexopathy	Idiopathic, trauma, tumor, radiation, compressive (TOS)
Mononeuropathy	
Suprascapular n.	Trauma, IBP
Dorsal scapular n.	Trauma, IBP
Long thoracic n.	Trauma, IBP
Musculocutaneous n.	Trauma, IBP
Median n.	
Anterior interosseous n.	Compression, trauma
Pronator teres syndrome	Compression, trauma
Carpal tunnel syndrome	Compression
Ulnar n.	
Cubital tunnel syndrome	Compression, trauma
Guyon's canal	Compression, trauma
Radial n.	
Spiral groove	Compression, trauma
Posterior interosseous	Compression, trauma
Superficial radial	Compression, trauma
MSK Disorders	
Rotator cuff injury	Overuse, trauma
Biceps tendinitis	Overuse, trauma
Adhesive capsulitis	Immobility, shoulder weakness
Lateral epicondylitis	Overuse, trauma

IBP = idiopathic brachial plexopathy; MSK = musculoskeletal; PNS = peripheral nervous system; n = nerve; TOS = thoracic outlet syndrome.

"tingling" or "pins and needles." Sensory loss refers to the absence of normal sensation, which patients may describe as "numbness" or "like Novocain." Paresthesias and sensory loss may occur together or independently, and either serves to suggest that a UE pain condition is a result of PNS disease rather than an MSK disorder. The distribution of paresthesias or sensory loss has localizing value similar to that described above for pain. However, in many cases of mononeuropathy or radiculopathy, paresthesias, sensory loss, and pain do not conform precisely to the known anatomic distribution of the affected nerve or nerve root. For example, a patient with a median mononeuropathy resulting from carpal tunnel syndrome may complain that the entire hand is numb. Thus, failure of sensory symptoms to localize clearly to a specific nerve or nerve-root distribution should not exclude the possibility of these disorders. The differential diagnosis of paresthesias and sensory loss needs to include central nervous system (CNS) disease, especially when pain is absent.

    b. **Motor symptoms.** Patients complaining of weakness should be asked to describe specific activities that cause difficulty. Problems with fine motor skills—e.g., buttoning buttons—indicates distal muscle weakness and suggests involvement of C8 or T1 roots, lower plexus, or nerves innervating hand muscles (median or ulnar nerves). Difficulty with arm and shoulder movements indicates proximal muscle weakness, suggesting involvement of the C5 or C6 roots, upper plexus, or nerves innervating proximal muscles (e.g., long thoracic, suprascapular, or axillary nerves). Patients with pain or sensory loss may misconstrue impaired motor performance as weakness. Careful attention to this possibility may be clarified during the exam, or by asking the patient to consider which factor chiefly limits his or her performance. CNS disorders can also produce weakness of either the proximal or distal musculature.

2. **Onset and precipitating factors.** The history should address the activities the patient was involved with at or just preceding the onset of symptoms and whether or not physical activities exacerbate the symptoms.
   a. **Physical activities.** Some physical activities predispose patients to development of specific PNS disorders. Heavy lifting might cause cervical disk herniation and resultant radiculopathy. Head turning often exacerbates pain or paresthesias associated with radiculopathy. Arm abduction or shoulder rotation exacerbates the pain of MSK shoulder disorders and also the pain associated with brachial plexopathy. Repetitive flexion and extension movements of the elbow or sustained elbow flexion may predispose to ulnar mononeuropathy at the elbow (cubital tunnel syndrome). Repetitive flexion and extension movements at the wrist or fingers may predispose to median mononeuropathy within the carpal tunnel, known as carpal tunnel syndrome (CTS). Repetitive pronation and supination may lead to hypertrophy of the pronator teres muscle and median nerve entrapment in the forearm (pronator teres syndrome). The radial nerve may be compressed in the axillary region by improper use of a crutch, or in the arm when pressure is applied by a tourniquet, a hard surface, or the body's weight. Radial nerve compression in the arm is especially likely to occur when the patient's level of consciousness is reduced by anesthesia, sedatives, or alcohol intoxication. Handcuffs or other tight-fitting objects at the wrist—e.g., watchbands or bracelets—may injure the median, ulnar, or superficial radial sensory nerves. The history should review the patient's occupation, hobbies, and recent changes in physical activity. Sporting activities, playing musical instruments, gardening, and knitting are examples of physical activities that might contribute to development of compressive nerve injuries.
   b. **Trauma** often causes UE pain and sensorimotor complaints. Even remote trauma may have a bearing on UE pain or sensorimotor symptoms. Examples include entrapment of a nerve by the callus of a healing fracture and development of a central cavity in the spinal cord (syringomyelia).
      (1) **Motor vehicle accident (MVA).** The severe trauma of an MVA may cause various PNS disorders, including vertebral fracture with direct spinal cord injury, nerve-root avulsion, radiculopathy, brachial plexus injury, peripheral nerve injury, or late development of syringomyelia. Arm traction or stretching the arm and neck in opposite directions may cause cervical root avulsions or a stretch injury to the brachial plexus. An MVA may cause more than one PNS disorder—e.g., cervical nerve-root avulsions and concomitant peripheral nerve injury. After an MVA, attention to multiple life-threatening injuries, or casting for multiple limb fractures, may preclude detection of PNS disorders until late in the course of recovery.
      (2) **Fractures and dislocations** may cause specific nerve injuries. Shoulder dislocation or fracture of the humerus may injure the axillary nerve. Fracture of the clavicle may injure components of the brachial plexus. Fracture of the humerus predisposes to radial nerve injury in the spiral groove, whereas fracture or dislocation of the radius may injure the posterior interosseous branch of the radial nerve. Fracture of the elbow predisposes to ulnar mononeuropathy, which may not manifest until years after the trauma, hence the name "tardy ulnar palsy." A wrist fracture may cause either median or ulnar mononeuropathy.
      (3) **Laceration.** When UE pain or sensorimotor symptoms begin after a skin laceration or puncture wound, direct injury to a nerve needs to be considered. Exploration is needed to determine if the nerve requires repair.
   c. **Physiologic compression sites.** The median and ulnar nerves have sites where the anatomical relationship between the nerve and normal ligamentous and bony structures makes the nerve vulnerable to physical compression. The site of common compression injury is at the wrist for the median nerve (carpal tunnel) and at the elbow for the ulnar nerve (cubital tunnel). At these locations, the nerves are particularly susceptible to compression injury, hence the term "physiologic compression

sites." A patient with UE sensorimotor symptoms, without any clear predisposing factors, is highly likely to have an abnormality of one of these nerves.

d. **Systemic illnesses.** Many systemic illnesses predispose to development of PNS disorders that may manifest as UE sensorimotor symptoms. A complete listing of systemic illnesses with PNS complications exceeds the scope of this chapter, but several common examples are given.

   (1) **Endocrine disorders.** Patients with diabetic polyneuropathy are more vulnerable to development of mononeuropathies at physiologic compression sites. Patients with hypothyroidism are prone to development of CTS.

   (2) **Rheumatologic disorders.** Several rheumatologic disorders predispose to UE nerve or nerve-root injury. Rheumatoid arthritis may cause degenerative spine disease leading to cervical radiculopathy. Patients with rheumatoid arthritis are also susceptible to CTS and posterior interosseous neuropathy. Systemic vasculitis may involve individual peripheral nerves in either the upper or lower extremities. Abrupt onset of a mononeuropathy is occasionally the presenting manifestation of systemic vasculitis. Primary amyloidosis and some hereditary forms are associated with CTS.

   (3) **Renal failure and dialysis.** Patients receiving chronic hemodialysis are particularly likely to develop CTS, owing to deposition of amyloid material (beta-2 microglobulin) within the carpal tunnel. Placement of arteriovenous fistulas for hemodialysis access may be associated with development of median or ulnar neuropathies and, less often, a severe distal ischemic injury to all UE nerves. Diabetic patients seem particularly prone to develop this severe UE nerve injury.

   (4) **Malignancy.** Patients with histories of cancer—particularly of the breast or lung—who develop UE sensorimotor complaints need to be evaluated for the possibility of metastases to the brachial plexus. Patients with histories of radiation therapy to the brachial plexus region can develop radiation-induced brachial plexopathies, which may be delayed many years after the radiation therapy.

3. **Other history.** The medical history should also include inquiries about symptoms of depression and a review of the social situation for factors that might influence the patient's symptoms. Specific questions should be asked regarding employment, accidents, work injuries, and possible litigation. Evidence of CNS disease should be sought, which might include seizures, disturbed consciousness, personality change, or problems with cognition, language, or vision.

B. **Physical examination**
1. **Motor examination**
   a. **Muscle inspection.** Muscles are inspected for evidence of atrophy and spontaneous muscle contractions. Muscle atrophy is present when reduction of the normal muscle bulk or contour is revealed by visual inspection or direct measurement of limb circumference. Atrophy of specific muscles helps localize the disorder. For example, atrophy of the thenar eminence alone suggests a disorder of the median nerve or the deep terminal branch of the ulnar nerve. Atrophy of the thenar and hypothenar areas and the interossei muscles should raise considerations of combined median and ulnar mononeuropathies, lower trunk brachial plexopathy, C8-T1 radiculopathy, or C8-T1 spinal cord disease. Inspection of the scapula when the arms are extended forward can reveal winging or elevation of one scapula, suggesting a long thoracic nerve mononeuropathy. Inspection of muscles also involves a careful search for fine muscle twitches visible through the skin, called fasciculations. These twitches may occur as isolated symptoms or findings in normal individuals. However, when present in conjunction with muscle weakness and atrophy, fasciculations are a sign of disease. The exam should include inspection for fasciculations in all four limbs, as well as in the back and abdomen. Fasciculations occur most commonly with anterior horn cell diseases—e.g., amyotrophic lateral sclerosis—but can also occur with diseases affecting the motor root, plexus, or peripheral nerve.

b. **Muscle strength ratings.** Muscle strength is assessed by manual muscle testing. The Medical Research Council strength rating scale is used (see Table 22-1). Muscle strength ratings are made for proximal and distal muscles in all four limbs, which may reveal weakness of which the patient was not aware. Muscles that should be tested bilaterally in the UE include muscles for arm abduction (deltoid and supraspinatus), arm external rotation (infraspinatus), elbow flexion (biceps), elbow extension (triceps), wrist flexion (flexor carpi radialis and flexor carpi ulnaris), wrist extension (extensor carpi radialis), finger flexion (flexor digitorum superficialis and flexor digitorum profundis), finger extension (extensor digitorum communis), finger spreading (interossei), thumb abduction (abductor pollicis brevis), and grip strength.

Patients with MSK disorders and patients with depression, psychological disturbances, or malingering may exhibit a type of weakness known as "breakaway" weakness, in which incomplete effort gives the appearance of weakness. Features suggesting breakaway weakness include pain complaints during testing, reasonable initial strength that diminishes, variability in motor performance on serial exams, improved strength with encouragement, and absence of other objective signs of motor impairment. When patients exhibit breakaway weakness as a result of a psychological disturbance or malingering, they often make facial expressions or contortions of the tested limb, which imply that great effort is being made.

c. **Muscle tone** is assessed by noting how easily the patient's limbs can be passively moved while the patient is asked to relax the limb tested. The tone is rated according to the Ashworth scale, in which normal tone is assigned a value of 1, and values 2–5 represent increasing degrees of abnormal stiffness. Muscle tone should be normal with all of the common PNS disorders causing UE pain and sensorimotor symptoms. Increased muscle tone should raise the question of a CNS disorder. When increased muscle tone occurs with UE weakness and atrophy, a compressive lesion of the cervical spine or amyotrophic lateral sclerosis needs to be considered.

2. **Reflexes** are tested bilaterally in all four limbs, including the brachioradialis (C5-C6), biceps (C5-C6), triceps (C7-C8), quadriceps (L2-L4), and soleus (S1) tendons. Reflexes are rated as normal, decreased, or increased. A significant reflex asymmetry suggests an abnormality of the nervous system. Radiculopathy involving a cervical root typically depresses the corresponding UE reflex on the affected side. Brachial plexopathy causes decreased reflexes corresponding to the part of the plexus involved. Radiculopathy of the C8 or T1 roots, or lower trunk brachial plexopathy, may exhibit normal UE reflexes. Mononeuropathies of the UE do not usually influence the UE reflexes, unless the nerve involved supplies the muscle tested in the reflex arc—e.g., musculocutaneous nerve mononeuropathy may cause a reduced biceps reflex. Reflexes are preserved in MSK disorders and increased in CNS disorders.

3. **Sensory examination.** The sensory examination involves testing of light touch, pain (pinprick), vibration, and joint position sensations in the upper and lower extremities. Particular attention is paid to cutaneous areas where there are sensory complaints.

4. **Maneuvers.** Several maneuvers may aid in the evaluation of UE sensorimotor complaints. Tinel's sign, originally used for assessment of regenerating nerve fibers, is now commonly used as an indication of paresthesias radiating in the nerve's cutaneous distribution. It is elicited by mild tapping over the nerve. It may be observed in association with regenerating nerve fibers, neuroma, or focal demyelinative nerve pathology, and even in normal individuals. Tinel's sign is easier to elicit from a diseased nerve than from a normal nerve, and thus it may help to localize an abnormal nerve. It is commonly used to assess for CTS by tapping over the median nerve on the volar surface of the wrist. In Phalen's maneuver, the wrist is flexed for up to 1 minute in an attempt to develop numbness or tingling in the median nerve distribution. A positive Phalen's maneuver provides supportive evidence for CTS. In Adson's maneuver, the arm is moved into an abducted and extended position, and the radial pulse is assessed. Although loss of the radial pulse

with this maneuver is alleged to indicate compression of the subclavian artery by a cervical rib, or hypertrophied or tight scalenus muscles, it is not a useful test, because it is subjective and may cause normal individuals to lose their radial pulse.

C. Laboratory studies

    1. Electrodiagnostic studies (EDS). Electrodiagnostic studies consist of nerve conduction velocity (NCV) studies and electromyography (EMG). These tests permit an objective and quantitative assessment of individual peripheral nerves and muscles. They can substantiate a clinically suspected diagnosis or reveal unsuspected abnormalities. With rare exceptions, all patients with symptoms of UE pain and sensorimotor symptoms should have EDS as part of the initial diagnostic evaluation. When performed in the first few days after onset of nerve injury, electrodiagnostic studies do not reveal as many abnormalities as when performed 7–10 days later. However, performing EDS early after injury can document preexisting abnormalities that may be important for complicated diagnostic cases or when medicolegal issues occur. Electrodiagnostic studies are further discussed in detail in Chap. 33.

    2. Radiologic studies

        a. Plain films. After trauma with neck or UE injury, cervical spine films or plain bone films are necessary to evaluate for fractures. When cervical radiculopathy is suspected, cervical spine films may reveal narrowing of specific neural foramina. Cervical spine films may also be useful in detecting a cervical rib, which should be investigated when clinical and EDS evidence suggests the neurogenic thoracic outlet syndrome. The patient with brachial plexopathy should have a chest film to evaluate for malignancy. If clinical evidence suggests Pancoast's syndrome, apical chest film views should be included to search for an apical tumor. Plain films may also be useful in evaluation of MSK disorders, by revealing evidence of degenerative arthritis or of calcifications within tendons.

        b. Magnetic resonance imaging (MRI). Radiologic evaluation of cervical radiculopathy is most often accomplished by MRI. Myelography combined with computerized tomography (CT) may also be used. MRI of the brachial plexus is often used to search for evidence of tumor as the cause of brachial plexopathy.

        c. Laboratory studies for investigation of systemic illnesses are obtained for patients with UE sensorimotor complaints, depending on individual case circumstances. Tests that may be useful include CBC with differential, chemistry panel, blood sugar, erythrocyte sedimentation rate (ESR), antinuclear antibody, urinalysis, serum immunofixation electrophoresis, thyroid function, and spinal fluid tests.

D. Unexplained symptoms. Occasionally, patients complaining of UE pain or sensorimotor symptoms present no objective evidence of a PNS disorder after thorough evaluation. For such patients, possible explanations for symptoms include CNS disease, depression, psychological factors, or malingering. The symptoms and signs of CNS and PNS diseases may overlap, particularly for slowly progressive conditions—e.g., brain tumor or multiple sclerosis. Evidence suggesting CNS disease includes painless weakness or sensory disturbance, upper motor neuron signs, altered consciousness or personality, or problems with cognition, language, or vision. Patients with depression may present with unexplained UE pain or sensorimotor symptoms. Some patients with unexplained UE symptoms may not have frank depression but some unhappiness or conflict in the psychosocial realm, which manifests as symptoms of neurologic dysfunction. Often such patients cannot recognize or accept relationships between their symptoms and their psychological states. Others have onsets of symptoms after accidents or injuries, and either the process of litigation or the power of suggestion from inquisitive physicians distorts the usual concept of wellness and perpetuates the symptoms. Patients with unexplained symptoms should have neurologic consultation, and may need to be followed and observed over time.

III. Diagnostic approach. Briefly, the history is used to form initial hypotheses about the cause of the symptoms, and these hypotheses are tested during the physical examination. Knowledge of PNS anatomy is essential for interpreting UE sensorimotor symptoms and signs. In almost all cases, EDS are performed to help localize a suspected PNS disorder or to exclude a PNS disorder. When a PNS disorder is present, electrodiagnostic studies help determine the severity and type of pathologic process. Additional diagnostic assessments may include radiologic studies or laboratory tests, depending on individual patient circumstances.

IV. **Selected disorders and criteria for diagnosis**
  A. **Peripheral nervous system disorders**
    1. **Mononeuropathy**
      a. **Median nerve**
        (1) **Carpal tunnel syndrome (CTS)**
          (a) **Anatomy and etiology.** CTS is an extremely common disorder caused by compression of the median nerve at the wrist within the unyielding space known as the carpal tunnel. Many disorders compromise this space, resulting in median nerve compression. The most common cause is flexor tenosynovitis, which may be associated with excessive physical use of the hands. Patients with primary carpal stenosis—i.e., a narrow carpal tunnel—may be especially prone to CTS. Other local factors causing CTS include vascular lesions, abnormal tendons, ganglion cysts, tumoral calcinosis, pseudoarthrosis, and infection. Systemic illnesses associated with CTS include endocrine disorders such as hyperparathyroidism, acromegaly, and hypothyroidism, and rheumatologic disorders such as rheumatoid arthritis, systemic lupus erythematosus, polymyalgia rheumatica, temporal arteritis, scleroderma, and gout. Other conditions predisposing to CTS include diabetic and other polyneuropathies, chronic hemodialysis, shunts for hemodialysis, and pregnancy.

          (b) **Clinical features** of CTS include numbness or tingling involving one or more of the first four digits (thumb through ring finger), although occasionally the entire hand is involved. There may be pain in the fingers or wrist, and at times in the forearm or shoulder. Patients often complain of being awakened at night by these symptoms, and physical activity involving use of the hands may exacerbate the symptoms. Patients may observe weakness and atrophy of the thenar muscle. Physical examination reveals decreased sensation in the volar aspect of the first four digits. Because the median nerve innervation frequently supplies only the lateral half of the ring finger, sparing of sensation on the medial half of the ring finger is a helpful sign. Advanced cases show weakness and atrophy of the abductor pollicis brevis. Tinel's and Phalen's signs may be present.

          (c) **Diagnosis** of CTS is established by clinical history, physical findings, and EDS results. The EDS findings vary with the severity of the disorder. In mild cases, the amplitude of the median compound muscle action potential (CMAP) and sensory nerve action potential (SNAP) are normal, and the latency values of the median SNAP and CMAP from the wrist are increased, with focal slowing of median NCV across the wrist. Slowing of NCV in proximal median nerve segments should not exclude the diagnosis of CTS. In some cases, there may be conduction block at the wrist level. In more advanced cases, the median CMAP and SNAP amplitude values decline, and fibrillation potentials may be demonstrated in the abductor pollicis brevis muscle, but not in other muscles, including median-innervated forearm muscles. The EDS results for the ulnar nerve in the same hand are normal.

        (2) **Pronator teres syndrome**
          (a) **Anatomy and etiology.** The pronator teres syndrome refers to presumed compression of the median nerve in the forearm where it passes between the two heads of the pronator teres muscle. This disorder is uncommon and is usually related to an occupation that involves repetitive pronation of the forearm. Such activity or hypertrophy of the pronator teres muscle may compress the median nerve. A fibrous band from pronator

teres to flexor digitorum superficialis, and local trauma, are other potential causes.

(b) **Clinical features.** The predominant symptom is pain in the volar forearm. Weakness of the abductor pollicis brevis and median distribution sensory complaints are not usually present, but occasionally occur. The pronator teres muscle itself remains strong. Examination may show tenderness in the region of the pronator teres muscle, and there may be a Tinel's sign over the pronator muscle.

(c) **Diagnosis** is established primarily by clinical features. Electrodiagnostic studies are often normal, but occasionally slow median NCV may be observed in the forearm segment.

(3) Anterior interosseous syndrome

(a) **Anatomy and etiology.** This relatively uncommon median nerve disorder involves compression of the anterior interosseous branch of the median nerve in the forearm, usually by a fibrous band from the pronator teres or the flexor digitorum superficialis muscles. Other forearm anomalies or forearm trauma may also cause the disorder. The anterior interosseous nerve (AIN) is a purely motor nerve that supplies the flexor pollicis longus (FPL), flexor digitorum (FD) I and II, and pronator quadratus (PQ) muscles.

(b) **Clinical features** include forearm or elbow pain combined with weakness of flexion of the distal phalanx of the thumb (FPL) and the index and middle fingers (FD), or weakness of some of these functions. Patients note inability to pinch the thumb and index finger together, but generally don't complain of weakness of pronation, because the major muscle involved with pronation, pronator teres, is unaffected.

(c) **Diagnosis** is established by the abovementioned clinical features and EDS results. The median NCV studies are normal, because the AIN does not contribute to the muscle assessed for median NCS, and median sensory fibers do not travel in the AIN. EMG shows fibrillation potentials confined to one or more of the above muscles supplied by the AIN. When AIN causes weakness confined to the FPL, EMG is extremely helpful for differentiating a partial AIN syndrome from rupture of the FPL tendon.

b. Ulnar nerve

(1) Cubital tunnel syndrome

(a) **Anatomy and etiology.** The most common cause of entrapment of the ulnar nerve in the elbow region is compression in the cubital tunnel. The floor of the tunnel is formed by the medial ligament of the elbow, and the roof is the aponeurosis of the flexor carpi ulnaris muscle. The ulnar nerve runs through this space, and then underneath the flexor carpi ulnaris muscle. Remote elbow trauma, with or without fracture, predisposes to later development of entrapment neuropathy in the elbow region (tardy ulnar palsy). However, many patients develop ulnar neuropathy from compression in the cubital tunnel without antecedent trauma. Repetitive movement at the elbow or prolonged flexion of the elbow may be predisposing factors.

(b) **Clinical features** include sensory complaints in the ulnar division of the hand (the fifth digit and the medial half of the fourth) and the ulnar-innervated portion of the hand and wrist. Sensory complaints may include decreased sensation, paresthesias, and pain. Pain may involve the medial forearm and elbow. Weakness involves the interossei, abductor digiti minimi, adductor pollicis, and flexor pollicis brevis. When weakness is chronic, atrophy may be present, and a clawhand deformity may develop. Most often, the flexor carpi ulnaris muscle remains strong. A diagnosis of ulnar neuropathy requires normal strength in C8-T1 muscles innervated by the median and radial nerves.

(c) **Diagnosis** is established by the characteristic history and physical findings, and EDS. Ulnar neuropathy at the elbow may show reduction of the ulnar CMAP and SNAP. There may be evidence of conduction block in motor fibers that can be localized to the elbow region. Ulnar NCV may be focally slow across the elbow. The EMG exam reveals fibrillation potentials and/or abnormal motor unit potentials (MUPs) in ulnar-innervated hand muscles. Usually the flexor carpi ulnaris does not show fibrillation potentials, although it may do so if its motor branch is also compressed.

(2) Compression at the wrist (Guyon's canal)

(a) **Anatomy and etiology.** Guyon's canal is a fibro-osseous tunnel connecting the pisiform and hamate wrist bones through which the ulnar nerve travels. As the ulnar nerve emerges from Guyon's canal, it divides into a deep terminal branch, which is purely motor and supplies all of the ulnar-innervated hand muscles, and a superficial terminal branch, which supplies sensation to the medial distal half of the palm and the palmar surfaces of the fourth and fifth digits. Sensation to the medial proximal half of the palm is supplied by the palmar cutaneous branch of the ulnar nerve, which arises in the midforearm and does not pass through Guyon's canal. Sensation to the medial dorsal half of the hand is supplied by the dorsal cutaneous branch of the ulnar nerve, which arises above the wrist and also does not pass through Guyon's canal. Factors predisposing to ulnar neuropathy at the wrist include chronic compression, which may occur in cyclists, and local trauma—e.g., wrist fracture.

(b) **Clinical features** vary depending on the precise level of abnormality. Compression of the entire ulnar nerve within Guyon's canal or of the two branches as they leave the canal causes weakness of all ulnar-innervated hand muscles and sensory loss in the superficial terminal branch distribution. Sensation of the dorsal medial hand and the proximal half of the medial palm is spared because sensation is supplied by other branches. Compression of the deep terminal motor branch may occur in isolation either before or after it supplies the hypothenar muscles, producing ulnar-innervated hand muscle weakness with no sensory loss. Finally, compression of only the superficial terminal branch causes sensory loss in its palmar distribution with normal hand strength.

(c) **Diagnosis** is established by clinical examination and EDS. The EDS findings vary depending on which of the abovementioned ulnar nerve branches is involved. If the superficial terminal sensory branch is involved, NCV studies will show a reduced or absent ulnar SNAP recorded from the fifth digit, but the SNAP from the dorsal ulnar cutaneous nerve remains normal. If the abnormality involves the deep terminal branch, ulnar CMAP amplitude may be reduced and there may be fibrillation potentials or abnormal MUPs in ulnar-innervated hand muscles.

c. Radial nerve

(1) Axilla or spiral groove compression

(a) **Anatomy and etiology.** The radial nerve may be compressed against the humerus by external pressure in the axilla or the spiral groove. Compression in the axilla can be caused by improper use of crutches. Compression in the spiral groove is likely to occur when an individual falls asleep with the arm hanging over a chair, or with a partner's head against the arm, and the effects of alcohol or sedatives prevent paresthesias from arousing the individual to move the arm. The term "Saturday night palsy" has been used for such a radial nerve palsy. A similar outcome may result from use of an arm tourniquet during surgery. The radial nerve may also be injured in the spiral groove by blunt trauma, by fractures of the humerus, and rarely by vigorous arm exercise.

(b) **Clinical features** are weakness of radial-innervated muscles and sensory loss on the dorsal aspects of the hand, thumb, and index and middle fingers. Radial-innervated muscles include triceps, brachioradialis, supinator, and the wrist and finger extensors. The triceps is affected by axillary compression but is spared by spiral groove compression. Weakness of wrist extensors causes wrist drop. Inability to stabilize the wrist and fingers as a result of radial-innervated extensor weakness frequently creates the false impression that ulnar-innervated hand muscles are weak.

(c) **Diagnosis** of radial mononeuropathy is confirmed by clinical features and EDS results that verify abnormalities confined to the radial nerve distribution. Nerve conduction studies show a reduced-amplitude radial CMAP and reduced or absent SNAP. The presence or absence of fibrillation potentials in triceps helps to localize the compression site (axilla or spiral groove).

(2) **Posterior interosseous nerve**

(a) **Anatomy and etiology.** The posterior interosseous nerve (PIN) is the purely motor termination of the radial nerve in the forearm. The PIN supplies the supinator muscle and the wrist and finger extensors. Entrapment of the PIN is relatively uncommon. When this occurs, it is usually at the level of the supinator muscle. Predisposing factors include vigorous use of the arm, fracture of the head of the radius, and other local traumas. Hypertrophied synovia of the elbow joint in patients with rheumatoid arthritis may compress the PIN.

(b) **Clinical features** are weakness of the wrist and finger extensors. Some patients have pain in the elbow or dorsal forearm. There are no sensory abnormalities apart from pain, because the posterior interosseous nerve is purely motor.

(c) **Diagnosis** is established by the abovementioned clinical features and EDS results. NCV studies show a reduced-amplitude radial CMAP and normal radial SNAP. The EMG exam shows fibrillation potentials and abnormal MUPs in the aforementioned radial-innervated muscles.

(3) **The superficial sensory branch**

(a) **Anatomy and etiology.** The superficial sensory branch of the radial nerve arises in the vicinity of the elbow and supplies sensation to the dorsolateral hand and the dorsal aspects of the first three digits. It may be injured at the wrist level by local trauma or compression from tight objects around the wrist, such as watchbands or handcuffs.

(b) **Clinical features** are purely sensory, with paresthesias and sensory loss in the radial sensory distribution.

(c) **Diagnosis** is made by the history, physical findings, and NCV evidence of a reduced or absent superficial radial SNAP.

d. **Axillary nerve**

(1) **Anatomy and etiology.** The posterior cord of the brachial plexus divides into the radial and axillary nerves. The axillary nerve travels below the shoulder joint and gives a branch innervating the teres minor muscle, which is an external rotator of the arm. The axillary nerve then courses behind and lateral to the humerus before dividing into anterior and posterior branches, which supply corresponding portions of the deltoid muscle. The posterior branch gives a cutaneous nerve that supplies the skin over the lateral deltoid. The axillary nerve may be injured by shoulder dislocation or fractures of the humerus. It may occasionally be the only nerve affected by idiopathic brachial plexopathy (see below).

(2) **Clinical features.** The main clinical manifestation is impaired shoulder abduction resulting from weakness of the deltoid. The supraspinatus initiates arm abduction, and so patients may retain limited arm abduction ability. Weakness of the teres minor muscle may be difficult to demonstrate on physical examination because of

the normal infraspinatus muscle function. Sensory loss may be demonstrated over the lateral portion of the deltoid muscle.

(3) **Diagnosis** is confirmed by finding weakness limited to the deltoid muscle and EMG abnormalities restricted to the deltoid and teres minor muscles. An axillary NCV study with surface recording from the deltoid muscle may show delay or reduced amplitude of the axillary nerve CMAP.

e. **Musculocutaneous nerve**

(1) **Anatomy and etiology.** The musculocutaneous nerve arises from the lateral cord of the brachial plexus and supplies the coracobrachialis, biceps, and brachialis muscles. It continues in the forearm as the purely sensory lateral antebrachial cutaneous nerve. Mononeuropathy of the musculocutaneous nerve is uncommon, but it may occur with shoulder dislocation, direct trauma or compression, or sudden extension of the forearm.

(2) **Clinical features** include impaired arm flexion resulting from weakness of the biceps and the other musculocutaneous-innervated muscles. The biceps reflex may be normal or reduced, depending on the severity of the biceps weakness. Sensory loss is present over the lateral forearm.

(3) **Diagnosis.** The clinical features of musculocutaneous neuropathy closely parallel those of C5 radiculopathy. Diagnosis is established by the abovementioned clinical features and EDS results that differentiate C5 radiculopathy from musculocutaneous nerve mono-neuropathy. The lateral antebrachial SNAP is reduced or absent in musculocutaneous neuropathy but normal in C5 radiculopathy. EMG shows involvement of only the abovementioned muscles supplied by the musculocutaneous nerve.

f. **Long thoracic nerve**

(1) **Anatomy and etiology.** The long thoracic nerve is a purely motor nerve arising from the ventral rami of the C5, C6, and C7 spinal nerves. It courses along with other brachial plexus components underneath the clavicle, then travels down the chest wall anterolaterally to supply the serratus anterior muscle. This large muscle fixes the scapula to the chest wall, providing general stability for the shoulder during arm movements. Injury of the long thoracic nerve may occur with trauma or with vigorous physical activities involving shoulder girdle movements. Long thoracic neuropathy may be caused by idiopathic brachial plexopathy.

(2) **Clinical features** of long thoracic mononeuropathy include pain and weakness in the shoulder. Patients have difficulty abducting the arm or raising it above the head. Winging of the scapula is demonstrated by having the patient extend the arms forward and push against a wall. The scapula elevates from the chest wall because the weak serratus muscle cannot hold it.

(3) **Diagnosis** is established by the abovementioned clinical features and EMG showing fibrillation potentials involving only the serratus anterior muscle. Long thoracic nerve NCS are technically difficult, and other NCS are normal.

g. **Suprascapular nerve**

(1) **Anatomy and etiology.** The suprascapular nerve is a purely motor nerve arising from the upper trunk of the brachial plexus and passing through the suprascapular notch on the upper border of the scapula to supply the supraspinatus and infraspinatus muscles. The suprascapular nerve is most often injured by trauma in which there is excessive forward flexion of the shoulder. It may be involved in idiopathic brachial plexopathy.

(2) **Clinical features** are pain in the posterior shoulder and weakness of the spinati muscles. The supraspinatus initiates arm abduction, whereas the infraspinatus externally rotates the arm.

(3) **Diagnosis** is established by clinical history, physical findings, and EDS. Routine NCV studies are normal, but motor NCV studies with recording from the supraspinatus muscle may show reduced ampli-

tude or prolonged latency relative to the unaffected side. The EMG exam shows abnormalities confined to the spinati muscles on the affected side.

h. Dorsal scapular nerve

(1) **Anatomy and etiology.** The dorsal scapular nerve (DSN) is a purely motor nerve arising from the upper trunk of the brachial plexus and passing through the scalenus medius muscle to supply the rhomboid and levator scapulae muscles. Injury to the DSN is relatively uncommon.

(2) **Clinical features** include pain in the scapular region and weakness of the rhomboid and levator scapulae muscles.

(3) **Diagnosis** is established by clinical features and EMG showing fibrillation potentials restricted to the muscles supplied by the DSN. There is no satisfactory NCS for the DSN.

2. Brachial plexopathy

a. Idiopathic brachial plexopathy

(1) **Anatomy and etiology.** Idiopathic brachial plexopathy, also known as Parsonage-Turner syndrome or neuralgic amyotrophy, is an uncommon condition believed to represent an immune-mediated neuropathy affecting various portions of the brachial plexus. An antecedent event such as an upper respiratory infection or immunization is present in about half of the cases.

(2) **Clinical features.** The main clinical features are abrupt onset of severe pain in the shoulder and proximal arm followed at a variable interval (hours to weeks) by shoulder and arm muscle weakness. The pain is exacerbated by movement of the arm, shoulder, or neck, which may give the false impression of an MSK disorder. Any combination of muscles innervated by nerves arising from the brachial plexus may be involved, but there is a predilection for proximal muscles. Muscles supplied by the axillary, suprascapular, long thoracic, radial, musculocutaneous, and anterior interosseous nerves are commonly involved, but other nerves can also be affected. Involvement may be extensive or restricted to a single nerve, and asymmetric bilateral involvement occurs in one-third of patients. Sensory loss or paresthesias may be present, but these features are relatively minor.

(3) **Diagnosis** is established by the characteristic clinical history, physical findings, and EDS. Patients with this disorder typically present early for evaluation and treatment of the severe pain. If EDS are performed early, abnormalities of MUP recruitment may be observed, but the studies may be otherwise normal. If EDS are repeated 7–10 days after weakness begins, the NCS show evidence of axonal injury, with the distribution varying according to the specific nerves involved. EMG shows fibrillation potentials in clinically weak muscles, and often in muscles that were not judged weak by physical examination. For this reason, EMG is essential for determining the extent of injury.

b. Neurogenic thoracic outlet syndrome

(1) **Anatomy and etiology.** The "true" neurogenic thoracic outlet syndrome (TOS) is a very rare disorder in which the lower trunk of the brachial plexus is compressed by an elongated transverse process of C7, a rudimentary cervical rib, or a fibrous band running from either of these to the first rib.

(2) **Clinical features** are weakness and wasting of the intrinsic hand muscles, most markedly affecting the abductor pollicis brevis muscle; pain involving the medial forearm or hand; and sensory loss involving the fourth and fifth fingers and the medial hand and distal forearm.

(3) **Diagnosis** is established by clinical features and characteristic EDS results. Radiographic evidence of an elongated C7 transverse process or a rudimentary cervical rib is helpful but not mandatory for diagnosis, because the structural problem may be a fibrous band that can be demonstrated only by surgical exploration. The NCV study results indicating neurogenic TOS are the combination of se-

verely reduced or absent median CMAP, normal median SNAP, reduced or absent ulnar SNAP, and mildly reduced or normal ulnar CMAP. The EMG exam shows fibrillation potentials in lower-trunk–innervated muscles, particularly those supplied by the median and ulnar nerves. In contrast to the rare and well-defined true neurogenic TOS is a condition commonly misdiagnosed as TOS, which has various UE sensorimotor symptoms but no consistent clinical history. Patients said to have this form of TOS have no objective neurologic abnormalities and no abnormalities on EDS. This form of TOS has been aptly referred to as "disputed" neurogenic TOS, and its existence as an entity remains controversial. Patients erroneously diagnosed with this type of TOS are often subjected to first-rib resection, and, unfortunately, severe brachial plexopathy may be a complication.

  c. Brachial plexopathy in patients with malignancy

   (1) Anatomy and etiology. Metastasis of tumor to the brachial plexus needs to be considered whenever a patient with a history of malignancy, especially breast or lung cancer, develops UE pain or sensorimotor symptoms. Brachial plexopathy is usually not the presenting feature of malignancy, except in Pancoast's syndrome, in which an apical lung carcinoma invades the lower trunk of the brachial plexus. For patients who have undergone prior chest wall radiotherapy, brachial plexopathy from radiation injury may occur months to many years after radiotherapy.

   (2) Clinical features of brachial plexopathy resulting from tumor invasion are pain, weakness, and sensory changes that may involve either the upper or lower plexus. Unlike idiopathic brachial plexopathy, malignant brachial plexopathy has a gradual onset of symptoms, and lymphedema of the arm is common. In Pancoast's syndrome, patients usually first have pain in the medial arm, and may develop sensorimotor abnormalities in the lower-trunk distribution. Horner's syndrome (ipsilateral ptosis, miosis, and facial anhidrosis) often results from a tumor invading the inferior cervical sympathetic ganglion. Malignant plexopathy may be more likely than radiation plexopathy to be painful and involve the lower trunk, but this generalization is not reliable.

   (3) Diagnosis. Patients with histories of malignancy and new onset of UE sensorimotor symptoms or pain should have EDS to exclude common conditions such as mononeuropathy or radiculopathy, which might cause symptoms identical to those of brachial plexopathy. The EDS can determine if there is evidence of brachial plexopathy and clarify the locations of abnormalities within the plexus. This information can help in planning and interpreting MRI studies of the plexus, which should be performed to look for evidence of tumor. Patients with lower-trunk plexopathy should have apical chest film views to look for an apical lung tumor. Myokymic discharges detected by EDS in patients with prior chest wall radiotherapy support a diagnosis of radiation plexopathy but do not conclusively exclude tumor metastases.

 3. Cervical radiculopathy. The clinical and electrodiagnostic features of cervical radiculopathy are mentioned above, and thoroughly reviewed in Chap. 22.

B. Musculoskeletal disorders share in common the predominant symptom of pain and an absence of other neurologic manifestations. In general, EDS are normal when MSK disorders are the cause of UE pain symptoms. However, it is common for an underlying neurologic disorder affecting the PNS to result in a secondary MSK disorder, in which case EDS may be abnormal as a result of the underlying neurologic disorder.

 1. Rotator cuff injury. The rotator cuff comprises the tendons of the supraspinatus, infraspinatus, teres minor, and subscapularis muscles, which fix the humeral head in the glenoid fossa during shoulder abduction and provide internal and external arm rotation. Rotator cuff inflammation (tendinitis) and tear are common causes of shoulder pain. Tendinitis results from repetitive minor trauma to the cuff, and tear may occur as a chronic stage of this degenerative process, or acutely from abrupt trauma. With tendinitis or tear, there is shoulder pain on arm abduction or on internal or external arm rotation. With tear, there may be weakness of rotator cuff functions, but EMG studies are negative. Plain films may reveal tendon or subacromial bursa calcifications. Ultrasound or an arthrogram of the shoulder may confirm a rotator cuff tear.

2. **Bicipital tendinitis.** Inflammation of the biceps tendon (tendinitis) causes pain and tenderness in the anterior shoulder region. The pain may be reproduced by supination of the forearm against resistance or by flexion and extension of the shoulder. There are no neurologic abnormalities, and the diagnosis is established clinically.

3. **Adhesive capsulitis (frozen shoulder).** Loss of motion at the shoulder joint may result in adhesion of the joint capsule to the humerus. Usually, shoulder pain from any cause leads to immobility and subsequent adhesive capsulitis. Alternatively, weakness of shoulder girdle muscles from either PNS or CNS disorders may cause this problem. Whatever the cause, the joint becomes stiff, and attempted motion causes severe shoulder pain. Muscle atrophy may result from PNS disease, or secondarily from disuse. The diagnosis is usually made by the clinical features.

4. **Lateral epicondylitis (tennis elbow).** Overuse of the extensor carpi radialis muscles (wrist extensors), or direct trauma to their tendinous insertion on the lateral epicondyle, may lead to inflammation, degeneration, or tear of the tendons. This produces pain localized over the lateral epicondyle, which may be exacerbated by use of the forearm-wrist extensor muscles.

V. **Referral.** Patients should be referred to a reliable electromyography laboratory for EDS, because this step is essential for accurate diagnosis. Subsequent diagnostic studies and management decisions depend on accurate diagnosis. The EDS are not only essential for diagnosis, but also estimate the severity of the abnormality. This information is helpful for prognosis and treatment decisions. Neurologic consultation for UE pain or sensorimotor symptoms is appropriate at any stage of the evaluation process if there are questions concerning diagnosis or management.

Recommended Readings

Cailliet R (ed). *Neck and Arm Pain. Pain Series* (2nd ed). Philadelphia: Davis, 1981.

Dawson DM. Entrapment neuropathies of the upper extremities. *N Engl J Med* 329:2013–2018, 1993.

Nakano KK. The entrapment neuropathies. *Muscle and Nerve* 1:264–279, 1978.

Pecina MM, Krmpotic-Nemanic J, Markiewitz AD (eds). *Tunnel Syndromes.* Boca Raton: CRC, 1991.

Stewart JD. *Focal Peripheral Neuropathies* (2nd ed). New York: Raven, 1993.

25

Approach to the Patient with Lower Extremity Pain and Paresthesias and Entrapment Neuropathies

Gregory Gruener

Lower extremity pain and paresthesias are common complaints. In general, peripheral nervous system disorders causing these symptoms result from specific mononeuropathies, lumbosacral radiculopathies, or plexopathies. Diagnosis of specific mononeuropathies rests on the motor, reflex, and sensory changes confined to a single nerve. The clinical signs are supplemented by electrodiagnostic studies. With appropriate diagnosis, and meticulous evaluation and management, gratifying results can be obtained.

The reemergence of the generalist in health care has resulted in at least two major effects in regard to the diagnosis and management of individuals with neuropathies. The first, as expected, is that such individuals will not be under the sole care of specialists. The second, somewhat unexpected, is that the specialist will not be replaced, but his or her role has now become more defined. A specialist will now have to develop a greater degree of proficiency in distinguishing neuropathies from radiculopathies, plexopathies, or other nonneurologic syndromes of pain, disturbed sensation, or weakness. However, this accuracy will have to take place in the setting of fewer and perhaps more carefully selected laboratory evaluations.

Fortunately, the recognition of neuropathies has always necessitated that adequate attention be placed on both the history and examination. Not only does this allow anatomical localization, but it helps to establish or rank potential etiologies. A well-thought-out assessment can then effectively and prudently guide further diagnostic evaluations.

This chapter will serve as a descriptive outline of common as well as some infrequent lower extremity neuropathies. Symptoms and findings are stressed and the most frequent etiological considerations reviewed. Throughout this section, the importance of bedside examination is stressed, but diagnostic tests are also reviewed and their usefulness discussed.

I. Evaluation

A. History. Various aspects of the history need to be taken into account in determining the etiology of a specific mononeuropathy, including the nature of its onset (abrupt or insidious), preceding events (injury, surgery, or illness), associated symptoms (fever, weight loss, or joint swelling), and aggravating or alleviating features (joint position or specific activities). Because the observed deficit can be similar regardless of the cause, historical information is instrumental in defining or limiting the possible etiologies of mononeuropathies.

B. Physical examination. Although motor and sensory symptoms and signs correspond to the distribution of a single peripheral nerve or its branch, the degree of the deficit can vary. Motor signs may be clinically absent, or varying degrees of weakness, atrophy, or fasciculations can be noted. Sensory symptoms likewise may not only be either positive (tingling, pricking, burning, etc.) or negative (hypesthesia), but also, although corresponding to the sensory distribution of a nerve, are frequently most pronounced in its distal distribution. Therefore, the sensory examination should begin with the patient's description of the area of involvement. This description may be more helpful than formal testing in identifying the pattern of sensory deficit. Finally, the course of the nerve should be evaluated in a search for local areas of discomfort or the presence of a Tinel's sign (pain or paresthesia in the cutaneous distribution of a nerve) elicited by light percussion over the nerve. The relationships of these sites of discomfort to adjacent anatomical structures can help in determining the etiology of the mononeuropathy.

C. Diagnostic studies. Further evaluation is often necessary not only to confirm the presence and severity of a mononeuropathy but also to help exclude more proximal sites of involvement (plexus or root) that may clinically masquerade as a mononeuropathy.

1. **Electrodiagnostic studies.** Electromyography (EMG) and nerve stimulation studies (NSS) are quite useful in the evaluation of mononeuropathies. They can aid in localization, define severity, detect bilateral but asymmetric processes, and provide prognostic information.

2. **Laboratory testing** is usually directed at the identification of a systemic or generalized disease that may predispose or be indirectly responsible for the mononeuropathy. Owing to the practical nature of this section, a full discourse on the multiple medical or systemic diseases that can "present" with mononeuropathies will not be provided. However, the readings provided at the end of the chapter can be consulted once an initial localization has been made and can provide a thorough listing of frequent as well as unusual causes of specific mononeuropathies.

3. **Imaging studies.** Radiologic testing is usually employed in an attempt to identify intrathoracic, abdominal, retroperitoneal, or pelvic masses that may lead to nerve-root or plexus injury. The role of imaging studies is less clear in delineating the causes of neuropathies that are localized to a limb, unless a focal site of involvement is suspected (entrapment or mass lesion). In such cases, testing is usually done by CT or, increasingly, by MRI, whereas routine x-ray studies now play a less significant role.

II. **Specific mononeuropathies**
   A. **Femoral and saphenous neuropathies.** Formed within the psoas by the fusion of the posterior divisions of the ventral rami of L2-L4 spinal nerves, the femoral nerve exits from its lateral border and descends between the psoas and iliacus muscles (which it may also innervate) and under the fascia of the iliacus. Emerging under the inguinal ligament, lateral to the femoral artery, it then divides into motor branches, which supply the quadriceps muscles, and sensory branches to the anterior thigh. One major division, the saphenous nerve, descends within Hunter's (adductor) canal, accompanying the femoral artery. At the medial and superior aspects of the knee, the saphenous nerve emerges from the canal and then, accompanying the saphenous vein, descends medially down the leg, ending at the medial aspect of the foot. The saphenous nerve supplies the sensory innervation to both the medial leg and foot.

   1. **Etiology.** Femoral neuropathies are usually caused by trauma from surgery (intrapelvic, inguinal, or hip operations), stretch or traction injuries (prolonged lithotomy position in childbirth), or direct compression (hematoma within the iliacus compartment). Although diabetes mellitus is described as a frequent etiology, such cases are usually misnomers and often represent restricted plexopathies or more widespread lesions with predominantly femoral nerve dysfunction. Saphenous neuropathies are most often attributable to injury during surgery (arterial surgery, saphenous vein removal, or knee operations).

   2. **Clinical manifestations**
      a. **History.** The initial complaint is one of leg weakness (as if the leg will "fold under") on attempting to stand or walk. Pain in the anterior thigh is a frequent accompaniment in cases resulting from iliacus hematoma and, when accompanied by the abrupt onset of leg weakness, should lead to its suspicion. A similar pattern of pain, but usually subacute in onset, can be observed in cases of "femoral neuropathy" occurring in diabetes mellitus. With the exception of pain, sensory involvement tends to be an infrequent and minimal symptom in femoral neuropathies.

      Because of its association with surgical injury, sensory loss in saphenous neuropathies may initially go unnoticed and often is of little concern. In some patients, however, pain is prominent, and in such cases it usually appears some time after the assumed injury to the nerve.

      b. **Physical examination**
         (1) **Neurologic.** A neurologic examination reveals weakness of the quadriceps muscles, absent or diminished patellar reflex, and sensory loss over the anterior thigh and, with saphenous nerve involvement, the medial leg/foot.
         (2) **General.** Examination or palpation within the inguinal region and, in cases of saphenous nerve involvement, the medial knee may be fruitful in identifying focal areas of pain and perhaps the site of in-

volvement. The close proximity of a surgical scar or point of injury may also provide additional etiologic information. In cases where retroperitoneal hemorrhage is suspected, peripheral pulses may be normal, but there is a characteristic posturing of the leg (held flexed at the hip, and attempts to extend or perform a reverse straight leg test exacerbate the pain).

3. Differential diagnosis. The most productive test for localization is evaluation of hip adduction strength. Its impairment suggests a more proximal process, either plexus or root, as the site of involvement, although a superimposed obturator neuropathy cannot be excluded.

4. Evaluation

  a. Electrodiagnostic. Nerve conduction studies (NCS) are not as helpful as EMG in evaluating patients suspected of having femoral neuropathies. EMG in such cases involves a careful search of both L2-L4 innervated muscles and paraspinal muscles, because they should not be involved in isolated femoral neuropathy.

  b. Imaging. Cases resulting from retroperitoneal hemorrhage or other mass lesion are best identified by CT or MRI scanning of the retroperitoneum.

B. Obturator neuropathy. Arising within the psoas muscle, from ventral divisions of L2-L4 spinal nerves, the obturator nerve exits from the psoas muscle at its lateral margin, descends into the pelvis, and exits through the obturator foramen. It innervates the adductor magnus, longus, and brevis, and also supplies sensation to the upper medial thigh.

1. Etiology. Isolated neuropathies of the obturator nerve are unusual. In cases resulting from pelvic or hip fracture, involvement of other nerves to the lower extremity or lumbosacral plexus also occurs. Both benign and malignant pelvic masses may also result in obturator neuropathy, as can surgical procedures performed on these masses or within the pelvis.

2. Clinical manifestations

  a. History. Leg weakness and difficulty in ambulation are the most common first complaints and usually overshadow sensory loss, if present.

  b. Physical examination

    (1) Neurologic. Motor evaluation shows weakness of hip adduction, and sensory loss may be demonstrable along the upper medial thigh. The patellar reflex should be intact.

    (2) General. Careful pelvic and rectal examinations to identify an intrapelvic tumor are needed in cases where obturator paralysis occurs without trauma.

3. Differential diagnosis. The clinical examination needs to be carefully directed at detecting, because of its infrequency, sensory or motor involvement other than what could be attributed to the obturator nerve. The presence of hip flexor or knee extensor weakness or an impaired patellar reflex suggests a lumbosacral plexopathy or L3-L4 radiculopathy. In addition, sensory loss, which extends below the knee, is also inconsistent with the sensory deficit of an obturator neuropathy.

4. Evaluation

  a. Electrodiagnostic. Once again, NCS are not as helpful as EMG studies in the evaluation of patients suspected of having obturator neuropathies. Evidence of involvement of other L2-L4 muscles or abnormalities on EMG on paraspinal muscles suggests a more proximal lesion.

  b. Imaging. In cases where obvious trauma is not a consideration, further evaluation may be needed. Here, imaging of the pelvic cavity by CT or MRI is helpful in identifying a mass or infiltrative lesion.

C. Lateral femoral cutaneous neuropathy. Dorsal divisions of the ventral primary rami of L2-L3 spinal nerves contribute to the lateral femoral cutaneous nerve, which emerges from the lateral border of the psoas major muscle. It then crosses laterally, to the depth of the fascia of the iliacus muscle, and over the sartorius muscle before passing under the lateral border of the inguinal ligament. Piercing the fascia lata, it divides into anterior and posterior branches that provide sensory innervation to the anterolateral aspects of the thigh. Anatomic variations are frequent in regard to its origin (it may arise as a branch of the femoral or genitofemoral nerve), its course after arriving at the inguinal ligament, and finally the extent of its sensory innervation.

1. **Etiology.** In most cases, entrapment/compression at or near the inguinal ligament is the assumed etiology. However, entrapment/compression at other sites, such as those of retroperitoneal masses, surgeries (especially those involving retroperitoneal structures, pelvis, or inguinal sites), and traumas to the thigh, may also injure the lateral femoral cutaneous nerve.
2. **Clinical manifestations**
   a. **History.** Pain, burning, or a "crawling" sensation with variable loss of sensation in the anterolateral thigh, exacerbated by walking or getting up and out of a chair, is a frequent presentation (meralgia paresthetica). Frequently, the patient rubs the thigh for relief, and this may also serve as a diagnostic clue.
   b. **Physical examination**
      (1) **Neurologic.** The area of sensory change is usually small and over the lateral aspect of the thigh.
      (2) **General.** Careful palpation along the inguinal ligament and anterior pelvic brim can usually detect a localized area of tenderness and may precipitate symptoms while also confirming the diagnosis.
3. **Differential diagnosis.** The primary differential is a femoral neuropathy. Lumbar plexopathy and L2 radiculopathy are also considerations, but are unlikely to be points of confusion. The limited sensory impairment, lack of motor involvement, and intact reflexes help in excluding these other possibilities.
4. **Evaluation.** Although clinical features usually provide enough support for a diagnosis, when there is uncertainty or preexisting disease that may complicate the issue (retroperitoneal mass), further testing may be needed.

   Unlike other entrapment syndromes, responsiveness to treatment also helps to confirm the diagnosis of a lateral femoral cutaneous neuropathy. With this in mind, injection of an anesthetic agent at the assumed exit point of the lateral femoral cutaneous nerve (medial to the anterior superior iliac spine and under the inguinal ligament) or at a site of local tenderness is a worthwhile approach. A response to such treatment not only supports the diagnosis but can also result in improvement of symptoms.
   a. **Electrodiagnostic.** The difficulty in eliciting a response by NSS in normal or control subjects has appropriately limited its application to patients believed to have lateral femoral cutaneous neuropathies. However, EMG studies play a role in evaluating patients with unusual or unclear symptoms, because the detection of clinically silent motor involvement implies involvement of more than the lateral femoral cutaneous nerve.
   b. **Imaging.** Unless there is a strong clinical suspicion of a retroperitoneal or pelvic mass resulting in lateral femoral cutaneous nerve entrapment, radiologic evaluation is not necessary. However, unexplained or concomitant gastrointestinal or urogenital symptoms should raise the suspicion of such a process.
D. **Sciatic neuropathy.** The sciatic nerve arises from the ventral rami of the L4-L5 spinal nerves, which, by way of the lumbosacral trunk, fuse with those from S1-S3. Passing along the inner wall of the pelvis, it exits through the sciatic notch and passes under the piriformis muscle, where it lies between the ischial tuberosity and greater trochanter. Remaining in this deep location, it descends into the thigh and, proximal to the knee, divides into the peroneal and tibial nerves. The sciatic nerve itself is clearly divisible into two trunks: the medial, which receives contributions from the L4-S3 rami and gives rise to the tibial nerve; and the lateral, whose contributions are from L4-S2 and from which the common peroneal nerve is derived. Although the sciatic nerve itself has no sensory branches, the lateral trunk provides innervation to the short head of the biceps femoris, and, by way of the medial trunk, semitendinosus, semimembranosus, and long head of the biceps femoris, and with the obturator nerve, the adductor magnus is also innervated.
1. **Etiology.** Possibly second to only the peroneal nerve, in regard to its frequency of involvement, is trauma, to which most sciatic neuropathies, whether involved at the glutei or the thigh, are secondary. This includes involvement secondary to injury to adjoining/neighboring structures from pelvic, hip, and femur fractures or gunshot wounds. Injection injuries are no longer as frequent a cause as in the past, but compression injuries are in-

creasing and often occur in the setting of prolonged immobility, such as in various operative procedures (e.g., cardiac bypass graft surgery). Miscellaneous causes include entrapment by fibrous constricting bands, local hematomas, or tumors.

Mention needs to be made of the so-called **piriformis syndrome.** As of this time, there are few cases that rigorously support the assumed pathogenesis of this syndrome, compression of the sciatic nerve by the overlying piriformis muscle, although it remains a frequent clinical diagnosis. Point tenderness of the sciatic nerve at the level of the piriformis muscle can also be observed in patients suffering from plexopathies or lumbosacral radiculopathies and does not necessarily confirm pathologic compression of the sciatic nerve by the piriformis muscle.

2. **Clinical manifestations**
   a. **History.** Complete lesions, which fortunately are infrequent, are associated with paralysis of hamstring muscles and all those muscles below the knee and with sensory loss in the tibial and peroneal distributions. Partial lesions, especially those of the lateral trunk, make up the majority of sciatic neuropathies and often present with foot drop.
   b. **Physical examination**
      (1) **Neurologic.** Although paralysis of varying degrees in muscles innervated by both the medial and lateral trunks can be present, involvement of muscles innervated by the lateral trunk tend to be the most frequent presentation. Sensory loss is variable, but restricted to the distribution of the sensory branches of the peroneal and tibial nerves. The muscle stretch reflexes of the hamstring and Achilles tendons can be depressed.
      (2) **General.** Palpation along the course of the nerve may help identify masses or locate points of pain and tenderness but, as mentioned earlier, do not entirely exclude more proximal nerve lesions.
3. **Differential diagnosis.** Care must be taken to ensure that a radiculopathy (especially L5-S1) is not masquerading as a sciatic neuropathy. The straight leg raise test, frequently positive in radiculopathies, can also be elicited in cases of lumbosacral plexopathies as well as sciatic neuropathies. However, a careful rectal and pelvic examination is indicated in suspected sciatic neuropathies, because involvement of the sacral plexus by pelvic masses may not otherwise be identified. Finally, isolated common peroneal or tibial neuropathies must be considered as causes of the patient's symptoms.
4. **Evaluation**
   a. **Electrodiagnostic.** Both NSS and EMG studies are useful in distinguishing sciatic mononeuropathies from L5-S2 radiculopathies or plexopathies, but they necessitate careful screening of paraspinal and gluteal muscles. However, just as the lateral division of the sciatic nerve can be the most involved clinically, EMG findings may demonstrate a similar pattern. In some sciatic mononeuropathies, a pattern of abnormal motor and sensory studies of the peroneal nerve, with normal tibial nerve studies, is not an entirely infrequent finding.
   b. **Imaging.** In cases where radiculopathies and plexopathies cannot be excluded, further neuroradiologic studies can provide useful information. In addition, in those cases where only sciatic nerve involvement is demonstrated, MRI with gadolinium may effectively "follow" the course of the nerve and help in identifying focal abnormalities.
E. **Peroneal neuropathy.** Arising from posterior divisions of the L4-S2 ventral rami of spinal nerves, the common peroneal nerve descends into the leg as the lateral division of the sciatic nerve. At the level of the popliteal fossa, it branches from the sciatic and moves toward the lower lateral portion of the popliteal fossa. Two cutaneous sensory branches arise at this point, one to the sural nerve and the other, the lateral cutaneous (sural) nerve of the calf, providing sensation to the upper lateral calf. Exiting laterally from the popliteal space, the peroneal nerve is in close juxtaposition to the fibula and winds below its head and then passes through a tendinous arch formed by the peroneus longus muscle. At the exit of the arch, it divides into the superficial and deep peroneal nerves. The superficial peroneal nerve descends adjacent to the peroneus longus and brevis, which it innervates, and in the distal third of the leg it pierces the fascia. Its terminal branches (medial and lateral) provide sensation

to the lateral dorsal surface of the foot. The deep peroneal nerve enters the extensor compartment of the leg and, with the tibial artery, descends on the interosseous membrane, innervating the tibialis anterior, extensor hallucis longus, and extensor digitorum longus muscles. The terminal portion of this nerve then passes under the extensor retinaculum at the ankle, where a lateral branch innervates the extensor digitorum brevis muscle and a medial branch provides sensory innervation to the first and second toes.

1. **Etiology.** Most cases are caused by external compression (anesthesia and casts) and trauma (blunt injury, arthroscopic knee surgery, and fractures) despite numerous, but less frequent, etiologies (tumor, constriction by adjacent structures, involvement in systemic disease, traction injuries from severe ankle strain, etc.).

2. **Clinical manifestations**
   a. **History.** Most patients present with foot drop, and sensory complaints are usually minimal or of no concern. Less prominent degrees of weakness or weakness affecting only intrinsic foot muscles may not elicit alarm in the patient. On reviewing the history, careful attention needs to be paid to potential episodes of trauma, compression, or unusual sustained postures that may have preceded the problem (squatting, kneeling, etc.).
   b. **Physical examination**
      (1) **Neurologic.** The characteristic presentation is foot drop, and in a complete lesion of the common peroneal nerve there is paralysis of ankle dorsiflexion, ankle eversion, and toe extension (dorsiflexion). Sensory loss occurs in the anterolateral lower leg and the dorsa of the foot and toes.
      (2) **General.** Palpation in the popliteal fossa and along the fibular head may elicit signs of tenderness or the discovery of a mass and further define the site of involvement, while suggesting possible etiologies. In addition, examination of the dorsa of the ankle and distal lateral leg, where the terminal branch of the deep peroneal nerve emerges, may reveal similar signs and suggest a distal injury. The most common sites at which focal pathologic processes can affect the nerve or its branches include the fibular head and its proximal neck, the outer compartment of the leg, and the superior and inferior extensor retinaculum at the ankle, beneath which branches of the peroneal nerve pass. However, the peroneal nerve also serves as a reminder that in cases of focal compression there can be variable fascicular involvement. Motor function of the deep or superficial component, only sensory dysfunction, or various combinations thereof may be the result of nerve compression at the fibular head.

3. **Differential diagnosis.** The primary differentials in these cases are other causes of foot drop. Involvement of the L5 root, the lumbosacral trunk, and the lateral division of the sciatic nerve can all produce foot drop.

4. **Evaluation.** The extent of evaluation depends on the history. In those cases where an identifiable episode of compression occurs, observation, after elimination of the compression, is often all that is needed. When disruption of the nerve (i.e., laceration) is suggested, the onset of the problem is insidious, or physical findings on EMG are inconclusive (incomplete common peroneal neuropathy), further evaluation is indicated.
   a. **Electrodiagnostic.** NCS can allow identification of both the site of involvement and the extent of axonal injury. Such studies may also need to be applied to the asymptomatic leg, because the discovery of bilateral but asymmetric nerve involvement suggests a systemic illness (diabetes) as the etiology. EMG further helps define the extent of axonal injury, or evidence of another cause of the patient's symptoms if abnormalities are found in other L4-L5 innervated muscles or paraspinal muscles.
   b. **Imaging.** X-ray studies can be useful when joint trauma or a mass is detectable on examination. However, CT and MRI are more useful in defining lesions of the nerve and delineating the relationship of adjacent structures to the nerve.

F. **Tibial neuropathy.** Ventral rami from L5-S2 spinal nerves contribute to the tibial nerve, which descends into the thigh as part of the medial trunk of the sciatic nerve. At the distal portion of the thigh, the sciatic nerve bifurcates into both the tibial and peroneal nerves. Now entering the calf, it descends to the depth of the gastrocnemius, which it innervates, and provides innervation to the soleus, tibialis posterior, flexor digitorum, and hallucis longus muscles as it continues its descent. Finally, at the level of the ankle, it divides into its terminal branches (plantar nerves), which provide innervation to all intrinsic foot flexor muscles as well as sensation to the sole of the foot.

1. **Etiology.** Tibial neuropathies are infrequent and result in part from the nerve's deep anatomic location. While occurring less frequently than peroneal neuropathies, severe ankle injuries can cause more proximal tibial nerve injuries. Surprisingly, major knee trauma infrequently results in severe tibial nerve injury.

2. **Clinical manifestations**
   a. **History.** Sensory loss is usually evident along the side of the foot and extending proximally if the tibial nerve's contribution to the sural nerve is involved. Weakness may not be noticed unless ankle plantar flexion is involved.
   b. **Physical examination**
      (1) **Neurologic.** Sensory loss is usually present along the sole of the foot. Weakness may be limited to intrinsic toe flexor muscles, or, with more proximal muscle involvement, ankle dorsiflexion and inversion weakness can also be found.
      (2) **General.** Careful palpation of the nerve's course, especially within the popliteal space, should be performed. The finding of a mass or precipitation of paresthesias or pain, in addition to helping localize the site of involvement, also suggests an etiology, because tumors involving the tibial nerve may increase its sensitivity to such maneuvers.

3. **Differential diagnosis.** Because of its infrequent occurrence, any suspicion of a tibial neuropathy should prompt a search for another cause or more proximal lesion. Radiculopathies, plexopathies, or sciatic neuropathies may present clinically as isolated tibial neuropathies. Careful examination of more proximal muscles and of reflexes, as well as a sensory exam, may help in identifying or suggesting these conditions as more appropriate diagnoses.

4. **Evaluation**
   a. **Electrodiagnostic studies** play a crucial role in identifying as well as ruling out tibial neuropathy. Involvement of other nerves on NSS, identification on EMG of muscles other than those innervated by the tibial nerve, or paraspinal muscle involvement suggests another etiology. At times, plantar nerve involvement may be identified as the cause of the sensory or motor deficits, rather than more proximal tibial lesions.
   b. **Imaging.** The identification of a mass or point of tenderness in cases of unclear etiology may necessitate MRI imaging to identify the anatomical structure of the nerve and its relationships to adjacent structures.

G. **Medial and lateral plantar neuropathies.** At the level of the ankle, the terminal portion of the tibial nerve lies medial to the Achilles tendon. As it descends, it passes under the flexor retinaculum, which comprises the roof of the tarsal tunnel. Within the tunnel, the tibial nerve divides into medial and lateral plantar nerves, which extend toward the foot, and a calcaneal or sensory branch, which provides sensation to the heel. Both plantar nerves then cross under the abductor hallucis muscle (which the medial plantar nerve innervates) and go on to innervate all the muscles of the sole of the foot as well as providing sensation to the sole of the foot and the toes (the medial nerve supplies the medial portion and the lateral nerve supplies the lateral portion) through their distal divisions, which give rise to the digital nerves. Muscles innervated by the medial plantar nerve include the flexor hallucis brevis and digitorum brevis. The lateral plantar nerve innervates the interossei, the flexor and abductor digiti minimi, and the adductor hallucis.

1. **Etiology.** The close proximity of the plantar nerves to osseous and fibrous structures results in their injury or compression as a direct result of disorders of those structures. At the level of the tarsal tunnel, external compression and ankle injury are the most frequent etiologies. A multitude of other less frequent structural abnormalities (i.e., synovial or joint changes and mass lesions) can also lead to nerve injury. Within the foot itself, the medial

and lateral plantar nerves are again susceptible to the effects of trauma or fracture of the foot bones.

2. **Clinical manifestations**
   a. **History.** The first recognition of disorder of these nerves occurs when sensory impairment develops, because foot pain or discomfort more frequently has an orthopedic origin. Sensory loss can be present in the sole and/or heel of the foot and at times can be precipitated by specific foot positions. Weakness of foot muscles usually produces no significant symptoms.
   b. **Physical examination**
      (1) **Neurologic.** Sensory loss in the distribution of the plantar nerves or their distal divisions (digital nerves) should be sought. If foot involvement is asymmetric, changes in foot muscle bulk may be appreciated, as can weakness, although usually only toe flexion can be reliably evaluated clinically.
      (2) **General.** Careful examination of the course of the nerve at the ankle and attempts to elicit a Tinel's sign by light percussion over its course help confirm the presence of a plantar neuropathy. Joint changes, deformity, or swelling may also help determine a site of nerve involvement.

3. **Differential diagnosis.** Here one needs to consider more proximal nerve (tibial) or root (S1) lesions that may also cause foot pain or paresthesias. Motor and reflex changes should aid in this distinction. Although polyneuropathies may enter into the differential, bilaterality, distal reflex depression, and sensory involvement of more than the plantar sensory nerve distribution should aid in the differential.

4. **Evaluation**
   a. **Electrodiagnostic studies** are helpful in demonstrating findings consistent with nerve entrapment (tarsal tunnel) and the sensory or motor changes that can be expected with involvement of medial or lateral plantar as well as calcaneal nerves. Because of the nature of such recordings, further study of asymptomatic or contralateral nerves is sometimes necessary for clear interpretation of electrodiagnostic findings. Once again, EMG may be needed to exclude more proximal difficulties (tibial neuropathies, sciatic neuropathies, or radiculopathies).
   b. **Imaging.** Studies of potential sites of involvement (ankle) are not usually indicated. However, in cases of significant discomfort or disability, such studies can identify orthopedic or joint abnormalities and guide their treatment.

H. **Iliohypogastric, ilioinguinal, and genitofemoral neuropathies.** We review the iliohypogastric, ilioinguinal, and genitofemoral nerves as a group because of the similarity of their origins, sites of innervation, and causes of dysfunction. These nerves arise from the L1 spinal roots (the genitofemoral nerve also has an L2 root contribution) and first pass through and then in close proximity to the psoas muscle in their intra-abdominal course. The iliohypogastric nerve emerges above the iliac crest and supplies sensation to an area of skin of the upper buttock and another near the pubis. The ilioinguinal nerve enters the inguinal canal at its lateral border and supplies the area above the inguinal ligament and the base of the genitalia. Both the iliohypogastric and ilioinguinal nerves also supply the muscles of the lower abdominal area. After the genitofemoral nerve emerges from the psoas muscle, it lies retroperitoneal and descends to the inguinal ligament while resting on the surface of the psoas. It supplies sensation to a small area over the proximal genitalia and anterior proximal thigh.

1. **Etiology.** Because of their location and course, neuropathies of these nerves are usually results of surgical procedures—especially inguinal herniorrhaphy. The development of neuralgias is also a not infrequent occurrence after injuries of these nerves.

2. **Clinical manifestations**
   a. **History.** Patients present with varying sensory complaints, including numbness, paresthesias, or pain within the ipsilateral inguinal and perineal areas. If the cause is related to surgery, these difficulties may be evident immediately following surgery or may not become evident for several weeks.

b. Physical examination
  (1) Neurologic. Iliohypogastric neuropathies are infrequent. They cause sensory loss over the suprapubic and upper buttock areas. Ilioinguinal impairments result in sensory loss over the inguinal area and the base of the genitalia, but typically resolve or result in minimal disability. In other cases, pain may appear both here and in the inferior abdomen and upper thigh and be worsened or precipitated by changes in leg position. Genitofemoral neuropathies usually accompany inguinal nerve involvement because of the close anatomic proximity of the genitofemoral and inguinal nerves. Symptoms and precipitating factors are similar as well, but sensory complaints may extend into the medial and proximal areas of the genitalia.
  (2) General. In ilioinguinal and genitofemoral neuropathies, areas of tenderness that often conform to the site of injury may be found in the inguinal region.
3. Differential diagnosis. In these cases, nerve involvement predominantly causes sensory impairment, and the differential diagnosis is directed at detecting other causes of sensory impairment outside the typical boundaries of these nerves, including abnormalities in the medial thigh (obturator nerve), anterior thigh (femoral nerve), and lateral thigh (lateral femoral cutaneous nerve), as well as dermatomal involvement caused by T12 or L1 radiculopathies. Because of these overlapping sensory innervations, the presence of motor deficits or reflex changes provides the strongest clue to the presence of one of these other disorders. Back pain, which may suggest a radiculopathy, or the absence of a prior operative procedure, which is the usual cause of such neuropathies, suggests another etiology.
4. Evaluation
  a. Electrodiagnostic studies play little role in the identification of these neuropathies. However, they become indispensable in helping to identify either more proximal lesions (i.e., plexus or root) or other neuropathies (femoral) that may clinically resemble these neuropathies in regard to sensory innervation.
  b. Imaging is employed only if there is suspicion of a radiculopathy or if a retroperitoneal, intra-abdominal, or pelvic lesion is suspected as a cause of the sensory symptoms.
I. Miscellaneous neuropathies. For the sake of completeness, the following nerves are briefly discussed. This grouping is based on both the infrequent occurrence of such neuropathies and the infrequency of isolated involvement of these nerves.
  1. Superior gluteal neuropathy. Arising from, and receiving its contributions from the L4-S1 components of, the sacral plexus, the superior gluteal nerve passes through the sciatic notch above the piriformis and innervates the gluteus medius and minimus. Its isolated involvement is unusual and is most often the result of an injury by a misplaced injection.
  2. Inferior gluteal neuropathy. The inferior gluteal nerve arises from the L5-S2 divisions of the sacral plexus and also exits through the sciatic notch. Its close proximity to the sciatic, pudendal, and posterior cutaneous nerves of the thigh results in their concomitant injury.
  3. Neuropathy of the posterior cutaneous nerve of the thigh. Arising from the S1-S3 components of the sacral plexus, the posterior cutaneous nerve of the thigh descends through the sciatic notch in close proximity to the sciatic nerve and supplies sensation to the posterior portion of the buttock and thigh. At times it is susceptible to local compression, but its isolated involvement is unusual.
  4. Pudendal neuropathy. Derived from the S2-S4 components of the sacral plexus, the pudendal nerve passes through the sciatic notch and then descends toward the perineum. Supplying muscles of the perineum, including the anal sphincter and erectile tissue, it also provides sensory innervation to the perineum. Its deep location provides it with significant protection, but prolonged compression can cause its dysfunction. Dysfunctions attributable to stretch injuries and related to prolonged labor may also occur, presenting with fecal and urinary incontinence.
III. Referral
  A. Indications for and purposes of neurologic consultation

1. Site of involvement unclear from examination or history
2. Identification of a diffuse disorder without a clear etiology or with a discrepancy between the severity of the underlying disease and the neuropathy
3. Progressive deterioration despite appropriate treatment
4. Problem precipitated by trauma or injury
5. Prior to embarking on a more costly or invasive evaluation (MRI imaging or nerve biopsy) or recommending a more aggressive intervention (surgery)
6. Confirmation of a diagnosis, etiology, and treatment plan
   B. EMG and NCS evaluation
   1. Basic tenets of such testing
   a. Testing is an extension of the clinical examination and not a replacement for a careful history and examination.
   b. Testing is intended to clarify the clinical question to be answered or addressed (i.e., carpal tunnel syndrome or a C6 radiculopathy).
   c. Sensitivity and specificity vary according to the etiology and process in question.
   2. Role in the evaluation of neuropathies
   a. Confirmation of diagnosis/characterization, localization, and quantification of a disease process
   b. Prognostication
   c. Detection of subclinical disease
   d. Planning of treatment or determination of the necessity for further evaluation or consultation

Recommended Readings

Brazis PW, Masdeu JC, Biller J. *Localization in Clinical Neurology* (3rd ed). Boston: Little, Brown, 1996.

Dawson DM, Hallet M, Millender LH. *Entrapment Neuropathies* (2nd ed). Boston: Little, Brown, 1990.

Medical Research Council of the U.K. *Aids to the Examination of the Peripheral Nervous System*. London: Baillière Tindall, 1986.

Mumenthaler M, Schliak H (eds). *Peripheral Nerve Lesions: Diagnosis and Therapy*. Stuttgart: Thieme, 1991.

Pećina MM, Krmpotić-Nemanić J, Markiewitz AD. *Tunnel Syndromes*. Boca Raton, FL: CRC, 1991.

Stewart JD. *Focal Peripheral Neuropathies* (2nd ed). New York: Raven, 1993.

26 Approach to the Patient with Failed Back Syndrome

Randall L. Braddom

Having at least one episode of low back pain (LBP) is practically universal in humans. It is estimated that approximately 20% of the population experience back pain annually, with a lifetime incidence of 60–90%. LBP can be acute or chronic. It can be so simple that it doesn't even require formal treatment. It can also be so severe and complex that it can devastate a patient's entire life. One of the most clinically challenging groups of back pain patients is those with **failed back syndrome (FBS).** For the purposes of this chapter, FBS is defined as back pain that persists to a chronic stage, regardless of the etiology and regardless of whether or not the patient has had surgery. The term "chronic" in this chapter refers to back pain that is not a result of cancer and that either persists longer than the typical time it takes for natural or postsurgical healing to occur or otherwise lasts longer than 6 months.

I. **Evaluation of the patient with failed back syndrome.** The most critical factor in helping patients with FBS is an efficient, cost-effective, and accurate evaluation. An inadequate evaluation leads to a less specific diagnosis. The less specific the diagnosis, the less treatment and the less likely the treatment is to work. Just about every available piece of information about the patient has to be factored into the final diagnosis, including the history, physical examination, psychosocial status, work status, current stressors, and whether or not compensation or secondary gain is a factor. Making the wrong diagnosis or providing the wrong treatment can greatly complicate the care of a patient with FBS. An inadequate history and physical can also result in inappropriate repetition of expensive medical tests.

A. **Back versus nonback causes of back pain.** The first step in evaluating the patient is to make sure that the LBP actually originates in the back and is not just being referred to the spine. Common abdominal problems that can present as back pain include penetrating peptic ulcer, cholelithiasis, cholecystitis, and aortic aneurysm. Malignancies of abdominal organs can also refer pain to the spine, as in the case of carcinoma of the head of the pancreas. Renal problems, including pyelonephritis and renal lithiasis, can cause flank and back pain. Retroperitoneal bleeding and neoplasms of many types also can cause back pain. Pelvic problems that are known to produce back pain symptoms include prostatitis and endometriosis. It is controversial whether or not other gynecologic problems (such as retroverted uterus) cause back pain. Even the best clinicians occasionally mistake a nonback cause of back pain for a spinal cause. Careful attention to the history and physical examination can reduce, but not completely eliminate, the tendency to make this clinical error.

1. **Rule out abdominal problems** that could cause referred back pain. Do a careful history and physical, and obtain appropriate laboratory studies. Imaging studies such as ultrasound, CT, and MRI can also be helpful in ruling out abdominal or pelvic pathology.

2. **Rule out pelvic and urologic problems** that can refer pain to the back. Rectal and vaginal examinations are particularly helpful.

3. **Rule out hip disease** referring pain to the back. Patients with severe osteoarthritis or aseptic necrosis of the hip can have referred pain to the back. The patient with hip disease rarely has only back pain, with no hip pain.

B. **Benign versus malignant cases.** Once it has been established that the back pain is not a result of a problem outside the back, the next step is to separate the patients into two categories: those with serious (progressive or life-threatening) causes of back pain and those with less serious causes. These two types of LBP are often referred to, respectively, as "malignant" and "benign" (with "malignant" being used beyond its usual sense—i.e., cancer). The most important practice is to look for "red flags."

1. **Fever** is a red flag in patients with LBP and can indicate the presence of infection such as osteomyelitis or diskitis, cancer of the spine or neighboring structures, collagen-vascular disorders, or other problems that require immediate attention.

2. **Pain that is worse when lying down** is a red flag and can indicate the presence of primary or metastatic cancer of the spine. Almost all types of back problems are less painful lying down, but cancer pain is the exception in that it is often worse lying down than in any other position.

3. **History of cancer** in a patient with back pain is a red flag and requires an evaluation to make certain that the cancer is not metastatic to the spine. The chance that the back pain represents a metastasis depends on the type of primary tumor. Bone scans are often a cost-effective way of ruling out bony metastasis. Patients who have had cancer in the past often neglect to mention it in the history, and you have to specifically quiz them about it. Some types of cancer, such as breast cancer, can metastasize to the spine a decade or more after the primary tumor was thought to have been eradicated.

4. **Generalized joint or soft tissue involvement** is a red flag and is observed in patients with collagen-vascular diseases. In these cases, the back pain represents only one part of a much larger syndrome. Such a patient requires treatment of the specific disease in addition to treatment of the back pain. If the history is suggestive of a collagen-vascular disease, an appropriate laboratory work-up should be done (such as ANA, sedimentation rate, rheumatoid factor, uric acid, synovial fluid analysis, etc.).

C. **Neurologic versus non-neurologic cases.** The next step in the evaluation process is to divide the patients into those with and without neurologic involvement (weakness, numbness, loss of reflexes, etc.). Cases having no neurologic dysfunction are typically purely musculoskeletal in nature. The prognosis and the nature of the treatment change dramatically when a neurologic deficit is present. The clinician has several tools to help make this distinction, as outlined below.

1. **History.** The history provides 80% of the diagnosis. If you can't diagnose the patient's back pain from the history, you probably have only a 20% chance of doing so from the physical examination and from imaging and laboratory tests. Some of the most important history questions are listed in Table 26-1.

2. **Evaluating strength.** One of the most important aspects of the physical examination is the assessment of the patient's strength.

   a. **Gait and functional testing.** Strength can often be inferred from observing the patient walk, as well as from such functional tests as walking on the heels, walking on the toes, and doing deep knee bends. Patients with weakness in the L5-innervated muscles typically have difficulty walking on their heels. Patients with weakness in the S1-innervated muscles often have difficulty walking on their toes. The latter test can be increased in sensitivity by having the patient stand only on the affected leg and then do 10–15 toe rises. The ability of the patient to do this on the affected side can be compared with the ability to do the same thing on the opposite side.

   b. **"Make and break" strength testing.** Although functional tests often give clues about strength, it is also usually necessary to test strength using manual muscle tests. Manual muscle testing uses the "make and break" system, in which the patient is asked to "make" one or more muscles do what they normally do and then the clinician attempts to "break" that position. For example, the elbow flexors can be tested by having the patient flex the elbow and then manually attempting to overcome the elbow flexors and forcibly extend the elbow. A numerical system is used to grade strength, with 5/5 indicating normal strength and 0/5 indicating a complete absence of muscle function.

   c. **Pitfalls in assessing strength.** There are many pitfalls in assessing strength. What appears to be visible muscle atrophy can at times be only a loss of subcutaneous fat (which can occur secondary to multiple injections or prolonged pressure). Pain inhibition of function can cause patients to appear to have weakness when they really have pain that prevents them from performing the muscle test. True strength cannot be

Table 26-1. Important history questions for patients with failed back syndrome.

Temporal factors
  How long since onset?
  Pain constant or intermittent?
  Time of day the pain occurs/worsens?
Had same problem in the past?
Sudden or gradual onset?
Trauma involved?
Character of the pain
  Burning, throbbing, aching, stabbing, etc.
  Severity of the pain
  Location of the pain
Exact location?
  Areas of radiation?
Position effects on the pain
  Worse standing, lying, sitting?
  Any change in position that makes it better?
Movement effects on the pain
  Better with movement?
  Worse with specific type of movement?
  Effect of coughing, sneezing
Environmental site of the pain
  Worse at work?
  Worse at home?
  Worse while driving?
Family history of back problems
Neurologic changes?
  Loss of sensation, strength?
  Loss of bowel, bladder, sexual function?
Current stressors?
Results of treatment to date?
Secondary gain factors?
Course (episodic, progressive, decreasing, fluctuating)?
History of cancer?
History of immunosuppression?
Presence of fever?
History of urinary tract infection?
Unexplained weight loss?

reliably assessed if the patient is unable or unwilling, because of pain or other factors, to give maximal muscle effort. Some patients consciously or unconsciously attempt to appear weak. This usually shows up as an obvious lack of effort on the manual muscle test, or as a "ratchety response" to muscle strength testing. It can also be detected as inconsistencies between the results of the manual muscle test and what is observed functionally. For example, a patient might claim to be unable to dorsiflex the foot during manual muscle strength testing and yet exhibit a normal heel strike and no foot drop or slap when walking. Patients are deemed to be "malingering" if they are consciously trying to appear to have weakness. Factitious weakness produced unconsciously by a patient is said to be a conversion reaction or hysterical paralysis. It is frequently difficult to distinguish between malingering and hysterical weakness, and sometimes a patient can have both.

  d. Assessing strength in radiculopathy
    (1) L5 is the most common radiculopathy level, and typically produces weakness in the anterior tibial, peroneus longus and brevis, posterior tibial, extensor digitorum longus and brevis, and extensor hallucis longus muscles. All of these muscles are located in the leg, except for the extensor digitorum brevis (EDB), which is located on the dorsum of the foot. (The EDB is the only intrinsic muscle of the foot that is innervated mainly at L5 and by the peroneal nerve.) The EDB is frequently injured by shoe trauma, and so weakness, atro-

phy, or electromyographic (EMG) changes observed only in the EDB must be interpreted with caution. Patients with L5 radiculopathy and weakness typically have a foot drop or slap. Some patients do not have a foot drop because the anterior tibial muscle (the one most involved in preventing a foot drop or slap) is innervated in some individuals mainly at L4. Although the hamstring muscles and the gluteus medius muscles have mainly L5 innervation, they typically are not as likely to show weakness in L5 radiculopathy as the more distal muscles noted above. Testing these muscles is still important, however, because finding weakness in the gluteus medius rules out a problem that is purely in the sciatic or the peroneal nerve, making the diagnosis of L5 radiculopathy more likely.

(2) **S1** is the second most common lumbosacral level of radiculopathy. Weakness that can result from S1 radiculopathy is often more difficult to detect than weakness in the muscles involved in L5 radiculopathy, mainly because of the inherent strength of the gluteus maximus and the gastrocsoleus complex. These muscles are so strong that relatively mild losses in strength are difficult to detect clinically. An EMG frequently shows abnormal muscle membrane irritability in the gastrocnemius, soleus, or gluteus maximus muscle when the physical examination shows no clinically evident weakness.

(3) **L4** is the third most common level of lumbosacral radiculopathy. L4 radiculopathy typically causes weakness of the quadriceps group and the hip adductor group. Some patients also have weakness of the anterior tibial muscle (this muscle is innervated by L4 and L5 levels, and the degree of innervation from each level varies from person to person).

3. **Evaluating gait.** Patients with low back pain frequently have abnormal gaits. This can result from either pain or weakness, but pain is the most common cause of abnormal gait in LBP cases.

   a. **Pain** can produce an abnormal walking pattern that is referred to as an "antalgic" gait. It represents a patient's attempt to avoid exacerbating pain during walking. Some of the most common manifestations of an antalgic gait include taking short steps on the affected side, holding the back stiffly in a specific position, or walking slowly and tentatively as if "walking on eggs."

   b. **Weakness** of the anterolateral muscles of the leg can result in a foot drop or slap gait. Patients often unconsciously compensate for a foot drop with a steppage gait in which the knee is raised higher during the swing phase of the gait to help clear the plantarflexed foot. They might also use vaulting to help clear the foot during the swing phase. Vaulting occurs when the patient goes up on the toes of the contralateral side during its stance phase in order to help clear the opposite leg during its swing phase. Severe L5 level weakness can affect the gluteus medius muscle, resulting in a drop of the contralateral pelvis on stance phase (Trendelenburg gait). Patients usually learn to compensate for this by leaning to the side of the affected limb during the stance phase of the gait (referred to as a compensated Trendelenburg gait). Patients with relatively severe weakness in the S1 muscles can exhibit a "weak calf limp," which is noted mainly at toe-off on the affected side. They can also lean back at the waist during the stance phase of the gait to avoid having the trunk fall forward as a result of a weak gluteus maximus.

4. **Sensory changes.** During the history, the patient's description of any sensory changes should be noted. Reproducible sensory changes should be outlined on the skin with a suitable marker. The modalities tested should be the typical ones of hot/cold, vibration, light touch, sharp/dull, and others as appropriate.

   Pitfalls in sensory testing include failing to document the specific area of sensory loss and confusing "real" or neurologic sensory change with "sclerotomal reference." Any soft tissue can refer pain or other sensations, but the pattern of this referral is not truly dermatomal. Dermatomal reference of pain or sensory change is typically observed in nerve injury such as radiculopathy. If the patient has a muscle strain or ligamentous strain in the low back, there can be referral of pain or unusual sensations into the lower limb. These sclerotomal reference sensations are not indicative of neurologic change or deficit and must be differentiated clinically from dermatomal references.

5. Reflexes

a. Muscle stretch reflexes (MSRs) should be assessed in every patient with LBP. The reflexes should be assessed for their symmetry, because radiculopathy is usually unilateral. Unfortunately, the most common radiculopathy (L5) has no reliable MSR. Some have touted the medial hamstring reflex for the L5 level, but it is not always reliable because some patients with obvious unilateral L5 radiculopathy do not have asymmetry of their medial hamstring reflexes. The S1 radiculopathy level can be assessed with the Achilles reflex (ankle jerk). The L4 radiculopathy level can be assessed with the patellar response (quadriceps muscles).

b. Normal superficial reflexes can also be used at times to assist in determining the level of radiculopathy. The cremasteric reflex is tested by scratching the proximal medial thigh and watching the ipsilateral testicle elevate. This helps check the L1 and L2 nerve-root levels. The rectal sphincter contracts if the skin around the anus is scratched, which checks levels S2, S3, and S4. If this reflex is simply observed, it is referred to as the anal wink reflex, and if it is elicited by palpation with a gloved finger in the anus, it is referred to as the anal reflex. The bulbocavernosus reflex can be used to check the S2, S3, and S4 levels. It is done by placing a gloved finger in the anus and then squeezing the glans penis. The normal response is rectal contraction. It is theoretically possible to elicit a clitorocavernosus reflex in women, although this is not commonly done. As an alternative in women, pulling the pubic hair causes a similar contraction of the anus. The plantar reflex that occurs when the lateral aspect of the sole of the foot is scratched provides a means of checking the S2, S3, and S4 root levels.

6. Palpation is felt by many to be the single most important aspect of the physical examination. The patient must undress sufficient to permit palpation of the entire low back, the buttocks, and the lower limbs. The palpation should identify areas of tenderness, trigger or tender points, areas of ropy muscle consistency, and areas of muscle atrophy.

7. Sciatic and femoral nerve stretch tests are among the most important means of identifying radiculopathy. Both the L5 and S1 roots are attached to the sciatic nerve. If these nerve roots are inflamed or irritable for any reason, stretching the sciatic nerve creates tension on them and elicits pain. The most commonly used sciatic nerve stretch tests are listed in Table 26-2.

The femoral nerve is attached to lumbar roots 2, 3, and 4. If any of these nerve roots is irritated or inflamed, stretching the femoral nerve causes pain. L4 radiculopathy typically gives a positive femoral nerve stretch test. The most common way to perform this stretch test is to have the patient lie supine and then flex the knee while attempting to place the heel on the buttock.

8. Assessing bowel, bladder, and sexual functions. The patient should be asked about recent changes in bladder, bowel, or sexual function. This is important because, for example, it is possible for a patient with an L5-S1 disk central herniation to have an isolated cauda equina syndrome that affects only the S2-S4 roots and produces only bowel, bladder, and sexual dysfunction. In this case, sensation and muscle strength in the lower extremities are normal.

9. Assessment for long tract signs should be done in every patient with neck or back pain. A spinal problem that encroaches on the spinal cord typically produces such long tract signs as loss of strength, loss of coordination, loss of sensation, and abnormal reflexes. These abnormal reflexes include Babinski's, Chaddock's, and Stranski's reflexes. Bowel, bladder, and sexual dysfunction can also be caused by spinal cord involvement. Because the spinal cord ends at the second lumbar vertebra level in adults, most low back problems typically do not produce spinal cord injury, but can cause cauda equina dysfunction.

D. The role of imaging studies in failed back syndrome. Radiographs and

Table 26-2. Sciatic stretch testing maneuvers and clinical signs.

Lasègue: This is also known as straight leg raising or SLR sign. Test maneuver is to slowly lift the patient's affected lower limb with the knee extended, while the patient is supine. Sign is positive if patient complains of pain in the low back radiating down the affected extremity. The sign is usually positive between 10 and 60 degrees of hip flexion. Don't confuse hamstring tightness with a positive straight leg raising sign, as pain induced by stretching the hamstring occurs frequently in normals beyond 60 degrees of hip flexion.

Braggard: The test maneuver is the same as for the SLR sign above. However, when the patient complains of pain in the lower extremity, lower the limb a few degrees until the pain stops, then dorsiflex the foot. The sign is positive if foot dorsiflexion reproduces the pain.

Bechterew: This is also known as the Flip Test. The test maneuver is to slowly raise the patient's leg while the patient is in the sitting position until the hip is at 90 degrees of flexion and the knee is fully extended. A positive sign is when low back and lower extremity pain occur.

Neri: Also known as the Buckle Sign. The test maneuver is to have the standing patient flex at the waist as if to touch the toes. A positive sign is when the knee of the affected side bends (or buckles).

Fajersztajn: This is also known as the Crossed Straight Leg Raising Sign. Test maneuver is to do the SLR sign as noted above on the unaffected lower limb. A positive sign is when raising the unaffected lower limb produces pain on the opposite (affected) side in the low back and lower limb.

Bonnets: Test maneuver is to flex the patient's hip and knee on the affected side with the patient supine. Then when the knee is as close to the chest as possible, adduct the hip. A positive sign is when pain occurs in the low back and affected lower limb.

Linder: Test maneuver is for the patient to actively extend the legs while sitting, then flex the neck. A positive sign is when the patient complains of pain or increased pain in the low back and affected lower limb.

Short step sign: Test maneuver is for the patient to walk. A positive sign is when the patient can take only a short step on the affected side (Braddom).

imaging studies are valuable for patients with back pain in general and also for patients with FBS. It should be remembered, however, that these studies represent only anatomy. There is no direct correlation between the anatomy of the back structures and what is occurring clinically. These studies are mere "shadows of reality" in the sense that they do not relate physiologic information. When FBS patients first present, they typically have already had numerous x-rays and imaging studies. It is usually sufficient in these cases to review all of the old films rather than to repeat the studies.

1. **False-positives.** Radiographs and images can show false-positives and false-negatives, with false-positive results being more common. For example, the degenerative changes of osteoarthritis and disk disease are common in plain films and MRIs of patients over 60 years of age, whether or not they have any back pain. CT and MRI scans done for other problems often show herniated or bulging disks in patients who have no back symptoms. Bulging disks are now known to be normal findings.
2. **Plain films** can be used to help identify fractures, malignancies, arthritis, congenital or acquired defects, and evidence of spinal instability.
3. **CT scanning** usually provides only axial images, although some newer equipment also provides sagittal views. It is excellent for bone detail as well as for detecting disk herniation with lumbosacral radiculopathy. CT plus myelography has replaced myelography as the gold standard for diagnosing herniated-disk-related radiculopathy.
4. **MRI scanning** is excellent for diagnosing herniated disks and provides sagittal views. MRI is an excellent imager of soft tissues, especially when combined with such contrast agents as gadolinium. For example, postsurgical MRI can be used in a case of back pain to determine if a nerve root is encased in scar tissue.
E. **Electrodiagnosis and the failed back syndrome.** Electromyography (EMG) and other electrodiagnostic studies are very helpful in evaluation of any patient suspected of having radiculopathy. Electrodiagnosis provides physiologic rather than anatomic information and in the proper hands presents few false-

positives. Because it reflects the actual physiology of the problem, it is often more useful than imaging studies in the diagnosis of radiculopathy.

1. **Limitations of electromyography.** It should be kept in mind that EMG detects only lower motor neuron and motor unit dysfunctions. EMG results cannot be expected to be abnormal in cases of upper motor neuron problems or back pain in which there is no neurologic dysfunction. Because it is a purely motor study, EMG can give false-negative results in cases of purely sensory radiculopathy. There are special problems in interpreting electrodiagnostic results for patients who have had one or more back surgeries. The surgical trauma itself can induce EMG changes in the paraspinal muscles. In these cases the EMG findings are most easily interpreted if preoperative studies are available for comparison.

2. **H reflex.** Special electrodiagnostic studies such as H reflex testing can increase diagnostic accuracy in cases of lumbosacral radiculopathy, especially at the S1 level. The H reflex uses the same pathway as the muscle stretch reflex, and it can be electronically timed across its sensory and motor pathways.

F. **Assessing risk factors in failed back syndrome.** There are clearly some types of individuals and some occupational groups who are more at risk for developing back pain than others. These individuals are also more at risk for developing the failed back syndrome. The risk factors most commonly cited in the literature include being white, increasing age up to age 55, living in a western state, smoking, prolonged driving of a motor vehicle, working at a job that requires heavy exertion, being under psychological stress, having osteoporosis, having a history of previous back injury, and being very obese. Although many of these risk factors cannot be changed, some can be eliminated or at least modified. Smoking is known to facilitate osteoporosis, which could partly explain its effect on the incidence of low back pain. It might also be a factor in that it serves as a marker for other unhealthy traits, such as lack of exercise, that can lead to back problems. It is somewhat puzzling that being white is a factor in back pain, but this could relate to some extent to the fact that osteoporosis is more common in whites. Anthropomorphic factors are not, however, as important in causing back pain as formerly thought. For example, obesity has to be almost morbid before it clearly increases the incidence of LBP.

G. **Assessing the psychogenic contribution to failed back syndrome.** Low back pain can be associated with psychological dysfunction, exaggeration of symptoms, and stressors in daily life. It is often difficult to determine which came first, the back pain or the psychological dysfunction. Depression, anxiety, and stress can exacerbate or even induce pain.

1. **Psychological tests for evaluation of failed back syndrome** patients commonly include the Minnesota Multiphasic Personality Inventory (MMPI), the Beck Depression Inventory, the Ransford Pain Drawing, the Hendler (Mensana) Back Pain Test, the Modified Somatic Perception Questionnaire, the McGill Pain Questionnaire, the Million Visual Analog Scale, the Dallas Pain Questionnaire, and the Oswestry Low Back Pain Disability Questionnaire. These and similar tests can be used to evaluate patients with FBS. A psychologist experienced in chronic pain cases often can provide valuable assistance in the interpretation of these tests or do a more general assessment of the patient's current mental status and personality. It is foolhardy for a surgeon to consider doing back surgery on an FBS patient without first obtaining some psychological data. A psychologist using such tests as the MMPI can usually predict whether a patient will be able to return to work after surgery more accurately than a surgeon who knows all the patient's physical data.

Table 26-3. Johnson's signs of hysterical weakness.

Slow motion
Exaggeration
Inconsistency
Ratchety response to muscle testing
"La belle indifference" for hysterical weakness, but appearance of great worry, concern, or
   even anger for malingering.

> **2. Signs of psychogenic involvement**
> > **a. Johnson's signs,** outlined in Table 26-3, represent the common findings in conscious (malingering) and unconscious (conversion reaction/hysteria) attempts by patients to appear weaker than they are or to have problems worse than those indicated by the clinical findings. Differentiating conscious from unconscious attempts to appear weak is difficult. One of the best differentiating signs is how upset patients are about their problems. In general, those with conversion reactions are relatively calm about their problems (the so-called "la belle indifference"), whereas those with conscious motives are typically animated (even hostile) and often "demand" services, procedures, diagnoses, and compensation. Unfortunately, there are a fair number of patients who appear to have a mixture of conscious and unconscious motivations to exaggerate their back pain. Understanding the psychogenic involvement is necessary not so much to assess blame, but to design an appropriate treatment strategy.
> > **b. Waddell's signs** of potential nonorganic involvement are listed in Table 26-4. Additional signs of potential nonorganic involvement are presented in Table 26-5.
>
> **II. Chronic pain versus chronic pain syndrome.** The next step in managing patients with FBS is to separate them into two broad pain categories that require vastly different treatments. One category is patients who have only chronic back pain and are otherwise leading essentially normal lives. The other category is patients who have developed an entire behavioral constellation of symptoms, characterized by excessive pain behavior, known as chronic pain syndrome (Table 26-6).
>
> **A. Chronic pain syndrome (CPS)** affects a patient's entire life. CPS patients often have depressed mood, sleep disturbances, somatic preoccupation, and reduced activity. They frequently also have reduced libido, fatigue, excessive use of drugs or alcohol, dependency on others, and secondary gain. Their disabilities are typically out of proportion to their impairments.
>
> **B.** CPS involves **learned pain behaviors.** Pain behaviors usually include grimacing, moaning, limping, rubbing a painful part, splinting, guarding, immobilization of a part, slow motion, bizarre gait, and ratchety response to muscle testing. Other items listed in Tables 26-3 and 26-4 (Johnson's and Waddell's signs)

Table 26-4. Waddell's nonorganic signs (three or more are significant).

Palpation tenderness: Widespread and nonanatomic, and tenderness to light touch.
Simulation tests: Painful motion is mimicked but not performed. Can be brought out by axial loading and rotation tests.
Distraction: Straight leg raising in the sitting position.
Regional disturbances: Weakness is nonorganic in its distribution and sensory loss is a stocking and glove pattern.
Overreaction: Excessive verbalization, grimacing, collapsing, and theatrics.

Table 26-5. Additional signs of psychogenic involvement in low back pain.

The "Everywheres"
Patient complains of pain or dysfunction in many or all body systems.
Clue here is that review of systems takes forever.

Multiple Doctor/Surgery Sign
Patient has pattern of "doctor shopping."
Patient complains about all previous physicians, but says "but I've heard so many nice things about you."

Straw that Broke the Camel's Back Syndrome
Patients who are at the end of their psychological rope have onset of minor back problems, which push them "over the edge" and they often never recover.
Observed most commonly in worker's compensation cases

High Ratio of Complaints to Findings Sign

Unusual Pain Drawing Sign

Table 26-6. Sternbach's six D's of chronic pain syndrome and their suggested treatment interventions.

Finding	Goal	Interventions
Dramatization of complaints	Reduce pain behavior; increase wellness behavior	Operant learning; eliminate reinforcement contingencies; inattention to pain behavior; reinforcement of well behavior
Drug misuse	Eliminate inappropriate medications	Detoxification; use medication logs; use pain cocktails to withdraw medications; time-contingent drug schedule
Dysfunction/disuse	Resume proper body mechanics and endurance	Remove unnecessary orthoses; proper nutrition; increase activity, strength, endurance, flexibility; pacing and quotas
Dependency	Reduce dependency on caregiver and health-care system	Cognitive therapy; self-management skills— relaxation, time management, assertiveness, anger management, stress management; counsel caregivers who enable dependency
Depression	Reduce depression; increase self-esteem, self-care, skills, activity level	Increase activity; fun socializing; counseling; psychotropic drugs
Disability	Back to work or substitute avocation	Vocational assessment; vocational counseling; physical capacity evaluation; work simulation; work training; work hardening

can also represent pain behaviors. Additional pain behaviors can include staying home from work, taking analgesic medications, voicing vivid descriptions of the pain, and seeking compensation.

C. Pain behavior does not require a **noxious stimulus.** CPS is usually initiated by a noxious stimulus. The pain behavior is then rewarded either externally by the patient's environment or internally by the patient's psyche. The pain behavior is thus reinforced and can now occur in the absence of a noxious stimulus.

   1. **External CPS reinforcers** include compensation, staying home from work, overzealous caretaking, prescription of medications, socialization with physicians, and attention from friends and relatives.

   2. **Internal CPS reinforcers** include relief from guilt, relief from fears of work, sex, and responsibility, and more pain.

D. CPS is more likely to occur in patients with certain **psychological syndromes** such as major depression, dysthymic disorder, somatization disorder, conversion disorder, and hypochondriasis. It should be differentiated from purely psychogenic pain. For patients with psychogenic pain, the pain typically occurs in multiple locations at different times, has been present fairly continuously since adolescence, and occurs without an evident somatic cause. Like CPS patients, those with psychogenic pain may have histories of abusive parents or spouses, multiple surgical procedures, alcohol or drug abuse (by patient or spouse), and frequent failures in jobs and in social life.

III. **Common causative factors in failed back syndrome.** A recent study (Long et al.; see Recommended Readings) of 1541 patients admitted to the Johns Hopkins Pain Treatment Program showed that two-thirds suffered from back pain. The typical back pain patient had undergone three spine operations and six myelograms, and was misusing medications. These authors were able to identify 78 patients out of this group for whom records and work-ups were sufficiently complete to allow in-depth studies of their cases. The following information, which is useful in managing FBS patients, was drawn from this study.

   A. **Psychiatric diagnoses** were common in this group of 78 patients.

   1. **Normal prepain personality** was found in only 34 of the 78 patients.

   2. **Maladaptive personality disorders** were found in 34 of the 78 patients.

   3. **Reactive depression** was observed in 67 of the 78 patients.

   4. **Definitive serious psychiatric diagnoses** could be made in 10 of the 78 patients.

B. A **wide range of diagnoses** was observed in this group of 78 patients.
   1. **Normal examinations** with no diagnoses were recorded in 16 of the 78 patients.
   2. **Minor spondylitic or postoperative changes** were observed in 16 of the 78 patients.
   3. **Epidural scarring** was present in 11 of the 78 patients.
   4. **Arachnoiditis** was felt to be causative in 10 of the 78 patients.
   5. **Other diagnoses,** in declining order of frequency, were traumatic neuritis, severe spondylosis, spinal stenosis, cancer, musculoskeletal abnormality, compression fracture, traumatic meningocele, lateral foraminal stenosis, tarsal tunnel syndrome, fractured hip, scoliosis, and disk herniation. In only 6 of the 78 patients was a new diagnosis established by the pain team.

C. **Surgery** was not indicated in most cases. Whether the patient had indications for surgery was assessed using the criteria of the American Association of Neurological Surgeons and the American Academy of Orthopedic Surgeons.
   1. **Clinical criteria for the first surgery** were met in only 25 of the 78 patients.
   2. **Clinical criteria for the second surgery** were met in only 18 of the 78 patients.
   3. The **most common justification for the third or subsequent surgeries** was treatment of ill effects of earlier surgeries, including arachnoiditis, retained foreign body, pseudomeningocele, meningitis, and operative injury of one or more lumbar roots.
   4. **Pseudoarthrosis** was found in fusions in nine of the 13 patients who underwent them.

IV. **Commonly misdiagnosed or unrecognized conditions that can lead to FBS.** There are several common conditions producing low back pain that frequently go unrecognized or are misdiagnosed.
   A. **Decompensation syndrome**
      1. This is a common condition, but one that physicians frequently miss. The "Catch-22" of our society is that machines have taken away almost all of our exercise, ironically causing us to turn to other machines as providers of exercise. Muscles, ligaments, bones, and joints all require activity to remain strong. The old adage "If you don't use it you lose it" is certainly true of the musculoskeletal system in general and of the low back in particular. Many people in our society no longer get the exercise needed to preserve their strength, especially truncal strength. Low back muscles tend to be more affected by decompensation than extremity muscles. This state of decompensation frequently results in the patient developing back pain, especially LBP. Many erroneously feel that such pain is a result of aging, but it does not occur in primitive societies in which the elderly are required to engage in vigorous activities.
      2. The **onset of pain** usually is insidious in decompensation syndrome. Patients are typically over 35 years of age and have histories of relative inactivity. Frequently they are obese or smoke tobacco (or both). Decompensation can be a vicious cycle in which patients get so little exercise in their daily lives that they get back pain, then exercise even less, then get more back pain, etc. Decompensation can be seen as a pure syndrome or as secondary to some other type of low back pain problem such as osteoarthritis. The Kraus-Weber tests can be used to help make the diagnosis. These tests require the patient to be able to do one sit-up, one hook lying sit-up, a leg lift for 10 seconds at 30 degrees of hip flexion while lying supine, a prone torso lift for 10 seconds, a prone leg lift for 10 seconds, and one slow toe touch in the standing position. If a patient is unable to do two or more of these, decompensation should at least be considered.
      3. **Treatment** consists of restoring the patient's back and abdominal muscle strength. The patient needs to exercise despite having pain, because the pain will gradually resolve as the patient gains strength. Exercises (such as those of the Kraus-Weber tests) can be done at home, or the patient can regain strength faster by working with a physical therapist, although this is typically not a long-term solution. Long-term treatment typically consists of getting the patient to be more active. Most patients will not typically do "calisthenics" or lift weights to strengthen themselves over a long period of time. To improve compliance with an exercise regimen, it is usually best to suggest that the patient take up a sport, walk 1–2 miles per day, or work out at a health spa or "Nautilus" outlet. Unemployed patients can be encour-

aged to start a vocation that requires exercise. Patients with decompensation pain must find ways to include sufficient, consistent exercise in their daily lives.

B. Lumbosacral spinal stenosis syndrome

1. Spinal stenosis occurs most commonly in the elderly, and is usually a combination of a congenitally narrow spinal canal and superimposed osteoarthritis and disk degeneration. This especially narrows the lumbar canal when the spine is in extension. Other causes of spinal stenosis include central disk herniation and any pathology that narrows the lumbosacral spinal canal.

2. Pain in the back or legs when standing is the hallmark of spinal stenosis, which is often referred to as pseudoclaudication or neurogenic claudication. The pain is typically relieved by stooping forward (flexing the spine) or by sitting down, because the caliber of the lumbosacral canal is greater in spinal flexion than in extension. Spinal stenosis is often confused with the intermittent claudication typically observed in peripheral vascular disease, but patients with spinal stenosis do not get relief by standing and resting. They must stoop or sit down to alleviate the pain. Relieving pain by flexing the spine while standing is known as the "stoop test." Most patients have no pain or neurologic changes unless they are standing. In more severe cases, the patient has sufficient pathology that pain is present even when the spine is in flexion or when sitting. Severe spinal stenosis can induce radiculopathy in one or more nerve roots, or even a cauda equina syndrome with secondary bowel and bladder dysfunction.

3. Spinal stenosis can be confirmed with **CT or MRI scans.** Severe cases involving radiculopathy or involvement of the sacral roots to the pelvic sphincters become evident on EMG studies. Most cases of spinal stenosis produce a transient embarrassment of the neural structures of the low back, which does not induce EMG abnormalities. Somatosensory evoked potential studies are often positive in spinal stenosis syndrome when the EMG is negative.

4. **Nonsteroidal anti-inflammatory drugs (NSAIDs)** are helpful in the majority of cases of spinal stenosis syndrome. General strengthening of the lumbosacral paraspinals and abdominal muscles is also helpful at times, although the reason is unclear. Some patients with severe or resistant cases require surgical decompression. Some patients refuse surgery and choose to learn to live with their symptoms. They can carry a cane stool (a cane that unfolds into a small stool) to allow them to sit intermittently as needed to relieve the pain. Others prefer to walk by stooping forward, with or without a walker. Some simply use wheelchairs when they are in situations that otherwise require long-term standing or walking.

C. Other conditions often unrecognized or misdiagnosed in FBS patients

1. **Myofascial pain syndrome (MPS)** can involve the lumbosacral paraspinals or the gluteal muscles. It is the "great imitator" in the sense that it can cause pain that mimics sciatica. Patients with MPS often are mistakenly thought to have radiculopathy and sometimes are even subjected to inappropriate operations. MPS can occur post-traumatically, secondary to a lumbar strain. In this scenario the patient with a simple muscle strain continues to have symptoms for more than the typical 6–8 weeks required for muscle healing.

2. **Osteoporosis** accounts for about 4% of low back pain in adults. Osteoporosis is simply a loss of bone that occurs with age, lack of exercise, and hormonal changes. There are two distinct types of osteoporosis pain. The most common type is the acute pain from a fracture of a vertebra, typically a compression fracture. These fractures are easy to recognize and are self-limited in the majority of cases. The second major type of osteoporosis back pain is chronic pain that is more or less continuous pain resulting from multiple small fractures. This type of osteoporosis pain is often unrecognized. The fractures typically are too small to show up on plain films but are visible on bone scans. The vertebrae of affected individuals are typically sufficiently osteoporotic that these microfractures occur continuously. Each of them hurts for 6 weeks, and usually enough of them are active at any given time to give the patient continuous pain. Treatment is aimed at preventing further fractures if possible and slowing or even stopping the loss of bone. The current treatments for osteoporosis and their advantages

and disadvantages are controversial and beyond the scope of this chapter. They include estrogen, estrogen-testosterone, didronel, calcium, vitamin D, fluoride, and many others. The frequency of fractures can be decreased by strengthening the spinal extensor muscles. Many experts believe that exercises involving spinal flexion are contraindicated in patients with severe spinal osteoporosis.

V. Referral

A. Neurologic deficit. Referral to a neurologist or neurosurgeon is indicated for any patient with a newly diagnosed moderately severe or progressive neurologic deficit in bowel or bladder function or with a loss of lower-extremity strength or sensation.

B. Chronic pain syndrome. A patient with chronic pain syndrome will not respond to the medical model of treatment, and should be referred to a pain center or other facility capable of a behaviorally based treatment program.

C. Red flags. Patients having red flags that might indicate that their back pain is a result of cancer or infection should be referred to a neurologist, neurosurgeon, or other specialist as appropriate, although most FBS patients will have already had these potential causes of back pain excluded.

D. Failure to respond to acute measures. The patient who has had back pain for 6 weeks or more, and who is not responding to primary efforts, should be referred to a physiatrist (specialist in physical medicine and rehabilitation) or other suitable practitioner (such as a neurologist or orthopedist) for continued evaluation and treatment.

Recommended Readings

Addison R, Schultz A. Trunk strengths in patients seeking hospitalization for chronic low back disorders. *Spine* 5:539–544, 1980.

Beck AT, et al. An inventory for measuring depression. *Arch Gen Psychiat* 4:561, 1961.

Braddom RL. Industrial rehabilitation: An overview. In Rehabilitation of the injured worker. *PM&R Clin N Amer* 3(3):499–511, August 1992.

Braddom RL, Johnson EW. Standardization of the H reflex and diagnostic use in S-1 radiculopathy. *Arch Phys Med Rehabil* 55:161–165, April 1974.

Charnley J. Orthopedic signs in the diagnosis of disc protrusion with special reference to the straight-leg-raising test. *Lancet* 1:156, 1951.

Deyo RA, Rainville J, Kent DL. What can the history and physical examination tell us about low back pain? *JAMA* 268:760–765, 1992.

Feinstein B, et al. Experiments on pain referred from deep somatic tissue. *JBJS* 36A:981–997, 1954.

Fordyce W. *Behavioral Methods for Chronic Pain and Illness*. St. Louis: Mosby, 1976.

Hall S, et al. Lumbar spinal stenosis: Clinical features, diagnostic procedures, and results of surgical treatment in 68 patients. *Ann Intern Med* 103:271–275, 1985.

Heithoff KB, Burton CV. CT evaluation of the failed back surgery syndrome. *Orthoped Clin N Amer* 16(3):417–444, 1985.

Herron LD, Pheasant HC. Prone knee-flexion provocative testing for lumbar disc protrusion. *Spine* 5:65–67, 1980.

Johnson EW, Worden RE, Burk RD. Diagnosis of hysterical weakness. Scientific Exhibit, American Academy of General Practice, Miami Beach, FL, April 17–20, 1961.

Katz JN, et al. The outcome of decompressive laminectomy for degenerative lumbar stenosis. *JBJS* 73-A:809–816, 1991.

Kraus H. *Diagnosis and Treatment of Muscle Pain*. Chicago: Quintessence, 1988.

Long DM, et al. Clinical features of the failed-back syndrome. *J Neurosurg* 69:61–71, 1988.

Margo K. Diagnosis, treatment and prognosis in patients with low back pain. *Amer Fam Phys* 49:171–179, 1994.

Pheasant HC, et al. The MMPI as a predictor of outcome in low-back surgery. *Spine* 4:78–84, 1979.

Powell MC, et al. Prevalence of lumbar disc degeneration observed by magnetic resonance in symptomless women. *Lancet* 2(8520):1366–1367, 1986.

Ransford AO, Cairns D, Mooney V. The pain drawing as an aid to the psychologic evaluation of patients with low-back pain. *Spine* 1:127–134, 1976.

Simons DG, Travell JG. Myofascial origins of low back pain. 3. Pelvic and lower extremity muscles. *Postgrad Med* 73:99–105, 1983.

Sinaki M, Mikkelsen BA. Postmenopausal spinal osteoporosis: Flexion versus extension exercises. *Arch Phys Med Rehabil* 65:593–596, 1984.

Sinaki M, Mokri B. Low back pain syndrome. In RL Braddom, *Textbook of Physical Medicine and Rehabilitation*. Philadelphia: Saunders, 1996.

Sternbach RA. *Pain Patients: Traits and Treatment*. New York: Academic, 1974.

Thompson JM. Diagnosis and treatment of muscle pain syndromes. In RL Braddom, *Textbook of Physical Medicine and Rehabilitation*. Philadelphia: Saunders, 1996.

Turner JA, et al. Surgery for lumbar spinal stenosis: Attempted meta-analysis of the literature. *Spine* 17:1–8, 1992.

Waddell G, et al. Nonorganic physical signs in low back pain. *Spine* 5:117–125, 1980.

Waddell G, et al. Chronic low back pain, psychological distress, and illness behavior. *Spine* 9(2):209–213, 1984.

Wiesel SW, et al. Acute low back pain: An objective analysis of conservative therapy. *Spine* 5:324–330, 1980.

Wiesel SW, et al. A study of computer-assisted tomography. I. The incidence of positive CAT scans in an asymptomatic group of patients. *Spine* 6:549–551, 1984.

Yunus MB, Kalyan-Raman UP, Kalyan-Raman K. Primary fibromyalgia syndrome and myofascial pain syndrome: Clinical features and muscle pathology. *Arch Phys Med Rehabil* 69:451–454, 1988.

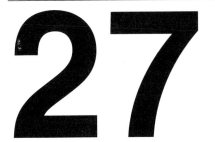

Approach to the Patient with Acute Sensory Loss

Oldrich J. Kolar

Acute sensory loss may result from pathologic processes involving sensory fibers in individual peripheral nerves (**mononeuropathy**), multiple individual peripheral nerves (**mononeuropathy multiplex**), multiple more or less symmetrically afflicted peripheral nerves (**polyneuropathy**), individual nerve roots (**monoradiculopathy**) or multiple nerve roots (**polyradiculopathy**), cervicobrachial or lumbosacral plexi (**plexopathy**), the spinal cord, the brainstem, the thalamus, or the cerebral hemispheres.

Acute sensory loss may be **transient, recurrent,** or **progressive.** Changes in the quality of sensory disturbances noticed over hours or days may suggest progressive neurologic affliction. In advancing processes involving the peripheral nervous system (PNS), increased sensation with or without discomfort to touch or to simple contact with bedsheets or clothing may in several hours or days be followed by progressive decreases in sensation modalities.

Localization of the pathologic processes resulting in acute sensory loss may be helpful in differential diagnostic considerations and in the proper selection of paraclinical investigations.

I. **Basic neuroanatomy of sensory innervation.** Sensory receptors are of two main types: exteroceptors and proprioceptors.

Exteroceptors, localized in the skin, represent superficial sensation modalities to pain, touch, cold, and warmth. The cutaneous sensory fibers run in sensory or mixed sensory and motor nerves. All the sensory neurons have their cell bodies in the dorsal ganglia with their central projections to the posterior roots.

Proprioceptors, localized in deeper somatic structures including tendons, muscles, and joints, transduce information about the positions of the extremities and the trunk; weight perception; direction of movements, force, and range of movements; pressure; touch; two-point discrimination; stereognosis; and vibration. The proprioceptive fibers, carried mainly in motor nerves, enter the gray matter of the dorsal horns, run in the ipsilateral dorsal columns of the spinal cord, and terminate in the gracile and cuneate nuclei of the medulla. The secondary afferent fibers from these nuclei cross the midline in the medulla and ascend in the brainstem as the medial lemniscus to the posterior thalamic complex. Unconscious proprioceptive information is carried through the spinocerebellar tracts in the lateral columns and in the cuneo- and rostrocerebellar tracts in the dorsal columns of the cord.

Decreased pain sensation resulting from compression of a **single root** can be detected in segments oriented longitudinally in the extremities and horizontally over the trunk. Overlapping in sensory zones from one nerve root to another is expressed more for touch than for pain. Similarly, there is also a 2–3-cm crossover in perception of sensory modalities at the midline over the chest and abdomen. Most fibers conducting pain and temperature sensation decussate over several segments by way of the ventral white commissure and ascend in the lateral columns of the cord as the spinothalamic tract.

Cutaneous **sensation from the face** is carried to the brainstem by the **trigeminal nerve.** After entering the pons, part of the sensory fibers descend as a bundle to form the spinal tract of the trigeminal nerve which reaches the upper cervical segment of the spinal cord. The spinal tract of the trigeminal nerve gives off fibers to the medially located nucleus of the spinal tract of the trigeminal nerve, which also descends into the upper cervical cord. The nucleus of the spinal tract of the trigeminal nerve receives fibers conducting sensations of pain, temperature, and light touch from the face and mucous membranes. Ascending fibers from the spinal nucleus travel mainly ipsilaterally in the trigeminothalamic tract and terminate in the thalamus. The spinothalamic tract has connections with the brainstem reticular formation. It joins the medial lemniscus at the midbrain level and terminates in the posterior complex of the thalamic nuclei.

The cortical projections of the posterior thalamic complex reach the postcentral cortex in a somatotropic arrangement similar to the precentral motor cortex with the face in the lowest area and the leg in the parasagittal region.

In addition to the postcentral cortex, the cortical thalamic projections also include the superior parietal lobule, which is considered to represent sensations of numbness and tingling over the contralateral or bilateral sides of the body. The fine sensory discrimination and fine location of pain, temperature, touch, and pressure require normal functioning of the sensory cortex.

II. **Examination of sensory modalities in acute sensory loss.** The sensory examination may represent the most difficult part of the neurologic examination. In patients indicating acute sensory loss, the location, extent, and quality of the sensory deficit may be decisive for optimal management of the neurologic disorder. Infrequently, patients complaining of numbness in the extremities actually refer to muscle weakness. Particularly at the early stage of an acute neurologic affliction resulting in sensory deficits, the patient may experience ill-defined sensations of tightness, pressure, or a "bandlike" feeling at the level of the upper chest, lower chest, waist, or extremities. If the patient complains of acute onset of a burning sensation usually associated with discomfort or pain, early involvement of the autonomic (sympathetic) nervous system should be considered.

Often, no sensory impairment can be demonstrated in individuals complaining of acute sensory disturbances. Conversely, the neurologic examination may detect sensory deficits of which the patient is unaware. The patient's alertness, willingness to cooperate, intelligence, and suggestibility may significantly influence the result of the examination. If the patient is tired following a lengthy examination, the evaluation of sensory modalities may show suboptimal reproducibility. The patient's eyes should be closed during the sensory examination.

Touch sensation is tested with a wisp of cotton. The stimulus applied to the area being tested should be compared with that applied to the contralateral area with expected normal sensation. A heavier stimulus usually has to be applied over cornified areas, particularly over soles and palms. Perception of a moving contact using cotton or the examiner's fingertips is more sensitive than perception of a stationary stimulus.

In testing of **pain sensation,** the patient is expected to indicate the intensity of the pinprick sensation in comparison with that in a corresponding area with normal pain sensation. The individual pinprick stimuli should be applied in intervals longer than 1 second to avoid excessive pain secondary to summation of the successive stimuli. If reproducible demarcation of the decreased sensation can be obtained, one has to determine whether the distribution is suggestive of nerve-root or peripheral nerve involvement. Should the pinprick sensation indicate a decrease or loss of pain sensation at a certain level of the chest or abdomen, the demarcation is determined more reliably by proceeding from the area of decreased or absent sensation to the level of normal sensation.

In testing **thermal modalities,** one should realize that their perception is relatively delayed. The test tube with cold and warm water should remain in contact with the tested skin area for several seconds. In the warm range, a normal individual recognizes differences between 35 and 40°C and in the cold range between 10 and 20°C. Exposure to temperatures below 10 and above 50°C may be confused with pain.

To determine the demarcation of the thermal sensation deficit, one should move the test tube from the areas of decreased sensation to the normal areas.

Position sense in fingers or toes is examined by holding the digit at the side opposite to the direction of movement, which is flexion or extension. The patient is asked to identify the directions of passive movements. In testing of lateralized postural sense in the extremities, the patient is asked to assume with the extremity being tested the position corresponding to that of the opposite limb as the opposite limb is passively manipulated by the examiner.

Vibration sense is a composite sensation requiring preserved touch and deep pressure sensation with fibers ascending in the dorsal columns of the spinal cord. Vibration and position senses are usually decreased together. A tuning fork with a low rate and long duration of vibration (128 dv) should be used for a routine examination. The tuning fork is placed over a bony prominence and the fork is moved quickly to the corresponding point on the opposite limb when the vibration is no longer perceived in the tested area.

In recording sensory disturbances, one should use the following generally accepted definitions. **Paresthesias** means abnormal sensations frequently described by the patient as tingling, prickling, or "pins and needles" occurring spontaneously. **Dysesthesias** refers to discomfort or pain triggered by painless stimuli such as soft touch or mild pressure.

Hyperesthesia indicates an abnormally increased sensitivity on examination of light touch, pinprick, or thermal sensation, which is not infrequently followed in the same area by **hypesthesia,** or decreased sensation. **Anesthesia** designates complete loss of sensation. **Thermohypesthesia,** which is decreased sensation for cold and warmth, may progress to **thermoanesthesia,** which indicates complete loss of thermal sensation. **Pallesthesia** refers to vibratory sense.

In practice, one may encounter individuals with **functional sensory loss.** However, it often is difficult to establish with certainty that the sensory impairment is functional. Functional sensory loss is frequently in a nonanatomic distribution. Demarcation of the losses of touch, pinprick, and vibration sensation is indicated exactly at the midline over the chest or abdomen or in the entire limb with sharp delineation of the sensory loss. Repeated examination usually reveals significant differences in the demarcation of the sensory deficits. Because examination of such patients may be rather time-consuming, it is helpful to provide them with a dermograph and ask them to draw a line demarcating the area of their sensory deficit themselves.

III. **Pathologic processes manifested by acute sensory loss.** Most patients with acute sensory impairment fall into three general diagnostic categories represented by (1) **infectious/parainfectious processes,** (2) **ischemic or hemorrhagic events,** and (3) **traumatic injuries.** Neurologic disorders secondary to metabolic or toxic affliction are rarely manifested by acute sensory loss.

   A. **Infectious or parainfectious neurologic diseases** are preceded by or associated with symptoms of acute, often febrile disease involving the upper respiratory or gastrointestinal system or the lower urinary tract. Parainfectious involvement of the nervous system follows the onset of clinical symptoms of the infectious process by 1–3 weeks.

   B. **Ischemic or hemorrhagic neurologic disorders** presenting with acute CNS or PNS afflictions usually occur in older individuals with vascular risk factors.

   C. **Traumatic lesions** of the CNS and PNS may manifest by acute sensory loss. CT or MRI scan of the brain or spine may indicate the extent to which the lesion involves the nervous system. Acute sensory loss may also, however, be demonstrated in the absence of radiologic abnormalities. Complications of surgical procedures, venipuncture, or intravascular injections should also be considered as potential causes of acute sensory loss, usually secondary to peripheral nerve damage.

IV. **Clinical aspects of acute sensory loss**

   A. **Acute sensory loss in the face.** Acute onset of facial paresthesias presenting as numbness, tingling, or an ill-defined discomfort is frequently encountered in clinical practice. If the paresthesias last only several seconds or minutes, or if the individual is young, tense, nervous, or exposed to stressful circumstances, often no specific pathology is identified. Paresthesias, especially in the perioral area, may be reproduced by hyperventilation. Basic laboratory evaluation including CBC with platelet count, serum glucose, electrolytes, and sedimentation rate, with clinical follow-up in 1 or 2 months, is indicated. The paresthesias usually regress completely.

   Some patients with acute onset of **idiopathic peripheral facial nerve (Bell's) palsy** may complain of numbness or abnormal sensation over the paretic facial muscles. In case of an isolated facial nerve involvement, the abnormal facial sensation ceases with regression of the muscle weakness.

   Should facial paresthesias persist over 1–2 days and become associated with pain and localized sensory deficits, thorough neurologic investigations are indicated.

   Pathologic processes involving the first division of the trigeminal nerve result in sensory impairment in the corresponding forehead area. Corneal, conjunctival, and sneeze reflexes are decreased or absent. Acute onset of dysesthesia followed after several days by hypesthesia to pain or light touch sensation may be an early manifestation of **herpes zoster infection.** If the patient has associated headaches, nausea, or vomiting, a CT scan is indicated to exclude associated intracranial hemorrhage.

Decreased or absent corneal reflex with alteration in sensory modalities in the ophthalmic division of the trigeminal nerve accompanying abrupt onset of fever, proptosis, chemosis, diplopia, and papilledema is suggestive of **cavernous sinus thrombosis.** Suppurative processes involving the upper half of the face, orbits, or nasal sinuses are usually present. Septic cavernous sinus thrombosis represents a life-threatening process requiring immediate hospitalization. CT, MRI, and MRV (magnetic resonance venography) are indicated. Sensory deficit in the area of the first division of the trigeminal nerve may also accompany acute onset of meningitis. If there are symptoms of meningeal involvement, cerebrospinal fluid (CSF) analysis with cultures is indicated.

A relatively sudden onset of numbness over the first two divisions of the trigeminal nerve associated with dysesthesia or hypesthesia to pinprick may represent a low-grade inflammatory process involving the cavernous sinus (Tolosa-Hunt syndrome). There is lateralized retro-ocular or periorbital pain and diplopia. The corneal reflex may be absent or decreased. Diplopia is most frequently secondary to involvement of the abducens nerve in the lateral wall of the cavernous sinus. MRI or MRV is indicated. Laboratory studies, including CBC with platelet count, sedimentation rate, ANA profile, luetic serology, coagulation profile, serum glucose, and CSF examination, may be unremarkable.

Patients with recurrent or chronic frontal or maxillary sinusitis may occasionally complain of numbness or a dull sensation in the area of the forehead or infraorbital region. Sensory disturbances are frequently associated with pain and decrease in pinprick or light touch sensation suggestive of symptomatic neuralgia of the ophthalmic or maxillary nerve. An ear, nose, and throat (ENT) consultation and aggressive treatment of the sinusitis usually result in complete regression of the neurologic symptomatology.

Decreased sensation in the first, second, or third division of the trigeminal nerve associated with a clinical history of acute injury involving the head requires a CT scan to exclude involvement of the trigeminal nerve secondary to skull fracture, contusion, or hematoma.

Acute onset of persistent sensory impairment usually presenting as numbness or ill-defined dysesthesia in the infraorbital area corresponding to the maxillary division may be an early sign of multiple sclerosis. If the sensory disturbances are persistent, extend over the entire half of the face or to the contralateral side, and become associated with discomfort or pain, and if the patient is young or middle-aged, a demyelinating process should be considered and a brain MRI is indicated. Absence of multifocal white matter disease on MRI, however, does not exclude the diagnosis of multiple sclerosis, particularly if no other etiology is established. In these patients, examination of visual-, brainstem-, and somatosensory-evoked potentials and CSF studies including CSF immunoglobulin G (IgG) index and isoelectric focusing to exclude the presence of oligoclonal bands are indicated.

Acute decrease or absence of pinprick, light touch, or thermal sensation in the area of the mandibular division of the trigeminal nerve may reflect inflammatory or traumatic events involving the mandible or fracture of the base of the skull in the area of the foramen ovale. Roentgenograms of the cranial base and mandible may be helpful in localizing the potential nerve damage.

Osteomyelitis of the mandible, usually complicating progressive dental pathology, may be manifested by a relatively abrupt onset of numbness with or without hypalgesia in the area of the chin suggestive of neuritis affecting the mental nerve. Acute presentation of the **numb chin syndrome** may represent a paraneoplastic manifestation in individuals with lymphoma, breast or prostate cancer, or melanoma. Orthodontic consultation should exclude malfitting dentures.

Abrupt onset of hypalgesia and thermoanesthesia over the entire half of the face accompanied by hypalgesia and thermoanesthesia over the contralateral half of the trunk and extremities indicates involvement of the lateral medulla. The acute sensory loss is often associated with dysphagia, dysarthria, vertigo, vomiting, ipsilateral cerebellar signs, and ipsilateral Horner's syndrome. The most frequent cause of the **lateral medullary (Wallenberg's) syndrome** is occlusion of the intracranial vertebral artery. Less common etiologies include vertebral artery dissection, hematoma, demyelination, metastatic disease, and abscess.

Acute onset of bilateral or unilateral facial numbness rapidly extending into the contralateral half of the face, and associated with or followed by progressive weakness of facial muscles, may be the earliest manifestation of an acute demyelinating polyneuropathy—the **Guillain-Barré syndrome (GBS).**

Particularly in individuals with histories of respiratory or gastrointestinal viral infections, immunizations, or surgical procedures preceding the onset of neurologic symptoms, the diagnosis of GBS should be considered.

Recurrent sensory disturbances in hemifacial distribution, particularly in older patients with clinical histories of arterial hypertension, cardiovascular disease, diabetes, and cigarette smoking, may represent a carotid artery territory transient ischemic attack (TIA). Patients may complain of numbness or a feeling of dullness or tingling involving the entire half of the face. The TIA episodes are of variable duration, usually lasting less than 20–30 minutes.

Loss of pain sensation and thermodysesthesia with preserved light touch sensation are suggestive of **syringobulbia.** In these patients, an expanding syrinx involving the spinal nucleus of the trigeminal nerve may be demonstrated by MRI.

The rostral part of the nucleus of the spinal tract of the trigeminal nerve represents the midline facial areas, whereas the sensation fibers from the lateral facial areas terminate in the more caudal part of the nucleus at the level of the medulla and spinal cord. In acute intraparenchymal processes involving the brainstem, facial sensory loss may occur in an "onionskin" distribution with decreased sensation in the central facial areas, indicating a pontine or pontomedullary lesion. Acute presentation of **"onionskin-like" sensation deficits** in the face may accompany acute brainstem encephalitis.

These patients usually develop flulike symptoms, headaches, nausea, dizziness, and facial numbness. In some instances, peripheral facial palsy may be observed. CSF examination frequently shows mild lymphocytic pleocytosis and normal or slightly elevated CSF protein. Involvement of the trigeminal nerve by tumor, vascular malformations, or connective tissue disease rarely presents with acute sensory loss in the face. If a space-occupying process in the area of the gasserian ganglion is suspected, MRI is indicated.

B. Acute sensory loss over the scalp and neck. Not infrequently, a tense and anxious patient may report acute onset of numbness in the "top of the head." Commonly, such patients also complain of discomfort or pain on combing the hair. Associated problems may include sleeping difficulties, generalized fatigue, lightheadedness, and recurrent biooccipital or diffuse pressurelike head-aches.

Some patients, after exposure to cold or with no obvious reasons, may experience the sudden onset of a lateralized discomfort or pain associated with decreased sensation in the occipital area. The pain has a tendency to radiate proximally into the ipsilateral parietal region. There may be discomfort on compression and decreased pinprick sensation in the distribution of the greater or lesser occipital nerves.

Acute sensory impairment in the area over the angle of the mandible, the lower part of the external ear, and the upper neck below the ear is suggestive of a neuropathy involving the great auricular nerve.

In cases of **acute sensory loss in the neck area** extending over two or three segments, MRI of the cervical spine is indicated. In the absence of a trauma, the presence of hyperintense signals at the corresponding spinal cord level is suggestive of an inflammatory demyelinating process. MRI of the brain not infrequently shows subclinical multifocal white matter disease. CSF examination, including cytomorphology, IgG index, and isoelectric focusing, is indicated.

C. Acute sensory loss over half of the face, trunk, and corresponding extremities. Acute sensory loss over the entire half of the patient's body is often a manifestation of a stroke. A traumatic CNS lesion should also be considered with a clinical history indicating injury.

Sensory loss in half of the body may be transient or permanent when indicative of irreversible tissue damage rostral to the upper brainstem up to the postcentral gyrus and parietal area of the cerebral hemisphere contralateral to the side of the sensory deficit.

Acute onset of numbness, tingling, prickling, or a crawling sensation starting in the lips, fingers, or toes and spreading in seconds over half of the body may represent a partial seizure with somatosensory manifestations. The abnormal sensation may follow a rather stereotypical pattern, usually lasting less than 1 minute. Onsets of focal seizures in adults frequently reflect focal pathologies such as tumors or vascular malformations involving the contralateral hemisphere. MRI and EEG are indicated. In patients with suspected intracranial vasculitis, magnetic resonance angiography (MRA) or cerebral angiography are indicated.

With a negative evaluation for focal sensory seizures in patients with recurrent hemisensory impairment, early symptoms of TIAs should be considered. The transient sensory impairment in TIAs usually lasts longer than sensory disturbances representing partial somatosensory epilepsy. The diagnosis of TIA is more probable if the episodic subjective hemisensory impairment is accompanied by motor deficits in the extremities.

A patient with an acute vascular event in the area of the nondominant, right parietal lobe may be unable to give a reliable history because of decreased ability to appreciate motor or sensory deficits in the contralateral extremities (**anosognosia**). Besides diminished light touch and pain sensations, ischemic lesions involving the contralateral postcentral gyrus may also cause decreased or absent perception of sizes and shapes of objects (**astereognosis**), inability to recognize numbers or letters drawn on the patient's skin (**agraphesthesia**), or altered **two-point discrimination.**

Acute onset of hemisensory impairment manifested by a tingling sensation, numbness, or ill-defined pain may accompany an acute vascular lesion involving the contralateral thalamus. Patients often have a midline demarcation of the sensory disturbances in the absence of reproducible abnormalities on examination. Patients may be unaware of the profound sensory loss in the involved areas. There may be a feeling of deformation and/or enlargement of the involved extremities. Thalamic paresthesias and pain are often disabling and difficult to treat.

D. **Clinical aspects of acute sensory loss in the area of the trunk.** Acute sensory loss with a horizontal sensory level over the chest or abdomen requires emergent evaluation in order to minimize residual neurologic impairment secondary to a potential spinal cord lesion. Particularly with a clinical history of a potential spinal cord injury, expedient decisions may be crucial in optimizing outcome.

A **complete transection of the spinal cord** is relatively easy to diagnose. Muscle weakness in both the lower or the upper and lower extremities is present. All forms of sensation are lost one to two segments below the level of the lesion. Absence of vibration sense at the spinous process below the lesion may be helpful in localizing the spinal cord damage. A zone of increased pinprick or light touch sensation at the upper border of the anesthetic zone may be established. Urinary and fecal incontinence are present. MRI of the spine, and neurologic referral if needed, should be urgently obtained.

In the case of an acute spinal cord lesion extending over the entire lateral half of the cord, a **syndrome of cord hemisection** (Brown-Séquard's syndrome) may be identified. There is loss of pain and thermal sensations one or two segments below the lesion on the contralateral side with muscle weakness in the lower extremity on the ipsilateral side of the spinal cord lesion. In post-traumatic transection or hemisection of the spinal cord, urgent MRI of the spine at the level of the sensory deficits is indicated, followed by neurosurgical consultation.

Acute loss of pain and temperature sensation may accompany occlusion of the anterior spinal artery. Light touch, position, and vibration senses remain intact. Anterior spinal artery syndrome may occur during aortic surgery or in advanced atherosclerotic disease of the aorta. It may also develop in the course of meningovascular syphilis, or as a manifestation of a collagen-vascular disease. MRI of the spinal cord; CSF examination, including VDRL, IgG index, isoelectric focusing; and basic laboratory studies with screening for collagen-vascular diseases and luetic serology are indicated. Dissociated sensory deficits may also occur in association with acute spinal cord infarction in the "watershed" areas (T1-T4 and T12-L1 levels).

Occasionally, following falls that involve landing on the buttocks, patients may develop loss of pain and temperature sensations with preserved tactile sensation one to two segments below the level of the expected spinal cord involvement. Expanding hematomas in the spinal cord gray matter compromise the ventral white commissure conducting fibers for pain and temperature sensation. Light touch and vibration senses remain intact. The dissociated sensory deficit may extend over several segments. MRI of the spine and neurosurgical referral should be urgently obtained.

Acute sensory loss for pain, soft touch, and temperature may be a manifestation of an acute spinal cord inflammatory process. In **acute transverse myelitis,** the sensory level is most frequently found at the T4-T6 and T10-T12 levels. Decreased or absent vibration and position senses below the level of the spinal cord involvement and functional alteration in sphincters with urinary and fecal incontinence are present. Symmetric, severe muscle weakness in the lower extremities may develop over hours. Viral diseases or vaccinations may precede the onset of neurologic symptoms by 1–3 weeks. **Acute myelitis** caused by viral infection, including poliomyelitis, herpes zoster, herpes simplex, and cytomegalovirus, is usually manifested by less severe sensory losses and less symmetric motor deficits in the extremities.

E. **Acute sensory loss in individual extremities** may be established in longitudinal zones corresponding to individual nerve roots, in various areas supplied by individual nerve roots, or in various areas supplied by individual nerves.

In the upper extremities, diminished or lost pinprick or light touch sensation over the thumb and the radial aspect of the arm is suggestive of involvement of the C6 nerve root. Decreased pinprick sensation over the ring and little fingers and the ulnar aspects of the forearm and arm is indicative of involvement of the C8 nerve root. If there is decreased pinprick sensation over the index and middle fingers, and sometimes over the radial aspect of the ring finger, damage of the C7 nerve root should be considered.

In the lower extremities, the acute loss of pinprick and light touch sensations involving the L1 nerve root may be established as a longitudinal zone at the level of the groin followed distally by the L2 and L3 nerve roots involving the anterior aspect of the thigh, extending proximally at the left above the buttocks.

Sensory deficits along the medial and lateral aspects of the shin correspond, respectively, to the L4 and L5 nerve roots. Involvement of the S1 and S2 nerve roots is manifested by decreased sensation in the posterior aspects of the thigh and calf.

Besides instances of acute sensory loss accompanying nerve-root involvement, localized sensory deficits suggestive of a peripheral nerve lesion may be also encountered. Dislocation of the shoulder joint, injuries of the humerus, or prolonged pressure, stretching, or traction involving the arm during anesthesia or sleep may result in lesions of the axillary nerve. Localized pinprick and light touch deficits over the lower portion of the deltoid muscle allow the examiner to identify the nerve involved.

1. Diminished or absent sensation over the palmar aspects of the first three and a half fingers and the dorsal aspects of the terminal phalanges of the second and third fingers and half of the fourth finger indicates damage of the median nerve. Acute sensory loss in the area of the median nerve is caused predominantly by injuries involving the arm, forearm, wrist, and hand, including stab and bullet wounds. Procedures requiring needle insertion, particularly in the cubital fossa, may also result in median nerve damage manifested by sensory deficits and pain, frequently with a burning, causalgic component. Rarely, prolonged compression during anesthesia or sleep may also cause an acute median nerve involvement manifested by sensory and motor deficits.

   Acute sensory impairment indicating ulnar nerve damage is manifested by paresthesias followed by decreased light touch and pinprick sensation over the fifth and ulnar half of the fourth finger, and the ulnar portion of the hand to the wrist. Fractures and dislocations of the humerus involving the elbow, lacerating wounds, and pressure on the nerve during anesthesia, or drunkenness are the most frequent causes of acute ulnar nerve damage.

   In patients with acute radial nerve lesions, the sensory deficit may be established over the posterior aspect of the arm if the nerve damage occurs in the axilla. Radial nerve affliction proximal to the spiral groove of the humerus leads to decreased sensation over the distal extensor aspect of the forearm. The superficial branch of the radial nerve gives origin to the dorsal digital nerve in the distal forearm supplying the skin on the dorsal and radial aspects of the hand and the dorsa of the first four digits. The radial nerve is probably the most commonly injured peripheral nerve. Injuries including dislocations and fractures of the shoulder, extended pressure on the nerve (particularly at the groove of the nerve), and fractures of the neck of the radius are the most frequent causes of radial nerve damage.

An acute lesion of the femoral nerve is manifested by decreased sensation over the anterior and medial aspects of the thigh and in the area of the saphenous nerve in the medial aspect of the lower leg. Acute femoral nerve injury may follow fractures of the pelvis and femur, dislocation of the hip, pressure or traction during hysterectomy, forceps delivery, or pressure in hematomas in the area of the iliopsoas muscle or groin. Paresthesia and sensory loss in the area of the saphenous nerve may occur as a result of injury in the area above the medial aspect of the knee in medial arthrotomy or as a complication of coronary artery bypass graft surgery.

Sensory loss in obturator nerve injury is found over a small area of skin over the medial aspect of the thigh. The nerve may be damaged during surgical procedures involving the hip or pelvis, in cases of obturator hernia, or secondary to iliopsoas hematomas.

Abrupt onset of tingling, numbness, and discomfort in the lateral and anterolateral aspects of the thigh is typical of involvement of the lateral femoral cutaneous nerve (meralgia paresthetica). Pinprick hyperesthesia is followed by hypesthesia for pain and soft touch. The discomfort or pain may be bilateral. The nerve may be damaged by compression by the inguinal ligament, in iliopsoas hemorrhage, or by tightly fitting garments on obese individuals.

2. Acute sensory impairment involving the outer aspect of the shin and over the dorsal, plantar, and inner aspects of the foot occurs in acute sciatic nerve lesions. The distribution of the sensory deficits reflects the areas of skin sensation supplied by the two branches of the sciatic nerve: the peroneal nerve and the tibial nerve. Acute sciatic nerve damage may occur in association with fractures or dislocations of the hip, hip joint surgery, other pelvic pathologies including gunshot wounds, or injections in the vicinity of the sciatic nerve.

With injury of the common peroneal nerve, at the level of the fibular head, impaired sensation in the lateral aspect of the shin and over the dorsum of the foot is established. Sometimes only the superficial branch of the peroneal nerve is damaged, presenting with decreased pinprick or light touch sensation in the more distal portion of the lateral aspect of the shin. A small patch of skin hypesthesia for pinprick or soft touch may be established between the first and second toes in instances of deep peroneal nerve lesion.

Acute damage of the **tibial nerve** results in sensory disturbances in the lateral calf supplied by its branch, the medial sural cutaneous nerve. Additional branches of the tibial nerve supply sensation to the skin of the lateral heel, the lateral aspect of the foot (sural nerve), and the sole, with the medial two-thirds of the sole being innervated by the median plantar nerve and the lateral third by the lateral plantar nerve.

3. The majority of peroneal nerve lesions are traumatic, including those caused by compression exerted at the upper and outer aspects of the leg, stretching of the hip and knee, or surgical procedures involving the knee joint. The tibial nerve is injured mostly in the popliteal fossa, at the level of the ankle or foot.

Acute sensorimotor deficits indicating multiple nerve involvement in the individual upper or lower extremities are suggestive of plexopathies. Acute onset of tingling, numbness, and pain, usually followed in several hours or days by muscle weakness and patchy hypesthesia in the area of the shoulder girdle and proximal arm muscles, is typical of brachial plexus neuritis (neuralgic amyotrophy). Acute brachial plexopathies may be caused by trauma in which the arm is hyperabducted or secondary to traction involving the arm, including birth injuries. Brachial plexus neuritis may occur in epidemic form. Brachial plexus neuritis may follow infections, vaccinations, or parenteral application of serum. Brachial plexopathy may occur as a complication of coronary bypass surgery. In some patients, no apparent etiology of plexopathy is established.

4. **Lumbosacral plexopathy** is recognized by sensorimotor deficits and pain in the lower extremities. In acute lumbar plexopathy, a common etiology other than trauma is retroperitoneal hemorrhage.

F. **Clinical aspects of acute sensory loss in both feet and/or both hands.** Some patients complain of tingling, prickling, numbness, or "stiffness" in the hands and feet. The acroparesthesia may be of variable duration, frequently is more pronounced at night, and may be associated with decreased sensation in the fingertips. The underlying pathology is usually of no imminent severity. Should the paresthesia increase in intensity and be accompanied by decreased ability to perform movements in the toes or fingers, close patient observation is indicated to exclude Guillain-Barré syndrome (GBS). Less frequently, the sensorimotor disturbances may start in both hands or be manifested by facial numbness. In some patients, the sensory disturbances are minimal in comparison with the severity of muscle weakness, or the ascending sensory deficits remain localized only in the lower extremities. In patients with GBS, deep sensory modalities, including position and vibration senses, are more impaired than superficial sensation.

Recommended Readings

Brazis PW, Masdeu JC, Biller J. *Localization in Clinical Neurology* (3rd ed). Boston: Little, Brown, 1996.

DeJong RN. *The Neurologic Examination* (4th ed). Hagerstown, MD: Harper & Row, 1979.

Folpe A, Lapham LW, Smith HC. Herpes simplex myelitis as a cause of acute necrotizing myelitis syndrome. *Neurology* 44:1955–1957, 1994.

Gilden DH, et al. Varicella-zoster virus myelitis: An expanding spectrum. *Neurology* 44:1818–1823, 1994.

Mayo Clinic and Mayo Foundation. *Clinical Examinations in Neurology* (6th ed). St. Louis: Mosby, 1991.

Van der Meche FGA. The Guillain-Barré syndrome: Plasma exchange or immunoglobulins intravenously. *J Neurol Neurosurg Psychiat* 57(Suppl):33–34, 1994.

Van der Meche FGA. Intravenous immunoglobulin in the Guillain-Barré syndrome. *Clin Exp Immunol* 94(Suppl 1):43–47, 1994.

Weber T. PCR as a diagnostic tool for the diagnosis of progressive multifocal leukoencephalopathy and CMV infections. In *Book of Abstracts, "Satellite Symposium": The Cerebrospinal Fluid in Neuroimmunology.* Amsterdam: Spinal Fluid Research Group, World Federation of Technology, 1994. P 4.

28

Approach to the Hyperkinetic Patient

Allison Brashear

The patient who presents with a **hyperkinetic movement disorder** experiences excessive movement. The patient may complain that it interferes with the activities of daily living, or the patient may be unaware of the problem and the family may prompt the evaluation. The correct diagnosis depends on the character of the movement—i.e., when it occurs, its speed, its location, and contributing factors. The more common disorders include dystonia, tremor, chorea, tics, myoclonus, and tardive dyskinesia (Table 28-1).

I. Dystonia

A. Definition. Dystonia is a disorder consisting of intermittent or sustained, often painful, twisting, repetitive muscle spasms that may occur in one part of the body (focal dystonia) or throughout the entire body (generalized dystonia).

  1. Initially, the movements may be triggered by a specific act, such as writing, and are made worse by movement of other parts of the body.

  2. There may be superimposed tremor or myoclonic jerks.

  3. The patient may use a "sensory trick"—a tactile stimulus—that can decrease the muscle contractions.

B. Classification

  1. Dystonia is classified by the part of the body affected (focal versus generalized dystonia), by the age of onset (adult-onset versus childhood-onset dystonia), and by contributing factors (idiopathic versus secondary dystonia).

  2. Psychogenic dystonia. Dystonia was once diagnosed as hysteria or malingering, and patients were often referred to psychiatry for evaluation. Differentiating psychogenic dystonia from idiopathic or secondary dystonia can be done only by a history and a physical. Sensory tricks and variations in weakness are common in idiopathic dystonia, and referral to a specialist may be needed to discern idiopathic dystonia from the psychogenic form. Clues to psychogenic dystonia include inconsistent movements and postures, false weakness and sensory complaints, and overt psychiatric disease.

C. Pathophysiology

  1. Idiopathic dystonia is not associated with any particular brain lesion. Secondary dystonia is most often observed in patients with lesions in the basal ganglia, such as the putamen, and their connections with the thalamus and cortex.

  2. Genetics. The prevalence of familial generalized dystonia is 1 in 160,000 in the general population, and in the Ashkenazi Jewish population it is 1 in 15,000 to 1 in 23,000. Familial idiopathic dystonia with autosomal dominant inheritance has been localized to chromosome 9q.

  3. Testing. Despite advances in genetics and symptomatic treatment for dystonia, there is no blood or radiologic test that confirms the diagnosis. A detailed neurologic history and examination comprise the best method of diagnosis.

D. Generalized dystonia. The spasms of generalized dystonia affect most of the entire body. They may present in one part of the body, particularly the foot, but rapidly spread to contiguous parts and usually involve the limbs, trunk, and neck. Generalized dystonia more commonly presents in children and young adults. Onset is typically in the legs and spreads to contiguous body parts.

E. Focal dystonia is isolated to one part of the body. See Table 28-2 for types and areas affected.

F. Etiology. Dystonia may be idiopathic (primary) or have a known cause (secondary).

  1. Idiopathic (primary) dystonia

Table 28-1. Hyperkinetic movement disorders.

Term	Clinical manifestations
Dystonia	Sustained muscular spasms that may be focal or generalized
Tremor	Rhythmic oscillation of agonist and antagonist muscles
Chorea	Quick, irregular, often semipurposeful movements
Tics	Sudden, fast, irregular movements, usually in the same muscle group
Myoclonus	Sudden, fast movements, usually repeated in the same body part
Tardive dyskinesia	Combined chorea and dystonic movements, usually in the face and lower jaw, but may be generalized; history of neuroleptic use

    a. Idiopathic dystonia has no known cause.

    b. Birth history is normal, and examination is normal except for dystonia, ceruloplasmin, and brain imaging.

    c. Types of idiopathic dystonia include focal and generalized forms. Regardless of a focal or generalized presentation, idiopathic dystonia can be autosomal dominant (most commonly localized to chromosome 9), X-linked, or sporadic.

  2. Secondary dystonia. The most common known metabolic defect causing secondary dystonia is Wilson's disease.

    a. Known metabolic defect. Wilson's disease is an inherited deficit in copper metabolism.

      (1) Neurologic symptoms affecting the basal ganglia, including bradykinesia, dysarthria, dystonia, tremor, ataxia, and abnormal gait, occur in 40–60% of patients. Spasmodic dysphonia (involving the vocal chords) is a common form.

      (2) Rare autosomal recessive disease located on the long arm of chromosome 13

      (3) Exclude with Kayser-Fleischer rings with serum ceruloplasmin and slit-lamp eye examination in patients younger than 50 years. Treatment can reverse the liver involvement in Wilson's disease and prevent severe neurologic sequelae.

      (4) Wing beating tremor is classically described in patients with Wilson's disease. This tremor is absent at rest and develops after the arms are extended.

    b. Other neurologic syndromes presenting as a secondary dystonia are those with **unknown metabolic defects,** including degenerative disease, a juvenile variant of Huntington's disease, dystonia with parkinsonian symptoms, early-onset Parkinson's disease, rapid-onset dystonia-parkinsonism, and dopamine-responsive dystonia (hereditary).

  3. Acquired dystonia. An acquired dystonia occurs as a result of an injury, treatment, or other disease process. These may include:

Table 28-2. Types of focal dystonia.

Term	Clinical manifestations
Blepharospasm	Involuntary spasms of the orbicularis oris (around the eyes), resulting in eye closure
Limb dystonia	Writer's cramp or intermittent spasms of the foot or hand
Oromandibular dystonia	Facial grimacing, sometimes isolated to jaw opening or closing; Meige's syndrome when eyes and lower jaw are both involved
Spasmodic dysphonia	Intermittent spasms of the vocal chords, resulting in a strain and strangle quality to the voice; rarely presents a breathy voice
Torticollis (cervical dystonia)	Involuntary twisting, turning, and tilting of the neck, often associated with pain and tremor

a. Prenatal injury resulting in an ischemic event manifesting as dystonia.
b. Exposure to toxins (carbon monoxide, manganese) resulting in structural changes to the basal ganglia.
c. Anoxic injury to the cerebral cortex or basal ganglia resulting in dystonic posturing.
d. Tardive syndrome from dopamine blockers (phenothiazine, metoclopramide). Tardive dystonia generally occurs during treatment or within 3 months of discontinuing therapy.
e. Focal brain pathology (stroke, tumor, demyelinating, postinfectious, post-traumatic). Any focal brain injury regardless of the cause may present as dystonia.
f. Peripheral nerve injury to the neck, arm, or leg may result in dystonic posturing of that body part. The reason why this causes dystonia has not been determined.
g. Psychogenic remains a diagnosis of exclusion. Irregular spasms, unusual triggers, and bizarre postures may be clues.

G. **Clinical manifestations of dystonia**
1. **Focal dystonia**
   a. **Blepharospasm** is a disorder that consists of uncontrollable involuntary spasms of the eyelids causing spontaneous closure. It often interferes with vision, resulting in functional blindness. It may be worsened by bright light or stress.
   b. **Oromandibular dystonia** consists of grimacing of the lower face, usually involving the mouth, jaw, and platysma muscle. If associated with blepharospasm, it is termed Meige's syndrome.
   c. **Spasmodic torticollis** or **cervical dystonia** consists of intermittent, uncontrollable spasms of the neck muscles, often associated with severe pain. The neck may involuntarily turn, tilt, or rotate forward, sideways, or backward.
   d. **Spasmodic dysphonia** involves only the vocal cords. There is hyperadduction of the cords, which produces an intermittent strain and strangle quality to the voice. Often patients also complain of a tightness in the throat during the spasms.
   e. **Occupational dystonia.** Writer's cramp is the most common and most underdiagnosed limb dystonia. Dystonic posturing may be noted in the hand or foot. Early in the course of the disease, the movement may be brought out by performing a specific task such as writing, typing, or playing a musical instrument.
2. **Hemidystonia** involves one side of the body and almost always results from a focal lesion (vascular, neoplastic, or traumatic).
3. **Generalized dystonia.** Spasms occur in two or more limbs, and usually also in the trunk and neck. Symptoms usually begin in the legs and progressively involve other parts of the body.

H. **Evaluation of dystonia**
1. **Focal dystonia**
   a. **Onset after 50 years of age**
      (1) MRI of the brain
      (2) Family history
      (3) Search for medication as a cause, such as phenothiazine or metoclopramide use.
   b. **Onset before 50 years of age**
      (1) MRI of the brain
      (2) Ceruloplasmin and slit-lamp examination for Kayser-Fleischer rings
      (3) Screen for medication as a cause.
2. **Hemidystonia**
   a. MRI of the brain to rule out structural causes (neoplastic, vascular, infectious, or traumatic)
   b. Ceruloplasmin and ophthalmologic examination with a slit lamp for Kayser-Fleischer rings
3. **Generalized dystonia**
   a. Family and medication history
   b. MRI of the brain
   c. Ceruloplasmin and ophthalmologic examination with a slit lamp for Kayser-Fleischer rings

II. Tremor

A. Definition. Tremor consists of rhythmic, oscillating movements of agonist and antagonist muscles. The movements are equal in amplitude and frequency. Symptoms are made worse by anxiety and disappear with sleep.

B. Classification

1. **Physiologic tremor** is a low-amplitude (8–12 Hz) tremor that is most prominent in outstretched hands and that under certain circumstances is present in all individuals.

2. **Essential tremor** is a postural or action-involved tremor that is rarely present at rest. The frequency is usually 4–12 Hz but may decrease with age.

3. **Cerebellar tremor** is most prominent in voluntary movements and has a frequency of 3–4 Hz. Patients perform poorly on finger-to-nose and heel-to-shin testing. The tremor may involve only the trunk in some patients.

4. **Rest tremor (parkinsonian tremor)** occurs at 3–7 Hz and is most obvious when the limb is fully supported and at rest. Rest tremor is reduced by action and intention.

C. Etiology

1. **Physiologic tremor** is exacerbated by excited mental states, metabolic derangements (endocrine and fever), drugs (thyroid, lithium, beta agonists, theophylline, and sodium valproate), alcohol withdrawal, and caffeine use.

2. **Essential tremor**
   a. The cause of essential tremor is unclear.
   b. Most patients have strong family histories.
   c. An association with Parkinson's disease and dystonia has been suggested.
   d. The diagnosis can be confirmed by suppression of the tremor by ingesting a small amount of alcohol. The lack of response does not exclude the diagnosis.

3. **Cerebellar tremor** is typically observed with a lack of feedback of the cerebellum to the motor cortex. The etiology of a cerebellar tremor may include a demyelinating disease (such as multiple sclerosis), a space-occupying lesion, or an ischemic, toxic, or infectious disorder.

4. **Rest tremor.** The cause of a resting tremor is generally considered to be in the central nervous system, but the exact anatomical lesion is unknown.

D. Evaluation

1. **Physiologic tremor**
   a. Medication (most common cause)
   b. Drug or alcohol withdrawal
   c. Assess for anxiety
   d. Thyroid functions should be performed to rule out hyperthyroidism.

2. **Essential tremor**
   a. Hyperthyroidism can worsen an existing essential tremor.
   b. Drug use such as lithium or sodium valproate or alcohol withdrawal can exacerbate an essential tremor.

3. **Cerebellar tremor.** Individuals presenting with a cerebellar tremor should be evaluated with an MRI of the brain, including the posterior fossa, to rule out a mass, ischemic, or demyelinating lesion as the cause.

4. **Resting tremor.** An individual presenting with a rest tremor should be given a trial of medication for Parkinson's disease. Rest tremor may be the presenting symptom of Parkinson's disease.

III. Chorea

A. Definition. Chorea is a hyperactive, fast, arrhythmic, often semipurposeful movement. It may affect the limbs, face, or trunk.

B. Classification

1. **Adult-onset chorea**
   a. **Positive family history**
      (1) **Huntington's disease**
         (a) Huntington's disease is a progressive neurodegenerative disease with autosomal dominant inheritance localized to chromosome 4.
         (b) Patients with positive family histories often present with chorea. The mean age is 40, but onset can occur anywhere from childhood to old age. Some patients may notice problems

with control of fine movements, dropping of objects, or incoordination before the onset of chorea.

(c) Cognitive deficits present with problems of concentration, attention, and coordination of spatial motor acts rather than problems of memory. Subtle findings, such as changes in job performance or interests, may be revealed when the patient presents to the physician. Memory problems are often short-term problems, and, unlike patients with Alzheimer's disease, patients with end-stage Huntington's disease may retain recognition of family and familiar surroundings.

(2) Wilson's disease. See sec. **I.F.2.a.**

b. **No family history.** A focal brain lesion, such as a mass, infection, or vascular lesion may cause chorea in someone without a family history of chorea. Hemiballismus is violent type of choreic movements occurring on one side of the body. Hemiballismus is most commonly associated with a vascular lesion of the subthalamic nucleus.

c. **Other causes of chorea**

(1) Pregnancy

(2) Encephalitis

(3) Drug induced: levodopa, oral contraceptives, anticonvulsants, lithium

(4) Metabolic and autoimmune: consider systemic lupus erythematosus, thyroid, and hypoparathyroidism

2. Childhood-onset chorea

a. **Positive family history**

(1) **Wilson's disease.** See sec. **I.F.2.a.**

(2) **Huntington's disease** may occur in children whose fathers have Huntington's disease.

(3) A history of rheumatic fever suggests a diagnosis of Sydenham's chorea.

b. **History of birth trauma or CNS infection.** Childhood-onset chorea may develop in children with a history of birth injury or as a result of encephalitis.

C. Evaluation

1. Positive family history

a. A positive slit-lamp examination for Kayser-Fleischer rings indicates Wilson's disease.

(1) Seek neurologic consultation for treatment.

(2) Seek genetic counseling.

b. A CT brain scan that shows atrophy of the caudate nucleus indicates Huntington's disease. Genetic counseling should be sought. Asymptomatic gene carriers and symptomatic cases can be confirmed by testing. Such testing should be performed in conjunction with psychological counseling and support.

2. Negative family history

a. CT scan of head

b. Birth history

c. History of drug use

d. Thyroid, calcium

e. Pregnancy test

f. CSF examination

IV. Tics

A. Definition. Tics are sudden brief movements or vocalizations that appear irregularly in a group of muscles. A tic may be a simple movement, such as a head jerk or shoulder shrug, or a complicated task that appears to mimic some voluntary act, such as an obscene gesture.

B. Types of tic disorders

1. Motor tics are abrupt, simple motor tasks, such as rapid head jerks.

2. Vocal tics are repetitive vocalizations, such as grunting and throat clearing.

3. Complicated motor and vocal tics

a. Complicated motor tics are semipurposeful movements.

b. Complicated vocal tics are repeated words or sentences. They may be made-up or obscene words.

4. Gilles de la Tourette's syndrome (TS)

a. TS patients exhibit multiple motor tics with one or more vocal tics.
b. Onset of symptoms occurs before age 21.
c. Symptoms persist for at least 12 months.
d. Behavioral disturbances
  (1) Obsessive-compulsive disorder (OCD) is characterized by repetitive stereotyped behaviors or thoughts.
  (2) Attention-deficit hyperactivity disorder (ADHD) (with or without hyperactivity) presents with poor attention span, restlessness, poor concentration, and decreased impulse control.
e. Learning disabilities. In addition to OCD and ADHD, some patients with TS have problems with classroom learning and academics.
f. Sleep disturbances include somnambulism, nightmares, insomnia, and restlessness. These disturbances may be related to treatment, environment, or superimposed psychiatric disease.
C. Etiology
  1. Tics involve **inherited changes in synaptic transmission.**
  2. The **dopamine hypothesis** suggests that tics result from an increased amount of hypersensitivity in the receptors.
  3. Tourette's syndrome. TS is generally hereditary. The gene and the biochemical defect are unknown. Data on TS suggest a sex-linked autosomal dominant inheritance with variable penetrance expressing as TS, OCD, or a mixed tic disorder.
  4. Other etiologies
    a. Tics may be observed after head trauma, toxin exposure, and encephalitis.
    b. Tics may occur in association with other primary neurologic disorders, such as Huntington's disease, Parkinson's disease, dystonia, and side effects of medications such as methylphenidate.
V. Myoclonus
  A. Definition. Myoclonus is defined as sudden, brief, involuntary jerks or contractions, either rhythmic or irregular, of single muscles or groups of muscles. It may occur at rest or in response to touch, auditory, or visual stimuli.
  B. Types of myoclonic disorders. Myoclonus can be divided into epileptic and nonepileptic types.
    1. Epileptic myoclonus comprises generally progressive degenerative disorders affecting the nervous system. Myoclonus may be observed in association with ataxia, dementia, or other seizure types.
      a. Progressive myoclonic epilepsy. Myoclonic and tonic-clonic seizures are exhibited by patients with progressive neurologic decline.
        (1) Progressive myoclonic epilepsy is associated with ataxia and dementia.
        (2) Neuropathologic studies can differentiate the subgroups of neurologic syndromes associated with myoclonus.
          (a) Myoclonic epilepsy with ragged red fibers (MERRF) presents in the second decade with myoclonic seizures and possibly hearing loss, optic atrophy, neuropathy, or hypoventilation. The diagnosis is triggered by detection of ragged red fibers on muscle biopsy.
          (b) Lafora's myoclonic epilepsy (Lafora's bodies) is an autosomal recessive storage disease diagnosed by skin biopsy. Dementia is always present and is accompanied by myoclonus and seizures. The mean age of presentation is 14 years, and the disorder may manifest as a behavioral change or school problem.
          (c) Baltic myoclonus (Unverricht-Lundborg disease) is an autosomal recessive inheritance with a mean age of presentation of 10 years. Myoclonus is always present, can be provoked by sound or touch, and may provoke a generalized seizure. There is no test for this disorder. There is the eventual development of gait ataxia, dysarthria, tremor, and mild dementia.
      b. Infections of the CNS
        (1) Creutzfeldt-Jakob disease presents with a rapid onset of dementia and associated myoclonic jerks. The characteristic EEG shows periodic lateralized epileptiform discharges (PLEDs).

(2) Subacute sclerosing panencephalitis (SSPE) is a rare sequela of measles infection. The onset usually occurs before age 2 years and is followed by a silent period of up to 8 years. Myoclonus is preceded by intellectual decline, personality changes, ataxia, and hyperactive reflexes. EEG shows PLEDs, and spinal fluid may demonstrate oligoclonal bands and antibodies to the measles virus.

   c. Drug-related conditions. Myoclonus has been noted in patients treated with levodopa, bromocriptine, tricyclic antidepressants, and narcotics.

   d. Toxic and metabolic conditions. Myoclonus may present in a confused patient as either large rhythmic movements or small irregular jerks and may be stimulus-induced. Myoclonic movements may be confused with seizures, particularly in an acutely ill patient, and ruling out seizures may require an EEG. The most common cause is severe renal or hepatic disease. Systemic infection or drug intoxication may also cause myoclonic jerks. Rarely, heavy metal intoxication can cause myoclonus.

 2. Nonepileptic myoclonus. Nonepileptic myoclonic disorders are nonprogressive. EEG correlation is found in some cases of epilepsy partialis continua and juvenile myoclonic epilepsy.

   a. Action myoclonus is induced by a voluntary movement or stimulus, such as a loud noise, and is commonly observed following hypoxic injury.

   b. Palatal myoclonus consists of regular, rhythmic movement of the palate that may spread to the throat, face, and diaphragm. Movement persists during sleep. The neuropathologic lesion involves the red nucleus, the inferior olive, and the dentate nucleus (triangle of Guillain-Mollaret). This lesion is often ischemic, but can be neoplastic, inflammatory, or degenerative.

   c. Segmental myoclonus may arise in an arm or leg secondary to a PNS or CNS trauma, infection, or inflammation. It also may accompany renal failure, neuropathy, or AIDS.

   d. Sleep myoclonus occurs shortly after going to or arousing from sleep. It may be confused with seizure, particularly in infants. This benign form of myoclonus may also be difficult to differentiate from infantile spasms. EEG remains normal.

   e. Epilepsia partialis continua manifests as regular myoclonic jerking associated with a cortical discharge and no change in the level of consciousness.

   f. Juvenile myoclonic epilepsy. Jerks in children may precede a seizure. A family history and abnormal EEG are diagnostic.

   g. Opsoclonus-myoclonus in children

   (1) Neural crest tumors may be seen on chest x-ray, or chest CT may be needed. Elevated catecholamine metabolites are present in the urine.

   (2) Opsoclonus-myoclonus may also occur in postinfectious syndromes.

VI. Tardive dyskinesia

 A. Definition. Tardive dyskinesia is a disorder manifested by involuntary movements in some patients after receiving prolonged neuroleptic drug therapy.

 B. Classification

 1. Classic form. Classic tardive dyskinesia presents as choreathetoid movements of the face, limbs, and trunk.

 2. Variable forms

   a. Tardive dystonia is manifested by spasms similar to those observed in torticollis, blepharospasm, or Meige's syndrome.

   b. Tardive akathisia presents as persistent motor restlessness.

 C. Etiology

 1. Tardive dyskinesia must be differentiated from other drug-induced syndromes.

   a. Acute extrapyramidal syndrome. Anticholinergic drugs improve acute extrapyramidal syndrome but leave a tardive syndrome unchanged or worse.

   b. Dopamine agonists and levodopa can cause hyperkinetic dyskinesias.

 2. Risk factors for tardive dyskinesia

   a. Age greater than 65 years

b. Severity may be greater in affective disorders than in schizophrenia.

c. Long-term use of antiemetic drugs, such as prochlorperazine and metoclopramide

d. The relationship between total dosage and duration is unclear.

VII. Referral

A. Dystonia. For diagnosis and planning of treatment, patients with focal or generalized dystonia should be referred to a neurologist with expertise in movement disorders.

B. Tremor

1. **Physiologic tremor** does not require neurologic evaluation.

2. **Essential tremor** may be diagnosed on clinical examination. Referral is recommended for those who do not respond to beta-blockers.

3. **Cerebellar tremor** requires no referral if symptoms follow the description in sec. **II.B.3.**

4. **Rest tremor.** Treatment can be initiated by the primary care physician. Refractory cases should be referred to a neurologist.

C. Chorea

1. **Huntington's disease.** Patients suspected of having Huntington's disease should be seen for a second opinion by a neurologist. Issues of genetic counseling and experimental clinical trials are best answered by a neurologist experienced in treating this disease.

2. **Other forms of chorea.** Drug-induced, metabolic, or pregnancy-associated chorea can be managed by a primary care physician. Refractory or unclear cases should be referred to a neurologist.

D. Tics. The majority of tics can be diagnosed and managed by the primary care physician. Referrals should be made for unclear or refractory cases.

E. Myoclonus. Most cases of myoclonus should be evaluated by a neurologist. An experienced neurologist can differentiate the epileptic and nonepileptic forms.

F. Tardive dyskinesia. Patients with tardive dystonia should be under the care of a psychiatrist. Antipsychotic medications should be adjusted to decrease the chance of further dystonia.

Recommended Readings

Bressman SB, Greene PE. Treatment of hyperkinetic movement disorders. *Neurol Clinic* 8(1):51–75, 1990.

Brown P. Myoclonus. *CNS Drugs* 3:22–29, 1995.

Butler I. Movement disorders of children. *Ped Neurol* 39(4):727–742, 1992.

Casey DE. Tardive dyskinesia. *West J Med* 153:535–541, 1990.

Hefter H. Wilson's disease. *CNS Drugs* 2:26–39, 1994.

Holds JB, et al. Facial dystonia, essential blepharospasm and hemifacial spasm. *Amer Fam Phys* 43(6):2113–2120, 1991.

Joseph AB, Young RR (eds). *Movement Disorders in Neurology and Neuropsychiatry.* Boston: Blackwell, 1992.

Regeur L, et al. Pharmacologic treatment of Gilles de la Tourette's syndrome. *CNS Drugs* 2:191–198, 1994.

Singer HS, Walkup JT. Tourette syndrome and other tic disorders: Diagnosis, pathophysiology, and treatment. *Medicine* 70(1):15–32, 1991.

Weisberg LA, Strub RL, Garcia CA. *Decision Making in Adult Neurology* (2nd ed). St. Louis: Mosby, 1993.

Winer WJ, Lang AE. *Movement Disorders.* New York: Futura, 1989.

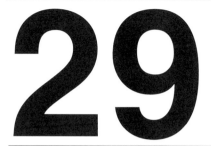

Approach to the Hypokinetic Patient
Robert L. Rodnitzky
Ergun Y. Uc

Hypokinesia is defined as a decrease in the normal amount, amplitude, or speed of automatic or volitional movements. The term **bradykinesia** is often used when the predominant movement abnormality is slowness, and the term **akinesia** is sometimes used to imply a severe reduction in the amount or amplitude of movement. In truth, it is rare for any of these three parameters of movement to be affected in isolation. Thus, the bradykinetic patient typically manifests a decreased amount and amplitude of movement in addition to a striking slowness of movement. Hypokinetic patients are often referred to as being parkinsonian because bradykinesia is so common in Parkinson's disease. However, bradykinesia is only one of four cardinal features of Parkinson's disease, the others being rigidity, rest tremor, and postural imbalance. Therefore, bradykinesia in the absence of these other features is not sufficient to make a diagnosis of Parkinson's disease. The term **parkinsonism** is used to infer a condition that is characterized by one or more of these cardinal signs and that clinically resembles idiopathic Parkinson's disease but is histologically different and often accompanied by additional neurologic signs and symptoms.

Both volitional movements, such as reaching for an object, and automatic movements, such as eye blinking or arm swinging while walking, can be referred to as hypokinesia. Surprisingly, when hypokinesia develops over a period of several months or longer, the patient and family members may be relatively unaware of the problem. A striking and remarkable decrease in the blink frequency often goes unnoticed until it is brought to the attention of the patient or family members. When hypokinesia begins to result in functional disability, patients then become aware of a problem in motoric function, but rather than attribute it to the speed or amplitude of their movements, they more commonly describe their difficulty as "weakness." Through careful questioning, the clinician can distinguish a history of weakness from one of hypokinesia. Once this distinction has been made, it is important to determine whether slowness or lack of movement is attributable to an extrapyramidal system disorder (e.g., Parkinson's disease) or to certain psychiatric disorders (catatonia or severe depression). One final differentiation that must be made is the differentiation between hypokinesia and neuromuscular disorders producing severe stiffness with associated slowness of movement.

Hypokinesia related to abnormalities of the motor system is seldom life-threatening except in extreme form when severe immobilization can result in serious complications such as sepsis or pulmonary embolism. Yet hypokinesia always merits serious attention because it often results in considerable functional and social disability.

I. Etiology of hypokinesia
A. Basal ganglia abnormalities.
Dysfunction of the basal ganglia is the most common cause of hypokinesia. Among basal ganglia disorders, those in which there is dysfunction of the striatum are most likely to produce a parkinsonian syndrome. Idiopathic Parkinson's disease (IPD), in which the nigrostriatal pathway is involved, is a classic example of striatal dysfunction, leading to hypokinesia. It is believed that the decrease in motor activity in this instance results from diminished excitatory drive of the motor cortex in turn resulting from dysfunction in the striatopalidal-thalamic pathways. Sometimes hypokinesia can be corrected by pharmacologic alteration of critical neurotransmitters found in these pathways or, less commonly, by stereotactic lesioning of component structures in hopes of restoring the critical balance of inhibitory and excitatory influences in motor systems.

There are various potential mechanisms whereby the basal ganglia or their neurotransmitter systems may become affected.

1. **Degenerative disorders** of the basal ganglia typically result in a loss of specific groups of cells often linked by neurotransmitter content or physiologic role.
2. **Pharmacologic agents** can result in hypokinesia by altering the release or reuptake of basal ganglia neurotransmitters or by blocking their receptors. This is especially true of those agents that affect the neurotransmitter dopamine.
3. **Vascular disorders** can result in isolated infarction affecting one or more basal ganglia. More commonly, hypokinesia results from a multi-infarct state consisting of multiple smaller ischemic lesions scattered throughout both hemispheres and diffusely affecting basal ganglia structures and their connections.
4. **Trauma** can result in basal ganglia dysfunction in several ways. Direct trauma such as a gunshot wound to the basal ganglia is one potential mechanism. Repetitive head trauma over a period of months or years often results in a parkinsonian state, presumably resulting from the cumulative effect of shearing forces on midbrain structures and blood vessels produced by rapid and severe blows to the head. This damage impairs the substantia nigra and its striatal projection fibers. This condition, which often occurs in boxers, is referred to as pugilistic encephalopathy.
5. **Toxins** may result in basal ganglia dysfunction as part of a generalized toxic encephalopathy, but even more commonly by targeting specific neurons in the basal ganglia or a connecting structure such as the substantia nigra.
6. **Central nervous system (CNS) infection** can impair basal ganglia function as a result of localized lesions such as abscesses involving these structures. Delayed onset of dysfunction can occur months to decades after a viral infection, as illustrated by the late appearance of parkinsonism after an epidemic form of encephalitis (encephalitis lethargica) that occurred early in the twentieth century.
B. **Psychiatric syndromes** can result in marked slowness or reduction in motor activity.
 1. **Depression** is classically associated with psychomotor retardation wherein spontaneous movement may be both reduced and slowed.
 2. **Catatonia** is characterized by severe reduction in spontaneous movement and a tendency to remain unmoving in a single position for a protracted period of time even when passively placed in that position by the examiner. This phenomenon is known as **waxy flexibility.**
C. **Metabolic disorders,** notably hypothyroidism, can result in global slowing of motor function.
D. **Neuromuscular disorders** that result in extreme muscle rigidity or stiffness retard the speed of movement, especially of axial and appendicular muscles, but seldom facial muscles.
II. **Clinical manifestations.** The clinical manifestations of hypokinesia result from different combinations of reduction in the speed, frequency, and amplitude of spontaneous or automatic movement.
A. **Hypomimia** is a decrease in facial expression. The diminished range of facial response to emotional stimuli gives rise to the term **expressionless facies.** The reduced eye blink rate results in an appearance resembling a constant stare.
B. **Diminished automatic movement** is noticeable as a decrease in gesticulation and head movement during conversation, a reduction in the automatic repositioning of limbs while sitting or reclining in bed, and a decrease in the amplitude of arm swinging while walking. In severe hypokinesia, the affected arm(s) may not swing at all, but rather be held in a semiflexed posture across the front of the trunk. In patients with asymmetric hypokinesia, as is often the case in Parkinson's disease, reduction in arm swinging is greatest on the most involved side.
C. **Impairment of repetitive movements** is particularly prominent in the hypokinetic patient. The patient may complain that activities such as handwriting and buttoning a shirt are particularly difficult. Not only are repetitive movements performed slowly, but the amplitude of each successive movement typically becomes progressively smaller. This may account for the progressively smaller letters (micrographia) observed when a hypokinetic patient is asked to write a long sentence or the increasing difficulty with the successive fine movements required to place a button through a buttonhole.

D. **Impaired initiation of movement** is manifested by difficulty in rising from a chair or hesitancy in taking the first step when attempting to walk. Many patients with Parkinson's disease have difficulty in simultaneously initiating two motor acts, such as standing up and shaking hands.

E. **Freezing** is a sudden involuntary cessation of a motoric act, usually walking, while other functions remain intact. This phenomenon is confined to basal ganglia disorders. Freezing may occur spontaneously or may be provoked by external circumstances such as attempting to turn in midgait or pass through a narrow space such as a doorway. Emotional stimuli such as anger and fear can provoke freezing, as can the prospect of entering a room filled with people. A variety of sensorimotor tricks, such as marching to a cadence, are effective in overcoming freezing.

F. **Hypophonia** is characterized by diminished amplitude and inflection of speech. In its most severe form it results in a muffled pattern of articulation. **Tachyphemia** is an excessively rapid speech pattern that is a common accompaniment of hypophonia, making speech even more unintelligible.

III. **Evaluation**
  A. **History**
    1. **Direct motoric symptoms of hypokinesia.** It is important to analyze carefully all motoric symptoms in the history, because what the patient describes as weakness or poor balance may actually be a manifestation of hypokinesia. Conversely, a complaint of slowness in performing motor functions, such as dressing, walking, eating, or writing, must be clarified to determine whether the slowing is actually a secondary phenomenon related to incoordination, weakness, or dementia. Specific symptoms that are particularly common in the hypokinetic patient should be recorded. These symptoms include difficulty in rising from a chair, hesitancy in initiating gait, and changes in the legibility and size of handwriting. If there have been frequent falls, it should be determined whether they are related to freezing. Because a change in facial expression may not be apparent to the patient, family members or friends should be asked to comment on this symptom.
    2. **Associated neurologic symptoms.** The identity of the underlying neurologic condition that has resulted in the hypokinetic state is often suggested by the constellation of other associated neurologic symptoms that the patient relates. Thus idiopathic Parkinson's disease (IPD) is suggested when hypokinesia is associated with the symptoms of rest tremor, stiffness (rigidity), and postural imbalance in the absence of other neurologic complaints. On the other hand, the association of hypokinesia with neurologic symptoms outside the motor realm usually suggests a condition other than IPD. Such symptoms include seizures, sensory loss, paresthesias, headache, early dementia, visual loss, apraxia, and early or severe autonomic symptoms such as impotence, orthostatic hypotension, or urinary incontinence. Another use-ful historical fact in differentiating IPD from other forms of parkinsonism is the sequence in which otherwise typical parkinsonian symptoms appear. Although postural imbalance and severe gait disturbance often appear late in the course of IPD, their appearance as presenting symptoms in the hypokinetic patient suggests a different etiology of parkinsonism.
    3. **Toxic exposure.** Exposure to the toxins manganese (observed in welders) and carbon monoxide must be ascertained, because both can result in parkinsonism. Less common toxins include mercury, carbon disulfide, methanol, and cyanide.
    4. **Medication usage.** Patients must be asked if they are currently taking or have recently received antidopaminergic drugs such as neuroleptics, reserpine, or metoclopramide. Additionally, any history of illicit drug use should be ascertained.
    5. **Family history.** Because idiopathic Parkinson's disease is a common disorder, it is not uncommon for patients to have family members who carry the same diagnosis. There appears to be only a mild contribution of heredity in this disorder. A family history of a hypokinetic disorder in more than one first-degree relative or a clear mendelian pattern of inheritance should raise the question of a neurologic disorder other than Parkinson's disease (although rare instances of autosomal dominant IPD have been reported). Heritable disorders that can mimic Parkinson's disease include Wilson's disease

(autosomal recessive), juvenile Huntington's disease (autosomal dominant), and essential tremor (autosomal dominant with variable penetrance).

6. **Psychiatric symptoms.** Determine whether there have been symptoms suggestive of depression such as suicidal thoughts, feelings of guilt or self-deprecation, or vegetative symptoms such as anorexia and disturbed sleep. If hallucinosis is present, it must be determined if it began early or late in the illness and whether it appeared in response to the institution or escalation of an antiparkinsonian drug. These symptoms are not present in early untreated IPD.

7. **Cognitive symptoms.** Document whether there have been any changes in memory, orientation, judgment, and intellectual functions. Severe, early abnormalities of this type may indicate a primary dementing disorder such as Alzheimer's disease or the presence of a multi-infarct state. Mild to moderate cognitive symptoms are present in most of the Parkinson's-plus syndromes, but are seldom the presenting symptom. Dementia appears in approximately 40% of patients with idiopathic Parkinson's disease, but usually only after time, when the illness is moderately advanced.

8. **Response to medications.** Determine if there has been a previous trial of therapy with dopaminergic agents and, if so, whether they produced an objective improvement. In a parkinsonian patient, absence of benefit from adequate dosages of dopaminergic drugs, especially levodopa, casts doubt on the diagnosis of IPD and suggests a diagnosis of secondary parkinsonism or one of the Parkinson's-plus syndromes. Equally important is determining whether, early in the illness, these medications produced psychiatric side effects such as hallucinations or autonomic symptoms such as severe orthostatic hypotension, the former suggesting the possibility of cortical Lewy body disease and the latter indicating possible multiple system atrophy (MSA). In IPD, psychiatric and autonomic side effects from dopaminergic drugs are not uncommon but usually appear when the illness is at least moderately advanced.

IV. **Physical examination**
   A. **The clinical findings of parkinsonism**
      1. **Gait and posture** should be evaluated by having the patient walk a distance of at least 20 ft in an area free of obstacles. In the parkinsonian patient, the length of stride is reduced. The arms do not swing and may be held flexed across the front of the trunk. The upright posture is commonly flexed in IPD. There may be difficulty in initiating gait, and turns may be accomplished with multiple small steps. The patient's feet may "freeze" in midgait.
      2. **Rising from a chair** is tested by asking the patient to rise with arms crossed in front of the body to prevent pushing off. The hypokinetic patient may require several attempts to succeed or may be totally unable to arise. If the patient is unable to rise without assistance, a judgment must be made as to whether the cause is weakness (which can be tested independently) or bradykinesia.
      3. **Postural reflexes** are evaluated by asking the patient to establish a comfortable base while upright and then, while standing behind the patient, applying a brisk backward sternal perturbation. A normal response is to take up to one corrective full step backward to prevent falling. When postural reflexes are impaired, more than one step is needed before balance is reestablished. When postural reflexes are absent, the patient continues to reel backward and falls if not checked by the examiner.
      4. **Rigidity.** If rigidity is present, it must be determined if it is predominant in axial muscles (e.g., neck or trunk), predominant in the limbs, or equally severe in both. Increased resistance to passive movement of the involved body part is easily appreciated when rigidity is severe. When subtle, rigidity can be reinforced by asking the patient to alternately open and close the fist of the hand not being tested. The presence of tremor in the same limb demonstrating rigidity gives rise to a rachetlike sensation referred to as **cogwheel rigidity.**
      5. **Tremor** may appear in one or more forms in patients with parkinsonism.
         a. **Rest tremor,** the hallmark of IPD and also present in some other forms of parkinsonism, is most commonly observed in the hands and to a slightly lesser extent in the lower extremities and mandible. Rest tremor rarely involves the head and never affects the voice. It appears at a fre-

quency of 4–5 Hz and is often at least temporarily extinguished by volitional movement. Because it is well known that rest tremor is enhanced by stress or anxiety, a subtle tremor can be uncovered by asking the patient to perform difficult mental arithmetic, a mildly stressful task. Rest tremor is the hallmark of IPD, and its absence casts some doubt on such a diagnosis but certainly does not rule it out.

b. **Action tremor** may also be present in Parkinson's disease as well as in other parkinsonian syndromes, especially those associated with cerebellar dysfunction. It can be present as a **postural tremor** while the arms are outstretched in front of the patient or as a **kinetic tremor** while the patient is performing a task such as the finger-to-nose test. Postural tremor alone, in the absence of parkinsonian signs, suggests a diagnosis of essential tremor (see Chap. 28, sec. **II**).

c. **Positional tremor.** Some tremors are particularly prominent when the involved body part is placed in a specific position. The **wing beating tremor** of Wilson's disease is an example of this phenomenon. This tremor is noted when the arms are abducted at the shoulders while flexed at the elbow.

6. **Bradykinesia** can be documented by simply observing the speed, amplitude, and amount of ordinary movements made by the patient, such as gestures or shifts in body position. Specific tasks such as the finger-to-nose test also provide opportunities to observe the speed of movement. Alternate motion tasks, such as tapping the index finger against the thumb, demonstrate slowness of movement and a progressive loss of amplitude as the movement is repeated.

7. **Facial expression.** The **diminished facial expression** typical of IPD is characterized by a constant neutral countenance with infrequent eye blinking. A **fixed facial expression,** often seen in progressive supranuclear palsy, consists of an unchanging expression such as surprise in which the forehead may be furrowed, the eyelids retracted, and the nasolabial folds deepened. **Myerson's sign** is present in Parkinson's disease and a variety of other basal ganglia disorders. It consists of persistent reflex eyelid blinking in response to repetitive finger taps applied to the glabella just superior to the bridge of the nose. In normal individuals there is rapid habituation to this stimulus so that no blinking occurs after the fourth or fifth tap.

B. **Nonparkinsonian neurologic signs.** Several neurologic findings are associated with one or more forms of parkinsonism.

1. **Apraxia** should be tested independently in both upper extremities. The patient should be asked to perform such tasks as saluting, throwing a kiss, or demonstrating how to use an imaginary toothbrush.

2. **Cortical sensory functions** such as graphesthesia, stereognosis, and tactile localization should be assessed.

3. **The alien limb phenomenon** can be detected by asking the patient to raise each limb individually while watching for a complimentary or interfering involuntary movement in one of the other limbs at rest.

4. **Ocular motility abnormalities** may be observed in some forms of parkinsonism. Inability to generate normal eye movements, especially downward, with preservation of the same movements when eliciting the oculocephalic reflex indicates a **supranuclear gaze palsy.** This finding is most characteristic of progressive supranuclear palsy (PSP) but can be found in other forms of parkinsonism as well. It is important to remember that limited upgaze is not an uncommon finding in the normal elderly patient, but impaired downgaze is always abnormal. Subtle abnormalities of saccadic eye movement can be uncovered by evoking saccades in the form of optokinetic nystagmus. In some basal ganglia disorders such as Huntington's disease, the saccadic excursion may be complete but the speed of eye movement is slowed. Lastly, it is important to check for the presence of **macro square-wave jerks.** This ocular movement abnormality consists of repetitive, alternate right then left, 5–10-degree horizontal deviations of the eyes from the midline. This finding is also associated with PSP.

5. **Reflex myoclonus** is elicited by tapping the arm or leg with the fingertip or a percussion hammer.

6. **Blood pressure measurements** must be measured in the recumbent and standing positions while recording the concurrent heart rate. Orthostatic hy-

potension is an early and common manifestation of MSA. It occurs later in the course of IPD, especially when dopaminergic or anticholinergic drugs are being used.

7. **Mental status evaluation** should include functions such as immediate and short-term recall, orientation, constructional praxis, calculation, and comprehension of three-step commands. The standardized Mini-Mental Test suffices for this purpose.

8. **Other neurologic signs.** In order to determine the full extent of involvement of the CNS, a complete neurologic examination should be performed to establish the presence of hyperactive or hypoactive stretch reflexes, sensory loss, cranial nerve dysfunction, cerebellar signs, pathologic reflexes (especially Babinski's sign), weakness, or muscle atrophy.

V. Laboratory studies

A. Neuroimaging studies

1. **Typical Parkinson's disease.** In classical IPD, for which the diagnosis is strongly suggested by the history and physical examination, neuroimaging is not necessary. Parkinson's disease is commonly somewhat asymmetric, but if symptoms or signs of parkinsonism are remarkably asymmetric, resulting in severe involvement on one side and virtually no involvement on the other, a CNS imaging study, preferably MRI, is indicated to evaluate for the possibility of a unilateral structural basal ganglia pathology such as a neoplasm, an arteriovenous malformation, an infarction, or the presence of brain hemiatrophy.

2. **Other forms of parkinsonism.** In patients with insufficient findings to make a diagnosis of IPD (e.g., patients with hypokinesia only) or with additional neurologic findings not usually seen in Parkinson's disease, a brain imaging procedure is indicated, preferably MRI. Not all degenerative forms of parkinsonism are associated with demonstrable MRI abnormalities, and those that are may demonstrate the characteristic abnormality infrequently or only in the advanced stages of the illness (see sec. **VII.C**). Therefore, a normal MRI or CT scan does not rule out syndromes such as PSP and MSA but usually does eliminate from consideration such conditions as normal pressure hydrocephalus (NPH), brain tumor, and stroke.

B. Laboratory and genetic tests are not useful in establishing a diagnosis of IPD but can be of benefit in diagnosing several other causes of parkinsonism (see sec. **VII**).

VI. Differential diagnosis (Fig. 29-1)

A. Idiopathic Parkinson's disease (IPD) is the most common cause of parkinsonism. It is a degenerative disorder of unknown but probable multifactorial etiology (environmental and hereditary). The predominant abnormality is in the substantia nigra pars compacta and the nigrostriatal pathway, leading to dopamine deficiency in the striatum. The wide spectrum of symptoms and the resistance of some symptoms (such as depression) to levodopa support pathologic observations that the degenerative process also involves other brainstem nuclei and subcortical structures.

1. **Clinical findings.** The cardinal symptoms are resting tremor, bradykinesia, rigidity, and impairment of balance. The onset is usually asymmetric, and tremor is the most common presenting sign. Postural instability, gait difficulty, and dysautonomia appear with progression of the disease. About 20% of patients develop dementia, but it is seldom severe and is never a presenting symptom. The incidence of IPD increases sharply with age, although it can present at any age. Arbitrarily, patients with onset between ages 21 and 39 are classified as young-onset IPD. They exhibit a more gradual progression of symptoms and can experience dystonia as an early sign. Levodopa-induced dyskinesias and motor fluctuations, which can occur in IPD at any age, are observed more frequently in this age group. The differential diagnosis of juvenile parkinsonism (before the age of 21) is broad and includes hereditary and metabolic conditions.

2. **Neuroimaging studies.** MRI and CT scans of the brain are usually unremarkable. PET scans show decreased fluorodopa uptake in the striatum.

3. **Neuropathology.** Lewy bodies (eosinophilic intracytoplasmic inclusions), mainly in the substantia nigra, are the pathologic hallmarks of this disorder.

4. **Other tests.** There is no specific test for the diagnosis of IPD.

B. Secondary parkinsonism can be induced by a wide spectrum of disease processes and other causes that affect the brain, especially the basal ganglia.

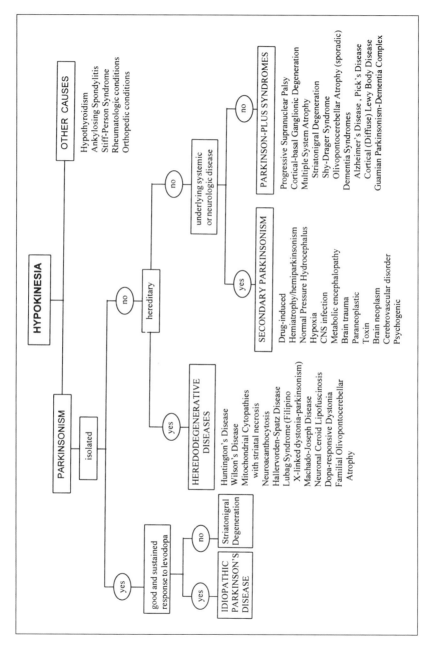

Figure 29-1. Algorithm for differential diagnosis of hypokinesia.

These causes include infection, cerebrovascular disorders, toxins, metabolic disorders, trauma, neoplasm, drug usage, hypoxemia, and hydrocephalus. Selected causes are as follows.

1. **Drug usage.** Neuroleptics and metoclopramide block striatal D-2 dopamine receptors whereas reserpine depletes dopamine from presynaptic vesicles. Each of these drugs can result in motoric symptoms indistinguishable from those of IPD. The "atypical" neuroleptic clozapine mainly blocks extrastriatal (D-4) receptors and does not cause parkinsonism. Another neuroleptic, risperidone, is reported not to cause parkinsonism in dosages under 5 mg per day. An underlying predisposition to Parkinson's disease may be in part responsible for the emergence of drug-induced parkinsonism. The resolution of drug-induced parkinsonism may take several months after discontinuation of the offending medication.

2. **Normal pressure hydrocephalus (NPH)**
   a. **Clinical findings.** NPH is a form of communicating hydrocephalus. Roughly one-third of patients with this disorder have histories of spontaneous or traumatic subarachnoid hemorrhage or meningitis, which may have led to impairment of CSF absorptive mechanisms over the surface of the brain. Although, as measured by lumbar puncture, CSF pressure is normal, there is excessive force on the walls of the dilated lateral ventricles, especially the frontal horn, leading to compression of surrounding structures. The clinical triad of NPH consists of gait apraxia ("magnetic gait"), subcortical dementia (which may later include cortical features), and urinary incontinence, often appearing late in the illness. The hesitant gait may resemble that observed in IPD, but the absence of rest tremor, the appearance of incontinence, and the absence of benefit from levodopa allow the two conditions to be distinguished. Early recognition of this syndrome is important because in some cases it can be reversed by shunting the ventricles.
   b. **Neuroimaging studies.** Enlarged lateral ventricles, especially the frontal and lateral horns, which are disproportionate to cortical atrophy, are observed. Proton density MRI images reveal periventricular hyperintensity, suggesting transependymal flow. In the elderly, separating this finding from nonspecific periventricular increased T_2 changes may be difficult. Isotope cisternography, although demonstrating impaired CSF absorption in some patients, is not considered a reliable predictor of response to shunting.
   c. **Other tests.** The Fisher test consists of removing 30–50 cc of CSF and watching for improvement in symptoms over the next 24 hours. It is a useful test and does not require sophisticated laboratory techniques. Intracranial pressure monitoring allows demonstration of periods of high CSF pressure (b waves) and is used widely as a predictor of response to shunting.

3. **Hemiatrophy-hemiparkinsonism** patients present at a relatively early age with markedly asymmetric parkinsonism affecting the side of the body manifesting hemiatrophy. There may be a history of abnormal birth and contralateral hemisphere hemiatrophy, both of which raise the possibility of an early childhood brain insult that later in life manifests as delayed-onset parkinsonism. The slow progression of this disorder, its occasional association with dystonia, and its striking asymmetry form the basis of its distinction from IPD.

4. **Toxins**
   a. **MPTP** (1-methyl-4-phenyl-1,2,3,6-tetrahydropyridine) is a toxin that was inadvertently self-administered by several substance abusers, resulting in an acute and severe parkinsonian state. The use of MPTP in the laboratory led to the most widely used animal model of IPD. New cases of human MPTP parkinsonism are rare.
   b. **Carbon monoxide (CO).** Parkinsonism may result from acute or chronic CO poisoning. This toxin causes globus pallidus or striatal necrosis. The onset can be immediately after the incident, but more commonly develops days to weeks after an initial recovery from coma. The history of CO-induced coma and poor or absent response to levodopa suggest the diagnosis.
   c. **Manganese** intoxication can result in a parkinsonian state and is also

frequently associated with unusual behavioral symptoms such as hallucinations and emotional lability, or with other movement disorders such as dystonia.

    d. Cyanide and **methanol** intoxication can also cause bilateral basal ganglia necrosis and parkinsonism.

5. Cerebrovascular disease. Either a lacunar state with multiple small infarcts of the basal ganglia or subacute arteriosclerotic encephalopathy affecting basal ganglia connections can lead to parkinsonism. In either condition, dementia is also common. Rest tremor is usually absent in these patients. Gait disorder can be very prominent and occasionally constitutes the only neurologic symptom, giving rise to the term "lower-body parkinsonism." The response to levodopa is limited.

6. Trauma. Pugilistic encephalopathy is a progressive neurologic syndrome characterized by parkinsonism, dementia, and ataxia and observed in boxers with a history of repeated head trauma. Treatment is usually unsatisfactory. Focal acute injury to the midbrain and substantia nigra and subdural hematoma are two other possible causes of post-traumatic parkinsonism.

7. Encephalitis. Approximately 50% of the survivors of the encephalitis lethargica epidemic of 1917–1925 developed parkinsonism, often as long as decades after the acute infection. This form of encephalitis has not reappeared in epidemic form since. Accordingly, new cases of postencephalitic parkinsonism are rare in the modern era.

C. Parkinson's-plus syndromes are a group of parkinsonian syndromes that are distinguished from IPD by the presence of additional prominent neurologic abnormalities. In these conditions there can be cerebellar, autonomic, pyramidal, oculomotor, cortical sensory, bulbar, cognitive, and psychiatric dysfunctions, as well as apraxia and movement disorders not typically observed in IPD, such as myoclonus, dystonia, or chorea. Any of these neurologic or psychiatric abnormalities can appear early in the course of the illness. Early falls with gait disturbance or postural instability, absence of rest tremor, early dementia, and supranuclear gaze palsy are signs that should always prompt consideration of a Parkinson's-plus syndrome. The parkinsonian components of these disorders, such as akinesia and rigidity, usually are not responsive to levodopa, although early transient responsiveness can be observed. The onset of these diseases generally occurs in the fifth or sixth decade of life, with an average survival of 5–15 years. The cause of death is usually intercurrent infection leading to pneumonia or sepsis. The etiopathogenesis of this entire group of disorders is largely unknown.

    Despite the apparent clinical differences between IPD and the Parkinson's-plus syndromes, differentiation between the two can be difficult. In a clinicopathologic study, 24% of patients who were clinically diagnosed with IPD were found to have a different type of parkinsonism at autopsy. In Parkinson's-plus syndrome, the head CT or MRI can be unremarkable, may show generalized cerebral or cerebellar atrophy, and may occasionally reveal focal changes in structures such as the caudate, putamen, cerebellum, or midbrain. Usually, CBC, blood chemistry, serology, EMG, and evoked potentials are not helpful. EEG may show a nonspecific abnormality such as slowing of the background activity. The specific features of individual Parkinson's-plus syndromes are described below.

1. Progressive supranuclear palsy (PSP)

    a. Clinical findings. Early onset of gait difficulty, loss of postural reflexes resulting in backward falls, and freezing of gait, coupled with supranuclear gaze palsy (initially downgaze), are suggestive of PSP. Axial rigidity and nuchal dystonia with extensor posture of the neck, generalized bradykinesia, "apraxia" of eyelid opening and closing, blepharospasm, furrowed forehead leading to a fixed facial expression, and a monotonous but not hypophonic voice are additional features suggesting the diagnosis. There is variable, but often mild, cognitive decline, especially in the executive functions. The presence of prominent bradykinesia in association with the typical fixed facial expression raises the possible diagnosis of Parkinson's disease in these patients, but the ocular motility abnormalities, the frequent absence of tremor, and the absence or loss of levodopa response suggest the correct diagnosis.

    b. Neuroimaging studies. Midbrain and, later, pontine atrophy are sometimes apparent on MRI or CT.

      c. Neuropathology. Globose neurofibrillary tangles are present, affecting mainly the cholinergic neurons of the basal ganglia and brainstem nuclei with apparent sparing of the cortex.

  2. Cortical-basal ganglionic degeneration (CBGD)

      a. Clinical findings. CBGD can present as a strikingly asymmetric or unilateral akinetic-rigid syndrome associated with limb apraxia, alien limb phenomenon, cortical sensory signs, stimulus-sensitive myoclonus, and postural or action tremor. Supranuclear gaze palsy, cognitive impairment, and pyramidal tract signs can also be observed.

      b. Neuroimaging studies. MRI or CT of the brain is abnormal in some patients and reveals asymmetric frontoparietal atrophy.

      c. Neuropathology. Neuronal loss and gliosis are found in the frontoparietal regions and substantia nigra pars compacta. Swollen achromatic neurons and basophilic nigral inclusions, which represent an overlap with Pick's disease, are characteristic.

  3. Multiple system atrophy (MSA) is a degenerative disorder that consists of three component syndromes: **striatonigral degeneration (SND), sporadic olivopontocerebellar atrophy (OPCA),** and **Shy-Drager syndrome (SDS).** These three syndromes can present individually or in various combinations.

      a. Clinical findings. In SND, akinetic-rigid parkinsonism is predominant, but tremor is seldom present. This syndrome usually is not responsive to levodopa because the degenerative process involves the postsynaptic dopamine receptors.

        In OPCA, cerebellar signs—especially ataxia and dysarthria—are the prominent findings, although they seldom exist in isolation. Other associated signs include gaze palsies, hyperreflexia, an extensor plantar response, and, most important, features of parkinsonism.

        In SDS, there is dysfunction of the autonomic nervous system (ANS), resulting in symptoms such as disabling orthostatic hypotension, bowel and bladder dysfunctions, and impotence. It is not clear whether these disorders are distinct entities or represent different clinical presentations of the same basic condition, but they commonly occur together and share pathologic features. From a diagnostic point of view, the syndrome of MSA should always be suspected in the hypokinetic patient with little response to levodopa who also manifests prominent autonomic or cerebellar dysfunction.

      b. Neuroimaging studies. MRI of the brain shows putaminal hypointensity in SND, probably resulting from excessive iron deposition in this structure. Cerebellar atrophy can be seen in OPCA.

      c. Neuropathology. Common to all the MSA syndromes is the presence of characteristic glial cytoplasmic inclusions. Especially in SDS, additional neuronal loss and gliosis are observed in the structures responsible for autonomic functions, such as the intermediolateral cell column of the spinal cord and the dorsal motor nucleus of the vagus.

  4. Dementia syndromes. Alzheimer's disease (AD), Pick's disease, and diffuse Lewy body disease (DLBD) are degenerative CNS diseases whose predominant manifestation is dementia. Although the degenerative process in these disorders has a predilection for certain cortical regions, subcortical structures may also be involved, leading to extrapyramidal manifestations including parkinsonism. The key to identifying a primary dementia disorder as a cause of parkinsonism is the early appearance of dementia, often antedating the onset of hypokinesia or rigidity.

D. Heredodegenerative diseases

  1. Wilson's disease is an autosomal recessive condition associated with impairment of copper excretion that results in copper accumulation in different organ systems, including the CNS, liver (cirrhosis), cornea (Kayser-Fleischer ring), heart, and kidney.

      a. Clinical findings. The age of presentation ranges from 5 to 50, peaking between 8 and 16. Neurologic symptoms are present at the onset of the disease in about 40% of patients. Extrapyramidal symptoms such as dystonia, rigidity, and bradykinesia are more common in children, whereas tremor and dysarthria are more likely to appear in adults. A variety of psychiatric symptoms can be seen in Wilson's disease. An especially important clue to the diagnosis is the presence of liver dysfunction such as cirrhosis or chronic active hepatitis, especially in young patients. The combination of bradykinesia and tremor in these patients may suggest Parkinson's disease, but the very young age of onset and the presence of psychiatric symptoms, liver dysfunction, or dystonia should prompt a search for laboratory signs of Wilson's disease. Because the consequences of Wilson's disease are preventable, and the neurologic symptoms are reversible with early treatment using copper chelating drugs, this condition should always be kept in the differential diagnosis of atypical parkinsonism, especially for patients below the age of 50.

   b. Neuroimaging studies. MRI of the brain shows ventricular dilation as well as cortical and brainstem atrophy. The basal ganglia, especially the putamen, can appear either hypo- or hyperintense on T_2 weighted studies, and hypodense on CT examinations. Occasionally there is the characteristic "face of the giant panda" appearance of the midbrain on MRI.

   c. Neuropathology. There is generalized brain atrophy. The putamen, globus pallidus, and caudate are cavitated and display a brown pigmentation reflecting copper deposition.

   d. Other tests. Plasma ceruloplasmin is the most useful screening test and is usually below 20 mg/dL (normal: 25–45 mg/dL). Plasma copper is decreased and urinary copper excretion is increased. Slit-lamp examination of the cornea reveals a Kayser-Fleischer ring in almost all neurologically symptomatic patients and represents a very specific but not pathognomonic finding. If one or more of these tests are normal and the diagnosis is in doubt, it should be confirmed by liver biopsy, which shows increased copper content.

2. **Huntington's disease (HD)** is a relentlessly progressive autosomal dominant disorder characterized by dementia, psychiatric disturbance, and a variety of movement disorders.

   a. Clinical findings. The major clinical components of HD are cognitive decline, various psychiatric abnormalities (personality changes, depression, mania, and psychosis), and movement disorder. Although chorea is the most common motoric symptom, bradykinesia usually coexists with chorea and may explain the occasional exacerbation of the motor impairment that occurs when control of the chorea is attempted with antidopaminergic medications. An abnormality of saccadic eye movement, particularly slow saccades, is often one of the earliest neurologic signs of this disorder. The typical age of onset is in the fourth or fifth decade, but 10% of the patients develop symptoms before age 20. Younger patients have usually inherited the disease from their fathers. They present with a combination of a progressive akinetic-rigid syndrome (the Westphal variant), dementia, ataxia, and seizures. It is these akinetic-rigid patients that are most likely to be misdiagnosed as having IPD, but the autosomal dominant inheritance pattern, the early age of onset, and the presence of seizures should suggest the correct diagnosis. There is an inverse correlation between age of onset and rapidity of progression. The duration of illness from onset to death is about 15 years for adult-onset HD and 8–10 years for patients with onset in childhood.

   b. Neuroimaging studies. Caudate atrophy is the principal finding on neuroimaging. It can be appreciated with either MRI or CT.

   c. Neuropathology. There is loss of medium spiny striatal neurons as well as gliosis in the cortex and striatum (particularly the caudate). This striatal neuronal loss accounts for the drastic decrease in the two neurotransmitters associated with these cells, gamma-aminobutyric acid (GABA) and enkephalin.

   d. Other tests. HD can be diagnosed and presymptomatic individuals can be identified with great certainty using DNA testing. The genetic abnormality has been localized to chromosome 4 and consists of an expansion of the usual number (11–34) of repeats of the trinucleotide sequence cytosine, adenine, guanine (CAG). The presence of 40 or more CAG repeats confirms the diagnosis of HD, and 32 or less excludes it. The status of those with 33–39 CAG triplets is uncertain. Because of the ethical, legal, and psychological implications of presymptomatic predictive testing, it should be carried out only by a team of clinicians and geneticists fully sensitive to these issues and aware of published guidelines.

3. **Other neurologic conditions** occasionally associated with parkinsonism include neuroacanthocytosis, Hallervorden-Spatz syndrome, Machado-Joseph disease, and familial calcification of the basal ganglia.

VII. Diagnostic approach

A. Clinical findings. Careful history-taking and physical examination are essential. A meticulous survey of medical and psychiatric histories, family history, and occupational or environmental exposure to toxins reveals most causes of secondary parkinsonism. Disease onset at a young age; a strong family history of the same disorder; early appearance of postural instability, gait disorder, dysautonomia, or dementia; lack of rest tremor; and lack of response to levodopa should be considered "red flags" that suggest a diagnosis other than IPD. The general physical examination is important because it may reveal signs of a systemic disease that is contributing to secondary parkinsonism. Neurologic examination establishes whether parkinsonism (rest tremor, bradykinesia, and rigidity) is isolated or associated with involvement of other neuronal systems in the CNS. The presence of aphasia, apraxia, supranuclear gaze palsy, cortical sensory loss, alien limb phenomenon, pyramidal signs, lower motor neuron findings, myoclonus, chorea, or dystonia indicates more widespread involvement of the CNS than is the case in IPD.

B. General laboratory tests

1. **CBC and peripheral blood smear.** Acanthocytes are found on a fresh peripheral blood smear in neuroacanthocytosis. Low hemoglobin and elevated reticulocyte counts consistent with hemolytic anemia may be present in Wilson's disease.

2. **Blood chemistry.** Abnormal liver function tests are found in Wilson's disease. Hypocalcemia, hypomagnesemia, and low parathormone are present in hypoparathyroidism. Elevated creatine phosphokinase (CPK) is associated with neuroacanthocytosis, and elevated serum lactate, suggesting lactic acidosis, is found in mitochondrial cytopathies. Low thyroxin and high thyroid-stimulating hormone (TSH) levels point to hypothyroidism.

3. **Serology.** Elevated erythrocyte sedimentation rate (ESR), C-reactive protein, or rheumatoid factor may be found in inflammatory or rheumatologic conditions which can induce hypokinesia by affecting the musculoskeletal system. Antibodies against glutamic acid decarboxylase or pancreatic islet cells are present in stiff-person syndrome.

C. Radiology

1. **Plain x-rays.** Spinal x-rays may reveal ankylosing spondylitis or osteoarthritis as the cause of mechanical limitation of movement.

2. **CT or MRI of the brain.** CT may demonstrate a neoplasm, cerebrovascular disease, hydrocephalus, basal ganglia calcification, atrophy, or sequelae of trauma. Contrast enhancement is recommended to evaluate for mass lesions. CT has some limitations, in that resolution is not always adequate to evaluate for density changes or storage materials in the basal ganglia, and brainstem or cerebellar cuts may suffer from bone artifacts. In these circumstances, MRI of the brain, although more expensive than CT, is more desirable. Several characteristic MRI patterns that are suggestive of specific hypokinetic disorders are as follows.

Many lacunae: vascular parkinsonism
Large ventricles, out of proportion to cerebral
    atrophy; transependymal flow: NPH
Caudate atrophy: Huntington's disease
Decreased T_2 signal in striatum: MSA
Homogeneous decreased T_2 signal or decreased T_2
    signal with a central hyperintensity ("Tiger's eye")
    in the globus pallidus: Hallervorden-Spatz syndrome
Striatal necrosis: Wilson's disease, Leigh disease,
    CO intoxication
Midbrain atrophy: PSP
Asymmetric frontoparietal atrophy: CBGD

D. Electrophysiology

1. **EKG.** Heart block may be present in mitochondrial cytopathy.

    2. EEG. Epileptic activity or focal slowing may appear with focal lesions (stroke or tumor). Slow background activity is observed in some primary dementias. Periodic triphasic complexes are present in Creutzfeldt-Jakob disease.

    3. NCV/EMG testing. Mild nerve conduction velocity (NCV) slowing suggestive of axonal polyneuropathy is observed in neuroacanthocytosis. Electromyography (EMG) findings consistent with myopathy may be present in mitochondrial cytopathy.

  E. Neuropsychological testing. If there is clinical suspicion of dementia, formal testing should be employed to plot the profile of cognitive decline.

  F. Cerebrospinal fluid (CSF) analysis. Elevated protein and pleocytosis can be detected in CNS infections. A large volume of CSF can be removed (Fisher's test) with observation for improvement in neurologic signs as one means of corroborating the diagnosis of NPH.

  G. Special diagnostic tests

    1. Huntington's disease. DNA testing can be done to measure CAG triplet expansion. Genetic and psychological counseling are advised before testing presymptomatic, at-risk individuals.

    2. Wilson's disease. Low ceruloplasmin, low serum copper, increased 24-hour urinary copper excretion, and Kayser-Fleischer ring on slit-lamp examination of the cornea are all suggestive of Wilson's disease. Liver biopsy for copper content is performed only if the diagnosis is in question.

    3. Normal pressure hydrocephalus (NPH). Intracranial pressure monitoring shows episodic appearance of high-pressure waves.

VIII. Referral. Patients with new-onset hypokinesia who have the following characteristics would benefit from referral to a movement disorders specialist.

Early onset—e.g., before 50 years of age

Early gait difficulty and postural instability

Prominent dementia

Positive family history

Supranuclear gaze palsy

Apraxia, alien limb phenomenon, cortical sensory loss, myoclonus, marked asymmetry of neurologic involvement

Bulbar, cerebellar, or pyramidal dysfunction

Marked dysautonomia

Absent, limited, or unsustained response to levodopa

Recommended Readings

Fisher CM. Hydrocephalus as a cause of disturbances of gait in the elderly. *Neurology* 32:1358–1363, 1982.

Giladi N, et al. Hemiparkinsonism-hemiatrophy syndrome: Clinical and neuroradiological features. *Neurology* 40:1731–1734, 1990.

Golbe LI. Young-onset Parkinson's disease: A clinical review. *Neurology* 41:168–173, 1991.

Golbe LI, Davis PH. Progressive supranuclear palsy. In *Parkinson's Disease and Movement Disorders*. Baltimore: Williams & Wilkins, 1993. Pp 145–161.

Hardie RJ, et al. Neuroacanthocytosis: A clinical, haematological and pathological study of 19 cases. *Brain* 114(Pt 1A):13–49, 1991.

International Huntington Association (IHA) and the World Federation of Neurology (WFN) Research Group on Huntington's Chorea. Guidelines for the molecular genetics predictive test in Huntington's disease. *Neurology* 44(8):1533–1536, 1994.

Koller WC, Silver DE, Lieberman A. An algorithm for the management of Parkinson's disease. *Neurology* 44(Suppl 10):S5–S52, 1994.

Purdon SE, et al. Huntington's disease: Pathogenesis, diagnosis and treatment. *J Psychiat Neurosci* 19(5):359–367, 1994.

Riley DE, et al. Cortical-basal ganglionic degeneration. *Neurology* 40:1203–1212, 1990.

Wenning GK, et al. Clinical features and natural history of multiple system atrophy: An analysis of 100 cases. *Brain* 117(Pt 4):835–845, 1994.

Yarze JC, et al. Wilson's disease: Current status. *Amer J Med* 92(6):643–654, 1992.

30

Approach to the Patient with Acute Muscle Weakness

Rahman Pourmand

Weakness is one of the most common complaints that leads a patient to consult a physician. Muscular weakness implies lack or diminution of muscle strength, which leads to an inability to perform the usual function of a given muscle or group of muscles. Muscle weakness should be differentiated from "fatigue," which is the subjective perception of weakness. In other words, weakness is the objective evidence of lack of strength, and fatigue is a subjective symptom.

After establishing "true" weakness, an etiologic search should be conducted. Muscular weakness has diverse etiologies. This chapter emphasizes the diagnostic evaluation and differential diagnosis of the leading neurologic causes of weakness, particularly as they relate to peripheral nervous system (PNS) involvement.

I. Evaluation

A. History. Determination of onset, course, and distribution of weakness and associated neurologic findings (such as cranial nerve involvement) is important. A history of recent febrile illness, changing of medications, or exposure to toxic agents should be elicited.

B. General physical examination. Examination of the skin is helpful in dermatomyositis or collagen vascular diseases, which can present with myopathic weakness. Signs of hyperthyroidism can be helpful in patients suspected of myopathy and/or myasthenia gravis (MG). Respiratory muscle dysfunction is paramount in the evaluation of any patient presenting with acute-onset muscle weakness.

C. Neurologic examination. Only the neurologic examination dealing primarily with the evaluation of acute muscle weakness resulting from PNS involvement is highlighted.

1. Distribution of weakness

    a. Proximal symmetric muscle weakness is usually observed in patients with primary muscle disease such as polymyositis/dermatomyositis (PM/DM) or in patients with acute polyradiculoneuropathy, such as the Guillain-Barré syndrome (GBS).

    b. Proximal asymmetric muscle weakness occurs in patients with acute brachial plexopathy or acute lumbosacral plexopathy. Also, acute focal myositis and MG may present with asymmetric limb weakness.

    c. Predominantly **distal asymmetric muscle weakness** occurs in patients with acute mononeuropathy such as foot drop secondary to peroneal nerve palsy or wrist drop resulting from radial nerve palsy. It is also observed with anterior horn cell involvement such as acute anterior poliomyelitis.

    d. Acute diffuse muscle weakness is found in patients with GBS, MG, periodic paralysis, or tick paralysis.

2. Muscle bulk. Muscle bulk is preserved in many adult neuromuscular diseases. Decreased muscle bulk is commonly present in patients with muscular dystrophy, motor neuron diseases (MND), and chronic neuropathies. Muscle bulk is usually normal during the acute stage of polymyositis, MG, MND, or acute polyneuropathy.

3. Muscle tone is often normal in patients with polymyositis or MG. Tone is decreased (flaccid) in MND and GBS.

4. Key muscles. Examination of selective muscles is key for differentiating upper and/or lower motor neuron type weakness. For example, neck flexor and hip flexor muscles are compromised early in MG and polymyositis (PM).

5. Sensory features. Sensory complaints are common in patients with polyneuropathy and/or plexopathy. The best examples are GBS and plexopathy, which present with sensory manifestations. Sensory examination is usually normal in patients with primary muscle disease and/or neuromuscular junction diseases.

6. **Muscle stretch reflexes (MSRs)** are normal in patients with neuromuscular junction diseases and/or primary muscle disease and are diminished or absent in patients with GBS, acute polyneuropathy, and/or acute MND.

II. **Laboratory studies** (Table 30-1)

A. **Blood tests.** If polymyositis is suspected, measurements of serum creatine kinase (CK), aldolase, erythrocyte sedimentation rate (ESR), lactic acid dehydrogenase (LDH), and serum glutamic-oxaloacetic transaminase (SGOT) are useful. If vasculitis is suspected, determinations of ESR, serum complement, antinuclear antibodies (ANA), antineutrophil cytoplasmic antibody (ANCA), and cryoglobulins are helpful. If MG is suspected, acetylcholine receptor (AChR) antibody titer and thyroid function tests are recommended. In conditions such as periodic paralysis, serum potassium and thyroid function tests are critical.

B. **Lumbar puncture (LP)** is indicated in patients suspected of having GBS, in which cerebrospinal fluid (CSF) may show protein elevation with minimal or absent pleocytosis (albuminocytologic dissociation). In the evaluation of patients with acute anterior poliomyelitis, LP may show lymphocytic pleocytosis and protein elevation.

C. **Electrodiagnostic studies (EDS).** Electromyography (EMG) and nerve conduction studies (NCS) are extremely useful in the evaluation of disorders of motor neurons, peripheral nerves, neuromuscular junctions, or muscles. The yield increases when an adequate history and careful clinical examination are available. The value of electrodiagnostic tests is discussed in Chap. 33.

D. **Muscle biopsy.** Muscle tissue can be obtained by open incision and/or needle puncture. The site of muscle biopsy should be identified by the physician performing the procedure in order to obtain the specimen from a weak but not atrophic muscle. Occasionally, two-site muscle biopsy is necessary to increase diagnostic yield. Specimen handling and interpretation of muscle biopsy by an experienced pathologist is crucial. Muscle biopsy is commonly indicated in acute PM/DM or acute vasculitis, and occasionally in periodic paralysis.

E. **Nerve biopsy** is commonly obtained from the sural nerve. This procedure

Table 30-1. Diagnostic differentiation among acute polyneuropathy, polymyositis, and myasthenia gravis.

Features	Polyneuropathy	Polymyositis	Myasthenia gravis
Clinical			
Weakness	Greater distal	Greater proximal	Greater oculobulbar
Fatigability	0	0	+
Wasting	0	0	0
Sensory loss	+	0	0
Muscle stretch reflexes	Decreased or absent	N	N
Fasciculations	±	0	0
Laboratory			
CSF protein	Increased	0	0
Needle EMG			
Fibrillations	+	+	±
Fasciculations	±	0	0
Number of potentials	Decreased	N	N
Slow NCVs	+	0	0
Muscle enzymes	N	Increased	N
AChR Ab	N	N	+ or increased
Muscle biopsy	Group atrophy or grouping	Necrosis, regeneration, inflammation	N*

0 = absent; + = present; ± = slight change; N = normal; AChR Ab = acetylcholine receptor antibody; *not necessary for diagnosis.

should be performed only when the clinical diagnosis remains in doubt and when the biopsy results will influence management. One of the leading indications for nerve biopsy is the suspicion of vasculitic polyneuropathy, particularly when presenting with a picture of mononeuritis multiplex or overlapping polyneuropathy.

III. **Differential diagnosis.** A useful approach for evaluation of acute muscle weakness associated with PNS involvement is to localize the site of lesion along the "motor unit," which consists of muscle fibers innervated by a single anterior horn cell. This discussion will be limited to the most frequent conditions causing acute muscle weakness, particularly those leading to generalized muscle weakness.

A. **Acute anterior horn cell disease.** Acute anterior poliomyelitis commonly affects children and is often caused by a group of polio viruses. Most persistent paralytic cases have been caused by type 1 polio virus. In the United States, oral polio vaccine strains represent a major source of acute paralytic poliomyelitis. It typically follows a prodrome of systemic symptoms such as fever, nausea, vomiting, constipation, muscle pain, and headaches. Muscle weakness develops a few days after the prodromal stage with asymmetric weakness of the lower extremities. Bulbar palsy and respiratory failure may occur. Tendon reflexes are decreased or absent. Some patients describe muscle pain in the acute stage. For confirmation of diagnosis, CSF examination is helpful. EMG is usually normal.

B. **Acute polyradiculoneuropathy.** Guillain-Barré syndrome (GBS) is an acute inflammatory demyelinating polyradiculoneuropathy. It begins with lower-extremity paresthesias followed by ascending symmetric muscle weakness. Proximal muscles are initially involved more often than their distal counterparts.

Muscle stretch reflexes are universally absent or diminished. Bifacial peripheral-type weakness is frequently observed. Labile blood pressure, tachycardia, and other autonomic disturbances may occur. Early in the course of the disease, the only EMG abnormality is absence of F waves as a result of proximal root involvement; later, the EMG shows changes consistent with segmental demyelination. CSF examination shows elevation of protein with minimal or no pleocytosis.

C. **Acute plexopathy**

1. **Acute idiopathic brachial plexopathy** is an uncommon disorder that is characterized by shoulder pain followed by weakness of shoulder girdle muscles. Pain is a very important part of this syndrome. There are familial and sporadic cases. A history of a preceding febrile illness resulting from viral infection and/or vaccination is common. Patients usually have good prognoses. The diagnosis is confirmed by clinical presentation and EMG.

2. **Other acute plexopathies.** Acute plexus lesions can also be observed in patients with closed and/or open trauma to the brachial plexus, such as in traction injuries. Neoplasia radiation and orthopedic procedures can cause plexus damage as well. Traumatic plexus injuries may follow gunshot wounds, needle punctures, and insertion of intravenous lines. Idiopathic lumbosacral plexopathy is a very rare entity. Diagnosis is confirmed by clinical features and EMG.

D. **Acute neuropathy**

1. **Guillain-Barré syndrome (GBS).** See sec. III.B.

2. **Lyme disease.** An acute demyelinating polyneuropathy can be observed in patients with Lyme disease. Lyme disease often presents with cranial neuropathies such as peripheral facial palsy and an ascending-type paralysis from the lower extremities, such as in patients with GBS. CSF is abnormal, showing elevation of protein, but in contrast to GBS there is a moderate degree of lymphocytic pleocytosis. Nerve conduction studies show evidence of demyelination.

3. **HIV infection.** An acute inflammatory demyelinating polyneuropathy similar to GBS is also observed in patients with HIV infection. CSF pleocytosis is common.

4. **Acute overlap polyneuropathy** is a form of acute generalized sensorimotor polyneuropathy commonly observed in patients with vasculitis. EMG examination shows evidence of asymmetric involvement of multiple nerves. Diagnosis is confirmed by EMG and nerve biopsy.

5. **Acute motor axonal neuropathy (AMAN)** was first recognized in northern China and was referred to as the Chinese paralytic syndrome (CPS). This

condition has many similarities to GBS. Pathologically, however, it is an axonopathy without inflammation and demyelination. CSF examination shows few cells but rising protein. Patients present with flaccid, symmetric paralysis of the lower extremities and areflexia. The clinical course is usually progressive and often causes respiratory failure. EMG shows evidence of normal motor conduction velocity and latencies, but the amplitudes of compound muscle action potentials are decreased. Sensory nerve action potentials and F waves are within normal ranges.

6. **Acute intermittent porphyria (AIP).** Weakness usually starts in the proximal upper extremities, but eventually all muscles become involved. Patients may become quadriparetic. Muscle tone is reduced. There is areflexia or hyporeflexia, except for ankle jerks, which may be preserved. Weakness of bulbar muscles is uncommon. Paresthesias and autonomic dysfunction are frequently present. Attacks of AIP usually are associated with abdominal pain and cramping. Confusion or seizures may occur. Attacks of AIP may be precipitated by fasting or by various drugs or infections. During attacks there are increases in urinary excretion of both delta-aminolevulinic acid (ALA) and porphobilinogen (PBG), determination of which should be supplemented by quantitative examination of urinary PBG excretion. The increase in PBG excretion (in milligrams per gram of creatinine) is greater than the increase in ALA excretion, whereas the reverse is true in other forms of porphyria. Between attacks and/or in the recovery phase, erythrocytes may show a low level of uroporphyrinogen I synthase. Nerve conduction velocity (NCV) studies show amplitude reduction of motor and sensory nerve action potentials, with preservation of conduction velocities and F waves. Needle examination shows evidence of denervation consistent with axonal neuropathy. The CSF is usually normal, but protein content may be elevated.

7. **Lead neuropathy** is predominantly a motor neuropathy. Weakness involves distal limb extensors, particularly in the upper extremities.

8. **Barium salt toxicity** may produce generalized weakness and areflexia. Muscle stretch reflexes are usually absent. Muscle fasciculations, perioral paresthesias, and dry mouth are common. Testicular pain is characteristic of patients with barium intoxication. Onset of weakness is usually associated with a low serum potassium level.

E. **Acute neuromuscular junction disorders**
1. **Presynaptic disorders.** Only selective disorders are considered. The Eaton-Lambert myasthenic syndrome, which has a more insidious presentation, is not discussed.
    a. **Botulism** is caused by the ingestion of toxins produced by *Clostridium botulinum*. This disease often presents with weakness of extraocular muscles followed by dysarthria and limb and respiratory muscle weakness. This diagnosis is suggested by a history of ingestion of contaminated food. Incremental responses are observed with repetitive nerve stimulation at high frequency rates. Nerve conduction studies are usually normal.
    b. **Tick paralysis** is a rare disease caused by the female tick (*Dermacentor andersoni*). Neurologic symptoms begin with walking difficulty and imbalance, followed by ascending flaccid paralysis and areflexia. Ocular and bulbar muscles may be involved. EMG shows reduced amplitudes of muscle action potentials and incremental response to a higher rate of stimulation, particularly during the acute stage. Some degree of slowing of conduction of motor and sensory nerves may be observed. A careful search for a tick in the scalp hair or pubic area is recommended.
    c. **Organophosphate poisoning** causes predominantly proximal lower-extremity muscle weakness. Extraocular and bulbar muscles may show signs of fatigue and weakness. Muscarinic symptoms such as miosis, increased salivation, and generalized fasciculations are often present. EMG is usually normal. Repetitive nerve stimulation may elicit incremental responses at higher rates of stimulation.
    d. **Drug-induced myasthenia gravis.** Certain medications adversely affect neuromuscular transmission. Weakness usually involves proximal limb muscles rather than ocular or bulbar muscles. Drug-induced MG may be associated with the use of kanamycin, gentamycin, procainamide, primidone, or hydantoins.

2. Postsynaptic disorders

a. Myasthenia gravis (MG). Adult onset of autoimmune acquired MG commonly begins with fluctuating and asymmetric weakness of extraocular and eyelid muscles followed by bulbar and limb weakness. Usual presenting features are uni- or bilateral and include eyelid ptosis followed by dysarthria, dysphagia, proximal limb weakness, and respiratory muscle dysfunction. There is also fatigability induced by repetitive exercise. Muscle tone, bulk, reflexes, and sensory examination are normal. Diagnosis is based on clinical examination, edrophonium (Tensilon) testing, single-fiber EMG, repetitive nerve stimulation, and determination of serum acetylcholine receptor (AChR) antibodies.

F. Primary myopathies

1. **Polymyositis/dermatomyositis (PM/DM).** Acute inflammatory myopathies usually begin with proximal symmetric weakness involving shoulder and hip girdle muscles. Muscle tone, bulk, and muscle stretch reflexes (MSR) are normal. There are no sensory deficits. PM is usually painless. If a typical skin lesion (erythematous rash in the periorbital, malar, forehead, or chest region, and particularly a scaly erythematous rash over the knuckles and extensor surfaces) exists with weakness, DM should be considered. Serum CK, aldolase, LDH, and SGOT are often elevated. ESR is usually high. NCVs and amplitudes are normal. Needle examination of the muscles shows increased numbers of spontaneous potentials such as fibrillations, positive sharp waves, bizarre high-frequency discharges, and small, polyphasic, short-duration, low-amplitude voluntary motor unit potentials. Muscle biopsy shows an inflammatory response involving the perimysium and endomysium, associated with muscle fiber necrosis and a variable degree of muscle fiber regeneration.

2. **Acute infectious myositis.** Postviral myositis is often associated with myalgia and weakness. In severe cases there is generalized weakness as well. Parasitic infections (trichinosis) and HIV infection can present with evidence of proximal muscle weakness.

3. **Acute toxic myopathy.** Acute alcoholic myopathy presents with generalized symmetric weakness. Hypermagnesemia also produces acute generalized weakness, particularly in alcoholic patients and in patients receiving hyperalimentation with magnesium. Amiodarone and L-tryptophan can cause acute myopathy, and L-tryptophan causes generalized myalgia, weakness, and eosinophilia.

4. **Acute periodic paralysis** is a group of primary muscle diseases associated with either normal potassium (normokalemic), elevated potassium (hyperkalemic), or low potassium (hypokalemic). Hyperkalemic periodic paralysis often follows the ingestion of a low- or high-carbohydrate diet after vigorous exercise. Hyperkalemic periodic paralysis presents with generalized weakness with sparing of cranial nerves and respiratory muscles. During attacks, MSRs are absent. Diagnosis is suspected on the basis of a history of intermittent weakness induced by exertion or a high-carbohydrate diet, family history, and measurement of serum potassium during attacks. EMG during an attack may show no abnormalities. A muscle biopsy may show a vacuolar myopathy, particularly if obtained during the attack. In highly suspected cases with normal potassium, a provocative test may induce the attacks.

5. **Acute steroid quadriplegic myopathy** is often observed in patients treated for status asthmaticus with high-dose steroids and neuromuscular blockade agents. After the status asthmaticus has been brought under control, patients remain weak and may even become ventilator-dependent. EMG shows evidence of neurogenic and myopathic features. Nerve conduction studies are normal. Muscle biopsy typically shows loss of myosin filaments on electron microscopy.

IV. Diagnostic approach. Diagnosis begins by first establishing the presence of muscle weakness and then determining if it reflects upper and/or lower motor neuron involvement. After exclusion of upper motor neuron weakness, further localization to the lower motor neuron is needed as suggested by the algorithm presented in Figure 30-1. Diagnosis often requires support by laboratory studies. Of these, the most confirmatory and cost-effective test is an EMG. Muscle biopsy is recommended for evaluation of PM/DM. Nerve biopsy is mainly indicated in cases of vasculitic neuropathy.

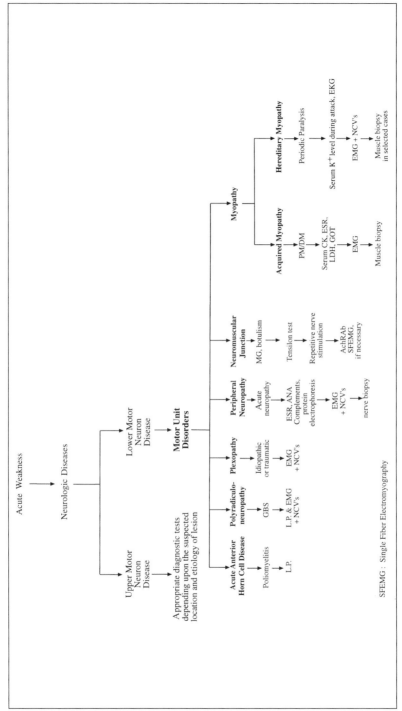

Figure 30-1. Diagnostic algorithm for selected patients presenting with acute muscle weakness resulting from neurologic disease. SFEMG = single fiber electromyography.

V. Referral. Patients with acute onset of generalized neuromuscular-type weakness need to be hospitalized, particularly those with acute paralysis and when GBS is suspected. If respiratory and/or bulbar muscles are compromised, patients need to be admitted to an intensive care unit. Other neuromuscular diseases can be diagnosed and treated in the outpatient setting. Most of these conditions can be taken care of by the primary care physician, but diagnosis often requires referral to a consulting neurologist.

Recommended Readings

Al-Lozi MT, et al. Rapidly evolving myopathy with myosin-deficient fibers. *Ann Neurol* 35:273–279, 1994.

Asbury AK, et al. Assessment of current diagnostic criteria for Guillain-Barré syndrome. *Ann Neurol* 27(Suppl):S21–S24, 1990.

Buruma OJS, et al. Periodic paralysis. In PA Vinken, GW Bruyn (eds), *Handbook of Clinical Neurology*. Amsterdam: North Holland, 1979. Pp 147–174.

Dalakas MC, et al. The postpolio syndrome. In F Plum (ed), *Advances in Contemporary Neurology*. Philadelphia: Davis, 1988. Pp 51–94.

Devere R, et al. Polymyositis: Its presentations, morbidity and mortality. *Brain* 98:637–666, 1975.

Gould DB, et al. Barium sulfide poisoning. *Arch Int Med* 132:891–894, 1973.

Hirano M, et al. Acute quadriplegic myopathy: A complication of treatment with steroids, nondepolarizing blocking agents or both. *Neurology* 42:2082–2087, 1992.

Hudgson P. Polymyositis and dermatomyositis in adults. *Clin Rheum Dis* 10:85, 1984.

Hughes JM, et al. Clinical features of type A and B food-borne botulism. *Ann Int Med* 95:442–445, 1981.

Kissel JT, et al. The spectrum of peripheral neuropathies with necrotizing angiopathy. *Ann Neurol* 14:122–123, 1983.

Leger JM, et al. The spectrum of polyneuropathies in patients infected with HIV. *J Neurol Neurosurg Psychiat* 52:1369–1374, 1989.

Oh SJ, et al. Diagnostic sensitivity of the laboratory tests in myasthenia gravis. *Muscle Nerve* 15:720–724, 1992.

Oosterhuis HJGH. Diagnosis and differential diagnosis. In H DeBaets, NJGH Oosterhuis (eds), *Myasthenia Gravis*. Boca Raton, FL: CRC, 1993. Pp 203–234.

Parry GJ. Peripheral neuropathies associated with human immunodeficiency virus infection. *Ann Neurol* 23(Suppl):S49–S53, 1988.

Pearn J. Neuromuscular paralysis caused by tick envenomation. *J Neurol Sci* 34:37–42, 1977.

Reik RJ. Peripheral neuropathy in Lyme disease. In Dyck PJ, Thomas PK (eds), *Peripheral Neuropathy*. Philadelphia: Saunders, 1993. Pp 1481–1511.

Ridley A. The neuropathy of acute intermittent porphyria. *Q J Med* 38:307–333, 1969.

Ropper AH, et al. Clinical features of the typical syndrome. In Ropper, Wiydicks, Truax (eds), *Guillain-Barré Syndrome*. Philadelphia: Davis, 1991. Pp 73–105.

Senanayake N, et al. Neurotoxic effects of organophosphorous insecticides: An intermediate syndrome. *N Engl J Med* 316:761, 1987.

Shankle R, et al. Acute paralysis from inhaled barium carbonate. *Arch Neurol* 45:579–588, 1988.

Swift TR, et al. Tick paralysis: Electrophysiological studies. *Neurology* 25:1130–1133, 1975.

Wadia RS, et al. Neurological manifestations of organo-phosphorous insecticide poisonings. *J Neurol Neurosurg Psychiat* 37:841–847, 1974.

Windebank AJ. Mental neuropathy. In PJ Dyck, PK Thomas (eds), *Peripheral Neuropathy*. Philadelphia: Saunders, 1993. Pp 1549–1570.

31

Approach to the Patient with Bladder, Bowel, or Sexual Dysfunction and Other Autonomic Disorders

Bhuwan P. Garg

I. Urinary incontinence

A. Introduction. A wide range of neurologic diseases are associated with urinary bladder dysfunction. Some common conditions are stroke, dementia, Parkinson's disease, multiple sclerosis, diabetes mellitus, and other neuropathies with autonomic involvement. Knowledge of normal bladder function is essential in understanding the urinary bladder pathology in neurologic disorders.

B. Anatomy and nerve supply. The urinary bladder is a hollow viscus with the primary function of urine storage with periodic evacuation. Micturition, an intricate and well-coordinated activity, is primarily a parasympathetic function. The sympathetic system is involved in urine storage and bladder capacity. Volitional control over micturition is exerted through the corticospinal pathways and spinal nerves innervating the external sphincter, periurethral muscles, and other abdominal and pelvic muscles. Cerebral cortex, basal ganglia, cerebellum, and brainstem pontine detrusor nuclei exert suprasegmental influence over the sacral spinal nuclei involved in urinary bladder innervation by means of the peripheral nerves.

   The various neuroanatomic connections that are important in urinary bladder control have been termed "circuits" (or "loops") by Bradley. The **first circuit** connects the dorsomedial frontal lobe to the pontine detrusor nucleus, with additional connections to the basal ganglia, and provides the volitional control over micturition. The **second circuit** (the spinobulbospinal pathway) is a reflex arc that starts in the sensory nerves of the urinary bladder and projects to the pontine detrusor nucleus and its outflow connections to the spinal sacral motor nuclei that make up the detrusor motor axons. This circuit constitutes the parasympathetic innervation. The **third circuit** is a spinal segmental reflex arc consisting of afferents from the detrusor muscle that synapse with the cells in the pudendal nucleus and its efferent nerve fibers to the striated sphincter muscles. The **fourth circuit** has a supraspinal component consisting of afferents running in the dorsal nerve of the penis and the posterior columns to the cerebral cortex and efferents by means of the corticospinal tracts to the sacral motoneurons. The spinal segment of this circuit is the sensory input from the external urethral sphincter and perhaps from muscle spindles in the other striated muscles of the periurethral area. The efferent arc of this circuit is formed by the axons of the alpha and gamma motoneurons in the sacral spinal cord that travel in the pudendal nerve and innervate the external urinary sphincter. Circuit 2 exerts brainstem control over micturition whereas circuits 1 and 4 provide the voluntary control. The sympathetic motor nerve supply to the bladder is carried by the hypogastric nerves, with the cell bodies situated in the intermediolateral column of the spinal cord extending from T11 to L2.

C. Clinical evaluation

   1. History. A careful and detailed history is essential (Table 31-1). The patient should be questioned regarding urinary incontinence, pattern of incontinence if present, changes in urinary habits, and frequency and urgency of urination. Desire to void, ability to initiate and terminate urination, force of urinary stream and urine volume, and sensations associated with urination are important aspects of the history. In spinal cord lesions, the level of lesion determines the symptoms and signs. Particular attention must also be paid to the drugs that the patient may be taking.

   2. Examination. Neurologic examination indicates the nature, site, and extent of the neuroanatomic lesion. The examination may also make it evident how

Table 31-1. Factors in history-taking for bladder, bowel, and sexual dysfunctions.

Bladder Dysfunction
Onset
  Acute, remittent, or progressive
Voiding
  Frequency: day and night
  Stream: slow, interrupted, or normal
  Initiation: voluntary or involuntary
  Termination: dribbling, abrupt, or normal
  Ability to stop on command
  Volume of urine passed
  Associated symptoms—e.g., headache, sweating
Sensation
  Sensation of bladder fullness
  Urge to void
  Passage of urine in urethra
  Effect of posture, cough, strain, etc.

Bowel Dysfunction
Continence or incontinence
Stool consistency
Constipation
Sensation of urge to void
Ability to discriminate between stool and flatus
Urgency, ability to hold
Drug use—e.g., laxatives, antacids

Sexual Dysfunction
Libido: normal or reduced
Erection: present or absent, duration, spontaneous, nocturnal, psychogenic
Ejaculation: normal, absent, or premature

Drug histories should be obtained for all patients.

much the patient can participate in his or her own care, such as in cases of dementia and Parkinson's disease. In frontal lobe lesions and suprasegmental spinal cord lesions, there are increased frequency and urgency of urination with reduced bladder capacity. Bladder sensation may be preserved in incomplete spinal cord lesions. This condition is termed neurogenic bladder. Table 31-2 presents clinical features of lower spinal cord lesions. In cauda equina lesions, if the motor nerves are preferentially involved, volitional voiding may be severely compromised even though bladder sensation may be largely preserved. This condition is called motor paralytic bladder.

  D. Laboratory evaluation. Laboratory studies are selected to clarify the nature of the bladder dysfunction and to detect any other associated abnormalities—e.g., renal dysfunction. MRI of the spine, and sometimes of the brain if indicated, is essential in the work-up of neurogenic urinary incontinence. Bladder neck obstruction must be excluded, especially in the motor paralytic type of bladder dysfunction. Consultation with a urologist is desirable in the evaluation and management of bladder dysfunction.

  1. Urine studies. Urinalysis and urine culture with appropriate sensitivity studies should be done. Patients with neurourologic dysfunction often may have associated urinary tract infection, which should be treated adequately and promptly with appropriate antibiotics.

  2. Renal function studies
    a. Blood urea nitrogen, creatinine, creatinine clearance, glomerular filtration rate, and other renal function studies, as indicated, should be obtained to detect impairment initially and subsequently.
    b. Intravenous pyelography is a useful test in the investigation and follow-up of patients with neurogenic bladder dysfunction.

  3. Urodynamic investigations
    a. Cystometry is an investigation of prime importance in the work-up of patients who have incontinence and voiding difficulties resulting from

Table 31-2. Features of lower spinal cord lesions.

Feature	Conus medullaris	Cauda equina
Location	S3–Cocc 1	L3–Cocc 1 roots
Onset	Often sudden and bilateral	Usually gradual and unilateral
Motor	Mild dysfunction; fasciculations may be present	Marked dysfunction; fasciculations are rare
Sensory	Symmetric, bilateral saddle-type distribution; mild pain if present	Asymmetric, unilateral saddle-type distribution; radicular pain may be present
Reflexes	Variable loss of Achilles tendon reflexes	Variable loss of patellar and Achilles tendon reflexes
Bladder	Paralytic, atonic bladder with increased capacity, incontinence	Paralytic, atonic bladder with increased capacity, incontinence, variable severity
Rectum	Patulous anus; decreased sphincter tone	Patulous anus; decreased sphincter tone; variable severity

neurologic causes. Cystometry provides information about the pressure-volume relationship on filling (bladder compliance), bladder capacity, volume at first sensation and at urge to void, voiding pressure, and the presence of uninhibited detrusor contractions. A normal adult bladder can usually be filled with 500 mL of fluid without the pressure rising to more than 10 cm of water. Urodynamic findings in various types of neurogenic bladder dysfunctions are listed in Table 31-3.

   b. **Micturating cystourethrogram (MCUG).** An MCUG is often combined with cystometry. Sphincter dyssynergia, position and opening of the bladder neck, and urethral anomaly and stricture as well as ureteric reflux can be visualized.

   c. **Cystourethroscopy** assesses the structural integrity of the lower urinary system, which consists of the urethra, bladder, and ureteral orifices. It does not examine the bladder during the voiding state and is not a useful test for diagnosis of functional disorders.

   d. **Retrograde urethrography** is used as a supplement to cystourethrography for delineation of urethral strictures, valves, diverticula, and false passages.

4. **Neurophysiologic studies.** Sphincter and pelvic floor electromyography (EMG) is a very specialized technique that is useful in experienced hands in detecting denervation potentials in selected muscles in lesions of the anterior horn cells in the spinal cord. Increased terminal latency on pudendal nerve stimulation may be observed in neuropathic causes of incontinence. Pudendal nerve conduction velocity (NCV) studies may also be abnormal in neuropathic causes. It is technically difficult to record from the urethral sphincter (mainly S3 innervation), and hence the anal sphincter (mainly S4 innervation) is often used instead.

E. **Management of urinary incontinence**
   1. **Incontinence with urgency**
      a. Patients who suffer from urinary incontinence with urgency usually have upper motor neuron signs on neurologic examination. Table 31-4 lists some causes of this type of incontinence. Frequency of micturition is often present in these patients, and bladder capacity is usually reduced.

Table 31-3. Urodynamic findings in various types of neurogenic bladder dysfunctions.

Spastic bladder	Atonic bladder	Sphincter dyssynergia
Decreased capacity	Increased capacity	Fluctuating voiding pressure
Reduced compliance	Increased compliance	Intermittent flow rate
Uninhibited detrusor contractions	Low voiding pressure and flow rate	

Table 31-4. Selected neurologic causes of urinary incontinence with urgency.

Alzheimer's disease
Parkinson's disease
Other diseases with dementia
Myxedema
Hydrocephalus
Bilateral frontal lobe lesions
Parasagittal tumors
Multiple sclerosis
Transverse myelitis
Cervical spondylosis
Spinal cord tumors
Spinal cord injury
Spinal cord compression
Syphilis
Sacral agenesis
Tethered cord syndromes
Myelomeningocele

The non-neurologic cause of urgency is usually a cystitis secondary to an infection or inflammation resulting from some other cause. Cystitis may be present in patients with neurogenic incontinence, and urinalysis and urine culture should be done when appropriate.

   b. Methods used in management

   (1) Bladder training. Timed bladder emptying, intermittent catheterization, and biofeedback techniques are used.

   (2) Pharmacotherapy. Many classes of drugs are useful. Such drugs include anticholinergics, musculotropics, calcium antagonists, beta-adrenergic agonists, and tricyclic antidepressants. (See Table 31-5 for doses.)

   (3) Surgical methods. Dorsal root rhizotomy, selective sacral root rhizotomy, peripheral bladder denervation, and cystoplasty to increase bladder capacity have all been used. Residual urine volumes should be checked in all patients, because large residuals predispose to further complications.

2. Atonic bladder with overflow incontinence is observed in cases of spinal shock, conus medullaris and cauda equina lesions, and neuropathies of various types (Table 31-6). It is also observed during the courses of some progressive neurologic diseases such as multiple system atrophy (MSA). The bladder capacity is increased.

The goal of therapy is to improve bladder tone and to reduce bladder capacity. The following methods are used.

   a. Credé's maneuver or Valsalva's maneuver may be used to empty the bladder.

   b. Intermittent self-catheterization is perhaps the mainstay of long-term treatment. Aseptic technique is taught to the patient to prevent infection.

Table 31-5. Drugs used for treating neurogenic bladder dysfunctions.

Class of drugs	Drug name	Dosage
Anticholinergics	Propantheline bromide	15–30 mg q4–6 hr
	Glycopyrrolate	1.0 mg bid or tid
Musculotropics	Oxybutynin	5 mg tid or qid
	Flavoxate	100–200 mg tid or qid
	Dicyclomine	20 mg tid
Calcium antagonists	Terodiline	12.5 mg bid or tid
Beta-adrenergic agonists	Terbutaline	5.0 mg tid
Tricyclic antidepressants	Imipramine	25 mg tid or qid

Table 31-6. Selected causes of atonic bladder.

Acute spinal shock
Acute transverse myelitis
Conus medullaris lesions
Cauda equina lesions
Peripheral neuropathy
Diabetes mellitus
Alcoholic neuropathy
Heavy metal toxicity
Guillain-Barré syndrome
Amyloid neuropathy
Tabes dorsalis
Multiple system atrophy
Friedreich's ataxia
Pelvic radiation
Acute intoxications (e.g., alcohol)
Plexopathy

    c. Pharmacotherapy is usually not an effective treatment modality. However, drugs such as bethanecol in a dosage range of 25–100 mg qid may be used, but often there are unacceptable side effects.

    3. Detrusor sphincter dyssynergia is a condition in which the external urethral sphincter fails to relax when there is constriction of the detrusor muscles during voiding. This failure may be intermittent and incomplete or may occur after a delay. There is often increased residual urine volume with low flow and an intermittent pattern of voiding (see Table 31-3). Urodynamic studies such as cystometry are useful in the diagnosis.

II. Fecal incontinence. The anatomy of the rectum, the anus, and the anal sphincters, and the associated neuromuscular reflex mechanisms, are important in maintaining fecal continence.

    A. Nerve supply. The innervation of the rectum parallels that of the urinary bladder. The external anal sphincter is innervated from sacral segments S2 to S4 by the pudendal nerves. The internal anal sphincter receives its innervation from the sympathetic system by means of the hypogastric plexus, with the nerve cell bodies being situated at the L1-L2 level. Somatic sensations of light touch, pain, and temperature reach the sacral cord through the pudendal nerves. In general, the parasympathetic system controls bowel emptying whereas the sympathetic system modulates rectal filling.

    B. Clinical evaluation

        1. History. A careful history is essential and should include an inquiry into the circumstances at the onset, alterations in bowel habits, and stool frequency, consistency, and mass (see Table 31-1). The patient should be questioned to establish whether there is preservation of rectal sensation as manifested by the ability to feel the pressure of fecal volume and the need to defecate, whether there is ability to differentiate between the passage of flatus and the passage of feces, whether the patient can voluntarily inhibit defecation, and whether there is urgency.

        2. Examination. The neurologic examination indicates the site and extent of the lesion responsible for bowel incontinence, as in the case of urinary incontinence. In upper motor neuron lesions rostral to the sacral cord, there is fecal retention, loss of voluntary control, increased anal sphincter tone, and inability to relax or contract the sphincter on command. Lesions of the sacral cord, conus medullaris, or cauda equina result in a weak and areflexic anal sphincter with a patulous anus. There may also be associated sensory loss. The extents of the sensory deficit and its recovery are important in determining bowel control.

    C. Laboratory evaluation. The laboratory studies used in the investigation of fecal incontinence are limited.

        1. Endoscopic studies. Proctoscopy and other endoscopic studies, as indicated, demonstrate structural abnormalities.

2. Radiologic studies
a. MRI of the spine is essential in spinal cord lesions.

b. Pelvic CT scans may be indicated for some patients with malformations and other structural abnormalities.

c. Barium enemas are helpful in demonstrating obstructions and also in some structural abnormalities.

3. Neurophysiologic studies.
Anal sphincter and puborectalis muscle EMG and pudendal nerve conduction studies, as discussed in the section on urinary incontinence, may provide discriminative evidence of the type of neurologic disorder (see Table 31-2).

D. Management of fecal incontinence.
First of all, overflow incontinence as a result of fecal impaction must be excluded. The history should have excluded overuse of laxatives or other medications such as magnesium-containing antacids as a cause of incontinence that will respond to cessation of the offending medication. Rectal prolapse, if present, should be treated.

1. Dietary management.
The goal is to increase the volume of the colonic contents and maintain them at a near normal consistency.

a. Diet high in fiber content

b. Docusate sodium to prevent stool hardening

c. Psyllium types of dietary fiber to decrease stool viscosity and increase volume

2. Techniques for achieving orderly defecation
a. Valsalva's maneuver and abdominal pressure work in some patients who have preservation of some rectal sensation and feel the urge to defecate.

b. Glycerine suppositories and digital stimulation of the rectum (using a gloved finger) work in some patients. They are most effective with the patient in the sitting position.

c. Neural stimulators. Anterior sacral root stimulators are under investigation.

d. Surgical intervention. Formation of a replacement sphincter and pelvic floor reconstruction may be considered in suitable cases.

III. Sexual dysfunction
A. Introduction.
The sexual response cycle of excitement, plateau, orgasm, and resolution is mediated through the integrated and coordinated activity of the somatic and autonomic nervous systems innervating the reproductive system. Sexual dysfunction in the male is better understood than that in the female.

Male sexual dysfunction may be manifested by diminished libido, impaired penile erection, or failure to ejaculate. Psychogenic causes of sexual dysfunction are common and may be the primary cause. Patients with organic sexual dysfunction often have secondary psychogenic factors. Depression and anxiety are the most common psychological causes of sexual dysfunction, whereas chronic ill health is probably the most common cause of organic sexual dysfunction. Organic causes of sexual dysfunction include vascular, endocrine, and neurologic abnormalities. Neurologic causes involve impairments of the somatic, sympathetic, and parasympathetic nervous systems.

B. Anatomy of and nerve supply to the sexual organs
1. Somatic motor and sensory nerve supply.
The pudendal nerve carries both the motor and sensory fibers that innervate the penis and clitoris. Motor nerve fibers that reach the pudendal nerve by way of the sacral plexus arise from cells in the medial part of the nucleus of Onufrowicz (Onuf's nucleus) situated at the sacral S2-S4 level. The sensory fibers also reach the same sacral levels. There are three branches of the pudendal nerve. The first branch, the inferior rectal nerve, innervates the external anal sphincter. The second branch, the perineal nerve, supplies the external urethral sphincter, the bulbocavernosus and ischiocavernosus muscles and other muscles of the perineum, as well as the skin of the perineum and scrotum in the male and labia in the female. The third branch is the dorsal (sensory) nerve of the penis or clitoris.

2. Parasympathetic nerve supply.
The parasympathetic nerves have their cell bodies in the sacral cord. The preganglionic fibers exit and travel with sacral ventral roots S2-S4 in the cauda equina and subsequently form the pelvic nerves that join the inferior hypogastric or pelvic plexus. The postganglionic fibers from this plexus innervate the erectile penile and clitoral

tissues, the smooth muscles in the urethra, and the seminal vesicles and prostate in the male and vagina and uterus in the female. They also innervate the blood vessels in the pelvic structures involved in sexual function.

3. **Sympathetic nerve supply.** The sympathetic nerves arise from cells in the intermediolateral cell column in the lower thoracic and upper lumbar spinal cord. The preganglionic fibers leave the cord at the T11-T12 level with the ventral nerve roots and enter the sympathetic chain and the inferior mesenteric and superior hypogastric plexus. The postganglionic fibers travel in the hypogastric nerves and innervate the same structures as do the parasympathetic nerves.

C. **Clinical evaluation**
   1. **History.** Tables 31-7 and 31-8 list various causes of diminished libido and erectile impotence, respectively. The history should be directed toward eliciting the appropriate information. Particular attention should be paid to the history of medications, alcohol intake, symptoms of leg claudication, and psychological symptoms.
   2. **Examination** may disclose evidence of liver dysfunction, testicular atrophy and hypogonadism, or vascular insufficiency. Neurologic examination should provide evidence of cerebral, spinal cord, or peripheral nerve dysfunction.
D. **Laboratory evaluation** of sexual dysfunction is an adjunct to clinical evaluation and is used to confirm a precise etiology and formulate a course of treatment.
   1. **Endocrine evaluation.** Fasting blood sugar and a glucose tolerance test if necessary, liver function tests, and appropriate endocrine tests such as thyroid function and prolactin level tests may be diagnostic. Consultation with an endocrinologist should be sought if necessary.
   2. **Neurophysiologic tests.** Specialized sleep studies, EMG (especially in suspected cases of MSA), and somatosensory evoked potentials in some cases of myelopathy may be useful in selected patients.
   3. **Vascular studies**
      a. Low-dosage injection of vasoactive agents such as papaverine into the corpora cavernosa of the penis may help distinguish vascular causes from other etiologies. The response to vasoactive agent injection is poor in erectile impotence resulting from vascular causes.
      b. Arteriography of the major leg and pelvic vessels may sometimes be indicated.
   4. **Psychiatric evaluation.** Psychiatric consultation should be obtained in appropriate cases.
E. **Management of sexual dysfunction.** Endocrine, metabolic, vascular, and psychogenic etiologies must be treated when present. Where drugs are the etiology, changes in medication may be beneficial. Other specialized treatment modalities consist of cavernosal unstriated muscle relaxant injection, penile

---

Table 31-7. Causes of diminished libido.

Chronic ill health
Addison's disease
Hypothyroidism
Hypogonadism
Excessive estrogen in males
Chronic hepatic disease
Drugs
  Reserpine
  Propranolol
  Cimetidine
  Tricyclic antidepressants
  Monoamine oxidase inhibitors
  Sedatives and narcotics
Alcohol
Depression
Anxiety

Drug history is important, and any medicine the patient is taking should be excluded as a cause.

Table 31-8. Causes of erectile impotence.

Conus medullaris lesions	Hyperprolactinemia
Cauda equina lesions	Antihypertensive medications
Spinal cord injury	Anticholinergic medications
Myelopathy	Antipsychotic medications
Multiple sclerosis	Antihistamines
Peripheral neuropathy	Alcohol
Diabetes mellitus	Syphilis
Amyloid neuropathy	Arteriosclerosis
Vitamin B_{12} deficiency	Excessive venous leakage (venous leakers)
Sacral plexus lesions	Depression
Multiple system atrophy	Anxiety
Pure autonomic failure	

Drug history is important, and any medicine the patient is taking should be excluded as a cause.

implants, sacral root stimulation, pharmacologic treatment, and use of a vibrator. Consultation should be obtained from physicians familiar with these techniques.

IV. Generalized autonomic failure

A. Introduction

1. Multiple system atrophy (MSA), initially described by Shy and Drager, is characterized by autonomic failure and motor abnormalities. It is often confused with Parkinson's disease, from which it must be distinguished. The onset of symptoms occurs in the fifth to the seventh decade of life. The condition may be more common than is usually recognized, with an estimated prevalence in the population of 5–15 per 100,000.

2. Pure autonomic failure is a clinical condition in which there is autonomic failure without other associated neurologic or motor abnormalities.

B. Clinical evaluation

1. Autonomic failure. Patients have orthostatic hypotension, urinary and rectal incontinence, loss of sweating, iris atrophy, and impotence. There is usually an atonic bladder and decreased rectal sphincter tone. Pupils may show alternating anisocoria. In men, sexual dysfunction is an early sign, first with failure of erection followed later by failure of ejaculation. MSA should be considered in patients with impotence who also have signs and symptoms of bladder and bowel dysfunction.

C. Motor abnormalities can be categorized into the following three types.

1. Striatonigral degeneration. Clinical features may superficially resemble those of Parkinson's disease. However, patients with MSA have a predominance of rigidity without much tremor. There is limb akinesia and rigidity without the classic cogwheel or lead pipe type of phenomenon that is commonly seen in Parkinson's disease. Patients have difficulty in standing, walking, and turning. Gait is slow and clumsy. There is progressive loss of facial expression with associated slurred speech, which is faint. Salivation is reduced. Patients have stooping posture with excessive cervical flexion, making forward gaze difficult.

2. Pyramidal and peripheral motor abnormalities. Spastic muscle tone may be difficult to detect in the presence of other extrapyramidal signs. Muscle stretch reflexes are increased, and primitive reflexes such as palmomental reflexes may be present. Conjugate extraocular movements may be restricted. There is often muscle atrophy of a mild nature, especially in the distal muscles, which is associated with fasciculations. Electromyography suggests involvement of the anterior horn cells.

3. Cerebellar dysfunction is characterized by a prominent truncal ataxia and gait disturbance that make it difficult for the patient to stand. Action tremor of mild to moderate intensity is present. Speech is markedly slurred and has a cerebellar quality. The cerebellar deficit resembles that seen in olivopontocerebellar atrophy (OPCA), although there is no associated optic atrophy, retinitis pigmentosa, chorea, or cataracts.

D. Laboratory evaluation

1. Orthostatic hypotension. Demonstration of orthostatic hypotension is crucial to the diagnosis of MSA. Blood pressure is measured in the supine and upright positions. A drop in the systolic blood pressure of 20 mm Hg or more, or a drop in the diastolic pressure of 10 mm Hg or more, in response to upright posture is abnormal. The patient may become symptomatic and complain of weakness, dizziness, or faintness, or may have a syncopal episode.

2. **Pharmacologic tests.** There is failure of the rise in plasma norepinephrine levels as a result of head-up tilt.

3. **Electromyography (EMG)** may show signs of denervation in limb muscles, suggesting involvement of the anterior horn cells.

4. **MRI.** Decreased signal intensity may be observed in the posterolateral aspect of the putamen on T2-weighted images. Cerebellar atrophy may be present in some patients even without any clinical cerebellar signs.

5. **Bladder, bowel, and sexual dysfunctions.** Evaluation and management of these abnormalities are as described in secs. **I, II,** and **III.**

E. **Management.** Only symptomatic treatment is available. Rigidity, bradykinesia, and motor symptoms usually do not respond to levodopa, although it may be worth a try. Side effects, especially accentuation of hypotension, must be kept in mind.

1. **Orthostatic hypotension**
   a. **Nighttime measures**
      (1) **Posture.** Elevation of the head of the bed by 6 to 12 in. at night is often helpful. Patients tolerate this rather uncomfortable position once they experience the benefits. Sitting on the edge of the bed for a short time after awakening in the morning may also minimize symptoms.
      (2) **Desmopressin (DDAVP)** is given at night as either a nasal spray or an intramuscular injection. A single dose of 5–40 µg is often sufficient to prevent nocturia and morning postural hypotension. It is best to start treatment in the hospital under close supervision to establish an appropriate dosage that does not cause side effects. Plasma sodium concentration and osmolality should be monitored on a regular, outpatient basis.
   b. **Daytime measures**
      (1) **Fludrocortisone** in oral doses of 0.1 mg/day, with adequate hydration and dietary intake of at least 150 mEq of sodium, is often helpful. Small, frequent meals prevent postprandial aggravation of orthostatic hypotension.
      (2) **Ephedrine or phenylpropanolamine** in a dosage of 12.5 to 75 mg tid as tolerated may be effective in some patients and is worth trying. Some patients may tolerate 5–10 mg tid of methylphenidate, although it may disturb sleep if the last dose of the day is given late in the evening.
      (3) **Elastic support garments** have long been used to treat orthostatic hypotension, and some patients find them beneficial. They rarely are of much long-term benefit.
      (4) **Mild exercise** may help by maintaining and improving muscle tone and thereby facilitating venous return.
      (5) **Bladder, bowel, and sexual dysfunctions** are managed as outlined in secs. **I, II,** and **III.**

V. **Acute autonomic dysfunction**
   A. **Autonomic crises.** Acute autonomic dysfunction is observed in many conditions, and a hypersympathetic state is most often encountered. Examples of such neurologic conditions are as follows.
      1. **Cerebral lesions:** ischemic stroke, cerebral hemorrhage, subarachnoid hemorrhage, Cushing response, intracranial mass lesion
      2. **Spinal cord lesions**
      3. **Peripheral nerve disease:** Guillain-Barré syndrome
      4. **Systemic diseases:** tetanus; porphyria, acute episode
      5. **Drug-related conditions:** neuroleptic malignant syndrome, sympathomimetic drug overdose, tricyclic antidepressant overdose
   B. **Autonomic dysreflexia** is a sympathetic storm observed in cases of spinal cord transection. The spinal cord lesion is usually above the midthoracic level. The episodes are paroxysmal and start several months following the acute

spinal cord injury as recovery occurs. The episodes are characterized by sudden onset of severe hypertension, headache, sweating and flushing, piloerection, and sometimes chills.

A precipitating cause can most often be identified and is a noxious stimulus. Urinary bladder distention and fecal impaction are common causes. Elimination of the precipitating cause often results in resolution of the episode. Prevention is the best therapy. Occasionally, drugs such as propantheline or oxybutynin, both of which have anticholinergic effects, may be used.

VI. Indications for referral

A. Referral to a specialist should be considered when bladder or bowel dysfunction is associated with complaints of numbness, tingling, pain, or weakness or when there is an abnormal neurologic examination. Thus, a 5-year-old boy with enuresis and a normal neurologic examination may not be a candidate for neurologic consultation, but if this patient also complains of back pain and has an abnormal neurologic examination, referral is appropriate.

B. Patients with autonomic dysfunction associated with an abnormal neurologic examination should be evaluated by a neurologist.

C. Patients with bladder, bowel, or sexual dysfunction who develop progressive neurologic dysfunction or do not respond to treatment are suitable candidates for referral to a specialist.

D. Patients with preexisting neurologic disease who develop bladder, bowel, or autonomic dysfunction are appropriate candidates for (re)evaluation by a neurologist.

E. Patients who develop bladder, bowel, or sexual dysfunction following trauma should be referred for evaluation by a specialist.

Recommended Readings

Bannister R. Multiple system atrophy and pure autonomic failure. In PA Low (ed), *Clinical Autonomic Disorders, Evaluation and Management*. Boston: Little, Brown, 1993.

Banwell JG, et al. Management of the neurogenic bowel in patients with spinal cord injury. *Urol Clin N Amer* 20:517–526, 1993.

Betts CD, et al. Erectile dysfunction in multiple sclerosis: Associated neurological and neurophysiologic deficits, and treatment of the condition. *Brain* 117:1303–1310, 1994.

Bradley WE. The diagnosis and treatment of patients with neurologic dysfunction of the urinary bladder. In PA Low (ed), *Clinical Autonomic Disorders, Evaluation and Management*. Boston: Little, Brown, 1993.

Fowler CJ. Electrophysiologic evaluation of sexual dysfunction. In PA Low (ed), *Clinical Autonomic Disorders, Evaluation and Management*. Boston: Little, Brown, 1993.

Garg BP. Disorders of micturition and defecation. In KF Swaiman (ed), *Pediatric Neurology, Principles and Practice* (2nd ed). St. Louis: Mosby, 1994.

Resnick WM, Yalla SV. Management of urinary incontinence in the elderly. *N Engl J Med* 313:800–805, 1985.

Rushton DN. Neurourology. In WG Bradley, et al. (eds), *Neurology in Clinical Practice, Principles of Diagnosis and Management*. Boston: Butterworth-Heinemann, 1991.

Rushton DN. Sexual and sphincter dysfunction. In WG Bradley, et al. (eds), *Neurology in Clinical Practice, Principles of Diagnosis and Management*. Boston: Butterworth-Heinemann, 1991.

Stewart JD. Evaluation of male sexual dysfunction. In PA Low (ed), *Clinical Autonomic Disorders, Evaluation and Management*. Boston: Little, Brown, 1993.

Walsh PC, et al. (eds). *Campbell's Urology* (6th ed). Philadelphia: Saunders, 1992.

Wein AJ. Practical uropharmacology. *Urol Clin N Amer* 18:269–281, 1991.

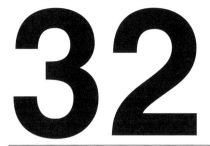

Approach to the Selection of Neuroimaging Studies
Buckley terPenning

I. Chronic headache. This chapter opens with one of the more contentious issues in neurology and radiology: Should the patient with chronic headache and normal neurologic examination be imaged? The answer to this question depends more on the resources available to the patient and physician and the expectations of the local community, including the local medical community, than on general guidelines currently available in print. Although this is the practical mode of decision making, it is not necessarily correct.

    A. Migraine. The following practice guideline has been issued by the Quality Standards Subcommittee (QSS) of the American Academy of Neurology:

> In adult patients that have been defined as migraine—including those with visual aura with no recent change in pattern, no history of seizures, and no other focal neurologic signs and symptoms, the routine use of neuroimaging is not warranted. In patients with atypical headache patterns, a history of seizures, or focal neurologic signs or symptoms, CT or MRI may be indicated.

    B. Nonmigranous or atypical headache. During their research, the QSS found six studies totaling 725 CT or MRI scans that uncovered a total of three potentially treatable lesions, for a 0.4% discovery rate. However, when two more studies from large tertiary referral centers were added to the sum, 43 potentially treatable lesions from a total of 1825 CT or MRI scans were uncovered, for a 2.4% discovery rate. Large tertiary centers may introduce a serious selection bias into this type of meta-analysis.

    Imaging with either CT or MRI is warranted when there has been a change in headache intensity or pattern or when there is an additional neurologic sign or symptom except for visual aura. Imaging is not warranted in the patient with stable chronic headache and a normal neurologic exam. But what about the 2.4% of patients with potentially treatable lesions? First, the rate is most likely to be closer to 0.4% of patients presenting to the clinic or emergency room. Second, the responsibility falls on the shoulders of the neurologic examiner to perform a complete history and physical exam (H&P). A noncontributory H&P often yields results when additional details are searched for and found. How often we were all enlightened or chagrined during morning rounds when the H&P of an intern appeared useless next to that of the chief resident, or both examinations yielded to the focused inquiry of the attending staff. A defensible, unbiased search for additional data that yields nothing provides a defensible clinical opinion that no other examination is required. Conversely, an additional physical or historical finding may allow the formulation of a working diagnosis that can be used to select CT or MRI as most appropriate. No other imaging exam, no matter how inexpensive and available, is appropriate for the work-up of headache.

    Appendix B lists the working diagnoses of potentially treatable conditions that may cause chronic headache, and the appropriate imaging modalities. If chronic headache is accompanied by global findings such as seizures or lethargy, you can select the imaging study most appropriate to the working diagnosis of the companion problem. MRI discloses lesions underlying headache with sensitivity that is equal to or better than that of CT, with one exception. CT is less expensive and more available than MRI for the focused work-up of sinus disease. It is adequate for following the progress of medically treated sinus disease and it is better than MRI for imaging the sinuses in the direct coronal plane if endoscopic sinus surgery is being considered. CT detects obstructive hydrocephalus as well as MRI, but if the cause lies in the posterior fossa or basal meninges, MRI is more likely to reveal that information. If meningitis or dural sinus thrombosis is suspected, additional coronal MRIs are helpful. Dural sinus thrombosis is best imaged by MRI with and without gadolinium contrast. Time-of-flight (TOF) magnetic resonance angiography (MRA) is very useful for imaging dural sinus thrombosis and can be performed (where available) during the same imaging session as MRI. Contrast MRI should be reserved for cases with evidence to support the strong possibility of tumor, inflammation including demyelination, infection, or dural sinus thrombosis.

II. **Acute headache**

A. **Subarachnoid hemorrhage.** If subarachnoid hemorrhage (SAH) is suspected, non-contrast CT (NCCT) is the preferred imaging study. NCCT reveals SAH 80–90% of the time if performed within 48 hours of ictus; the usefulness of NCCT diminishes to a sensitivity no better than 50% by day 7 post ictus. A negative CT scan should be examined for downward mass effect if a diagnostic lumbar puncture is planned to diagnose SAH by the presence of xanthochromia in the cerebrospinal fluid (CSF). The work-up of spontaneous (i.e., nontraumatic) SAH calls for four-vessel cerebral angiography, because 75–80% of spontaneous SAHs are caused by intracranial aneurysms, with arteriovenous malformations, hypertension, tumors, and various vasculopathies causing the other 20–25%. Cerebral angiography is associated with a 1% incidence of neurologic deficit and a 0.5% incidence of a persistent neurologic deficit. Angiography demonstrates an aneurysm in 85–90% of studies. If a cerebral angiogram is negative, it is usually repeated. A second angiogram increases the sensitivity of the search to 90–97%. Angiography is required prior to surgery for aneurysm clipping. Although aneurysms can now be seen with MRA and digital subtraction spiral-CT angiography, these modalities do not have sufficient resolution to show the relationship of small perforating arteries to the dome of the aneurysm. The advantage of both MRA and CT angiography is that the image of the arterial tree can be rotated to best display the neck of the aneurysm for clipping, and this can be done after the examination is over without exposing the patient to additional risk. TOF MRA is not adequately sensitive to aneurysms smaller than 5 mm. Remember that all angiographic techniques reveal only the aneurysm lumen. MRI can show the aneurysm dome, and any clot lining the dome, better than CT can. In the case of some large aneurysms, this may have significant implications for the operative approach.

B. **Intracerebral hemorrhages (ICHs)** are readily imaged by CT, and in the acute setting this may be the only available modality. CT is adequate for most solitary ICHs, but small petechial hemorrhages such as those caused by vasculitis or vasculopathy can be missed, as can posterior fossa ICHs that may be hidden by bone artifacts. Routine MRI (axial T1, T2, and intermediate images) is highly sensitive for ICHs—even for small petechial foci. Contrast MRI is useful if hemorrhagic cerebral metastases are suspected.

C. **Arterial dissection.** Carotid or vertebral arterial dissection may require angiographic examination for diagnosis. If the patient is stable, MRI with MRA is the safest and most efficient study. However, artifacts often appear as false narrowing at bends in the arteries on MRA. MRI is most sensitive to areas of ischemia or infarction. Cerebrovascular reserve may be estimated by transcranial doppler or by single-photon emission computed tomography (SPECT) of the brain using hexamethylpropylene amine oxime (HMPAO) or some other first-pass blood flow agent both with and without a carbonic anhydrase inhibitor challenge. CT angiography is useful where available, but currently it does not replace either MRA or conventional angiography.

D. **Intracerebral vasculitis** is a difficult working diagnosis. The yield on angiography is low (6%) despite the moderately high sensitivity of angiography for vasculitis (70%), probably because of the low prevalence of intracranial vasculitis. MRI is believed to be highly sensitive but poorly specific for vasculitis. Therefore, in cases in which vasculitis is suspected, a normal MRI is strong evidence against vasculitis. An abnormal MRI that does not reveal another etiology may lead to angiography.

III. **Facial pain.** Candidates for MRI have failed standard therapies for their particular maladies. The good soft-tissue contrast of MRI can screen for multiple causes of trigeminal neuralgia, hemifacial spasm, and other neuralgias. Intracranial vascular impingement of the trigeminal nerve at the root entry zone, primary tumors of the fifth nerve or Meckel's cave, posterior fossa lesions, and multiple sclerosis all have been implicated as causes of trigeminal neuralgia. MRI is sensitive for all of these lesions. Other vascular compression syndromes can be imaged by MRI as well. In MRI, image orientation, pulse sequences, and contrast decisions are best tailored to each patient.

IV. Neck pain

   A. Nonradicular neck pain. A small proportion of patients with nonradicular neck pain require imaging for possible etiologies that are discussed in sec. **IV.B.**

   B. Radicular neck pain is most often a result of degenerative disk or joint disease, but tumor or infection is also possible. MRI gives the best overall depiction of alignment, disk position, cord detail, and vertebral body composition and morphology. MRI does not optimally visualize the neural foramina because they course obliquely to the sagittal plane in the cervical spine. Although one can image perpendicular to these foramina with MRI, these extra acquisitions currently require too much additional time to be routinely practical. Axial views of the foramina are routinely acquired using T1- or gradient-echo-sensitive sequences, but these views often demonstrate false narrowing of foramina if the plane of imaging does not pass directly through the widest extent of the foramen. One approach is to combine standard sagittal and axial MRI views of the cervical spine with oblique cervical spine plain films for specific examination of foraminal cross sections.

   Contemporary cervical myelography always includes a postmyelographic CT examination of the affected cervical levels. A good cervical myelogram can replace the MRI and plain film combination referred to above for the evaluation of most radicular neck disease, but the test is invasive and is very insensitive for diskitis/osteomyelitis, lateral disk herniation, or paravertebral soft tissue lesions such as cellulitis or tumor.

   C. Myelopathy. Cervical myelopathy most frequently results from stenosis caused by disk or joint degenerative disease, or both. Occasionally, spinal instability causes stenosis resulting in myelopathy. Other causes include multiple sclerosis, syrinx, intrinsic cord tumor, metastatic disease, and, rarely, epidural hematoma.

   MRI best demonstrates the width of the central canal and spinal cord in sagittal views. Axial views may be obtained through regions of pathology. Myelographic CT may substitute for MRI in most respects. Plain films are not nearly as useful as CT or MRI except for assessing instability.

   D. Instability in the cervical spine occurs as a result of rheumatoid arthritis, remote neck trauma, or trisomy 21 (Down syndrome). Cervical spine instability is the one condition in which plain films give the best evaluation for a potentially correctable lesion: a standard spine film series of AP, lateral, oblique, and odontoid views is augmented by films obtained with the patient in maximum cervical flexion and extension while under physician observation. The levels and extent of instability and the surgical approach can be evaluated from these studies. MRI may complement these studies by examining the cord at the level of instability. Although this is often requested in cases of suspected cord atrophy, MRI does not affect the subsequent management of such patients and should not be ordered routinely. CT may be of value in examining the intactness of individual vertebral bodies in cases of dysmorphic vertebrae.

V. Low back pain

   A. Patient selection. Both CT and MRI examinations of the lumbar spine result in a large number of false-positive findings. Add to this the fact that, of all adults suffering low back pain (LBP), 50% resolve in 1 week, 80% in 2 weeks, and 90% in 3–7 weeks. The conclusions are that (1) the only patients who should be imaged are those who have failed conservative therapy and who are being considered for surgery (approximately 2% of patients with low back pain) and (2) the radiographic findings ought to be interpreted with respect to the clinical presentation.

   B. Modality selection. MRI is most sensitive for most of the causes of LBP, including disk disease, degenerative facet disease, tumor, and infection. NCCT is limited to the LBP patient who cannot lie still enough for MRI, and to evaluation of cortical margins or neural foramina that are indistinct on MRI. Myelography and postmyelographic CT are used when MRI is equivocal, nonexplanatory, or contraindicated. Plain films of the lumbar spine are limited in utility to the acute trauma setting.

C. Specific conditions. MRI is superior to CT for degenerative disk disease (DDD) because of its multiplanar capabilities. CT has a slight advantage over MRI for disclosing degenerative joint disease (DJD) because it has better resolution for bone margin and foraminal width. Tumor is best detected by MRI and may be imaged in two or three planes. Contrast-enhanced MRI examination for tumor is advantageous only when it follows an unenhanced MRI study and when fat-suppressed T1 images are used to diminish the bright marrow signal. Early diskitis or osteomyelitis is best disclosed by a slightly increased T2 signal. Indium 111–WBC imaging also picks up early infection, as does gallium 67, although gallium 67 is less sensitive and less specific than indium 111–WBC. Diskitis or osteomyelitis is usually more advanced by the time it reveals itself on delayed technetium 99m or CT imaging. Plain films may be the least sensitive modality for diskitis or osteomyelitis. MRI has the added advantage of being able to demonstrate cellulitis or abscess.

VI. Myelopathy

A. MRI is the most sensitive imaging study for cord pathology. However, two shortcomings of MRI must be mentioned. First, patient motion can seriously degrade MRI images, and second, MRI is presently one of the most expensive imaging studies. Image acquisition requires a relatively long period of time compared with CT or plain films. Each level of spine imaging requires the separate placement of a surface coil over the area examined. If a total spine MRI is requested, the result is that patients tire. Fatigue plus pain make it very difficult for most patients to cooperate fully during very long imaging sessions. Because imaging for myelopathy is often performed on an emergency basis, the time impact on other scheduled patient examinations is considerable. MRI is very sensitive for myelopathy, but it is not specific. MRI is useful for detecting surgically correctable lesions; otherwise, most diagnoses and treatments are made and followed clinically.

B. Imaging approach. Performing sagittal T1- and T2-weighted gradient echo images at each of three levels is an acceptable quick screening study for detection of potential surgically correctable spinal lesions. Ideally, the study should be checked by a radiologist before the patient is released, and additional images of abnormal areas can be acquired. Suspicious or unclear areas might best be examined clinically and the patient brought back for additional focused examination. The initial examination can be more complete and focused if the imaging request is limited to the one or two most suspicious regions—either cervical, thoracic, or lumbar spine. As mentioned, a negative spine MRI may require examination of the brain: both cerebral multiple sclerosis (MS) and amyotrophic lateral sclerosis may present in a fashion similar to that of myelopathy. Metastatic disease of the spine in a nonemergent setting is best approached with technetium 99m bone uptake imaging. Areas considered for surgery, including radiosurgery, may then be examined by MRI with and without contrast.

C. Etiologies. Central canal stenosis can be imaged by MRI, CT, or plain films. Epidural disease such as tumor, abscess, or hematoma can be detected by CT or MRI. Intrinsic tumor or syrinx can also be imaged by CT or MRI. MS is demonstrated with high sensitivity by T2-weighted MR images. Cord atrophy is a sequel of MS if the disease is severe enough. Other conditions, such as acute disseminated encephalomyelitis and transverse myelitis, do not always appear abnormal on MRI. Contrast-enhanced MRI is useful for demonstrating active MS plaques, tumor, and occasionally transverse myelitis. There is some discussion as to whether MRI enhancement has any prognostic value for transverse myelitis.

D. Failed back syndrome (FBS). Recurrent LBP after spinal surgery may occur in 15–25% of patients and is commonly associated with epidural fibrosis or disk reherniation. Differentiation of reherniation from epidural scarring is best demonstrated by comparing T1-weighted images from contrast-enhanced MRI with T1-weighted images from unenhanced images in the sagittal and axial planes through the affected areas. Scar tissue is readily enhanced, whereas disk tissue is not. The distinction is important, because a reherniated disk may be reoperated whereas a scar generally is not. T2-weighted images are also obtained, because infection can be a cause of protracted postoperative pain. The timing of postsurgical MRI examination is important. For the first 2–3 postoperative months, the T1 image of the operated level often appears similar to the preoperative image because an anterior epidural signal similar to that from a disk is present in the diskectomy bed. For this reason, as well as for patient management reasons, MRI examinations for FBS are best carried out at least 3 months after surgery. T2 images are also obtained as part of this work-up, because infection can be an occasional cause of postoperative pain. Arachnoiditis is another, less common cause. Granulation tissue associated with diskitis, osteomyelitis, or arachnoiditis appears as abnormal contrast enhancement.

VII. **Alterations in consciousness and cognition**
   A. **The role of imaging** in a patient who presents with alterations in consciousness and cognition is to detect a potentially correctable lesion such as a bleed, compressing mass, or herniation. Basilar artery thrombosis is also potentially treatable with intra-arterial thrombolysis in the proper setting. Nonsurgical conditions such as meningitis, cerebral vasculitis, metabolic derangements including alcohol-related derangements, encephalitis, acute disseminated encephalomyelitis, and neurosyphilis are also potentially correctable. NCCT imaging in the acute period is fast, widely available, and highly sensitive to clinically sensitive mass effects. A negative NCCT scan is sufficient to permit lumbar puncture (LP), which is required in the further work-up of potential medically correctable causes of impaired consciousness or cognition. Although MRI may permit exquisite visualization of some structural abnormalities associated with progressed diseases, such as parahippocampal atrophy in Alzheimer's disease or mammillary atrophy in Wernicke-Korsakoff syndrome, diagnoses of dementia, as well as of stupor and coma from infectious, toxic, or metabolic causes, are formed on the basis of clinical and laboratory data. Although MRI may be able to locate herpes simplex encephalitis (HSE) classically to a frontotemporal area of edema, if a patient with suspected HSE is not receiving treatment while being imaged, the chances of recovery are expected to be poorer than if therapy were initiated immediately. For most treatable causes of dementia, the patient's response to treatment confirms the diagnosis more readily than does the appearance of an MR image. There is no correlation between generalized loss of brain volume (atrophy) on CT or MRI and dementia.
   B. **Transcranial Doppler** ultrasonography may confirm basilar artery thrombosis in the acute period. This examination can be done with portable equipment and is compatible with an intensive care setting. Dense thrombus in the affected arteries may occasionally be detected by NCCT, but unreliably. MRA can detect interruption of flow in the affected arteries, but some intensive care equipment, such as a ventilator, is not transportable into the MR suite. Angiography is both diagnostic and potentially therapeutic if intra-arterial thrombolysis is available. An NCCT study is required prior to any thrombolysis to detect hemorrhagic infarction, a contraindication to most subsequent thrombolyses.

VIII. **Dysphagia.** The causes of dysphagia are legion. Videofluoroscopy is the primary modality used to evaluate deglutition disorders. The diagnosis of these disorders—even those resulting from neurologic causes—is overwhelmingly based on clinical information. Central nervous system causes of dysphagia include stroke, MS, Alzheimer's disease, progressive supranuclear palsy, Huntington's disease, amyotrophic lateral sclerosis, and Parkinson's disease. Of these, only previously undetected MS requires neuroimaging to explain the patient's symptoms. MRI is the most sensitive modality for imaging of MS. Contrast may enhance acute MS plaques.

IX. **Seizure**
   A. **Neonatal seizure** is often caused by perinatal hypoxic-ischemic injury (HII), intracranial hemorrhage, CNS infection, or neuronal migration anomalies. One other cause of neonatal seizures is maternal drug abuse. Other less common causes are inborn errors of metabolism and benign neonatal convulsions. MRI is important in the diagnosis of HII, hemorrhage, and migration abnormalities, and it is usually necessary to image the patient to exclude these conditions even if the working diagnosis points elsewhere; CT is less sensitive but useful if MRI is not available. For all types of neonatal seizure, MRI would subject some neonates to unnecessary sedation, with the possibility of patients picking up hemorrhage or ischemic change in a few unsuspected cases. Supportive care would likely not be affected by the additional data.
   B. **Childhood seizure** may be as prevalent as 0.5% of the population. Most febrile seizures and absence seizures need no imaging studies. Those seizures that may be caused by focal lesions are the best candidates for neuro-

imaging. Other seizure activity of uncertain etiology that persists unexpectedly or changes in pattern may also reveal itself on imaging. Infantile spasms (with or without West's syndrome) generally do not require imaging, but those spasms that are lateralizing may have underlying seizure foci. Patients suffering intractable seizures with foci are candidates for epilepsy surgery. Patients with Lennox-Gastaut syndrome present with a variety of seizure patterns most often caused by diffuse processes. Occasionally, however, one of these patients is found to have a seizure focus that is amenable to epilepsy surgery. Although the condition termed "benign partial seizures" does not itself require imaging studies, the pattern of seizures is similar to that caused by a tumor, and so an MRI baseline study is usually obtained. Generalized seizures, complex partial seizures, and seizures accompanying infection and trauma are all best imaged by MRI. Also, MRI gives additional information in the first 2 years of life about the maturity of brain myelination. MRI is less sensitive than CT for calcium, and so dystrophic calcifications of TORCH syndrome or brain dysmorphisms and suspected skull fractures should be imagined by CT.

The search for a seizure focus when epilepsy surgery is being planned starts with an EEG. MRI is then performed to confirm or clarify the EEG localization. If the results are still equivocal, interictal or postictal blood flow imaging using the blood flow marker HMPAO imaged by single-photon emission computed tomography (SPECT) may show regional or focal blood flow abnormalities. EEG, MRI, and SPECT results are correlated with one another to locate a seizure focus. If results are still equivocal, further physiologic imaging can be done in the form of positron emission tomography (PET), in which radiolabeled glucose is administered and taken up by the brain. Focal abnormalities in the local cerebral metabolic utilization of glucose appear on PET images and can be correlated with MRI, EEG, and SPECT information.

C. **Adult-onset seizure** may be the first manifestation of a tumor. Glioma, meningioma, and metastasis can all present in this manner. Vascular abnormalities such as cavernous angioma and arteriovenous malformation (AVM) can also initially present in this way. Other sources of seizure in the adult include encephalitis, meningitis, stroke, hypertensive encephalopathy, and vasculitis. MRI is the best imaging modality for demonstrating findings suggestive of all these conditions except vasculitis. A normal MRI is believed to rule out the presence of vasculitis, but the abnormalities of vasculitis on MRI have little specificity, and an angiogram is necessary.

For seizures caused by renal failure, metabolic derangements, or toxic agents, correcting the abnormality often obviates the need for imaging, except when the seizure activity does not respond to the correction. Alcohol-related seizures are one exception to this guideline because of the prevalence of trauma among alcohol-addicted patients. The patient with alcohol-related seizures is in the same category as a more obviously post-traumatic patient: cerebral edema, contusions, hematoma of the brain or its coverings, and skull fracture should be looked for acutely. NCCT is the best imaging modality for these lesions in the acute period. It is accepted that MRI performed after the patient is stabilized may detect small cerebral contusions and deep shear injuries not apparent on CT.

X. **Hearing loss** is divided into conductive (prelabyrinthine) and sensorineural (postlabyrinthine) categories for purposes of diagnosis and treatment.

A. **Conductive hearing loss** involves the external or middle ear and is best examined by thin-section NCCT (1.0–1.5 mm) through the petrous temporal bone in axial and direct coronal sections. Congenital middle ear deformities, cholesteatoma, serous otitis, and tympanic paragangliomas are some of the major potentially correctable causes of conductive hearing loss that can be diagnosed by CT.

B. **Sensorineural hearing loss (SNHL)** involves the cochlea, cochlear nerve, brainstem, or cortical connections. SNHL is best examined by means of axial and coronal T1- and T2-weighted images. Thin-section T2-weighted images through the internal auditory canals (IAC) may be as good as or better than contrast-enhanced T1-weighted images for detecting acoustic neuromas (schwannomas). Other major causes of SNHL include unknown causes likely to be results of vascular insufficiency or postviral damage to inner ear structures. Masses other than acoustic neuromas may impinge on the IAC, including meningiomas, fifth- or seventh-nerve neuromas and inflammatory petrosal cholesterol granulomas or cysts. MS may rarely present with hearing loss.

C. **Tinnitus** may be nonpulsatile or pulsatile. Nonpulsatile tinnitus may be caused by otosclerosis, acoustic neuroma, cerebellopontine angle masses, or Ménière's syndrome. All but the last may be diagnosed by MRI or CT. Pulsatile tinnitus may be caused by an AVM of the brain, dura, or face, by an aberrant jugular bulb or carotid artery, by a vertebral or carotid fistula, or by a paraganglioma of the skull base or middle ear. These conditions are best demonstrated by MRI, except vertebral and carotid fistulae, which may require MRA if they are small.

XI. **Vertigo**

A. **Causes.** Imaging alternatives are usually directed by the larger problem of which vertigo is a symptom. Vertigo caused by drugs or toxins requires no imaging. Vertigo resulting from trauma or stroke is addressed by working up the larger problem. Vertigo can be a symptom of cortical, cerebellar, or medullary stroke. Masses of the cerebellopontine angle and cerebellum, otomastoiditis, and labyrinthitis all have been implicated as causes of vertigo. Vascular compression of the eighth nerve is one cause of vertigo that may show up on MRI and may possibly appear abnormal on MRA. If posterior circulation aneurysm is revealed on MRI or MRA, conventional angiography is indicated prior to surgical clipping. One diagnosis of exclusion is Ménière's syndrome, or endolymphatic hydrops, which causes recurrent attacks of tinnitus, hearing loss, and vertigo accompanied by a sense of pressure in the ears. MRI of Ménière's syndrome does not show any abnormality except in isolated cases when special techniques are used.

B. **Imaging.** MRI is likely to reveal cortical or brainstem stroke as well as tumor of the posterior fossa or skull base. Otitis and mastoiditis reveal themselves as increased, bright fluid signals on T2-weighted images. Labyrinthitis may or may not appear this way, owing to the fineness of the structure involved. Occasionally, labyrinthitis may show enhancement on MRI. Routine axial T1, spin-density, and T2 images are sufficient to screen for causes of vertigo. Coronal T2 images are occasionally helpful. Contrast examination may be used to follow up if there are any equivocal findings. Vascular insufficiency to the labyrinth is usually not apparent, even on angiography. However, MRA may be useful in determining if there is a more extensive vertebrobasilar problem.

XII. **Vision**

A. **Good vision** requires proper functioning of cranial nerves II, III, IV, and VI and of tracts that extend from the frontal lobes (visual pursuit) ventrocaudally to the superior colliculi (visual-motor coordination). Therefore, any disturbance of brain function has a high likelihood of manifesting itself as some visual disturbance. Unfortunately for the neurodiagnostician, visual disorders caused by ocular globe pathologies (refractive, cataractous, and retinal pathologies) are highly prevalent in the population.

B. **Neuro-ophthalmologic disorders** may manifest themselves as double vision if tumors or vascular aneurysms impinge on the third, fourth, or sixth cranial nerve. Unequal pupil sizes or pupillary reflexes occur when large mass effects shift the brain downward and stretch or press the third nerve against the tentorium. Visual loss may be caused by orbital tumors, chiasmatic tumors, or stroke anywhere along the optic tracts or radiations, including the calcarine (visual) cortex. Monocular loss of acuity may be caused by an orbital inflammation or mass, or by a vascular pathology affecting the ophthalmic artery or carotid artery. Loss in the form of homonymous hemianopia is characteristic of many parieto-occipital AVMs and strokes.

C. **Imaging** of neuro-ophthalmologic disorders relies heavily on MRI, which has great soft-tissue sensitivity to disorders of brain parenchyma and ocular globe. In addition, individual cranial nerves can be visualized, as well as arteries and veins that supply the globe, run concurrently with nerves, or drain the orbit. MRA greatly assists in the evaluation of these vascular structures. Orbital pathology, which may be manifested as proptosis, "frozen eye," or monocular loss of visual acuity, can be imaged by axial and coronal MRI using T1, spin-density, and T2 images, and occasionally fat-suppressed T1 images. Axial MR images of neuro-ophthalmologic disorders include images of the brain from base of skull to vertex.

CT examination is acceptable for orbital pathology, in which case axial and direct coronal images are obtained similar to MRI. The intracoronal fat allows orbital pathology to stand out distinctly in CT images. CT is superior to MRI only for orbital trauma in which thin bone walls of the orbit are demonstrated by CT better than MRI. A "blow-out fracture" of the orbital floor requires that direct coronal CT images be obtained; the fracture may be missed on axial images.

XIII. **Transient ischemic attack (TIA)**
   A. **Imaging** of TIA should begin with brain imaging. All too frequently, stroke or ischemic-like symptoms may be caused by a brain tumor, usually metastasis. Intracranial hemorrhage may cause mild or transient neurologic symptoms. Ischemic brain lesions are demonstrated by CT in about 40%, and by MRI in about 70%, of TIA patients. New lesions may not be evident in either study for about 24 hours. The imaging work-up of the TIA patient then proceeds with duplex ultrasonography (DU) of the carotid arteries. DU refers to the simultaneous acquisition of sonographically acquired carotid artery images plus Doppler-acquired data concerning the flow dynamics of the blood within the carotid. There are many discussions about the accuracy of DU compared with angiography with its high resolution for anatomic detail. DU lies in the 80–90% range for accuracy in judging carotid stenosis compared to angiography, so it is an excellent screening tool for selecting patients for angiographic examination in order to confirm their status with respect to surgery. MRA is now being used as a screening test to assign appropriate patients to angiography. MRA appears to have an accuracy for estimating carotid stenosis similar to that of DU. The usefulness of MRA lies in its ability to obtain this information at the time that the initial brain MRI is performed on the patient who presents with TIA.
   B. **Cerebral blood flow** studies may be performed to assess cerebrovascular reserve (CR). Cerebrovascular reserve refers to the ability of the cerebral arteries to dilate in response to increased need or decreased perfusion, and it is mediated by pCO_2 levels. CR can be measured by assessing cerebral blood flow increase in response to increasing brain CO_2. Arterial pCO_2 is most conveniently elevated by the intravenous administration of acetazolamide, a carbonic anhydrase inhibitor. Blood flow imaging using the blood flow marker HMPAO imaged by SPECT may show hemispheric blood flow diminution ipsilateral to the stenotic carotid artery. If this flow increases after acetazolamide administration, the patient has CR. If the flow does not increase, this implies that the cerebral vasculature is already maximally dilated in response to the diminished carotid inflow. Such patients may be in greater need of intervention than those with sufficient CR. Blood flow can also be estimated using transcranial Doppler ultrasonography or xenon CT.

XIV. **Stroke** usually requires CT imaging in the acute period to determine the presence or absence of intracranial hemorrhage. Investigation of etiology does not usually progress beyond noninvasive cardiac, laboratory, or carotid DU studies. Minor stroke is treated much the same as outlined for TIA above. As previously mentioned, stroke may not become apparent on MRI or CT during the first 24 hours, depending on severity. MRI diffusion imaging, which actually measures the motion of diffusing tissue water, shows the earliest changes of cerebral infarction, which appear as early as 45 minutes post ictus. In the absence of demonstrable carotid disease on DU, further work-up by MRA or conventional angiography may be warranted to determine other etiologies of stroke.

XV. **Trauma**
   A. **Penetrating trauma of the head, including depressed fractures of the face and skull,** requires that patients receive CT imaging of the head as soon as they are stable enough. Foreign bodies, intracranial hematomas, orbital injuries, and fractures of the skull base all are best imaged by CT, and their presence or absence determines the course of treatment. Fractures of the face or orbits are also imaged in the direct coronal plane as soon as the patient is able to cooperate. Blunt injury to the head or face requires neck imaging as well (see sec. **XV.C**). Follow-up CT is obtained to assess the results of surgery and whenever intracranial bleeding is suspected. MRI is sometimes obtained after the acute period to assess any subtle brain contusions or shear injuries, but there is some discussion as to whether this information materially affects the course of treatment. MRI complements CT examination of the orbits. Whereas CT can demonstrate the status of the orbital rim, walls, floor, optic nerve canal, and orbital fissures, MRI can reveal the status of the optic nerve, extraocular

muscles, orbital fat, and globe. Both CT and MRI studies of the orbit are performed in the axial and coronal planes.

B. **Closed head trauma** requires that patients receive CT or MRI as soon as they are stable. Patients who are initially imaged with CT often are imaged with MRI after the acute period. Although both modalities show cerebral contusions, edema, or hematoma, MRI shows subtle (petechial) hemorrhage, small contusions, and deep white matter shear injuries better than CT. MRI is relatively insensitive to fractures and subarachnoid hemorrhages; if MRI is the initial study, plain skull films can be used as a simple means of assessing the presence or absence of any suspected skull fracture.

C. **Cervical spine imaging.** Any patient with closed head trauma or neck trauma should undergo a plain film study of the spine consisting of AP, lateral, odontoid, and oblique views of the spine. If these views are normal, flexion and extension lateral plain film views of the spine should be performed under a physician's guidance to assess cervical spine stability. If pain or splinting prevents the patient from flexing or extending, this should be considered abnormal, and the plain films should be reviewed again, any suboptimal views repeated, or a neck CT scan obtained. There is beginning to be a movement toward obtaining a neck CT scan for any trauma patient requiring a head CT. This is being done in centers that have access to a spiral CT scanner, which can obtain such views quickly. Incremental CT scanners, especially older models that require more tube cooling, take too long to easily obtain an entire spine study. Newer, spiral model CT imagers can scan the entire cervical spine in less time than it would take to obtain the five plain film spine series. Any CT study is helpful at the level of any fracture or instability that shows up on plain spine films.

MRI in cervical trauma is most helpful when there are symptoms or a strong suspicion of spinal cord damage. Myelopathies, radicular signs, plain film signs of hyperextension injury such as prevertebral hematomas, teardrop vertebral fractures, widened anterior disk spaces, and cervical CT scans demonstrating cervical canal narrowing or bone or missile fragments within the spinal canal are all indications that a cervical spine MRI should be obtained in order to assess the cord. Cord edema presents an abnormally bright signal on spin-density and T2 sagittal images. Cord and epidural hematomas exhibit characteristic MRI blood signals on sagittal T1- and T2-weighted images. Axial images should be obtained through any pathology demonstrated on sagittal view.

Recommended Readings

Harris KG, et al. Diagnosing intracranial vasculitis: The roles of MR and angiography. *AJNR* 15:317–330, 1994.

North American Symptomatic Carotid Endarterectomy Trial Collaborators. North American Symptomatic Carotid Endarterectomy Trial: Methods, patient characteristics and progress. *Stroke* 22:711–720, 1991.

Otsubo H, et al. Neuroimaging for investigation of seizures in children. *Ped Neurosurg* 18:105–116, 1992.

Report of the Quality Standards Subcommittee of the American Academy of Neurology. Practice parameter: The utility of neuroimaging in the evaluation of headache in patients with normal neurologic examinations (summary statement). *Neurology* 44:1353–1354, 1994.

Thorne RP, Curd JG. A systematic approach to disorders of the cervical spine. *Hosp Pract (Off Ed)* 28(6):49–58, 1993.

Vanderburgh DF, Kelly WM. Radiographic assessment of discogenic disease of the spine. *Neurosurg Clin North America* 4:13–33, 1993.

Weir B. *Aneurysms Affecting the Nervous System.* Baltimore: Williams & Wilkins, 1987. Pp 570–603.

Yukunori K, et al. Intracranial aneurysms: Diagnostic accuracy of three-dimensional, Fourier transform, time-of-flight MR angiography. *Radiology* 193:181–186, 1994.

33

Approach to the Selection of Electrodiagnostic, Spinal Fluid, and Other Ancillary Testing
Paul W. Brazis

Neurophysiologic electrodiagnostic studies define alterations in the functions of the nervous system that may not be visualized by imaging procedures. The major areas of study include electroencephalography (EEG), nerve conduction studies (NCS) and electromyography (EMG), and evoked potentials. The clinical usefulness of these examinations is here discussed, followed by brief descriptions of other ancillary neurologic tests such as polysomnography and the multiple sleep latency test, and finally the indications, contraindications, and clinical worth of performing lumbar puncture (LP) for cerebrospinal fluid (CSF) analysis.

Electroencephalography (EEG)

I. **Introduction.** EEG involves recording of the spontaneous electrical activity of the brain from the scalp and activity elicited by activation procedures, including sleep, hyperventilation, and photic stimulation. Small metal disks containing conductive gel are attached to the scalp and ear lobes according to a system of measurements and are connected by flexible wires to a recording instrument that amplifies the brain activity about a million times. The EEG is sampled on moving paper or on a computer simultaneously from 16 or 21 pairs of electrodes (derivations) in selected combinations (montages).

II. **Normal EEG activity**
   A. **EEG rhythms.** The EEG is a composite of several different types of activity, each with characteristic factors of frequency, amplitude, morphology, reactivity, topography, and quantity. The frequency bands of activity are as follows.
   1. **Delta activity** (<4 Hz)
   2. **Theta activity** (4–<8 Hz)
   3. **Alpha activity** (8–13 Hz)
   4. **Beta activity** (>13 Hz)
   B. The most characteristic feature of a normal EEG in an adult during relaxed wakefulness is the **alpha rhythm,** which occurs over the posterior regions of the head while the eyes are closed. Judgments of normality for various EEG activities depend on the age and state of alertness of the subject as complex changes in EEG patterns occur throughout life and patterns evolve when going from wakefulness through different stages of sleep.
   C. **Activation procedures** are used to elicit abnormal activities that may not occur spontaneously.
   1. **Hyperventilation** for 3 minutes is most effective for activating generalized seizure activities, such as the spike-wave paroxysms of absence (petit mal) seizures. Hyperventilation may less frequently activate focal abnormalities (e.g., slowing) and focal epileptiform activity. Hyperventilation is contraindicated in a patient with cardiac infarction, recent subarachnoid hemorrhage, or significant pulmonary disease.
   2. **Photic stimulation** consists of repetitive brief flashes of light generated by an electronic apparatus and delivered at frequencies of 1–30 Hz. This procedure evokes responses over the occipitoparietal regions (photic driving). The most frequent abnormal response is diffuse paroxysms of spike-wave complexes (photoparoxysmal or photoconvulsive response) that often indicate a seizure propensity.
   3. **Sleep recordings** are most useful for recording paroxysmal abnormalities in patients with epilepsy. Sleep may activate focal or generalized epilepti-

form activity. Sleep deprivation on the night before the study may facilitate sleep, and the deprivation itself may activate epileptiform activity.

III. Abnormal EEG activity. Many EEG changes are nonspecific, but some are highly suggestive of specific entities, such as epilepsy, herpes encephalitis, and metabolic encephalopathies. In general, neuronal damage or dysfunction is suggested by the presence of **slow waves** (activity in the theta or delta range) in a focal or diffuse location, while the presence of **sharp waves** or **spikes** (epileptiform activity) in a focal or diffuse pattern suggests a seizure tendency. Localized slowing is highly sensitive and significant for local neuronal dysfunction or focal brain damage but is quite nonspecific because it cannot distinguish the pathologic type of lesion. Thus, cerebral infarction, tumor, abscess, and trauma may all cause similar focal EEG changes. Diffuse slowing also indicates organic rather than psychiatric disease but again is nonspecific because such slowing may occur with any significant toxic, metabolic, degenerative, or even multifocal disease process. The EEG is also useful in following the courses of patients with altered states of consciousness and may, in certain circumstances, provide prognostic information. Finally, the EEG is important in the determination of brain death.

A. Epilepsy

1. Some types of interictal EEG patterns are termed "epileptiform" because they have a distinct morphology and occur in a high proportion of EEGs from patients with seizures but rarely in records from asymptomatic patients. Such patterns include **sporadic spikes, sharp waves,** and **spike-and-slow-wave complexes.** Not all spike patterns indicate epilepsy: 14- and 6-Hz positive spikes, sporadic sleep spikes, wicket spikes, 6-Hz spike-wave complexes, and the psychomotor variant pattern are all spike patterns that are of no proven clinical significance. Interictal findings must always be interpreted with caution because, although certain patterns of abnormality may be evidence useful in supporting a diagnosis of epilepsy, even epileptiform discharges, with few exceptions, are poorly correlated with the frequency and likelihood of recurrence of epileptic seizures. One must always treat the patient and never "treat" the EEG.

2. A substantial portion of patients with unquestioned epilepsy have normal EEGs. However, epileptiform activity has a high correlation with clinical epilepsy. Only about 2% of nonepileptic patients exhibit epileptiform EEG activity, in contrast with 50–90% of patients with epilepsy, depending on the circumstances of recording and on whether more than one EEG has been obtained. The most conclusive proof of an epileptic basis for a patient's episodic symptoms is obtained by recording an electroencephalographic seizure during a typical behavioral episode.

3. The EEG helps establish whether the seizure originates from a limited or focal area of the brain **(focal or partial seizures)** or involves the brain as a whole from the onset **(generalized seizures).** This distinction is important because of the different possible causes of these two basic epilepsy types and because the clinical manifestations of both types may be similar.

4. In general, the epileptiform activity on the EEG may be helpful in classifying the patient's seizure type.

   a. Generalized seizures of nonfocal origin usually are associated with bilaterally synchronous bursts of spikes and spike-wave discharges.

   b. Consistently focal epileptiform activity correlates with partial or focal epilepsy.

      (1) Anterior temporal spikes correlate with complex partial seizures.

      (2) Rolandic spikes correlate with simple motor or sensory seizures.

      (3) Occipital spikes correlate with primitive visual hallucinations or diminished visual function.

5. EEG analysis may permit further discrimination of several relatively **specific electroclinical syndromes.**

   a. Hypsarrhythmia refers to a high-voltage, arrhythmic EEG pattern with a chaotic admixture of continuous, multifocal spike-wave and sharp-wave discharges and widespread, high-voltage, arrhythmic slow waves. This infantile EEG pattern usually occurs in association with infantile spasms, myoclonic jerks, and mental retardation (West's syndrome) and usually indicates severe diffuse cerebral dysfunction. **Infantile spasms** consist of tonic flexion or extension of the neck, body, or extremities with the arms flung outward, and typically last 3–10 seconds. The EEG and clinical findings do not correlate with a specific disease entity but reflect a severe cerebral insult occurring before 1 year of age.

   b. **3-Hz spike-and-wave activity** is associated with typical absence attacks **(petit mal epilepsy).** This pattern most often occurs in children between the ages of 3 and 15 years and is enhanced by hyperventilation and hypoglycemia. These bursts are typically accompanied by clinical signs, such as staring, brief clonic movements, unresponsiveness, and motor arrest.

   c. **Generalized multiple spikes and waves** (polyspike-wave pattern) are typically associated with myoclonic epilepsy.

   d. **Generalized slow spike-and-wave patterns** at a frequency of 1–2.5 Hz occur in children between the ages of 1 and 6 years who have some underlying diffuse cerebral dysfunction. Most of these children are mentally retarded and have poorly controlled seizures. The clinical triad of mental retardation, severe seizures, and the slow spike-and-wave pattern is called the **Lennox-Gastaut syndrome.**

   e. **Central-midtemporal spikes** occur in childhood and are associated with **benign rolandic epilepsy.** These seizures are often nocturnal and consist of focal clonic movements of the face or hand, tingling in the side of the mouth, tongue, cheek, or hand, motor speech arrest, and excessive salivation. The spells are easily controlled with anticonvulsants and disappear by 12–14 years of age.

   f. **Periodic lateralized epileptiform discharges (PLEDs)** are high-voltage, sharply contoured complexes that occur over one cerebral hemisphere with a periodicity of one complex every 1–4 seconds. These complexes are not necessarily epileptiform and correlate with acute destructive cerebral lesions, including infarction, rapidly growing tumors, and herpes simplex encephalitis (HSE).

6. **Focal slowing (delta activity)** in the interictal period usually indicates an underlying structural lesion of the brain as the cause of the seizures. However, such focal slowing may be a transient aftermath of a partial seizure and may not indicate a gross structural lesion. Such slowing may correlate with a clinical transient postictal neurologic deficit (Todd's phenomenon) and subsides within 3 days after the ictus.

7. The EEG can make a critical contribution to the diagnosis of a patient who is obtunded when prolonged epileptiform discharges with only brief interruptions are recorded, signifying **nonconvulsive status epilepticus.**

8. **Ambulatory EEG monitoring** is the recording of an EEG in a freely mobile patient outside of the EEG laboratory, similar to Holter monitoring for electrocardiogram (ECG) recording. The main indication is to determine whether a spell is a seizure or some other phenomenon, especially in patients whose spells occur at unusual times or in association with specific events or activities. The yield depends on the type of patient selected, but the absence of EEG seizure activity during a spell does not fully exclude a seizure disorder, because surface electrodes may not record some mesial temporal, basal frontal, or deep midsagittal seizure discharges.

9. Patients with intractable focal seizures are sometimes candidates for surgical removal of the area of abnormality. Precise identification of the epileptogenic brain area requires special inpatient monitoring facilities for **simultaneous closed-circuit television (CCTV) and EEG recording.** Prolonged CCTV-EEG monitoring is also often used to document whether a patient's clinical spells are epileptic or functional (psychogenic).

B. Altered states of consciousness

1. For most causes of acute encephalopathy (e.g., toxic-metabolic disease), the EEG changes are nonspecific, consisting of diffuse slowing. There is, however, a generally good correlation between the degree of EEG abnormality and the clinical state.

2. An abnormal EEG confirms an organic, rather than a psychogenic, cause for a patient's altered state of consciousness. It is also required to document unrecognized epileptic activity as a cause of depressed consciousness (nonconvulsive status epilepticus).

3. Certain EEG patterns increase the likelihood of **specific metabolic disorders.**

      a. Prominent **generalized fast (beta) activity** in the EEG of a comatose or obtunded patient should raise the suspicion of drug intoxication.

      b. Broad **triphasic waves** that are bilaterally symmetric and synchronous and have a frontal predominance may occur during an intermediate stage of hepatic encephalopathy. However, such a pattern may also occur with other metabolic disorders.

      c. Severe generalized voltage depression may suggest hypothyroidism if anoxia and hypothermia can be excluded.

      d. Patients with uremia, uremic patients undergoing hemodialysis, and patients with hyponatremia may exhibit paroxysmal spike-wave discharges and a photoparoxysmal response to photic stimulation, in addition to the diffuse slow-wave abnormality.

      e. Focal epileptiform activity is common in hyperosmolar coma.

4. Cerebral hypoxia produces diffuse nonspecific slow-wave abnormalities that may be reversible. More severe hypoxia may cause EEG abnormalities that may be paroxysmal and associated with clinical myoclonus. An EEG obtained 6 hours or more after a hypoxic insult may demonstrate patterns of prognostic value in determining the likelihood of neurologic recovery. A poor neurologic outcome is suggested by the presence of the following abnormalities.

      a. Alpha coma refers to the apparent paradoxical appearance of monorhythmic alpha frequency activity in the EEG of a comatose patient. However, in contrast to normal alpha activity, that observed in alpha coma is generalized, often most prominent frontally, and completely unreactive to external stimuli.

      b. The **burst-suppression pattern** consists of occasional generalized bursts of medium- to high-voltage, mixed-frequency slow-wave activity, sometimes with intermixed spikes, with intervening periods of severe voltage depression or cerebral inactivity. The bursts may be accompanied by generalized myoclonic jerks.

      c. The **periodic pattern** consists of generalized spikes or sharp waves that recur at a relatively fixed periodity of one to two per second. The periodic pattern is usually accompanied by myoclonic jerks.

      d. Electrocerebral silence. See sec. **III.C.1,** below.

5. Infectious disease processes of the CNS produce predominantly diffuse and nonspecific slow-wave activity. However, certain EEG patterns assist in the diagnosis of specific infectious etiologies.

      a. The EEG is extremely important in the initial assessment of **herpes simplex encephalitis (HSE),** often showing abnormalities before lesions detected by CT or MRI are recognized. A majority of patients show temporal or frontotemporal slowing that may be unilateral or, if bilateral, asymmetric. **Periodic sharp complexes** over one or both frontotemporal regions add relative specificity to the EEG findings. These diagnostic features usually appear between the second and fifteenth days of illness and are sometimes detected only on serial tracings.

      b. Subacute sclerosing panencephalitis (SSPE) has a distinctive EEG pattern of periodic bursts of stereotyped slow-wave and sharp-wave complexes occurring at intervals of 3–15 seconds.

      c. Creutzfeldt-Jakob disease is associated with a relatively specific EEG pattern of diffuse high-voltage di- and triphasic sharp-wave complexes occurring at a periodicity of approximately one per second.

C. Brain death

  1. Because the EEG is a measure of cerebral—especially cortical—function, it has been widely used to provide objective evidence of loss of that function. With cortical death, the EEG demonstrates complete loss of brain-generated activity—**electrocerebral silence.** The determination of electrocerebral silence is technically demanding and requires strict adherence to a standard special recording protocol.

  2. Rarely, temporary and reversible loss of cerebral electrical activity may be observed immediately following cardiorespiratory arrest, overdose of CNS depressants, and severe hypothermia. Therefore, electrocerebral silence in these circumstances does not indicate irreversible cortical dysfunction.

  3. Patients in a chronic vegetative state, with preserved brainstem function, may have an isoelectric EEG, probably reflecting total neocortical death.

4. Thus, the establishment of **brain death** (cerebral plus brainstem death) requires the following criteria.
   a. Irreversible structural brain damage
   b. Apneic coma
   c. Loss of brainstem reflexes and signs of brainstem function
   d. Electrocerebral silence on EEG (best viewed as a confirmatory test)

Nerve Conduction Studies (NCS) and the Electromyogram (EMG)

I. Introduction

   A. Nerve conduction studies (NCS) comprise a simple and reliable method of testing peripheral nerve function. An impulse initiated by electrical stimulation of the nerve travels along motor, sensory, or mixed nerves, and the conduction characteristics of the impulse are assessed by recording potentials either from the muscle innervated by the motor nerve or from the nerve itself.

   B. The **motor unit** consists of a single lower motor neuron and all of the muscle fibers it innervates. **Motor nerve conduction studies** are techniques used to assess the integrity of the motor unit. Information about the function and the structural status of the motor neuron, nerve, neuromuscular junction, and muscle is acquired. Quantitative information can be obtained regarding the location, distribution, time course, and pathophysiology of lesions affecting the peripheral nervous system (PNS). Prognosis, response to treatment, and the status of repair of the motor unit may also be obtained. For motor conduction studies, recording electrodes are placed on the skin over the motor point of a muscle and over the tendon of the muscle and stimulating electrodes are placed over the skin along the course of the nerve to be tested. The response of the muscle to electrical stimulation can be measured by recording the compound muscle action potential (CMAP), which is the summation of the electrical potentials of all muscle fibers that respond to stimulation of the nerve. The time it takes for the electrical impulse to travel to the muscle (latency) can be measured, and by stimulating the nerve at various locations and measuring the distance the stimulus travels, motor nerve conduction velocities are attained. Motor nerve conduction studies can be used for the following purposes.

   1. To obtain objective evidence of disease of motor units
   2. To identify and localize sites of compression, ischemia, and other focal lesions of nerves that can be manifested by conduction block, slow conduction at the site of the lesion, or abnormal conduction proximal or distal to the lesion
   3. To detect widespread involvement of nerves in patients who present with involvement of a single nerve (i.e., mononeuropathies)
   4. To differentiate peripheral neuropathies from myopathies and lower motor neuron cell disease (e.g., amyotrophic lateral sclerosis) in patients with weakness
   5. To detect disease prior to development of significant clinical signs (e.g., familial neuropathies)

   C. Diseases of the neuromuscular junction (e.g., myasthenia gravis) can be assessed by **repetitive stimulation of motor nerves.** With fatigability of the neuromuscular junction, if a CMAP is recorded and compared with subsequent CMAPs, a decline in amplitude of the potential may be observed as progressively fewer muscle fibers respond to the stimuli, even though the nerve is stimulated at rates that a normal muscle could endure for long periods.

   D. Sensory nerve conduction studies are obtained by recording the action potential evoked in a cutaneous nerve by electrical stimulation. Selective sensory nerve conduction studies can be performed by stimulating nerves that have only sensory components (e.g., the sural nerve) or, alternatively, by selectively stimulating only the sensory components of a mixed nerve. The latter can be done by isolating the sensory components anatomically (i.e., stimulating the digits of the hand and recording over the mixed nerve at the wrist or elbow) or stimulating the mixed nerve and recording over the digits where only sensory axons are present for the most part. Sensory nerve conduction studies may be valuable for the following purposes.

   1. In diffuse disorders affecting the sensory system, for determining which population of sensory nerves is involved (e.g., small fibers carrying pain and temperature sensation or large fibers conveying proprioception), determining whether the disorder is predominantly affecting the axon or the myelin of the peripheral nerve, or determining whether the peripheral sensory nerves are involved at all

2. In focal neuropathies, for demonstrating a site of injury or block, particularly when only sensory nerves are affected

3. For confirmation or quantification when sensory abnormalities appear earlier than motor changes in peripheral neuropathies or before objective clinical signs

4. For predicting whether a lesion is proximal or distal to the dorsal root ganglion (e.g., for differentiating brachial plexus from nerve-root injury)

E. The **electromyogram (EMG)** is usually performed along with nerve conduction studies and yields complementary information. A needle electrode is inserted into the muscles of interest and the action potentials generated by groups of muscle fibers (the **motor unit potentials** or **MUPs**) are observed and recorded. The muscle is tested at rest, with slight contraction, and with stronger contraction. Normally, the muscle is silent at rest. In **active neuropathic processes** or in severe or inflammatory myopathies, spontaneous action potentials from single muscle fibers (fibrillation potentials) may occur. In certain neurogenic processes, especially motor neuron disease, spontaneous contractions of groups of muscle fibers (fasciculation potentials) may be observed. Characteristic changes in MUP parameters and recruitment may occur in neurogenic or myopathic processes. In **neuropathic conditions,** the MUPs are often of increased amplitude, duration, and degree of polyphasia with poor recruitment of fibers with increased effort, whereas in **myopathic processes,** the MUPs may be of decreased amplitude and duration with increased polyphasia and rapid recruitment. Single muscle fiber action potentials may be studied by a technically more difficult method, **single-fiber electromyography.**

F. In general, EMG and NCS are used to study and diagnose patients with motor neuron disease (e.g., amyotrophic lateral sclerosis), processes affecting the plexi or nerve roots, entrapment neuropathies, peripheral polyneuropathies, diseases of the neuromuscular junction (e.g., myasthenia gravis), and diseases of the muscle. Because it involves electrical shocks and the insertion of needles into multiple muscles, the EMG/NCS study is uncomfortable. The study is safe as long as electrical safety techniques are applied; a bleeding tendency may limit the EMG study.

II. **EMG/NCS abnormalities**

A. The EMG/NCS study is essential for evaluation and electrophysiologic diagnosis of **motor neuron disease** (e.g., amyotrophic lateral sclerosis). In general, nerve conduction studies are normal except perhaps for some decrease in the CMAP amplitudes (because the disease is purely motor, sensory conduction studies are normal). Needle EMG shows diffuse evidence of neurogenic damage from anterior horn cell injury, including abnormal spontaneous activity (fibrillations and fasciculations), abnormal MUP parameters (large, wide, polyphasic MUPs), and poor recruitment of MUPs with effort. Often the EMG study indicates active neurogenic damage even in muscles or limbs that appear to have little or no clinical involvement. The needle exam may also provide information about prognosis, and the EMG may assist in the diagnosis of other diseases of the anterior horn cells, such as the postpolio syndrome and the spinal muscular atrophies.

B. **Radiculopathies** comprise a constellation of symptoms and signs resulting from transient or permanent damage of the nerve at the anatomic level where the nerve exits the spinal canal in the spinal foramina. Nerve conduction studies are generally normal. The EMG shows evidence of neurogenic changes (e.g., fibrillations and MUP changes) in muscles innervated by a specific root, with other muscles innervated by uninvolved roots being spared. The pattern of neurogenic changes depends on the severity of the process, the duration of the disease, and the degree of neurogenic repair (reinnervation). The EMG study can be helpful in several ways, as follows.

1. The EMG study is useful for identifying the location of disease and confirming that it is at the level of the root. In studies of patients with surgically demonstrated cervical or lumbosacral radiculopathies, the EMG is abnormal

only about 90% of the time. Thus, a normal study does not preclude the presence of a radiculopathy.

2. EMG provides further localization by determining which root or roots are affected.
3. The EMG study is useful in determining if there is *active* denervation (indicated by the presence of fibrillation potentials).
4. EMG can determine the time elapsed since the onset of the radiculopathy (whether it is acute, subacute, chronic, or old).
5. EMG may give some information about the severity of the radiculopathy.
6. EMG may reveal other abnormalities that explain the patient's symptoms.
7. EMG may help to determine if an abnormality on an MRI scan or myelogram has any physiologic significance.

C. Brachial and lumbosacral **plexopathies** and **entrapment neuropathies** (e.g., carpal tunnel syndrome, ulnar neuropathies at the elbow, and peroneal neuropathies at the fibular head) are localized and diagnosed with EMG/NCS.

D. **Peripheral polyneuropathies** are often investigated by EMG/NCS. The electrophysiologic characteristics of the neuropathic disorder serve as additional sources of information to help characterize the disease and allow a narrowing of the differential diagnostic possibilities. EMG/NCS allows evaluation of the amount of motor and sensory involvement, determines whether the lesion is primarily the result of damage to the myelin sheath or to the axon, indicates whether the lesion is focal or diffuse, determines whether the process is distal or proximal, and gives information concerning the severity and temporal profile of the process. Prolonged distal sensory and motor latencies, slowed conduction velocities, abnormalities of sensory responses and MUPs, and "neurogenic" EMG changes occur. When abnormal, the study confirms the presence of a neuropathy, but it should be noted that small fiber sensory neuropathies (i.e., those affecting only sensory nerve fibers conveying pain and temperature sensation) are often associated with normal studies. EMG/NCS can separate a generalized sensorimotor peripheral polyneuropathy from multiple mononeuropathies at sites of common compression (e.g., median and ulnar neuropathies at the wrist). Peripheral polyneuropathies may be divided by electrophysiologic patterns into the following categories.

1. Uniform demyelinating mixed sensorimotor neuropathies, including certain hereditary neuropathies, metachromatic leukodystrophy, Krabbe's disease, and Tangier disease
2. Segmental demyelinating motor sensory polyneuropathies, including inflammatory neuropathies (e.g., Guillain-Barré syndrome) and neuropathies associated with gammopathies, hypothyroidism, carcinoma or lymphoma, AIDS, Lyme disease, and certain toxins
3. Axonal motor sensory polyneuropathies, including porphyria, certain hereditary neuropathies, lymphomatous neuropathies, and certain toxic neuropathies
4. Axonal sensory neuronopathy or neuropathies, including certain hereditary neuropathies, primary amyloidosis, Sjögren's syndrome, paraneoplastic neuropathies, and neuropathies caused by drugs or vitamin B_{12} deficiency
5. Mixed axonal demyelinating sensorimotor polyneuropathies resulting from uremia or diabetes mellitus
6. Axonal sensorimotor polyneuropathies, including neuropathies caused by nutritional deficiencies, alcohol, sarcoidosis, connective tissue diseases, toxins, heavy metals, and drugs

E. **Diseases of the neuromuscular junction** may be diagnosed by repetitive stimulation studies. Repetitive stimulation of motor nerves is used chiefly in the diagnosis of **myasthenia gravis (MG).** In this disease, a characteristic progressive decline in amplitude of the first few responses to stimulation is revealed at a stimulation rate of two per second. The defect may be further characterized by the way it is altered after a brief contraction of the muscle. In some MG patients with normal repetitive stimulation studies, the diagnosis may be assisted by single fiber EMG. Repetitive stimulation studies are also invaluable in the diagnosis of the **Eaton-Lambert myasthenic syndrome.** In the myasthenic syndrome, the initial action potential evoked in the rested muscle by a single maximal nerve stimulation is greatly reduced in amplitude. A further reduction in amplitude may occur with repetitive stimulation at low rates, but striking facilitation (enlargement of the MUPs) occurs during stimulation at higher rates. Unusual fatigability of the peripheral neuromuscular system may occasionally be demonstrated in other diseases, such as amyotrophic lateral sclerosis, but this abnormality is of little diagnostic value.

F. Electrodiagnostic studies show a wide variety of abnormalities in patients with **myopathies.** The NCS is essentially normal, except for occasional reductions in CMAP amplitudes. The EMG may reveal fibrillation potentials in severe myopathies or in inflammatory myopathies (e.g., polymyositis). "Myopathic" MUPs are of decreased amplitude and duration with increased polyphasia and rapid recruitment out of proportion to the degree of contraction effort. EMG studies usually are not sufficient to identify a specific disease, but the pattern of findings can be associated with groups of muscle disorders. Toxic and endocrine myopathies may produce little or no EMG abnormalities. An EMG/NCS examination can:

1. Distinguish neurogenic from myopathic disorders as causes of weakness.
2. Provide clues to the etiology of a myopathy.
3. Provide estimates of the severity and acuteness of the process.
4. Assess the activity and course of the disease.
5. Provide important information on the distribution of involvement to guide selection of a biopsy site (muscle biopsy must not be performed on a muscle that has been needled but in a corresponding muscle in the opposite extremity).
6. Detect abnormalities even if not clinically apparent.

Evoked Potentials

I. Introduction. Evoked potentials are electrical signals generated by the nervous system in response to sensory stimuli. The timing and location of these signals are determined by the sensory system involved and the sequence in which different neural structures are activated. Identical sensory stimuli are presented repeatedly while a computer averages the time-locked low-voltage responses from the brain or spinal cord and unrelated electrical noise and background EEG activity are averaged out.

II. Visual evoked potentials (VEPs)

A. Disorders of central visual pathways are tested by **VEPs,** which are the cortical responses to visual stimuli. Stroboscopic flashes of light or, more commonly, black-and-white checkerboard patterns evoke potentials over the occipital lobes that are detected by scalp electrodes. The major positive deflection at a latency of approximately 100 msec (the **P100 response**) is most useful for clinical applications. Delays in this latency suggest damage to visual conducting pathways.

B. Unilateral prolongation of the P100 response implies an abnormality anterior to the optic chiasm (usually in the optic nerve) on that side. Bilateral P100 delay can be caused by bilateral lesions either anterior or posterior to the chiasm or by a lesion within the chiasm itself.

C. Uses of VEPs

1. VEPs may aid in the detection of a clinically "silent" lesion in a patient suspected of having multiple sclerosis (MS). The VEP is a sufficiently sensitive indicator of optic nerve demyelination that it can reveal asymptomatic and clinically undetectable lesions. VEPs reveal abnormalities in 70–80% of patients with definite MS who do not have histories of optic neuritis or visual symptoms. Abnormalities are not specific for MS and may be abnormal in a variety of other diseases, including certain ocular diseases, compressive lesions of the optic nerve, nutritional and toxic optic neuropathies including pernicious anemia, and diffuse CNS diseases such as adrenoleukodystrophy and some spinocerebellar degenerations.
2. The VEP is helpful in distinguishing functional (e.g., psychogenic) visual impairment from true blindness or bilateral optic nerve disease. A normal VEP strongly favors functional illness. It should be mentioned, however, that rare patients have been described with blindness from severe bilateral destruction of the occipital lobes who had essentially normal VEP studies. Also, some patients with functional problems can voluntarily suppress the VEP response by such strategies as transcendental meditation, concentration beyond the plane of the checks, or ocular convergence.

3. VEPs may be of some assistance in evaluating vision in pediatric patients—for example, in assessing high-risk infants or in the detection of amblyopia.

III. Brainstem auditory evoked potentials (BAEPs)

A. BAEPs are a series of evoked potentials elicited by auditory clicks and generated by sequential activation of the brainstem auditory pathways. Although five waveforms (I–V) are usually resolved, the most stable and important waveforms are I, III, and V. The I–III interpeak latency is a measure of auditory conduction of the more caudal segment of the brainstem (acoustic nerve to lower pons), whereas the III–V interpeak latency is a measure of conduction in the more rostral pontine and lower midbrain pathways. The I–V interpeak latency is a measure of the total conduction time within the brainstem auditory pathways.

B. Abnormality is measured by prolongation of interpeak latencies, especially asymmetric prolongations, as well as reduction in amplitude or absence of certain waveforms. A prolonged I–III interpeak latency indicates a lower pontine lesion, whereas a prolonged III–V interpeak latency indicates a lesion of the upper pons–lower midbrain levels.

C. BAEPs may be clinically helpful in the following circumstances.

1. BAEPs, like VEPs, may be very sensitive to white matter disease and may help confirm or document a lesion within the brainstem, even if there are no brainstem signs or symptoms, when MS is suspected clinically and the patient has a lesion outside the brainstem. Approximately 50% of patients with definite MS exhibit abnormal BAEPs. However, VEPs and SEPs (see sec. **IV**) are more sensitive than BAEPs in detecting abnormalities in MS patients. Other demyelinating processes affecting the brainstem, such as central pontine myelinolysis, metachromatic leukodystrophy, and adrenoleukodystrophy, may also cause BAEP abnormalities.

2. A **posterior fossa tumor or other mass** within or outside of the brainstem can produce abnormal BAEPs by either direct involvement of the brainstem auditory pathways or secondary brainstem compression. BAEPs are very sensitive screening procedures for acoustic neuromas and other cerebellopontine angle tumors.

3. BAEPs may assist in the determination of **brain death.** Preservation of wave I with loss of all subsequent response supports brainstem death in the comatose patient. The BAEP does not, however, provide any information about cortical function in the comatose patient.

4. BAEPs may be used to assess **hearing in young children** and in patients otherwise unable to cooperate for standard audiometry. BAEP testing can estimate hearing threshold and may distinguish conductive hearing loss from sensorineural hearing loss.

IV. Somatosensory evoked potentials (SEPs)

A. Following electrical stimulation of a peripheral nerve (usually the median or ulnar nerve at the wrist or the tibial nerve at the ankle), recording electrodes placed over the spine and scalp reveal a series of electrical potentials that correspond to sequential activation of neural structures along the dorsal column–lemniscal pathway. These **somatosensory evoked potentials (SEPs)** are named according to their polarities and their times of occurrence in normal individuals. Because SEP latencies vary significantly with body height and limb length, absolute latency values are of limited use; interpeak latencies, which measure the time intervals between successive peaks in the sensory pathways, are incorporated in clinical studies.

B. SEPs yield information concerning PNS abnormalities, but are not as effective as standard NCS in identifying and localizing peripheral disorders. Therefore, although SEPs have been used to study plexopathies and radiculopathies, their use is limited for these conditions.

C. Uses of SEPs

1. SEPs can be used to confirm the presence of a clinically "silent" spinal cord lesion in a patient suspected of having MS. Median SEPs are abnormal in about two-thirds of patients with definite MS; lower-limb SEPs have somewhat greater abnormality rates, probably because of the greater length of white matter traversed. Prolonged central conduction times do not necessarily indicate demyelination, because abnormal interpeak latencies may occur with hereditary spastic paraplegia, olivopontocerebellar atrophy, and subacute combined degeneration resulting from vitamin B_{12} deficiency.

2. Abnormally large ("giant") cortical SEPs are characteristic of some relatively rare neurologic conditions, such as progressive myoclonic epilepsy, late infantile ceroid lipofuscinosis, and some other disorders associated with myoclonus.
3. SEPs may be helpful in demonstrating intact central sensory pathways in patients with functional (e.g., hysterical) sensory loss.
4. SEPs have been especially helpful in monitoring spinal cord function during surgery (e.g., surgery for correction of spinal scoliosis).

Other Ancillary Neurologic Studies

I. **Polysomnography**
   A. Polysomnography consists of continuous monitoring of multiple biological variables during nocturnal sleep. Eye movements (electro-oculography), EEG activity, submental EMG, the ECG, and limb movements are routinely monitored. Respiration is monitored with intraesophageal pressure gauges, intercostal surface EMG, rib cage and abdominal strain gauges, oronasal thermistors or CO_2 detectors, ear or finger oximetry, and other means of determining the presence of central, peripheral, or mixed apnea syndromes. A microphone attached to the throat may detect snoring. Each 30-second epoch of the polysomnogram is scored as awake, stage I–IV non-REM (rapid eye movement) sleep, or REM sleep.
   B. Polysomnography is used to investigate two types of problems: sleep complaints (i.e., too much or too little sleep) and risk factors or specific syndromes induced by or linked to sleep or specific sleep states. These disorders include:
      1. Sleep apnea syndromes, which may be obstructive, central, or mixed
      2. Narcolepsy
      3. Idiopathic CNS hypersomnia
      4. Periodic movements of sleep and sleep-related myoclonus
      5. REM behavioral disorder
      6. Disorders of the sleep-wake cycle
      7. Parasomnias, such as sleepwalking, nightmares, night terrors, and head banging

II. **Multiple sleep latency test**
   A. The multiple sleep latency test consists of five 20-minute attempts, once every 2 hours, to fall asleep throughout the day. The aim is to determine the sleep latency and whether or not REM sleep episodes are recorded during the nap. Patients should be withdrawn from sleep-related medications for 10–15 days. The study usually follows polysomnography because knowledge of the patient's previous night's sleep is required for appropriate interpretation. During the study, the EEG, submental EMG, ECG, and eye movements are monitored. Normal patients have mean sleep latencies greater than 10 minutes and fewer than two sleep onset REM periods during the study.
   B. The multiple sleep latency test is designed to evaluate:
      1. The complaint of **excessive daytime somnolence** by quantifying the time required to fall asleep. Pathologic sleepiness is manifested by a mean sleep latency of less than 5 minutes.
      2. The possibility of **narcolepsy** by checking for abnormally short latencies to REM sleep. The occurrence of two or more sleep onset REM periods during the study is strong evidence for narcolepsy, as long as sleep apnea and withdrawal from stimulants and alcohol have been ruled out.

Lumbar Puncture

I. **Introduction.** Lumbar puncture (LP) should be considered only after a thorough evaluation of the patient and serious consideration of the potential value and hazards of the procedure.
II. **Indications for cerebrospinal fluid (CSF) examination and LP are as follows.**
   A. CSF examination is key to the diagnosis and management of various **CNS infections,** including acute and chronic meningitis and encephalitis. In many patients with fever of unknown origin, even in the absence of meningeal signs, an early LP is commonly of value, especially because meningeal signs may be minimal or absent in very young or elderly patients. Meningeal infection should

especially be sought in patients with fever and impaired sensorium or an immunocompromised state (e.g., AIDS patients). If a patient presents with unexplained acute confusion, stupor, or coma, even if afebrile, CSF examination is necessary for evaluation for meningoencephalitis. In most clinical settings, a CT scan of the brain should be performed before the LP to rule out a possible intracranial mass (e.g., hemorrhage or abscess), which would make LP a potentially lethal procedure. However, in an extremely ill patient in whom acute meningitis, such as meningococcal meningitis, is suspected, LP should be done without delay to avoid losing valuable time in beginning appropriate therapy.

B. In patients with suspected **subarachnoid hemorrhage,** an urgent CT scan is indicated to evaluate for the presence of blood. However, in approximately 10% of patients with subarachnoid hemorrhage, CT fails to reveal blood, and a spinal tap is indicated. If the diagnostic LP shows subarachnoid blood or xanthochromia, a cerebral angiogram is needed to determine the source of the hemorrhage.

C. In patients with **unexplained dementia,** CSF examination may be necessary to evaluate for CNS vasculitis, infection, or granulomatous disease. The CSF should always be examined in a patient with dementia and a positive fluorescent treponemal antibody absorption (FTA-ABS) study. Also, patients with radiographic hydrocephalus may require a CSF study to exclude chronic meningitis as an etiology for the symptomatic hydrocephalus.

D. CSF examination is usually not warranted, and may be dangerous, in most patients with stroke. However, CSF analysis may assist in the etiologic diagnosis of **unexplained stroke in young or middle-aged patients** who lack atherosclerotic risk factors. Such etiologies as CNS vasculitis, meningovascular syphilis, and AIDS may be diagnosed.

E. CSF studies may aid in the diagnosis of **MS,** although there is no specific CSF marker for this disease. Elevated CSF IgG levels, with normal serum IgG, and the presence of oligoclonal bands in the CSF are characteristic, but not specific, for MS. Elevated CSF gammaglobulin may also occur in neurosyphilis, viral meningoencephalitis, and subacute sclerosing panencephalitis.

F. CSF analysis is often necessary in evaluating patients admitted with an **initial tonic-clonic seizure or status epilepticus,** after appropriate neuroimaging, to exclude an active CNS infection or hemorrhage.

G. Lumbar puncture is necessary to confirm the clinical suspicion of **carcinomatous or leukemic meningitis.** Often, multiple LPs are needed. The typical CSF pattern is a pleocytosis with elevated protein, low glucose, and a positive cytology for malignancy.

H. CSF studies may aid in the diagnosis of certain **inflammatory or demyelinating neuropathies,** such as the Guillain-Barré syndrome or chronic idiopathic demyelinating polyradiculoneuropathy. The CSF protein is often elevated without an abnormal cellular response.

I. Although LP is generally contraindicated in patients with papilledema, LP is indicated to document increased intracranial pressure in a patient suspected of having **idiopathic intracranial hypertension (pseudotumor cerebri)** after neuroimaging studies have been proven to be normal. The spinal fluid is under increased pressure but is otherwise normal in this entity, except for occasional decreased CSF protein levels. Also, LP is required to document low CSF pressure in rare low-pressure syndromes in a patient whose headaches occur on standing and are relieved by lying down.

J. Lumbar puncture can be used to deliver **intrathecal antibiotics and chemotherapy** in the treatment of certain CNS infections and meningeal malignancies, respectively. Also, LP is required in certain diagnostic procedures, such as myelography or cisternography.

III. **Contraindications for lumbar puncture**

A. LP is contraindicated in any patient with **increased intracranial pressure,** except idiopathic intracranial hypertension, because of the real danger of cerebral herniation and death.

B. LP is contraindicated if there is **suppuration in the skin or deeper tissues overlying the spinal canal** because of the danger of inducing a purulent meningitis.

C. LP is dangerous in the presence of **anticoagulation therapy or a bleeding diathesis.** Also, heparin should not be reinstituted for a minimum of 2 hours after an LP is performed. In general, LP is hazardous if the platelet count is be-

low 50,000, or especially if it is below 20,000. In such cases, platelet transfusions should be initiated if possible prior to the LP.
  D. LP should not be performed when a **spinal mass** is suspected unless the procedure is part of a myelogram with neurosurgical assistance readily available. A dramatic deterioration in spinal cord or cauda equina function can occur after LP.
IV. **Complications of lumbar puncture**
  A. **Brain herniation and death** may occur if an LP is performed on a patient with increased intracranial pressure from a cerebral mass lesion. LP is contraindicated in any patient suspected of having an intracranial mass.
  B. **Headache of low-pressure type** may occur in up to 10% of patients after an LP ("spinal headache"). This type of headache occurs only on standing and is relieved by lying down. It is usually self-limiting, but may require an epidural autologous blood patch for relief. Post-LP headache is most common in young women with lower-body mass. The occurrence of post-LP headache is unrelated to CSF opening pressure, cells, and protein; patient position during LP; duration of recumbency after LP; and amount of CSF removed.
  C. **Diplopia,** which usually results from unilateral or bilateral cranial nerve VI palsies, may occur rarely and is usually self-limiting.
  D. **Aseptic meningitis** may occur rarely and is characterized by posterior neck pain, headache, and neck stiffness. This process is usually self-limiting.
  E. **Spinal epidural, subdural, and subarachnoid hematomas** may occur, especially in patients on anticoagulants or with bleeding diatheses. Such hematomas are usually self-limiting and may cause local pain and meningeal irritation. However, epidural hematoma may rarely cause a flaccid and potentially irreversible paraplegia that requires emergency surgical evacuation.
V. **General comments on evaluation of lumbar puncture results**
  A. The normal **CSF pressure** is 70–180 mm of water in the lateral recumbent position. Pressures should be greater than 200 mm of water to be considered elevated. In an obese patient with possible idiopathic intracranial hypertension, the pressure should be greater than 250 mm of water to establish this diagnosis.
  B. The normal **CSF glucose** is approximately two-thirds of the serum glucose, which must be drawn at the time of the LP. Hypoglycorrhachia (low CSF glucose) with few white cells suggests a fungal infection, with many white cells a bacterial infection, and with abnormal (malignant) cells a meningeal malignancy.
  C. The **CSF protein** may be increased (>100 mg/dL) in many CNS infectious and malignant processes. Causes of elevated CSF protein with normal neuroimaging studies include myxedema, inflammatory demyelinating polyneuropathies, diabetic polyneuropathy, neurofibromas within the CSF pathways, resolving subarachnoid hemorrhages, gliomatosis cerebri, CNS vasculitis, and any process that causes spinal compression or obstruction of CSF flow.
  D. Normally, the CSF can contain up to five lymphocytes or mononuclear cells per cubic centimeter. A **pleocytosis** causes CSF clouding when there are at least 200 cells/cc. An increased WBC count occurs with subarachnoid infections, hemorrhages, chemical meningitis, or meningeal neoplasms. Also, it should be noted that a pleocytosis may occur for approximately 24 hours after a generalized seizure episode.
  E. If initial spinal fluid appears **bloody,** one must attempt to determine whether the source of the blood is a traumatic tap or a subarachnoid hemorrhage. If the initial tube of fluid is bloody and subsequent tubes are progressively clear, it is most likely that the tap was traumatic. One should then *immediately* centrifuge the fluid to see if the supernatant is clear, which suggests a traumatic tap. If the supernatant fluid is xanthochromic (yellow-tinged), it is likely that the blood has been present in the CSF for a few hours. Xanthochromia occurs approximately several hours after a subarachnoid hemorrhage, reaches its greatest intensity at the end of 1 week, and clears in approximately 2–4 weeks. Xanthochromia can also be observed in jaundice and hypercarotenemia.

Referral

All clinical neurophysiologic tests should be performed and interpreted by clinicians with expertise and special training in clinical neurophysiology. Laboratories performing these studies must follow the clinical and technical guidelines that have been published by neurophysiologic societies, the American Academy of Neurology, and other organizations. Strict adherence to these guidelines is mandatory to ensure patient safety and meaningful clinical interpretation.

Neurology consultation is suggested whenever LP reveals abnormalities suggesting CNS infection, increased or decreased intracranial pressure, or subarachnoid hemorrhage.

Recommended Readings

Aminoff MJ. *Electrodiagnosis in Clinical Neurology* (2nd ed). New York: Churchill-Livingstone, 1986.

Brown WF, Bolton CF. *Clinical Electromyography* (2nd ed). Boston: Butterworth-Heinemann, 1993.

Daly DD, Pedley TA. *Current Practice of Clinical Electroencephalography* (2nd ed). New York: Raven, 1990.

Donofrio PD, Albers JW. AAEM minimonograph #34. Polyneuropathy: Classification by nerve conduction studies and EMG. *Muscle and Nerve* 13:889–903, 1990.

Fishman RA. *Cerebrospinal Fluid in Diseases of the Nervous System* (2nd ed). Philadelphia: Saunders, 1992.

Kimura J, Dickins QS. Electrodiagnosis of neuromuscular disorders. In WG Bradley, et al. (eds), *Neurology in Clinical Practice*. Boston: Butterworth-Heinemann, 1991. Pp 452–467.

Kuntz KM, et al. Post-lumbar puncture headaches: Experience in 501 consecutive procedures. *Neurology* 42:1884–1887, 1992.

Members of the Department of Neurology, Mayo Clinic and Mayo Foundation for Medical Education and Research. *Clinical Examinations in Neurology* (6th ed). St. Louis: Mosby, 1991.

Parkes JD. Disorders of sleep. In WG Bradley, et al. (eds), *Neurology in Clinical Practice*. Boston: Butterworth-Heinemann, 1991. Pp 1479–1506.

Pedley TA, Emerson RG. Electroencephalography and evoked potentials. In WG Bradley, et al. (eds), *Neurology in Clinical Practice*. Boston: Butterworth-Heinemann, 1991. Pp 429–451.

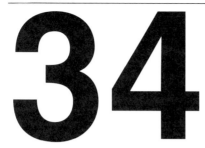

Approach to Common Office Problems of Pediatric Neurology

David W. Dunn
Hema Patel

Delayed Development

I. **Definition.** The child with developmental delay has failed to meet expected milestones in one or more areas. This can be determined with a screening test such as the Denver Developmental test, with more specific intelligence tests such as the Wechsler Intelligence Scale for Children (WISC III), or with achievement tests such as the Wide Range Achievement Tests–Revised (WRAT-R) or the Peabody Individual Achievement Tests. Both tests of intelligence and tests of achievement require referral to a psychologist or other professional trained to administer these assessments. The causes of delay fall into two main categories: nonprogressive and progressive retardation.

II. **Static encephalopathy.** Nonprogressive causes of retardation or delay are also called static encephalopathies. The child may have delays obvious at birth or may fail to reach milestones at the expected rate. The child continues to progress, although at a reduced rate, and does not lose any previously acquired skills. Such children do not reach a level of normal functioning. However, their developmental curves seem to parallel those of children without difficulties in acquiring milestones.

III. **Etiologies of static encephalopathies**

A. **Nonprogressive delays involving multiple functional areas.** Chromosomal disorders, brain malformations, intrauterine infections, and perinatal insults to the brain are potential etiologies of static encephalopathies. This may also follow acquired damage to the brain from meningitis, encephalitis, hypoxia, and head trauma.

B. **Nonprogressive delay in a single functional area.** A nonprogressive motor delay can be observed in some children with cerebral palsy and in some children with congenital myopathies. Nonprogressive isolated speech delay can accompany deafness, autism, and developmental speech disorders.

IV. **Progressive retardation.** The child with progressive retardation first stops acquiring new skills and then loses developmental milestones. The differential is extensive, including degenerative, metabolic, infectious, and mass lesions. It is the constellation of symptoms and signs with which the child presents that determines the evaluation. Some children may have disorders involving the CNS diffusely. They have dysfunctions in both cognitive and motor areas. In the beginning of the illness, there may be predominantly motor or cognitive symptoms and signs, but with time the patient progressively loses function in other areas. In some children the regression may be limited to a single area of the neuromuscular systems. As examples, children with cerebellar degenerative disorders may have progressive loss of coordination with preservation of cognitive function, and children with certain muscular dystrophies may have deterioration limited to motor skills.

V. **Etiologies of degenerative disorders**

A. **Isolated involvement of the CNS**

1. **Disorders involving predominantly white matter** present with spasticity and motor regression. There is prominent demyelination on MRI. Examples include metachromatic leukodystrophy, globoid cell leukodystrophy, Alexander's disease, Canavan's disease, Pelizaeus-Merzbacher disease, and adrenoleukodystrophy.

2. **Disorders involving predominantly gray matter** start with seizures or loss of cognitive function. In this category are found the aminoacidurias, or-

ganic acidurias, lactic acidemias (such as Leigh disease), Tay-Sachs disease, ceroid lipofuscinosis, and Rett's disorder.

3. **Disorders with prominent abnormalities of posture or movement.** Disorders that involve dystonia include torsion dystonia, Wilson's disease, Hallervorden-Spatz syndrome, and Niemann-Pick disease type C. With juvenile Huntington's disease and juvenile parkinsonism, there may be rigidity and chorea or tremor. Chorea is a prominent component of Lesch-Nyhan syndrome.

4. **Disorders with prominent ataxia.** Ataxia may be a component of many of the degenerative and metabolic disorders. It is most pronounced in ataxia-telangiectasia, Refsum's disease, abetalipoproteinemia, Friedreich's ataxia, and the many other familial ataxia syndromes (see Gilman, Bloedel, and Lechtenberg).

5. **Disorders with prominent peripheral nervous system (PNS) involvement.** In globoid cell and metachromatic leukodystrophies, there is a demyelinating neuropathy. With neuroaxonal dystrophy, there is a combination of dementia, hypotonia, and areflexia. The child with Fabry's disease has an angiectatic skin rash and a painful sensory neuropathy.

B. **Disorders involving both the CNS and other organs**

1. **Disorders with prominent dysmorphic features** all have coarse facial features in common. In this category are the mucopolysaccharidoses, the mucolipidoses, the sialidoses, and GM_1 gangliosidosis.

2. **Disorders with both organomegaly and CNS involvement.** Hepatomegaly is a major feature in most of the mucopolysaccharidoses, galactosemia, Pompe's disease, Zellweger syndrome, GM_1 gangliosidosis, and Niemann-Pick disease. Splenomegaly is more prominent in type 2 Gaucher's disease.

VI. **Evaluation**

A. **History.** For the child with a static encephalopathy, the history and examination may be all that is needed for the appropriate diagnosis. An example is the child who was a very premature infant and who suffered multiple complications including intraventricular hemorrhage, and now presents with spastic quadriparesis and cognitive delay. The history involves a careful review of complications of pregnancy, labor, and delivery, subsequent injuries and illnesses, and a detailed family history. The developmental history documents both when milestones were met and when symptoms and signs began. By means of the history, one can usually assign the child to a progressive or nonprogressive category. Difficulties arise when the child has a severe metabolic disorder that manifests in the neonatal period and when the child has a slowly progressive disorder and is seen at a time at which there is a falling away from the normal developmental curve but no loss of milestones. In the first case, the diagnosis is suspected when there is no clear etiology for the encephalopathy that occurred in the neonatal period. In the second case, a repeated evaluation may be necessary.

B. **Examination.** The standard pediatric and neurologic examination helps place the condition into a category that makes laboratory assessment more efficient. Referral to an ophthalmologist is helpful. Optic atrophy is observed in many of the leukodystrophies; macular or retinal pigmentary degeneration occurs in ceroid lipofuscinosis, abetalipoproteinemia, Refsum's disease, and certain mucopolysaccharidoses; cherry red spots are present in Tay-Sachs disease, sialidosis, and some cases of Niemann-Pick disease and GM_1 gangliosidosis; lens opacities are found in galactosemia, Wilson's disease, Marinesco-Sjögren syndrome, and homocystinuria; corneal opacities accompany certain storage diseases; and the Kayser-Fleischer ring helps in the diagnosis of Wilson's disease.

C. **Laboratory**

1. **Nonprogressive encephalopathies** should not require extensive workups. Neuroimaging helps define brain malformations and is important for ruling out hydrocephalus and mass lesions. Chromosomal studies are necessary if the etiology is not obvious from the history. Assessment of vision and hearing are essential for appropriate developmental and educational planning.

2. **Progressive encephalopathies.** Appropriate studies are determined by the history and examination. A CT or MRI scan may be necessary to rule out hydrocephalus or mass lesion. MRI also documents the demyelination that accompanies leukodystrophies. EEG is necessary for the evaluation of seizures. Thyroid function studies should be obtained if there are coarse fa-

cial features. Urine should be checked for amino acids and organic acids if the child has seizures and cognitive delays. Urine is checked for reducing substances when there is hepatomegaly or cataracts suggesting galactosemia. A urine screen for mucopolysaccharides should be performed if there are coarse facial features or organomegaly. Slowing of nerve conduction and delays in evoked response tests are observed in association with leukodystrophies. Abnormal or absent electroretinograms are characteristic of retinitis pigmentosa and tapetoretinal degenerative disorders. The definitive diagnosis for many of these disorders requires demonstration of enzyme deficiencies in leukocytes or cultured fibroblasts.

Nonepileptiform Paroxysmal Events

In this section we review intermittent, transient, recurrent episodes of neurologic dysfunction. Between episodes, the child is usually normal. The most common disorders are headaches, seizures, and syncope. Both headaches (Chaps. 20, 21) and seizures (Chap. 6) are covered elsewhere in this text.

I. **Evaluation**
   A. **History.** The description should be obtained from the child and from witnesses to the event. Review the situation immediately prior to the episode, asking specifically about any potential trigger. Ask the child to describe how he or she felt before and after the episode. Witnesses can provide detailed descriptions of the episode. The history is reviewed for predisposing conditions and any family history of paroxysmal disorders.
   B. **Examination.** Between episodes, the examination is usually normal. For possible syncopal episodes, blood pressure is measured with the child both supine and standing. If it seems that there was a trigger for the event, repeating this precipitant may help with the diagnosis.
   C. **Laboratory.** If there is a possibility of epilepsy, serum glucose and calcium tests and an EEG are necessary. An ECG, Holter monitoring, and cardiac ultrasound are parts of the work-up for syncope. Neuroimaging is essential if headaches and loss of function occur during the same episode.
II. **Diagnostic approach based on major symptom**
   A. **Episodic loss of function with a clear-cut precipitant**
      1. **Breath-holding spells.** The triggers for breath-holding spells are pain, anger, frustration, surprise, and fright. In the cyanotic form, the child cries, holds the cry in expiration, becomes cyanotic, and loses consciousness. The child may become rigid and may exhibit a few clonic movements. The entire episode is brief, usually less than 60 seconds. In the pallid form, the child does not cry, becomes pale and apneic, and loses consciousness. In both forms, there can be urinary incontinence and profound bradycardia. These episodes are most common between 6 months and 3 years of age, and are not associated with any increased risk of epilepsy or learning disability. They usually cease within 2–3 years. The family history is often positive for similar episodes in first-degree relatives.
      2. **Syncope** is the result of a sudden decrease in brain perfusion, most commonly from a vasovagal reflex. Syncope is more frequent in adolescents than in younger children. It typically occurs after prolonged standing or sudden standing. It rarely occurs while the child is sitting and does not happen when the child is lying down. The triggers may be emotional situations, embarrassment, a Valsalva's maneuver, or a sudden change in position. The child first notes lightheadedness or dizziness, or may fall without warning. Loss of muscle tone and loss of consciousness occur simultaneously. The child may exhibit a few clonic jerks during the period of decreased consciousness. The period of alteration in consciousness is usually less than 1 minute long.
      3. **Reflex epilepsies.** See Chap. 6. Potential triggers are flashing lights, startling events, and, rarely, somatosensory or auditory stimuli or complex activities such as reading.
   B. **Episodic movement disorders**
      1. **Weakness.** Periods of weakness with recovery between episodes may occur in association with myasthenia gravis (MG). Periods of weakness are also characteristic of the periodic paralyses. These paralyses are autosomal dominant disorders in which weakness may be triggered by rest following

exertion, carbohydrate loads, cold exposure, or stress. The serum potassium level may be low, mildly elevated, or normal.

2. **Ataxia.** Intermittent ataxia occurs with seizures, migraine, and metabolic disorders including Hartnup disease, a form of maple syrup urine disease (MSUD), and certain urea cycle abnormalities. There is also a familial periodic ataxia that may be responsive to acetazolamide.

3. **Chorea.** There are both kinesiogenic and dystonic forms of chorea. The kinesiogenic form is precipitated by movement or a startling event and lasts less than 5 minutes. The dystonic form can be precipitated by fatigue, caffeine, or alcohol and may last up to 4 hours. Both forms are familial.

4. **Other movements.** Three disorders seen only in children are spasmus nutans, shuddering attacks, and paroxysmal torticollis. Spasmus nutans begins at 3–30 months of age and consists of episodes of monocular nystagmus, head tilt, and head bobbing. The episodes last for seconds to a few minutes. Shuddering attacks are brief shaking spells usually observed in infants. The infant remains alert throughout the episode. Shuddering attacks may be associated with later onset of essential tremor. Paroxysmal torticollis occurs during the first 2–3 years of life. The episodes may last for a few minutes or as long as several weeks. The child may vomit but remains alert during the episode. This condition can evolve into benign paroxysmal vertigo.

C. **Episodic sensory disturbances**

1. **Transient visual loss** is an uncommon symptom in childhood. With epilepsy, there are almost invariably other symptoms at the time of the visual loss or a history of seizure immediately prior to the loss. Transient visual loss can be the aura of childhood migraine, although this aura is more common in older people. Transient visual loss during headache should raise the possibility of a mass lesion causing increased intracranial pressure. A graying-out of vision can be part of a hyperventilation syndrome or presyncope.

2. **Episodic numbness or paresthesias.** Episodes of numbness may be the sole manifestation of a partial complex seizure, and can occur as an aura in childhood migraine. Tingling of the hands or, less often, the feet, along with shortness of breath, suggest a hyperventilation syndrome.

3. **Vertigo** is distinguished from incipient syncope by rotational symptoms. An acute onset of vertigo that persists for over an hour suggests labyrinthitis; otitis media; drug exposure, including aminoglycosides, alcohol, anticonvulsants, hypnotics, tranquilizers, and aspirin; trauma causing an inner ear fistula, or tumors of the inner ear or the vestibular portion of the eighth cranial nerve. Recurrent episodes of vertigo may follow meningitis and head injury. Basilar artery migraine may cause vertigo and a throbbing occipital headache. Partial complex seizures may feature vertigo and a brief alteration of consciousness. Benign paroxysmal vertigo affects preschool children and causes brief episodes of vertigo not associated with alteration of consciousness or headache. Some of these children later develop migraines.

Headaches

I. **Differential diagnosis of headaches**

A. **Acute headaches**

1. **Febrile children.** Headaches are commonly associated with systemic febrile illnesses and infectious processes involving the head and neck. With uveitis, the pain is periorbital, and with otitis media, the pain is in the temporal region. The pain of sinusitis may be localized directly over the sinus or may be more diffuse, usually in the frontal or retro-orbital region. The pain should resolve within 3 days of starting appropriate antibiotic therapy. The combination of fever, headache, nuchal rigidity, and alteration in level of consciousness suggests meningitis. Other causes include cervical adenopathy and retropharyngeal abscess.

2. **Afebrile children.** In an afebrile child with a normal neurologic examination, an acute onset of headaches could be the beginning of childhood migraine or tension-type headache, but the diagnosis cannot be made without follow-up. Other possibilities include hypertensive headache, hydrocephalus, leukemic meningitis, and drug use. The drugs most often associated with headache are diet pills containing phenylpropanolamine and CNS stim-

ulants such as amphetamines. Headache plus neurologic abnormalities suggests a mass lesion or a subarachnoid hemorrhage. In children, subarachnoid hemorrhage is usually a result of head trauma, with arteriovenous malformations (AVMs) and aneurysms being much less common causes.

B. Chronic headaches

1. Abnormal neurologic examination. Headaches may be the first symptoms in children with increased intracranial pressure from mass lesions. Within 4 months of the onset of headaches, 90% of children with mass lesions have definite abnormalities on neurologic examination. If CT or MRI is normal, possibilities are chronic meningitis and pseudotumor cerebri (also called idiopathic intracranial hypertension, or IIH). On lumbar puncture (LP), the opening pressure is elevated in both chronic meningitis and pseudotumor cerebri, with abnormal cerebrospinal fluid (CSF) cell count only in chronic meningitis. The usual symptoms of pseudotumor cerebri in children are headache, vomiting, diplopia, and blurred vision. Although this condition has been associated with several disorders, the most frequently encountered are cerebral venous thrombosis, otitis media or mastoiditis, corticosteroid use, thyroid dysfunction, vitamin A excess, and tetracycline use. Treatment is essential to prevent potential visual loss.

2. Normal neurologic examination. The most common causes of chronic headache in children are migraine and tension-type headaches. Throbbing vascular-type headaches can also be caused by hypertension and AVMs. Nonvascular headaches may be caused by disorders of the nasal sinuses, the muscles of the head and neck, the cranial periosteum, or the cervical or cranial nerves. With acute sinusitis there may be frontal headaches or facial pain. With temporomandibular (TM) joint dysfunction there may be temporal headaches, especially after eating. Occipital neuralgia causes lancinating pains starting in the neck and spreading to the top of the head. Ocular problems are relatively uncommon causes of frontal or temporal headaches. Increasingly severe headaches should prompt a reevaluation of the diagnosis and a consideration of mass lesion as a possible cause.

II. Classification and clinical manifestations of the most common chronic headaches

A. Migraine affects 2–5% of elementary school children and 5–10% of teenagers. Initially, the sex ratio is equal, but by the teenage years, twice as many girls are affected. More than 75% of children with migraine have positive family histories. Common triggering factors are stress, sleep deprivation or excess, menstrual periods, upper respiratory tract infections, and skipping of meals. Migraine attacks may follow minor head trauma. Migraine may occasionally be triggered by chocolates, nitrates or nitrites, monosodium glutamate, or dairy products. In comparison with adults, children are less likely to have classical auras or unilateral headaches. They more commonly have bilateral throbbing headaches with associated nausea and vomiting. Most children try to find a quiet, dark room and go to sleep to get rid of the headache. Cyclic vomiting and benign paroxysmal vertigo may be migraine equivalents in children. Younger children may have ophthalmoplegic migraine with ptosis and a complete 3rd nerve palsy, including on occasions pupillary dilatation. Acute confusional migraine, a confusional state followed by throbbing headaches, is more common in teenagers. Adolescents also may have basilar migraine, with ataxia or other brainstem signs including alterations in consciousness, followed by throbbing occipital headaches.

B. Tension-type headaches

1. Episodic tension-type headache is probably the most common type of headache. The childhood form is similar to the adult form. Such headaches occur more often in the afternoon or evening and are associated with stress or with excessive exertion or fatigue. They may be occipital or frontal, or may involve the entire head, and are described as a steady ache or sensation of pressure. They generally respond well to mild analgesics or rest.

2. Chronic tension-type headache is similar in character to the episodic form but occurs daily for more than 180 days per year. Such headaches are not responsive to standard medications. They can be disabling and can cause excessive school absences. These headaches have been called psychogenic headaches in the past and are best considered a somatoform disorder. The "sick role" should be discouraged, and the child should be pushed to take part in normal activities. Instead of medication, self-relaxation techniques and behavioral therapies are used to help the child cope with these headaches.

III. Evaluation

A. History. An assessment of headaches involves a history of the headaches over time and a description of a typical individual headache. Important factors include changes in frequency or intensity, triggers, time of occurrence both seasonally and during the day, and those factors that cause worsening or improvement during the headaches. The description of an individual headache includes prodrome, auras, location and quality of the pain, associated symptoms, and the postheadache period. If the child has more than one type of headache, a description of a typical headache should be solicited for each type.

B. Examination. A complete neurologic examination is essential. In addition, tenderness over the sinuses, clicks in or misalignment of the TM joint, decreased visual acuity, and cervical lymphadenopathy are important clues to etiology. The blood pressure must be recorded and the skull auscultated for cranial bruits.

C. Laboratory. For typical headaches, little is needed. If the child has fever and a headache, studies are obtained to determine the source of the fever. An LP should be performed if meningitis cannot be confidently excluded by history and examination. For the child with an acute headache but no fever, MRI of the brain may be necessary. If the child is not imaged, follow-up is necessary to ensure that no signs of increased intracranial pressure occur. If the child has chronic headaches, neuroimaging is needed if the headaches worsen, if there are atypical features, if the child has complicated migraine, or if abnormal neurologic signs appear. EEG may be indicated for the child with confusional migraine or hemiplegic migraine. For the child with chronic tension-type headaches, eye and ENT evaluations may be necessary. MRI of the brain may be required to help assure the family that there is no life-threatening illness, and psychological testing may be helpful to determine appropriate therapy.

Enuresis

I. Clinical description. Urinary continence is usually obtained by 2–3 years of age. Occasional wetting during the first few years after toilet training is considered a normal variant. Nocturnal enuresis is a common problem that affects boys more than girls. Approximately 10% of 6-year-olds and 1% of 18-year-olds have nocturnal enuresis at least once per month.

II. Evaluation

A. History. A history of pain on urination, past urinary tract infections, trouble initiating or maintaining a forceful urinary stream, or chronic dribbling all suggest disorders of the urinary tract. Back pain or difficulties in walking may indicate a spinal cord or cauda equina lesion. Symptoms that might represent a frontal cerebral dysfunction or nocturnal seizures include lethargy, apathy, or confusion the morning after the episode of enuresis. Headaches, visual loss, and growth disturbances suggest a frontal lobe lesion with a neurogenic bladder. Part of history-taking is a developmental evaluation. A child with significant delays might be expected to be incontinent if the developmental level is less than 2½ years of age.

B. Examination. On physical examination, the presence of a fatty mass, tuft of hair, or hemangioma in the midline overlying the lower spine, or sacral dimple often signals the presence of a tethered cord or a lipoma involving the cauda equina. In addition, absence of ankle jerks or weakness in the muscles of the feet suggests cord lesions. Observing the urinary stream may help diagnose anomalies of the urinary system.

C. Laboratory. Laboratory studies should include urinalysis and culture. An MRI scan of the lumbosacral spine should be obtained if there is any indication of cord problems, and either MRI or CT of the head should be done if there is a suggestion of hydrocephalus or mass lesion involving the frontal lobe. An EEG should be obtained if there are additional symptoms or signs of nocturnal seizures. Intravenous pyelography (IVP) and cystoscopy should be performed if there has been a history of urinary tract infections or if there are signs or symptoms of anomalies involving the urinary tract.

III. Differential diagnosis. In most cases, enuresis is best considered a developmental problem and not a true illness. Less than 5% of children with enuresis have organic lesions. Occasionally, enuresis may be associated with transient regression following hospitalization, the absence of a parent, or the birth of a new sibling, or with excess rigidity or battles between parent and child over the establishment of toilet control.

Motor Disorders

Many of the motor disorders observed in childhood are similar to those in adults. In this section we discuss those disorders occurring only, or predominantly, in children.

I. Motor development. The following list indicates the average ages for reaching motor milestones.

2 months: lifts head for several seconds while prone, hands usually fisted
4 months: head steady while in sitting position, reaches and grasps objects
6 months: rolls prone to supine, transfers objects hand to hand
10 months: sits without support, thumb and two finger grasp
12 months: walks, pincher grasp
18 months: climbs stairs with help, feeds self and throws toys
24 months: runs, balances on one foot for 1 second, builds tower of 4–6 blocks
3 years: walks on toes and heels, balances for 5 seconds, slow alternating movements
4 years: walks with arms still at side, smooth finger-to-nose, draws square
5 years: walks with limited arm swing, smooth and accurate finger-to-nose, balances 10 seconds
6 years: balances for 13–16 seconds, unsteady heel-to-knee movement, awkward rapid alternating movements
8 years: balances more than 20 seconds, smooth rapid alternating movements
9 years: no mirror movements

II. Weakness. The causes of weakness are similar in children and adults. This differential of weakness in adults is covered in Chap. 30, Approach to the Patient with Acute Muscle Weakness. A major area of difference is in the child under 1 year of age. The child with hypotonia and weakness is often called a floppy infant. The causative lesion may be located anywhere from brain to muscle.

A. Evaluation

1. **History.** The diagnosis may be suggested by the presence of similar neuromuscular disorders in other family members, by known asphyxia or seizures at birth, or by complications of delivery. Lethargy or poor responsiveness indicates CNS dysfunction. Variations in the degree of weakness may occur in neuromuscular junction disorders.

2. **Examination.** The presence of brisk or normal reflexes and fisting are clues to CNS damage. Dysmorphic features and organomegaly also indicate possible CNS dysfunction. A level with normal function proximally and weakness distally occurs with spinal cord damage. Disorders of the lower motor unit cause depressed to absent reflexes. Fasciculations may be seen in the tongue but are harder to find in the extremities. Joint contractures (arthrogryposis) may accompany both upper and lower motor unit lesions. An examination of the mother can be helpful. A diagnosis of myotonic muscular dystrophy or myasthenia gravis can be made easier in the mother.

3. **Laboratory.** Creatine kinase is elevated in inflammatory and rapidly progressive muscular dystrophies. Electromyography (EMG) and nerve conduction studies (NCS) help distinguish among neuropathies, neuromuscular junction disorders, and myopathies. With myasthenia, there is an improvement in strength after administration of neostigmine (0.04 mg/kg/dose) or edrophonium chloride (0.2 mg/kg/dose). A muscle biopsy is necessary for an adequate diagnosis of myopathy.

B. Etiologies of the floppy infant syndrome

1. **Central hypotonia**

a. **Acquired central hypotonia.** Infants who have ischemic or hypoxic damage in the perinatal period and who are destined to have cerebral palsy may be hypotonic and weak. Increased tone first appears distally and may cause persistent fisting of the hands. At the same time, there is decreased truncal tone, causing poor head control. There are steady increases in reflexes, tone, and strength. Spinal cord lesions may be associated with complicated breech deliveries.

b. Chromosomal anomalies and metabolic-degenerative disorders. Hypotonia with mild weakness is a feature of Down syndrome and the Prader-Willi syndrome. Weakness and hypotonia may be prominent in early-onset disorders such as GM_1 gangliosidosis and Zellweger syndrome (cerebrohepatorenal syndrome).

2. Lower motor unit disorders

a. Anterior horn cell disorders. Acute infantile spinal muscular atrophy (Werdnig-Hoffmann disease) and chronic infantile spinal muscular atrophy are degenerative disorders presenting with profound weakness, areflexia, and fasciculations in the tongue. Both are progressive, with the acute form leading to death in 1 year and the chronic form often stabilizing for long periods, allowing some children to live into the young adult years. In addition, there is a neurogenic form of arthrogryposis, presenting with weakness, areflexia, and joint contractures, that is usually not associated with progressive weakness.

b. Neuropathies are rare in young children. Neuropathies may be components of diffuse leukodystrophies, or may result from Guillain-Barré syndrome. Familial dysautonomia (Riley-Day syndrome) causes failure to thrive, hypotonia, decreased reflexes, and absence of tears. The diagnosis can be confirmed by the absence of the flare response to intradermal histamine.

c. Neuromuscular junction disorders. Transient neonatal myasthenia occurs in infants whose mothers have myasthenia. The infant's weakness resolves over 4–6 weeks. There are several congenital myasthenic syndromes, with ptosis, ophthalmoplegia, breathing or feeding trouble, and generalized weakness, that begin in the first 2 years of life. Referral to a research center is necessary for exact diagnosis. Infant botulism causes a similar picture with the additional findings of nonreactive or poorly reactive pupils, constipation, poor feeding, and hypotonia. Diagnosis is confirmed by the identification of *Clostridium botulinum* and botulinus toxin in the feces.

d. Myopathies. There are many different disorders of muscle affecting children, and referral to a specialized clinic is often warranted. Duchenne's muscular dystrophy begins by 2–3 years of age with hip weakness, enlarged calves, and marked elevation of serum creatine kinase. The congenital myopathies, diagnosed on the basis of changes revealed on muscle biopsy (e.g., nemaline rod, central core, and myotubular myopathies), may present with pronounced weakness in the neonatal period or with very slowly progressive hip and shoulder weakness. Pompe's disease, a glycogen storage disease, starts in the first few months of life with both weakness and cardiac failure. Some of the mitochondrial myopathies may also be associated with cardiac disease. A severe form of myotonic muscular dystrophy may begin in the neonatal period in an infant who has the gene for this disorder and whose mother is affected. The infant has both weakness and mental retardation.

e. Connective tissue disorders. Children with Ehlers-Danlos syndrome and Marfan syndrome have hypotonia with normal reflexes and normal or only mildly diminished strength.

III. Ataxia

A. Definition. Ataxia is an impairment of balance and an incoordination of volitional movement. Sensory ataxia involves disruption of the vestibular connections to the caudal vermis of the cerebellum or sensory pathways in the spinal cord connecting to the brainstem and cerebellum. Motor ataxia is observed in association with cerebellar damage or damage to the frontopontocerebellar fibers.

B. Evaluation

1. History. The first step is assessment of the course of the ataxia. The ataxias can be initially divided into acute-onset, chronic progressive, chronic nonprogressive, and intermittent forms. A history of recent infections or exposure to toxins is helpful in evaluating the acute ataxias. Symptoms of increased intracranial pressure and family histories of ataxia may be found in the chronic progressive ataxias. Patients with chronic nonprogressive ataxias may have histories of trauma, meningitis, lead poisoning, or hypoglycemia.

2. **Examination.** Cerebellar hemisphere damage produces ipsilateral limb ataxia and nystagmus, and rostral vermis damage causes gait and truncal ataxia. Involvement of sensory pathways in the spinal cord is indicated by Romberg's sign.

3. **Laboratory.** CT or MRI should be performed in most cases of acute ataxia and all cases of chronic ataxia. Patients with acute ataxias should be given toxicology screens, LPs, and tests for urinary catecholamines. Metabolic studies that can be helpful in children with chronic ataxias include tests for urinary amino acids and serum levels of ammonia, vitamins A and E, cholesterol, triglycerides, lipoproteins, phytanic acid, and biotin.

C. **Etiologies of ataxia in children**
   1. **Acute-onset ataxia**
      a. **Intoxications.** Ataxia may follow ingestion of alcohol, sedative drugs, or anticonvulsants.
      b. **Infections.** Ataxia may be observed both acutely and during recovery from bacterial meningitis. Viral cerebellitis has been associated with mumps and the enteric viruses. A postinfectious cerebellar ataxia may occur at the end of a course of chickenpox. The prognosis is excellent, with most patients recovering completely. Ataxia may also be a prominent part of Fisher's syndrome (a variant of Guillain-Barré syndrome).
      c. **Paraneoplastic disorders.** A relatively acute-onset ataxia may accompany neuroblastoma. The patient has a combination of ataxia, opsoclonus, and myoclonus. The tumor may be found in the abdomen or mediastinum.
   2. **Chronic progressive ataxia**
      a. **Tumors.** The posterior fossa is the most common location of brain tumors in children. The child with a medulloblastoma presents with headaches, vomiting, and gait ataxia. The child with a cerebellar astrocytoma usually has ipsilateral limb ataxia and a good prognosis for cure. Brainstem gliomas cause a combination of cranial nerve palsies, spasticity, and ataxia. Hydrocephalus may also cause progressive gait unsteadiness.
      b. **Degenerative disorders.** There are a large number of hereditary ataxias, which may require referral to a specialty center for diagnosis. One of the more common is Friedreich's ataxia. It begins at the end of the first decade and causes scoliosis and pes cavus, truncal ataxia, decreased reflexes, and reduced vibratory and position senses in the legs. Ataxia-telangiectasia is an autosomal recessive disorder. The child first develops ataxia, and then, by 3–6 years of age, telangiectasias. The patient has frequent infections and low levels of IgA and IgE.
      c. **Metabolic disorders.** Ataxia, abdominal pain, and failure to thrive as a result of fat malabsorption are symptoms of abetalipoproteinemia. Wilson's disease may cause ataxia, dystonia, learning and behavioral disturbances, and hepatic damage. Other metabolic disorders causing ataxia include vitamin E deficiency, biotin-responsive multiple carboxylase deficiency, and urea cycle defects.
   3. **Chronic nonprogressive ataxia**
      a. **Malformations** include the Dandy-Walker malformation (a dilation of the fourth ventricle and hypoplasia of the cerebellar vermis), Chiari type 1 malformation (downward displacement of the cerebellar tonsils), and Joubert's syndrome (vermal agenesis, hyperpnea, pendular eye movements, and delay).
      b. **Acquired cerebellar damage.** Ataxia may follow head trauma or meningitis. It has also been reported as a sequela of severe hypoglycemia and lead poisoning. With ataxic cerebral palsy, there is usually spasticity or dystonia, and ataxia.
      c. **Clumsy child syndrome** is also called developmental dyspraxia or, in the *Diagnostic and Statistical Manual of Mental Disorders, Fourth Edition* (DSM-IV), developmental coordination disorder. These children

have poor handwriting and trouble dressing. They run awkwardly and fall frequently. Their poor performance in sports may lead to a lowering of self-esteem.

4. Intermittent ataxias

a. Migraine. Basilar artery migraine occurs most often in adolescent girls. Ataxia, vertigo, and vomiting may last from minutes to several hours. There is usually a throbbing occipital headache associated with the ataxia.

b. Metabolic disorders are rare. The intermittent form of MSUD causes intermittent ataxia, is diagnosed by finding branched chain keto acids in the urine, and is treated with thiamine. Other examples include acetazolamide-responsive familial periodic ataxia, urea cycle defects, and Hartnup disease, a disorder of amino acid transport.

c. Epilepsy. Rarely, either partial complex or generalized seizures may have ataxia as a major sign, usually accompanied by some clouding of consciousness or clonic movements.

IV. Chorea

A. Definition and evaluation. See Chap. 28.

B. Etiologies of chorea in children

1. **Acute-onset chorea.** Intoxication with stimulants, anticonvulsants, oral contraceptives, antihistamines, lithium, and the phenothiazines may cause chorea. Chorea may occur after infarcts of the basal ganglia, and may follow surgery utilizing deep hypothermia.

2. **Subacute onset of chorea.** Sydenham's chorea follows streptococcal infections by several weeks. The child slowly develops chorea, hypotonia, and emotional lability. Recovery may take months. Chorea can be a symptom of childhood lupus, endocrine disorders including hyperthyroidism and Addison's disease, and tumors involving the basal ganglia.

3. **Chronic chorea.** Static chorea and athetosis following kernicterus is now relatively uncommon. A progressive chorea may be observed with Lesch-Nyhan syndrome, chorea acanthocytosis, juvenile Huntington's disease, and ataxia-telangiectasia.

V. Tics

A. Definition and evaluation. See Chap. 28.

B. Etiology

1. **Isolated tics.** Tics are common in children. Approximately 25% of children have tics, usually involving facial muscles and lasting for more than 1 month but less than 1 year. Chronic motor tics, which last for more than 1 year, are uncommon, and are thought by some to be a variant of Tourette's disorder.

2. **Tourette's disorder** is common, affecting 4–5/10,000. This is an autosomal dominant disorder of varying severity that affects boys more often than girls. It usually begins as a motor tic involving facial muscles. These first symptoms appear between 4 and 7 years of age. With time, the child develops multiple motor tics and vocalizations consisting of throat-clearing sounds, coughing, snorting, barking, or multiple other odd sounds. Coprolalia, part of the original description, is relatively rare in children but can be debilitating when present. Behavioral problems are often more disruptive than tics. These children have a high incidence of attention-deficit problems, obsessive-compulsive disorder (OCD), and emotional lability. The tic disorder changes with time, with two-thirds becoming asymptomatic or much improved.

VI. Dystonia

A. Definition and evaluation. See Chap. 28.

B. Etiologies of childhood dystonia

1. **Acute dystonia.** Phenothiazine exposure is the most common cause of acute dystonia, although cases have been associated with lithium, antihistamines, and anticonvulsants. Acute torticollis may follow trauma to muscles in the neck and may accompany cervical adenitis or retropharyngeal abscess.

2. **Chronic dystonia**

a. Isolated torticollis. Congenital torticollis suggests an anomaly of the cervical spinal column or fibrosis following a hematoma in the sternocleidomastoid muscle. Acquired torticollis may result from bone abnormalities including tumor, infection, subluxation, and basilar impression,

from a superior oblique muscle palsy, or from tumors of the cerebellum or spinal cord.
   b. **Generalized dystonia.** Torsion dystonia is a familial disorder that most often begins in the feet and progresses over months or years to involve the rest of the body. The child with hemiplegia may develop dystonia in the involved extremity. Dystonia may be a part of Wilson's disease, Hallervorden-Spatz syndrome, and Niemann-Pick disease type C. Paroxysmal dystonic choreoathetosis is an autosomal dominant disorder with abnormal movements lasting up to a few hours.

Abnormal Head Size, Scoliosis, and Neurocutaneous Disorders

I. **Abnormal head size**
   A. **Definition.** Macrocephaly is defined as a head size greater than the ninety-eighth percentile and microcephaly as a head size less than the second percentile.
   B. **Etiologies**
      1. **Macrocephaly.** In familial macrocephaly, one parent has a head size greater than the ninety-eighth percentile. In these cases, the child's development and neurologic examination are usually normal. Rarely, bone overgrowth in the chronic anemias or cranioskeletal dysplasias may cause macrocephaly. Chronic subdural effusions following trauma or meningitis cause enlargement of the head, as do all forms of progressive hydrocephalus. The most common forms of hydrocephalus are communicating hydrocephalus from obstruction of the arachnoid villae, obstruction at the fourth ventricle in the Dandy-Walker malformation, and lateral and third ventricular enlargement from aqueductal stenosis. Megalencephaly results from storage diseases which cause progressive retardation and macrocephaly. In the first year of life, large supratentorial tumors may cause macrocephaly from the bulk of the tumor.
      2. **Microcephaly.** If the small head size is proportional to the body size, endocrine disorders or syndromes (see *Smith's Recognizable Patterns of Human Malformation*) should be suspected. Premature closure of the sutures, craniosynostosis, may prevent appropriate brain growth and, when multiple sutures are involved, requires surgical correction. Primary failure of brain growth may be familial, either autosomal dominant with mild delay or autosomal recessive with more severe delay, or may be the result of a chromosomal anomaly. Acquired brain damage with subsequent microcephaly may follow intrauterine infections, hypoxia or ischemia, trauma, or postnatal CNS infection.
   C. **Evaluation**
      1. **History.** Developmental delay is expected with congenital and static problems, and progressive loss of milestones is characteristic of storage disorders and evolving mass lesions. Symptoms of increased intracranial pressure, headache, irritability, vomiting, and lethargy may accompany pancraniosynostosis, hydrocephalus, and tumors.
      2. **Examination.** Both the child's and the parents' head sizes are measured. Serial measures can be helpful. A head size that continues to parallel the normal curve is less worrisome, whereas a head size that crosses percentiles is of more concern. A bulging fontanel, widened sutures, failure of upgaze, and hyperactive reflexes are signs of increased intracranial pressure. Areas of abnormal retinal pigmentation on funduscopic examination suggest intrauterine infection as an etiology for microcephaly.
      3. **Laboratory.** CT or MRI should be performed on almost all children with abnormal head size to assess brain structure. CT with bone windows can be utilized to evaluate sutures in the child with microcephaly. Chromosomal studies are obtained if there are dysmorphic features or brain malformations, and metabolic studies are required if there is megalencephaly and progressive loss of milestones.
II. **Scoliosis**
   A. **Definition.** Scoliosis is defined as an abnormal curvature of the spine. In children it is idiopathic in approximately 70% of cases.
   B. **Clinical manifestations.** In practice, scoliosis may first be found on a routine screening examination often performed in schools or as a part of well child

care, or may be detected on regular examinations of children at risk for scoliosis. Examples of the latter are children with cerebral palsy, various neuromuscular disorders, and neurofibromatosis.

C. **Etiologies**

1. **Abnormalities of bone.** Congenital anomalies such as hemivertebra or fused ribs may cause an early-onset scoliosis. Diastematomyelia is a congenital midline bone spur that may cause both scoliosis and spinal cord dysfunction below the level of the lesion. A sharp angulation of the spinal column resulting from bone anomaly may be observed in neurofibromatosis.

2. **Lower motor unit disorders.** Scoliosis may be a complication of myopathies. The diagnosis is suggested by associated weakness and can be confirmed by muscle biopsy. Progressive scoliosis may contribute to increasing respiratory insufficiency. Scoliosis may also accompany neuropathies such as peroneal muscular atrophy (Charcot-Marie-Tooth disease) or the postpolio syndrome.

3. **CNS disorders.** Scoliosis is a frequent finding in children with spastic quadriparetic, athetoid, or dystonic cerebral palsy. It may become a fixed deficit in children with torsion dystonia, and it is observed in the spinocerebellar ataxias. Spinal cord tumors and syringomyelia may present with scoliosis, lower motor unit signs at the level of the lesion, and spasticity below the level of the lesion.

4. **Idiopathic scoliosis** most often affects adolescent girls, with a girl-boy ratio of approximately 8:1. The neurologic examination is otherwise normal, and patients can be followed with regular examinations.

D. **Evaluation**

1. **History.** Back pain, bowel or bladder problems, and leg or foot weakness suggest spinal cord involvement and require immediate evaluation. Progressive weakness or clumsiness indicates neuromuscular disorders or spinocerebellar degeneration.

2. **Examination.** The screening examination starts with the child standing straight. Scoliosis may cause tilting of the hips or unequal heights of the shoulders. With the child bending forward to touch the toes, there may be a hump over the ribs on one side. A midline patch of hair or a mass over the spinal column suggests diastematomyelia. Café-au-lait spots are a sign of neurofibromatosis. A complete neurologic examination is essential because of the multiple levels of involvement that may be associated with scoliosis.

3. **Laboratory.** The basic screen is the posteroanterior (PA) film of the spine. Any suggestion of a spinal cord lesion on neurologic examination or the presence of bowel or bladder dysfunction should lead to an MRI of the spine. If the child has diffuse weakness or decreased tendon reflexes, EMG, NCS, and muscle biopsy may be needed.

III. **Neurocutaneous disorders.** In the neurocutaneous disorders, there are both skin and brain involvement. The two most common disorders are neurofibromatosis, with a prevalence of 1/5000, and tuberous sclerosis, with a prevalence of 1/10,000.

A. **Neurofibromatosis type 1 (NF1)**

1. **Definition.** NF1 (von Recklinghausen's disease) is an autosomal dominant disorder with a gene locus on chromosome 17. About 50% of the cases are new mutations. Using the National Institutes of Health (NIH) criteria, one can make a diagnosis of NF1 if there are two or more of the following seven items: café-au-lait spots, neurofibromas, axillary freckling, characteristic bone anomalies, optic nerve glioma, iris (Lisch) nodules, and a definite diagnosis of NF1 in a first-degree relative.

2. **Evaluation**

a. **History.** In half the cases, there is a family history of NF1, although determining such a history may require asking about birthmarks or tumors as well as NF. Many of the children with NF1 have mild delay or learning disabilities. A history of constipation and headaches is also common. A history of decreased vision or growth problems suggests optic nerve glioma.

b. **Examination.** Isolated café-au-lait spots are common in the normal population. Children with NF1 should have six or more spots at least 5 mm in diameter. The café-au-lait spots are found most often on the trunk. The freckling in NF1 is in the axillary and inguinal regions. Plexiform neurofibromas are ropy cords of tumor that may lead to distortion of involved structures. Dermal neurofibromas have a purplish or red overlying skin discoloration and are soft tumors. Kyphoscoliosis occurs in 2% of patients with NF1, and pseudoarthrosis occurs in 0.5–1%. Hypertension may result from renal artery stenosis or pheochromocytoma. A repeat neurologic examination is needed to watch for CNS tumors. A slit-lamp examination by an ophthalmologist is required to find iris hamartomas (Lisch nodules).

   c. **Laboratory.** If there is a family history of neurofibromatosis, chromosomal studies can be used for an early diagnosis. MRI scans are obtained if there is any suggestion of CNS dysfunction or any change in visual acuity that suggests optic nerve glioma. Areas of increased signal are often found in the basal ganglion on MRI of the brain in children with NF1.

3. **Natural history.** The child with NF1 may have café-au-lait spots, plexiform neurofibroma, or glaucoma in infancy; increased head size, pseudoarthrosis, and growth delay in the toddler years; iris nodules, freckling, learning disabilities, headaches, and constipation in the elementary school years; and neurofibromas, scoliosis, and hypertension in the adolescent years.

4. **Differential diagnosis.** Four or fewer café-au-lait spots may be a normal variant. Single neurofibromas and optic nerve gliomas may be observed in children without other evidence of NF1. If a child presents during infancy with more than five café-au-lait spots, there is a 50–60% chance that additional signs of NF1 will develop.

B. **Neurofibromatosis type 2 (NF2)** is an autosomal dominant disorder with a gene locus on chromosome 22. It is much less common than NF1. The primary features are schwannomas involving the vestibular portion of the eighth cranial nerve and meningiomas and gliomas in the CNS. Café-au-lait spots are fewer in NF2 than in NF1. Symptoms develop more often in the adolescent or young adult years.

C. **Tuberous sclerosis**
1. **Definition.** Primary features of tuberous sclerosis are facial angiofibromas, multiple ungual fibromas, cortical tubers, subependymal nodules or giant cell astrocytomas, multiple calcified subependymal nodules protruding into the ventricles, and retinal astrocytomas.

2. **Evaluation**
   a. **History.** Children with tuberous sclerosis are at increased risk for seizures, autism, and developmental delay. Delay is most often seen in those children with tuberous sclerosis who develop infantile spasms or partial seizures with an onset prior to 2 years of age.
   b. **Examination.** Skin lesions observed in tuberous sclerosis are hypopigmented macules, angiofibromas over the bridge of the nose, and shagreen patches, which are raised, thickened, leathery lesions found most often on the trunk. Signs of increased intracranial pressure suggest a giant cell astrocytoma at the intraventricular foramen (foramen of Monro). Cardiac failure is observed in association with cardiac rhabdomyomas. An abdominal mass or hypertension may accompany angiomyolipomas of the kidney and renal cysts.
   c. **Laboratory.** A CT scan is effective in demonstrating the calcified periventricular nodules of tuberous sclerosis and can show the giant cell astrocytoma that may cause hydrocephalus. Renal function studies and renal scans are used for detecting the possible renal tumors or polycystic changes in tuberous sclerosis. Echocardiography establishes the diagnosis of cardiac rhabdomyomas.

3. **Natural history.** Cardiac tumors, hypopigmented macules, infantile spasms, and delay may occur in the first year of life; hydrocephalus from giant cell astrocytomas may occur at any time; and renal complications occur more often in the adolescent years. The facial angiofibromas are usually present by the elementary school years.

4. **Differential diagnosis.** Band heterotopia may be distinguished from subependymal nodules by the continuous nature of the band heterotopia and the more isolated nodules of tuberous sclerosis. Familial polycystic kidneys occur in families with no other stigmata of tuberous sclerosis.

D. **Other neurocutaneous disorders**
1. **Vascular skin lesions.** Sturge-Weber syndrome consists of a port-wine-col-

ored stain involving the upper eyelid and other areas of the face, and a hemangioma of the ipsilateral surface of the brain that causes seizures and contralateral hemiplegia. In Klippel-Trénaunay-Weber syndrome there are cavernous hemangiomas and hypertrophy of the extremity under the hemangiomas. Telangiectasias starting first on the conjunctiva and later involving the face, neck, elbows, and knees are signs of ataxia-telangiectasia.

2. **Pigmentary changes.** Incontinentia pigmenti presents with linear, whorled, hyperpigmented skin lesions, and, in 20–30% of affected children, alopecia and seizures, delay, and spasticity. In hypomelanosis of Ito, there are linear streaks of hypopigmentation and, in 75% of cases, seizures and delay. A linear hyperkeratotic, verrucous, hyperpigmented nevus is found on the forehead in the linear sebaceous nevus sequence. These children often have seizures, delay, and ipsilateral brain malformation.

3. **Neurotrichosis (hair anomalies).** Menkes disease is an X-linked recessive disorder with seizures, hypertonia, brain infarcts, and short, coarse, easily broken hair. Serum copper and ceruloplasmin are low. Other disorders with hair abnormalities include biotin deficiency, argininosuccinicaciduria, and the Pollitt syndrome. All three are characterized by seizures, delay, and alopecia or easily broken hair.

Behavioral Disorders

I. **Definitions.** Behavioral disorders are commonly observed in the practice of child neurology. Some disorders, such as adrenoleukodystrophy, may present as learning and behavioral disorders. In other disorders, the behavioral component may seem to be the main problem. Examples include the child with tuberous sclerosis and severe autism and the child with Tourette's disorder who has well-controlled tics but severe attentional problems and emotional lability. In this section we discuss two common problems: autism and attention-deficit hyperactivity disorder (ADHD).

II. **Autism**
   A. **Definition.** In DSM-IV, autism is defined as a combination of impairment in social interaction, impairment in communication, and a restricted, repetitive, stereotyped pattern of behavior, interests, or activities that begins prior to 3 years of age and cannot be more appropriately classified as another pervasive developmental disorder.
   B. **Clinical manifestations**
      1. **Social interaction.** Autistic children fail to develop normal awareness of others, empathy, and adequate peer interactions.
      2. **Communication.** Speech may be very delayed, or the child may be mute. Echolalia is common.
      3. **Unusual behaviors.** The child with autism has repetitive stereotypic behaviors, unusual preoccupations, and an inflexible adherence to routine.
   C. **Evaluation**
      1. **History.** After delineating the various components of autism, the history should be reviewed for neurologic disorders, such as fragile X syndrome and tuberous sclerosis, that have been associated with autism, and for complications such as mental retardation (observed in 75% of children with autism) and seizures (observed in 25%).
      2. **Examination.** Dysmorphic features, skin lesions, and CNS abnormalities may suggest an underlying brain disorder that might be the etiology for autism.
      3. **Laboratory.** If the child has delay in language, a hearing screen should be obtained. The basic laboratory work-up should include CBC, glucose, electrolytes, thyroid function studies, ammonia, urine for amino acids and organic acids, chromosomes, neuroimaging, and EEG.
   D. **Differential diagnosis.** The child with mental retardation has communication and social skills commensurate with his or her level of development. Rett's disorder is distinguished from autism by regression beginning at 6–9 months of age. Rett's disorder affects only girls, causes loss of hand function, and leads to an acquired microcephaly. Asperger's disorder is thought by some to be a mild form of autism in which there is impaired social interaction and abnormal pat-

terns of behavior, with normal language and cognitive development. With disintegrative psychosis, there is a definite regression beginning after 2 years of age.

III. **Attention-deficit hyperactivity disorder (ADHD)**

A. **Definition.** In DSM-IV, ADHD is defined as having symptoms of inattention, hyperactivity, and impulsiveness, starting prior to 7 years of age, and exhibited both at home and at school. The symptoms cause significant impairment and are not caused by any other psychiatric disorder.

B. **Clinical description.** Children with ADHD usually have trouble paying attention in school and following serial instructions at home. They have difficulty sitting still at mealtimes and in the classroom. They are described as constantly interrupting and speaking out of turn. They may suffer injuries from impulsive behaviors. Some children have only inattention and not hyperactivity. Oppositional defiant disorder and learning disorders are often comorbid conditions.

C. **Evaluation**

1. **History.** The time of onset of the disorder is important. Problems of temperament begin in the first months of life, and ADHD more often begins around 3–4 years of age. Barbiturates, benzodiazepines, and theophylline may cause symptoms of hyperactivity. Symptoms of sadness, fearfulness, or anxiety suggest other psychiatric causes for the attention deficit. A developmental assessment is needed, because children with mental retardation and pervasive developmental disorders may have inattention and hyperactivity as a component of their disorders.

2. **Examination.** The neurologic examination may be normal or may show "soft signs." Soft signs are developmental findings that are normal at one age but abnormal at a later stage of development. They are often inconsistent and are of concern only if they fit an overall pattern of delay.

3. **Laboratory.** Basic chemistries are seldom helpful. Some researchers have noted changes in thyroid function studies in a few children with ADHD, and elevated lead levels have been found occasionally. EEG and neuroimaging are indicated only if additional abnormalities are present on examination.

D. **Differential diagnosis.** A normally active child may appear hyperactive to an excessively strict, controlled parent or to an overly rigid school system. This is particularly true for the child with an active temperament—a congenital style of behavior that is a source of distress when the child's fit with the environment is poor. Symptoms of ADHD that are present only in a single setting should suggest problems in that area. The child with symptoms only at school may be incorrectly placed, being either too advanced for the class or too far behind to keep up. If the ADHD is present only at home, a chaotic home environment or stresses within the family should be considered. Other psychiatric disorders to consider in the differential diagnosis include anxiety disorders, depression, pervasive developmental disorders, and substance abuse.

Referral

Much of the assessment and follow-up of children with delayed development can be performed by the family practitioner or pediatrician. It is often necessary to refer to a psychologist for specific intellectual and achievement testing, and to have vision and hearing screening performed. If the child develops a progressive form of retardation, we suggest referral to a child neurologist or a geneticist, because many of these disorders are rare and difficult to diagnose. The child neurologist or geneticist may also have new information about possible treatments for these disorders.

The child with nonepileptiform paroxysmal events (such as headaches) or enuresis can have evaluation and follow-up with the primary physician. We would refer to a child neurologist only if the diagnosis is unclear or the child fails to respond to conventional treatment.

Because of the multitude of disorders that may cause motor problems in childhood, we suggest referral for an initial evaluation in all cases of progressive motor disorders and for most cases of static disorders. Many disorders of acute onset can be rapidly diagnosed and do not need to be evaluated by a child neurologist. For chronic and progressive conditions, the child neurologist may be able to make beneficial suggestions for treatment.

In children with microcephaly or macrocephaly, an initial evaluation should provide clues to directions for referral. Children with hydrocephalus or craniosynostosis need referral to a neurosurgeon. If there are dysmorphic features, evaluation by a geneticist may be helpful. If the child has progressive scoliosis, orthopedic evaluation is important to monitor for appropriate surgical corrections. The child with neurofibromatosis may benefit from evaluation and periodic follow-up in a specialty clinic, where counseling and follow-up can be obtained for the variety of complications of this illness. Similarly, the child who has tuberous sclerosis may benefit from evaluation in a specialty clinic or by a child neurologist.

In cases of behavioral disturbance, many of the developmental problems can be handled on an outpatient basis without referral to a specialist. Children with autism present many difficult behavioral problems and usually benefit from evaluation by a specialist in child psychiatry or child neurology. We would refer children with ADHD only if they fail to respond to initial treatment or if they have complicating factors such as severe learning disabilities or oppositional defiant disorder. A child psychiatrist or child neurologist can help with ongoing therapy.

Recommended Readings

Adams RD, Lyon G. *Neurology of Hereditary Metabolic Diseases of Children.* New York: McGraw-Hill, 1982.

Aicardi J. *Epilepsy in Children* (2nd ed). New York: Raven, 1994.

Babikian P, Corbett J, Bell W. Idiopathic hypertension in children: The Iowa experience. *J Child Neurol* 9(2):144–149, 1994.

Cohen DJ, Leckman JF. Developmental psychopathology and neurobiology of Tourette's syndrome. *J Am Acad Child Adolesc Psychiatry* 33(1):2–15, 1994.

Diagnostic and Statistical Manual of Mental Disorders (4th ed). Washington, DC: American Psychiatric Association, 1994.

Dunn DW, Epstein LG. *Decision Making in Child Neurology.* Toronto: Decker, 1987.

Fenichel GM. *Clinical Pediatric Neurology: A Signs and Symptoms Approach.* Philadelphia: Saunders, 1993.

Gay CT, Bodensteiner JB. The floppy infant: Recent advances in the understanding of disorders affecting the neuromuscular junction. *Neurol Clinics* 8(3):715–726, 1990.

Gillberg C, Coleman M. *The Biology of the Autistic Syndromes* (2nd ed). New York: Cambridge University Press, 1992.

Gilman S, Bloedel J, Lechtenberg R. *Disorders of the Cerebellum.* Philadelphia: Davis, 1981.

Gomez MR. *Tuberous Sclerosis* (2nd ed). New York: Raven, 1988.

Hahn YS, et al. Head injuries in children under 36 months of age. *Childs Nerv Syst* 4:34–40, 1988.

Jones KL. *Smith's Recognizable Patterns of Human Malformation* (4th ed). Philadelphia: Saunders, 1988.

Menkes JH. *Textbook of Child Neurology* (4th ed). Philadelphia: Lea & Febiger, 1990.

Percy AK. The inherited neurodegenerative disorders of childhood: Clinical assessment. *J Child Neurol* 2(2):82–97, 1987.

Rothner AD. Headaches in children: A review. *Headache* 18:156–162, 1979.

Tusa RJ, Saada AA, Niparko JK. Dizziness in childhood. *J Child Neurol* 9(3):261–274, 1994.

35

Approach to Ethical Issues in Neurology

Michael P. McQuillen

Clinical ethics—the business of being human in the interchange between physician and patient—has been an integral part of that interchange for as long as there has been a profession of medicine. Until the past few decades, however, it was assumed that being a physician meant being ethical; that everyone's ethics were the same (or at least of equivalent worth); and that there was no underlying theory or set of standards necessary for ethical decision-making. In part, this state of affairs was a reflection of the simplicity of life in general and of medicine in particular. With advances in technology, more options became possible—options to evaluate new forms of treatment (research) as well as to utilize proven diagnostic and therapeutic modalities (with their inherent risk-benefit relationship). Questions of *who* should make *which* decisions in *what* circumstances began to be asked. Particular judgments no longer stood in isolation, but rather led to the formulation of **rules** that could govern in similar situations; a recognition of the **principles** on which such rules might be based; and the development of a theory underlying the principles—much as an understanding of anatomy, biochemistry, pathophysiology, and other basic sciences made it possible to clarify approaches to the complicated problem of stroke, for example. Other theorists appealed directly to **conscience,** developed and refined in reflection on individual cases without the formality of the process just described. Underlying it all, however, was the realization that ethical problems arise in almost any clinical situation and that such problems should be addressed as systematically as any dimension of the given clinical situation. This realization called forth a new academic discipline (biomedical or clinical ethics) out of what previously had been purely philosophical, and in a sense impractical, thought (ethics).

From the start, this discipline found fertile ground in neurology, where ethical theory met real-life problems such as "brain death," the "vegetative state" and other conditions of incapacity, neurogenetic diseases, and a whole gamut of issues at the end of life. Early on, this meeting generated encounters with the law, and the recognition that what is ethical may not be legal, and vice versa. To plow the field, one must first understand the background of ethical theories, then develop a structured approach to the recognition and solution of ethical problems, and finally understand how that approach helps to deal with particular problems and how an effective interface with the law can be developed.

I. **Ethical theories.** Before accepting any ethical theory as a basis on which practical judgments can ultimately and validly be made, one should inquire whether the theory is adequate to the task by virtue of its satisfying certain criteria, and then look to the basis of the theory to determine its usefulness and applicability. No one theory satisfies every clinical situation. Some are better adapted to one circumstance and others to another, whereas yet additional circumstances demand a hybrid of complementing theories.

A. **Criteria of an adequate theory.** Beauchamp and Childress set forth a series of questions that should be answered in the affirmative with regard to any particular theory, if that theory is to be regarded as adequate and helpful with clinical conundra. Their questions include the following.

1. **Is it clear?** Is the language in which the theory is formulated clear, or is it so complex as to muddle the situation?

2. **Is it coherent?** A necessary (although not sufficient) criterion of an adequate theory, missing when elements of the theory are in contradiction, is coherency.

3. **Is it complete, or at least comprehensive?** Does the theory deal with all of the major questions raised in diverse clinical circumstances, or are there important concerns on which the theory is silent?

4. **Is it simple?** Does the theory set forth only enough norms so that it can be used without confusion by clinicians, or are there so many that the answer gets lost in practice?
5. **Can it explain and justify the conclusions reached with its help,** or does it simply set forth in other words a preexistent, intuitive belief?
6. **Does its use yield new insights,** or does it only serve to repeat old convictions?
7. **Is it practical?** In short, does it provide a useful answer to the clinical problem, or one that is attractive in theory only?

B. **Types of ethical theories**
   1. **Utilitarianism.** The theory of utilitarianism looks at the consequences of acts, and holds that an action is good if it produces more benefit than harm. Problems arise, however, when one attempts to establish definitions of "benefit" and "harm"; of the relation between the individual who is acting and the society in which that individual acts; and of single actions each in isolation or of classes of actions governed by rules that appeal to the principle of utility.
   2. **Obligation-based theory.** The test of this theory is the **categorical imperative** of Immanuel Kant: the reason for an action should apply to everyone, and in all situations; moral rules are absolute. Problems arise when such rules—often abstract and legalistic, rather than relational—are found to be in conflict with each other in specific sets of circumstances.
   3. **Virtue-based, or character, ethics.** This approach looks to the person who is acting, and to the motives and desires that propel his or her actions. Because even the most virtuous person can act wrongly—even for the best of reasons—a viable ethical theory cannot rest on character alone.
   4. **Rights-based ethics or liberal individualism.** Rights are justified claims that an individual or group is entitled to make on a society at large. Such claims, while protecting the interests of an individual, at the same time may impose a corresponding obligation on others. Rights may be **positive rights** (requiring actions by others) or **negative rights** (precluding such actions). An overemphasis on rights may neglect the legitimate demands of the society at large.
   5. **Communitarian ethics.** In contrast to the focus of rights on the individual, communitarians look to the needs of society at large. Prescinding from *how* such needs may be articulated *by whom*, an overemphasis on this aspect of morality may neglect the legitimate interests of the individual.
   6. **An ethics of care.** Sometimes referred to as **feminist ethics,** the focus of this approach is on a caring, attached relationship between persons, and on the implications of such a relationship. Impartiality and balance may suffer as a consequence, with the result being a less complete and practical system than obtained with other theories.
   7. **Casuistry.** This term evokes an image of Jesuitical sophistry, but really refers to the need to make decisions according to the particulars of any given situation. Every detail of the case is examined and weighed, and a judgment is reached often by analogy to similar cases. The connection between cases provides a maxim to rule the case—but which maxim is given the most credence in any particular situation, and why?
   8. **Ethics based on principles, or "common morality."** A "bottom-up" approach to validating particular judgments looks to rules that govern such judgments, and from rules to the principles from which they are derived. Four such principles are woven into "common sense" morality—an ethics that grows out of the nature of human beings, one that is simply put as "do good and avoid evil." The principles in question are as follows.

      Autonomy: respect for the autonomous choices of other persons
      Nonmaleficence: the obligation not to inflict harm intentionally
      Beneficence: actions taken for the benefit of others
      Justice: a fair, equitable, and appropriate distribution of goods in society

      Critics of the principlist approach refer to its elements as a mantra without substance; one which does not offer a schema for resolving conflict when more than one principle applies; a ritualistic incantation without a unifying, overriding theory to govern its use. When all is said and done, similar objections can be leveled against *any* ethical theory. The heart of the matter is to recognize the (ethical) problem and to admit with honesty which approach to solving it should be used, and why.

II. **A case method approach to clinical ethics.** John Fletcher and his colleagues have developed a case method approach to the recognition and solution of ethical dilemmas that mimics standard decision-making in medicine. The elements of their method are as follows.

A. **Assessment.** What is the nature of the medical problem, and the relevant context in which it occurs? What are the options for therapy, their foreseeable risks and benefits, their short- and long-term prognoses, and the costs and resources/mechanisms for payment? What do the patient/family/surrogate decision-makers want? What does the patient need, and what other needs may compete with that need? Are there any institutional/societal/legal factors impinging on the patient/problem? What are the ethnic/cultural/religious backgrounds from which the problem has arisen?

B. **Identification of ethical problems.** Which ethical problems—ranked in order of importance—are self-evident and/or hidden? Which ethical theories are most relevant to such problems? Are there analogous cases in medicine or law, and if so how do they apply? Which guidelines are most appropriate?

C. **Decision-making and implementation.** What are the ethically acceptable options for solving the problem(s), and which are most acceptable? What justification(s) can be given for the preferred resolution(s) of the problem(s)? How can the preferred resolution(s) of the problem(s) be accomplished? Is ethics consultation necessary or desirable? Is judicial review necessary or desirable?

D. **Evaluation** is an ongoing process that seeks to recognize missed opportunities and correct unworkable solutions. The process carries a preventive dimension that may propose changes in policy or provide educational opportunities to minimize the chance that similar problems will recur in the future.

III. **Approaches to particular problems**

A. **Decision-making.** At the heart of any interaction between physician and patient is the matter of *who* decides *what* shall be done, and *when.* The physician brings to this interaction experience, knowledge, skill, and a set of personal values that may or may not be the same as, or even compatible with, those of the patient. In years gone by, the physician's judgment ruled supreme. Today that judgment is tempered not only by a primacy of respect for the wishes of the patient but also by the rules and regulations of various healthcare plans as well as by statutory and case law.

1. **The primacy of the patient.** Competent patients with the capacity for decision-making can and should make certain decisions regarding their treatment—even before the fact, anticipating the future through advance directives (e.g., "living wills" and durable powers of attorney for healthcare decisions—"healthcare proxies"). Because many neurologic illnesses are chronic and inexorably disabling, often leaving patients without the capacity to decide, it is wise to introduce discussion of advance directives early in the course of care of such patients. (Indeed, federal regulations now require patients to be asked, on admission to hospitals, whether they have executed or wish to execute advance directives.) Obviously, a bond of trust should first be established, so that patients do not interpret such discussions as plans to abandon them at the ends of their lives. (This element is missing in the federal requirement just mentioned.) It is important to emphasize that minds may change as situations evolve.

2. **Surrogate decision-making.** When capacity is lost, a surrogate may be called on to make decisions for the patient. Unless previously identified (in a healthcare proxy), the appropriate surrogate may be selected according to a hierarchy spelled out in state law. In extreme circumstances, a court-appointed surrogate may be necessary. Surrogates may strive to determine what the patient would have wanted **(substituted judgment standard)** or to decide what is best for the patient **(best interests standard).** The former standard is generally thought to be better, avoiding as it does conclusions made by one person (the surrogate) about another's "quality of life." Courts may require "clear and convincing evidence" of what the patient would have wanted in the circumstance in question; but because such evidence rarely exists, and because people often change their minds, requirements of this sort are most impractical. In all instances, it is wise to seek consensus, and to continue to act in favor of life until that consensus is reached. It may take time to develop

consensus, even when a surrogate has previously been appointed, especially when capacity is lost suddenly and without warning (e.g., after a stroke).

3. **"Managed care" plans.** The spiraling costs of healthcare, among many contributing factors, have fueled a process of "healthcare reform"—much of which is basically about money. Because an immediate effect of physician decisions is the expenditure of money, a feature common to many proposals for such reform is a process requiring approval before such decisions can be implemented. Sometimes the process has at its center a "gatekeeper"—often a primary care physician, who may be guided by situation-specific protocols. The rewards built into the system are key to its ethical dimension: under traditional fee-for-service medicine, the more physicians did, the more they were paid, whereas, under "managed care," the less they do, the more they are paid. The concept of "managed care" emphasizes the physician's obligation to *all* patients covered by a given plan—indeed, to society at large. Nevertheless, any decision made by a physician should be made in the patient's best interest. No test should be done, no treatment instituted, without that interest in the forefront of the physician's mind. If the system stands in the way of such decisions, the physician should oppose the system on behalf of the patient, vigorously but also fairly—i.e., not "gaming" the system with fabrications and the like. "Managed care" plans that reward physicians with incentives that limit or compromise care (e.g., by restricting the time that can be spent with a patient, denying access to appropriate consultants, requiring the use of generic drugs, etc.) should be avoided.

B. **"Brain death."** An unwanted consequence of the development of more effective intensive care was the recognition that patients whose brains had suffered complete and irreversible loss of all function could continue to manifest adequate cardiovascular, renal, and gastrointestinal functions, as long as pulmonary function was supported by a ventilator. The presence of death—previously identified by the absence of heart action and breathing—could no longer be affirmed in such patients. This state of affairs called for the development of a new set of criteria by which the presence of death could be recognized. Once those criteria are satisfied, the patient is considered dead—an unsettling conclusion for many to whom a warm body with a strong pulse, whose chest is moving in rhythm with a machine, cannot be dead and must only be asleep.

1. **"Whole brain" criteria.** Death of the whole brain is recognized in a normothermic body in which loss of brain function results from an identifiable, irreversible, structural lesion in the absence of sedative-hypnotic drugs or another, potentially reversible, metabolic condition. Clinical examination for death of the whole brain requires the absence of brainstem reflexes (e.g., oculocephalic and ice water caloric stimulation evokes no eye movement, pupils are dilated and fixed to light, and corneal responses are not present) and the absence of ventilatory movement when the ventilator is stopped after a period of ventilation with 100% oxygen, even though the pCO_2 rises above 60 mm Hg without ventilation. Recognition must be affirmed by a second examination, separated in time from the first by a variable interval that depends on such factors as age and clinical cause; the interval may be specified by local statute or hospital policy. As with the use of cardiorespiratory criteria to recognize the presence of death, the patient is considered dead when the criteria are satisfied—i.e., when the second examination affirms the findings of the first. Several **confirmatory tests** are helpful when the clinical condition is compromised (e.g., when a patient has been in barbiturate coma after head injury) and may be required in certain circumstances (e.g., in children under the age of 1 year). However, such tests are neither necessary nor sufficient to affirm the presence of death.

2. **"Brainstem" criteria.** In the United Kingdom (UK), emphasis has been placed on the fact that the clinical examination on which the criterion of "brain death" is based looks only at the function of the brainstem, and not at the whole brain function; higher cortical function is irrelevant in UK practice. This means that a person whose brainstem has irreversibly ceased to function but whose cerebral hemispheres are still working—a person with the so-called "locked-in syndrome"—can be declared dead in the UK even though the cerebral hemispheres are still functioning. Partly for this reason, many "brain death" policies and procedures in the United States require a confirmatory test to demonstrate that higher brain function is or must be ab-

sent (e.g., an isoelectric EEG, cerebral angiography showing no flow within the cranium, etc.).

3. **"Higher brain" death.** Certain philosophers (e.g., Robert Veatch, among others) have called for a new definition of death, one that holds that death is the permanent loss of that which is essential to the nature of a human being: consciousness and cognition. Prescinding from the difficulty of establishing the criteria by which death, so defined, might be recognized, certain very practical problems arise when one considers the implementation of such a definition—e.g., can someone in the end stages of Alzheimer's disease, still breathing and with normal vegetative functions, be buried?

4. **Ethical considerations**

   a. **Telling the family.** Once the physician has recognized the presence of death using "brain death" criteria, the fact of that recognition should be conveyed to the family and others with ethical standing in the case. The physician should be aware that statutory or case law (as in New Jersey and New York, respectively) may make allowance for the family to reject the use of "brain death" criteria on religious grounds, in which case the physician may be required to rely on traditional (cardiorespiratory) criteria for death. As in every interchange between physician and patient (including the extended patient—family and others), the physician should convey the fact gently, with compassion, and, if necessary, repeatedly until it is understood and accepted. Although the family and others should not be burdened by being asked for their permission to discontinue the ventilator (and thus to permit cardiovascular death to ensue within a short time), the physician should be sensitive to reactions of denial and the like. The family should be given time to assimilate and accept the sorrowful fact, and the physician should be very sensitive to different ethnic and cultural heritages, and unresolved issues from the past, that may determine how long it will take for acceptance. Terms such as "brain death" and "life support" should be avoided because they convey erroneous information: when someone is dead, the person—not just the brain—is dead, and there is no longer any life to support.

   b. **After "brain death."** In addition to solving the problem of inappropriate and theoretically interminable use of a scarce resource (the intensive care bed), recognizing the death of a person whose body can continue to be kept "alive" permits a utilitarian judgment for the benefit of others. This is true in two instances: organ donation and the continued nurturing of an unborn child beyond the point of viability inside the body of a mother who has died. Permission for either action must be sought in the standard fashion (see sec. **III.A**). Considerations of justice weigh heavily in these situations, and different ethical theories come to different conclusions with regard to either action.

C. **The "vegetative state."** In a situation regarded by some as a fate worse than death, a certain proportion of patients who have incurred overwhelming damage to their cerebral hemispheres (from anoxia after cardiac arrest or from massive brain trauma or stroke) may—after a period of coma—evolve into a state of "wakefulness without awareness" accompanied by sleep-wake cycles and essentially intact brainstem and autonomic functions. Other patients may reach this state at the end of a chronic degenerative process. A Multi-Society Task Force published its consensus on the clinical, diagnostic, and prognostic features of this condition—a consensus with the particulars of which some physicians disagree. At the heart of the matter are the issues of whether the patient in a "vegetative state" is truly unaware of all stimuli and has no conscious thought; when the condition can be regarded as persistent and, finally, permanent; and what, if any, impact may be had by a variety of therapeutic efforts, at what cost. Some regard these issues as incapable of anything but arbitrary resolutions. The Task Force felt that any motor response in a "vegetative state" patient was primitive, random, and/or reflex and, as such, could not be interpreted as evidence of cognition. Further, they relied on imaging and pathologic studies to exclude any anatomic substrate for consciousness.

   1. **Withholding/withdrawing.** It is generally accepted that patients with the capacity to make decisions for themselves are not obliged to accept all treatments, diagnostic studies, and the like, and may reject any treatment or study even if such rejection results in death. With patients in the "vegetative

state," such decisions devolve on surrogates, duly identified (see sec. **III.A.2**). Most commonly, a burdens-benefits analysis is employed in making a decision to reject. Such decisions should never be made with the intent of causing death, but may be made even when the probability is that death will ensue. The obligations of the physician in this process are threefold: to reach medical certainty, as far as such certainty is possible; to convey that certainty, as gently and as often as necessary to ensure understanding and acceptance, to the decision-maker; and to respect and implement the decision, as long as it does not violate the conscience of the physician. From an ethical point of view, **withholding** is more problematic than **withdrawing,** because the former does not give the patient the benefit of a therapeutic trial. It is imperative that all involved parties recognize (and behave accordingly with such recognition) that it is not *care* that is being withheld or withdrawn, but rather a burdensome treatment or diagnostic study without sufficient benefit to the patient. The natural tendency to avoid such patients, to visit them less often, and even not to speak as though they might understand, should be steadfastly eschewed.

2. **Nutrition and hydration.** Given the deep meaning of food and water in human society, it is no wonder that some have balked at the withholding or withdrawing of these essentials as symbolic of abandonment of the patient. Others have equated the nutrition and hydration given to a patient in the "vegetative state"—generally through a gastrostomy tube, with all of its attendant paraphernalia and cost—with any other therapy that may be rejected (for reasons previously given). Clearly, it is licit to withhold nutrition and hydration for the benefit of the patient—such as when the intent is to minimize excess gastric or pulmonary secretions, incontinence, and the like; but when the intent is to cause death, some regard this not as a benefit to the patient but rather as the beginning of a "slippery slope" that leads inexorably to the elimination of "absolutely worthless human beings."

3. **Other considerations.** In making judgments about level of care in patients in the "vegetative state" or with other devastating, irremedial neurologic conditions, the physician is increasingly called on to consider questions of **distributive justice.** These questions arise in such matters as access to intensive care, "managed care" decisions, and even conservation of individual and group resources. The ethical physician owes primary responsibility to the patient, unless both have knowingly entered into a contract that permits limitation of care on such bases. This is not to demean the need for the physician to be in constant communication with the patient or surrogate, in a gentle yet persistent effort to convince them of the wisdom of a considered position that may differ from theirs.

D. **Neurogenetic diseases.** There has been a literal explosion in the understanding of heritable neurologic disorders since a marker for the gene for Huntington's disease was identified on chromosome 4 in 1983.

1. **Diagnostic testing.** Research as well as testing in commercial laboratories can provide the physician with DNA and non-DNA information that is helpful in the diagnosis of more than two dozen disorders of the central and peripheral nervous systems (including various genetic myopathies) at present, with the likelihood that information about more diseases—and even about such considerations as behavioral traits—will be available in the near future. Such testing may yield information pertinent not only to the diagnosis of an existing condition, but also in the presymptomatic (or even prenatal) situation, as well as with regard to carrier detection. Some, but by no means all, institutions employ extensive counseling systems, before and after testing, to ensure thorough, informed decision-making for testing as well as appropriate support after results are made known to the patient or the guardian/surrogate.

2. **Ethical considerations.** Because the information garnered through diagnostic testing for neurogenetic diseases in essence belongs to the patients being tested, it is important to their decision-making that they understand all of the implications of testing and are prepared—with support from their physicians—to deal with those implications. For example, knowledge that one is a carrier of a neurogenetic disease may permit more responsible parenthood. Prenatal recognition that a neurogenetic disease is present in a developing infant may permit the infant's parents to prepare to shoulder the

burden of the disease, or to elect termination of the pregnancy. Because certain neurogenetic diseases (e.g., Huntington's disease) are associated with a higher rate of suicide than obtains in the population at large, presymptomatic diagnosis may enhance the risk of suicide, especially in a person who has experienced the ravages of the disease in an affected family member. Confirmation of the diagnosis of a neurogenetic disease may help the patient cope with the disease, because certainty is always easier to deal with than uncertainty. Caution must be exercised to prevent misuse of information from diagnostic testing by employers and insurers (especially healthcare insurers), who might exclude persons with proven neurogenetic diseases arbitrarily, without reference to the impact (presently or in the future) of their particular diseases on their specific job performance or to its call on pooled healthcare resources. With regard to the latter issue, competing considerations of justice enter in, and may require the person being tested to disclose the results of testing. In the last analysis, the physician requesting the test, as well as the person being tested, should be aware of and informed about these various aspects of testing before proceeding. Genetic testing should never be done as part of the "routine" evaluation of a patient without such considerations first being taken into account and explored.
   3. **Gene therapy.** A promise for the future is the hoped-for ability to insert or replace missing or defective genes in the cells of persons affected by neurogenetic diseases. When the manipulation is directed at the affected cells, the procedure is termed **somatic cell therapy;** when it is directed at the initial fusion of sperm and ovum (or at those precursors of new human life themselves), it is termed **germ cell therapy.** Somatic cell therapy raises issues common to research (see sec. **III.G**). Germ cell therapy, with its implications for future generations, raises a whole set of other considerations beyond the scope of this chapter.
E. **Static or progressive disorders with intact cognition.** There is a whole spectrum of neuromuscular and spinal cord diseases that share in common the absence or loss of various degrees of motor functions (and hence, basically, of independence) and intact higher cortical functions. Notable examples of these diseases include spinal muscular atrophies; muscular dystrophies; and spinal cord dysraphisms (e.g., meningomyeloceles), injuries, and other illnesses (e.g., multiple sclerosis).
   1. **Truth-telling** becomes exceptionally painful for the physician when confronted by a healthy mind in a body presently or predictably about to be robbed of its normal function. Maintaining hope and thwarting inevitable depression, without making false and empty promises, is an art not easily learned and yet one that carries manifold rewards from the patient and from the family for whom, indeed, life goes on. Truth, although painful for physician and patient alike, is a reliable ally in the practice of this art. Physicians must be exceedingly sensitive to, and must take time to care for, the emotional dimensions of the states in which their patients find themselves. As difficult as it may be not to do so, the physician must never abandon a patient in such a state, especially in circumstances in which breathing becomes progressively more difficult.
   2. **Problems at the end of life.** Despite all attempts at describing life on a ventilator, the patient may not be able to understand what such a life might be like unless a trial of assisted ventilation is undertaken, after which the problem of withdrawing such assistance enters the scene. Minimizing suffering during withdrawal (e.g., with sedative-analgesic medications) runs the risk of suppressing what ventilatory function the patient still has; but as long as the intent is to relieve the suffering, and not to cause a more rapid demise, the use of such medications is appropriate (see sec. **III.H**). In all such circumstances, the physician should call on colleagues with complementing skills—nurses, social workers, physiotherapists, hospice caregivers, etc.—to carry out the healthcare decisions reached by the patient, properly informed.
F. **Static or progressive disorders with impaired cognition.** Absence or loss of that which makes us uniquely human—consciousness and related higher neurologic functions—poses several dilemmas for the physician, who must deal with surrogates or even the courts in attempting to resolve those dilemmas. The paradigmatic clinical conditions range from anencephaly at one end

of life to end-stage Alzheimer's disease at the other, with varying degrees of mental retardation and behavioral disorders, all of diverse causes, in between.

1. **Limiting care.** Until a new definition of death (see sec. **III.B.3**) is accepted, persons afflicted with these conditions remain human beings, as difficult as it may be to recognize that fact at any given clinical moment. One may argue whether some human beings have more of a right to healthcare resources than others, but this is a societal decision that must not be invoked at the bedside of a particular patient by the patient's physician without agreement by the decision-maker for the patient. On the other hand, the focus of decision-making should properly be on compassionate care, not high-technology cure, once it is clear that one is dealing with a definitive, irreversible process.

2. **Making decisions.** Surrogate decision-making according to a substituted judgment standard (see sec. **III.A.2**) is particularly problematic when the patient has never had the capacity for independent judgment (e.g., an infant with anencephaly or a patient with severe mental retardation at any age). There is a sorry chapter in American jurisprudence in this regard—the one dealing with involuntary sterilization justified by the more subjective best interests standard. This standard is often employed in dealing with unwanted, sometimes self-injurious, behavior by means of medication, restraints, institutionalization, and even "psychosurgery." Extreme caution must be the rule, with compassion as a guide.

3. **Involvement of family.** Family members, and others bearing responsibility for the care of those who lack the capacity to make decisions for themselves, should be intimately involved with decision-making for patients in this category, unless there is a valid reason for them not to be involved. When capacity has been present and is now lost (as in the end stages of Alzheimer's disease), attention should be paid to healthcare proxies if previously executed, bearing in mind that people change their minds even as circumstances change. Very few of us can truly be aware of what it is like to become demented, nor can we truly know what decisions we would make for ourselves if and when we reached such a state. The burden of dementia falls on those who care for the demented, not on the demented themselves.

G. **Research in neurology.** The practice of neurology was once described by Dr. Labe Scheinberg under the aphorism, "diagnose—then adios!" The last decade of the twentieth century has been called the "decade of the brain" because of the remarkable advances in the understanding and treatment of neurologic diseases. The move from Scheinberg's aphorism to a brave and wonderful new world occurred in large measure because of research. Often such research involved the use of human subjects (because no appropriate animal models existed), posed significant risks (in searching for elusive benefits), and raised the specter of a conflict of interest (between the physician caring for patients and conducting meaningful research by enrolling patients in controlled clinical trials).

1. **Valid versus invalid research.** The sine qua non of valid research is peer review—approval of a research proposal by a thoughtful, responsible, knowledgeable group of peers who judge the question as worthy of being asked, the answer as likely to be forthcoming, and the hoped-for benefit as worth the predicted risk. The availability of external funding makes it possible to conduct approved research honestly and openly, without employing the subterfuge of paying for research under the guise of accepted patient care. The process that effects valid research involves institutional review boards and other oversight bodies to ensure its validity at every step along the way.

2. **Consent issues.** Patients with devastating illnesses are particularly vulnerable to any offer of hope, even when that offer wears the cloak of a research hypothesis. The offer of hope may come in the form of a controlled clinical trial, in which the decision as to which treatment (for example, active medication or placebo) the patient is to receive is made by the parameters of the trial, not by the physician. The physician who refers his or her patient for enrollment in such a trial must agree that the trial is necessary; that there is not, as yet, any proven approach that would guarantee benefit to the patient; and that the risks of the trial are balanced by the benefit the patient can expect. If there is no expected benefit for the patient, then, at the very least, society should benefit from the expected gain in knowledge that will come

from the trial. Consent is especially problematic for children and for others without the capacity to give their own consent. Some have gone so far as to take the position that nontherapeutic research should not be done on such patients, whereas others emphasize a broader debt to society that can be paid only by advancing knowledge through research.

H. Chronic pain. Diverse neurologic conditions are commonly associated with pain, often requiring hefty doses of potent analgesics for relief—doses of medications that may suppress respiration, lower blood pressure to dangerous levels, and have other unwanted effects. The ruling principle here is that of the "double effect": the unwanted (indirect, merely permitted) effects (in this instance, possible aspiration or even death) are allowed as long as the primary (direct, intended) effect (in this instance, the relief of pain) is desirable and cannot be achieved in any other way. It is important to remember that pain may be physical and identifiable, or metaphysical and existential. Adequate relief of both kinds of pain is at the heart of "comfort care," which may be elected by patients at any stage of their lives, especially at the end of a terminal illness.

IV. Interface with the law. Many of the most notable, landmark cases in the recent history of biomedical or clinical ethics have dealt with patients with neurologic problems. Thus, in the matter of surrogate decision-making with regard to the withholding or withdrawal of medical treatment, *Quinlan* (see *Garger* v. *New Jersey*) and *Belchertown State School* v. *Saikewicz* set the standards of substituted judgment for once-competent and never-competent patients, respectively; *Conroy* affirmed the fact that autonomy remains intact, even when a person is no longer able to assert that right or even appreciate its effectuation; and *Cruzan* v. *Director, Missouri Department of Health* acknowledged the right of states to require stringent ("clear and convincing") evidence of the prior wishes of a once-competent person as applicable to their current status. The physician should be aware of such cases, should try to discern their relevance to the situation at hand (see sec. **II**), and should recognize that the impact of such cases (in terms of setting precedents) is limited to the jurisdiction in which the decision was rendered but may (in terms of argument) be of probitive value in other jurisdictions.

V. Referral. The vast majority of ethical dilemmas can and should be dealt with by the physician and the physician's colleagues (nurses, social workers, clergy, etc.) in the care of patients—perhaps with the help of ethics consultation and the expertise of hospital administrators and attorneys. In solving such dilemmas, the physician should keep in mind at all times the general principles of decision-making, of truth-telling, and of involvement of family (see secs. **III.A**, **III.E**, and **III.F.3**). The physician should not hesitate to seek the guidance and assistance of senior, more experienced clinicians in dealing with these issues at a practical level. Generally, recourse to the courts should be a last resort, because the legal process takes interminable time and often is insensitive to the important nuances of specific clinical situations.

Recommended Readings

American Academy of Neurology Code of Professional Conduct. *Neurology* 43:1257, 1993.

American Medical Association Council on Ethical and Judicial Affairs. *Code of Medical Ethics*. Chicago: American Medical Association, 1994.

Beauchamp TL, Childress JF. *Principles of Biomedical Ethics*. New York: Oxford University Press, 1994.

Bernat JL. *Ethical Issues in Neurology*. Boston: Butterworth-Heinemann, 1994.

Brody B. *Life and Death Decision Making*. New York: Oxford University Press, 1988.

Brody H. *The Healer's Power*. New Haven, CT: Yale University Press, 1992.

Cassell EJ. *The Nature of Suffering and the Goals of Medicine*. New York: Oxford University Press, 1991.

Faden RR, Beauchamp TL. *A History and Theory of Informed Consent*. New York: Oxford University Press, 1986.

Fletcher JC, et al. (eds). *Introduction to Clinical Ethics*. Charlottesville, VA: Elliewood Copies, 1994.

Holmes HB, Purdy LM (eds). *Feminist Perspectives in Medical Ethics*. Bloomington, IN: Indiana University Press, 1992.

Jonsen AR, et al. *Clinical Ethics*. New York: Macmillan, 1986.

Lynn J (ed). *By No Extraordinary Means: The Choice to Forgo Life-Sustaining Food and Water*. Bloomington, IN: Indiana University Press, 1989.

Multi-Society Task Force on PVS. Medical aspects of the persistent vegetative state (parts I and II). *N Engl J Med* 330:1499 and 1572, 1994.

Pellegrino ED, Thomasma DC. *For the Patient's Good: The Restoration of Beneficence in Health Care*. New York: Oxford University Press, 1988.

President's Commission for the Study of Ethical Problems in Medicine and Biomedical and Behavioral Research. *Defining Death: Medical, Ethical, and Legal Issues in the Determination of Death*. Washington: US Government Printing Office, 1981.

President's Commission. *Making Health Care Decisions: The Ethical and Legal Implications of Informed Consent in the Patient-Practitioner Relationship*. Washington: US Government Printing Office, 1982.

President's Commission. *Deciding to Forego Life-Sustaining Treatment: Ethical, Medical, and Legal Issues in Treatment Decisions*. Washington: US Government Printing Office, 1983.

Quill TE. *Death and Dignity: Making Choices and Taking Charge*. New York: Norton, 1993.

Veatch RM. The impending collapse of the whole-brain definition of death. *Hastings Cent Rep* 23(4):18–24, 1993.

Veatch RM. The whole-brain oriented concept of death: An outmoded philosophical formulation. *J Thanatol* 3:13–30, 1975.

Treatment

36

Ischemic Cerebro-vascular Disease

José Biller
André Durocher

Cerebrovascular disease comprises a heterogeneous group of diseases that herald their presence by producing symptoms and signs resulting from either ischemia or hemorrhage within the CNS. The term **stroke** is most commonly used by both physicians and laypersons to refer to any one of this diverse group of disorders, and connotes the idea that the onset of symptoms is abrupt and leaves a lasting physical or cognitive disability.

Cerebrovascular disease is the third leading cause of death, after cardiovascular disease and cancer, and a primary cause of long-term disability in much of the industrialized world. Cerebrovascular disease is a major cause of chronic disability and the most common neurologic condition requiring hospitalization. The focus of this chapter is to outline the general approach to the diagnosis and management of ischemic stroke.

Of the 500,000 new or recurrent strokes in the United States each year, approximately 80–85% result from **cerebral infarction.** Ischemic stroke may result from (1) large-artery stenosis or occlusion, (2) small-artery occlusion (lacunes), (3) cardioembolism, (4) hemodynamic (watershed) infarcts, (5) nonatherosclerotic vasculopathies, (6) hypercoagulable disorders, and (7) infarcts of undetermined cause.

Ischemia sets in motion a cascade of biochemical alterations leading to lactic acidosis, influx of calcium and sodium, and efflux of potassium culminating in cell death. The pathogenesis of ischemic strokes can be conceptualized as a permanent lack of blood flow to a focal region of the brain, thus depriving it of needed glucose and oxygen. The normal cerebral blood flow (CBF) is 50–55 mL/100 g/min. The threshold for synaptic transmission failure occurs when the CBF drops to about 8–10 mL/100 g/min. At this level, neuronal death can occur. The brain region with a CBF level from 8–18 mL/100 g/min has been referred to as the **ischemic penumbra.** Rational treatment of patients with ischemic cerebrovascular disease depends on accurate diagnosis. The etiology of an ischemic stroke must first be established through careful history-taking, detailed physical examination, and paraclinical investigations.

A basic work-up, to be done in all patients with ischemic stroke, should include complete blood count (CBC) with differential and platelet count, erythrocyte sedimentation rate (ESR), prothrombin time (PT), partial thromboplastin time (PTT), plasma glucose level, blood urea nitrogen, serum creatinine, lipid analysis, luetic serology, urinalysis, chest roentgenography, and electrocardiography (ECG). Computed tomography (CT) should also be performed on all patients because it may detect hemorrhagic lesions that can mimic an ischemic stroke. Magnetic resonance imaging (MRI) is superior to CT for cerebral ischemia, particularly in the evaluation of ischemic areas in the posterior fossa.

The emphasis in screening should be on noninvasive testing for evaluating carotid artery disease, including Doppler imaging, B-mode scanning, duplex scanning, and transcranial Doppler imaging. Cardiac investigations to determine whether emboli have cardiac sources are advised in selected circumstances. Two-dimensional echocardiography for older patients with ischemic stroke should be limited to those patients with clinical clues of heart disease. Two-dimensional echocardiography should be considered for all patients less than 45 years old with otherwise unexplained ischemic stroke. Transesophageal echocardiography should be used for selected individuals, particularly for evaluation of mitral and aortic prosthetic valves or vegetations, whenever there is a need for better visualization of the left atrial appendage or interatrial septum, or when a right-to-left shunt is suspected.

Most patients with ischemic stroke have cerebrovascular atherosclerosis, and therefore the mechanism of ischemia results from thrombotic vascular occlusion, embolization of atherosclerotic debris, or hemodynamic disturbances causing focal hypoperfusion in areas in which the circulation is inadequate. The results of the North American Symptomatic Carotid Endarterectomy Trial (NASCET) and the European Carotid Surgery Trial (ECST) have emphasized the need for accurate quantification of the degree of extracranial internal carotid stenosis. Although magnetic resonance angiography (MRA) complements the information obtained with MRI, and frequently delineates the pathoanatomic substrate of the stroke, the gold standard for establishing the extent of vascular disease remains conventional angiography or intra-arterial digital subtraction angiography.

I. Natural history and prognosis

A. Ischemic stroke resulting from large-artery atherosclerotic disease.
Large-artery atherothrombotic infarctions almost always occur in patients who already have significant risk factors for cerebrovascular atherosclerosis such as arterial hypertension, cigarette smoking, diabetes, asymptomatic carotid bruits, asymptomatic carotid stenosis, and transient ischemic attacks (TIAs). A TIA is defined as a temporary focal neurologic deficit, presumably related to ischemia of the brain or retina, lasting less than 24 hours. Yet most TIAs last only a few minutes. TIAs involving the anterior or carotid circulation should be separated from those involving the posterior or vertebrobasilar circulation. The following symptoms are considered typical of TIAs in the carotid circulation: ipsilateral amaurosis fugax, contralateral sensory or motor dysfunction limited to one side of the body, aphasia, contralateral homonymous hemianopia, or any combination thereof. The following symptoms represent typical TIAs in the vertebrobasilar system: bilateral or shifting motor or sensory dysfunction, complete or partial loss of vision in both homonymous fields, or any combination of these symptoms. Isolated diplopia, vertigo, dysarthria, and dysphagia should not be considered TIAs, but in combination with one another, or with any of the other symptoms just listed, they should be considered vertebrobasilar TIAs. Preceding TIAs occur in about 50% of patients with atherothrombotic brain infarctions. A TIA is a risk factor for stroke. The independent risk of a subsequent stroke is at least three times greater for patients with histories of TIAs than for those who have not suffered TIAs.

Atherosclerosis tends to occur in areas of reduced shear, such as the lateral aspect of the carotid artery bulb. It primarily affects the larger extracranial and intracranial vessels. About 80% of ischemic strokes occur in the **carotid or anterior circulation,** and 20% in the **vertebrobasilar or posterior circulation.**

The mechanism of large-artery atherothrombotic infarction is either **artery-to-artery embolization** or **in situ formation of a thrombus** in the setting of preexisting arterial stenosis. Artery-to-artery embolism is a common mechanism of cerebral ischemic events. Embolism from ulcerated carotid atherosclerotic plaques is the most common cause of cerebral infarction. In situ thrombosis occurs in the proximal carotid, distal vertebral, and basilar arteries. Such a circumstance may arise in association with hypercoagulable states. Episodes of dehydration may also trigger these events.

B. Ischemic strokes resulting from small-vessel or penetrating artery disease (lacunes).
Long-standing arterial hypertension affects primarily the smaller penetrating intracranial vessels. It induces hypertrophy of the media and deposition of fibrinoid material into the vessel wall (fibrinoid necrosis), which eventually leads to occlusion. Lacunes are small ischemic infarctions in the deep regions of the brain or brainstem that range in diameter from 0.5–15.0 mm and result from occlusion of the penetrating arteries—chiefly the anterior choroidal, middle cerebral, posterior cerebral, and basilar arteries.

C. Ischemic stroke resulting from cardioembolism.
Embolic occlusion of intracranial vessels can be caused by material arising proximally—most commonly from the heart, from the aorta, from the carotid or vertebral arteries, and rarely from systemic veins. Embolism of cardiac origin accounts for about 15% of all ischemic strokes. Emboli from cardiac sources frequently lodge in the middle cerebral artery territory, are often large, and often have the worst outcomes. Although most types of heart disease may produce cerebral embolism, certain cardiac disorders are more likely to be associated with emboli (Table 36-1). Identification of a potential embolic cardiac source is helpful for management. However, finding a potential cardiac source is not by itself sufficient to diagnose an embolic cerebral infarct, because many cardiac problems may coexist with cerebrovascular atherosclerosis.

D. Ischemic stroke resulting from hemodynamic mechanisms.
Another

Table 36-1. Common sources of cardiac emboli.

Acute myocardial infarction
Left ventricular aneurysm
Dilated cardiomyopathy
Cardiac arrhythmias
   Atrial fibrillation
   Bradytachyarrhythmia
Valvular heart disease
   Rheumatic mitral valve disease
   Calcific aortic stenosis
   Mitral valve prolapse (MVP)
   Infective and nonbacterial thrombotic endocarditis
   Prosthetic heart valves
Intracardiac tumors
Intracardiac defects with paradoxical embolism
   Atrial septal defect (ASD)
   Patent foramen ovale (PFO)
   Atrial septal aneurysm (ASA)

mechanism of ischemic CNS damage is decreased systemic perfusion pressure, which causes diminished blood flow to the brain in a diffuse manner. This occurs most commonly in the setting of cardiac pump failure, or systemic hypotension. This type of insult is most critical in border-zone territories or so-called "watershed areas" in the most distal regions of supply of the major arterial territories. Border-zone ischemia may result in several characteristic syndromes, depending on whether the ischemia is in the border-zone territory of all three major arterial systems (anterior, middle, and posterior cerebral arteries), the territory between the anterior and middle cerebral arteries, or the territory between the middle and posterior cerebral arteries. Watershed infarcts are often bilateral but may be unilateral when there is preexisting ipsilateral vascular disease causing focal hypoperfusion in the most distal territory. Other mechanisms whereby watershed infarcts develop include microemboli and hematologic abnormalities.

E. **Ischemic stroke resulting from nonatherosclerotic vasculopathies.** Several nonatherosclerotic vasculopathies can predispose to ischemic stroke. These vasculopathies include, among others, cervicocephalic arterial dissections, moyamoya, fibromuscular dysplasia, and cerebral vasculitis. Together, these uncommon conditions represent 5% of all ischemic strokes. They are relatively more common in children and young adults.

F. **Ischemic stroke resulting from hypercoagulable disorders.** Alterations in hemostasis have been associated with an increased risk of ischemic stroke. These conditions include deficiencies in the anticoagulant proteins such as antithrombin III, protein C, protein S, and heparin cofactor II; disorders of fibrinogen or of the fibrinolytic system; and secondary hypercoagulable states encountered in the nephrotic syndrome, polycythemia vera, sickle cell disease, thrombotic thrombocytopenic purpura, and paroxysmal nocturnal hemoglobinuria. These disorders account for 1% of all strokes, and for 2–7% of ischemic strokes in young patients.

G. **Ischemic stroke resulting from undetermined causes.** Despite extensive work-up, in up to 40% of ischemic strokes an etiology cannot be determined. This percentage is possibly higher in patients under 45 years of age. It is possible that some of these strokes are caused by cardioembolic or hematologic events not demonstrable by our present means of investigation. The risk of recurrence of these strokes appears to be slightly less than that of ischemic strokes of other types.

II. **Prevention.** The prevention of strokes follows three main avenues: control of modifiable risk factors, pharmacologic therapy, and surgical intervention. Knowledge and control of modifiable risk factors are of paramount importance in prevention of primary and secondary strokes. Treatable or modifiable risk factors include hypertension, diabetes mellitus, cigarette smoking, hyperlipidemia, excessive alcohol intake, obesity, and physical inactivity. Other risk factors include age and gender, cardiac disease, TIAs, prior strokes, asymptomatic carotid bruit/stenosis, high hemoglobin/hematocrit, increased fibrinogen, use of oral contraceptives, and possibly race/ethnicity.

A. Hypertension predisposes to ischemic stroke by aggravating atherosclerosis and accelerating heart disease. Arterial hypertension is the most important modifiable risk factor for stroke, increasing the relative risk three- to fourfold. Blood pressure treatment resulting in a drop in mean diastolic BP of 5 mm Hg over 2–3 years is associated with a 40% reduction in risk of stroke.

B. Diabetes mellitus increases the risk of ischemic cerebrovascular disease two- to fourfold compared with the risk of nondiabetics. In addition, diabetes increases morbidity and mortality after stroke. There is presently no evidence to suggest that tighter diabetic control decreases the risk of stroke or recurrent stroke.

C. Cigarette smoking is an independent risk factor for ischemic stroke in men and women of all ages. More than 5 years may be required before a reduction in stroke risk is observed after cessation of smoking.

D. Hyperlipidemia. Some studies have shown a significant positive relationship between serum cholesterol levels and death resulting from nonhemorrhagic stroke. This relationship has not been consistent, however, possibly because different risks are associated with different lipoprotein subtypes. People with high serum lipoprotein A levels have a higher risk of ischemic stroke. Additional studies may hold clues to the potential value of lipid-lowering agents in reducing the risk of ischemic stroke.

E. Excessive alcohol use. There is a J-shaped association between alcohol consumption and ischemic stroke; lower doses (up to two drinks a day) offer a reduced risk, and higher doses elevate the risk. Moderate alcohol intake may elevate high-density lipoprotein concentration.

F. Obesity and physical inactivity. Obesity exerts an independent increase in risk of stroke in men under the age of 63. This increase is greater in cigarette smokers and in patients with hypertension, elevated blood glucose, or hyperlipidemia. There is some evidence that physical activity can reduce the risk of stroke.

III. Treatment. Ischemic stroke is approached as a medical emergency. Any patient with an acute ischemic stroke should be admitted to a hospital for evaluation and treatment. This is best accomplished in an **intensive care unit** or **stroke unit.** Management must be individualized according to pathophysiology.

A. General measures

1. Medical measures

a. Respiratory tract protection and infection. The airway of an obtunded patient should be protected. Some critically ill patients need ventilatory assistance. Aspiration and atelectasis should be prevented. Nosocomial pneumonia frequently complicates stroke and is a leading cause of mortality in the second to fourth weeks following cerebral infarction. Risk factors for nosocomial pneumonia in stroke patients include advanced age, prolonged hospitalization, serious medical comorbidity, immunosuppression, and endotracheal intubation. Dysphagia is common after stroke. Failure of the swallowing process increases the risks of aspiration, malnutrition, and dehydration. The risk of pneumonia is increased by aspiration, which is observed in up to 25% of unilateral hemispheric strokes and 70% of bilateral hemispheric or brainstem strokes. A meticulous history, and examination of the oral, pharyngeal, and esophageal stages with a modified barium swallow using videofluorography, are often recommended. Oral ingestion of food or liquids is often precluded in the first 24–48 hours. Nasogastric feedings are often necessary. Some patients may require gastrostomies to maintain adequate nutritional intake.

b. Urinary tract infections. Urinary bladder dysfunction may complicate stroke, particularly basal ganglia, frontoparietal, and bilateral hemispheric strokes. There are three major mechanisms for the occurrence of urinary incontinence after an acute ischemic stroke: (1) disruption of the neuromicturition pathways, which results in bladder hyperreflexia and urgency incontinence; (2) stroke-related cognitive and language deficits, with normal bladder function; and (3) concurrent neuropathy or medication use, resulting in bladder hyporeflexia and overflow incontinence.

Urinary tract infections are an important cause of hyperpyrexia following stroke. They contribute to almost one-third of stroke-related deaths and are present in almost half of the patients in autopsy series. Incontinent or comatose patients should be catheterized, preferably with a condom catheter in men or a closed Foley catheter in women. Many patients require the use of an indwelling catheter, which is associated with a risk of infection. In addition, even continent patients can have postvoiding residuals, which also increase the likelihood of urinary tract infections.

c. **Electrolytic and metabolic disturbances**
   (1) **Electrolytic disturbances.** Stroke patients are at risk for developing electrolytic disturbances resulting from reduced oral intake, potentially increased gastric and skin losses, and ADH secretion derangements. Levels of ADH are increased after stroke. In some cases, inappropriate ADH secretion places the patient at risk of hyponatremia. Possible mechanisms include damage to the anterior hypothalamus and a prolonged recumbent position. In most cases, these alterations do not persist beyond the first week after stroke.
   (2) **Hyperglycemia** in acute stroke is a common phenomenon and correlates with a poor outcome. Experimental studies in animals indicate that hyperglycemia increases the extent of ischemic brain damage. High serum glucose levels result in increased anaerobic metabolism, raised lactic acid production in ischemic brain tissue, and cellular acidosis. Despite current controversy, we recommend that hypotonic solutions or fluids containing glucose be avoided.

d. **Venous thromboembolism** is a common complication in patients with acute ischemic stroke. The risk is highest in the early weeks after ictus but remains significant in the chronic phase. In the absence of prophylactic measures, deep venous thrombosis develops in about 60–75% of patients with hemiplegia, and lethal pulmonary embolism occurs in less than 3%. Prevention includes the use of pressure gradient stockings, pneumatic compression stockings, low-dosage subcutaneous heparin (5000 units q8–12h), adjusted-dosage heparin, low-molecular-weight heparin (LMWH) and low-molecular-weight heparinoids.

e. **Cardiac events** constitute an important cause of death after acute stroke, because 40–70% of these patients have baseline **coronary artery disease.** About 15% of the deaths following ischemic strokes are from fatal arrhythmias or myocardial infarctions. Up to 30% of patients have ST segment depression on the ECG in the first 48 hours after the event, and 35% have ventricular couplets or tachycardia. Other changes include Q–T interval prolongation, T-wave inversions, or increases in T-wave duration and amplitude. Patients with lesions of the left cerebral hemisphere, especially the insular area, tend to have more cardiac disturbances.

f. **Cerebral autoregulation** is lost during an acute ischemic stroke. The blood pressure should be measured frequently during the first few days after ischemic stroke. Transient blood pressure elevation following acute cerebral infarction and normalization over days without treatment are common. Mild to moderate hypertension may be compensatory, and rapid lowering of the blood pressure is generally not recommended. Exceptions to this rule include patients with hypertensive encephalopathy and cerebral ischemia secondary to aortic dissection.

g. **Pressure sores.** Surveys suggest that 3–10% of patients in acute care hospitals have pressure sores. Stroke patients, like other patients with reduced mobility, are at increased risk. Altered level of consciousness, peripheral vascular disease, and malnourishment are also contributing factors. Pressure sores develop most often over bony prominences— sacrum, ischium, trochanters, and the areas around the ankles and heels. Positioning should be changed frequently to reduce pressure and shear forces. Flotation beds help reduce the risk. Treatment includes debridement and moist dressing. Surgical treatment is sometimes necessary.

Cellulitis in the surrounding skin and systemic infections require antibiotic therapy.

h. Depression can be an aggravating factor causing increased disability. Depression affects half of all stroke patients, and it often fulfills the criteria for major depression. Depression occurs in the first few weeks after stroke, but is maximal between 6 and 24 months. Patients with left frontal strokes appear to be more susceptible than those with right hemisphere or brainstem strokes. Depression also correlates with severity of neurologic deficit and quality of available social support. Finally, although depressed patients gain some benefit from rehabilitation, its effects are not sustained. Treatment for poststroke depression is the same as that for endogenous depression.

2. Neurologic measures. Approximately 30% of patients with acute ischemic strokes worsen after the initial presentation, but deterioration after stroke or "stroke in evolution" does not necessarily indicate propagating thrombus or recurrent embolism (Table 36-2).

a. Brain edema is the most common cause of deterioration and early death during the first week after an acute cerebral infarction. Young patients and patients with large infarctions are most affected. Massive cerebral edema complicates about 10% of large hemispheric strokes. Edema develops within several hours after an acute ischemic insult to the brain and peaks after 24–96 hours. Ischemic brain edema is initially cytotoxic and later vasogenic. Cytotoxic edema involves predominantly the gray matter, whereas vasogenic edema involves predominantly the white matter. There is no specific pharmacologic agent that has been proven effective against ischemic cerebral edema. Physicians often make the erroneous assumption that depressed consciousness in patients with large cerebral infarctions is caused solely by increased intracranial pressure and inappropriately begin "conventional" intracranial hypertension therapies such as hyperventilation to maintain pCO_2 at 25–30 mm Hg (useful in the first 24 hours), osmotherapy with mannitol supplemented by nonosmotic diuretics, and corticosteroids. Corticosteroids have not been proven to be useful in the management of ischemic cerebral edema and may even be detrimental. Mannitol does not cross the blood-brain barrier and may accentuate compartmentalized pressure gradients between abnormal and normal brain regions. Hypernatremia, hypokalemia, and hypocalcemia can result from excessive osmotherapy. In addition, excessive osmotherapy can result in intravascular volume depletion and arterial hypotension. Normal saline is administered to prevent intravascular depletion. Appreciating the role of brain tissue shifts, surgical evacuation of life-threatening supratentorial infarctions by hemicraniectomy may need to be considered. In cases of cerebellar infarction with mass effect, when fourth ventricular compression and hydrocephalus are the primary concerns, some neurosurgeons

Table 36-2. "Evolution" of stroke: Causes.

Thrombosis of a stenotic artery
Thrombus propagation
Recurrent embolism
Collateral failure
Hypoperfusion resulting from hypovolemia, decreased systemic
    pressure, or decreased cardiac output
Hypoxia
Brain edema
Seizures
Metabolic evolution of ischemic insult
Pneumonia
Urosepsis
Medication effects
Herniation syndromes
Hemorrhagic transformation

prefer to do a ventriculostomy; however, this procedure is associated with a risk of upward cerebellar herniation through the free edge of the tentorial incisura. For this reason, other neurosurgeons favor posterior fossa decompressive surgery for such patients.

b. **Hemorrhagic transformation** occurs in about 40% of all ischemic infarcts, and of these, 10% show secondary clinical deterioration. Hemorrhagic transformation often occurs in the first few weeks following stroke, most often in the first 2 weeks. Risk factors for hemorrhagic transformation include large strokes with mass effect, enhancement on contrast CT, and severe initial neurologic deficits.

c. **Seizures** occur in 4–6% of ischemic infarctions, mostly in carotid territory cortical infarcts. Infarcts in the posterior circulation are infrequently associated with seizures. Cardioembolic strokes have been found to be more epileptogenic than atherothrombotic ones, but several studies have found no significant difference. Seizures associated with lacunar infarcts are extremely rare. **Partial seizures** are more common than generalized tonic-clonic seizures. Many seizures occur within 48 hours of the onset of symptoms. In general, seizures are self-limited and respond well to medication. Patients whose seizures occur in the first few days after the ischemic event do not have increased mortality. Status epilepticus is unusual.

3. **Rehabilitation.** Prevention of complications is the first stage of rehabilitation. Patients requiring inpatient rehabilitation are transferred to the appropriate rehabilitation facility. Long-term prognosis of stroke depends on severity and type of neurologic deficit, stroke etiology, medical comorbidity, premorbid personality, family constellation, home environment, type of community and available services, and the rehabilitation team. About 50–85% of long-term stroke survivors are able to walk independently, with most of the recovery taking place in the first 3 months. About two-thirds of long-term survivors eventually become independent for activities of daily living, and about 85% of surviving patients eventually return home.

B. **Specific measures**

1. **Medical therapy.** At present, general measures and use of antithrombotic agents (antiplatelet agents or anticoagulants) remain the mainstays of medical therapy for acute ischemic stroke.

a. **Antiplatelet agents** that are beneficial include aspirin and ticlopidine. These agents are indicated for secondary prevention of stroke.

(1) **Aspirin** is the standard medical therapy currently used for prevention of stroke and recurrent stroke. The mechanism of action of aspirin is an irreversible inhibition of platelet function by inactivation of cyclooxygenase. Meta-analyses have shown that aspirin reduces the combined risk of stroke, myocardial infarction, and vascular death by approximately 25%. The range of acceptable management includes daily doses of 30–1300 mg of aspirin. The main side effect is gastric discomfort. Gastrointestinal hemorrhage occurs in 1–5% of cases. Enteric-coated preparations are generally best tolerated by patients.

(2) **Ticlopidine** reduces the risk of death or nonfatal stroke by 12% in comparison with aspirin. Ticlopidine acts primarily by irreversibly inhibiting the adenosine diphosphate pathways of the platelet membrane. Ticlopidine also reduces plasma fibrinogen levels and increases erythrocyte deformability. The recommended dosage of ticlopidine is 250 mg bid. Ticlopidine has more side effects than aspirin, including diarrhea, nausea, dyspepsia, and rash. These side effects tend to occur during the first few months of therapy. The dosage can be temporarily reduced to lessen the side effects for a few weeks, then brought back to 250 mg bid. A more important adverse reaction is reversible neutropenia, which occurs in 2.4% of the cases and is severe in 0.8%. This reaction can be encountered during the first 3 months of treatment, and for this reason a CBC must be obtained every 2 weeks during this period. The drug must be discontinued if the neutrophil count falls below 1200/μl.

(3) **Other agents.** There is no persuasive evidence from current or past trials that patients benefit from the use of sulfinpyrazone, su-

loctidil, or dipyridamole, although a recent study concluded that both low-dose aspirin and high-dose dipyridamole alone were superior to placebo, and that the combination was significantly superior to each drug alone.

The CAPRIE study assessed the relative efficacy of clopidogrel (75 mg daily), a novel platelet antiaggregant, and aspirin (325 mg daily) in reducing the incidence of nonfatal stroke, nonfatal myocardial infarction (MI), or vascular death among almost 20,000 patients who survived a recent ischemic stroke, recent MI, or had symptomatic atherosclerotic peripheral arterial disease. The results of this study show that clopidogrel was more effective than aspirin in reducing the combined risk of ischemic stroke, myocardial infarction, or vascular death in patients with atherosclerotic disease.

b. Anticoagulants

(1) **Prevention.** Oral anticoagulation with warfarin is indicated for primary and secondary prevention of stroke in patients with nonvalvular atrial fibrillation (AFib). Several recent multicenter studies suggest that in this clinical situation warfarin is the most effective drug for stroke prevention unless the patient has lone AFib. Warfarin is also indicated for prevention of stroke in patients with rheumatic atrial fibrillation or mechanical heart valves.

(2) **Treatment.** Guidelines for anticoagulant therapy in the setting of an acute ischemic stroke are not well defined. Although convincing statistical proof is still lacking, intravenous heparin is often utilized by some physicians for patients with recent TIAs; TIAs of increasing severity, frequency, or duration; "strokes in evolution" resulting from large-vessel atherosclerosis; ischemic symptoms associated with an intraluminal thrombus; cervicocephalic arterial dissections; cerebral venous thrombosis; and ischemic strokes associated with hypercoagulable states. Intravenous heparin is also used as an interim measure during evaluation of symptomatic patients prior to surgery or initiation of maintenance medical therapy. A good argument can be made for the use of heparin to prevent recurrence of recent nonseptic cardioembolic cerebral infarctions. If a decision is made to use heparin, one should carefully balance the risks (the potential side effects) against the possible benefit, recognizing that there has never been a proven benefit of heparin. When it is given, many neurologists do not use a bolus, and aim to keep the PTT between one and a half and two times the control level. Many physicians have attested to having observed improvement during the time heparin is administered, but no cause-and-effect relationship between heparin administration and clinical improvement can be established.

2. **Surgical therapy.** Precise determination of vessel stenosis has significant potential in the routine clinical assessment of patients with ischemic cerebrovascular disease. Carotid endarterectomy (CEA) is recommended for secondary prevention in selected patients and is indicated for symptomatic patients with carotid territory TIAs or minor strokes with 70–99% stenosis. Among symptomatic patients with less than 30% stenosis, medical therapy with platelet antiaggregants is recommended. The utility for symptomatic patients with 30–69% carotid artery stenosis has not yet been determined. The ACAS study found CEA to be of benefit in patients who were less than 80 years old and had degrees of asymptomatic carotid stenosis of 60% or higher. Overall, the 30-day ipsilateral stroke or death rate among surgically treated patients was only 2.3%. However, selection of asymptomatic patients for CEA remains controversial; some experts recommend surgery only when the degree of stenosis is greater than 80%. Emergency CEA in acute stroke is highly controversial.

3. **Experimental therapies** directed specifically toward reducing infarct volume consist mainly of attempts to improve cerebral perfusion to the area of ischemia by reopening the occluded vessel with the use of thrombolytic

agents, by using cytoprotective agents (e.g., calcium channel entry blockers, excitatory amino-acid antagonists, and free radical scavengers such as the 21-aminosteroids) aimed at salvaging neurons around the area of infarction that are subject to the so-called penumbral ischemia, and by interrupting programmed cell death (or "apoptosis") by using neurotrophins or calpain inhibitors.

a. **Thrombolytics.** Results of current open and randomized trials have provided evidence of the tolerance of thrombolytic agents in acute ischemic stroke. Urokinase, streptokinase, and tissue plasminogen activator (t-PA) have been used intravenously and intra-arterially. A recent NINDS rt-PA study showed that treatment with intravenous t-PA within 3 hours of onset of ischemic stroke improved clinical outcome (minimal or no disability on the clinical assessment scales) at 3 months. However, treatment did not lessen death rates. The incidence of symptomatic intracerebral hemorrhage was 10 times greater in patients given t-PA (6.4% in the treatment group compared with 0.6% in the placebo group). Most hemorrhages occurred within 36 hours of treatment. Recent trials of intravenous streptokinase within 4 to 6 hours of acute ischemic stroke were associated with increased morbidity and mortality.

b. **Defibrinogenating agents.** Ancrod, an enzyme extracted from the venom of the Malayan pit viper, lowers fibrinogen and blood viscosity, inhibits erythrocyte aggregation, indirectly stimulates thrombolysis by t-PA upregulation, and possibly causes local vasodilation by acting on the prostacyclin-stimulating factor. It also has a weak anticoagulant effect at high dosages. Its potential as a treatment for ischemic stroke is being evaluated. Preliminary studies indicate that it can be used safely in stroke patients. A trial of ancrod in acute or progressing ischemic stroke is under way.

c. **Anticoagulants.** Low-molecular-weight heparins (LMWH) and heparinoids have been evaluated for the prophylaxis or treatment of venous thromboses and as alternatives to heparin in cases of heparin-induced thrombocytopenia. Their potential advantages over standard heparins include increased bioavailability and longer half-lives. They also possess better antithrombotic activity through more efficient inhibition of coagulation factor X, and fewer bleeding side effects because of better preservation of platelet function. One randomized controlled trial of nadroparin calcium (Fraxiparin) as a treatment for acute ischemic stroke has been completed. The primary endpoint was poor outcome defined as the total of all-cause mortality and dependency with respect to activities of daily living during the 6 months after randomization. Poor outcome at 3 months was a secondary endpoint. The study showed no significant difference in poor outcome at 3 months. At 6 months, there was a significant dose-dependent reduction in the rate of poor outcome in favor of nadroparin. The heparinoid Organon 10172 has been evaluated in ischemic stroke patients within 24 hours of presentation in phase I and II trials. Few bleeding episodes were reported, and the compound appeared safe overall. Encouraging functional outcomes were observed at 3 months. A multicenter trial is currently under way.

d. **Inhibitors of neutrophil adhesion/migration.** Intercellular adhesion molecules (ICAMs) are molecules to which leukocytes adhere and that facilitate their migration through endothelium. Some of these molecules are expressed in the cerebral vasculature during ischemia. Neutrophils in particular can contribute to tissue injury by obstructing capillaries and possibly by liberating cytotoxic products. Prevention of neutrophil adhesion by infusion of monoclonal antibodies directed at ICAMs improved neurologic outcome in animal models of transient ischemia. Their efficacy in ischemic stroke is currently being investigated.

e. **Cytoprotective agents.** The sudden decrease in blood flow after ischemia provokes a cascade of events eventually leading to cell death. These events include the release of excitatory amino acids with secondary opening of ion channels, leading to an increase in intracellular calcium concentration, activation of enzymes, and generation of free

Table 36-3. Current status of medical management of cerebral ischemia: Results of selected therapies.

Therapy	Conclusion
Antithrombotic Agents	
Aspirin	Positive
Ticlopidine	Positive
Dipyridamole	Controversial
Sulfinpyrazone	Negative
Suloctidil	Negative
Clopidogrel	Positive
Warfarin	Positive*
Heparin	Under investigation
LMWH (Fraxiparin)	Positive
LMWH/heparinoids	Under investigation
Reperfusion Therapy	
Streptokinase	Negative
t-PA	Positive (within 3 hr)
r-pro-Urokinase	Under investigation
Hemorheological Therapy	
Hemodilution	Negative
Pentoxifylline	Negative
Ancrod	Under investigation
Cerebral Protection	
Nimodipine	Negative
Tirilazad	Negative
EAA antagonists	Under investigation
Neurotrophins	Further evaluation needed
Calpain inhibitors	Further evaluation needed
Other Agents	
Gangliosides	Negative
Barbiturates	Negative
Prostacyclins	Negative
Opiate antagonists	Negative
Aminophylline	Negative
Beta-adrenergic receptor blockers	Negative
Vasopressor therapy	Negative
Anti-ICAM antibodies	Under investigation
Naftidrofuryl	Under investigation

*For primary and secondary prevention in patients with nonvalvular atrial fibrillation. Under investigation for secondary prevention of noncardioembolic infarcts.

radicals. Several agents have been shown in vitro and in animal studies to interfere at one step or another with this cascade, thus potentially protecting the cells from ischemia.

(1) **Calcium channel blockers.** Cerebroselective calcium channel blockers such as nimodipine have been tested in acute stroke. The benefits of nimodipine administration for patients with acute ischemic stroke remain unproven.

(2) **Excitatory amino-acid antagonists.** In the last few decades, several observations have provided support for the hypothesis that endogenous excitatory amino-acid (EAA) neurotransmitters play a major role in the pathogenesis of cerebral ischemia. In animals, EAA antagonists have been shown to reduce the size of an infarct after occlusion of a major artery. From preliminary studies, some of these compounds appear to be safe in humans, but their efficacy has not been demonstrated. Several clinical trials are under way. Optimal protective regimens may require blockading of both NMDA and non-NMDA receptors.

(3) **Free radical scavengers.** Free radicals produced during ischemia can degrade polyunsaturated lipids, which are building blocks of cellular membranes, by lipid peroxidation. The CNS appears particularly susceptible to free radical injury. The 21-aminosteroid compounds inhibit lipid peroxidation by scavenging free radicals. Tirilazad is one such compound, and has been shown in experimental animal models to decrease damage secondary to global ischemia. Its clinical application is uncertain.

(4) **Neurotrophins** are factors that are known to promote cell growth in certain neuronal populations. Recent studies have shown that some of these factors, when given intraventricularly to animals during ischemia, reduce infarct size. The mechanism of action is still unknown, but could be related to interaction with the excitatory amino acids.

(5) **Calpain inhibitors.** Calpains are cytosomal enzymes that are normally quiescent but become activated by increases in intracellular calcium concentration. These enzymes have many proteins as their targets, and thus their activation can cause considerable damage. In experimental models of stroke in animals, intra-arterial infusion of calpain inhibitors given after onset of ischemia significantly reduced infarct size compared with controls. The value of calpain inhibitors in humans has not been established.

f. **Other agents.** The use of naftidrofuryl is presently under investigation. Treatments with gangliosides, barbiturates, prostacyclins, opiate antagonists, aminophylline, beta-adrenergic receptor blockers, vasopressor therapy, and iso/hypo/hypervolemic hemodilution have been ineffective (Table 36-3).

Recommended Readings

Adams HP Jr, et al. Studies of Org 10172 in patients with acute ischemic stroke. *Haemostasis* 22:99–103, 1992.

Antiplatelet Trialists' Collaboration. Collaborative overview of randomised trials of antiplatelet therapy—I: Prevention of death, myocardial infarction, and stroke by prolonged antiplatelet therapy in various categories of patients. *Br Med J* 308:81–106, 1994.

Atrial Fibrillation Investigators. Risk factors for stroke and efficacy of antithrombotic therapy in atrial fibrillation: Analysis of pooled data from five randomized controlled trials. *Arch Intern Med* 154:1449–1457, 1994.

Barnett HJM, Eliasziw M, Meldrum HE. Drugs and surgery in the prevention of ischemic stroke. *N Engl J Med* 332(4):238–248, 1995.

Biller J, Love BB, Gordon DL. Antithrombotic therapy for ischemic cerebrovascular disease. *Semin Neurol* 4(11):353–367, 1991.

Brandstater ME, Roth EJ, Siebens HC. Venous thromboembolism in stroke: Literature review and implications for clinical practice. *Arch Phys Med Rehabil* 73:S379–S391, 1992.

CAPRIE Steering Committee. A randomised, blinded trial of clopidogrel versus aspirin in patients at risk of ischaemic events (CAPRIE). *Lancet* 348:1329–1339, 1996.

Cerebral Embolism Study Group. Immediate anticoagulation of embolic stroke: A randomized trial. *Stroke* 14:668–676, 1983.

Chimowitz MI, Mancini JGB. Asymptomatic coronary artery disease in patients with stroke: Prevalence, prognosis, diagnosis and treatment. *Stroke* 23:433–436, 1992.

Donnan GA, Davis SM, Chambers BR, et al., for the Australian Streptokinase (ASK) Trial Study Group. Streptokinase for acute ischemic stroke with relationship to time of administration. *JAMA* 276:961–966, 1996.

European Atrial Fibrillation Trial Study Group. Secondary prevention in non-rheumatic atrial fibrillation after transient ischaemic attack or minor stroke. *Lancet* 342:1255–1262, 1993.

European Carotid Surgery Trialists' Collaborative Group. MRC European Carotid Surgery Trial: Interim results for symptomatic patients with severe (70–99%) or with mild (0–29%) stenosis. *Lancet* 337:1235–1243, 1991.

European Stroke Prevention Study (ESPS-2) Working Group. ASA/Dipyridamole is superior to either agent alone and to placebo. *Stroke* 27:195, 1996.

Executive Committee for the Asymptomatic Carotid Atherosclerosis Study. Endarterectomy for asymptomatic carotid artery stenosis. *JAMA* 273(18):1421–1428, 1995.

Fisher M. Potentially effective therapies for acute ischemic stroke. *Eur Neurol* 35:3–7, 1995.

Hass WK, et al. A randomized trial comparing ticlopidine hydrochloride with aspirin for the prevention of stroke in high-risk patients. *N Engl J Med* 321:501–507, 1989.

Hobson RW, et al. Efficacy of carotid endarterectomy for asymptomatic carotid stenosis. *N Engl J Med* 328:221–227, 1993.

Kay R, Wong KS, Yu YL, et al. Low molecular-weight heparin for the treatment of acute ischemic stroke. *N Engl J Med* 333:1588–1593, 1995.

Loftus CM, Biller J. Acute cerebral ischemia. Part I: Pathophysiology and medical treatment. *Contemp Neurosurg* 16(25):1–6, 1994.

Marsh EE, et al. Use of antithrombotic drugs in the treatment of acute ischemic stroke: A survey of neurologists in practice in the United States. *Neurology* 39:1631–1634, 1989.

Multicenter Acute Stroke Trial–Italy (MAST-I) Group. Randomized controlled trial of streptokinase, aspirin, and combination of both in treatment of acute ischemic stroke. *Lancet* 346:1509–1514, 1995.

National Institute of Neurological Disorders and Stroke rt-PA Stroke Study Group. Tissue plasminogen activator for acute ischemic stroke. *N Engl J Med* 333:1581–1587, 1995.

North American Symptomatic Carotid Endarterectomy Trial Collaborators. Beneficial effect of carotid endarterectomy in symptomatic patients with high-grade carotid stenosis. *N Engl J Med* 325:445–453, 1991.

Powers WJ. Acute hypertension after stroke: The scientific basis for treatment decisions. *Neurology* 43:461–467, 1993.

Robinson RG, Lipsey JR, Price TR. Diagnosis and clinical management of post-stroke depression. *Psychosomat* 26(10):769–778, 1985.

Sandercock PAG, et al. Antithrombotic therapy in acute ischaemic stroke: An overview of the completed randomised trials. *J Neurol Neurosurg Psychiat* 56:17–25, 1993.

Scheinberg P. Stroke: The way things really are. *Stroke* 25:1290–1294, 1994.

Sherman DG, et al. Antithrombotic therapy for cerebrovascular disorders. *Chest* 102:529S–537S, 1992.

Siesjo BK. Pathophysiology and treatment of focal cerebral ischemia. Part I: Pathophysiology. *J Neurosurg* 77:169–184, 1992.

Siesjo BK. Pathophysiology and treatment of focal cerebral ischemia. Part II: Mechanisms of damage and treatment. *J Neurosurg* 77:337–354, 1992.

Wardlaw JM, Warlow CP. Thrombolysis in acute ischemic stroke: Does it work? *Stroke* 23:1826–1839, 1992.

Zeiler K, Kollegger H. Risk factors associated with ischaemic stroke: Implications for disease prevention. *CNS Drugs* 1(2):132–145, 1994.

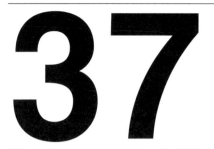

Hemorrhagic Cerebrovascular Disease
Harold P. Adams, Jr.
Birgitte H. Bendixen

Hemorrhagic stroke (hemorrhagic cerebrovascular disease or intracranial hemorrhage) is a life-threatening condition that is second only to cardiac disease as a medical cause of sudden death (death that occurs within 24 hours of onset of symptoms). The 1-month mortality of hemorrhagic stroke approaches 40–50%. In 10% of cases, the patient does not survive long enough to reach a hospital or dies shortly after arriving at an emergency room. Many survivors of hemorrhagic stroke have major disabilities.

Head injury is the most common cause of intracranial bleeding but is usually not included in this group. Hemorrhagic strokes include nontraumatic bleeding that occurs primarily in the brain (intraparenchymal or intracerebral hemorrhage), the ventricles (intraventricular hemorrhage), the subarachnoid space (subarachnoid hemorrhage, or SAH), or the subdural space (subdural hematoma). Bleeding may simultaneously involve the brain, ventricles, and subarachnoid space.

Hemorrhages account for approximately 15–20% of the 400,000 strokes that occur annually in the United States. Although the incidence of stroke, including hypertensive hemorrhage, has declined during the last 30 years, the rate of SAH, largely resulting from ruptured aneurysms, has not dropped. Although the risk of hemorrhagic stroke increases with advancing age, children and young adults are also affected. Because ischemic strokes are relatively uncommon in children and young adults, hemorrhagic strokes are more prominent in these age groups. Even when trauma is excluded, hemorrhagic stroke is more common among men than among women. The incidence of hemorrhagic stroke is higher among Americans of African or Asian ancestry than among those of European heritage.

I. **Causes of hemorrhagic stroke.** Intracranial hemorrhage is a manifestation of an underlying disease. In most cases, the most likely cause of hemorrhagic stroke can be identified.

   A. **Occult craniocerebral trauma.** Trauma is a potential cause of intracranial hemorrhages—typically subdural or epidural hematomas or parenchymal contusions. A history of injury may be lacking when a patient is found unconscious and other clues must be sought—e.g., lacerations or soft-tissue swelling. Conversely, a patient who has a primary hemorrhage may suffer secondary trauma. For example, a patient with an SAH may have a secondary seizure and suffer a fall. In such circumstances, observers and the patient should be carefully quizzed about the course of the illness and whether the neurologic symptoms were present before the injury.

   B. **Hypertension.** Either acute or chronic hypertension can predispose to bleeding. Chronic hypertension causes degenerative changes in the brain's penetrating arteries. Sudden severe hypertension, complicating acute glomerulonephritis, eclampsia, or sympathomimetic drug use presumably overwhelms the brain's autoregulatory responses and a vessel ruptures. The most common sympathomimetic drugs are cocaine, methamphetamine, and phenylpropanolamine. Up to 50% of sympathomimetic drug users are found to have underlying saccular aneurysms or arteriovenous malformations, with resulting SAHs or lobar hemorrhages, respectively. The most common locations for hypertensive hemorrhage are the putamen, thalamus, pons, and cerebellum. Hypertension should be considered as a cause of a hematoma located in deep gray matter structures if the patient has a history of hypertension. Other findings of hypertension, such as retinopathy, renal failure, or left ventricular hypertrophy, help support the diagnosis. Hemorrhagic stroke frequently is attributed to arterial hypertension because of the presence of an elevated blood pressure detected on arrival at an emergency room. However, markedly elevated blood pressure frequently is common among acutely ill patients with intracranial bleeding and should not lead automatically to a diagnosis of hypertensive hemorrhage. Hypertension is not a common cause of primary SAH.

C. **Saccular aneurysms.** Rupture of saccular aneurysms is the leading cause of nontraumatic SAH and is an important cause of intracerebral hemorrhage. Approximately 1–5% of adults harbor intracranial aneurysms, a minority of which will rupture during life. Approximately 25% of affected patients have multiple aneurysms. These patients have a higher-than-expected incidence of coarctation of the aorta, fibromuscular dysplasia, and polycystic kidney disease. A small percentage have family histories of cerebral aneurysms. Approximately 85% of saccular aneurysms are in the carotid circulation. The most common sites are the junction of the anterior communicating and anterior cerebral arteries, the origin of the posterior communicating artery, and the bifurcation of the middle cerebral artery. The most common locations in the posterior circulation are the bifurcation of the basilar artery and the origin of the posterior inferior cerebellar artery.

D. **Other aneurysms.** Infective, neoplastic, and traumatic aneurysms are rare etiologies of intracranial bleeding. They usually are located in peripheral branch arteries and are smaller than saccular aneurysms. Dolichoectatic (fusiform) aneurysms are tortuous, elongated arterial enlargements most commonly found in the basilar arteries of patients with extensive atherosclerosis in other vascular beds. They cause symptoms of ischemic stroke or compression of brainstem structures; hemorrhage is an unusual complication. Spontaneous or traumatic dissecting aneurysms of intracranial arteries, particularly of the basilar and distal vertebral arteries, are potential causes of atypical SAH.

E. **Vascular malformations** are a leading cause of hemorrhagic stroke, particularly among children and young adults. These lesions are classified as arteriovenous malformations (AVMs), venous angiomas, cavernous angiomas, and telangiectasias. They can arise in any part of the brain. Although familial cases, such as with hereditary hemorrhagic telangiectasias, are reported, most are sporadic. Nonhemorrhagic symptoms, which typically antedate hemorrhage, include seizures, recurrent headaches, and progressive neurologic impairments. Patients with large malformations may hear turbulent blood flow, and a cranial bruit may be auscultated.

F. **Amyloid angiopathy (congophilic angiopathy)** is an important cause of lobar hemorrhage in the elderly. Up to 70% of these patients have clinical dementia or Alzheimer's disease. Amyloid is deposited in leptomeningeal and cortical arterioles. The hemorrhage is typically located at the junction between gray and white matter, most commonly in the frontal or parietal lobe. The risk of recurrent hemorrhage is high. The presence of concomitant amyloid angiopathy is thought to underlie some of the cerebral hemorrhages observed in patients receiving thrombolytic therapy for acute myocardial infarction.

G. **Vasculitis.** Multisystem or isolated CNS vasculitis rarely causes hemorrhage. Bleeding is most commonly associated with necrotizing arteritides, such as polyarteritis nodosa.

H. **Bleeding disorders.** Intracranial hemorrhage complicates several coagulation disorders such as hemophilia, sickle cell disease, thrombocytopenia, and leukemia. The use of thrombolytic drugs, heparin, hirudin, oral anticoagulants, and antiplatelet agents may be complicated by bleeding. The severity of bleeding is greater and the prognosis is poorer than among patients who have spontaneous hematomas. Approximately 1% of patients who receive thrombolytic drugs for treatment of acute myocardial infarction have complicating intracranial hemorrhages. Thrombolytic drug therapy, combined with heparin, hirudin, or aspirin, may be associated with an increased risk of hemorrhage. Intracranial hemorrhagic transformation is a potentially life-threatening side effect of thrombolytic drugs given to patients with major ischemic strokes.

Bleeding can complicate treatment with heparin, particularly among patients who have had large acute ischemic strokes. The degree of increased risk conferred by the use of heparin is not known, and no specific dosage or regimen has been found to be associated with a higher or lower risk. Intracranial hemorrhage is a side effect of oral anticoagulants. Bleeding should be considered in any patient who develops acute neurologic signs while taking oral anticoagulants even if there is no other evidence of bleeding. Hemorrhages are more likely to occur in patients who are elderly, who have histories of stroke, and who have poorly controlled hypertension. The risk of intracranial bleeding is increased when the prothrombin time (PT) is excessively prolonged.

I. **Venous thrombosis** is an uncommon cause of intracranial bleeding, and its course differs from those of most hemorrhagic strokes. Patients present with the combination of worsening headaches, seizures, altered consciousness, and focal neurologic signs. Venous thrombosis most commonly develops in the peripartum period and among persons who are dehydrated or have malignancies, recent cranial operations, or otolaryngologic infections.

J. **Brain tumors.** Hemorrhage can be the initial neurologic presentation and occasionally the first finding of a highly vascular primary brain or metastatic tumor. The most common hemorrhagic metastatic tumors are choriocarcinomas, melanomas, and carcinomas of the lung, kidney, or breast. The leading primary brain tumor is glioblastoma. Many patients have histories of evolving neurologic symptoms such as headaches or personality changes before the bleeding event. The presence of considerable brain edema in the first few hours following hemorrhage or multiple hemorrhagic lesions prompts consideration of an underlying tumor.

II. **Presentations of hemorrhagic stroke**
   A. **History**
      1. Hemorrhagic stroke is usually a sudden, dramatic event. Observers or the patient often relate the circumstances surrounding the onset of symptoms. Headache, of any quality and location, is usually described as intense. A headache accompanied by transient loss of consciousness or one that is of cataclysmic onset is the premier symptom of SAH; it is often described as "the worst headache of my life." Accompanying symptoms include nausea, vomiting, prostration, photophobia, phonophobia, and nuchal rigidity.
      2. Disturbed consciousness is common, and prolonged unresponsiveness occurs in patients who have major bleeds. Transient alteration in alertness at the time of bleeding may be secondary to temporarily increased intracranial pressure (ICP). Disorientation or confusion is common. Although focal or generalized seizures can occur, recurrent seizures and status epilepticus are uncommon.
      3. Focal neurologic symptoms reflect the location of the hematoma. Patients with cerebellar hemorrhages often have subacute courses. They complain of headache, dizziness (vertigo), disturbed balance, nausea, and vomiting. Subsequently, signs of brainstem compression or increased ICP appear, including cranial nerve palsies, motor impairments, and disturbed consciousness. Although most patients with SAH do not have focal neurologic symptoms, features suggesting the location of an aneurysm can be detected; the most common symptom is diplopia secondary to a third nerve palsy.
   B. **Examination**
      1. Assessment of the vital signs and the ABCs of emergent care are the first steps in the examination (Table 37-1). Vital signs are measured frequently, and close neurologic monitoring is required. The airway must be secured in patients with altered consciousness, seizures, vomiting, or prominent weakness. Patients with severe hemorrhages often have respiratory abnormalities that lead to hypoxia, hypercapnia, or acidosis.
      2. Electrocardiographic abnormalities and cardiac arrhythmias can be detected. Arterial hypertension is common. A bruit auscultated over the head or neck suggests an AVM. Multiple ecchymoses or petechiae point to infective endocarditis, recent trauma, or an underlying coagulation disorder. Evidence of cervical spine, facial, or cranial injury, such as Battle's sign (basilar skull fracture), is sought. Neck pain or tenderness may represent an associated cervical spine fracture. The neck should not be flexed to check for signs of meningeal irritation until the possibility of a cervical spine fracture is eliminated.
      3. Meningeal irritation results from blood in the subarachnoid space. Nuchal rigidity (Brudzinski's sign) may not be present in patients whose hematomas are restricted to the parenchyma or in comatose patients. A stiff neck is prominent in most persons with SAH but may take several hours to appear. Ocular hemorrhages (subhyaloid, conjunctival, or retinal) develop in a minority of persons, but they are highly specific for serious hemorrhages. Because the course of the illness is usually quite short, papilledema is not commonly observed.

Table 37-1. Physical examination of patients with suspected intracranial hemorrhage.

Vital signs
  Airway
  Breathing
  Respiratory pattern
  Heart rate
  Blood pressure
Cardiovascular examination
General medical examination
  Petechiae
  Ecchymoses
  Bleeding elsewhere
Signs of craniocerebral trauma
  Battle's sign
  Raccoon eyes
  Optic hemorrhage
  Scalp lacerations
  Skull tenderness
Signs of meningeal irritation
  Brudzinski's sign
  Kernig's sign
Ocular signs
  Subhyaloid hemorrhage
  Papilledema
Level of consciousness
Glasgow Coma Scale
Other neurologic findings
  Language deficits
  Articulation abnormalities
  Motor deficits
  Sensory loss

    4. Assessment of consciousness is the most important component of the neurologic examination because it strongly correlates with the severity of hemorrhage. The patient's level of consciousness is rated as alert, drowsy, stuporous, or comatose. Although the easily performed Glasgow Coma Scale was originally developed to assess patients with head injuries, it is directly applicable to persons with acute nontraumatic brain diseases, including hemorrhage. The remainder of the neurologic examination is aimed at detecting the abnormalities specific for different locations of hemorrhage.

III. Differential diagnosis of hemorrhagic stroke
    A. Imaging of the brain—computed tomography (CT) in particular—greatly expedites the diagnosis of hemorrhagic stroke. The differential diagnosis is not extensive. The brief duration, clinical severity, and prominent focal neurologic signs are relatively specific. The leading alternative diagnosis is acute ischemic stroke. Although there are no truly unique features, patients with hemorrhagic stroke generally are more severely ill than those with ischemic stroke. Their symptoms are usually more severe than those observed in occlusions of single arteries (as in ischemic stroke). Headaches, alterations in consciousness, nausea and vomiting, and photophobia and phonophobia also are more prominent in hemorrhagic stroke.

    B. Craniocerebral trauma is another alternative. Differentiation of traumatic bleeding from spontaneous hemorrhage can be difficult when a patient is comatose and no history is available. In general, hemorrhages located deep in the brain are not the results of trauma. Conversely, multiple small cortical petechiae in the frontal, temporal, and occipital poles are usually caused by injuries.

    C. In contradistinction to that of intracerebral hemorrhage, differential diagnosis of SAH is broad (Table 37-2). Although patients with SAH usually seek medical attention because of the severity of their complaints, physicians can be misled.

Table 37-2. Misdiagnoses in patients with acute SAH.

Migraine headache	Tension headache
Sinusitis	Viral meningitis
Flu	Hypertensive crisis
Eclampsia	Head injury
Cervical spine injury	Cervical herniated disk
Alcohol intoxication	Drug intoxication

The diagnosis of SAH is missed in approximately 25% of cases, most commonly among the least seriously ill patients. Failure to recognize a ruptured aneurysm has serious consequences because of the risk of potentially fatal recurrent hemorrhage and the availability of therapies that are effective when administered early. The only way to avoid missing an SAH is to maintain a high index of suspicion. Patients who have the sudden onset of a severe headache ("the worst headache of my life") or a headache associated with a loss of consciousness should be evaluated for SAH. The absence of focal neurologic deficits or meningeal irritation does not preclude the diagnosis. Atypical features include severe neck, face, shoulder, eye, or ear pain. Occasionally a ruptured aneurysm in the posterior fossa presents with neck or back pain as the primary complaint.

IV. **Diagnostic studies.** The goals of the emergent evaluation are to confirm intracranial hemorrhage as the cause of the neurologic symptoms and to look for acute complications (Table 37-3). These seriously ill patients are at risk for a variety of neurologic and medical side effects. The most frequent neurologic problems are brain edema, hydrocephalus, increased ICP, and seizures. The most serious early medical complications are myocardial ischemia, cardiac arrhythmias, gastrointestinal bleeding, respiratory abnormalities, and fluid and electrolyte disturbances. Obtunded patients with possible craniocerebral trauma should have x-rays of the cervical spine to eliminate occult fracture before they are moved.

Table 37-3. Diagnostic studies for patients with acute hemorrhagic stroke.

Emergent Studies

CT of the brain
Chest x-ray
Lateral cervical spine x-ray (if a neck injury is suspected)
Electrocardiogram
Arterial blood gases (if hypoxia or respiratory failure is suspected)
CBC
Serum electrolytes
Blood glucose
CSF examination (if subarachnoid hemorrhage is suspected and no blood is seen on CT)

Subsequent Studies

CT of the brain with and without enhancement
MRI of the brain with and without enhancement
MRA
Arteriography
Transcranial Doppler imaging
CBC
Platelet count
Fibrinogen
Prothrombin time (PT)
Partial thromboplastin time (PTT)
Serum electrolytes
Hepatic and renal studies
Blood glucose
Erythrocyte sedimentation rate (ESR)
Blood cultures
Urine and blood screens for illicit drugs
Brain and meningeal biopsy

A. CT is the single most important diagnostic test. It is available in most medical centers, is relatively inexpensive, and can be performed quickly. The yield of unenhanced CT scans among patients with hemorrhagic stroke is extraordinarily high. When CT is performed within 24 hours of the onset, blood density can be detected in almost 100% of patients with intraparenchymal hematomas and in approximately 95% of those with SAH. CT might miss a small collection of subarachnoid blood in a patient with a mild hemorrhage or if the bleeding is restricted to the posterior fossa. If CT is performed several days after the onset, its yield drops because the collection of blood may have been reabsorbed. CT also detects early complications, including brain edema and hydrocephalus. The location of blood is also used to guide further diagnostic studies and provides clues to the likely cause of hemorrhage. CT also provides prognostic information; for example, large amounts of subarachnoid blood are predictive of vasospasm and ischemic stroke after SAH.

B. Magnetic resonance imaging (MRI) can also detect intracranial bleeding and provide additional data about the likely cause. It also provides information about the age of the hematoma. However, it has few advantages over CT in the acute setting and thus is an ancillary emergent diagnostic study.

C. Examination of cerebrospinal fluid (CSF) identifies bleeding within the subarachnoid space, but its importance has declined with the advent of CT. There is little reason to do a lumbar puncture (LP) if CT demonstrates bleeding. Conversely, CSF examination is important if SAH is suspected and CT does not show blood. It can detect bleeding among alert persons who have mild signs. The risk of neurologic complications, such as herniation, is low in an alert patient who has no focal signs and no mass lesion on CT. Determining whether the source of bloody CSF is an intracranial hemorrhage or a traumatic LP (bloody tap) may be difficult. Bloody CSF from an SAH generally does not clear in sequentially collected tubes. Xanthochromia (yellowing) of the CSF supernatant after centrifugation is the most reliable sign, but it may take 12 hours to develop. A physician should immediately centrifuge a bloody CSF specimen to check for xanthochromia, because a delay of several hours may give a false-positive result. The CSF findings evolve, and if the LP is delayed by several days, only slightly yellow fluid, an elevated CSF protein, or an inflammatory response that suggests a viral meningitis may be detected.

D. Additional screening studies for determining the etiology of hemorrhage are performed on a case-by-case basis after the patient has been stabilized. Contrast-enhanced CT or MRI provides evidence of the cause of bleeding, such as an aneurysm or AVM. Magnetic resonance angiography (MRA) is becoming a useful screening tool for detecting aneurysms or vascular malformations.

E. Arteriography is a critical component of evaluation, especially in cases of SAH. Although it is invasive, arteriography is generally safe for patients with hemorrhagic stroke. It is the best means of detecting a saccular or small peripheral aneurysm or a vascular malformation. Besides detecting the aneurysm, arteriography also provides information about the adjacent vascular anatomy and the presence of vasospasm—findings that influence decisions about surgery. Arteriography provides information about the presence, location, and extent of cerebral vasculitis.

V. Treatment

A. Prevention. Several treatments, selected on the basis of potential cause, can lower the risk of hemorrhagic stroke. Either acute or chronic sustained elevations of blood pressure can lead to intracranial bleeding, but antihypertensive drugs can lower the risk of this complication effectively. Care in the use of antithrombotic or thrombolytic drugs should lessen the likelihood of adverse intracranial bleeding. Management of inherited or acquired disorders of coagulation also prevents hemorrhage. Surgical treatment of an unruptured AVM or saccular aneurysm is a very effective prophylactic measure. Treatment can prevent recurrent rupture of one of these lesions.

B. Referral and admission. Hemorrhagic stroke is a very expensive illness. Not only are healthcare costs high, but the secondary economic consequences, including lost productivity, are also considerable. Thus, the most cost-effective therapy is prevention.

Patients with hemorrhagic stroke are critically ill. Inpatient care is warranted because intracranial hemorrhage is potentially life-threatening and is accompanied by many serious complications. The facilities and personnel required for successful care of these very ill patients are not available in most hospitals. Admission to a specialized treatment facility that has monitoring capabilities or an intensive care unit usually is needed. The high-risk nature of hemorrhagic stroke means that most patients should be transferred to centers that have neurologic and neurosurgical expertise. Primary care physicians should not attempt to manage these patients but should refer them to specialized treatment centers as soon as possible.

C. **General management**

1. Management includes measures for control of acute medical and neurologic complications (Table 37-4). Endotracheal intubation and ventilatory assistance may be required. Hypoxic patients should receive supplemental oxygen. Access for intravenous administration of drugs and fluids is required, and normal saline or lactated Ringer's solution is infused slowly. Hypotonic solutions should generally be avoided to minimize edema. Cardiac monitoring to detect arrhythmias and frequent assessments of vital signs and neurologic status are performed. Hypoglycemia or markedly elevated blood sugar should be treated.

2. Markedly elevated blood pressure can worsen the bleeding. The blood pressure is volatile during the first few hours but usually declines as agitation, pain, seizures, and vomiting are controlled. The level of blood pressure that mandates medical treatment is not known. However, a rule of thumb is not to initiate therapy unless the systolic blood pressure is greater than 240 mm Hg or the diastolic pressure is greater than 130 mm Hg. Responses to antihypertensive drugs are exaggerated, and the best drugs for this setting have not been determined. The goal should be slow and cautious lowering of the blood pressure. Drugs that dilate cerebral vessels are avoided because of the risk of increased ICP. Excessive sedation should also be avoided because it may obscure the patient's neurologic status. Continuous monitoring of arterial pressure is required if a parenteral drug is given. Short-acting parenteral drugs are preferred because the dosage can be titrated in response to the patient's blood pressure and neurologic status.

3. Symptoms such as headache, agitation, and vomiting warrant treatment. Patients who have had seizures are given anticonvulsants, but prophylactic administration of anticonvulsants to patients who have not had seizures is controversial. Because of concerns that the stress of a seizure might cause rebleeding, many physicians give anticonvulsants to patients who have ruptured aneurysms.

4. Management of increased ICP is important. Impaired venous return, agitation, fever, hypoxia, hypercapnia, and hypoventilation aggravate increased ICP and should be managed. Elevation of the patient's head, control of pain and agitation, modest fluid restriction, and avoidance of potentially hypo-osmolar fluids, such as 5% dextrose in water, are early measures. Neither conventional nor large dosages of corticosteroids help. Intubation and hyperventilation are prescribed when a patient is deteriorating and are complemented by infusion of 20% mannitol in a dosage of 0.5–1 gm/kg. Mannitol's effects appear within 20 minutes, and its duration of action is approximately 4–6 hours. Recurrent dosages of mannitol may be needed to prevent rebound in ICP increases, although a hyperosmolar state can develop. Monitoring of intracranial pressure is frequently used

Table 37-4. Emergent management of patients with hemorrhagic stroke.

ABCs of emergent care
  Frequent measurements of vital signs and blood pressure
  Frequent neurologic assessments
  Airway support
  Cardiac monitoring
Intravenous access
  Slow infusion of normal saline or lactated Ringer's solution
Treatment of elevated blood pressure
Symptomatic treatment of pain, vomiting, or seizures

to guide treatment in such a critical situation. Furosemide may also be helpful.

D. Surgical evacuation of the hematoma. A critical early decision regards the need for surgical evacuation of the hematoma. Removal of a large hematoma can save a patient's life. The location and size of the hematoma and the patient's neurologic status, course, and general health affect such a decision. Surgery is recommended when a large (>2.5 cm) cerebellar hematoma threatens to compress the brainstem or obstruct CSF outflow. A ventricular catheter is used to drain CSF if the patient has secondary hydrocephalus. This effectively controls increased ICP and helps forestall a craniotomy. Patients with small-to-moderate-sized hematomas of the cerebral hemispheres that do not exhibit mass-related signs usually do not need surgery. Patients with large superficial hemispheric hematomas often are treated operatively. The usefulness of surgical treatment of a large hematoma located in the lobar white matter, thalamus, or basal ganglia has not been established.

E. Inpatient care

1. Emergent management is continued after admission. Treatment is limited to bed rest until the patient is stable. Close nursing care, monitoring, and regular assessments of the patient's neurologic status and vital signs are continued. Patients not admitted to intensive care units often are housed in quiet, dark rooms. Liquids and food are not given by mouth until the patient's ability to swallow safely is confirmed. A modest fluid restriction is continued for patients who have large hematomas. Other patients, including most of those with SAH, do not need such a limitation. Close observation and management of intravenous fluids are necessary.

2. Incontinence or the need for accurate measurement of urine output often leads to insertion of an indwelling bladder catheter. Because of the risk of infection, the catheter should be removed as quickly as possible. Bedridden patients receive measures to forestall deep-vein thrombosis and pulmonary embolism, including alternating-pressure stockings. Because heparin might worsen bleeding, it usually is not prescribed. There may be situations, such as pulmonary embolism, in which anticoagulation is needed. Passive and active range of motion exercises help avoid orthopedic complications. Care in avoiding pulmonary complications is part of general management. When the patient is stable, increased activity, mobilization, and rehabilitation begin.

F. Cause-specific treatments. Treatment of the cause of hemorrhage is key. For example, an underlying coagulopathy should be corrected, and the effects of an antithrombotic drug should be reversed.

1. Vascular malformations. Patients with ruptured vascular malformations usually undergo definitive therapy to prevent recurrence of hemorrhage. Because the risk of early rebleeding is low, treatment is usually delayed until the hematoma has been reabsorbed. The decision of whether or not to perform surgery is influenced by the size and location of the malformation and the number and caliber of feeding arteries. Lesions in neurologically eloquent areas and those that are deep in the brain may not be surgically approachable. A high-flow malformation is also a problem because a hyperperfusion state leading to brain edema and hemorrhage can follow surgery. A staged procedure with preliminary endovascular placement of balloons, microemboli, or a sclerosing agent may be needed before surgical excision. Small, deep, vascular malformations may be treated with focused, high-intensity radiation, which leads to secondary fibrosis of the vessels over a 2-year period. Very large malformations may not be treatable by any of the currently available modalities.

2. Aneurysms. Patients with ruptured aneurysms are vulnerable to recurrent hemorrhage and ischemic stroke (Table 37-5). Recurrent aneurysmal rupture is a largely fatal event that peaks during the first 24 hours, when the risk of recurrence is approximately 4%. The aggregate risk of recurrent hemorrhage during the first 10 days approaches 20%. The second hemorrhage has greater morbidity and mortality. The symptoms of rebleeding are the same as those of the initial hemorrhage; CT demonstrates more blood.

3. Aneurysmal rebleeding. Several therapies are aimed at avoiding recurrence of hemorrhage. The most effective is direct surgical obliteration of the aneurysm. The timing of surgery is influenced by the patient's condition, the location of the aneurysm, the presence of serious comorbid diseases, the pres-

Table 37-5. Treatment of patients with aneurysmal SAH.

Prevention of Early Recurrent Hemorrhage
Intracranial surgery
Clipping of aneurysm
Wrapping of aneurysm
Trapping of aneurysm
Carotid ligation
Endovascular placement of a balloon
Antifibrinolytic drugs
Antihypertensive drugs
Bed rest

Prevention of Vasospasm and Ischemic Stroke
General
Avoid hypotension and dehydration
Avoid use of antifibrinolytic drugs
Lower increased ICP
Intracranial operation
Surgical lavage of subarachnoid space
Instillation of thrombolytic drugs
Nimodipine or other calcium blocker
Tirilazad
Angioplastic dilation of narrowed arteries

ence of vasospasm, and the preferences of the surgeon. Most neurosurgeons favor early surgery. Very seriously ill patients and those with relatively inaccessible aneurysms are stabilized before surgery is undertaken. In such circumstances, several medical therapies are prescribed. Antifibrinolytic drugs (aminocaproic acid or tranexamic acid) effectively reduce the risk of rebleeding, but because of a higher rate of brain ischemia they do not reduce mortality or improve the likelihood of a favorable outcome. Endovascular placement of a balloon or occlusive compound within the aneurysm is being tested.

4. **Vasospasm and ischemic stroke.** Vasospasm is a localized or generalized arterial process that occurs almost exclusively in association with aneurysmal SAH. Thick collections of blood in the subarachnoid space trigger progressive arterial narrowing that peaks 7–10 days after the SAH and gradually abates over the next 7–10 days. Vasospasm is more likely to occur with severe hemorrhages or when CT shows evidence of extensive subarachnoid blood. The arterial narrowing leads to hypoperfusion, which causes ischemia that can progress to infarction. The symptoms of vasospasm are worsening headaches, altered consciousness, and focal neurologic signs that can wax and wane. Transcranial Doppler imaging can detect alterations in velocities before the signs of neurologic worsening appear. These studies are performed at regular intervals during the high-risk period. Arteriography is the most definitive means of diagnosing vasospasm following SAH.

Potential treatments include measures that prevent or reverse the arterial narrowing or prevent ischemic stroke. Avoiding the administration of antifibrinolytic and antihypertensive drugs, controlling increased ICP, and controlling hyponatremia and dehydration may lessen the risk of infarction following SAH. Nimodipine is efficacious in improving outcome after SAH. It is unclear if it has any effect on vasospasm. It protects the brain from the consequences of ischemia because it can be given before ischemia begins. Nimodipine is relatively safe, although hypotension can occur. The 21-aminosteroid tirilazad may also reduce the risk of ischemic stroke after SAH. It and several other promising therapies are currently being tested.

Hypervolemic hemodilution and drug-induced hypertension are frequently prescribed for patients who develop ischemic symptoms. Although no controlled trials have demonstrated the efficacy of this regimen, several series have reported improvement, and it is widely prescribed. Hypervolemic hemodilution and drug-induced hypertension are very vigorous interventions, and monitoring is critical, because myocardial ischemia, congestive heart failure, and pulmonary edema are potential complications. This regimen can cause recurrent rupture of an aneurysm that has not been operatively clipped. Angioplastic dilation of narrowed arteries is performed when a patient does not respond to medical interventions.

Recommended Readings

Adams HP Jr, et al. Pitfalls in the recognition of subarachnoid hemorrhage. *JAMA* 244:794–796, 1980.

Adams HP Jr, et al. Computed tomographic findings and clinical correlates in recent aneurysmal subarachnoid hemorrhage: A preliminary report of the Cooperative Aneurysm Study. *Neurology* 33:981–988, 1983.

Broderick J, et al. Lobar hemorrhage in the elderly: The undiminishing importance of hypertension. *Stroke* 24:49–51, 1993.

Broderick J, et al. Management of intracerebral hemorrhage in a large metropolitan population. *Neurosurgery* 34:882–887, 1994.

Fisher CM. Clinical syndromes in cerebral thrombosis, hypertensive hemorrhage, and ruptured saccular aneurysm. *Clin Neurosurg* 22:117–147, 1995.

Kase CS. Intracerebral hemorrhage: Non-hypertensive causes. *Stroke* 17:590–594, 1986.

Kassell NF, et al. The International Cooperative Study on the Timing of Aneurysm Surgery. II. Surgical results. *J Neurosurg* 73:18–36, 1990.

Lisk DR, et al. Early presentation of hemispheric intracerebral hemorrhage. Prediction of outcome and guidelines for treatment allocation. *Neurology* 44:133–139, 1994.

Mayberg MR, et al. Guidelines for the management of aneurysmal subarachnoid hemorrhage: A statement for health care professionals from a special writing group of the Stroke Council, American Heart Association. *Stroke* 25:2315–2328, 1994.

Mendelow AD. Spontaneous intracerebral haemorrhage. *J Neurol Neurosurg Psychiat* 54:193–195, 1991.

Ropper AH, Gress DR. Computerized tomography and clinical features of large cerebral hemorrhages. *Cerebrovasc Dis* 1:38–42, 1991.

Vermeulen M, van Gijn J. The diagnosis of subarachnoid hemorrhage. *J Neurol Neurosurg Psychiat* 50:365–372, 1990.

Epilepsies in Children
Hema Patel
David W. Dunn

Approximately 3% of the United States population can be expected to have **epilepsy** at some time during their lives. Among children, 3–4% have a febrile seizure during the first 6 years of life, 2% have a single afebrile seizure, and 0.5% have recurrent afebrile seizures.

I. Classification. Accurate characterization of epilepsy has practical significance. The differentiation between partial and generalized seizures is important for the correct choice of antiepileptic drug (AED) therapy, determination of etiology, and prognosis. The most widely used classification describes epilepsies and epileptic syndromes with particular reference to age of onset, etiology, site of seizure onset, and prognosis. Refer to Chap. 39 for clinical descriptions of the different types of seizures.

   A. Localization-related epilepsies and syndromes are characterized by partial seizures arising from a focal cortical area with occasional progression to a generalized seizure. If this progression is rapid, the initial focal nature may be masked. A simple partial seizure is associated with intact consciousness, whereas during a complex partial seizure, consciousness is impaired. Electroencephalography (EEG) shows focal epileptiform discharges overlying the epileptogenic region. A simple partial seizure may progress to a complex partial seizure. During any focal seizure (simple or complex partial), the focal epileptic excitation may spread diffusely, resulting in a secondarily generalized tonic-clonic seizure.

   1. Idiopathic epilepsies with age-related onset are common epileptic syndromes that comprise about one-fourth of all epilepsies with onset before 13 years of age. They are characterized by genetic predisposition; focal (localization-related) seizures and EEG abnormalities; normal intellect, neurologic examination, and neuroimaging and laboratory studies; and an excellent prognosis.

   a. Benign focal epilepsy of childhood with centrotemporal spikes (BFECTS). This disorder was previously known as benign rolandic epilepsy.

   (1) BFECTS comprises 75% of the benign focal childhood epilepsies.

   (2) Age of onset is 8–10 years.

   (3) Clinical features include unilateral motor seizures mainly involving facial grimacing and twitching, inability to speak, salivation, and occasional progression to a generalized tonic-clonic seizure. Seizures are usually nocturnal, during sleep.

   (4) EEG shows frequent, unilateral or bilateral, high-amplitude centrotemporal spikes that are activated by sleep. If an initial EEG is normal, a repeat sleep-deprived EEG to include sleep should be obtained.

   (5) Treatment is usually unnecessary after the first or even the second seizure. AED therapy may be initiated after a second documented seizure. All major AEDs have been reported to be successful even in small dosages. Carbamazepine is the drug of choice. Valproic acid is also effective. Phenobarbital and phenytoin, although effective, have the disadvantages of sedative and cosmetic side effects. It may be preferable to maintain AED therapy up to 14–16 years of age. Seizures spontaneously resolve by that time.

   (6) Prognosis is excellent. Approximately 13–20% of patients have only a single seizure. Seizures usually resolve within 1–3 years of onset and no later than 16 years of age. About 1–2% persist into adult life.

b. Benign childhood epilepsy with occipital spike waves (BEOSW)
   (1) BEOSW comprises 25% of the benign focal childhood epilepsies.
   (2) Age of onset is 4–5 years, with girls being affected more frequently than boys.
   (3) Clinical features include frequent, brief (a few seconds to 2–3 minutes) diurnal seizures characterized by visual illusions (multicolored circles or spots) or blindness, followed by postictal headaches. Consciousness may be preserved, but it is impaired if the seizure secondarily generalizes. BEOSW is often misinterpreted as basilar (Bickerstaff's) migraine.
   (4) EEG exhibits occipital paroxysms of high amplitude, often bilateral sharp/spike slow-wave complexes attenuating with eye opening. Generalized or centrotemporal spike waves are observed in one-third of all cases.
   (5) Treatment is similar to that for BFECTS.
   (6) Prognosis. There is some controversy regarding the benign nature of BEOSW. Clinical remission rates vary from 60–90%.
c. Benign focal childhood epilepsies that have not yet achieved international acceptance
   (1) Benign childhood epilepsy with affective symptoms presents with brief seizures characterized by screaming, automatisms (chewing), autonomic disturbances (pallor, sweating, and abdominal pain), and speech arrest occurring in the first decade with remission within 1–2 years and excellent response to treatment. EEG shows focal epileptiform discharges in the frontotemporal and parietotemporal electrodes.
   (2) Benign childhood epilepsy with somatosensory evoked spikes
   (3) Benign childhood epilepsy with frontal and with midline spikes
2. Symptomatic partial (localization-related) epilepsies. Most localization-related epilepsies are symptomatic or acquired. The clinical manifestation of the seizure depends on the anatomic location of the epileptogenic focus. Temporal lobe seizures (complex partial seizures) are the most common type of symptomatic partial seizures.
B. Generalized epilepsies and syndromes are characterized by seizures that are generalized from onset with initial involvement of both hemispheres. These seizures are usually associated with impairment of consciousness, and the EEG patterns are generalized and bilateral, reflecting involvement of both hemispheres. They include absence seizures, atypical absence seizures, myoclonic seizures, atonic seizures, generalized tonic-clonic seizures (GTCS), tonic seizures, clonic seizures, and infantile spasms.
1. Idiopathic epilepsies with age-related onset. In these disorders, which are listed below in order of age of appearance, the seizures and EEG abnormalities are generalized from the very onset. Intellect, neurologic examination, and neuroimaging and laboratory studies other than EEG are normal (idiopathic). There is a genetic predisposition with no other identifiable etiology.
   a. Benign neonatal familial convulsions. This is a rare, autosomal dominant epilepsy with a genetic defect localized to chromosome 20q. Seizures occur on the second or third day of life and are relatively refractory to AED therapy. Other causes of neonatal seizures, such as infection or metabolic, toxic, or structural abnormalities, should be excluded.
   b. Benign neonatal convulsions. Seizures occur on the fifth day of life without known etiology. The prognosis is good with no seizure recurrence and normal subsequent psychomotor development.
   c. Benign myoclonic epilepsy in infancy
      (1) Age of onset is 1–2 years.
      (2) Clinical features are brief, generalized myoclonic seizures in an otherwise normal child, usually with a positive family history of epilepsy.
      (3) EEG shows brief, generalized bursts of spike-polyspike wave activity.
      (4) Treatment. Valproic acid is the drug of choice. Clonazepam may be

used if valproic acid is ineffective. Seizures are exacerbated by phenytoin and carbamazepine.

  (5) Prognosis. Response to treatment is good. Occasionally, some psychomotor delay and behavioral abnormalities may persist.

  d. Childhood absence epilepsy (pyknolepsy). See Chap. 6.

  e. Juvenile absence epilepsy. See Chap. 6.

  f. Juvenile myoclonic epilepsy (impulsive petit mal) of Janz. See Chap. 6.

  g. Epilepsy with GTCS on awakening. See Chap. 6.

 2. Symptomatic and/or cryptogenic epilepsies. These disorders, which are listed below in order of age of appearance, include generalized epilepsy syndromes that are secondary to known or suspected disorders of the CNS (symptomatic) or to disorders whose causes are hidden or occult (cryptogenic).

  a. West's syndrome (infantile spasms), salaam convulsions

   (1) Etiology. Approximately 30–40% of cases are cryptogenic. In symptomatic cases there is evidence of previous brain damage (mental retardation, neurologic and radiologic evidence, or known etiology). See Table 38-1.

   (2) Age of onset. Onset occurs in infancy (peak 4–6 months).

   (3) Clinical features comprise the triad of infantile spasms, mental retardation, and hypsarrhythmia. Several infantile spasms occur in clusters, frequently during drowsiness and on awakening. They are characterized by brief nodding of the head associated with extension or flexion of the trunk, and often of the extremities, and they occur rapidly, suggestive of a startle reaction. They may be flexor (salaam attacks), extensor, or mixed spasms. They are almost always associated with arrested development.

   (4) EEG shows hypsarrhythmia—chaotic, high-amplitude, disorganized background with multifocal spikes. Intravenous pyridoxine (vitamin B_6) should be administered in a dosage of 100 mg during the EEG to exclude pyridoxine-dependent infantile spasms.

   (5) Treatment

    (a) Treat underlying conditions as identified.

    (b) Adrenocorticotropic hormone (ACTH). Opinions vary regarding dosage and duration of ACTH therapy, ranging from high-dosage therapy (160 units/m^2/day) to low-dosage therapy (20–40 units/day). We recommend starting at 40 units/day intramuscular and continuing for 3–4 weeks, or for a shorter period if an early positive clinical response is observed. The dosage is then slowly decreased over 6–9 weeks by 20% per week. If seizures recur during withdrawal, the dosage should be increased to the previous effective level. ACTH therapy is initi-

---

Table 38-1. Causes of secondary generalized epilepsy syndromes (infantile spasms and Lennox-Gastaut syndrome).

Idiopathic/Cryptogenic

Symptomatic
Perinatal factors: hypoxic-ischemic encephalopathy, hypoglycemia, hypocalcemia
Infections: intrauterine infections (toxoplasmosis, rubella, cytomegalovirus, herpes), meningoencephalitis
Cerebral malformations: holoprosencephaly, lissencephaly, Aicardi's syndrome
Vascular: infarction, hemorrhage, porencephaly
Neurocutaneous syndromes: tuberous sclerosis, Sturge-Weber syndrome, incontinentia pigmenti, others (e.g., neurofibromatosis)
Metabolic diseases: nonketotic hyperglycinemia, pyridoxine deficiency, aminoacidopathies (phenylketonuria, maple syrup urine disease)
Degenerative disorders: neuronal ceroid lipofuscinosis (Batten disease)
Chromosomal disorders: Down syndrome, Angelman's syndrome (happy puppet syndrome: abnormality in chromosome 15q11-13, seizures, developmental delay, dysmorphic features, paroxysms of inappropriate laughter)

ated in the hospital under the guidance of a pediatric neurologist. Parents should be taught the injection technique with systematic rotation of injection site.

(c) **Side effects of ACTH therapy** are irritability, hyperglycemia, hypertension, sodium and water retention, potassium depletion, weight gain, gastric ulcers, occult GI bleeding, and diabetic ketoacidosis.

(d) **Laboratory tests prior to initiation of ACTH therapy** include serum electrolytes, BUN, serum creatinine, glucose, urinalysis, CBC, chest x-ray, and tuberculin skin test.

(e) **Laboratory tests performed weekly during ACTH therapy** include serum electrolytes, blood glucose, stool guaiac, and monitoring of weight and blood pressure.

(f) **Concomitant management.** Antacid gel and/or histamine$_2$ receptor antagonist (cimetidine) should be administered during ACTH therapy.

(6) **Alternative treatment**

(a) **Prednisone** may be substituted when ACTH cannot be administered because parents cannot or will not learn to give injections. It is administered orally at 2–3 mg/kg/day for 3–4 weeks and gradually withdrawn in a schedule similar to ACTH withdrawal.

(b) **Valproic acid** is initiated at 10–15 mg/kg/day in three divided doses and is increased according to the clinical response. Usually, high therapeutic levels of 75–125 μg/ml are required to achieve seizure control.

(c) **Benzodiazepines.** Clonazepam at 0.03 mg/kg/day is administered in two or three divided doses and gradually increased to 0.1 mg/kg/day. Common side effects include extreme somnolence and excessive oral secretions. Nitrazepam at a dosage of 0.5–1.5 mg/kg/day has also been tried but is not commercially available in the United States.

(d) **Ketogenic diet** requires hospitalization for initiation under the expertise of a pediatric neurologist and an experienced dietitian. To be effective, it should be maintained for at least 1 year. Hypoglycemia, vomiting, and dehydration are common associated problems.

(e) **Vigabatrin** has been used in Europe with some success but is not yet approved in the United States.

(f) **Vitamin B$_6$.** The efficacy of this vitamin has not been confirmed.

(g) **Excisional surgery** of the region of cortical abnormality defined by EEG, MRI, and positron emission tomography (PET) is being performed in children with infantile spasms intractable to medical therapy, but only in specialized centers.

(7) **Prognosis.** West's syndrome has a high morbidity, with a 90% incidence of mental retardation. From 25–50% of the cases evolve into Lennox-Gastaut syndrome, with infantile spasms transforming to other seizure types (GTCS, and myoclonic and tonic seizures) over subsequent years. Favorable prognostic indicators are as follows.

(a) Cryptogenic spasms, which have a better prognosis than cases in which there are preexisting neurologic conditions

(b) Normal development and neurologic examination before the onset of spasms

(c) Short duration of seizures before control

b. **Lennox-Gastaut syndrome**

(1) **Etiology.** A significant number of patients have histories of infantile spasms. From 10–40% of cases are cryptogenic. In 60–90% of symptomatic cases, a specific cause—usually perinatal insult—is found (see Table 38-1).

(2) **Age of onset** is 1–7 years.

(3) **Clinical features** comprise seizures of multiple types that are often frequent and intractable to medical treatment—commonly tonic, atonic, or atypical absence seizures but also myoclonic, GTCS, and partial seizures. Seizures usually are associated with severe psychomotor retardation.

(4) **EEG** exhibits slow background activity and generalized, bisynchronous arrhythmic, sharp-and-slow-wave discharges (1–2 Hz) activated by sleep.

(5) **Treatment.** Sedative AED therapy should be avoided if possible, because AEDs may increase seizure frequency by decreasing alertness in patients.

 (a) **Valproic acid monotherapy** is effective against all the different types of seizures associated with Lennox-Gastaut syndrome. However, these seizures are often intractable, and valproic acid may have to be used in combination with phenytoin, ethosuximide, phenobarbital, primidone, carbamazepine, or even benzodiazepines (clonazepam, Tranxene), depending on the types of seizures.

 (b) **Ketogenic diet** may be effective in occasional patients with otherwise intractable seizures.

 (c) **Lamotrigine and gabapentin** have been recently approved for use in adults in the United States. Trials involving small numbers of patients have shown these drugs to be potentially effective in children with Lennox-Gastaut syndrome. Clobazam is not currently approved in the United States but, like other benzodiazepines, has been occasionally effective.

 (d) **ACTH** has been found to be effective in some patients.

 (e) **Psychological support** for the child and family are often helpful.

 (f) **Referral to occupational therapy** for protective helmets to prevent head injuries in patients with drop attacks.

 (g) **Surgical procedures** such as corpus callostomy and hemispherectomy have been tried, with variable results.

 (h) **Felbamate** was found to be effective but is no longer used because of reported severe side effects such as aplastic anemia and acute liver failure.

c. **Myoclonic seizures** are difficult to differentiate from nonepileptic myoclonus. However, characteristic epileptiform discharges associated with myoclonic jerks in myoclonic epilepsy help distinguish the two. Valproic acid in high dosages may be effective. It may have to be used in combination with clonazepam, lorazepam, nitrazepam, or the ketogenic diet.

 (1) **Early myoclonic encephalopathy.** Etiology is not known. Other causes of symptomatic myoclonic epilepsy, including inborn errors of metabolism (particularly nonketotic hyperglycinemia), hypoxic ischemic encephalopathy, and dysgenetic brain disorders, should be excluded. Early myoclonic encephalopathy is characterized by onset of medically intractable myoclonic seizures in early infancy, burst suppression on EEG, and very poor prognosis including death or profound neurologic impairment.

 (2) **Severe infantile myoclonic epilepsy** occurs before 2 years of age in previously normal children. It is characterized by myoclonic seizures and GTCS with characteristic spike/polyspike-wave activity on EEG, followed by other seizure types including absence, tonic, and partial seizures. Later, neurologic impairment, including mental retardation and ataxia, become evident.

 (3) **Symptomatic myoclonic epilepsy** is associated with specific progressive neurologic diseases such as Lafora's disease, Baltic myoclonus (Unverricht-Lundborg disease), neuronal ceroid lipofuscinosis (Batten disease), sialidoses, mitochondrial encephalomyopathies, and Ramsay Hunt syndrome.

C. **Epilepsies and syndromes undetermined as to whether focal or generalized**

 1. **Neonatal seizures**

 a. **Clinical features.** Neonatal seizures are more fragmentary than seizures in older children. GTCS do not occur in neonates. Common causes are outlined in Table 38-2. Some types of seizures are almost always associated with electrographic changes. They can be classified as follows.

 (1) **Seizures associated with electrographic signatures** include fo-

Table 38-2. Common causes of neonatal seizures.

Trauma: subdural hematoma, intracerebral hemorrhage
Asphyxia
Congenital abnormalities: lissencephaly, holoprosencephaly
Metabolic: hypocalcemia, hypomagnesemia, hypoglycemia, hyponatremia, hypernatremia
Infections: meningitis, encephalitis (herpes), abscess, cytomegalovirus, toxoplasmosis
Drug withdrawal: heroin, barbiturate, methadone
Pyridoxine dependency
Amino-acid disturbances: urea cycle disorder, nonketotic hyperglycinemia
Neurocutaneous and genetic syndromes: tuberous sclerosis, phenylketonuria, galactosemia
Benign familial epilepsy

cal clonic seizures, focal tonic seizures, some myoclonic seizures, and, rarely, apnea. These seizures are usually associated with focal structural lesions (infarction or hemorrhage), infections, or metabolic abnormalities (hypoglycemia or hypocalcemia).

(2) **Seizures not associated with electrographic signatures** include generalized tonic seizures, some myoclonic seizures, and subtle seizures (oral-buccal-lingual movements, bicycling movements, and some rhythmic ocular movements such as horizontal eye deviation). These seizures are usually observed in lethargic, comatose neonates with poor prognoses, such as those with severe hypoxic ischemic encephalopathy.

b. **Evaluation.** Neonatal seizures should be treated in a neonatal intensive care unit by experienced personnel including a pediatric neurologist and a neonatologist.

(1) **History and examination.** A detailed history, including illness during pregnancy, maternal drug and alcohol abuse, perinatal history, and family history, should be obtained. A general physical examination, including evaluation of the skin and the anterior fontanelle, and neurologic and ophthalmologic exams, should be performed.

(2) **Laboratory data.** Serum glucose; electrolytes; magnesium; calcium; phosphate; BUN; serum creatinine; ammonia; arterial blood gas; CBC; lumbar puncture to rule out infection and subarachnoid hemorrhage; urinalysis for amino acids, organic acids, and ketones; maternal and infant titers for toxoplasmosis, rubella, cytomegalovirus, and herpes (TORCH); and VDRL are usually indicated. Additional studies, such as CSF lactate, plasma amino acids and very-long-chain fatty acids, and leukocyte and fibroblast enzyme studies, may be indicated if metabolic disorders are suspected. Head ultrasound at bedside to rule out intracranial hemorrhage, and a non-contrast-enhanced CT scan of the head when the neonate is stable, can be performed. EEG is especially useful for the diagnosis of subclinical seizures.

c. **Treatment**

(1) **Treatment of underlying cause.** Treatment begins with the underlying cause of the seizures, such as a CNS infection or specific metabolic abnormality (hypoglycemia, hypocalcemia, or hypomagnesemia).

(2) **Phenobarbital** is the initial drug of choice. A loading dose of 20 mg/kg is given intravenously, with additional 5–10 mg/kg boluses as needed to control clinical seizures and attain therapeutic serum levels of 20–40 μg/ml. Maintenance doses of 2–4 mg/kg/day given in bid dosing are sufficient because phenobarbital has a relatively long half-life in the neonate. Close cardiorespiratory monitoring is important because IV administration of phenobarbital may be associated with respiratory depression and hypotension.

(3) **Phenytoin** is added if a phenobarbital level of 40 μg/ml is not sufficient to control seizures. An IV loading dose of 20 mg/kg results in serum levels ranging from 15–20 μg/ml. Thereafter, a maintenance dose of 3–4 mg/kg/day is administered in bid dosing. It is infused

slowly with cardiac monitoring, because it may cause cardiac arrhythmias and prolonged Q–T intervals.

(4) Diazepam is administered by continuous IV infusion in isotonic saline at 0.1–0.3 mg/kg/hour. Lorazepam has similar efficacy.

(5) IV pyridoxine (100 mg) administered during EEG monitoring causes cessation of seizures and normalization of the EEG within minutes in the rare patient with pyridoxine-dependent seizures.

2. **Acquired epileptic aphasia (Landau-Kleffner syndrome)** is characterized by acquired aphasia, including verbal auditory agnosia, rapid reduction of spontaneous speech, and behavioral and psychomotor disturbances. Seizures (generalized and focal) and EEG abnormalities including multifocal spikes and spike-wave discharges are rare and usually remit before the age of 15 years. However, the ultimate outcome is still unclear.

D. Special syndromes
 1. **Situation-related seizures**
  a. **Febrile seizures**
   (1) Incidence. Febrile seizures occur in 2–5% of young children.
   (2) Age of onset ranges from 3 months to 5 years (peak 6 months to 2 years), familial.
   (3) Clinical features, which usually manifest within the first few hours of acute infection, include upper respiratory infections, otitis media, and gastrointestinal infections. Intracranial infections and other defined causes such as dehydration and electrolyte imbalance should be excluded.
    (a) Simple febrile seizures present as single, brief GTCS without associated evidence of intracranial infection or defined cause.
    (b) Complex febrile seizures are prolonged (more than 15 minutes), have focal features (focal onset or Todd's paralysis postictally) and occur at a rate of more than one seizure within 24 hours.
   (4) Evaluation. Lumbar puncture (LP) is indicated unless the possibility of meningitis can be confidently eliminated clinically. LP should be performed in all children less than 18 months of age, because they may not always exhibit meningeal signs in the face of meningitis. If in doubt, err on the side of performing the LP. Serum electrolytes and glucose tests should be performed.
   (5) Acute treatment of seizure
    (a) The patient should be admitted overnight for observation if the seizure was prolonged or multiple.
    (b) Phenobarbital in an IV loading dose of 15–20 mg/kg is administered slowly at the rate of 1 mg/kg/min, followed the next day by a maintenance dose of 3–5 mg/kg/day in bid dosing.
    (c) Some pediatric neurologists use oral or rectal diazepam (0.1–0.3 mg/kg) only when fever is present and have found it to be effective in reducing the risk of recurrent febrile seizures. Potential side effects include lethargy, irritability, and ataxia.
    (d) Any underlying infection or fever should be treated.
   (6) Long-term treatment of seizure
    (a) Daily phenobarbital treatment reduces the risk of recurrent febrile seizures and may be indicated for patients with complex febrile seizures, abnormal underlying neurologic exams, family histories of nonfebrile seizures, recurrent febrile seizures, or febrile seizures at less than 1 year of age.
    (b) Valproic acid is the second choice because of increased incidence of side effects including liver toxicity in this age group. Carbamazepine and phenytoin are ineffective in the treatment of febrile seizures.
   (7) Prognosis. Approximately 33% of children with febrile seizures have at least one recurrence, and 9% have three or more seizures. Remission occurs by 6 years of age in approximately 90% of children.
    (a) A risk factor for recurrence is early age (less than 1 year) at initial seizure.
    (b) Risk factors for developing epilepsy include complex febrile

seizures, underlying developmental or neurologic abnormalities, and family history of nonfebrile seizures.

b. Seizures related to identifiable situations. Such situations include stress, hormonal changes, use of drugs (theophylline, stimulants, or neuroleptics), use of alcohol, and sleep deprivation.

2. Isolated apparently unprovoked epileptic events

3. Epilepsies characterized by specific modes of seizure precipitation include seizures occurring in response to discrete or specific stimuli (reflex epilepsy), such as reading epilepsy, hot water epilepsy, and arithmetic epilepsy.

4. Chronic progressive epilepsia partialis continua of childhood (Kozhevnikov's epilepsy) syndrome is thought to be a result of chronic encephalitis (Rasmussen's encephalitis). The cause is unknown. It is characterized by partial motor seizures, often associated with myoclonus, that are resistant to treatment, and it results in progressive hemiplegia with unilateral brain atrophy and mental retardation.

II. Evaluation. Details regarding histories, physical examinations, and studies such as electroencephalography and neuroimaging are discussed in Chap. 6. Important aspects of the evaluation with respect to children are outlined below.

A. It is important to determine if the paroxysmal events in question are in fact epileptic. They should be differentiated from **nonepileptic paroxysmal events** in children (see Chap. 34).

B. Specific predisposing factors for childhood seizures

   1. Birth history

   a. Prenatal. Duration of pregnancy, complications (e.g., toxemia or premature labor), medications, and alcohol and drug abuse

   b. Perinatal. Complications of labor and delivery, use of vacuum or forceps, birth weight, and Apgar scores

   c. Postnatal. Care received in nursery (including intensive respiratory care), and problems such as intraventricular hemorrhage and exchange transfusions

   2. Developmental history. Learning disabilities, attention deficit, and developmental regression (loss of previously attained developmental milestones) that may be associated with a degenerative disease

C. Physical examination is an extension of information obtained in the history. In addition to the physical examination described in Chap. 6, specific aspects in children include:

   1. Head circumference. Microcephaly and macrocephaly are associated with various neurologic disorders.

   2. Height and weight abnormalities may be secondary to endocrine disorders related to midline CNS tumors.

   3. Dysmorphic features associated with storage diseases or brain malformations

   4. Skin. Neurocutaneous disorders: café-au-lait spots suggest neurofibromatosis, hypopigmented macules and adenoma sebaceum are observed in tuberous sclerosis, and facial hemangiomas are seen in Sturge-Weber syndrome.

   5. Hair. Broken hair and alopecia suggest metabolic disorders (biotinidase deficiency, Menkes' syndrome, and argininosuccinic aciduria).

   6. Mental status and behavioral pattern. Evaluate development. Loss of previously attained milestones may be indicative of a neurodegenerative disease, whereas delays in achieving developmental milestones reflect static encephalopathies (e.g., cerebral palsy). Presence of anxiety, depression, and family conflict may lead to possible diagnosis of psychogenic seizures.

   7. Systemic exam. Organomegaly may suggest a storage disease or an inborn error of metabolism.

D. Laboratory testing. In addition to EEG and MRI of the head, other important studies in children include:

   1. Chemical and metabolic screening. Electrolytes, glucose, calcium, magnesium, hepatic and renal function tests, and toxic screening for possible drug ingestion. Elevation of serum prolactin and serum creatine kinase may help distinguish seizures from nonepileptiform paroxysmal disorders. However, they must be obtained within 30 minutes after an episode and then be compared with baseline values. Thyroid functions should be obtained because seizures are rarely associated with thyrotoxicosis. Specific metabolic or neurodegenerative disorders may be diagnosed by tests such as urinalysis for amino acids, organic acids, lysosomal enzymes (mucopolysaccharidosis and Batten disease), and very-long-chain fatty acids (peroxisomal disorders such as adrenoleukodystrophy).

2. **Lumbar puncture (LP)** is indicated if there are signs suggestive of acute CNS infection or inflammation (e.g., fever or stiff neck). LP is indicated for all children less than 1 year of age with history of fever and seizures, because clinical signs of CNS infection may be absent. LP should also be performed on all febrile patients with new-onset seizures.

3. **Chromosomal analysis** is indicated if dysmorphic features suggest chromosomal abnormalities.

4. **Skin biopsy** is performed to diagnose certain metabolic diseases such as Batten disease.

5. **Simultaneous prolonged video-EEG monitoring** in an epilepsy unit may help determine the exact nature of paroxysmal events if they cannot be defined by routine EEGs.

III. Treatment

  A. **Single seizure.** Approximately 9% of the population will have a seizure sometime during their lives, and about 3% will have more than one seizure. The risk of recurrence is highest in the first year after a single seizure. It is low if the patient has a normal neurologic exam, a single GTCS with a negative family history, a normal neuroimaging study, and a normal or mildly slow EEG.

  1. **Indications for treatment**
     a. Clear-cut epileptiform abnormalities on EEG
     b. Lesions on CT or MRI
     c. Abnormal neurologic exam suggesting prior brain damage
     d. Active CNS infection (encephalitis, meningitis, or abscess)
     e. Status epilepticus as the first seizure
     f. Certain types of seizures, including infantile spasms, Lennox-Gastaut syndrome, and focal seizures
     g. Unprovoked or asymptomatic single seizure with history suggesting that one may have occurred earlier

  2. **Treatment is not indicated** when seizures are provoked by a correctable metabolic disturbance (glucose or electrolyte abnormalities), sleep deprivation, exposure to drugs or alcohol, febrile illness, or physical or emotional stress. In such cases the underlying disturbance should be corrected.

  B. **General principles of treatment**
  1. **Choice of appropriate drug** should be based on the clinical description of the seizures (Table 38-3). This choice may be influenced by other factors, such as the patient's age, economic circumstances, and child-bearing poten-

Table 38-3. Drugs for treatment of epilepsy.

Type of seizures	First-line drug(s)	Second-line drugs
Partial		
Simple partial, complex partial, GTCS	Carbamazepine, phenytoin	Phenobarbital (<4 years), valproic acid, primidone, gabapentin or lamotrigine (>16 years), felbamate
Generalized		
Absence (typical, atypical)	Ethosuximide, valproic acid	Clonazepam, acetazolamide
Myoclonic	Valproic acid	Clonazepam, phenobarbital, primidone, acetazolamide, chlorazepate
Tonic-clonic	Valproic acid, phenytoin	Phenobarbital, primidone, carbamazepine
Atonic	Valproic acid, felbamate	Phenobarbital, clonazepam, clorazepate
Infantile spasms	ACTH	Prednisone, valproic acid, felbamate, ketogenic diet

tial (e.g., phenytoin is preferred in the child-bearing age group because it has the least teratogenic side effects).

2. **Monotherapy.** Start with one drug beginning at one-third to one-half the recommended dosage and gradually increase it until seizures are controlled or intolerable side effects appear. Approximately 75–80% of children should respond to monotherapy. If the first drug is ineffective, start a second AED and, after therapeutic levels are achieved, gradually withdraw the first drug.

3. **Polypharmacy** is indicated only if monotherapy with at least two first-line AEDs fails and should be initiated only after consultation with a pediatric neurologist. Problems with polypharmacy include drug interactions, difficulties in acquiring therapeutic levels of either drug despite use of very high dosages, and increased risks of toxicity.

4. **Simplify medication schedule.** Decreasing the number of doses will improve compliance. For the older child, phenobarbital and phenytoin may be given in single nighttime doses. However, carbamazepine and valproic acid have shorter half-lives and should be given in at least two or three divided daily doses.

5. **Avoid sedative anticonvulsants** such as benzodiazepines—especially for patients with secondary generalized epilepsy syndrome—because increased sedation may result in increased seizure frequency.

6. **Maintain a seizure diary.** Record seizure frequency, medication dosages and levels, and occurrence of side effects, if any.

7. **Anticonvulsant level** should be checked just prior to a dose, preferably the morning dose to obtain the lowest (trough) level. It is helpful to monitor the level at a consistent time in order to avoid misinterpretation of fluctuations. CBC and serum glutamic-oxaloacetic transaminase (SGOT) are checked every 1–2 months initially and then every 6 months after a steady dosage has been established. AED blood level should be checked:

   a. After starting a medication, to aid in initial titration of dosage to achieve a therapeutic level.
   b. After making a major change in drug dosage.
   c. If seizures recur on the usual dosage of AED.
   d. If seizures persist despite "correct therapy."
   e. If symptoms of toxicity develop.
   f. If noncompliance is suspected.

8. **Repeat EEG** during therapy if there is a change in the character of the seizures, or if the child has been seizure-free for a significant period, to help decide if medications can be withdrawn.

C. **Drug therapy.** The following information serves as a broad guideline for commonly used AEDs in children. Details regarding their metabolism, side effects, and interactions are discussed in detail in Chap. 39.

1. **Phenytoin (Dilantin)**
   a. **Indications.** Focal seizures (simple and complex partial seizures, partial seizures with secondary generalization), status epilepticus, and generalized epilepsy manifested by GTCS
   b. **Dosage.** 3–8 mg/kg/day in a single dose or two divided doses
   c. **Serum half-life.** 24 ± 12 hours
   d. **Metabolism.** Hydroxylated by liver. Phenytoin has nonlinear elimination kinetics. Therefore, small increases in dosage after therapeutic levels of 10–20 μg/ml have been achieved result in large increases in plasma levels and toxicity.
   e. **Therapeutic blood level.** 10–20 μg/ml
   f. **Formulation.** Capsules: 30 and 100 mg; Infatabs: 50 mg; suspension: 125 mg/5 ml and 30 mg/5 ml. Dilantin suspension is not recommended for routine use because it is unreliable.
   g. **Side effects.** Dosage-related side effects are nystagmus, ataxia, and drowsiness. Gingival hypertrophy requiring more frequent dental cleaning, hirsutism, coarsening of features, blood dyscrasias, Stevens-Johnson syndrome, and megaloblastic anemia may also occur. Fetal hydantoin syndrome is characterized by craniofacial anomalies, hypoplasia of distal phalanges, intrauterine growth retardation, and mental deficiency. It occurs not only in children exposed to phenytoin in utero, but also in those exposed to other AEDs such as phenobarbital, primidone, mephobarbital, and phensuximide.

2. Carbamazepine (Tegretol)
   a. Indications. Focal seizures (simple and complex partial seizures, partial seizures with secondary generalization) and generalized epilepsies manifested by GTCS
   b. Dosage. Start at 5 mg/kg/day and increase by 5 mg/kg/day every 3–4 days to a maximum of 15–20 mg/kg/day in two or three divided doses. Check levels at that time and then titrate dosage further if needed to achieve therapeutic blood levels.
   c. Serum half-life. 12 ±6 hours
   d. Metabolism. Hepatic conversion to epoxide and other metabolites
   e. Therapeutic blood level. 4–12 μg/ml
   f. Formulation. Tablets: 200 mg; chewable tablets: 100 mg; elixir: 100 mg/5ml
   g. Side effects. Dosage-related side effects are sedation, blurred vision, and leukopenia. Agranulocytosis, aplastic anemia syndrome of inappropriate antidiuretic hormone secretion (SIADH) may also occur. There is a 0.5% risk of spina bifida with first-trimester exposure to carbamazepine. Developmental delay may also result.
   h. If oral administration is contraindicated, Tegretol elixir (100 mg/5 ml) can be given rectally, diluted 1:1 with water in an enema at a dosage of 10–20 mg/kg to attain therapeutic levels.

3. Phenobarbital
   a. Indications. Focal seizures (simple and complex partial seizures, partial seizures with secondary generalization), GTCS of generalized epilepsy (in which it may exacerbate absence, atypical absence, and myoclonic seizures), febrile seizures, and status epilepticus
   b. Dosage. 3–8 mg/kg/day in a single daily dose or two divided doses
   c. Serum half-life increases with age. It is 20–65 hours for patients less than 10 years old and 64–140 hours for those more than 15 years old. Therefore, children require higher maintenance dosages of 4–8 mg/kg/day as opposed to adults, who need only 1–2 mg/kg/day.
   d. Metabolism. Hydroxylation by the liver
   e. Therapeutic blood level. 15–40 μg/ml
   f. Formulation. Tablets: 15, 30, 60, and 100 mg; elixir: 20 mg/5 ml
   g. Side effects. Paradoxical hyperactivity, sedation, learning disabilities, personality changes, and Stevens-Johnson syndrome

4. Valproic acid (Depakene/Depakote)
   a. Indications. Primary generalized epilepsy (absence, myoclonic, GTCS), secondary generalized epilepsy syndrome (infantile spasms, Lennox-Gastaut syndrome), complex partial seizures, and febrile seizures
   b. Dosage. Start at 10–15 mg/kg/day and gradually increase to a maximum of 60 mg/kg/day in three divided doses.
   c. Serum half-life. 10 ±6 hours
   d. Metabolism. Hepatic
   e. Therapeutic blood level. 40–100 μg/ml
   f. Formulation. Depakote (divalproex sodium): enteric-coated tablets, 125, 250, and 500 mg; sprinkles, 125 mg. Depakene (sodium valproate): capsules, 250 mg; elixir, 250 mg/ml.
   g. Side effects. Dose-related side effects are nausea, vomiting, and gastric irritation, which can be minimized by the use of the sprinkles, the enteric-coated preparation, or administration after meals. Other side effects include weight gain, alopecia, tremor, thrombocytopenia, and liver failure. Liver failure is more common in children less than 2 years of age. It can be a fulminant progressive failure or a subacute gradually progressive failure. Valproic acid is therefore contraindicated in children with preexisting hepatic damage, organic acidurias, or carnitine deficiency. A 10% solution of carnitine (Carnitor) should be administered at 50 mg/kg/day in two or three divided doses in conjunction with valproic acid for children on long-term, high-dosage therapy with poor nutrition (e.g., cerebral palsy). Baseline liver function and serum ammonia should be checked prior to starting valproic acid and at least four to six times monthly while this medication is being given. There is a 1.5% risk of neural tube defects such as spina bifida and, less commonly, myelomeningocele in the fetus when valproic acid is used during pregnancy.

    h. If oral administration is contraindicated (e.g., paralytic ileus), Depakene elixir (250 mg/5 ml) can be given rectally, diluted 1:1 with water in an enema at a dosage of 20 mg/kg to attain therapeutic levels of 40–50 μg/ml.

  5. Ethosuximide (Zarontin)
    a. Indication. Absence seizures
    b. Dosage. 20–40 mg/kg/day in two or three divided doses
    c. Serum half-life. 30 ±6 hours
    d. Metabolism. Hepatic
    e. Therapeutic blood level. 40–80 μg/ml
    f. Formulation. Capsules: 250 mg; elixir: 250 mg/5 ml
    g. Side effects. Anorexia, nausea, hiccups, and hallucinations

  6. Primidone (Mysoline)
    a. Indications. GTCS and focal seizures (simple and complex partial seizures, partial seizures with secondary generalization)
    b. Dosage. 10–25 mg/kg/day in two divided doses
    c. Serum half-life. 12 ±6 hours
    d. Metabolism. Hepatic conversion to phenobarbital and PEMA (phenylethylmalonamide)
    e. Therapeutic blood levels. Primidone, 5–12 μg/ml; phenobarbital, 15–40 μg/ml
    f. Formulation. Tablets: 50 and 250 mg; suspension: 250 mg/5 ml
    g. Side effects. Sedation, tremor, behavioral changes, and skin rash

  7. Clonazepam (Klonopin)
    a. Indications. Myoclonic, focal (simple and complex partial), absence, and atonic seizures
    b. Dosage. 0.03–0.10 mg/kg/day in two or three divided doses
    c. Serum half-life. 22–33 hours
    d. Metabolism. Hepatic
    e. Therapeutic blood level. 40–70 ng/ml
    f. Formulation. Tablets: 0.5, 1, and 2 mg
    g. Side effects. Drowsiness, blurred vision, ataxia, and drooling

  8. Clorazepate (Tranxene)
    a. Indications. GTCS, focal seizures, and secondary generalized epilepsy syndrome
    b. Dosage. 0.3–3.0 mg/kg/day, increased to a maximum of 60 mg/day
    c. Serum half-life. 50–150 hours (prolonged in obesity)
    d. Metabolism. Converted to desmethyldiazepam (active form) in stomach within 20 minutes of oral administration
    e. Therapeutic blood level. Not established
    f. Formulation. Tablets: 7.5 mg
    g. Side effects. Drowsiness, dizziness, ataxia, and drooling

  9. Newer antiepileptic medications available in the United States include felbamate (Felbatol), lamotrigine (Lamictal), and gabapentin (Neurontin).

D. Psychosocial issues. The patient's family should be advised in regard to the following concerns.

  1. Risk factors to be avoided are fatigue, sleep deprivation, and medications that may lower the seizure threshold. Seat belts and bicycle helmets should be worn to prevent head injuries that may lead to seizures.

  2. Febrile illness must be treated promptly.

  3. Bathtubs should be avoided; only showers should be taken. Activities such as climbing of heights, swimming without supervision, driving, contact with heavy machinery and fire, and other activities that could be potentially dangerous in the event of a seizure should be avoided.

  4. Parents should guard against overprotection, which may develop out of fear and anxiety. Unnecessary limitations prevent the child from taking the risks that are necessary for him or her to become an independent person and develop self-confidence.

  5. Parents must inform schoolteachers (as well as baby-sitters) about the child's seizures. This allows teachers to be prepared to deal with seizures in the classroom and the reactions of classmates.

  6. Participation in activities such as sports and exercise should be permitted. If certain activities must be restricted because of poor seizure control, substitute exercise programs must be found.

7. A medication schedule that avoids school hours should be planned, because it is often inconvenient and embarrassing for a child to take AEDs at school.

8. Teachers should be expected to provide information about frequency of seizures during school hours, changes in the child's behavior that may indicate side effects, unexplained changes in school performance that may reflect increases in frequency or severity of seizures, and abnormal behavioral and social problems that may require referral for counseling.

9. Referral to services such as the Epilepsy Foundation of America or local support groups for counseling should be recommended.

IV. Status epilepticus

A. Definition. One or more seizures lasting for more than 30 minutes without full recovery of consciousness between seizures

B. Types

1. Generalized convulsive status epilepticus is characterized by persistent GTCS. In children, it is associated with a higher morbidity and mortality than in adults. We will therefore focus on the treatment of this type of status epilepticus.

2. Nonconvulsive status epilepticus includes cases of absence status and complex partial status and is often described as "twilight state."

C. Precipitating factors. Status epilepticus may be an initial unproved event or may occur as a result of:

1. Abrupt discontinuation of or changes in anticonvulsants (noncompliance).

2. Acute intercurrent infections such as meningitis and encephalitis.

3. Acute metabolic/toxic disturbances such as electrolyte disturbances, hypoglycemia, hyperpyrexia, and lead intoxication.

4. Acute cerebral insult such as subarachnoid hemorrhage, subdural hematoma, anoxia, hypoxia-ischemia, and depressed skull fractures.

D. Prognosis. Approximately 15% of all epileptic patients experience an episode of status epilepticus at some time in their lives. Morbidity is higher in children than in adults (approximately 10–25%), including most commonly hemiplegia and mental retardation. Recurrent status epilepticus is also more common in children.

E. Treatment

1. Confirmation of diagnosis of status epilepticus. The longer the seizure continues, the more difficult it is to control and the greater the possibility of permanent brain damage. One should be certain that the patient is in status epilepticus and is not merely postictal.

2. General measures

a. Position the child's head on one side to allow drainage of secretions. Loosen clothing and place a soft object (e.g., a pillow) under the head to avoid injuries during seizures.

b. Establish airway patency and ventilation by gentle suctioning to avoid enhancing seizure activity by overstimulation. A plastic airway should be inserted and taped securely. Wooden tongue blades and hard objects should not be used, because they can cause injuries to the mouth and teeth.

c. Oxygen administration by nasal cannula and quick initiation of general anesthesia with endotracheal intubation may prove necessary.

d. Monitor vital signs, including heart rate, blood pressure, and temperature (fever may be indicative of an infective process).

e. Place an IV line (preferably two, one with normal saline). Blood should be obtained at this time for CBC, electrolytes, calcium, magnesium, glucose, liver function tests, AED levels, toxicology screening, and blood cultures.

f. IV glucose (50% solution) at 2 ml/kg should be administered.

g. Consider lumbar puncture (LP) later in any febrile child—especially if less than 18 months of age—because meningitis may occur without clinical signs of neck stiffness.

h. Obtain a history surrounding the status epilepticus, as well as general and neurologic exams. Subsequent evaluation and treatment are often determined by prior history. In a patient with known seizures in whom status epilepticus may have been caused by AED withdrawal, the treatment of choice is reinstatement of the same drug.

3. Drug treatment involves administration of a drug for immediate termination of the seizure and a second drug for maintenance therapy. The initial treatment is similar regardless of the type of seizure. Maintenance treatment varies depending on the type of epilepsy. The protocol has been outlined in Table 38-4.

a. **Benzodiazepines**

(1) **IV Lorazepam (Ativan)** is recommended as a first-line treatment in a dosage of 0.05–0.10 mg/kg at a rate of 1–2 mg/minute to a maximum of 5 mg. Its advantages are rapid onset of action, prolonged antiepileptic activity compared with diazepam, and less respiratory depression after previous administration of anticonvulsants such as phenobarbital.

(2) **IV Diazepam** (0.2–0.5 mg/kg/dose, maximum of 5 mg) may also be used. Its disadvantages include short duration of action (less than ½ hour), high incidence of respiratory depression, and tendency to precipitate tonic status in patients with Lennox-Gastaut syndrome.

b. After IV lorazepam has been administered, give **IV phenytoin** slowly, at 18–20 mg/kg, not to exceed 1 mg/kg/minute or a total of 50 mg/minute. This will result in therapeutic levels of 18–20 μg/ml. Disadvantages of phenytoin include cardiac arrhythmias and hypotension requiring close ECG and blood pressure monitoring. Intramuscular administration is avoided because of unpredictable absorption and muscle irritation. Intravenous extravasation can result in phlebitis and tissue necrosis. Poor absorption occurs in children, resulting in difficulty in maintaining steady therapeutic levels, especially when the patient is switched to the oral form for maintenance. It should be administered in normal saline, because it precipitates in glucose solutions.

c. If seizures persist, **IV phenobarbital** is administered at 15–20 mg/kg at a rate of 50 mg/minute. In neonates, this may be administered as a single dose. In older children, it may be divided into aliquots of 10 mg/kg to avoid respiratory depression, until seizures stop or a maximum loading

Table 38-4. Management of generalized tonic-clonic status epilepticus in children.

Time from start of treatment	Procedure
0 minutes	Verify diagnosis of status epilepticus. Monitor cardiorespiratory function. ECG, pulse oximetry, and stabilize. EEG if possible. Insert oral airway, administer oxygen if needed. Insert IV catheter with normal saline. Draw AED levels, glucose, electrolytes, calcium, magnesium, BUN, CBC, arterial blood gas.
5 minutes	Start IV normal saline. Administer 50% glucose at 2 ml/kg.
10–30 minutes	IV lorazepam, 0.1 mg/kg, at 1–2 mg/min to maximum of 5 mg. Start IV phenytoin 18–20 mg/kg, at a rate not to exceed 1 mg/kg/min or 50 mg/min with ECG and blood pressure monitoring.
31–60 minutes	If seizures still persist, administer IV phenobarbital at a rate not to exceed 50 mg/min until seizures stop or give a loading dose of 20 mg/kg.
>60 minutes	If seizures still persist, available options include: (1) IV diazepam: continuous infusion, 50 mg diluted in 250 ml normal saline or D5W at 1 ml/kg/hr (2 mg/kg/hr) to achieve blood levels of 0.2–0.8 μg/ml. (2) IV pentobarbital: initial loading dose of 5 mg/kg followed by maintenance infusion of 1–3 mg/kg/hr (with EEG monitoring) to produce "burst suppression" pattern on EEG. Decrease infusion rate 4–6 hours later to check for reappearance of seizures. If seen, repeat procedure. If not, taper over 12–24 hours.
	If seizures are still not controlled, general anesthesia with halothane and neuromuscular blockade is instituted by an anesthesiologist.

dose of 20 mg/kg has been administered. Disadvantages of phenobarbital include hypotension and respiratory depression.

   d. A more detailed history and neurologic exam should be performed at this time. Evaluate the initial blood work. Prior to initiating additional therapies, it is preferable to order a CT without contrast enhancement and an LP to look for causes such as intracranial structural lesions or infections.

   e. Refractory status epilepticus. If seizures persist for 60 minutes and the patient fails to respond to loading doses of phenytoin and phenobarbital, the following drugs can be administered.

      (1) Diazepam drip (50 mg) diluted in 250 ml of normal saline or D5W in continuous infusion at a rate of 1 ml/kg/hour to achieve blood levels of 0.2–0.8 μg/ml.

      (2) Pentobarbital coma. Initial IV loading dose of 5 mg/kg followed by a maintenance dose of 1–3 mg/kg/hour, titrating dosage to achieve a "burst suppression" pattern on EEG

      (3) Phenobarbital may also be used by administering additional IV boluses of 5–10 mg/kg with EEG monitoring until seizures stop and a "burst suppression" pattern is obtained on EEG. The disadvantage of phenobarbital coma is that, because of a longer half-life, its effect takes longer to wear off. The recommended duration of coma is 48–72 hours. During this time, the patient is rechecked for seizures by decreasing the infusion rate. If seizures persist, the procedure is repeated. If they are adequately controlled, medication is slowly withdrawn. Administration of coma requires an ICU setting with controlled mechanical ventilation and close cardiac monitoring.

   f. If seizures are still not controlled, **general anesthesia** with halothane and neuromuscular blockade is recommended.

V. Medication withdrawal. Although there is no consensus on how long the patient should remain seizure-free before drug withdrawal is considered, a seizure-free period of 2–4 years is recommended. Relapse rates are higher in adults than in children. Children with febrile seizures have a 97% chance of outgrowing them by age 6 years. There is an 80–85% chance of remission in children with absence seizures.

  A. Favorable factors associated with lower relapse rate

    1. Reasonable ease of seizure control

    2. Normal neurologic exam and developmental milestones

    3. Normal EEG at time of withdrawal

    4. Early onset (less than 8 years)

    5. Certain seizure types: febrile seizures, absence seizures, GTCS

  B. Unfavorable factors associated with increased chances of recurrence

    1. Seizures of long duration before successful establishment of control

    2. Abnormal EEG at time of medication withdrawal

    3. Abnormal neurologic exam

    4. Later age of onset (more than 9 years)

    5. Certain seizure types: focal seizures, jacksonian epilepsy, infantile spasms, Lennox-Gastaut syndrome

VI. Surgical therapy. Procedures that resect or disconnect epileptogenic areas can reduce or eliminate seizures in patients with medically intractable epilepsy. These procedures are performed in specialized epilepsy centers. Extensive preoperative evaluation includes video-EEG monitoring to identify seizure focus, neuropsychiatric evaluation, neuroimaging studies (MRI, SPECT, and PET), intracarotid sodium amytal test (Wada's test), and even invasive studies (subdural and depth electrodes) if indicated. The most common types of epilepsy surgery in children are as follows.

  A. Resective surgery. Removal of the epileptogenic area (e.g., temporal lobectomy)

  B. Corpuscallosotomy. Interruption of the anterior two-thirds of the corpus callosum, effective in atonic seizures, tonic seizures, and GTCS.

  C. Hemispherectomy. One cerebral hemisphere is disconnected from the rest of the brain and a limited area is resected. It is performed in early-onset or congenital hemiplegia in which seizures arise from one side of the brain.

Recommended Readings

Aicardi J. *Epilepsy in Children.* New York: Raven, 1983.

Aicardi J, Chevrie JJ. Convulsive status epilepticus in infants and children: A study of 239 cases. *Epilepsia* 11:187–197, 1970.

Commission on Classification and Terminology of the International League Against Epilepsy. Proposal for revised classification of epilepsies and epileptic syndromes. *Epilepsia* 30:389–399, 1989.

Dodson WE, Pellock JM (eds). *Pediatric Epilepsy: Diagnosis and Therapy.* New York: Demos, 1993.

Gilman JT, Duchowny M. Childhood epilepsy: Current therapeutic recommendations. *CNS Drugs* 1(3):180–192, 1994.

Gumnit RJ. *The Epilepsy Handbook: The Practical Management of Seizures* (2nd ed). New York: Raven, 1995.

Levy RH, et al. (eds). *Antiepileptic Drugs* (3rd ed). New York: Raven, 1989.

Wyllie E (ed). *The Treatment of Epilepsy: Principles and Practice.* Philadelphia/London: Lea & Febiger, 1993.

39

Epilepsies in Adults
Omkar N. Markand

I. Definitions

A. An **epileptic seizure** is a transient and reversible alteration of behavior caused by a paroxysmal, abnormal, and excessive neuronal discharge.

B. Epilepsy is usually defined as two or more seizures not directly provoked by intracranial infection, drug withdrawal, acute metabolic changes, or fever. Antiepileptic drug (AED) therapy is usually initiated after at least two epileptic seizures have occurred—i.e., when a diagnosis of epilepsy has been made.

II. Classifications.
There are two classifications: one of seizure types and one of epilepsies or epileptic syndromes. Accurate diagnosis of the type(s) of epileptic seizures the patient has and categorization of the patient's epilepsy (or epileptic syndrome) are essential for proper selection of AED therapy and for prognosis.

A. Classification of epileptic seizures is based on the patient's behavior during seizures and on the associated EEG characteristics. Epileptic seizures are classified into two main types: partial and generalized.

1. Partial (focal) seizures arise at specific loci in the cerebral cortex, and are associated with focal interictal and ictal EEG changes. Clinically, a partial seizure may range in intensity from a disorder of sensation without loss of consciousness to a generalized convulsion.

a. Simple partial seizures. Consciousness remains intact. Such seizures may be motor seizures (focal motor twitchings or jacksonian seizures), sensory seizures (numbness or tingling involving parts of the body), autonomic seizures, or seizures with psychic symptoms.

b. Complex partial seizures. Consciousness is impaired during complex partial seizures. Previously, these seizures were called psychomotor seizures or temporal lobe seizures. They constitute the most common type of seizure in adults. Approximately 85% have epileptogenic focus in the temporal lobe, whereas the remaining 15% are of extratemporal origin (usually frontal).

c. Secondarily generalized (tonic-clonic) seizures. During any focal seizure (simple or complex partial), the epileptic excitation may spread widely to the entire brain, resulting in a generalized tonic-clonic convulsion.

2. Generalized seizures are characterized by generalized involvement of the brain from the outset and have no consistent focal areas of ictal onset. They are of many subtypes.

a. Absence seizures were formerly known as "petit mal" seizures. The dominant feature is a brief loss of consciousness with no or minimal motor manifestations (e.g., twitching of the eyelids). During the seizure the EEG shows 3-Hz generalized spike-wave discharges.

b. Myoclonic seizures are brief jerks involving part of the body or the entire body.

c. Clonic seizures are rhythmic twitchings of the body.

d. Tonic seizures are brief attacks of stiffness in part of the body or the entire body.

e. Atonic seizures are losses of posture with resultant drop attacks.

f. Tonic-clonic seizures are generalized convulsions or "grand mal" seizures. It is important to emphasize that there are tonic-clonic ("grand mal") seizures that are generalized from the outset and those that are secondarily generalized (that start as focal seizures and then become generalized). The second type is the most common in adults. The presence of an aura, focal manifestations during the seizure, and postictal focal deficits favor a secondarily generalized tonic-clonic seizure.

Confusion may arise in differentiating between absence seizures and complex partial seizures. Both may present with a brief loss of awareness or altered responsiveness, and in both there may be automatic activities of various kinds. Diagnosis is aided by EEG findings (generalized spike-wave discharges in absence seizures and focal epileptiform abnormalities in complex partial seizures). Correct diagnosis is critical for instituting proper AED therapy.

B. Classification of epilepsies or epileptic syndromes. Classifying the seizure type, although useful, is of limited value because seizures usually appear as part of a cluster of other symptoms and signs that include etiology, site of seizure onset, age, precipitating factors, response to medication, and prognosis. Hence, in diagnosing a patient with an epilepsy or an epileptic syndrome, it is critical that all these features be taken into account.

    1. Localization-related (focal, or partial) epilepsies or epileptic syndromes are disorders in which a localized origin of the patient's seizures can be established. The patient suffers from focal and/or secondarily generalized tonic-clonic seizures. EEG shows focal epileptiform discharges overlying the epileptogenic focus.

        a. Most localization-related epilepsies are **acquired** or **symptomatic.** Temporal lobe epilepsy is the common localization-related epilepsy encountered in adults.

        b. There are some age-related **idiopathic** or **primary** localization-related epileptic syndromes; the best known is benign rolandic epilepsy of childhood.

    2. Generalized epilepsies or epileptic syndromes are disorders that involve one or more types of generalized seizures. EEG shows generalized epileptiform abnormalities.

        a. Primary generalized epilepsies are characterized by generalized seizures without any identifiable etiology. Genetic factors predominate in these epilepsies. Common syndromes include absence epilepsy and juvenile myoclonic epilepsy.

        b. Secondary generalized epilepsies are characterized by various types of generalized seizures resulting from acquired cerebral diseases (e.g., seizures secondary to ischemic-hypoxic encephalopathy or following severe cerebral trauma or intracranial infection) or from inborn errors of metabolism (lipidoses, progressive myoclonus epilepsy, etc.). Patients usually have varying degrees of cognitive and neurologic deficits, and their seizures are often drug-resistant. Within this category are two age-related syndromes: **West's syndrome** (infancy) and **Lennox-Gastaut syndrome** (childhood).

III. Evaluation. It is essential to establish that the patient's spells or "episodes" are indeed epileptic seizures. Nonepileptic disorders that result in transient, reversible alterations of behavior or function—e.g., syncope, migraine, breath-holding spells, anxiety episodes, transient ischemic attacks (TIAs), hypoglycemic episodes, and narcoleptic-cataplectic attacks—must be differentiated from epileptic seizures. Moreover, there are psychogenic seizures or pseudoseizures that are conversion reactions characterized by episodes of motor activity and loss of consciousness but not associated with ictal EEG patterns.

A. A **history** of the episodes, obtained not only from the patient but also from one or more observers, is perhaps the most essential element in making the diagnosis of epileptic seizures and differentiating them from nonepileptic disorders. The history may also aid in determining the type of epileptic seizures.

B. Physical and neurologic examinations may help detect the underlying cause of the brain disorder responsible for the epilepsy by uncovering evidence of a focal cerebral lesion or some other organic disorder, such as tuberous sclerosis or neurofibromatosis.

C. Neuroimaging. Although computerized tomography (CT) of the head with and without contrast is performed on most patients suspected of having epilepsy, magnetic resonance imaging (MRI) of the head is the imaging procedure of choice. MRI is particularly sensitive in detecting hamartomas, cavernous hemangiomas, and low-grade gliomas and in providing evidence for mesial temporal sclerosis in patients with temporal lobe epilepsy.

D. Electroencephalography (EEG) is the most informative test for confirming the diagnosis of epilepsy, proper classification of the seizure type, and even the epileptic syndrome, and also aids in selecting antiepileptic therapy. It is uncommon for an actual seizure to occur during an EEG study except when the patient suffers from absence or myoclonic seizures. Hyperventilation may help precipitate an absence seizure. In the event that an actual seizure is recorded during an EEG study, the type of ictal EEG pattern accompanying the seizure establishes the diagnosis of epilepsy beyond a doubt and provides critical information necessary to classify the type of seizure.

The usefulness of EEG is largely dependent on the interictal epileptiform abnormalities (spikes, sharp waves, or spike-wave discharges). These abnormalities constitute interval discharges that certainly have a high correlation with clinical seizures but do not automatically imply epilepsy. Generalized epileptiform abnormalities occur in generalized epilepsies, whereas focal abnormalities suggest focal or localization-related epilepsies.

Not all epileptic patients exhibit interictal epileptiform abnormalities; about 50% show such abnormalities in a routine awake-and-asleep EEG that includes hyperventilation and intermittent photic stimulation. The yield increases with repeated EEG studies, using sleep deprivation and extra recording electrodes. On the other hand, 1–2% of healthy people without clinical seizures exhibit epileptiform abnormalities in EEG studies. Hence, an interictal EEG alone can neither prove nor rule out a diagnosis of epilepsy. Similarly, the presence of interictal epileptiform abnormalities in the EEG does not automatically warrant AED therapy, and the absence of such abnormalities is not sufficient grounds for discontinuing AED treatment.

E. Intensive video-EEG monitoring. Patients with drug-resistant epilepsy may require intensive monitoring that consists of simultaneous use of closed-circuit television, videotape, and EEG to provide detailed clinical and EEG correlation of epileptic episodes. This is an expensive and time-consuming technique and thus is left to the discretion of the consulting neurologist. Only 5–10% of patients suspected of having epilepsy may require this technique to characterize and classify their epileptic episodes. Video-EEG monitoring is most helpful in the evaluation of those patients who have frequent episodes that are suspected to be of the nonepileptic type. These episodes are not accompanied by the characteristic ictal pattern in the simultaneously recorded EEG.

IV. Basic principles in managing epileptic patients

A. AED therapy should be initiated only when the diagnosis of epileptic seizures is well established. If the patient's episodes are yet to be clearly defined and there is reasonable doubt of their being epileptic in nature, it is prudent to wait until the diagnosis of epilepsy can be confirmed.

B. AED therapy is rarely indicated following a single tonic-clonic seizure. Treatment is postponed until a second seizure occurs and the diagnosis of recurrent seizures or epilepsy is made. This is particularly true if a single tonic-clonic seizure was related to sleep deprivation, physical or mental stress, drug or alcohol withdrawal, or use of psychotropic drugs (e.g., cocaine). On the other hand, a strong family history, an aura, abnormal cognitive and neurologic examinations, a lesion on neuroimaging examination, and the presence of epileptiform abnormalities in the EEG may require prompt initiation of therapy.

C. Monotherapy is preferable to the use of multiple drugs because of fewer toxic side effects, less likelihood of drug interactions, and better compliance. The chosen AED (Table 39-1) should be slowly increased until seizures are controlled or until clinical signs of toxicity develop. If seizures are not adequately controlled at the maximum tolerable dosage, a second AED is slowly introduced, and after it attains therapeutic levels the first drug is gradually withdrawn. Monotherapy adequately controls new-onset epilepsy in 50–75% of patients.

D. Only if monotherapy with two or more first-line AEDs has been unsuccessful, **polytherapy** using a combination of two AEDs may become necessary. This decision should be made in consultation with a neurologist. One should avoid using more than two AEDs simultaneously. If a combination of two AEDs in a compliant patient with blood levels in the therapeutic range fails to provide adequate control of epileptic seizures, **referral to an epileptologist or an epilepsy center** is indicated for further evaluation and management.

E. Avoid using AEDs with sedative/hypnotic side effects unless first choice AEDs don't work. These drugs include phenobarbital, primidone, and clonazepam.

Table 39-1. Antiepileptic drugs (AEDs) of choice for specific types of seizures and epilepsy syndromes.

Types of seizures or syndromes	Recommended AED(s)*		
	First choice	Second choice	Possibly useful
Partial (Focal) Epilepsies			
Simple partial seizures	PHT/CBZ	VPA	PB/PRM
Complex partial seizures	PHT/CBZ	VPA	PB/PRM
Secondarily generalized tonic-clonic seizures	PHT/CBZ/VPA	PB/PRM	. . .
Primary Generalized Epilepsies			
Primary generalized tonic-clonic seizures	VPA/PHT/CBZ	PB/PRM	. . .
Absence epilepsy without motor seizures	ESM	VPA	CLZ
Absence epilepsy with generalized tonic-clonic seizures	VPA	ESM	CLZ
Myoclonic seizures	VPA	CLZ	. . .
Myoclonic seizures with absence or tonic-clonic seizures	VPA	CLZ	PHT/CBZ
Secondary Generalized Epilepsies			
Usually multiple seizure types—e.g., tonic, absence, myoclonic, clonic, atonic, tonic-clonic	VPA	PHT/CBZ	CLZ/PB/PRM, ketogenic diet

*AEDs separated by virgules are roughly equal in efficacy. The choice of specific AED for a given patient should be based on factors such as toxicity and cost. Sedative AEDs are generally considered to be second-line drugs. PHT = phenytoin; CBZ = carbamazepine; VPA = valproate; PB = phenobarbital; PRM = primidone; CLZ = clonazepam; ESM = ethosuximide.

Often a patient on polytherapy including one of the aforementioned sedative AEDs is best served by a very gradual withdrawal of the sedative AED while the dosage of the other AED is maximized. Such changes in medication must be made in consultation with a neurologist. Discontinuation of sedative/hypnotic AEDs is followed not only by a reduction in side effects but also often by better control of seizures.

F. Avoid using less well-known AEDs. Acquire experience with the use of a few major AEDs, such as phenytoin, carbamazepine, valproic acid, and ethosuximide.

G. Avoid complicated drug schedules. Most AEDs have long elimination half-lives (Table 39-2) and thus can be prescribed in a single daily dose or two divided daily doses. Exceptions are valproic acid and carbamazepine, which need to be given in two or three divided daily doses. When multiple AEDs are given, they have shorter elimination half-lives than when given in monotherapy, and thus require larger dosages and multiple dosing.

H. Any change in the drug schedule should be made gradually, and the effects of the change should be assessed over a long period of time. Because of the long biological half-lives of many AEDs, it takes several days to several weeks before a steady state is reached after any change in schedule.

I. After a properly chosen AED is started, it should not be discarded unless a hypersensitivity reaction occurs or there is inadequate benefit on the maximum tolerable dosage, not just on the dosage that produces blood levels within a therapeutic range.

J. Regularity in taking the daily doses needs to be stressed; medication is best taken at the time of meals for easy remembrance. For most AEDs, an occasional missed dose can be made up by taking an additional dose within the same 24-hour period. It is also convenient for the patient to put the medication in a plastic pill box with divided compartments, and to ensure at bedtime that the entire day's medication has been taken.

K. Advise the patient to maintain a **seizure diary.** Such a diary provides an accurate record of the frequency of seizures and assists in evaluating the effectiveness of the therapy.

Table 39-2. Pharmacokinetics of common antiepileptic drugs (AEDs).

AED	Elimination half-life (hours)	Time to steady state (days)	Therapeutic level (µg/ml)	Protein binding (%)	Maintenance dosage (mg/kg)	Usual daily adult dosage (mg)	Usual adult dosage range (mg/day)	Elimination route[a]
Phenytoin	10–35[b]	7–21	10–20	70–90	4–10	300–400 in one or two divided doses	300–600	H
Carbamazepine	10–25[c]	3–7	4–12	65–90	10–30	200–400 tid	600–2000	H
Valproic acid	8–12	1–3	40–100	80–95	15–60	250–500 tid-qid	750–3000	H
Ethosuximide	20–60	7–14	40–100	0	15–30	250–500 bid	250–1000	H75, R25
Phenobarbital	50–120	14–21	15–40	30–50	1–5	60–120 qid	60–300	H75, R25
Primidone[d]	6–12	3–7	5–12	0	10–20	250 tid-qid	750–1250	H
Clonazepam	20–40	7–14	0.02–0.07	40–50	0.03–0.10	1–2 tid-qid	0.5–6.0	H

[a]H = hepatic; R = renal. Numbers are approximate percentages for each route.
[b]Elimination half-life is concentration-dependent; at higher levels the half-life is longer.
[c]Elimination half-life is longer in the initial 2–4 weeks of therapy before self-induction becomes significant.
[d]Primidone therapy produces three active metabolites: primidone, phenobarbital, and phenylethylmalonamide (PEMA).

L. Stress to the patient the need for constant **medical follow-up.** Once the patient has been well established on AED therapy and the seizures have been brought under satisfactory control, the patient should be followed at 6–12-month intervals. Evaluate the patient for any evidence of drug toxicity or development of progressive neurologic disorder at the follow-up visits. CBC, liver function tests, and serum calcium are also obtained every 6–12 months to detect untoward effects of AEDs on bone marrow and liver. A patient well controlled on drug therapy may suffer a **"breakthrough" seizure** during periods of physical or mental stress, sleep deprivation, or infection. Appropriate treatment of such precipitants, rather than increases in dosage or changes in the AED, is indicated.

M. Generic substitution for brand-name AEDs can reduce the cost of medication, but the bioavailabilities of generic and proprietary AEDs are not the same. Generic preparations are required by the FDA to provide bioavailabilities within ±20% of those of the corresponding proprietary formulations, but some patients may be sufficiently sensitive to these fluctuations that replacing one with the other leads to either loss of seizure control or signs of neurotoxicity. This problem applies primarily to phenytoin and carbamazepine. The proprietary phenytoin (Dilantin) is more slowly absorbed than generic phenytoin, so that blood levels are maintained with less fluctuation and no more than one or two daily doses are required. Similarly, brand-name carbamazepine (Tegretol) is absorbed more slowly than the generic formulation. The patient should avoid switching between formulations of AEDs. When a generic AED is used, the formulation by the same manufacturer should be refilled.

N. Therapeutic drug levels are rough guides to the ranges that in the majority of patients provide best seizure control while avoiding dosage-related side effects. They are not to be followed rigidly in a given epileptic patient. Some patients may attain complete seizure control at low "therapeutic" levels, and increasing the dosage to attain idealized levels is not indicated. On the other hand, there are patients who require higher than "therapeutic" levels for control of their seizures and tolerate such levels without significant untoward side effects. In such patients it is fully justified to maintain phenytoin level as high as 20–30 μg/ml, valproic acid level as high as 100–150 μg/ml, and carbamazepine level as high as 12–15 μg/ml. Anticonvulsant blood levels are indicated:

1. To determine the baseline plasma-dosage level.
2. When the patient is suspected of being noncompliant.
3. When the patient fails to respond adequately to the usual dosage of an AED.
4. When symptoms and signs of clinical toxicity are suspected.
5. When there is a question of drug interaction.
6. To establish the correct dosage of an AED in a patient with diseases affecting absorption, metabolism, or excretion (i.e., hepatic, renal, or gastrointestinal disorders).

O. Most AEDs have linear or first-order elimination kinetics. This means that progressive increases in dosages are associated with proportional increases in blood levels. Major exceptions are phenytoin and valproic acid. Phenytoin has nonlinear kinetics, particularly after a blood level of 12–15 μg/ml has been attained. With further dosage increments, a disproportionately higher level occurs. It is, therefore, very important that increases in phenytoin dosages be made in smaller steps (30 mg/day or so) when the blood levels are higher than 15 μg/ml. This is also true when the dosage of phenytoin is reduced because of high levels or clinical toxicity.

Valproate binding to serum protein is nonlinear, and higher concentrations of valproate exceed the capacities of binding sites. Hence, at high blood levels, free valproate is disproportionately higher than the bound fraction. It is the free fraction that relates to drug effectiveness and presence of drug toxicity.

V. General management
A. Educate the patient and family members regarding epilepsy, its causes, its significance, and the necessity of continuing medication for several years despite prompt control of seizures with AEDs, taking the medication regularly, and not discontinuing it suddenly without medical advice.
B. Emphasize the need to regularize the time and duration of sleep, because sleep deprivation tends to potentiate seizures.

C. Alcohol in any form is best avoided or used in small amounts (e.g., one drink) because of possible interactions with most AEDs.

D. Drugs that lower the seizure threshold (e.g., tricyclic antidepressants and phenothiazines) or those that can cause drug interactions (increasing or decreasing the levels of AEDs) should be used with caution.

E. Encourage the patient to make the adjustments that are necessary for leading a normal life as much as possible. Moderate exercise does not affect seizure frequency. Encourage a regular exercise program. Participation in highly competitive sports increases the risk of physical injury and needs to be individualized by considering the risk of a particular sport against the patient's needs. Swimming may be permitted under supervision for a patient with good control of seizures. Bathing in a bathtub is to be avoided; taking a shower is recommended instead.

F. Most adults who have epilepsy are able to maintain competitive employment and should be encouraged to do so. This improves their self-esteem and their acceptance in the mainstream of society. There are, however, some realistic limitations on the types of work a patient with epilepsy can be permitted to do. Certain occupations, such as working with heavy machines, working above ground level, working close to water or fire, driving trucks or buses, and flying planes, may be off limits for reasons of personal and public safety. There are still scores of jobs, such as secretary, lawyer, physician, accountant, and stockbroker, that are acceptable.

G. Some women have increased frequency of seizures just before or during **menstruation**—probably related to hormonal changes and water retention. These patients may benefit from intermittent use of acetazolamide at 250–500 mg/day, starting 2–4 days before the onset and then continuing during menstruation. Alternatively, this period may be covered by additional doses of the AED or use of a benzodiazepine such as lorazepam for a few days.

H. Family members or caregivers should be educated regarding proper management of the patient when a seizure occurs. During a grand mal seizure, the patient should be helped to lie on the ground, a bed, or a couch and should be turned on one side or placed in the prone position so as to avoid aspiration. An object such as a spoon or a finger should *not* be thrust into the patient's mouth. It is simply a myth that the tongue can be swallowed during a seizure. Pushing a hard object into the mouth often results in broken teeth. The patient must be closely watched and the sequence of events observed during the seizure, which may help determine what type of seizure it is.

I. In a patient with a known history of seizures, an isolated self-limiting seizure does not constitute a need to call for an ambulance and have the patient rushed to an emergency room. However, if the seizure lasts longer than 15 minutes or if the patient suffers repeated seizures without regaining consciousness between them, prompt transfer to a nearby hospital becomes essential.

J. Driving. Most states have laws denying driving privileges to patients with uncontrolled epilepsy but permit driving once the seizures have been brought under control by AEDs. In a few states, doctors are required to report cases of epilepsy. The period of time that the patient must remain seizure-free before being permitted to drive varies from 3 months to 2 years, depending on the state. Rare patients who have only nocturnal seizures or who have only simple partial seizures (i.e., without loss of consciousness) may be exempted from driving restrictions. Some states require the treating physician to certify at regular intervals that the patient has continued to remain seizure-free before reissuing the driving permit.

There is no consensus as to how long the patient should be advised not to drive after suffering a "breakthrough" seizure following a long seizure-free period. If such a seizure follows a known precipitant such as infection, mental or physical stress, prolonged sleep deprivation, or poor compliance, observation for at least 3–6 months is required before driving is again permitted.

VI. Selection of AEDs. Table 39-1 lists AEDs that are effective for treating various epilepsies and epileptic syndromes.

A. Symptomatic partial (localization-related) epilepsies. For simple partial, complex partial, and secondarily generalized tonic-clonic seizures, several AEDs, including phenytoin, carbamazepine, phenobarbital, and primidone have very similar antiepileptic potencies but differ significantly in toxicity. **Carbamazepine** and **phenytoin** are the first-line drugs because they have fewer side effects. Primidone and phenobarbital are more often associated with neurotoxicity and thus are considered second-line AEDs. There are very small differences in overall effectiveness and basic mechanism of action between carbamazepine and phenytoin. **Phenytoin** is relatively inexpensive, is better tolerated in the initial period of therapy, and can be used in a single daily dose or two divided daily doses. However, it has a high incidence of chronic dysmorphic side effects, such as hirsutism, coarsening of facial features, and acneiform eruptions. **Carbamazepine** has side effects that are most bothersome at the start of therapy, but these effects can be minimized by starting the therapy at a low dosage and increasing it slowly over 3–4 weeks. Carbamazepine has no dysmorphic effects and hence is better accepted by adolescent and young adult female patients. Its shorter half-life usually necessitates using carbamazepine in three or four divided doses. Cognitive side effects with chronic use of phenytoin or carbamazepine have been found to be equally frequent in recent studies.

Most physicians recommend that carbamazepine be used initially, especially in young women. If carbamazepine is ineffective, phenytoin is added, and once therapeutic levels of phenytoin have been achieved, carbamazepine is gradually withdrawn. If monotherapy fails to achieve satisfactory control, combination therapy is tried—carbamazepine plus valproate, phenytoin plus valproate, phenytoin plus primidone, carbamazepine plus primidone, or phenytoin plus carbamazepine. Combination therapy is more likely to result in cognitive and other side effects.

Even with adequate AED therapy, only 40–60% of patients with symptomatic partial epilepsy, particularly those with complex partial seizures (the most common type of seizures in adults), attain full control of their seizures.

B. Primary generalized epilepsies (PGE). Most patients with PGE have either absence, myoclonic, or tonic-clonic seizures, and most suffer from more than one type of seizure, although one type may dominate. Depending on seizure type(s), several epileptic syndromes are identified under the heading of PGE. The best example is juvenile myoclonic epilepsy, which is characterized by myoclonic seizures in the early hours after waking, but most patients also have occasional tonic-clonic seizures. Less often, even absence seizures may occur. Other syndromes include primary tonic-clonic seizures (contrasted with secondarily generalized tonic-clonic seizures, which are part of focal epilepsies), which also tend to occur in the morning hours and hence are termed "awakening grand mal" seizures. Absence seizures as the dominant manifestation of PGE commonly occur in childhood, but in rare cases they may start in adolescence or early adulthood (juvenile absence epilepsy syndrome).

Valproate is the drug of choice for PGE manifesting as primary grand mal seizures, juvenile myoclonic epilepsy, photosensitive seizures, or combined absence–grand mal epilepsy. The advantage of valproate is that it is effective against many seizure types comprising PGE.

Rare juvenile or adult patients who have absence seizures unaccompanied by myoclonic or tonic-clonic seizures can be treated with either **ethosuximide** or valproate. Ethosuximide is preferred because of its lesser toxicity. The longer half-life of ethosuximide allows it to be taken in only one or two divided daily doses.

Appropriate AED therapy is generally more effective in various syndromes of PGE. Good seizure control is possible in as many as 70–90% of patients with PGE.

If valproate fails, carbamazepine, phenytoin, or primidone can be tried for primary tonic-clonic seizures as monotherapy or in combination with valproate. Carbamazepine, primidone, and phenytoin not only are ineffective for absence seizures but may even exacerbate them.

Clonazepam is an effective AED for myoclonic and absence seizures but has certain drawbacks. It has a high incidence of sedative and cognitive side effects, and patients develop a tolerance to its antiepileptic potency after several months of therapy. It is, therefore, considered a second-line drug for PGE. In patients with myoclonic or absence seizures, clonazepam may be added to valproate if the latter by itself fails to be fully effective.

C. Secondary generalized epilepsy, which is secondary to multifocal or diffuse cerebral disorders (static or progressive), occurs mostly in children and less often in adults. Patients have multiple seizure types, including atypical absence seizures, myoclonic seizures, tonic seizures, tonic-clonic seizures, drop attacks, etc.

In general, response to any AED is poor, with only 20–40% of patients attaining acceptable seizure control. Such patients commonly end up on polypharmacy, which not only fails to provide better seizure control than the use of one or two AEDs, but may even exacerbate certain types of seizures (absence seizures, myoclonic seizures, and drop attacks).

Valproate is the mainstay AED for secondary generalized epilepsy and may be used as monotherapy or in combination with phenytoin, carbamazepine, or clonazepam. When drug combinations are prescribed, appropriate dosages should be used to avoid sedation, which tends to exacerbate minor seizures in such patients.

VII. Using AEDs. Selected pharmacokinetic characteristics of the seven most commonly used AEDs are listed in Table 39-2.

A. Phenytoin

1. **Indications.** Phenytoin is effective for all types of focal epilepsies (simple partial, complex partial, and secondarily generalized tonic-clonic seizures) and for primary and secondary generalized epilepsies manifesting with tonic-clonic seizures. It is also one of the major AEDs used for controlling generalized convulsive status epilepticus.

2. **Preparations.** Proprietary 100-mg and 30-mg capsules (Dilantin) are sustained-release preparations. The proprietary 50-mg preparation (Infatab) and generic phenytoin are both prompt-release preparations. Because of different bioavailabilities, switching from one formulation to another is to be avoided. Phenytoin is also available for parenteral use during status epilepticus.

3. **Administration.** Phenytoin is usually started at a daily dosage of 300 mg/day. Long elimination half-life permits either a single daily dose or at the most two divided daily doses. After 1–2 weeks, when the steady state has reached the trough level, plasma levels should be obtained for further manipulation of the dosage.

   In those patients for which promptness is needed, an oral loading dose of 15 mg/kg can be used, followed by 300 mg/day. Alternatively, the patient can be given 300 mg three times on the first day, 300 mg twice on the second day, and 300 mg/day thereafter. With such loading treatment, adequate therapeutic levels can be established in 2–3 days. Phenytoin is not recommended for intramuscular use because of its slow and erratic absorption when administered by this route.

4. **Nonlinear elimination kinetics.** A unique characteristic of phenytoin is its nonlinear kinetics resulting from saturation of hepatic microsomal enzymes. Increases in dosage in the therapeutic window of 10–20 μg/ml should be made with 30-mg capsules. Giving a 100-mg capsule to a patient with a blood level of 15 μg/ml on a daily dosage of 300 mg can lead to levels of over 20 or even 30 μg/ml and introduce a risk of toxicity.

5. **Side effects.** Frequent side effects include **coarsening of the facies** caused by thickening of the subcutaneous tissue around the eyes and nose, **facial and body hirsuties** in women (30%), and **gum hyperplasia** (30%). These cosmetic effects are particularly concerning to young women and require consideration of an alternative therapy—e.g., carbamazepine. Phenytoin is also associated with **idiosyncratic reactions** including **skin rash** (2–5%) and, in rare cases, even **Stevens-Johnson syndrome.** Other rare reactions include **lupus-like syndrome** (positive antinuclear antibodies), **blood dyscrasias, pseudolymphoma,** and **hepatitis.**

   Several dosage-related side effects also occur. Higher dosages result in neurotoxicity characterized by **nystagmus, ataxia, drowsiness,** and **behavioral disturbances.** Other side effects include a megaloblastic anemia resulting from folic acid deficiency, low protein-bound thyroxine, hypocalcemia, osteoporosis, and mild elevation in serum alkaline phosphatase. Many of these side effects do not require discontinuation of phenytoin; neurotoxicity is treated by reductions in dosage, and other side effects are countered by supplements of folic acid (1 mg/day), vitamin D, and calcium.

6. **Drug interactions.** Certain drugs utilize the same hepatic microsomal enzymes used for degradation of phenytoin. Such drugs increase phenytoin

levels by **competitive inhibition.** These drugs include sulthiame, *p*-amino-salicylic acid (PAS), cycloserine, isoniazid (INH), dicumarol, disulfiram (Antabuse), chloramphenicol (Chloromycetin), methylphenidate (Ritalin), cimetidine, phenothiazine, phenylbutazone, propoxyphene, salicylates, and valproic acid. Starting any one of these drugs may increase phenytoin levels and cause toxicity.

Phenytoin induces microsomal hepatic enzymes and increases biotransformation of certain drugs, reducing their levels and effectiveness. Phenytoin decreases the effectiveness of estrogens, dicumarol, cycloserine, corticosteroids, digitalis, and other drugs.

B. Carbamazepine

1. **Indications** are similar to those of phenytoin—i.e., all types of partial (focal) epilepsies and generalized tonic-clonic seizures.

2. **Administration.** Carbamazepine is available only for oral use. Carbamazepine induces its own metabolism, called **autoinduction.** The elimination half-life is initially 20–40 hours, but elimination increases after 2–4 weeks of initiation of therapy and the half-life decreases to 10–20 hours. To avoid untoward neurotoxicity, it is very important to start with a small dosage, usually 100 mg bid in an adult. The dosage is gradually increased over 3–4 weeks, and most adults ultimately need a daily dosage of 600–1000 mg given in three divided doses. Blood levels are determined after 3–4 weeks of starting therapy for further dosage adjustments.

   Elimination half-life of carbamazepine decreases further to 8–12 hours with concomitant therapy with enzyme-inducing AEDs (phenobarbital, phenytoin, or primidone), and larger amounts, given in four divided daily doses, are required.

3. **Side effects.** Common dosage-related side effects, which are more bothersome in the initial period of therapy, include **sedation, blurred or double vision,** and **dizziness.** These side effects are most apparent when therapy is begun with higher dosages or if the dosage is increased too rapidly at the start of therapy. Other side effects of carbamazepine include **allergic skin rashes, hyponatremia,** and **hematologic alterations.**

   The hematologic side effects of carbamazepine have received inordinate publicity. Severe complications such as aplastic anemia and agranulocytosis are extremely uncommon. On the other hand, a usually benign leukopenia occurs in 10–20% of patients. A total white cell count of 3000/μl and an absolute granulocyte count of 1000/μl are well tolerated and do not indicate reduction or discontinuation of carbamazepine.

   Hyponatremia is most likely to occur following several weeks or months of carbamazepine therapy. It is considered to be a result of inappropriate secretion of antidiuretic hormone (ADH), but this is controversial. Asymptomatic hyponatremia in the range of 125–135 mEq/L may be followed. If the condition becomes symptomatic or if serum sodium concentration drops below 125 mEq/L, fluid restriction is instituted. If this fails, dosage reduction or a trial of another AED may be required.

4. **Drug interactions.** Carbamazepine, like phenytoin, is an inducer of hepatic microsomal enzymes. Several drug interactions of carbamazepine are similar to those of phenytoin.

   Enzyme inducers—phenobarbital, phenytoin, and primidone—tend to stimulate biotransformation of carbamazepine and to lower the carbamazepine level, requiring higher dosages of carbamazepine to be given in more daily divided doses. On the other hand, the intermediary metabolite, carbamaze-pine-10-11-epoxide, increases in proportion and may contribute to additional neurotoxic side effects.

   Erythromycin markedly inhibits metabolism of carbamazepine. **Cimetidine** and **propoxyphene** have similar but lesser effects. These drugs should be avoided, because carbamazepine levels may rise, with resultant clinical toxicity.

C. Valproic acid

1. **Indications.** Valproic acid has a broad antiepileptic range.

   a. Valproic acid has antiabsence efficacy similar to that of ethosuximide. Patients who have absence seizures and also suffer from convulsive attacks are best treated with valproate.

   b. Valproic acid is the drug of choice for PGE, including juvenile myoclonic epilepsy, primary generalized epilepsy manifesting with grand mal seizures, and photosensitive epilepsy.

    c. Valproic acid is also the drug of choice for secondarily generalized epilepsy syndromes, although satisfactory seizure control is attainable in only one-third of patients with these syndromes.

    d. Valproic acid is also effective for treating complex partial seizures, although probably less so than carbamazepine, phenytoin, and primidone. It is indicated as an add-on agent for complex partial or secondarily generalized seizures, especially for those from a frontal lobe focus.

2. Preparations. Depakene is the form of valproic acid that is available in tablets and syrup. It has more rapid absorption and a high incidence of gastric disturbances than Depakote. Divalproex sodium (Depakote) is a stable coordination compound comprised of sodium valproate and valproic acid in a 1:1 molar relationship. It is available in the form of delayed-release tablets (Depakote tablets) and sprinkle capsules. Depakote tablets cause less gastric disturbance and have slower gastrointestinal absorption than Depakene, and therefore are the form preferred for adults.

3. Administration. In adults, valproic acid is usually started as a dose of 250 mg. Depakote tablets are given once or twice a day. The dosage is gradually increased by 250 mg every week until seizures are controlled or side effects occur. The usual adult dosage is 1–2 g/day, which should be given in three or four divided daily doses because of a relatively short elimination half-life.

    Smaller daily dosages (blood levels of 40–60 μg/ml) are usually needed for patients with PGE (absence epilepsy, juvenile myoclonic epilepsy, or primary tonic-clonic seizures) than for patients with secondary generalized epilepsy, for whom dosages of up to 4.0 g or 60 mg/kg and blood levels of 100–120 μg/ml may be necessary for adequate seizure control.

    When used with such enzyme-inducing AEDs as phenytoin, carbamazepine, phenobarbital, and primidone, valproic acid must be given in much larger dosages because of increased metabolism resulting in shortening of elimination half-life.

4. Side effects. Nausea and vomiting are common initial side effects, particularly if a large starting dose is given or if the dosage is increased too rapidly. Gastric irritation may be reduced by taking valproic acid immediately after meals. A common dosage-related side effect is **tremor** associated with high blood levels. Valproic acid is relatively free of cognitive and behavioral side effects. Some patients suffer excessive **hair loss** or **weight gain** as a result of increased appetite.

    The risk of valproic acid causing hepatic toxicity has been overstated in the past. Patients above the age of 6 years without underlying liver disease and not taking any other hepatotoxic drug have almost never developed serious toxic hepatitis. Another rare idiosyncratic effect is **pancreatitis.** Mild **hyperammonemia** is common, particularly with high dosages. It is renal rather than hepatic in origin and is not a reason to discontinue therapy unless lethargy occurs.

    Valproic acid is also reported to produce **thrombocytopenia,** interference in the platelet aggregation, and an increased tendency toward bleeding.

    Baseline CBC, platelet count, and liver function (SGOT) tests should be performed. These tests are repeated after 2–4 weeks of therapy and then every 6–12 months. If the patient is to undergo surgery, these tests are obviously repeated prior to surgery. Routine ammonia levels do not predict rarely occurring serious hepatic complications and thus serve no purpose.

5. Drug interactions are common. Valproic acid inhibits metabolism of many AEDs. It consistently increases phenobarbital levels (resulting in toxicity), and hence phenobarbital dosages should be reduced by 20–40% when valproic acid is added. Valproic acid decreases the total (free plus bound) phenytoin level without changing the free level owing to competition for protein binding sites. These changes do not necessitate changes in phenytoin dosages.

D. Ethosuximide continues to be the drug of choice for PGE of the pure absence type, which is more common in children than in adults. (Remember that absence-like seizures in adults are often brief complex partial seizures that are not helped by ethosuximide.) Ethosuximide is also ineffective against convulsive seizures.

Ethosuximide can be started at a dosage of 250 mg bid and gradually increased every 1–2 weeks until the seizures are controlled or side effects occur. Even though the elimination half-life is long enough to permit a single daily dose, it is better to use two divided daily doses to reduce gastrointestinal toxicity.

Significant side effects are rare with ethosuximide. **Gastrointestinal upset, hiccups,** and **hallucinations** may occur when high dosages are used.

E. **Phenobarbital** is the oldest and the least expensive of the commonly used AEDs.
1. **Indications.** Phenobarbital is effective in treating simple partial, complex partial, and secondarily generalized tonic-clonic seizures. It is also used in controlling generalized convulsive status epilepticus. Although often used in patients with secondary generalized epilepsy syndromes, it may exacerbate certain types of seizures (e.g., absence, tonic-clonic, and myoclonic seizures) in such patients.
2. **Administration.** Because of its very long elimination half-life, phenobarbital can be used in a single daily dose. The usual adult dosage is 1–3 mg/kg. Patients should be warned not to terminate phenobarbital abruptly, because such termination often produces withdrawal convulsions even in patients without seizure disorders, and does so more frequently in patients with epilepsy.
3. **Side effects.** The undesirable chronic side effects limiting the use of phenobarbital are its **sedative effects** and the **paradoxical hyperactivity** it produces in children. Idiosyncratic reactions such as **skin rash** are uncommon.

F. **Primidone** is converted to three active antiepileptic blood metabolites—primidone, phenobarbital, and phenylethylmalonamide (PEMA)—but only the first two are usually measured.
1. **Indications.** Primidone monotherapy is as effective against all types of partial seizures as phenytoin or carbamazepine, but primidone is less well tolerated by patients because of its clinical toxicity—especially during the initial period of therapy.
2. **Administration.** Primidone can only be given orally. It appears to be better tolerated in adults when started at a very small dosage of 50 mg at night for three days; larger initial dosages have resulted in hypersomnolence in some patients. The dosage is then increased to 125 mg/day, and is further increased in steps of 125 mg at weekly intervals up to an initial target daily dosage of 750–1000 mg/day. Although the elimination half-life of its major metabolite, phenobarbital, is long, that of primidone itself may be as short as 6–8 hours, which requires that it be given in three divided doses.
3. **Side effects.** The major side effect is **sedation,** which initially may be severe but can be avoided if the drug is introduced in small doses and if increments are made very slowly. Other side effects are similar to those of phenobarbital and include **dizziness, allergic rash, behavioral and cognitive changes, ataxia, respiratory depression,** and **impotence.**

G. **Clonazepam**
1. **Indications.** This benzodiazepine is useful in the treatment of primary and secondary generalized epilepsies manifesting with absence, myoclonic, and other minor motor seizures. Because of its sedative side effects and because patients develop a tolerance to its antiepileptic effectiveness after several months of therapy, clonazepam is a second-line drug that usually is used in combination with other AEDs for difficult-to-treat patients.
2. **Administration.** Clonazepam is administered once daily starting with a small dosage of 0.01–0.03 mg/kg (usually 0.5–1.0 mg in adults), which is gradually increased by 0.5 mg every 5–7 days to a maximum daily dosage of 0.2 mg/kg.
3. **Side effects** include **drowsiness, dizziness, blurred vision, ataxia,** and **personality changes.**

H. **Newer AEDs.** After a lapse of more than a decade, three new AEDs have been introduced in the United States: felbamate (Felbatol), gabapentin (Neurontin), and lamotrigine (Lamictal). Use of these drugs may be entrusted to the referring neurologist or epileptologist.

After enthusiastic use in patients with complex partial seizures (CPS) and secondary generalized epilepsy, **felbamate** has fallen in repute because of its recently recognized untoward side effects of aplastic anemia and liver toxicity besides its well-known side effects of weight loss, insomnia, and gastrointestinal symptoms.

Gabapentin is approved as an add-on AED for patients with partial or secondarily generalized tonic-clonic seizures. Its greatest advantages include entirely renal clearance, lack of drug interactions, lack of protein binding, and absence of serious side effects.

Lamotrigine is approved by the FDA but is still not available for use at the time of this writing.

VIII. **Status epilepticus**

A. **Definition.** Status epilepticus is defined as continuous seizure activity persisting for at least half an hour, or two or more sequential seizures repeating within half an hour without full recovery of consciousness between seizures.

B. **Types.** Any type of seizure may manifest as status epilepticus, but the common forms include the following.

1. **Generalized convulsive status epilepticus (GCSE)** presents as repeated major motor convulsions without full recovery of consciousness between seizures. In the past, the term "status epilepticus" implied essentially this form of status.

2. **Nonconvulsive status epilepticus** produces a continuous or fluctuating "epileptic twilight" state. This includes patients with absence status and complex partial status.

3. **Simple partial status epilepticus** is characterized by repeated focal motor seizures, epilepsia partialis continua, and focal impairment of function (e.g., aphasia) without accompanying alteration of consciousness.

C. **Etiology of GCSE.** GCSE is the most common and most serious type of status epilepticus. Unconsciousness associated with convulsive major motor seizures are the cardinal features. The motor activity may vary in symmetry and form depending on the previous history of seizures, duration of status, duration of treatment, and associated brain pathology. GCSE occurs mainly in the following settings.

1. **Acute cerebral insult** or **acute encephalopathies** account for half of the cases of GCSE. These disorders include meningitis, encephalitis, head trauma, hypoxia, hypoglycemia, drug intoxication (e.g., cocaine), drug withdrawal, and strokes or metabolic encephalopathies.

2. GCSE may occur in patients with **previous history of epilepsy** on the basis of remote neurologic insults. Common precipitants of GCSE include changes in AEDs, sudden discontinuation or reduction in AEDs, systemic infections, physical and emotional stresses, and sleep deprivation.

3. GCSE may occur as an **initial unprovoked epileptic event** in an otherwise normal person. Such "idiopathic" patients may account for one-third of all GCSE patients.

D. **Prognosis.** GCSE is an emergency associated with substantial morbidity and mortality; the overall mortality may be as high as 30% in adults. GCSE associated with acute neurologic insults has the poorest prognosis, which essentially depends on the underlying cerebral etiology.

When GCSE is the first epileptic event in an otherwise neurologically intact patient, or when it occurs in a patient with a previously known history of epilepsy but has a benign or reversible etiology (e.g., hypoglycemia or drug/alcohol withdrawal), the prognosis is good if therapy is instituted promptly.

Without adequate and prompt treatment, GCSE may progress to a state of electromechanical dissociation in which the patient becomes increasingly unconscious or encephalopathic from the ongoing status but the convulsive activity becomes increasingly subtle even though the EEG continues to show an ictal pattern. Patients with this condition, which is often termed "subtle status epilepticus," are considered to be candidates for an aggressive therapy, as are those with overt GCSE.

E. **Management of GCSE.** The treatment protocol outlined in Table 39-3 is useful in the management of GCSE.

1. **Diagnose status epilepticus** by observing either continued seizure activity or one additional generalized convulsion in a patient who presents with a history of GCSE.

2. **Assess vital functions** and systemic abnormalities, and stabilize the vital functions as much as possible.

a. **Maintain an adequate airway and oxygenation.** This usually can be accomplished with an oral airway. The airway should be suctioned peri-

Table 39-3. Treatment protocol for status epilepticus in adults.

Time (min)	Treatment
0–5	Diagnose status epilepticus by observing either continued seizure activity or one additional seizure.
	Assess vital functions, insert oral airway, and give O_2.
6–10	Establish IV infusion line with normal saline. Monitor temperature and BP. Draw blood for electrolytes, glucose, Ca, Mg, AED levels, CBC, BUN, and SGOT.
	Administer 100 mg of thiamine followed by 50 ml of 50% glucose IV push.
11–15	Give lorazepam 0.1 mg/kg IV push at a rate of <2 mg/min, *or* give diazepam 0.2 mg/kg IV at a rate of <5 mg/min. Diazepam can be repeated until seizures stop or a total of 20 mg has been given.
16–45	Whether or not lorazepam or diazepam stops the seizures, proceed to administer phenytoin 20 mg/kg IV no faster than 50 mg/min.
	Monitor BP and ECG during phenytoin infusion, and if hypotension or ECG changes occur, slow the infusion or temporarily withhold the phenytoin.
	If seizures continue, an additional 5–10 mg/kg of phenytoin can be given.
46–59	If seizures continue, perform elective endotracheal intubation before giving phenobarbital 20 mg/kg IV push at a rate of <100 mg/min.
60–90	If status persists, start barbiturate coma by either giving more phenobarbital or starting pentobarbital.
	Start pentobarbital with a dose of 5 mg/kg IV to produce suppression-burst pattern on EEG, and continue at 0.5–3.0 mg/kg/hr to maintain seizure-free state or suppression-burst pattern on EEG.
	Slow rate of infusion periodically to determine if seizures have stopped. Monitor EEG, BP, ECG, and respiratory function.

odically to maintain patency. Oxygen should be administered by means of a nasal cannula or with a mask and a bag-valve-mask ventilator. If, after bagging, respiratory assistance is still needed, endotracheal intubation should be considered.

b. **Assess blood pressure** and maintain it at a normal or high-normal level during prolonged GCSE. Use vasopressors if necessary.

c. **Establish an IV infusion line** using normal saline. Blood should be drawn initially for CBC, blood sugar, BUN, serum electrolytes (including calcium and magnesium), and AED levels, and both urine and blood should be obtained for toxicology screening.

d. **Assess oxygenation** by oximetry or periodic arterial blood gas determination.

e. **Monitor rectal temperature.** Body temperature may increase to a high level during prolonged status epilepticus as a result of increased motor activity.

f. If hypoglycemia is documented or if it is impossible to obtain prompt blood sugar determination, **administer 50 ml of 50% glucose** by IV push. In adults, **thiamine** (100 mg) is always given before glucose to protect the patient from exacerbation of Wernicke's encephalopathy in a thiamine-deficient patient.

g. Acidosis commonly develops during GCSE. However, bicarbonate therapy is usually not necessary, because the acidosis responds promptly once the seizure activity is controlled.

h. In rare patients with GCSE resulting from hyponatremia (serum sodium less than 120 mEq/L), hypocalcemia, or hypomagnecemia, appropriate electrolytes are administered by IV drip.

3. **Drug therapy for control of GCSE.** The goals of therapy are rapid termination of the clinical and EEG evidence of seizure activity and subsequent maintenance of a seizure-free state.

a. **Benzodiazepines.** If the patient is actively convulsing, administer either diazepam or lorazepam, which are effective in rapidly terminating GCSE. This is followed by the use of a long-acting AED such as phenytoin to prevent recurrence of convulsions.

Lorazepam is administered at 0.1 mg/kg IV at a rate of less than 2 mg/min. **Diazepam** is given at 0.2 mg/kg at a rate less than 5 mg/min. The dose of diazepam can be repeated if the seizures do not stop after 5 minutes. Up to a total of 20 mg of diazepam may be administered.

Some prefer lorazepam over diazepam. Diazepam enters the brain exceedingly rapidly and is very prompt in terminating GCSE. However, it is extremely lipid-soluble and is quick to redistribute to body fat stores with the result that the blood and brain concentrations drop, allowing seizures to recur in 15–30 minutes. Lorazepam has relatively rapid effectiveness and yet has a prolonged duration of action against status epilepticus. Both diazepam and lorazepam can produce serious respiratory depression or hypotension, particularly when given in combination with barbiturates.

b. Phenytoin. If seizures are still continuing after the administration of one of the benzodiazepines, IV administration of phenytoin should be promptly initiated. Even if the benzodiazepines have been successful in terminating the seizure activity, phenytoin is usually needed to prevent recurrence of convulsions, especially following the use of diazepam.

The usual loading dose of phenytoin is 20 mg/kg, given through a syringe into the IV port close to the patient at a rate less than 50 mg/min. Injection is preferably performed by a physician. Blood pressure and ECG are continuously monitored throughout the infusion. The rate of infusion should be slowed or temporarily stopped if sufficient hypotension develops or if the ECG shows widening of Q–T interval or development of arrhythmias. Some prefer diluting phenytoin in 100 mg of saline solution, but most recommend administering it undiluted because the drug may precipitate in IV solutions—particularly glucose.

If the standard loading dose of 20 mg/kg of phenytoin fails to stop GCSE, an additional 5–10 mg/kg may be given. Some patients may require high blood levels (30–40 μg/ml) before the seizure terminates. Phenytoin is effective in 40–90% of GCSE patients.

Phenytoin should be used cautiously in elderly patients, patients with known cardiac abnormalities, and patients with low baseline blood pressure.

c. Phenobarbital is generally the next choice in adults if the GCSE fails to respond to phenytoin. Close attention to the respiratory status is required, especially if the patient has already received one of the benzodiazepines. Respiratory assistance, including endotracheal intubation, usually becomes necessary at this stage, and the physician must be prepared for this eventuality.

The usual dose of phenobarbital is 20 mg/kg given intravenously at a rate less than 100 mg/min. Sedation, respiratory compromise, and hypotension are potential side effects requiring attention. Use of phenobarbital is likely to be effective at stopping GCSE in 40% of patients who require a third AED.

4. Management of refractory GCSE

a. Consultation with a neurologist is recommended in managing GCSE if the patient continues to exhibit altered consciousness and the administration of a benzodiazepine and phenytoin fails to control seizures.

b. If the triple therapy fails to control GCSE, the patient requires **general anesthesia** to eliminate not only clinical seizures but also electrical discharges indicative of continuing seizure activity. This is best accomplished by barbiturate coma induced by either phenobarbital or pentobarbital.

Pentobarbital is preferred because of its shorter half-life. It is started intravenously with a loading dose of 5 mg/kg, followed by a maintenance dosage of 0.5–3.0 mg/kg/hr to maintain a suppression-burst pattern on the EEG or bring about cessation of the ictal pattern, whichever occurs first.

Phenobarbital can be used as an alternative in additional doses of 5–10 mg/kg at 30-minute intervals until the seizure activity stops both clinically and on the EEG. The rate of infusion is then adjusted to maintain a seizure-free state.

Barbiturate coma is almost always associated with significant hypotension, which requires the use of **pressor agents.**

5. **Additional diagnostic studies.** When the seizures have been stopped or sufficiently controlled and the patient's vital signs have been stabilized, additional diagnostic studies, such as **chest x-rays, lumbar puncture (LP), brain imaging,** and **EEG,** are performed to evaluate the cause of the GCSE and the effectiveness of the antiepileptic therapy.

6. **Long-term antiepileptic therapy.** After the episode of GCSE has been brought under control, most patients need continuation of some form of AED therapy.

Long-term AED therapy is indicated when GCSE is caused by a structural brain lesion or when the patient has a previous history of epileptic seizures. When GCSE constitutes the patient's first seizure and no cause is found, the decision to initiate long-term AED therapy should be individualized, but most physicians initiate long-term treatment under such circumstances. If the GCSE was caused by an acute CNS involvement such as metabolic encephalopathy, meningoencephalitis, or cerebrovascular compromise, antiepileptic therapy is continued for a short period of 3–6 months.

F. **Treatment of other types of status epilepticus.** Other forms of status epilepticus do not pose the same emergency situation that GCSE poses. **Complex partial status epilepticus** has been reported to result in long-term neurologic deficits (e.g., permanent memory impairment) and should be treated promptly by benzodiazepines followed by IV phenytoin and even phenobarbital. Barbiturate coma is rarely indicated.

The treatment of absence status or simple partial status (focal motor seizure or epilepsia partialis continua without loss of consciousness) is not standardized. **Absence status** is best treated by IV benzodiazepine followed by oral valproate therapy. **Simple partial status** responds to phenytoin, usually in large dosages to maintain blood levels as high as 30 µg/ml. Benzodiazepines and phenobarbital are not desirable because of their sedative side effects.

IX. **Epilepsy and pregnancy**

A. **Major problems.** Pregnancy in a woman with epilepsy is considered to constitute a high risk for the following reasons.

1. **Increased frequency of seizures** occurs in over one-third of pregnant women, especially during the second and third trimesters.

2. A major factor for exacerbation of seizures is the **alteration of the pharmacokinetics of AEDs,** with significant decreases in the serum concentrations of phenytoin, carbamazepine, phenobarbital, valproate, and primidone.

3. The incidence of **fetal malformation** is two to three times higher in mothers with epilepsy than in controls. Most of this effect is a result of fetal exposure to AEDs. The overall incidence of major birth defects (oropalatal clefts, urogenital and congenital heart anomalies, and neural tube defects) in infants of epileptic mothers is about 7%.

All major AEDs have potential teratogenic effects, and there is no evidence that any one is safer than any other. Valproate and carbamazepine, however, are more likely to be associated with spina bifida and other neural tube defects. The incidence of birth anomalies has been higher in women on polytherapy than in those on monotherapy.

4. **Hemorrhagic disease** is reported in 7% of newborns delivered by women who have received hepatic enzyme-inducing AEDs (phenobarbital, primidone, phenytoin, and carbamazepine) because of their effect in decreasing the vitamin K–dependent clotting factors.

B. **Management guidelines.** Management of pregnancy in an epileptic woman is a therapeutic challenge that requires the physician to keep the patient free of seizures while minimizing the adverse effects of seizures and AEDs on the course of pregnancy and the fetus. The major guidelines, which preferably are initiated before the patient becomes pregnant, are as follows.

1. AEDs may be withdrawn before pregnancy if the patient has remained free of seizures for several years.

2. Counsel the patient about the higher incidence of fetal malformation but assure her that most pregnant women (more than 90%) exposed to AEDs still bear normal offspring.

3. For a woman who is longing to bear a child, select the best drug for the pa-

tient's seizure type and use monotherapy. Because of the relatively high inci- dence of neural tube defects with valproate (1–2%) and with carbamazepine (0.5–1.0%), avoid these AEDs if at all possible and replace them with other AEDs *before* the patient becomes pregnant.

4. Do not stop AED therapy after the pregnancy has been diagnosed. The risk of fetal malformation is highest during the first 4–8 weeks of pregnancy. It is usually too late to protect the fetus by the time pregnancy is confirmed. Stopping or changing the drug may induce more frequent and more violent seizures, with adverse consequences on both the mother and the fetus.

5. Monitor the AED serum level every month and adjust the dosage accord- ingly. Avoid both low and high blood levels.

6. If the patient is on valproate or carbamazepine, obtain serum **alpha-feto- protein** at 15–16 weeks of gestation to be followed by high-definition **ultra- sound imaging** of the fetus at 18–20 weeks to detect spina bifida or neural tube defects. **Amniocentesis** is indicated only if the alpha-fetoprotein level is high and the ultrasound is unable to provide positive exclusion of a neural tube defect.

7. Supplemental vitamins including folic acid (3–5 mg/day) are prescribed dur- ing the entire pregnancy. Give oral vitamin K_1 (phytonadione) to the mother at 20 mg/day during the last month of pregnancy.

8. Administer vitamin K_1 (1 mg, IM) to the neonate immediately after birth.

9. Unless the infant becomes symptomatic, breast feeding is allowed. Most AEDs, with the possible exception of ethosuximide, do not reach sufficient concentrations in the breast milk to pose a serious concern for the infant.

C. **Prevention of pregnancy by oral contraceptives in sexually active women**

1. Oral contraceptives do not exacerbate epilepsy despite the warnings on package inserts.

2. The major concern in using oral contraceptives is the higher failure rate in women taking hepatic enzyme-inducing AEDs (phenytoin, carbamazepine, phenobarbital, primidone, etc.). Breakthrough bleeding may be a warning of decreased contraceptive efficiency. Patients may, therefore, need a medium- dosage oral contraceptive rather than the "mini-pill."

3. Valproate, which is not an enzyme-inducer, is unlikely to cause failure of oral contraception.

X. **Discontinuation of AEDs.** The decision to discontinue AEDs in a patient who has been seizure-free for several years depends on many prognostic factors. The re- lapse rate after AED withdrawal is around 30–40% in adults with chronic epilepsy.

A. **Prognostic factors**

1. **Types of epilepsies**

   a. Some childhood epilepsies (e.g., benign rolandic epilepsy and childhood absence epilepsy) usually remit during adolescence.

   b. **PGE** patients with onset in adolescence or adulthood have good prog- noses. They often remit, but many require lifelong therapy.

   c. Patients with localization-related epilepsies (simple partial seizures, complex partial seizures, and secondarily generalized tonic-clonic seiz- ures) have a high recurrence rate (40–50%) after discontinuing AEDs— especially adults with complex partial seizures, for which the relapse rate may approach or exceed 50%.

   d. Patients in whom seizures occur in the setting of an acute cerebral insult (e.g., trauma, infection, or stroke) may not develop chronic epilepsy. Such patients should be considered for withdrawal of AED after a seizure-free period of 3–6 months.

2. **EEG findings** obtained just before discontinuation of AED therapy are use- ful predictors of the outcome. If the EEG shows epileptiform abnormalities, the relapse rate is four to five times higher than if the EEG is normal or min- imally abnormal. Hence, most physicians consider continuing AEDs if the EEG continues to show paroxysmal abnormalities.

3. **Other predictors of outcome.** A high frequency of seizures and a long du- ration before seizures are controlled by AEDs carry less favorable prog- noses. Similarly, patients who have structural abnormalities responsible for seizures, who have mental retardation or neurological deficits are more likely to have recurrence of seizures after discontinuation of AEDs.

4. **Duration of seizure-free period.** There is no consensus as to how long the patient should remain seizure-free before drug withdrawal is considered.

Most physicians recommend a seizure-free period of 2–5 years, but such recommendations must be individualized because of the serious socioeconomic impact resulting from recurrence of seizures.

B. General guidelines for withdrawing AEDs

1. Adult patients with PGE who have remained seizure-free for 2–5 years and whose EEGs show no paroxysmal abnormalities are good risks for withdrawal of therapy.
2. Women who wish to raise families and who have been seizure-free for several years should be considered for withdrawal of medication to avoid possible ill-effects of the AEDs on their fetuses.
3. On the other hand, most adults with complex partial seizures with or without secondarily generalized tonic-clonic seizures probably need long-term, if not lifelong, AED therapy unless continuation of the medication and the seizure-free state are possible only at the cost of unpleasant side effects.

C. AED withdrawal mode and precautions

1. AEDs must be withdrawn slowly, typically over 3–6 months or even longer, especially barbiturates and benzodiazepines.
2. Patients on more than one AED should have the less or least effective drug withdrawn before the first-line drug. Only after the patient has remained seizure-free on only one drug for several months is the final drug withdrawn.
3. During the withdrawal period, the patient is advised to follow a restricted lifestyle (no driving or hazardous occupational or recreational activities) to minimize the consequences should the seizures recur.
4. If the seizures recur, the patient is promptly placed on an adequate dosage of an appropriate AED, which then probably needs to be continued on a lifelong basis.
5. During the withdrawal period, attention needs to be paid to such lifestyle issues as getting adequate sleep, avoiding alcohol, and avoiding anxiety that might cause recurrence.

XI. Counseling for psychosocial problems. Patients with epilepsy face many personal and psychosocial difficulties that require counseling. Driving restrictions, concerns regarding pregnancy, and possible transmission of epilepsy to the offspring are some of the concerns that need to be addressed. Employers usually regard epileptic employees as high accident risks and often terminate their jobs when seizures occur at work. Epileptics have difficulties in getting auto and life insurance. All these adversities lead to economic hardships, emotional problems, dependence, and poor self-esteem. It is important to detect these problems, respond to them promptly, and refer patients to neurologists, to psychiatrists, or to social workers or nurses for further management and counseling.

Patients should also be put in touch with local support groups, state epilepsy associations, and the Epilepsy Foundation of America.

XII. Referral to epilepsy centers for comprehensive care, experimental AEDs, or surgical treatment. Patients requiring comprehensive care may be referred to local epilepsy clinics or centers equipped with multidisciplinary teams capable of providing psychosocial and vocational counseling in addition to the appropriate medical therapy.

About 15–25% of patients with epilepsy who have medically intractable seizures may be helped by referral to regional epilepsy centers, which may conduct ongoing clinical trials of new AEDs. Such patients often require combination therapy with two or more AEDs, which is best handled by an epileptologist in the epilepsy center or clinic.

Patients who have complex partial or secondarily generalized tonic-clonic seizures should be referred for at least 2 years to an epilepsy center for presurgical evaluation to determine whether they are suitable candidates for resective surgery (anterior temporal lobectomy, selective amygdalohippocampectomy, or corticectomy).

Recommended Readings

Bleck TP. Convulsive disorders: The use of anticonvulsant drugs. *Clin Neuropharm* 13:198–209, 1990.

Callaghan N, Garrett A, Goggin T. Withdrawal of anticonvulsant drugs in patients free of seizures for two years: A prospective study. *N Engl J Med* 318:942–946, 1988.

Commission on Classification and Terminology of the International League Against Epilepsy. Proposal for revised clinical and electroencephalographic classification of epileptic seizures. *Epilepsia* 22:489–501, 1981.

Commission on Classification and Terminology of the International League Against Epilepsy. Proposal for revised classification of epilepsies and epileptic syndromes. *Epilepsia* 30:389–399, 1989.

Delgado-Escueta AV, Janz D. Consensus guidelines: Preconception counseling, management and care of the pregnant woman with epilepsy. *Neurology* 42(suppl 5):149–160, 1992.

DeLorenzo RJ, et al. Status epilepticus in children, adults, and the elderly. *Epilepsia* 33(suppl 4):S15–S25, 1992.

Dodson WE. Level off. *Neurology* 39:1009, 1989.

Engel JE Jr. *Seizures and Epilepsy.* Philadelphia: Davis, 1989.

Gumnit RJ. *The Epilepsy Handbook: The Practical Management of Seizures* (2nd ed). New York: Raven, 1995.

Hauser WA. Status epilepticus: Epidemiologic considerations. *Neurology* 40(suppl 2):9–13, 1990.

Leppik IE. Status epilepticus: The next decade. *Neurology* 40(suppl 2):4–9, 1990.

Leppik IE, et al. Double-blind study of lorazepam and diazepam in status epilepticus. *JAMA* 249:1452, 1983.

Levy RH, et al. (eds). *Antiepileptic Drugs.* New York: Raven, 1989.

Levy RJ, Krall RL. Treatment of status epilepticus with lorazepam. *Arch Neurol* 41:605, 1984.

Mattson RH, et al. Comparison of carbamazepine, phenobarbital, phenytoin, and primidone in partial and secondarily generalized tonic-clonic seizures. *N Engl J Med* 313:145–151, 1985.

Mattson RH, et al. A comparison of valproate with carbamazepine for the treatment of complex partial seizures and secondarily generalized tonic-clonic seizures in adults. *N Engl J Med* 327:765–771, 1992.

Reynolds EH, Shorvon D. Monotherapy or polytherapy for epilepsy. *Epilepsia* 22:1–10, 1981.

Scheuer ML, Pedley TA. The evaluation and treatment of seizures. *N Engl J Med* 323:1468–1474, 1990.

Theodore WH, Porter RJ. Removal of sedative-hypnotic antiepileptic drugs from the regimen of patients with intractable epilepsy. *Ann Neurol* 13:320–324, 1983.

Therapeutics and Technology Assessment Subcommittee of the American Academy of Neurology. Technology assessment: Generic substitution for antiepileptic medication. Position statement, 1989.

Treiman DM. The role of benzodiazepines in the management of status epilepticus. *Neurology* 40(suppl 2):32–42, 1990.

Working Group on Status Epilepticus. Treatment of status epilepticus. *JAMA* 270:854–859, 1993.

40 Multiple Sclerosis
Galen W. Mitchell

Multiple sclerosis (MS) is a primary demyelinating disease of the central nervous system (CNS). This disorder appears to be **immune-mediated,** although the actual development of the disease and the subsequent clinical course are probably influenced by genetic and environmental factors along with many factors that have not yet been determined. MS represents a very important neurologic disorder by virtue of prevalence, chronicity, induced disability, and tendency to affect young adults. The goal of this chapter is to provide an overview of MS with general information for patient counseling and insights into diagnosis, disease forms, clinical course, and therapy.

I. **Epidemiology.** The estimated number of MS patients in the United States is between 250,000 and 350,000. MS is a disorder of young adults, with the onset of disease occurring most frequently between the ages of 20 and 35 years in females and 35 and 45 years in males. The prevalence of MS is one and a half to two times higher in females than in males and is much more common in whites than in other races. Although there are no definite mendelian patterns of inheritance for MS, first-degree relatives of an index case have a 10- to 20-fold increased risk of contracting the disorder. This genetic risk is borne out in studies of twins, where the monozygotic concordance rate is approximately 30%, compared with 5% in dizygotic twins. Furthermore, human leukocyte antigen (HLA) studies show a subtle but significant correlation between MS and different HLA antigens within various ethnic groups. Together, these facts suggest that there is a **genetic predisposition** toward developing the disorder but that noninherited factors play a more dominant role.

II. **Pathogenesis.** The exact pathogenesis of MS remains elusive, but substantial clinical and laboratory data suggest an autoimmune process. Although MS patients have significant abnormalities in humoral immune function, the disorder appears to be primarily mediated through T cells. The target of the autoimmune disorder is the **myelin sheath,** which surrounds axons in the CNS. This myelin is important for saltatory conduction along the axons. Demyelination frequently occurs in localized areas, resulting in the pathologic lesions called **plaques.** These plaques are usually located deep in the **cerebral white matter,** near the ventricles, but they can occur anywhere, including the gray matter, cerebellum, brainstem, spinal cord, and proximal nerve roots. This almost limitless variation of distribution is responsible for the variety of clinical presentations. The pathologic appearance of the plaque changes with repeated episodes of demyelination and chronicity. In an early active plaque, there is breakdown of the blood-brain barrier with demyelination but relative sparing of the axons. Perivascular infiltrates of lymphocytes, macrophages, and occasionally plasma cells are present in small veins and venules. Demyelination may spread outward from the plaque, especially along these vessels. Perivascular and interstitial edema may be prominent. At the edge of the plaque there is hyperplasia of oligodendrocytes and activated astrocytes. These hyperplastic oligodendrocytes are probably involved in remyelination, but thin myelin sheaths noted on electron microscopy suggest that this remyelination is often suboptimal and incomplete. In older plaques, oligodendroglia disappear, astrocytes show hypertrophy and hyperplasia ("sclerosis"), and axonal loss occurs.

III. **Clinical features.** Areas of CNS demyelination or plaques can result in conduction abnormalities with **delayed or blocked conduction,** impaired response to repetitive stimulation, or ephaptic conduction. Delayed or blocked conduction and impaired response to repetitive stimulation may result in negative signs or symptoms. Depending on the extent of the conduction defect and the location of the lesion in the CNS, the patient may develop visual loss, numbness, weakness, ataxia, or nearly any loss of function attributable to a CNS lesion. Ephaptic conduction may result in positive signs and symptoms including pain, seizures, and paroxysmal syndromes. The variations of positive and negative signs and symptoms that a patient may develop further contribute to the complexity of the clinical disorder.

A. Presenting symptoms. Patients with MS may present with a wide variety of neurologic symptoms. The most common symptoms at onset are weakness and sensory disturbances in one or more limbs, with each accounting for 25% of the patients. Approximately 20% of patients present with visual loss in one eye and 15% each with disorders of micturition and cerebellar ataxia. About 10% of patients present with a variety of other symptoms. These percentages are approximations and vary among reports. It is common for patients to present with multiple symptoms, which explains why these percentages total more than 100%.

B. Clinical course. Approximately 20–30% of MS patients have benign disorders. Some of these patients have only a few exacerbations, after which the disorder appears to resolve. Others, typically with predominantly sensory exacerbations, have recurrent events over years, without significant residual defects. More characteristically, not all exacerbations fully resolve, and the patient accumulates neurologic dysfunction over time. About 10% of patients have very malignant courses with severe disabilities within months to a few years, and in some cases even within weeks or days.

C. Disease forms. There are several forms of MS. Approximately 35% of patients have an **exacerbating/remitting** form of the disease with neurologic dysfunction that frequently builds over days to weeks, reaches a plateau, and then resolves over weeks to months. In some cases the exacerbation is maximal within minutes to hours. Some patients have only partial or no recovery from their exacerbations and accumulate disability in a stepwise manner. Their disorders are classified as **exacerbating/progressive MS,** which accounts for approximately 45% of all MS cases. Over time, in a subset of patients who were initially exacerbating/remitting or exacerbating/progressive, a course develops that is predominantly progressive in a more linear manner. This form of the disease is referred to as **secondary chronic progressive MS.** In a final subset of patients, the disorder exhibits a near-linear progressive course from the onset and is termed **primary chronic progressive MS.** These patients are typically older at disease onset and their dysfunctions manifest primarily as insidiously progressive spastic paraparesis with ataxia and bladder dysfunction. It is of note that, even in the primary chronic progressive form of the disorder, a substantial number of patients stabilize after several years. Regrettably, there may be severe residual disability prior to stabilization.

D. Prognosis is difficult to make in newly diagnosed MS patients. The most reliable prognostic factor is the form of the disease. Patients with discrete exacerbations with significant recovery have the best prognosis. In this group, there is a trend toward better outcome when the onset of disease is at a younger age and the symptoms are restricted to one region of the CNS. This is especially true if the symptoms are predominantly sensory. Patients who begin with a chronic progressive disorder usually undergo a much more severe course. These patients usually have disease onset later in life and are more frequently of male gender. Overall, the **"Kurtzke 5-year rule"** is reasonably reliable. This rule states that the absence of significant motor or cerebellar dysfunction at 5 years correlates with limited disability at 15 years.

IV. Diagnosis. An accurate diagnosis of MS is extremely important, because this disorder mimics many diseases of the CNS. Unfortunately, the diagnosis cannot be achieved reliably through any single paraclinical study. Rather, the entire clinical syndrome must be evaluated with a careful clinical history and examination. The resulting findings direct further laboratory studies to eliminate other disorders or to support the diagnosis of MS by paraclinical studies such as MRI, evoked potentials, and cerebrospinal fluid (CSF) tests. Optimally, the clinician should understand the relative importance, specificity, and sensitivity of each symptom, sign, and paraclinical study for each clinical form of MS at various points of time in the clinical course. Patient evaluation by this approach allows an experienced clinician to obtain a diagnosis with greater than 95% accuracy in many cases.

A. Clinical aspects of diagnostic importance

1. **Age.** The peak age range of disease onset is between 20 and 45 years. It is very rare for MS to start before age 14 or after age 60. Careful consideration must be given to other disorders in patients who present with MS-like symptoms in atypical age groups.
2. **Character of signs and symptoms**
   a. **Lesion localization.** Symptoms should suggest a CNS origin. Examples of exceptions include patients who present with an infranuclear cranial nerve palsy or monoradiculopathy resulting from plaque formation over the exit of the cranial nerve or nerve root within the CNS.
   b. **Onset features and course.** Most symptoms develop over hours to days, plateau, and then begin to decline. On occasion, the symptoms are maximal within seconds or minutes. Consideration should be given to an infarct in these cases, especially if localization suggests a vascular territory. For all but chronic progressive patients, the most consistent history is of relapses and remissions involving various areas of the CNS at different points in time. For primary chronic progressive patients, such a history is rarely obtained, making their diagnosis more difficult. These patients usually have an insidiously progressive spinocerebellar syndrome that may mimic several other disorders, including mass or compressive lesions, infectious diseases, metabolic disorders, inherited spinal cerebellar syndromes, and degenerative diseases. Presentation with aphasia, dementia, psychosis, acute anxiety, movement disorders, and intense pain is unusual in MS.
3. **Differential diagnosis.** Early on, a subset of patients with many CNS disorders have symptoms suggestive of the various forms of MS. A partial listing includes systemic lupus erythematosus, antiphospholipid antibody syndrome, Sjögren's syndrome, primary CNS vasculitis, sarcoidosis, Lyme disease, tropical spastic paraparesis, progressive multifocal leukoencephalopathy, subacute sclerosing panencephalitis, acute disseminated encephalomyelitis, postinfectious demyelination, vitamin B_{12} deficiency, adrenomyeloneuropathy, idiopathic and inherited spinocerebellar syndromes, CNS mass lesions, and paraneoplastic syndromes. Because of the potential overlapping symptoms and findings, a clinician must always pursue a complete evaluation of a suspected MS patient and never force a diagnosis of MS in the setting of atypical features or findings.
B. **MRI studies.** Overall, the cranial MRI is the most sensitive paraclinical study available for diagnosis of MS. Lesions are most frequently detected with proton density–weighted images (first echo of a T2-weighted sequence).
   1. **Frequency of MRI abnormalities in MS**
      a. **Definite MS.** 85–97%
      b. **Suspected MS.** 60–85%
   2. **MRI abnormalities**
      a. MRI images typically reveal multiple focal **periventricular** areas of increased signal that are irregular in shape and less than 2.5 cm long. Unfortunately, none of these characteristics is specific to lesions secondary to MS. For example, in older normal control populations, it is common for MRI to reveal multiple, punctate, nonspecific areas of increased T2 signal in the deep white matter.

      Abnormalities more suggestive of demyelination are multiple lesions, some of which are greater than 5 mm in size, are ovoid in shape, and/or abut the body of the lateral ventricle. In MS it is also common to find lesions that involve the corpus callosum or that are infratentorial in location.
      b. Gadolinium-enhancing lesions are transient and reflect the local temporary **blood-brain barrier breakdown** that occurs in active plaque. These contrast-enhanced MRIs reflect acute disease more accurately than do nonenhanced studies.
      c. Atrophy is common in longstanding disease.
C. **CSF examination** is frequently performed in evaluation of MS patients. Certain patterns of CSF abnormalities are highly suggestive of this disorder. These patterns, however, are not specific to MS and may be observed in association with other inflammatory or infectious disorders.
   1. The appearance of the CSF and the opening pressure are normal.
   2. **Cell count.** The red blood cell count is normal. A mild lymphocytosis is typical, with more than one-third of the patients having more than 5 cells/mm³.

In the unusual event that more than 50 cells/mm^3 are noted, consideration should be given to an infectious process.

3. **Protein.** The CSF protein is usually mildly elevated, with greater than one-fourth of the patients having protein levels greater than 54 mg/dl. A protein level higher than 100 mg/dl is very rare.

4. **Myelin basic protein.** Myelin is destroyed in MS plaque. Approximately 30% of CNS myelin is myelin basic protein (MBP). MBP is released with the destruction of myelin, and its presence in the CSF is one of the most reliable indicators of current demyelination, with the level being proportional to the extent of myelin destruction. This elevated level is observed during the first 2 weeks after a substantial exacerbation in 50–90% of patients, then disappears with time. MBP is not disease-specific and may be present in any process involving myelin destruction, such as an infarct or CNS infection.

5. **Immunoglobulin.** The CSF immunoglobulin (primarily IgG, but also IgM and to a lesser extent IgA) is elevated (to a value greater than 12% of total protein) in 60–80% of MS patients. This increase results mainly from an abundance of plasma cells producing immunoglobulin in the brain and spinal cord. A smaller component of immunoglobulin arises from normal transfer from the serum and increased entry through a disturbed blood-brain barrier.

   a. **IgG synthesis rate.** The IgG synthesis rate represents a calculated estimate of the synthetic rate of IgG within the intrathecal space. It is increased to more than 3 mg/day in 80–90% of MS patients but rarely exceeds 130 mg/day. This rate correlates with MRI plaque burden and decreases with adrenocorticotropic hormone (ACTH) or glucocorticoid therapy. The rate is increased in 12% of the normal population and in 30–50% of patients with CNS infections.

   b. **IgG index.** The IgG index is a calculation [(CSF IgG/serum IgG)/(CSF albumin/serum albumin)] that reflects the increased IgG in the intrathecal space. It is increased (to a value greater than 0.7) in 86–94% of MS patients and is often the first CSF abnormality observed early in the disease.

6. **CSF oligoclonal bands (OCBs)** are discrete bands that are frequently detected in the CSF of MS patients. Most data indicate that OCBs are not directed against specific antigens and are not involved in pathogenesis of disease. They are present in 30–40% of possible and 90–97% of definite MS patients. OCBs are also observed in other chronic inflammatory diseases of the CNS, in infectious disorders, and in 7% of normal controls. Although the prevalence of OCBs increases when CSF is sampled later in the course of the disease, these bands are not related to current disease activity or therapy. The pattern of bands varies from patient to patient. In a single patient, the pattern tends to be relatively stable with some minor changes and addition of bands over a period of time. The bands found in MS are usually observed only in the CSF, when paired CSF and serum samples are evaluated simultaneously. This differs from the typically paired OCBs found in many other conditions such as inflammatory neuropathies, neoplasms, and systemic immune responses.

D. **Evoked potentials** provide electrophysiologic evidence of conduction blocks or delays caused by demyelination. These studies were very important in documenting widespread lesions prior to the availability of MRI. They still play an important role in the diagnosis of MS in some patients.

1. **Visual evoked potentials (VEPs).** Demyelination frequently occurs in the optic nerves and optic chiasm in MS patients. Whereas some patients develop symptoms consistent with optic neuritis, others have no associated visual symptoms. VEPs evaluate conduction defects in the visual pathways. In the majority of patients with **prior demyelination** of the optic nerve, the VEPs remain abnormal.

   VEPs are abnormal in approximately 40, 60, and 85% of possible, probable, and definite MS patients, respectively.

2. **Somatosensory evoked potentials (SSEPs)** detect conduction defects in the somatosensory pathways. The study involves stimulation of the large myelinated fibers of the peroneal, tibial, or median peripheral nerve while recording over the contralateral sensorimotor cortex.

SSEPs are abnormal in approximately 50, 70, and 80% of possible, probable, and definite MS patients, respectively.

3. **Brainstem auditory evoked potentials (BAEPs)** evaluate conduction disturbances in the auditory pathways after auditory stimulation.

BAEPs are abnormal in approximately 30, 40, and 70% of possible, probable, and definite MS patients, respectively.

V. **Therapy.** The complex, highly variable signs and symptoms observed in MS patients result in a clinical disorder that is often a challenge to treat. Therapy for MS is both symptomatic and immune-modulating. **Symptomatic therapy** involves treatment of fatigue, spasticity, neurobehavioral disorders, paroxysmal disorders, pain, bladder dysfunction, and cerebellar dysfunction. **Immune-modulating therapies** are directed at altering the clinical course. This may involve treatment of acute exacerbations or the overall progression of the disease.

A. **Symptomatic therapy.** Patients with mild or early disease may have limited neurologic dysfunction and require minimal therapy. In these patients, the main therapy is limited to counseling and education. In more severe cases or later in the clinical course, patients often have many symptoms that respond to treatment.

1. **Spasticity** is very common in severe or longstanding MS. Patients complain of tightness or stiffness of affected limbs or trunk and reflex spasms. These spasms may be provoked by a variety of stimuli or may occur spontaneously. Spasticity makes ambulation difficult, causes fatigue, may make transfer arduous, may interfere with sleep, and may cause pain. During an exacerbation or with an otherwise asymptomatic urinary tract infection, there may be a significant increase in spasticity. Treatment of the underlying disorder often returns the spasticity to baseline. Range of motion exercises around each joint in the spastic limb may decrease spasticity and prevent fibrosis of the muscle. **Pharmacologic agents** are usually required when a substantial amount of strength is wasted in overcoming the spastic component to ambulate or when the patient is too weak to ambulate, and yet spasticity causes discomfort and difficulty with transfers. Overmedication should be avoided in ambulatory patients, because a small amount of extensor spasticity is beneficial for weight-bearing purposes in weak lower limbs.

a. **Baclofen** is the most effective agent for reducing spasticity, especially of spinal cord origin. The medication may be started at a low dosage of either 10 mg at bedtime or 10 mg bid and slowly increased weekly or biweekly by 10 mg/day as tolerated or needed. When the dosage is too high, patients notice a decline in strength. At that point, decreasing the dosage by 10 mg/day usually offers the optimal level of function and maximal treatment of spasticity without significant induction of weakness. For patients with spastic paraplegia, ambulation is not an issue and higher dosages are often tolerated and necessary. The maximum dosage recommended by the manufacture is 80 mg/day in four divided doses, but higher dosages are prescribed by many physicians. In addition to the aforementioned dosage-related weakness, the most common side effects are sedation, dizziness, and confusion. When the drug is discontinued, the dosage should be gently tapered off, because abrupt withdrawal may result in confusion and seizures.

b. **Benzodiazepines** provide benefit in a subset of patients with severe spasticity that is refractory to baclofen. Addition of small dosages of diazepam to baclofen may result in a synergistic effect. Usual dosages are 0.5–1.0 mg bid-tid. If patients are intolerant to baclofen, diazepam may be used alone. The dosage may be started at 1–2 mg bid-tid and gradually increased to a maximum of 20–30 mg/day. Dependence may develop, so the drug is withdrawn gradually when discontinued.

c. **Dantrolene** may be used for spasticity when baclofen and benzodiazepines are ineffective. Weakness induced by the drug limits its usefulness for many patients already compromised with motor impairment. For the rare patient in whom strength is preserved in the presence of severe spasticity, the drug may provide benefit. Other patients who are good candidates have severe weakness, no useful function of the legs, and spasticity that contributes to flexion contracture, discomfort, and difficulties with transfer and activities of daily living. In this situation, the loss of strength is of less consequence. The dosage is usually started at 25 mg/day and gently increased to 100 mg qid if needed. **Liver functions** must be monitored, because liver toxicity is a rare but potentially fatal complication of this medication. The risk is highest in females, in patients over 35 years old, and when the dosage is greater than 200 mg/day. Other side effects include diarrhea at higher dosages and, occasionally, pericarditis or pleuritis. Although dantrolene usually has little effect on cardiac or smooth muscle, it should be used with care for patients with myocardial disease.

   d. When these pharmacologic agents are contraindicated because of complications or do not control spasticity, **surgical intervention** may be considered. Surgical procedures include percutaneous radiofrequency foraminal rhizotomy, sciatic neurectomy, tenotomy, neurectomy, myelotomy, and intramuscular neurolysis. Intrathecal baclofen delivered by a subcutaneous pump is an effective alternative for some patients. Again, this therapy should be reserved for patients with severe spasticity that is unresponsive to oral therapy or for patients in whom oral agents have resulted in severe complications. The pump is expensive, requires frequent dosage adjustments (especially during the first several months), and requires refilling every 1–3 months. Furthermore, the battery has a limited life and requires replacement along with the pump (not the catheter) every few years.

2. Fatigue and heat sensitivity. The majority of MS patients complain of fatigue, which varies from mild to severely disabling. This symptom may be further potentiated by spasticity, depression, a current infection, sleep disorders, or interruptions of sleep by nocturia resulting from bladder dysfunction. After these causes have been treated, patients should be instructed to conserve energy through time management, economy of effort, and simplification of work. A subset of patients complain of extreme fatigue and even exacerbation of focal neurologic symptoms in hot environments, with increased body temperature during exertion or with a febrile illness. Heat-sensitive patients should be advised to decrease ambient temperature to comfortable levels, dress lightly to enhance heat dispersion, and treat fevers aggressively.

   a. Amantadine provides a modest reduction in fatigue in the majority of patients. The dosage is 100 mg bid. The medication is discontinued if there is no benefit after 1 month.

   b. Pemoline may be used for patients undertaking short-term projects or activities in which fatigue may cause significant dysfunction. The stimulant effects and abuse potential of this medication preclude its long-term use. The initial dosage of 18.75 mg every morning may be increased to 37.5 mg or more.

   c. Experimental medications. Preliminary trials with the potassium channel blockers 4-aminopyridine and 3,4-diaminopyridine have shown promise in improving the level of function and decreasing fatigue and heat sensitivity. These medications have the potential for several complications and need further evaluation to establish their efficacy and safety for chronic use.

3. Neurobehavioral disorders. Patients with MS may have several neurobehavioral disorders, including depression, euphoria, emotional lability, dementia, cognitive impairment, and, in rare instances, bipolar disease, extreme anxiety, and psychosis. Recognition of these disorders is important because some are amenable to therapy, which can decrease disability and improve the patient's quality of life.

   a. Depression is common in MS. The reported prevalence varies considerably, with a probable range of 25–50%. The etiology of the depression is most likely multifactorial, having biological, psychological, and social elements. All factors should be considered, and therapy should be tailored to each patient. When the depression appears to be a reaction to the illness, the patient may benefit from counseling and treatment of the MS. Although actual investigation of drug efficacy in MS is limited, in many patients a trial of antidepressants should be considered.

      (1) Desipramine is a reasonable therapeutic choice because it has fewer anticholinergic side effects than do other antidepressants.

The drug may be started at 25 mg at bedtime and increased gradually over a period of weeks to 75–100 mg/day. If there is no effect after 4–6 weeks, the dosage may be raised to 150–200 mg/day in divided doses.

   (2) **Alternative antidepressants** include amitriptyline, doxepin, trazodone, and imipramine. Imipramine provides treatment for both bladder dysfunction and depression in patients with spastic bladders.

   (3) **Electroconvulsive therapy** may have only a limited role in treating MS, because it has been complicated by exacerbations in anecdotal cases.

   b. **Other neurobehavioral disorders** include euphoria, pathologic laughing and crying, anxiety, and psychosis. **Euphoria** is defined as a persistent change in mood consisting of cheerfulness and optimism. This mood may persist in spite of the patient's awareness of very suboptimal circumstances including severe disability. No treatment is required. **Emotional lability** is common in MS patients. This disorder ranges from mild giggling or tearing to pathologic laughing and crying or, in severe cases, complete emotional incontinence. Usually the patient is aware of the lability and these emotional outbursts are socially distressing. Amitriptyline improves emotional control in many patients. This drug may be given at bedtime, starting at 25 mg and increasing the dosage as needed, with the majority of patients responding to less than 100 mg. If amitriptyline is ineffective, a trial of levodopa or bromocriptine is merited.

   Extreme anxiety is rare in MS. Alprazolam at a dosage of 0.25–0.50 mg bid-tid may decrease the symptoms. An alternative medication is diazepam. Both of these drugs have abuse potentials and should be prescribed with care and withdrawn gradually when discontinued. Although rare, psychosis is sometimes observed in MS patients. This psychosis is typically an agitated depression or a complication of steroid therapy rather than an isolated phenomenon. Antipsychotic drugs are used as in the psychiatric population.

4. **Paroxysmal disorders** typically present as intense ephaptic events lasting seconds to minutes, with a tendency to recur in a stereotypic manner. These events occur in 1–4% of MS patients without associated epileptiform activity on EEG. Some are unique to MS and occasionally are the presenting symptoms. They may occur either during exacerbations or in isolation. They frequently last weeks to months and then spontaneously resolve. A careful inquiry for the presence of these disorders is important, because they can cause the patient significant discomfort or dysfunction. The majority of paroxysmal disorders respond to anticonvulsant agents, with carbamazepine being the usual drug of choice.

   a. **Trigeminal neuralgia (TN)** consists of triggered and nontriggered paroxysmal episodes of facial pain in the trigeminal distribution. TN occurs in 1–2% of MS patients. The pain of TN is similar in MS and non-MS patients except that in MS patients it has a higher incidence, occurs at a younger age, and is more often bilateral. Also, there is an increased incidence of atypical TN, with longer episodes of intense pain superimposed on persistent facial discomfort, among MS patients. Carbamazepine, used alone or in combination with baclofen or phenytoin, gives complete relief in some patients and reduces pain in the majority of patients. When TN is refractory to these medications, the orally active antipsychotic agent pimozide may be considered. This medication should be used with care, because the majority of MS patients exhibit adverse effects including lethargy, impaired concentration, hand tremors, involuntary movements during sleep, and slight parkinsonian features. When there are serious drug complications or a lack of pain control with conservative management, surgical intervention should be considered.

   b. **Other paroxysmal sensory or painful symptoms** include a variety of sensations such as burning paresthesias, severe or aching pain, unpleasant quivering sensations, spontaneous Lhermitte's-like phenomenon, and itching. The majority of these episodes last seconds to a few minutes and most frequently involve the extremities, although they may affect any part of the body. **Paroxysmal itching** differs from the other sensations in that the episodes last as long as 30 minutes and sometimes occur in a dermatomal distribution, especially over the shoulders and neck. All of these paroxysms usually respond to low-dosage carbamazepine.

c. **Tonic spasms** are severe spasms that last seconds to minutes, beginning in the limbs or trunk and spreading upward or downward, sometimes crossing the midline. Many times, an intense pain or unpleasant sensation starts at a "trigger zone" and precedes or accompanies the spasm. In other patients, the spasms occur without discomfort. These spasms may occur spontaneously or may be provoked by movement, tactile stimulation of a "trigger zone," or hyperventilation. In an individual patient, the tonic spasm, with or without the pain, recurs in a very stereotypic pattern. These episodes may occur as part of an exacerbation or when the patient is stable. Tonic spasms should be differentiated from flexor spasms. Tonic spasms are more intense, usually are associated with severe pain, spread in a stereotypic manner, and are not correlated with the same degree of underlying spasticity. Whereas flexor spasms are best treated with baclofen, tonic spasms usually respond to carbamazepine at dosages of 200–400 mg/day. If carbamazepine does not provide relief, a typically less effective alternative is phenytoin.

d. **Paroxysmal dysarthria and ataxia** present as episodes that usually last less than 1 minute but may recur several times in one day. In some patients, the episodes are precipitated by anxiety or hyperventilation. The ataxia may result in falls, and the dysarthria may be so severe that the speech is uninterpretable. Although the dysarthria and ataxia are always present, there may be other associated symptoms, including diplopia, numbness, and weakness. Carbamazepine is almost always effective, with isolated cases responding to phenytoin or acetazolamide.

e. **Diplopia** may occur with dysarthria and ataxia or in isolation. With isolated diplopia, the episodes last seconds to a few minutes and may occur up to 100 times a day. Carbamazepine is the drug of choice.

f. **Other paroxysmal disorders** include akinesia in one or more limbs, lasting a few seconds and frequently recurring several times a day; weakness usually of a leg or hand, lasting 10–20 seconds to a few minutes with resultant unexpected falls or dropping of objects; and paroxysmal hemiataxia and crossed paresthesia.

5. **Pain.** Although pain is rarely a presenting symptom in MS, it commonly develops during the course of the disease, affecting over 50% of the population. The paroxysmal pain syndromes that respond best to anticonvulsant-type medications have already been discussed. More commonly, patients develop chronic pain that includes dysesthetic pain, back pain, and painful leg spasms. The typical burning or aching dysesthetic pain responds best to antidepressant-type drugs such as amitriptyline and imipramine. This pain is difficult to control with most patients refractory to therapy even with dosages as high as 100 mg/day. A combination of aggressive physical therapy and nonsteroidal anti-inflammatory agents provides partial relief in most patients with chronic back pain. Addition of antidepressant-type medications may be required. Patients who are resistant to therapy and debilitated by severe pain may require intrathecal morphine, intrathecal phenol, or neurolytic procedures such as dorsal rhizotomy.

6. **Bladder dysfunction.** Patients with MS frequently develop neurogenic bladder at some point during the illness. In many, bladder dysfunction persists and causes major social concerns. This dysfunction may be the result of an uninhibited small capacity or a flaccid neurogenic bladder. The symptoms of an uninhibited neurogenic bladder are primarily irritative, whereas those of a flaccid neurogenic bladder are primarily obstructive. There is a substantial amount of overlap between the symptomologies of these disorders, and a clinical history is frequently insufficient for diagnosis. Because both conditions can accompany MS, the optimal approach is for the patient to undergo a **urologic evaluation** to determine the exact bladder dysfunction. This is especially true because the therapies for these disorders are directly antagonistic.

a. **Uninhibited neurogenic bladder.** Patients with uninhibited small-capacity bladders are prone to frequent urination. When this is not feasible, the patient may transiently decrease fluid intake to decrease the frequency. To reduce the likelihood of incontinence, patients should void on a routine schedule, every 3–4 hours. Anticholinergic agents constitute the primary medical therapy. Propantheline bromide may be started at 15 mg qid and then gradually increased until the symptoms are controlled or the side effects of blurred vision, dry mouth, constipation, sedation, and confusion preclude further increases. Oxybutynin is an alternative anticholinergic with similar side effects. This medication is started at 5 mg bid and is increased to a maximum of 5 mg qid. The anticholinergic side effects of other medications such as tricyclic antidepressants may be beneficial, especially when they provide multiple benefits such as treatment of the neurogenic bladder, pain, and/or neurobehavioral problems. Finally, desmopressin and maprotiline have provided benefits with decreased side effects in preliminary trials. All medications with substantial anticholinergic actions may cause urinary retention, and thus urinary residual volume should be monitored after initiation of therapy. Intermittent **catheterization** may be performed in combination with the medication if the patient develops elevated residual urine volumes. When medications are ineffective, most patients resort to intermittent catheterization. An indwelling Foley, condom (male), or suprapubic catheter may be used for patients who have no available assistance and cannot perform intermittent catheterization.

   b. **Flaccid neurogenic bladder** is less common in the MS population. Patients should attempt to void every 3–4 hours, with complete bladder emptying often requiring double or triple voiding. Trials of the cholinergic agents carbachol and bethanechol chloride are merited, but benefits are usually limited and usage is complicated by urinary retention accompanied by prostatic hypertrophy, and bladder-sphincter dyssynergia, and a spastic external urethral sphincter. Combining a cholinergic antagonist with an alpha-adrenergic blocker such as phenoxybenzamine or an antispasmodic such as diazepam, baclofen, tizanidine, or chlorpromazine may improve bladder function in some patients. Unfortunately, response to medical therapy is usually inadequate and straight catheterization is required at 4–6-hour intervals. If the patient cannot perform intermittent catheterization and assistance is not available, more permanent measures may be taken as with the uninhibited bladder.

   c. **Urinary tract infections.** Patients with neurogenic bladders frequently develop bacterial bladder infections. Such infections can contribute to the symptoms of bladder irritability and may result in transient lower-extremity weakness and spasticity, resembling an exacerbation. Patients on immunosuppressive agents may develop life-threatening urinary **sepsis.** To decrease the risk of infection, patients should maintain adequate hydration to purge the bladder and dilute the bacterial population. They should also concentrate on emptying the bladder thoroughly, because residual volumes of more than 50 ml are complicated by a threefold increase in bacteriuria. Antibiotic selection by urine culture with organism sensitivity is preferable to empiric therapy because the latter predisposes to resistant organisms. Preventive therapy is often required in patients with recurrent infections. There are several methods of promoting bacteriostasis. Acidification of the urine may be achieved with vitamin C (1 g qid) or cranberry juice. Other citrus juices, including orange juice, should be avoided because they tend to raise the urine pH. Methenamine hippurate or methenamine mandelate may be given to generate formaldehyde salts. If these methods fail, a prophylactic antibiotic such as sulfamethoxazole or trimethoprim is required.

7. **Cerebellar dysfunction** is common, especially in the chronic progressive form of MS. Upper-extremity ataxia and tremors may be so severe that activities of daily living are impossible and nursing home care is required. This dysfunction is especially resistant to therapy. In spite of reported benefits in small trials, isoniazid, carbamazepine, primidone, and glutethimide all provide only marginal control in most patients. Other medications that have been used with little success are baclofen, clonazepam, propranolol, choline, and lecithin. In summary, there is no effective medical therapy to date. Surgical intervention is controversial and has included stereotaxic thalamotomy and deep brain stimulation. Exacerbations have occurred after

surgery, and it is difficult to predict the response of tremors to surgical procedures. When a patient begins to develop significant cerebellar dysfunction, consideration should be given to more aggressive immune-modulating therapy.

B. Immune-modulating therapy. Although the exact pathogenesis of MS is unknown, it appears to be multifactorial with a substantial autoimmune contribution. This has prompted numerous clinical trials of immune-modulating agents in an attempt to alter the disease's course. Available therapies remain inadequate and have the potential for substantial complications.

1. Treatment of exacerbations

   a. Indications for therapy. Exacerbations are common in patients with active exacerbating/remitting or exacerbating/progressive MS. There are few data to support changes in long-term clinical course or disability with treatment of exacerbations. Rather, the advantage of therapy is to expedite recovery from an exacerbation, allowing the patient to return to a higher level of function more quickly than if the exacerbation were allowed to run its natural course. It is our experience that many patients initially show an excellent response to treatment but the benefit is lost after several interventions. In light of these factors, not all exacerbations should be treated. We typically reserve therapy for patients who exhibit definite changes in functional status, usually related to significant declines in visual, motor, or cerebellar function.

   b. Therapy. Acute exacerbations are usually treated with **methylprednisolone** or **ACTH.** There are no definitive data to indicate which drug is more effective. However, methylprednisolone is probably superior because it is usually given over a shorter period of time and because the cortisol response to ACTH is not consistent and may be delayed. Furthermore, the endogenous steroid production of ACTH may never reach the range generally recommended for inflammatory autoimmune diseases. The optimal dosages and treatment schedules are not well studied. Most treatment protocols for acute exacerbations indicate 25–60 units of ACTH given intramuscularly or infused over an 8-hour period and tapered gradually over a 2–4-week course. Intravenous methylprednisolone may be given in dosages of 500–1000 mg each morning for 5 days. This may be followed by prednisone administered in a dosage of 60 mg every morning for 3 days and then decreased by 10 mg every 3 days on a relatively rapid taper. The prednisone appears to help prevent immediate relapses after the methylprednisolone is discontinued. Exacerbations may be treated with oral prednisone without the preceding methylprednisolone. We are now more reluctant to treat in this manner, however, because the optic neuritis trial showed benefit from methylprednisolone followed by oral prednisone but increased relapse rates for optic neuritis after treatment with oral prednisone alone. Treatment with glucocorticoids is avoided in pregnant patients. Severe exacerbations in such patients have been treated successfully with plasma exchange in isolated cases. Finally, consideration may be given to the use of plasma exchange and IV bolus cyclophosphamide in patients with fulminant disease for which glucocorticoids have provided no benefit.

2. Prevention of exacerbations and progression. Immune-modulating agents are commonly used in MS in an attempt to alter the natural history of the disorder. The majority of immunosuppressive agents are controversial, with published data both supporting and disproving their efficacy. In each patient treated, the risk/benefit ratio must be carefully weighed by both the clinician and the patient, and full agreement must be reached after the patient has been completely informed. The complex nature of choosing these medications for particular disease forms and particular patients makes it difficult to make prudent decisions without substantial background information and expertise. These decisions are more optimally made by clinicians specializing in the treatment of MS.

   a. Interferon-beta (IFN-β) has been shown to reduce the number and severity of exacerbations as well as the total lesion load as detected by cranial MRI in a randomized, double-blind, placebo-controlled trial of exacerbating/remitting MS patients. The medication was generally well tolerated, with the most common side effects being a flulike syndrome of fever and myalgias during the first weeks to months of therapy and injection-site reactions throughout the clinical trial. Other side effects, including mild lymphopenia and elevation of serum transaminases, were also noted but rarely caused withdrawal of treatment. IFN-β has been approved and licensed as Betaseron for exacerbating/remitting and mild to moderate MS by the FDA. This medication is expensive and requires subcutaneous injections every other day. Within the exacerbating/remitting disease group, it is difficult to ascertain which specific patients respond best to the medication and how long it should be administered. These questions are currently being addressed in open-label trials. If a patient has been stable without a significant exacerbation for 1–2 years, we typically defer initiation of IFN-β therapy unless the patient strongly desires such treatment. Although not a cure, IFN-β is the first agent shown to affect positively the natural history of MS without leading to unacceptable adverse effects. Evaluation of an intramuscular form of IFN-β is currently in progress, and studies of Betaseron in chronic progressive MS are planned for the near future. Investigations of other IFN-β products and different administration protocols are likely to follow.

   b. **Other agents.** There are several other agents that have been evaluated in various MS populations. Azathioprine, cyclophosphamide, and cyclosporine provide benefits in individual patients, but the adverse effects of these agents preclude their use in the patient population at large. Methotrexate and cladribine have shown some promise in the treatment of chronic progressive MS, and further investigation of these drugs is merited. Many other agents and approaches are being considered or are under investigation. A partial list includes interferon-alpha, Copolymer 1, intravenous immunoglobulin, T-cell vaccination, immunization with T-cell receptor peptides, and induction of oral tolerance with myelin. Through the tremendous efforts of many investigators and participation in clinical trials by many patients, there has been substantial progress in the understanding and treatment of MS in the last few years. The development of optimal immune-modulating therapies for the future will require the continued collaboration of clinical and laboratory scientists.

VI. **Management of MS patients by primary care physicians.** Physicians with specialized training in MS are often more adept than primary care physicians in obtaining an accurate diagnosis of the disease. This is especially true because there are many disorders of the nervous system that can mimic MS and the diagnosis cannot be achieved reliably through any single paraclinical study. However, after diagnosis, primary care physicians may play a very important role in patient care. Early in the disease, many patients exhibit little or no neurologic dysfunction, and one of the more important physician services is patient education and emotional support, as well as making the patient aware of the excellent state and national MS organizations available for the same purposes. Later, referrals to physical and occupational therapists often result in substantial decreases in disability and improvements in the quality of life. Recognition of the previously discussed symptoms often allows them to be managed at the primary care level. This is frequently preferable, because multiple visits and frequent medication and dosage adjustments may be required and the primary care physician is often in closer proximity to the patient than the neurologist. Decisions concerning the use of immune-modulating agents for exacerbations or disease progression are usually better made by the clinician specializing in the treatment of MS. However, the primary care physician may provide vital services, because their implementation often requires careful patient monitoring for various systemic and organ-related complications.

Recommended Readings

Beck RW, et al. A randomized, controlled trial of corticosteroids in the treatment of acute optic neuritis. *N Engl J Med* 326:581–588, 1992.

Beck RW, et al. The effect of corticosteroids for acute optic neuritis on the subsequent development of multiple sclerosis. *N Engl J Med* 329:1764–1769, 1993.

Betts CD, Dmellow MT, Fowler CJ. Urinary symptoms and the neurological features of bladder dysfunction in multiple sclerosis. *J Neurol Neurosurg Psychiat* 56:245–250, 1993.

Bever CT. The current status of studies of aminopyridines in patients with multiple sclerosis. *Ann Neurol* 36:S118–S121, 1994.

Bornstein MB, et al. A placebo-controlled, double-blind, randomized, two-center, pilot trial of Cop 1 in chronic progressive multiple sclerosis. *Neurology* 41:533–539, 1991.

Canadian Coop MSS. The Canadian cooperative trial of cyclophosphamide and plasma exchange in progressive multiple sclerosis. *Lancet* 337:441–446, 1991.

Goodkin DE, et al. Low-dose (7.5 mg) oral methotrexate reduces the rate of progression in chronic progressive multiple sclerosis. *Ann Neurol* 37:30–40, 1995.

Herndon RM, Brooks B. Misdiagnosis of multiple sclerosis. *Semin Neurol* 5:94–98, 1985.

INF-B Multiple Sclerosis Study Group. Interferon beta-1B is effective in relapsing-remitting multiple sclerosis—clinical results of a multicenter, randomized, double-blind, placebo-controlled trial. *Neurology* 43:655–661, 1993.

Minden SL, Schiffer RB. Affective disorders in multiple sclerosis: Review and recommendations for clinical research. *Arch Neurol* 47:98–104, 1990.

Mitchell GW. Update on multiple sclerosis therapy. In J Biller (ed), *The Medical Clinics of North America: Contemporary Clinical Neurology*. Philadelphia: Saunders, 1993 (77:1). Pp 231–249.

Mitchell GW, Whitaker JN. Immunotherapy for neuroimmunologic disorders. In SH Appel (ed), *Current Neurology*. St. Louis: Mosby, 1994. Pp 73–109.

Moulin DE, Foley KM, Ebers GC. Pain syndromes in multiple sclerosis. *Neurology* 38:1830–1834, 1988.

Offenbacher H, et al. Assessment of MRI criteria for a diagnosis of MS. *Neurology* 43:905–909, 1993.

Paty DW, et al. Interferon B-1b is effective in relapsing-remitting multiple sclerosis. 2. MRI analysis results of a multicenter, randomized, double-blind, placebo-controlled trial. *Neurology* 43:662–667, 1993.

Poser CM. The epidemiology of multiple sclerosis: A general overview. *Ann Neurol* 36:S180–S193, 1994.

Rodriguez M, et al. Plasmapheresis in acute episodes of fulminant CNS inflammatory demyelination. *Neurology* 43:1100–1104, 1993.

Runmarker B, Andersen O. Prognostic factors in a multiple sclerosis incidence cohort with 25 years of follow-up. *Brain* 116:117–134, 1993.

Sipe JC, et al. Cladribine in treatment of chronic progressive multiple sclerosis. *Lancet* 344:9–13, 1994.

Tourtellotte WW, et al. The long march of the cerebrospinal fluid profile indicative of clinical definite multiple sclerosis; and still marching. *J Neuroimmunol* 20:217–227, 1988.

Weiner HL, et al. Intermittent cyclophosphamide pulse therapy in progressive multiple sclerosis—Final report of the Northeast-Cooperative-Multiple-Sclerosis-Treatment-Group. *Neurology* 43:910–918, 1993.

Yudkin PL, et al. Overview of azathioprine treatment in multiple sclerosis. *Lancet* 338:1051–1055, 1991.

41

Movement Disorders
Eric Siemers

Movement disorders are frequently categorized as **hypokinetic** or **hyperkinetic.** The clinical features of the various disorders based on this categorization can be found in Chaps. 28 and 29. The hypokinetic movement disorders are comprised essentially of the various causes of parkinsonism. Biochemically, the abnormality of movement is in large part a result of a relative deficiency of dopaminergic neurotransmission within the striatum of the basal ganglia. Conversely, many of the hyperkinetic movement disorders respond to blockading of dopaminergic transmission by receptor antagonists or other methods. A few disorders, including essential tremor and dystonia, do not appear to be mediated by changes in dopaminergic transmission; these disorders are generally grouped with the hyperkinetic movement disorders. This chapter summarizes the treatment strategies for a variety of movement disorders.

I. **Hypokinetic movement disorders**
   A. **Idiopathic Parkinson's disease (IPD)** accounts for about 80% of all cases of parkinsonism, with the other 20% falling into the general category of **Parkinson's-plus syndromes.** This distinction is of some practical significance, because patients with IPD are generally more responsive to antiparkinsonian medications and, at least early in the course of the disease, given adequate treatment, can be expected to have very few limitations on activities of daily living. Each of the medications discussed below helps to compensate for the loss of dopamine-containing cells in the substantia nigra, which is the primary cause of the motoric symptoms.
      1. **Long-term management strategies** in the treatment of IPD are important considering that the life expectancy of these patients is now nearly the same as that of age-matched controls. The point of greatest importance and uncertainty is whether the medications used for symptomatic improvement also affect the rate of progression of the underlying degenerative process. Two medications may have, but have not been proven to have, such effects. In a large prospective investigation known as the Deprenyl and Tocopherol Antioxidative Therapy of Parkinsonism (DATATOP) study, deprenyl was shown to delay the need for initiation of levodopa. Whether this finding was a result of a protective effect of deprenyl (i.e., slowing of the rate of disease progression) or was simply caused by a therapeutic effect has become a focus of some controversy. Conversely, data obtained primarily in vitro have suggested that the use of levodopa can possibly hasten the progression of the disease, perhaps through the generation of free radicals. For this reason, the introduction of levodopa is sometimes delayed in the management of IPD, even though it is clearly the most effective medication for relieving symptoms. These concepts, although not proven, may influence the choice of antiparkinsonian medications for a given patient at a given point in the course of the disease.
      2. **Deprenyl or selegiline (Eldepryl)** is an inhibitor of monoamine oxidase (MAO) and at prescribed dosages is specific for the B isozyme.
         a. **Deprenyl has a very modest therapeutic effect,** which is imperceptible for most patients when the drug is used as monotherapy. It is most frequently used as an initial treatment, not for improvement in symptoms but for its possible protective effects. It is effective as an adjunct to treatment with levodopa. The addition of deprenyl to levodopa permits levodopa dosages to be lowered about 25% and also prolongs the effect of each dose. The emergence of dyskinetic movements (see **I.A.5.c**) after

the addition of deprenyl to levodopa frequently can be treated most effectively by lowering of the dosage of levodopa. The currently recommended dosage is given in Table 41-1. Recent studies have suggested that
5 mg/day may be equally efficacious.

  b. **Adverse effects of deprenyl** are relatively infrequent when the drug is
  used early in the disease. Occasional patients report insomnia, which
  can be minimized by using the recommended regimen of one tablet in the
  morning and one at noon. Any of the other "dopaminergic" adverse effects that can occur with most antiparkinsonian medications may be associated with deprenyl. These effects include gastrointestinal upset,
  orthostatic hypotension, worsening or onset of dyskinetic movements,
  and development of mental status changes such as hallucinations that
  are usually visual, paranoia, and agitation. The tyramine or "wine and
  cheese" reaction associated with the use of nonspecific MAO inhibitors
  has not been associated with the use of deprenyl when given at the recommended dosage. This reaction is mediated by inhibition of MAO A in
  the liver and therefore would not be expected. As with other MAO inhibitors, patients taking deprenyl should not receive meperidine (Demerol) for pain control. There have been reports of the "serotonin syndrome" in patients taking deprenyl with a specific serotonin reuptake
  inhibitor (SSRI) for depression.

3. **Amantadine (Symmetrel)** has been used for many years in the treatment of
mild to moderate Parkinson's disease. The mechanism of action, although
not well understood, may be to inhibit the reuptake or enhance the release
of dopamine. Amantadine also has anticholinergic effects.

  a. **Amantadine can be used as initial therapy for IPD,** particularly for
  those patients who have mild to moderate bradykinesia along with mild
  to moderate tremor. The use of amantadine with deprenyl for patients
  with early disease can provide very acceptable results. Amantadine can
  also be used as an adjunctive treatment for patients taking other medications such as levodopa. Several sources indicate that amantadine is effective for only 6–12 months, which probably is related to the loss of effective symptom control with amantadine as the disease progresses;
  however, if amantadine is discontinued, symptoms often worsen unless
  another more potent medication is substituted. The usual dosage range
  for amantadine is given in Table 41-1.

  b. **Adverse effects of amantadine** are generally mild. Gastrointestinal upset is unusual. Mental status changes occur infrequently, perhaps related
  to the anticholinergic effects of the drug. Amantadine is excreted renally,
  and thus the dosage should be reduced in patients with renal insufficiency and the drug should be avoided in those with renal failure. A macular rash sometimes accompanied by edema of the lower extremities,
  known as livedo reticularis, is sometimes observed in association with
  amantadine. Although this rash is of primarily cosmetic significance,
  many patients do not wish to continue the medication should it occur.

4. **Anticholinergic drugs** have been used for many years in the treatment
of IPD, and were used even before their mechanism of action was understood. Many anticholinergic medications are available; the two that are used
most commonly are trihexyphenidyl (Artane) and benztropine (Cogentin).

Table 41-1. Antiparkinsonian medication regimens.

Drug	Total daily dosage (mg)	Frequency
Deprenyl	10	bid (see text)
Amantadine	200–400	bid-qid
Trihexyphenidyl	4–8	bid-qid
Benztropine	2–4	bid-qid
Levodopa	300–2500	tid-q90min
Sinemet CR	400–1600	bid-q3h
Bromocriptine	7.5–40	tid-q3h
Pergolide	0.75–6.0	bid-q3h

Diphenhydramine (Benadryl) is currently used only infrequently for Parkinson's disease because of its sedative side effect and the availability of better tolerated medications.

a. **Anticholinergics are frequently used early in the course of IPD** and seem to be particularly effective in controlling tremor. They may also be effective for patients with more advanced disease, but in these cases their use may be limited by adverse effects, as discussed below (sec. **b**). As listed in Table 41-1, the dosage ranges used for trihexyphenidyl and benztropine are quite narrow, and for this reason these drugs require little titration.

b. **Adverse effects of anticholinergic medications** include dry mouth, impaired visual accommodation, urinary hesitancy, and constipation. Patients with moderate to advanced IPD sometimes have associated memory loss and thus may be quite sensitive to the cognitive changes and memory disturbances associated with anticholinergic medications. The adverse cognitive effects of anticholinergics are the most common causes of their limited use for patients with moderate to advanced disease.

5. **Levodopa** has revolutionized the treatment of IPD. This medication is the precursor of dopamine. It is absorbed from the small intestine by a carrier-mediated process, and is similarly transported across the blood-brain barrier by the carrier for large neutral amino acids. Once in the brain it is converted to dopamine by the enzyme dopa decarboxylase. Particularly early in the course of the disease, this medication can provide almost complete relief of symptoms. For patients with more advanced disease, the use of levodopa can be complicated by response fluctuations, as discussed in sec. **c**.

a. **Available preparations of levodopa** include standard (now known as "immediate-release") carbidopa/levodopa (Sinemet, Atamet) and a controlled-release preparation (Sinemet CR). Carbidopa inhibits dopa decarboxylase and does not cross the blood-brain barrier. The inhibition of peripheral dopa decarboxylase markedly reduces the required total daily dosage of levodopa and minimizes the gastrointestinal upset associated with it. A minimum of 75 mg/day of carbidopa is required. Carbidopa/levodopa preparations are available as 10/100, 25/100, and 25/250 (mg carbidopa/mg levodopa) tablets and as 25/100 and 50/200 tablets for the controlled-release preparation.

b. **Levodopa generally relieves all of the cardinal signs of IPD:** bradykinesia, tremor, and rigidity. A lack of response to levodopa suggests a possible diagnosis of one of the Parkinson's-plus syndromes. Other associated symptoms, including hypophonia, dysphagia, and loss of postural reflexes, improve less reliably. For patients with advanced disease, levodopa may still provide relief of bradykinesia, but postural reflexes may remain substantially unchanged, thus increasing the likelihood of falls. Occasionally, tremor worsens, particularly when treatment with levodopa is initiated. With continued use of the drug or further increases in dosage, the tremor may subsequently subside. Treatment with carbidopa/levodopa is usually initiated using one 25/100 standard-release tablet tid or one 50/200 controlled-release tablet bid.

c. **Response fluctuations** occur in patients with moderate to advanced disease. Although the plasma half-life of levodopa is only about 2 hours, the effect of the medication lasts much longer in patients with mild disease, perhaps as a result of the storage of levodopa or dopamine by the remaining dopaminergic neurons. Later in the course of the disease, the control of motor disability is dependent on the minute-to-minute availability of levodopa from the blood. As patients progress, they first may develop "wearing off," the gradual loss of medication effectiveness prior to the next dose. They later may develop the "true on/off phenomenon," the sudden and unexpected wearing off of medication effectiveness. Conversely, higher blood levels of levodopa may cause dyskinetic movements in patients with moderate to advanced disease. Dyskinetic movements are usually choreoathetoid movements and most commonly involve the head and neck. The movements may, however, be quite diverse and involve foot, leg, trunk, or oral-buccal-lingual movements. Mild dyskinetic movements are usually well tolerated by patients because they occur when the medications are effectively controlling the bradykinesia. Patients with moderate to severe IPD may have periods of dyskinesia after each dose of carbidopa/levodopa, followed by either gradual or sudden wearing off. Treatment of response fluctuations is discussed in sec. **I.A.8.**

   d. **Adverse effects of levodopa** are representative of those of dopaminergic excess. When carbidopa/levodopa is initiated, gastrointestinal upset can occur, even with usually sufficient dosages of carbidopa. This effect can be minimized by having patients take carbidopa/levodopa after meals or by supplying them with supplemental carbidopa. GI upset usually gradually resolves with continued use of the drug. Changes in mental status can occur, especially in patients with moderate to advanced disease. These changes may take the form of overt psychosis, paranoia, sexual preoccupation, or intermittently agitated behavior. Visual hallucinations that can be quite vivid may occur, frequently in the form of people or animals. Early in the course of the disease, the patient may retain insight into the nature of the hallucinations, but later in the course they may become quite bothersome and, not infrequently, frightening. Mental status changes are usually dosage-dependent, but may continue in some patients after antiparkinsonian medications are discontinued. Anecdotal reports of acceleration of the growth of melanomas have been made, and thus levodopa should be used only with extreme caution in patients with such malignancies.

6. **Dopamine receptor agonists** are medications that directly stimulate dopamine receptors. Two of these medications—bromocriptine and pergolide—are currently available in the United States, and several others are undergoing clinical trials. There are several different dopamine receptor subtypes. Bromocriptine and pergolide act differently at receptors of different subtypes, but the clinical relevance of this finding is not clear at this time. Studies have shown that individual patients may respond more favorably to either of the two drugs.

   a. **All of the cardinal manifestations of IPD may be improved by dopamine receptor agonists.** These agents have been reported to be useful in the treatment of de novo IPD, but are more widely prescribed as adjuncts to levodopa. The plasma half-lives of these drugs are substantially longer than that of levodopa, and thus few patients report wearing off between doses. In order to minimize gastrointestinal upset, the dosage of a receptor agonist should be gradually increased to a minimum therapeutic level over 2–3 weeks. The therapeutic dosage ranges for bromocriptine and pergolide are listed in Table 41-1. Pergolide is approximately 10 times as potent as bromocriptine on a per-milligram basis.

   b. **Adverse effects of dopamine receptor agonists** are generally similar to the dopaminergic effects discussed in sec. **I.A.5.d.** Patients occasionally have difficulty with GI upset despite a gradual increase in dosage. In such cases the dosage can be increased even more slowly or adjunctive treatment with promethazine (Phenergan) can be given. Changes in mental status can be dealt with as discussed in sec. **I.A.9.** Bromocriptine occasionally causes stuffy nose, and pergolide can cause stuffy nose or pedal edema.

7. **Surgery** has played a very limited role in the treatment of Parkinson's disease since the introduction of levodopa in the late 1960s. However, several recent studies have addressed the role of stereotactic pallidotomy or thalamotomy for selected patients. The results of the studies to date have been positive; additional studies will be necessary to define clearly the optimal clinical indications for the use of this treatment modality.

8. **Treatment of response fluctuations** frequently requires combination therapy. Response fluctuations include the development of choreoathetoid dyskinetic movements after medications (usually levodopa), the gradual loss of medication effect (wearing off), or the sudden and unexpected loss of medication effect (true on/off phenomenon). Dyskinetic movements may be improved by lowering the dosage of levodopa. Wearing off can be improved by the use of Sinemet CR, the addition of deprenyl, or the addition of a dopamine receptor agonist. Patients not infrequently develop complex pat-

terns of response fluctuations that are best treated by a physician experienced in the use of combination therapy for IPD.

9. **Psychoses and hallucinations** are adverse effects that can occur in association with virtually any antiparkinsonian medication. These effects are usually improved simply by lowering the dosages of antiparkinsonian medications, if possible. If worsening of motoric symptoms make such a reduction impossible, the judicious use of neuroleptic medications may be necessary. In order to avoid exacerbation of the parkinsonism, neuroleptics with the least possible extrapyramidal side effects should be chosen. These drugs include thioridazine (Mellaril) and atypical neuroleptics such as clozapine (Clozaril) or olanzapine (Zyprexa).

10. **Constipation** is a concern for virtually every patient with parkinsonism and on rare occasions can cause significant morbidity and even mortality. Bulk laxatives alone are usually not sufficient to treat the constipation. Milk of magnesia, taken up to seven nights per week, can be helpful. Agents that stimulate gut motility, such as bisacodyl (Dulcolax), can be added if necessary. Metoclopramide (Reglan) should not be given, because it worsens parkinsonism, but cisapride (Propulcid) has no such ill effect.

11. **Contraindicated medications** for patients with IPD generally are those with antidopaminergic activity, including most antiemetics (promethazine is preferable when an antiemetic is needed). Metoclopramide (Reglan) can markedly worsen parkinsonism. As discussed above (sec. **I.A.2.b**), it is recommended that patients taking deprenyl not take meperidine (Demerol) or antidepressants of the SSRI class.

B. **Parkinson's-plus syndromes** represent degenerative conditions other than idiopathic Parkinson's disease that cause parkinsonism. Most of these syndromes have clinical features in addition to the parkinsonism, and for some of these disorders the parkinsonism may not be the primary source of disability. There are several of these conditions, all of which are rare; those specifically discussed in sec. **I.B.1–3** are most common or most amenable to treatment.

1. **Shy-Drager syndrome** is characterized by autonomic failure in addition to parkinsonism. A lack of response to antiparkinsonian medications and the onset of autonomic failure prior to the parkinsonism are both consistent with a diagnosis of Shy-Drager syndrome. Specific treatment of Shy-Drager syndrome is directed at the various autonomic symptoms.

   a. **Orthostatic hypotension** is frequently of greatest concern and can be worsened by most antiparkinsonian medications. Treatment may include nonpharmacologic measures such as the use of elastic stockings and raising the head of the bed 8 inches at night. Caffeine in the morning and after meals is reportedly effective. Indomethacin, 25 mg tid, can also improve orthostasis for some patients. Treatment with fludrocortisone (Florinef), usually at dosages of 0.1–0.3 mg/day, may be required. Pedal edema may become problematic as a result. The alpha adrenergic agonist midodrine (Pro-amatine) has recently become available and is reportedly effective. Dosages of these agents adequate to prevent syncope when standing may also cause significant hypertension when recumbent. In this case, the use of a short-acting antihypertensive medication at bedtime may be necessary.

   b. **Urinary frequency or incontinence** should be evaluated with a urologic examination and cystometry, because other causes of urologic dysfunction, such as prostate enlargement, are common in this age group. Treatment such as oxybutynin (Ditropan) for a spastic bladder or bethanechol (Urecholine) for a hypotonic bladder may provide relief. Surgical treatment of impotence may be necessary.

2. **Progressive supranuclear palsy** is named for the disturbance of volitional gaze that occurs in addition to parkinsonism. One of the primary sources of disability for these patients is a profound loss of balance with axial rigidity. Dementia is also usually present.

   a. **Treatment** of progressive supranuclear palsy is extremely limited. Antiparkinsonian medications may have no effect, in which case they should be discontinued. Occasionally they provide some relief.

   b. **Antidepressant medications** have been reported to be effective, but only for a minority of patients.

   c. Given the lack of effective pharmacologic management, the use of **phys-**

ical therapy and other nonpharmacologic modalities becomes of greater importance.

3. **Striatonigral degeneration** is characterized by parkinsonism—usually without a rest tremor and without additional features to suggest an alternative diagnosis. A mild postural tremor may be present. This condition is differentiated chiefly by the relative lack of response to antiparkinsonian medications, although in some cases high dosages of dopamine receptor agonists may be of some benefit.

4. Other degenerative causes of parkinsonism include **olivopontocerebellar atrophy (OPCA), multiple system atrophy (MSA), cortical-basal ganglionic degeneration (CBGD),** and **diffuse Lewy body disease,** among others. A vascular form of parkinsonism may exist. The diagnosis and treatment of each of these entities is difficult and is generally attempted by neurologists with particular expertise in movement disorders and degenerative diseases.

II. **Hyperkinetic movement disorders**

A. **Chorea** can be caused by a variety of disorders of the basal ganglia. Treatment of the choreiform movements themselves is essentially identical regardless of the cause. Huntington's disease involves treatment of symptoms in addition to chorea and is discussed separately.

1. **Huntington's disease (HD)** is an autosomal-dominant degenerative disorder of the CNS that causes loss of primarily medium-sized spiny neurons in the striatum. The neurotransmitters gamma-aminobutyric acid (GABA) and enkephalin are among a number of others whose levels decline. Dopaminergic input from the substantia nigra is preserved. Symptomatic treatment is directed at the major clinical features discussed below. Clinical trials of medications designed to slow the underlying pathophysiologic process are likely to begin in the near future.

a. **Choreiform movements** can be reliably controlled by neuroleptics that have prominent extrapyramidal effects. Most commonly, haloperidol (Haldol) is prescribed, but others may be equally effective. Relatively low dosages (less than 5 mg/day for haloperidol) are usually required, although patients occasionally require much higher dosages. The involuntary movements can almost always be improved by neuroleptics, but these medications must be used judiciously in patients with HD. Neuroleptics may worsen the loss of postural reflexes observed in HD, can be associated with worsening depression, can cause worsening of the parkinsonism that accompanies juvenile and advanced adult HD, and may cause an overall worsening of the patient's functional status. For these reasons, neuroleptics should be used only when choreiform movements interfere with activities of daily living, and the lowest possible dosages should be prescribed. Benzodiazepines can also have some effectiveness in this regard and may help with agitation.

b. **Depression** affects at least 30–50% of patients with HD and can respond very adequately to treatment. The SSRI fluoxetine (Prozac) has been specifically demonstrated to be effective. It is not uncommon for the required dosage of fluoxetine to be as high as 60 mg/day.

c. **Dementia** is the third major symptom associated with HD and is seen in more advanced stages of the disease. At this time no specific treatment has been shown to have any practical benefit. The future use of "cognitive enhancers" developed to treat Alzheimer's disease could be considered.

2. Other causes of chorea include **Sydenham's chorea (St. Vitus' dance), hyperthyroidism, systemic lupus erythematosus (SLE), chorea acanthocytosis,** and other degenerative disorders such as **dentatorubropallidoluysian atrophy (DRPLA).** Regardless of the underlying cause, the movements can be improved with the use of neuroleptics. The risk of tardive dyskinesia should be noted if prolonged treatment is anticipated. Benzodiazepines can be of some benefit. The major point of concern in these cases is identification of the correct underlying diagnosis, because symptomatic treatment is relatively straightforward.

B. The tics associated with **Tourette's syndrome (TS)** vary from simple head movements or vocalizations to more complex ritualistic behaviors and coprolalia. **Obsessive-compulsive behavior** has been associated with TS, and **at-**

tention-deficit disorder (ADD) as well as other more difficult-to-define behavioral abnormalities may be particularly problematic in children.

1. **Simple motor tics** can usually be treated successfully using neuroleptics with extrapyramidal effects. Haloperidol is frequently used first. Pimozide (Orap) was developed specifically for use in TS, and may cause less sedation than does haloperidol. Trifluoperazine (Stelazine) and thiothixene (Navane) can also be effective. A given neuroleptic may appear to become ineffective over time, in which case substitution of a different neuroleptic can subsequently improve control. Low dosages of these medications (less than 10 mg/day for haloperidol) are usually required, although the necessary dosage may vary widely among patients and at different times for a given patient. More complex tics respond less reliably; the distinction between complex ritualistic tics and frankly obsessive behaviors can sometimes become difficult. The usual adverse effects of neuroleptics can occur; in particular, sedation or depression may be problematic. Although the risk of tardive dyskinesia appears low for patients with TS, this long-term adverse effect must be considered.

2. **Treatment of obsessive-compulsive behavior** associated with TS is identical to that of the purely psychiatric condition. Clomipramine (Anafranil) and SSRIs such as fluoxetine (Prozac) may be used in this regard. The major adverse effects of clomipramine are sedation and anticholinergic effects.

3. **Attention deficit disorder (ADD)** and other behavioral disorders in children may be difficult to control. Use of CNS stimulants such as methylphenidate (Ritalin) may improve ADD, but may worsen motor tics. Occasionally motor tics will occur first during a trial of medication for ADD, but no actual causal relationship between CNS stimulants and TS has been established. The diverse behavioral abnormalities sometimes exhibited by children with TS not infrequently require family counseling and other nonpharmacologic approaches.

C. **Tardive dyskinesia (TD)** is a consequence of long-term treatment with dopamine receptor antagonists. Neuroleptics are the main cause of this disorder, but antiemetics—particularly metoclopramide (Reglan)—may also cause TD. Oral-buccal-lingual movements are often observed, and a wide variety of other hyperkinetic movements are not uncommon.

1. The **pathophysiology** of tardive dyskinesia is not completely understood. A probably incomplete explanation is that the response of TD to medications is consistent with the presence of upregulated dopamine receptors on neurons in the striatum. Thus, the involuntary movements characteristically worsen, or may first appear, just after the causative agent is discontinued, and initially may improve after the drug is restarted or the dosage is increased. Conversely, restarting a dopamine receptor antagonist or raising its dosage is likely to worsen the underlying condition ultimately. **Thus, treatments with dopaminergic drugs cause immediate changes in clinical state that are opposite to their long-term effects.**

2. **Many drugs have been reported to improve TD,** but well-designed prospective studies of large numbers of patients have not been performed for all of them. In general, anticholinergic medications worsen hyperkinetic movement disorders. They have been reported to be effective in treating dystonia when it appears as a tardive movement disorder. Amantadine and dopamine receptor agonists have been suggested as means of "downregulating" dopamine receptors, but a clear demonstration of clinical benefit from this pharmacologic manipulation is lacking.

   a. **Drugs that presynaptically suppress dopaminergic neurotransmission** have the greatest degree of effectiveness with the least likelihood of worsening the underlying condition. Reserpine or tetrabenazine (not available in the United States) have been most widely used in this regard. Dosages of reserpine generally range from 0.10–0.25 mg tid. This medication has several potential adverse effects, including parkinsonism, depression, orthostatic hypotension, and peptic ulcer disease. Despite these limitations, when carefully titrated, reserpine can provide substantial relief of symptoms.

   b. **Benzodiazepines** may also prove useful for patients with mild symptoms, consistent with studies showing a loss of GABA receptors in animal models of TD. Long-acting agents such as clonazepam (Klonopin) (usually 1.5–3.0 mg/day) provide the most consistent relief of symptoms. The usual potential adverse effects, including sedation and depression, can occur.

   c. **Neuroleptics,** used in the lowest possible dosages, may be necessary if symptoms markedly interfere with activities of daily living. Dosages of haloperidol as low as 0.25 mg/day may provide some relief of symptoms. When withdrawn, the neuroleptic should be reduced gradually over as much as 2 years. Once the neuroleptic has been withdrawn, every attempt should be made to avoid the future use of medications that can result in TD.

   d. **Vitamin E** has been reported to improve symptoms in several recent studies. Given at a dosage of 400 IU tid with meals, this treatment has few if any adverse effects.

   e. A **long-term strategy** is important in the treatment of TD. For many patients, combination therapy is most effective. The use of a benzodiazepine with either reserpine or a low dosage of a neuroleptic may be necessary. Gradual improvement after a neuroleptic has been discontinued may occur for up to 2 years; the eventual rate of remission is about 60%. For some elderly patients, the decision can be made simply to continue to suppress the movements with additional neuroleptic, but this strategy is reliably effective for only several months.

D. Dystonia can arise from any of several secondary causes or can be idiopathic. Structural lesions most commonly involve the putamen but may be found in other parts of the basal ganglia. Several inherited diseases with known metabolic deficits have been identified as causes of dystonia. Dopa-responsive dystonia (also known as dystonia with diurnal variation, or the Segawa variant) and Wilson's disease are examples of this group. Idiopathic dystonia may be generalized or restricted to a particular muscle group. In patients with idiopathic dystonia, the basal ganglia shows no gross or microscopic abnormalities, and no specific biochemical abnormality that accounts for the motor symptoms has been determined. As might be expected, given this lack of understanding of the relevant neurochemistry, a wide variety of medications have been used and reported to be effective for some patients. The use of botulinum toxin (Botox) injections for focal and segmental dystonia has greatly advanced the treatment of these forms of the disorder.

   1. **Dopa-responsive dystonia** usually becomes apparent during childhood and may first cause changes in gait. Patients with this rare form of dystonia have markedly fewer symptoms after first awakening and become progressively more symptomatic throughout the day. The importance of this disorder is that it is exquisitely sensitive to small doses of levodopa. Prolonged treatment is only rarely complicated by the response fluctuations that accompany Parkinson's disease. A brief trial of levodopa (Sinemet) for childhood-onset dystonia is frequently recommended in order to exclude this disorder.

   2. **Medical management of idiopathic dystonia or dystonia resulting from secondary causes** can be attempted with the medications listed in Table 41-2. None of these medications provides complete relief of symptoms. Combinations of medications, such as a benzodiazepine with an antidepressant (which also provides control of pain) may be beneficial. The use of high-

Table 41-2. Medications used in the treatment of dystonia.

Class	Example	Dosage (mg/day)
Anticholinergics	Trihexyphenidyl	6–100
Dopaminergics	Levodopa	≤300
	Bromocriptine	7.5–40
Antidopaminergics	Haloperidol	2–20
Benzodiazepines	Diazepam	5–20
GABA agonists	Baclofen	15–60
Antidepressants	Amitriptyline	25–150
Anticonvulsants	Carbamazepine	300–1200

dosage anticholinergic medications such as trihexyphenidyl requires specific comment. Extremely high dosages of anticholinergic drugs have been reported to benefit more than 50% of patients in some trials. In order to reach dosages of more than 20 mg/day, a gradual increase of 2–5 mg/week is necessary. Usual adverse effects of anticholinergic medications can be minimized by very gradual increases in dosage. Children tolerate dosages of trihexyphenidyl as high as 20 mg/day much better than adults. In addition to the usual anticholinergic adverse effects, high dosages of these medications can cause losses of memory and difficulties in concentration, especially for adults. A dosage of more than 60 mg/day of trihexyphenidyl may take months to achieve.

3. **Botulinum toxin injections** are the first line of treatment for many patients with focal and segmental dystonia and may be used for some patients with generalized dystonia. Injections are made directly into the affected muscle and must be repeated at an average interval of 3 months. Guidance with electromyography is necessary for some muscle groups. Although these injections pose little technical difficulty for many of the most commonly affected muscle groups, they are best performed by clinicians experienced in the identification of the appropriate muscles and knowledgeable regarding the usual necessary dosages of the toxin.

E. **Tremor** is the most common movement disorder and may result from a variety of different causes. The identification of the underlying cause is of primary importance in determining the appropriate treatment regimen.

1. **Essential tremor** occurs with posture or action, may improve with small amounts of alcohol, and in about 50% of cases exhibits an autosomal-dominant inheritance pattern. The underlying cause is unknown, although recent studies have suggested abnormalities of cerebellar output pathways. Generally it is not possible to eliminate the tremor, and the goal of therapy should be to normalize activities of daily living. Most patients respond well to the medications listed below, but in a few cases the tremor may be quite resistant to any medical management.

   a. **Beta-adrenergic receptor antagonists** have been used most extensively to treat essential tremor. Their effect is due to antagonism of beta-2 receptors on muscle spindles peripherally. For this reason, beta antagonists that are not selective (i.e., for beta-1 receptors) are preferred. Specifically, propranolol (Inderal), either as the standard or the long-acting formulation, has been shown to be effective. Potential adverse effects of beta-adrenergic antagonists are well known and include congestive heart failure, worsening of obstructive lung disease, masking of signs of hypoglycemia for diabetics, and worsening of perfusion impeded by peripheral vascular disease. Water-soluble, renally excreted agents that are usually given once daily do not readily cross the blood-brain barrier and thus may not cause adverse CNS effects. If adverse CNS effects such as depression or nightmares occur with propranolol, substitution of nadolol (Corgard) can be used. Dosages of beta antagonists can be titrated by following the resting heart rate.

   b. **Primidone (Mysoline)** is an anticonvulsant that for unclear reasons may improve essential tremor. When primidone is used for essential tremor, it is given in a much lower dosage than when it is used as an anticonvulsant. Treatment is usually started at 25 mg every hour of sleep (qhs) and frequently can be maintained at 50 mg qhs. Increases in dosage above 150 mg/day do not usually provide further improvement. Patients with essential tremor appear to be quite sensitive to the ataxia that is usually associated with higher dosages of primidone. Drowsiness may also occur, particularly when treatment is first initiated.

   c. **Carbonic anhydrase inhibitors** including methazolamide (Neptazane) and acetazolamide (Diamox) have recently been shown to have some effectiveness for essential tremor. Several relatively mild but uncomfortable adverse effects, including paresthesias and taste alterations, may occur.

   d. **Benzodiazepines** may be used if other forms of therapy do not provide sufficient control of symptoms. Only partial improvement can be expected. Long-acting agents such as clonazepam (Klonopin) can be used, but many patients prefer to use shorter-acting agents such as alprazolam

(Xanax) on an as-needed basis. Potential adverse effects include sedation, ataxia, and tolerance.

e. **Surgery** can be used in select cases when activities of daily living such as eating are severely affected despite medical management. Stereotactic thalamotomy has been demonstrated to improve tremor from several different causes. Surgery can be performed only unilaterally, providing improvement of the contralateral extremities.

2. **Other causes of tremor** include Parkinson's disease and dystonia. Treatment of tremor associated with Parkinson's disease is discussed above (sec. **II.A**). Beta receptor antagonists can also be effective if the tremor has a significant postural component. The tremor associated with dystonia is usually postural and responds to treatment for essential tremor. Rubral tremor is usually caused by lesions of the cerebellar outflow pathways in the brainstem. Ataxia is also frequently present. A coarse tremor at rest, affecting posture and action, is characteristic of rubral tremor. Treatment of this type of tremor is usually quite difficult, but treatment with beta receptor antagonists and benzodiazepines can be attempted.

F. **Wilson's disease** is a rare autosomal recessive disorder characterized by low plasma levels of the copper-binding protein ceruloplasmin. Loss of the binding protein causes deposition of copper in the liver, iris, and basal ganglia. A variety of movement disorders can accompany Wilson's disease, including dystonia, chorea, and parkinsonism. Symptomatic treatment of the movement disorder is as discussed above. More important is the prevention of additional copper deposition and worsening of end-organ damage.

1. **Penicillamine (Cuprimine)** is the most commonly used chelating agent for copper. For reasons that are not well understood, symptoms may worsen transiently just after the drug is begun. Excretion of tissue copper stores can be followed with 24-hour urine copper measurements. These values initially rise and then fall as total body stores of copper are mobilized. Several potentially serious adverse effects are associated with penicillamine and should be familiar to the prescribing physician. These effects include aplastic anemia, agranulocytosis, thrombocytopenia, membranous glomerulopathy, Goodpasture's syndrome, myasthenia gravis, hepatitis, pemphigus vulgaris or foliaceus, and a lupus erythematosus-like syndrome with a positive antinuclear antibody. Because of the potential hematologic and renal adverse reactions, a CBC, platelet count, and urinalysis are recommended every 2 weeks for the first 6 months of therapy and monthly thereafter. Total daily dosages of 750–1500 mg are usually used. Other chelating agents, such as triethylene tetramine (Trien) and dimercaprol (BAL), have also been used for patients who do not respond to penicillamine.

2. **Zinc** can be used to inhibit the absorption of copper from the gut. Dosages of 225 mg qid and 50 mg tid with meals have been employed. Recent studies have suggested that patients may be treated with zinc alone, rather than in combination with penicillamine, if their laboratory measurements and examinations remain normal. Whether patients may worsen after initiation of zinc has been a subject of recent debate.

3. A **low-copper diet** is also important for patients with Wilson's disease. Foods containing large amounts of copper include shellfish, liver, nuts, chocolate, and mushrooms.

III. **Long-term management strategies for treatment of movement disorders**

A. **Hypokinetic movement disorders,** including idiopathic Parkinson's disease, are frequently most difficult to treat early in the course of the illness just after symptoms reach medical attention and again later during the advanced stages of the disease. **Key issues regarding the newly diagnosed Parkinson's patient** include whether deprenyl or other agents may have protective effects and whether the initiation of some therapeutic agents such as levodopa should be delayed. Consultation with a neurologist regarding these issues may be helpful just after diagnosis. Similarly, **development of response fluctuations** or other problems associated with more advanced IPD may require consultation with a neurologist. Patients with stable IPD adequately controlled by medication usually need to be seen by a neurologist no more than once or twice per year. Patients with parkinsonism caused by other degenerative disorders usually do not respond well to antiparkinsonian medications and thus require specialized care.

B. **Hyperkinetic movement disorders** are a heterogeneous group of disorders each of which may be treated differently. **Consultation is frequently necessary** to establish the correct diagnosis. After establishing a diagnosis, considering the rarity of many of these disorders, consultation may be helpful in instituting an effective medication regimen. **Once an initial therapy has been established, its effectiveness should be reviewed at least once or twice per year.** Some of these disorders (e.g., Huntington's disease) are progressive degenerative conditions that require treatment of different symptoms at different points during the course of the illness. Others, such as dystonia, may wax and wane, but do not show overall changes in severity. Conditions such as TD and possibly TS may improve over the lifetime of the patient. **Consultation may become necessary when the current treatment no longer provides acceptable control.** The treatment of essential tremor with a beta-adrenergic receptor antagonist or primidone is usually straightforward; however, a minority of patients may be quite resistant to, or suffer adverse effects of, many potential therapeutic agents. These patients may therefore be candidates for referral.

Recommended Readings

Adler LA, et al. Vitamin-E treatment of tardive dyskinesia. *Am J Psychiat* 150:1405–1407, 1993.

Bannister R. Multiple-system atrophy and pure autonomic failure. In PA Low (ed), *Autonomic Nervous Disorders*. Boston: Little, Brown, 1993.

Braun V, Richter HP. Selective peripheral denervation in patients with spasmodic torticollis. *Stereotact Funct Neurosurg* 57:113–122, 1991.

Busenbark K, et al. The effect of acetazolamide on essential tremor—An open label trial. *Neurology* 42:1394–1395, 1992.

Calne DB. Drug therapy—Treatment of Parkinson's disease. *New Engl J Med* 329:1021–1027, 1993.

Diederich N, Goetz CG, Comella CL. New approaches in the treatment of the dystonias. *Klin Wochenschr* 68:935–941, 1990.

Fletcher NA, et al. Successful treatment of childhood onset symptomatic dystonia with levodopa. *J Neurol Neurosurg Psychiat* 56:865–867, 1993.

Goetz CG, et al. Neurosurgical horizons in Parkinson's disease. *Neurology* 43:1–7, 1993.

Greene P, Cote L, Fahn S. Treatment of drug-induced psychosis in Parkinson's disease with clozapine. *Adv Neurol* 60:703–706, 1993.

Hallett M. Classification and treatment of tremor. *JAMA* 266:1115–1117, 1991.

Huber SJ, Paulson GW. Efficacy of alprazolam for essential tremor. *Neurology* 38:241–243, 1988.

Hutton JT, Morris JL. Long-acting carbidopa-levodopa in the management of moderate and advanced Parkinson's disease. *Neurology* 42:51–56, 1992.

Jankovic J, Schwartz K, Donovan DT. Botulinum toxin treatment of cranial-cervical dystonia, spasmodic dysphonia, other focal dystonias and hemifacial spasm. *J Neurol Neurosurg Psychiat* 53:633–639, 1990.

Koller WC, Silver DE, Lieberman A. An algorithm for the management of Parkinson's disease. *Neurology* 44(suppl 10):S1–S52, 1994.

Lewitt PA. Therapeutics of Tourette syndrome—New medication approaches. *Adv Neurol* 58:263–270, 1992.

Marsden CD, Fahn S (eds). *Movement Disorders 3*. Oxford, England: Butterworth-Heinemann, 1994.

Montgomery EB. Pharmacokinetics and pharmacology of levodopa. *Neurology* 42:17–22, 1992.

Muenter MD, et al. Treatment of essential tremor with methazolamide. *Mayo Clinic Proc* 66:991–997, 1991.

Parkinson Study Group. Effect of deprenyl on the progression of disability in early Parkinson's disease. *N Engl J Med* 321:1364–1371, 1989.

Parkinson Study Group. Effects of tocopherol and deprenyl on the progression of disability in early Parkinson's disease. *N Engl J Med* 328:176–183, 1993.

Robertson MM, Eapen V. Pharmacologic controversy of CNS stimulants in Gilles de la Tourette's syndrome. *Clin Neuropharmacol* 15:408–425, 1992.

Rodnitzky RL. The use of Sinemet CR in the management of mild to moderate Parkinson's disease. *Neurology* 42:44–50, 1992.

Stern MB, Koller WC. *Parkinsonian Syndromes.* New York: Marcel Dekker, 1993.

Weiner WJ, Lang AE. *Movement Disorders: A Comprehensive Survey.* Mt. Kisco, NY: Futura, 1989.

Whitehouse PJ. Cholinergic therapy in dementia. *Acta Neurol Scand* 88(suppl 149): 42–45, 1993.

42

Dementia
Martin R. Farlow

Dementia is defined as a decline in memory and at least one other cognitive deficit that impairs the patient's ability to function in the activities of daily living. Behavioral abnormalities are common and contribute to the impairment of function. There are no treatments that have been demonstrated to reverse the neurodegenerative processes in the vast majority of patients with this syndrome. Therapeutic approaches have concentrated on identifying those few patients with reversible etiologies and on palliating disabling symptoms for as long as possible in patients with progressive disease. Recently, tacrine has been used effectively in some patients for treatment of the primary symptoms—memory loss and cognitive disturbance—of Alzheimer's disease.

I. **Dementia (reversible causes).** The current percentage of dementia patients whose disorders have reversible underlying etiologies is relatively small (approximately 5%). However, in elderly patients with no reversible underlying etiologies, as many as 40% have modifiable abnormalities the correction of which can slow progression and/or temporarily improve the patient's ability to function.

A. **Structural lesions causing dementia.** Space-occupying masses and/or abnormalities in brain structure that are treatable may be identified by brain imaging studies, including computed tomography (CT), magnetic resonance imaging (MRI), positron emission tomography (PET), and single-photon emission computed tomography (SPECT). Unfortunately, neurosurgical interventions in many of these patients may halt deterioration but not significantly improve clinical symptoms.

1. **Normal pressure hydrocephalus (NPH).** Patients with ataxia, urinary incontinence, dementia, and ventricular enlargement out of proportion to sulci on CT or MRI should be referred for neurosurgical evaluation and possible placement of a ventriculoperitoneal (VP) shunt. Patients whose symptoms improve after lumbar puncture (LP) are particularly likely to improve after shunting. Ataxia and incontinence are more likely to improve than memory. Overall, one-third of patients improve, one-third remain unchanged, and one-third continue to have progressive symptoms.

2. **Subdural hematomas and hygromas.** Chronic subdural hematomas and hygromas can be asymptomatic, cause cognitive impairment, or cause frank dementia in the elderly. Neurosurgical evaluation is required. Increases in the size of the fluid collection and progressive clinical impairment are indications for surgical intervention. Surgery often does not improve cognition but stops progression of cognitive impairment.

3. **Frontal, temporal, and parietal lobe tumors.** Large meningiomas, gliomas, and metastases to the brain that occupy substantial space and/or cause substantial edema in the adjacent frontal, temporal, or parietal lobe can cause dementia. Such tumors should be treated by neurosurgical excision, or by biopsy and radiation and/or chemotherapy, as appropriate for the tumor type and location. The prognosis for significant recovery from cognitive impairment and clinical dysfunction after such treatments in patients older than 65 years of age is guarded.

B. **Metabolic abnormalities associated with dementia.** Relatively subtle deviations from the normal range of metabolic parameters can cause or significantly exacerbate mental impairment in elderly patients. A history of fluctuat-

This work was supported by NIA grant AG10133-04.

ing deficits suggests a metabolic cause for dementia. Changes in mental status are generally reversible with correction of the underlying etiology of the metabolic disturbance or appropriate supplementation.

1. **Hypokalemia and hyperkalemia.** Hypokalemia most commonly occurs during antihypertensive therapy using diuretic drugs in elderly patients. It can be treated by stopping the diuretic, supplementing potassium, or switching to a potassium-sparing diuretic such as spironolactone. Steroids also can cause hypokalemia in the elderly, and patients should be supplemented with potassium if necessary. Hyperkalemia may result from oversupplementation of potassium and use of potassium-sparing antihypertensive agents. The offending agents should be discontinued.

2. **Hyponatremia and hypernatremia.** Hypernatremia is most commonly observed in association with dehydration and is often found in physically impaired patients who are dependent on caregivers for their oral intake. In dehydrated patients, both free water and electrolytic deficits should be calculated and corrected, and body weight and electrolytes should be monitored frequently and adjusted as necessary. Relatively minor hyponatremia with serum sodium (Na^+) at 120–130 mg/dl can significantly impair cognition in the elderly. Treatment of hyponatremia can totally reverse the mental impairment. Hyponatremia with Na^+ less than 120 mg/dl should be corrected over 3 or more days, because overrapid normalization may precipitate CNS demyelination.

3. **Hypocalcemia and hypercalcemia.** Abnormalities in serum calcium levels may be associated with hypoparathyroidism or hyperparathyroidism, antihypertensive therapy, cancer, and renal diseases. The underlying etiology should be determined and treated when possible.

4. **Hypoglycemia and hyperglycemia.** Many patients with diabetes mellitus have dementias with varying degrees of reversibility. The long-term effects of diabetes mellitus can contribute to microvascular ischemic changes in the brain as well as accelerate atherosclerosis in the major vessels supplying the brain. Both can potentially cause irreversible vascular dementia. Many diabetes patients have very high blood glucose levels (greater than 300–400 mg/dl) and variable mental status changes during the day. These subtle deficits can be difficult to recognize and control. Similarly, some patients may have periods of confusion associated with unrecognized hypoglycemia. Treatment of glucose abnormalities requires careful monitoring of blood glucose levels and correction by adjustments in diet and in dosages of oral hypoglycemic agents, or by insulin injections as necessary to achieve normalization of blood glucose level.

C. **Endocrine abnormalities that cause dementia.** Chronic endocrine diseases can cause cognitive impairments and dementia in elderly individuals with few, if any, of the other physical findings associated with deficiency or excess hormonal state. Detection and correction of these conditions can lead to complete reversal of dementia, including return to normal activities of daily living.

1. **Thyroid disease**
   a. **Hypothyroidism.** In the elderly, hypothyroidism should be treated initially with levothyroxine (T_4) at a dosage of 0.025 mg/day. The dosage may be increased by 0.025-mg increments at monthly intervals, with routine monitoring of T_4 and thyroid-stimulating hormone levels. The dosage should be increased until symptoms improve and until T_4 levels are in the therapeutic range. If the initial T_4 thyroid level is very low in an elderly patient, supplemental steroids, such as prednisone (Deltasone) at 5.0–7.5 mg/day, may be given for the first 2 weeks after levothyroxine is initiated.
   b. **Hyperthyroidism.** An endocrinologist should generally be consulted and appropriate therapy begun, including propranolol to decrease pulse rate and anxiety, medical therapy with methimazole or with radioactive iodine, or surgical excision of the thyroid gland. Most mental status changes associated with thyroid disease are highly reversible.

2. **Diabetes mellitus.** See sec. **I.B.4.**

3. **Hypoparathyroidism and hyperparathyroidism.** See sec. **I.B.3.**

D. **Dementia secondary to systemic organ failure.** The CNS is dependent on the functions of all of the major organ systems. Mild abnormality in systemic organ functions in the elderly patient can cause mental status changes including confusion, disorientation, and memory loss.

1. **Pulmonary disease.** Both acute illnesses (such as pneumonia) and chronic obstructive lung disease can cause hypoxemia resulting in dementia. Supplemental oxygen by nasal cannula or ventimask can improve cognitive functions. Various diseases of the lungs, particularly small-cell cancer, can metastasize or have distal effects on the brain and cause dementia. The underlying tumor should be the focus of treatment.

2. **Hepatic disease.** Diseases of the liver, such as the various forms of hepatitis and cirrhosis (hereditary and alcoholic), can cause dementia. Dementia in such cases is often associated with elevated blood ammonia levels. The underlying liver disease is the focus of treatment. Cognitive improvement results from lowering ammonia levels using lactulose or neomycin, or both.

3. **Cardiac disease.** Cardiac dysfunction can contribute to the process of dementia in different ways. Congestive heart failure (CHF) may decrease the blood supply to the brain. Enlarged heart chambers and valvular diseases may promote formation of thrombi that may embolize to the brain. Arrhythmias may decrease blood flow to the brain. Treatment of the underlying cardiac disease should be the focus.

4. **Renal disease.** Chronic or acute renal failure can cause uremic encephalopathy. Dialysis and transplants have decreased the frequency of this illness. Renal patients are more prone to fluctuating mental status changes resulting from a variety of metabolic abnormalities. Aluminum may occasionally accumulate in some patients, causing dialysis dementia. Chelation by deferoxamine can reverse some symptoms associated with cognitive decline.

E. **Chronic CNS infections.** Infectious diseases that cause systemic illness often directly or indirectly affect CNS function. In elderly patients, urinary tract infections and upper respiratory infections can secondarily cause declines in cognitive function that clear after effective antibiotic treatment. In the elderly, chronic meningitis or encephalitis can be caused by syphilis, tuberculosis, cryptococcus, and other fungal infections. Symptoms include intermittent fevers, night sweats, headache, stiff neck, papilledema, nuchal rigidity, rapidly progressive dementia, ataxia, and urinary incontinence (see Chap. 2). Therapy should be appropriate to the identified causative organism.

F. **Epilepsy (partial complex status).** Symptoms or signs of intermittent confusion, staring spells, lip smacking, and automatisms suggest the possibility of intermittent partial status epilepticus. Ictal activity should be demonstrated by electroencephalography. Diazepam or lorazepam should be given for acute suppression of seizures. Phenytoin, carbamazepine, or valproic acid can be given for longer-term treatment of the seizure disorder.

G. **Side effects of medications taken for chronic illnesses in the elderly.** As many as 75% of elderly patients take three or more medications, several of which have the potential to cause side effects of chronic confusion and deficits in cognition and memory. The worst offenders are anticholinergic drugs such as bethanecol and oxybutynin, antihypertensives, antidepressants, and antianxiety and antipsychotic medications. Anticonvulsants, sleep medications, and analgesics also frequently cause declines in mental function. Excessive dosages and numbers of medications are probably the most common reversible causes of dementia in the elderly. Medications should be titrated to the lowest dosage levels sufficient for control of symptoms, and if they are not clearly effective, they should be eliminated.

II. **Dementia (irreversible causes).** The vast majority of patients with dementia have underlying etiologies that are not reversible (Alzheimer's disease, Pick's disease, and vascular dementia). Treatment strategies for the neurodegenerative dementias have focused on control of disturbances in behavior, development of neuroprotective agents to slow progression of the disease, and use of antiacetylcholinesterase therapy to improve symptoms of memory loss and other deficits in cognition.

A. **Treatment of behavioral symptoms.** The treatment of agitation, depression, anxiety, and sleep disorders in patients with dementia can be challenging. Drugs that improve behavioral symptoms may worsen the dementia. Some drugs may have paradoxical effects, worsening behavioral disturbances. Dosage ranges that provide effective control of behavioral symptoms vary widely in individual patients, and so frequent adjustments in therapy may be necessary to control such symptoms.

1. **Agitation, hallucinations, delusions, and bizarre or violent behaviors.** Changes in the patient's environment that may have precipitated the aberrant behavior should be identified and modified, if possible. All antipsychotics at equivalent dosages have equal potential for positive therapeutic effects. Some are less commonly used in dementia patients because of potential side effects such as sedation and orthostatic hypotension. Target behavioral symptoms for potential improvement should be identified before therapy is begun. Therapy might start with haloperidol at 0.5–1.0 mg, loxapine at 5.0 mg, or thiothixene at 1.0–2.0 mg, as necessary, with frequency up to three or four times a day. The dosages can be adjusted upward as necessary to control behavior and downward as necessary to minimize side effects. Trazodone at a dosage of 50–100 mg before going to bed and, if necessary, an additional 50 mg bid, can be used for agitation but may be excessively sedating in some patients. The roles of risperidone (Risperdal) and clozapine (Clozaril) in treatment of agitation in patients with dementia are still being investigated.

2. **Anxiety, phobias, and excessive activities.** When caregivers of patients with dementia describe symptoms suggestive of anxiety, phobias, or excessive activities (constant pacing, hand washing, etc.), several questions should be asked. Is this behavior disturbing to the patient? Is it interfering with the patient's activities of daily living? Are behavioral symptoms making it difficult for the caregiver to manage the patient? Lorazepam at a dosage of 0.5–1.0 mg tid and alprazolam at a dosage of 0.25–1.0 mg tid may be used to control these symptoms, but in dementia patients these drugs may be excessively sedating. A useful alternative medication is buspirone at dosages of 5 mg tid up to 10 mg qid. Patients need to be monitored for excessive sedation.

3. **Depression.** Symptoms of depression are present in at least 25% of patients with Alzheimer's disease, often in the early stages of the illness. Few double-blind, placebo-controlled trials of antidepressants in this population have been reported. A double-blind trial using imipramine did not show any benefits in comparison with a placebo. Imipramine has anticholinergic effects that may have worsened the dementia. Nortriptyline at an initial dosage of 10 mg qhs is commonly used and anecdotally is effective in patients with dementia. The newer antidepressants fluoxetine, sertrulin, and paroxetine have fewer side effects in the general population. In the elderly, they are anecdotally effective at dosages lower than those used in young adults (fluoxetine 10 mg/day, sertraline 25 mg/day, and paroxetine 10 mg/day). In moderate to severe dementia patients, these drugs may cause agitation. If agitation occurs, the dosage should be cut by 50% or an alternative antidepressant should be substituted.

4. **Insomnia.** Disturbances in the sleep-wake cycle can contribute to depression, anxiety, and agitation in the patient with dementia. A dementia patient who is active in the middle of the night puts extraordinary stress on the caregiver. Daytime napping should be discouraged. Chloral hydrate given one-half hour before bedtime at a dosage of 500–1000 mg is often effective in restoring a normal sleep-wake cycle and may be given for 1–2 weeks. Useful alternatives include triazolam (10–15 mg qhs) or diphenhydramine (25–50 mg qhs).

B. **Treatment of Alzheimer's disease (neuroprotective approach).** Currently there is no approved therapy that delays the degenerative processes of Alzheimer's disease. However, several promising approaches to keeping neurons in the brain alive and retarding the clinical progression of the disease are being investigated.

1. **Free radical generation may cause neuronal death in Alzheimer's disease.** The Deprenyl and Tocopherol Antioxidative Therapy of Parkinsonism (DATATOP) study suggests that L-deprenyl may have cut the rate of progression of extrapyramidal symptoms in patients with Parkinson's disease by 50%—possibly by a neuroprotective effect that decreases formation of free radicals. Clinical trials investigating the utility of L-deprenyl in Alzheimer's disease are in progress.

2. **Inflammation in Alzheimer's disease.** Retrospective studies have suggested that patients with rheumatoid arthritis taking nonsteroidal medications have a decreased prevalence of Alzheimer's disease. A preliminary double-blind, placebo-controlled pilot trial using indomethacin suggested significant retardation in progression of Alzheimer's disease. The ultimate role of immunosuppression in the treatment of Alzheimer's disease remains to be defined.

3. **Estrogens may benefit cognition in elderly women.** It has been suggested that supplemental estrogen therapy in postmenopausal women may delay the onset of Alzheimer's disease. The potential benefits of estrogen therapy in women at risk for and affected with Alzheimer's disease are currently being investigated.

C. **Symptomatic therapy for memory and cognitive deficits of Alzheimer's disease.** Tacrine is the only drug currently approved in the United States for treating the primary symptoms of Alzheimer's disease. Symptomatic improvements occur in no more than 40% of patients who are able to tolerate the maximum approved daily dosage of 160 mg. Tacrine potentially can cause several adverse effects, and thus it is important for families and caregivers to know the advantages and disadvantages of tacrine therapy and to develop realistic expectations.

1. **Rationale for cholinergic therapy of Alzheimer's disease using tacrine.** Progression in Alzheimer's disease is associated with marked neuronal loss in the basal nucleus of Meynert (the primary cholinergic nucleus of the brain) and consequently decreased levels of acetylcholine in the areas of the cortex to which it projects. Tacrine is an active inhibitor of acetylcholinesterase in the CNS. Blocking this enzyme raises levels of acetylcholine in the brain. Use of this drug appears for some patients to improve memory and cognition.

2. **Who to treat.** It has been shown that patients with mild to moderate symptoms of dementia respond to tacrine. These patients typically have Mini-Mental State Exam (MMSE) scores of 10–26 (see Fig. 2-1). In general they are still able to express themselves verbally and to take tests using pencil and paper. They have memory and cognitive deficits but still are able to cooperate in being evaluated by the physician. These patients should have reliable caregivers who can guarantee that their medication is taken properly four times each day.

3. **Who not to treat.** Tacrine has not been demonstrated to be effective in patients with questionable or very early dementia or in those who are more severely affected in the later stages of the illness. Because it has the potential to cause hepatotoxicity, tacrine should not be used in patients with known liver disease. Caution should be exercised in prescribing this drug for those with symptoms of peptic ulcer or heart disease. Either condition may theoretically be exacerbated by therapy with tacrine.

4. **Baseline for treatment.** Before therapy is started it is important that the physician and the patient's caregiver establish a baseline for the current level of function. Brief interviews of the patient with questions directed at memory, orientation, and cognition may suffice, but a standardized neuropsychological instrument such as the MMSE may help quantitate the severity of cognitive deficits. History from the caregiver should help establish the patient's capabilities in performing activities of daily living. In practice, the caregiver's opinion about global change in the patient's cognitive status in two large previous trials of tacrine was at least as useful as the physician's evaluation or neuropsychological tests in judging treatment benefits.

5. **Protocol for using tacrine.** Tacrine should be started at an initial dosage of 10 mg qid for 6 weeks, and then advanced every 6 weeks thereafter by 10 mg qid until a maximum dosage of 40 mg qid is achieved. If side effects occur, the daily dosage can be reduced or advanced at a slower rate.

6. **Potential side effects of tacrine therapy.** In general, the two major types of adverse effects of tacrine therapy are hepatotoxicity and cholinergic side effects. These reactions tend to occur at different times in the course of the therapy, with hepatotoxicity occurring early and cholinergic problems occurring later.

   a. **Liver toxicity.** Tacrine is a known hepatotoxin that in controlled trials has caused at least some elevation in alanine aminotransferase levels in 50% of patients, elevations greater than three times the upper limits of normal in 25%, and those greater than 10 times the upper limits of normal in 7% of treated subjects. However, 95% of liver function elevations occurred during the first 3 months of tacrine therapy. For this reason it is recommended that serum glutamate pyruvate transaminase (SGPT) levels be checked every other week for 18 weeks and every 3 months thereafter. If SGPT levels remain less than three times the upper limits of normal, the titration schedule should be continued. If SGPT levels are at least three times the upper limits but less than five times the upper limits of normal, the dosage should be reduced by one-half until levels of SGPT are less than three times the upper limits of normal, and then the daily dosage of tacrine should be advanced at a slower rate.

b. Cholinergic toxicity. When tacrine therapy is initially started and when dosage is increased, there may be marked but often temporary cholinergic side effects, including facial flushing, dyspepsia, nausea, vomiting, anorexia, and diarrhea. These symptoms often diminish after a few days at the new, higher dosage. If they persist, a temporary reduction in dosage may be necessary. Many patients are not able to achieve the maximum dosage of 160 mg/day because of cholinergic side effects. Cholinergic effects on the gastrointestinal system may be decreased by giving tacrine with food to delay absorption, antacids for dyspepsia, and kaolin pectin for diarrhea. In patients with more severe cholinergic effects, anticholinergic drugs such as glycopyrrolate may be used temporarily. It is important that the physician be persistent in efforts to achieve the highest possible daily dosage of tacrine, because the probability of cognitive benefits in treated patients increases in direct proportion to total daily dosage.

c. Other side effects of tacrine. Tacrine therapy can cause skin rash, but this is relatively uncommon. Rashes are treated by withdrawal of the medication. There have been several case reports of increased extrapyramidal symptoms, increased rigidity, or bradykinesia during therapy with tacrine. If these symptoms are mild, some may be acceptable if the patient receives cognitive benefits. If bradykinesia and rigidity are disabling, a dosage reduction or withdrawal of the medication should be initiated.

7. Withdrawal of tacrine. In patients taking tacrine with significant side effects during dose titration, treatment can be immediately discontinued. If the physician or caregiver believes it should be restarted, the same dosage can be given if less than one month has passed since the therapy was halted. Otherwise, the patient should be rechallenged starting at 10 mg qid. Alzheimer's disease is a progressive illness, and even the best responders to tacrine therapy deteriorate with time. In these patients, withdrawal of therapy may be considered. There is potential for marked increases in cognitive deficits in some patients after the drug is discontinued. To minimize the potential for withdrawal effects, patients should be tapered off the drug over a 2-week period.

8. Patients who fail to respond to or cannot tolerate the side effects of tacrine. Tacrine is the only drug approved for treatment of cognitive deficits and memory loss in Alzheimer's disease. However, there are several other drugs that are now in experimental clinical trials for therapy of dementia. Most trials use a double-blind, placebo-controlled design, which implies that a participating subject may be on a placebo. Drug trials for Alzheimer's disease require considerable commitment from the patient's caregiver. Referral for a clinical trial can generally be arranged through a local university medical center or the Alzheimer's Association.

9. Predictors of response to tacrine therapy. There currently are no predose clinical, demographic, or biological characteristics that can predict which patients will benefit from taking tacrine. The best determinants of who will get positive clinical responses are sufficient dosages, adequate plasma levels, and "normalizing" effects on the CNS, as indicated by less slowing on EEG and increased parietal metabolism on PET.

D. Therapies for other irreversible dementias. No medication that improves the primary deficits in cognition and memory that occur in other dementias has been shown convincingly to be effective by double-blind, placebo-controlled trials. Some evidence, however, suggests that appropriate therapies may be helpful in at least some of these patients.

1. **Diffuse Lewy body disease** may be the primary cause of symptoms or contribute significantly to symptoms in 10% of all patients with irreversible dementia. There is considerable overlap of this entity with Alzheimer's disease. There are two recent case reports that suggest that tacrine may actually be more effective in patients with diffuse Lewy body disease than in those with Alzheimer's disease. The protocol for evaluation and treatment is the same as that described in sec. **II.C.5.**

2. **Frontal lobe dementia (including Pick's disease).** Frontal lobe dementias occur in a surprisingly large percentage of the population (5–10%) and exhibit considerable overlapping with Alzheimer's disease. Early symptoms often are behavioral abnormalities and language problems. Memory deficits typically occur during the later stages of the illness. Behavioral disorders should be treated as described in sec. **II.A.** Because of the overlap with Alzheimer's disease, it is reasonable to run a trial of tacrine if there are significant deficits in memory and cognition.

3. **Vascular dementia.** Currently, there are no drugs that have been approved for treatment of vascular dementia. Accurate diagnosis is important for determining the etiology and preventing or delaying progression of the disease.

   a. **Ischemic vascular dementia** may occur in 5–15% of the population and may occur jointly with Alzheimer's disease in another 10%. Control of hypertension and use of aspirin may help prevent progression of dementia in patients with multiple infarctions. In patients with elevated levels of cholesterol and triglycerides, reduction should be encouraged by changes in diet and use of a drug such as niacin, gemfibrozil, or lovastatin. There is, however, no evidence that reduction in cholesterol modifies the course of the disease. Tacrine therapy may be a consideration, particularly in the substantial numbers of patients in whom Alzheimer's disease and ischemic vascular dementia may coexist.

   b. **Multiple infarctions secondary to emboli.** Occasionally, dementia occurs after repeated embolic strokes. Treatment involves stopping or decreasing new infarctions by identification of the embolic source and appropriate treatment. Carotid source emboli may be treated medically with aspirin or ticlopidine or, if there is more than 70% stenosis, surgically by carotid endarterectomy. Cardiac source emboli usually require full anticoagulation with heparin and then long-term therapy with warfarin. If the etiology is infective endocarditis, the patient should not be anticoagulated, but antimicrobial therapy should target the underlying infection.

   c. **Amyloid angiopathy** is suggested by intermittent parenchymal hemorrhages of the brain. Angiography shows no evidence of aneurism or arteriovenous malformation (AVM). In a small number of these cases with positive family history, the cause is hereditary cerebral hemorrhage with amyloidosis of the Dutch type (HCHWA-D) or hereditary cerebral hemorrhage with amyloidosis in Islandic kindred (HCHWA-I). There is no treatment but aspirin, and nonsteroidal therapy should be specifically avoided.

   d. **Vasculitis.** The diagnosis of vasculitis is suggested in dementia patients with diffuse brain disease when there is elevation of Westergren sedimentation rate to greater than 75 mm/hr without other identified cause and elevation of cerebrospinal fluid (CSF) protein to greater than 75 mg/dl with fewer than 10 cells/mm^3. Angiography shows characteristic areas of narrowing in the small vessels, which confirm the diagnosis. Patients with vasculitis should be treated aggressively with high-dosage intravenous steroids followed by tapering oral steroid therapy. Steroid therapy may potentially improve memory and cognitive deficits dramatically.

   e. **Emotional incontinence in vascular dementia.** Many patients with multiple infarcts located in the frontal lobes or interrupting frontal lobe tracts may exhibit peculiar verbal outbursts that may be triggered by even the most minor emotional stimulus. These emotional verbal outbursts may have characteristics of both crying and laughter. They are involuntary and can be very disturbing to patients and their families, often leading to avoidance of social activities. Low dosages of tricyclic antidepressants are often very effective in controlling these symptoms.

Recommended Readings

American Psychiatric Association. Dementia of the Alzheimer's type (chapter). In *Diagnostic and Statistical Manual of Mental Disorders* (4th ed). Washington: American Psychiatric Association, 1994.

Arnold SE, Kumar A. Contemporary Clinical Neurology: Reversible dementias. *Med Clin N Amer* 77(1):215–230, 1993.

Burke WJ, et al. L-deprenyl in the treatment of mild dementia of the Alzheimer type. Preliminary results. *J Am Geriatr Soc* 41:367–370, 1993.

Cohn CK, et al. Double-blind, multicenter comparison of sertraline and amitriptyline in elderly depressed patients. *J Clin Psychiat* 51:12(suppl B), 28–33, 1990.

Farlow M, et al. A controlled trial of tacrine in Alzheimer's disease. *JAMA* 268:2523–2529, 1992.

Farlow MR. Tacrine in the treatment of Alzheimer's disease. *Res Staff Phys* 39(12): 39–43, 1993.

Friedland RP. Alzheimer's disease: Clinical features and differential diagnosis. *Neurology* 43(suppl 4):S45–S51, 1993.

Gardner ME. Treatment of depression in patients with senile dementia of the Alzheimer's type. *Consult Pharm* 7:739–741, 1992.

Gottlieb GL, Kumar A. Conventional pharmacologic treatment for patients with Alzheimer's disease. *Neurology* 43(suppl 4):S56–S63, 1993.

Henderson VW, et al. Estrogen replacement therapy in older women. *Arch Neurol* 51:896–900, 1994.

Jones BN, Reifler BV. Alzheimer's and related dementias: Depression coexisting with dementia. *Med Clin N Amer* 78(4):823–840, 1994.

Knapp MJ, et al. A 30-week randomized controlled trial of high-dose tacrine in patients with Alzheimer's disease. *JAMA* 271:985–991, 1994.

Kunik ME, et al. Pharmacologic approach to management of agitation associated with dementia. *J Clin Psychiat* 55:2(suppl), 13–17, 1994.

Leibovici A, Tariot PN. Agitation associated with dementia: A systematic approach to treatment. *Psychopharmacol Bull* 24(1):49–53, 1988.

Levy R. Alzheimer's disease and Lewy body dementia. *Brit J Psychiat* 164(2):268, 1994.

Levy R, et al. Lewy bodies and response to tacrine in Alzheimer's disease. *Lancet* 343:176, 1994.

Paganini-Hill A, Henderson VW. Estrogen deficiency and risk of Alzheimer's disease in women. *Am J Epidemiol* 140:256–261, 1994.

Reifler BV, et al. Double-blind trial of imipramine in Alzheimer's disease patients with and without depression. *Am J Psychiat* 146:45–49, 1989.

Reynolds CF III, et al. The nature and management of sleep/wake disturbance in Alzheimer's dementia. *Psychopharmacol Bull* 24(1):43–48, 1988.

Rogers J, et al. Clinical trial of indomethacin in Alzheimer's disease. *Neurology* 43: 1609–1611, 1993.

Salzman C. Treatment of agitation, anxiety, and depression in dementia. *Psychopharmacol Bull* 24(1):39–42, 1988.

Schneider LS, Olin JT, Pawluczyk S. A double-blind crossover pilot study of *l*-deprenyl (selegiline) combined with cholinesterase inhibitor in Alzheimer's disease. *Am J Psychiat* 150:321–323, 1993.

Skelton WP III, Skelton NK. Alzheimer's disease: Recognizing and treating a frustrating condition. *Post Grad Med* 90(4):33–41, 1991.

Watkins PB, et al. Hepatotoxic effects of tacrine administration in patients with Alzheimer's disease. *JAMA* 271:992–999, 1994.

Wilcock GK, Scott MI. Tacrine for senile dementia of Alzheimer's or Lewy body type. *Lancet* 344:544, 1994.

43

I. Bacterial meningitis. The initial signs and symptoms of bacterial meningitis are fever, stiff neck, headache, lethargy, confusion or coma, nausea and vomiting, and photophobia. Examination of the cerebrospinal fluid (CSF) demonstrates an elevated opening pressure (>180 mm H_2O), a decreased glucose concentration (<40 mg/dl), a polymorphonuclear pleocytosis, and an elevated protein concentration. The diagnosis is made by demonstrating the organism with Gram's stain or in culture. Bacterial meningitis is a neurologic emergency, and initial treatment is empiric until a specific organism is identified.

A. Therapeutic approach

1. Dexamethasone therapy. The American Academy of Pediatrics recommends the consideration of dexamethasone therapy in infants and children 2 months of age and older with proven or suspected bacterial meningitis on the basis of CSF examination, a Gram's-stained smear of the CSF, or antigen test results. In clinical trials, dexamethasone improves the outcome of meningitis. In infants and children with *Haemophilus influenzae* type b (Hib) meningitis, dexamethasone therapy reduces the incidence of moderate or more severe sensorineural hearing loss and reduces meningeal inflammation. In experimental models of bacterial meningitis, dexamethasone decreases the leakage of serum proteins into the CSF, minimizes damage to the blood-brain barrier, and decreases production of inflammatory cytokines. Dexamethasone also decreases brain edema and intracranial pressure. The pathophysiology of bacterial meningitis is the same in infants, children, and adults. For this reason, dexamethasone therapy should also be considered in adults with proven or suspected bacterial meningitis.

The recommended dosage of dexamethasone is 0.15 mg/kg IV q6h for the first 4 days of therapy. The initial dose of dexamethasone should be given 20 minutes prior to the initial dose of antimicrobial therapy for maximum benefit. The concomitant use of an IV H-2 receptor antagonist is recommended with dexamethasone to avoid gastrointestinal bleeding.

2. Antimicrobial therapy. If bacterial meningitis is suspected, antimicrobial therapy must be initiated immediately. This should be done prior to the performance of a computed tomography (CT) scan or a lumbar puncture (LP). Initial antimicrobial therapy is empiric and is determined by the most likely meningeal pathogen based on the patient's age and underlying condition or predisposing factors. The most likely etiologic organisms of bacterial meningitis in **neonates** (up to 27 months old) are group B streptococci, enteric gram-negative bacilli (*Escherichia coli*), and *Listeria monocytogenes*. Empiric therapy for bacterial meningitis in the neonate should include a combination of ampicillin and cefotaxime or an aminoglycoside. Empiric therapy of community-acquired bacterial meningitis in **infants and children** should include coverage for Hib, *Streptococcus pneumoniae*, and *Neisseria meningitidis*. A third-generation cephalosporin (ceftriaxone or cefotaxime) and vancomycin are recommended as initial therapy for bacterial meningitis in children in whom the etiologic agent has not been identified. Cefuroxime, also a third-generation cephalosporin, is not recommended for therapy of bacterial meningitis in children because of reports of delayed sterilization of CSF cultures associated with hearing loss in children treated with cefuroxime. Empiric therapy for community-acquired bacterial meningitis in **adults** (aged 15–50 years) should include coverage for *S. pneumoniae* and *N. meningitidis*. Penicillin G, ampicillin, or a third-generation cephalosporin can be used for initial therapy. If penicillin or ampicillin is used, CSF isolates of pneumococci or meningococci should be tested for penicillin susceptibility. Cefotaxime or ceftriaxone is recommended for relatively resistant strains of pneumococci (penicillin minimal inhibitory concentrations [MICs] of 0.1–1.0 μg/ml). For highly penicillin-resistant pneumococcal meningitis (MICs ≥2.0 μg/ml), a combination of vancomycin and a third-generation cephalosporin is recommended; however, there are a few reports documenting failure of vancomycin in pneumococcal meningitis, indicating the importance of careful monitoring of these patients. Initial therapy for meningitis in the **postneurosurgical patient** should be directed against gram-negative bacilli, *Pseudomonas aeruginosa*, and *Staphylococcus aureus*. A third-generation cephalosporin is recommended for treatment of gram-negative bacillary meningitis. Ceftazidime is the only cephalosporin with sufficient activity against *P. aeruginosa* in the CNS. Vancomycin should be added until infection with staphylococci is excluded. In infants, children, and adults with CSF ventriculoperitoneal shunt infections, initial therapy for meningitis should include coverage for coagulase-negative staphylococci and *S. aureus*. The assumption can be made that the organism will be resistant to methicillin; therefore, the initial therapy for a shunt infection should include a combination of intravenous vancomycin and oral rifampin. Intrashunt or intraventricular vancomycin may also be required to eradiate the infection. In the **immunocompromised patient,** the infecting organism can be predicted on the basis of the type of immune abnormality. In patients that are neutropenic, initial therapy for bacterial meningitis should include coverage for *L. monocytogenes*, staphylococci, and enteric gram-negative bacilli. Patients with defective humoral immunity and those who have had splenectomies are unable to mount an antibody response to a bacterial infection or to control an infection caused by encapsulated bacteria. These patients are at particular risk for meningitis caused by *S. pneumoniae*, Hib, and, less commonly, *N. meningitidis*. The most common organisms causing meningitis in the **older adult** (aged 50 years or older) are *S. pneumoniae* and enteric gram-negative bacilli; however, meningitis caused by *Listeria* and Hib are increasingly recognized. The recommended initial therapy for meningitis in the older adult is either ceftriaxone or cefotaxime in combination with ampicillin. Table 43-1 lists empiric antimicrobial therapies for bacterial meningitis by age group, and Tables 43-2 and 43-3 list the recommended antimicrobial therapies for bacterial meningitis in neonates, infants and children, and adults by organism.

3. **Treatment of raised intracranial pressure.** Raised intracranial pressure is an expected complication of bacterial meningitis and should be anticipated. Treatment of raised intracranial pressure is as follows.

   a. **Elevation of the head of the bed** 30 degrees

   b. **Hyperventilation** to maintain $PaCO_2$ between 27 and 30 mm Hg

   c. **Mannitol**

      (1) **Children.** 0.5–2.0 g/kg infused over 30 minutes, and repeated as necessary

Table 43-1. Empiric antimicrobial therapies for bacterial meningitis.

Age group	Antimicrobial agent
Neonates (≤4 weeks old)	Ampicillin plus cefotaxime or an aminoglycoside
Infants and children (>4 weeks old)	Ceftriaxone or cefotaxime plus vancomycin
Adults (15–50 years old)	
Community-acquired	Penicillin G or ampicillin or third-generation cephalosporin*
Postneurosurgical	Ceftazidime plus oxacillin or vancomycin plus aminoglycoside
Immunocompromised	Ceftazidime plus ampicillin
Older adults	Third-generation cephalosporin plus ampicillin

*Consideration should be given to the addition of vancomycin to penicillin for cephalosporin-resistant pneumococcal meningitis.

Table 43-2. Recommended antimicrobial therapies for bacterial meningitis in neonates and in infants and children by organism.

	Total daily dose		
Organism	Neonates (<1 week)	Neonates (1–4 weeks)	Infants and children (>4 weeks)
Haemophilus influenzae type b (Hib)	Cefotaxime 100 mg/kg/ day q12h	Cefotaxime 150 150 mg/kg/day q8h	Ceftriaxone 100 mg/kg/ day IV in a once or twice daily dosing regimen, or cefotaxime 225 mg/kg/day IV in divided doses q6h
Streptococcus pneumoniae	Penicillin G 50,000– 150,000 U/ kg/day q8h	Penicillin G 150,000– 200,000 U/kg/day q6h	Penicillin G 250,000– 400,000 U/kg/day IV in divided doses q4–6h
Group B streptococci	Ampicillin 100–150 mg/ kg/day q12h plus amika- cin 15 mg/kg/ day q12h, or gentami- cin 5 mg/kg/ day q12h	Ampicillin 200 mg/ kg/day q8h plus amikacin 30 mg/kg/day q8h, or gentamicin 7.5 mg/kg/ day q8h	Ampicillin 150–200 mg/ kg/day q4–6h plus amikacin 20 mg/kg/ day q8h, or gentamicin 5 mg/kg/day q8h
Listeria monocytogenes	Ampicillin	Ampicillin	Ampicillin
Neisseria meningitidis	Penicillin G 50,000– 150,000 U/ kg/day q8h, or ampicillin 100–150 mg/ kg/day q12h	Penicillin G 150,000– 200,000 U/kg/day q6h, or ampicillin 200 mg/ kg/day q8h	Penicillin G (same dosage as for *S. pneumoniae*), or ampicillin 150–200 mg/kg/day IV in divided doses q4–6h
Enteric gram-negative bacilli	Cefotaxime (same dosage as for Hib)	Cefotaxime (same dosage as for Hib)	Ceftriaxone or cefotaxime (same dosage as for Hib)
Staphylococcus aureus	Oxacillin 50– 100 mg/kg/ day q6h	Oxacillin 100–200 mg/ kg/day q6h	Oxacillin 200–300 mg/ kg/day q4h
Methicillin-resistant staphylococci	Vancomycin 20–30 mg/kg/ day q12h	Vancomycin 40 mg/kg/ day q6h	Vancomycin 40 mg/kg/ day in divided doses q6h plus oral rifampin 20 mg/kg/day; may also add intrashunt or intraventricular vancomycin 20 mg once daily

      (2) Adults. 1.0 g/kg bolus injection and then 0.25 g/kg q2–3h. A dosage of 0.25 g/kg appears to be equally as effective in lowering ICP as a dosage of 1.0 g/kg, with the major exception that the higher dosage has a longer duration of action. Serum osmolarity should not be allowed to rise above 320 mOsm/kg.

   d. Pentobarbital
      (1) Loading dose. 10 mg/kg over 30 minutes
      (2) 5 mg/kg/h for 3 hours, supplemented with 200-mg IV boluses if no burst-suppression pattern is obtained on EEG
      (3) Maintenance dosage. 1 mg/kg/h by constant IV infusion
  4. Seizure activity is such a common complication of bacterial meningitis in

Table 43-3. Recommended antimicrobial therapies for bacterial meningitis in adults by organism.

Organism	Antimicrobial agent
Streptococcus pneumoniae	Penicillin G 20–24 million U/day IV in divided doses q4h, or ampicillin 12 g/day q4h, or ceftriaxone or cefotaxime
Neisseria meningitidis	Penicillin G or ampicillin
Gram-negative bacilli (except *P. aeruginosa*)	Ceftriaxone 2–4 g/day IV in divided doses q12h, or cefotaxime 8–12 g/day q4h
Pseudomonas aeruginosa	Ceftazidime 6 g/day q8h
Haemophilus influenzae type b	Ceftriaxone or cefotaxime
Staphylococcus aureus (methicillin-sensitive)	Oxacillin 9–12 g/day IV in divided doses q4h
Staphylococcus aureus (methicillin-resistant)	Vancomycin 1 g IV q12h
Listeria monocytogenes	Ampicillin 12 g/day IV in divided doses q4h
Enterobacteriaceae	Ceftriaxone or cefotaxime

adults, especially pneumococcal meningitis, that prophylactic anticonvulsant therapy is not unreasonable.

a. **Prophylactic therapy.** Phenytoin is administered at a dosage of 18–20 mg/kg at a rate no faster than 50 mg/min. Phenytoin can prolong the Q–T interval or lead to hypotension, and therefore should be administered intravenously while monitoring ECG and BP. If either of these side effects is observed, the rate of administration should be decreased. It is recommended that phenytoin be administered no faster than 25 mg/min in the elderly. A standard maintenance dosage is 100 mg q8h. A serum concentration of 20–25 μg/ml should be maintained.

b. **Status epilepticus**
   (1) Diazepam (5–10 mg in adults; 0.2–0.3 mg/kg/dose in children) or lorazepam (0.1 mg/kg in adults; 0.05 mg/kg in children) is administered intravenously.
   (2) Phenytoin is administered in a dose of 18–20 mg/kg as described above (see sec. **I.A.4.a**).
   (3) If a dose of 18–20 mg/kg of phenytoin fails to control seizure activity, an additional 500 mg of phenytoin should be given.
   (4) If phenytoin fails to control seizure activity, phenobarbital is administered intravenously at a rate of 100 mg/min to a loading dose of 20 mg/kg. The loading dose of phenobarbital in children is also 20 mg/kg. The most common adverse effects of phenobarbital loading are hypotension and respiratory depression. Obviously, prior to phenobarbital loading, the patient should be intubated and mechanically ventilated. The primary reason for failure to control seizure activity is that either anticonvulsants are administered in subtherapeutic dosages or, as is the case for phenobarbital, the rate of administration is too slow.

5. **Fluid management.** A majority of children with bacterial meningitis are hyponatremic (serum sodium concentration <135 mEq/L) at the time of admission. For this reason, fluid restriction to correct serum sodium is important. The initial rate of intravenous fluid administration is limited to approximately one-half of normal maintenance requirements, or about 800–1000 ml/m²/day. A 5% dextrose solution with one-fourth to one-half normal saline and 20–40 mEq/L potassium is recommended. The volume of fluids administered can be gradually increased when the serum sodium concentration rises above 135 mEq/L.

B. **Expected outcome.** Despite appropriate antimicrobial therapy, patients with bacterial meningitis are very sick. Prognosis is dependent on age, underlying or associated conditions, time from onset of illness to institution of appropriate antimicrobial therapy, and the infecting organism. Pneumococcal meningitis has the worst prognosis, and a poor prognosis is associated with the extremes of age—that is, the very young and the very old have significantly higher rates of morbidity and mortality than older children and younger adults.

C. Referral. Patients who are comatose should be seen by a neurologist.

D. Prevention. Rifampin is recommended for all close contacts with a patient who has meningococcal meningitis and is given in divided doses at 12-hour intervals for 2 days as follows: adults, 600 mg; children, 10 mg/kg; neonates (<1 month), 5 mg/kg. A single oral dose of ciprofloxacin (750 mg) has also been demonstrated to be efficacious in adults in the eradication of the carrier state in meningococcal infection.

For prophylaxis of Hib meningitis, rifampin is recommended not only for all close contacts with the patient but also for the patient, because the organism usually is not eradicated from the nasopharynx by systemic antimicrobial therapy. Rifampin in the following dosages is recommended: adults, 20 mg/kg/day orally for 4 days; children, 20 mg/kg/day orally (maximum 600 mg/day) for 4 days; and neonates (<1 month), 10 mg/kg/day for 4 days. Rifampin is not recommended for pregnant women.

The FDA has approved only the Hib conjugate vaccines HbOC and PRP-OMP for administration to children younger than 15 months of age. Patients should be vaccinated with Hib conjugate vaccine as follows.

1. All infants should be vaccinated at ages 2, 4, and 6 months.

2. Unvaccinated children 12–14 months of age should receive one dose plus a booster dose after 15 months of age.

3. Unvaccinated children 15–60 months of age should receive a single dose and do not require a booster.

4. Children older than 5 years of age should be vaccinated on the basis of disease risk.

5. Rifampin prophylaxis should be given to children who come in contact with patients who have Hib meningitis regardless of whether or not they have been vaccinated with the Hib vaccine.

II. Herpes encephalitis. Encephalitis is inflammation of the brain parenchyma. Herpes simplex virus (HSV-1) is the principal cause of herpes virus encephalitis. Initial infection occurs either after exposure to infected saliva or respiratory secretions, with the virus gaining access to the CNS along the olfactory nerve and tract into the limbic lobe, or as a result of a reactivation of latent virus from the trigeminal ganglion. Virus is transmitted from infected people to other people only through close personal contact. The typical clinical presentation is a several-day history of fever and headache, followed by memory loss, confusion, olfactory hallucinations, and seizures. The hallmark sign is a focal neurologic deficit suggestive of a structural lesion in the frontotemporal area. The EEG is often abnormal, demonstrating periodic sharp-wave complexes from one or both temporal regions on a background of low-amplitude activity. The abnormalities on the EEG arise from one temporal lobe initially, but typically spread to the contralateral temporal lobe over a period of 6–10 days. A CT or MRI scan may show an area of abnormality in the temporal lobe with mass effect. On CT scan there is a low-density lesion within the temporal lobe with mass effect. On MRI scan, the infection appears as an area of decreased signal intensity on T1-weighted images and increased signal intensity on T2-weighted images. Examination of the CSF demonstrates a lymphocytic pleocytosis (with an average WBC count of 50–500 cells/mm^3), an elevation in the protein concentration, and a normal glucose concentration. Because this infection produces areas of hemorrhagic necrosis, the CSF may demonstrate RBCs or xanthochromia. The necessity of a brain biopsy in making the diagnosis of HSV-1 encephalitis is controversial. Several other infectious diseases have clinical presentations similar to that of HSV-1 encephalitis, including brain abscess (bacterial, fungal, or parasitic), brain tumor, Rocky Mountain spotted fever, togavirus encephalitis, and acute disseminated encephalomyelitis. If the clinical presentation, CSF, and EEG abnormalities are strongly suggestive of HSV-1 encephalitis, therapy for this infection should be initiated without brain biopsy. If the diagnosis is unclear, a brain biopsy should be performed.

A. Therapeutic approach

1. Antiviral activity. Acyclovir is the antiviral drug of choice for HSV-1 encephalitis. It is given at a dosage of 10 mg/kg q8h (30 mg/kg/day) intravenously, with each infusion lasting more than 1 hour, for a period of 10–14 days. Intravenous acyclovir can cause transient renal insufficiency secondary to crystallization of the drug in renal epithelial cells. For this reason, it is recommended that acyclovir be infused slowly over a period of 1 hour and that attention be paid to adequate IV hydration of the patient.

   2. **Anticonvulsant therapy.** Seizure activity, either focal or focal with secondary generalization, occurs in two-thirds of patients with HSV-1 encephalitis. Anticonvulsant therapy is indicated if seizure activity develops, and the following drugs are recommended.

      a. Lorazepam at dosages of 0.1 mg/kg for adults and 0.05 mg/kg for children, or diazepam at 5–10 mg for adults and 0.2–0.3 mg/kg/dose in children

      b. Phenytoin at a dosage of 18–20 mg/kg at a rate no faster than 50 mg/min. The daily maintenance dosage of phenytoin should be determined by serum levels.

   3. **Therapy for raised intracranial pressure (ICP).** Raised ICP is a common complication of herpes encephalitis and is associated with a poor outcome. Raised ICP should be aggressively treated as outlined for bacterial meningitis in sec. **I.A.3.**

   B. **Expected outcome.** In untreated HSV-1 encephalitis, mortality is higher than 70%, and only 2.5% of patients return to normal function following recovery. Patients treated with acyclovir have a significantly lower mortality of 19%, and 38% of these patients return to normal function.

   C. **Referral.** Patients who present with altered levels of consciousness or in comas have poor prognoses. Because the clinical diagnosis of herpes encephalitis typically requires interpretations of the neurologic presentation, the EEG, neuroimaging studies, and CSF, the diagnosis of this severe and devastating neurologic illness should be made in consultation with a neurologist and/or a neurosurgeon and an infectious disease specialist.

III. **Herpes zoster (shingles)**

   A. **Therapeutic approach.** Oral acyclovir (800 mg five times a day) accelerates the rate of cutaneous healing and reduces the severity of acute neuritis, but does not reduce the incidence or severity of postherpetic neuralgia. This therapy is most beneficial if it is initiated within 48 hours after the onset of the disease.

   B. **Side effects.** Oral acyclovir therapy has not been associated with renal dysfunction. This is an uncommon and reversible side effect of intravenous acyclovir. Oral acyclovir may cause dizziness, nausea, and headaches.

IV. **Lyme disease** is caused by the spirochete **Borrelia burgdorferi**, which is transmitted by the bite of an infected tick. Lyme disease is endemic in the coastal Northeast from Massachusetts to Maryland (particularly in New York), in the upper Midwest in Minnesota and Wisconsin, and on the Pacific coast in California and southern Oregon. Lyme disease is typically classified into three stages. Stage I is characterized by the classic appearance of erythema migrans, an annular erythematous cutaneous lesion with central clearing. This lesion appears within 3 days to 1 month after a tick bite and may be associated with headache and stiff neck along with constitutional symptoms. Stage II Lyme disease is characterized by cardiac involvement, meningitis, and cranial and peripheral neuropathies and radiculopathies. The most common neurologic abnormality during stage II Lyme disease is meningitis. The clinical picture is typical of a viral meningitis with symptoms of headache, mild stiff neck, nausea, vomiting, low-grade fever, and photophobia. These symptoms may be associated with a unilateral or bilateral facial nerve palsy or with symptoms of radiculopathy (paresthesias and hyperesthesias with or without focal weakness). Stage III (late or chronic) Lyme disease is associated with a progressive encephalopathy characterized by impaired memory, impaired concentration, and fatigue. There may also be a sensorimotor axonal polyradiculoneuropathy. A rare and late syndrome is a progressive encephalomyelitis. The only distinct clinical marker of Lyme disease is the typical erythema migrans lesion. Unfortunately, not all patients develop this lesion, and in some cases it goes unrecognized. It is standard practice to run a serologic test for antibodies against *B. burgdorferi* when Lyme disease is suspected. Most laboratories use an enzyme-linked immunosorbent assay (ELISA) technique. False-positive serologies are a problem with this test for two reasons.

   1. Tests can be performed on identical sera in several different laboratories with several different results. Because these tests are not well standardized, it is recommended that the physician use a laboratory that is reliable in performing this

test. A positive test may indicate only exposure to *B. burgdorferi* rather than active infection. People who live in high-risk areas may have measurable antibodies without having Lyme disease.
2. False-positive serologies can occur with rheumatoid arthritis, Rocky Mountain spotted fever, infectious mononucleosis, syphilis, tuberculous meningitis, and leptospirosis.

The CSF is generally abnormal in CNS Lyme disease. CSF should be examined for cell count, glucose, protein, and the intrathecal production of anti–*B. burgdorferi* antibodies. The Centers for Disease Control (CDC) requires the following for a diagnosis of Lyme disease: erythema migrans at least 5 cm in diameter or one or more late disease features (neurologic, rheumatologic, or cardiac) with laboratory isolation of the spirochete, detection of *B. burgdorferi* antibodies in serum or CSF, or a rising antibody titer on acute and convalescent serum samples. Most physicians, however, would opt to treat any patient with a clinical presentation or course suggestive of Lyme disease and possible exposure to a tick.

A. Therapeutic approach. Parenteral antibiotics are indicated for patients with neurologic involvement in Lyme disease, as follows.

Ceftriaxone is the drug of choice for neurologic Lyme disease. The adult dosage is 2 g/day, which may be given in a single daily dose, and the dosage for children is 75–100 mg/kg/day (up to 2 g/day). Treatment is given for at least 2 weeks, and should be continued for an additional 2 weeks if the response to treatment is slow or there is a severe infection. The major side effects of ceftriaxone are gastrointestinal disturbance (including *Clostridium difficile* colitis), hypersensitivity reaction, and cholelithiasis.

Alternatives to ceftriaxone are penicillin G and cefotaxime. Penicillin G is administered at an adult dosage of 3–4 million units (miU) q4h for 10–14 days or at a child dosage of 250,000 U/kg/day in divided doses. The major side effect of penicillin G is hypersensitivity reaction. Cefotaxime is given at dosages of 2 g tid for adults and 120–200 mg/kg/day (q6h) for children. The major side effects of cefotaxime are hypersensitivity reaction and gastrointestinal disturbance as well as inflammation at the injection site.

B. Expected outcome. Patients with neurologic complications of stage II Lyme disease (meningitis, cranial neuropathies, and peripheral neuropathies) should improve clinically within days, although improvement of facial weakness and radicular symptoms may take weeks. Patients with encephalopathies associated with stage III Lyme disease may fail to improve and continue to complain of fatigue and memory impairment. The longer the neurologic symptoms go untreated prior to initiation of parenteral antibiotic therapy, the greater the risk that they will persist.

C. Prevention. The deer tick is the usual vector of Lyme disease in the Northeast and Midwest. People who pursue outdoor occupational or recreational activities should be able to recognize the deer tick. Protective clothing may help decrease the risk of infection. Transmission of infection is unlikely if the tick has been attached for less than 24 hours. Pets that are permitted to roam in tick-infested areas should be fitted with tick-repellant collars and inspected for ticks.

V. Cryptococcal meningitis. Initiation of therapy for cryptococcal meningitis is based on examination of the CSF with the findings of a lymphocytic pleocytosis, a decreased glucose concentration, and a positive CSF cryptococcal antigen assay.

A. Therapeutic approach. The standard therapeutic regimen for cryptococcal meningitis is amphotericin B alone (in AIDS patients) or in combination with flucytosine (in immunocompetent patients). Amphotericin B is administered intravenously at 0.3 mg/kg/day, for a total of at least 1.0–1.5 g. Flucytosine is given orally at 150 mg/kg/day, divided into four daily doses. In either case, treatment is continued for at least 6 weeks.

B. Side effects. The most important adverse effect of amphotericin B is renal dysfunction, which occurs in 80% of patients. The incidence of nephrotoxicity is reduced by the combination regimen of amphotericin B and flucytosine. Renal function should be monitored two or three times weekly during the first month of therapy and once a week thereafter until therapy is discontinued. Serum creatinine, blood urea nitrogen, serum potassium, sodium and magnesium, bicarbonate, and hemoglobin concentrations should be monitored. Renal toxicity appears to be reduced or prevented by careful attention to the serum sodium concentration at the time of administration of amphotericin B.

Flucytosine is generally well tolerated; however, bone marrow suppression with anemia, leukopenia, and/or thrombocytopenia may develop. These hematologic abnormalities occur more often when serum concentrations of the drug exceed 100 µg/ml; therefore, serum concentrations of flucytosine should be monitored and the peak serum concentration kept well below 100 µg/ml. The current recommended dosage of 150 mg/kg/day may be too high, and a dosage of 75–100 mg/kg/day may be adequate. Gastrointestinal symptoms, including nausea, vomiting, diarrhea, and severe enterocolitis as well as drug-induced hepatitis, have been reported in association with the use of flucytosine.

VI. **Neurosyphilis in immunocompetent patients.** In immunocompetent patients, the clinical presentation of neurosyphilis falls into one or more of the following categories: (1) asymptomatic neurosyphilis, (2) meningitis, (3) meningovascular syphilis, (4) dementia paralytica, and (5) tabes dorsalis. The diagnosis of neurosyphilis is based on CSF abnormalities. In neurosyphilis, there is often a mild CSF mononuclear pleocytosis, mild elevation in the CSF protein concentration, and a positive CSF-VDRL test. A nonreactive CSF-VDRL does not rule out neurosyphilis. The CSF-VDRL test is nonreactive in 30–57% of patients with neurosyphilis.

   A. **Therapeutic approach.** The regimen recommended by the CDC for treatment of neurosyphilis is IV aqueous penicillin G at 12–24 million U/day (2–4 million U q4h) for 10–14 days. An alternative regimen is IM procaine penicillin at 2.4 million U/day and oral probenecid at 500 mg qid, both for 10–14 days.

   B. **Expected outcome.** The serum VDRL titer should decrease after successful therapy of neurosyphilis. The serum fluorescent treponemal antibody absorption test (FTA-ABS) test and the microhemagglutination-*T. pallidum* (MHA-TP) test remain reactive for life. The CSF-WBC count should be normal 6 months after therapy is completed. If on reexamination of the CSF, the WBC count remains elevated, retreatment is indicated.

VII. **Tuberculous meningitis**

   A. **Clinical presentation.** Tuberculous meningitis presents as an acute meningitis syndrome or as a slowly progressive dementing illness. The intradermal tuberculin skin test is helpful when positive. Radiographic evidence of pulmonary tuberculosis is found more often in children with tuberculous meningitis than in adults with tuberculous meningitis. The classic abnormalities on CSF examination are decreased glucose concentration, elevated protein concentration, and a polymorphonuclear or lymphocytic pleocytosis. Acid-fast bacilli are often difficult to demonstrate by CSF testing. The CSF pleocytosis is typically neutrophilic initially, but then becomes mononuclear or lymphocytic within several weeks. A CSF tuberculostearic acid assay may be obtained from the CDC. This test has high sensitivity and high specificity.

   B. **Therapeutic approach.** The CDC recommends a regimen of isoniazid (5–10 mg/kg/day up to 300 mg/day), rifampin (10–20 mg/kg/day up to 600 mg/day), and pyrazinamide (15–30 mg/kg/day up to 2 g/day). If the clinical response is good, pyrazinamide is discontinued after 8 weeks and isoniazid and rifampin are continued for an additional 10 months. Ethambutol is added, and the course of treatment is extended to 1–2 years in immunocompromised patients. The American Academy of Pediatrics recommends addition of streptomycin at 20–40 mg/kg/day to the above regimen for the first 2 months. Pyridoxine may be administered at a dosage of 25–50 mg/day to prevent the peripheral neuropathy that can result from use of isoniazid. Corticosteroid therapy is recommended when clinical deterioration occurs after treatment has begun. Dexamethasone can be administered at a dosage of 0.3–0.5 mg/kg/day for the first week of treatment and followed by oral prednisone.

VIII. **Neurocysticercosis.** A diagnosis of neurocysticercosis should be considered in patients who have seizures and exhibit neuroimaging evidence of cystic brain lesions. Cysticercosis is acquired by ingesting the eggs of the *Taenia solium* tapeworm shed in human feces. This occurs most often in areas where drinking water is contaminated with human feces.

   A. **Principal forms.** Neurocysticercosis presents in parenchymal, ventricular, subarachnoid, and racemose forms. In the parenchymal form, single or multiple cysts are found in the gray matter in the cerebrum and cerebellum. The most common clinical manifestation of parenchymal neurocysticercosis is new-onset seizure activity. In the ventricular form, single or multiple cysts are adherent to the ventricular wall or free in the CSF. Cysts are most common in the area of the fourth ventricle. In subarachnoid neurocysticercosis, cysts are found in the subarachnoid space or fixed under the pia and burrowed into the cortex. In the racemose form, cysts grow, often in clusters, in the basilar cisterns and obstruct the flow of CSF.

B. Therapeutic approach

  1. Cysticidal therapy consists of praziquantel at a dosage of 50 mg/kg/day for 15 days or albendazole taken orally at 15 mg/kg/day for 8 days.

  2. Corticosteroids. Cysticidal therapy frequently causes an inflammatory response with an increase in the CSF protein concentration and a CSF pleocytosis. This may result in an exacerbation of signs and symptoms. The incidence of an inflammatory response is reduced by the concomitant use of corticosteroids. Prednisone at 30–50 mg/day can be given with praziquantel for 15 days.

  3. Side effects. Phenytoin and carbamazepine lower serum praziquantel levels. If one of these anticonvulsants is used with praziquantel, it is recommended that oral cimetidine be added at a dosage of 800 mg bid. Phenytoin and carbamazepine lower serum praziquantel levels by inducing the cyto-chrome P-450 liver enzyme system. Cimetidine inhibits the P-450 cyto-chrome enzyme system, and in this way increases serum levels of praziquantel.

  4. Surgical therapy. Intraventricular cysts require surgical therapy, and when they obstruct the flow of CSF with resulting hydrocephalus, an intraventricular shunting device is indicated.

C. Expected outcome. The prognosis of patients with parenchymal neurocysticercosis is very good with cysticidal therapy. Cystic lesions should disappear within 3 months of treatment. The mortality is higher in patients with increased intracranial pressure, hydrocephalus, or the racemose form of the disease.

D. Prevention. Humans can acquire cysticercosis by eating food handled and contaminated by *T. solium* tapeworm carriers. Persons at high risk for tapeworm infection who are employed as food handlers should be screened for intestinal parasites. Improved sanitation can decrease the incidence of cysticercosis from contaminated food or drinking water.

Recommended Readings

Barry M, Kaldjian LC. Neurocysticercosis. *Semin Neurol* 13:131–143, 1993.

Coyle PK. Neurologic Lyme disease. *Semin Neurol* 12:200–208, 1992.

Kent SJ, et al. Tuberculous meningitis: A 30-year review. *Clin Infect Dis* 17:987–994, 1993.

Lebel MH, et al. Dexamethasone treatment for bacterial meningitis: Results of two double-blind, placebo-controlled trials. *NEJM* 319:964–971, 1988.

Marra CM. Syphilis and human immunodeficiency virus infection. *Semin Neurol* 12:43–50, 1992.

Meyding-Lamade U, Hanley DF, Skoldenberg B. Herpesvirus encephalitis. In W Hacke (ed), *NeuroCritical Care*. Berlin: Springer-Verlag, 1994. Pp 455–467.

Newton RW. Tuberculous meningitis. *Arch Dis Child* 70:364–366, 1994.

Pfister HW, Roos KL. Bacterial meningitis. In W Hacke (ed), *NeuroCritical Care*. Berlin: Springer-Verlag, 1994. Pp 377–397.

Reik L, et al. Neurologic abnormalities of Lyme disease. *Medicine* 58:281–294, 1979.

Roos KL, Tunkel AR, Scheld WM. Acute bacterial meningitis in children and adults. In WM Scheld, RJ Whitley, DT Durack (eds), *Infections of the Central Nervous System*. New York: Raven, 1991. Pp 335–409.

Skoldenberg B. Herpes simplex encephalitis. *Scand J Infect Dis* 78:40–46, 1991.

Sotelo J, Guerrero V, Rubio F. Neurocysticercosis: A new classification based on active and inactive forms. A study of 753 cases. *Arch Intern Med* 145:442–445, 1985.

Sugar AM, Stern JJ, Dupont B. Overview: Treatment of cryptococcal meningitis. *Rev Infect Dis* 12:S338–S348, 1990.

Whitley RJ, Gnann JW. Drug therapy: Acyclovir: A decade later. *NEJM* 327:782–789, 1992.

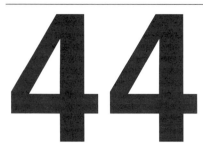

Neurologic Complications in AIDS
Bruce A. Cohen

I. **General considerations.** Neurologic symptoms and signs occur in 50–60% of AIDS patients during the course of the disease and are the presenting manifestations in 5–10%. By the time of neuropathologic evaluation, 90–100% of AIDS patients have abnormalities of the nervous system that may affect any level of the neuraxis. Neurologic manifestations may result from effects of the human immunodeficiency virus (HIV) itself or from opportunistic processes. Acute meningitis, meningoencephalitis, or polyneuritis may mark HIV seroconversion, but conventional antibody-based HIV testing may not become positive for several months after these syndromes occur. Patients with such syndromes should be tested with direct viral or antigen based assays or retested for HIV 3–6 months after the occurrence. In approaching the AIDS patient with neurologic manifestations, the following basic postulates can facilitate diagnosis and therapy of opportunistic neurologic complications.

A. Most opportunistic complications appear after significant immunosuppression has occurred, as reflected by CD4 lymphocyte counts of 200/mm³ or less.

B. Neurologic presentations of opportunistic infections in AIDS patients may be subtle and lack classic textbook features.

C. The imaging modality of choice in most instances of neurologic involvement is magnetic resonance imaging (MRI). However, most imaging patterns are nonspecific.

D. Multiple concurrent pathologies in the nervous system are common, occurring in one-third or more of patients. Vigilance during therapy is important, and reevaluation to detect concurrent conditions should be considered when abrupt or atypical changes in condition occur, or the anticipated responses are not observed.

E. Opportunistic processes may develop rapidly, with changes in imaging, laboratory, and clinical parameters over short intervals.

F. Diagnosis requires neuropathologic assessment in many instances, and thresholds for biopsy in AIDS patients with neurologic manifestations should be low. Treatment strategies in AIDS are continuously and rapidly evolving. The National Institutes of Health (NIH) sponsors AIDS Clinical Trials Units (ACTU) through the Division of AIDS of the National Institute of Allergy and Infectious Diseases (NIAID). In patients with neurologic conditions for which satisfactory therapies have not yet been established, referral to neurologic protocols available at ACTUs should be considered when feasible. Entities causing neurologic complications in AIDS are summarized in Table 44-1.

II. **Conditions attributed to HIV**

A. **HIV encephalopathy (HIVE)**

1. **Natural history.** HIV encephalopathy (HIV dementia, AIDS dementia complex, HIV encephalitis) affects 15–20% of AIDS patients, usually appearing after significant immunosuppression has developed. On occasion, it may represent the presenting manifestation of AIDS. HIVE is gradually progressive, with median survival of about 6 months following diagnosis. The pathogenesis is not presently understood. Clinical impairment is disproportionate to the degree of neuropathology demonstrated at autopsy, and noncytolytic perturbations of neuronal function are currently considered important in the pathophysiology.

2. **Clinical features.** A clinical triad of cognitive impairment, behavioral changes, and motor impairment characterizes HIVE. Cognitive features include slowness of thought, cognitive perseveration, and impairment of recall

Table 44-1. Entities causing neurologic complications in AIDS.

Encephalopathy	Meningitis
Diffuse:	HIV
HIV	Cryptococcus
PML	Syphilis
CMV	Tuberculosis
VZV	Lymphoma
Syphilis	CMV
Toxoplasmosis	HSV
Aspergillus	VSV
Toxic (medications)	Other fungi
Metabolic (hypoxia, sepsis, etc.)	**Neuropathy**
	HIV
Focal:	Toxic (dideoxynucleosides, etc.)
Toxoplasmosis	CMV
PML	Lymphoma
Lymphoma	Syphilis
Cryptococcus	B_{12} deficiency
CMV	**Myopathy**
HSV	HIV
VZV	Toxic (AZT)
Syphilis	CMV
Tuberculosis	Toxoplasmosis
Fungal abscess	Cryptococcus
Nocardia asteroides	Pyogenic
Pyogenic abscess	

Myelopathy
HIV
CMV
HSV
VZV
Syphilis
Lymphoma
Tuberculosis
Toxoplasmosis
Cryptococcus
B_{12} deficiency
Nocardia asteroides
Pyogenic abscess

memory with relative preservation of recognition. Patients become apathetic and withdraw from social interaction. They may initially be thought to be depressed. A few patients may present with atypical psychoses. Motor features include hyperreflexia and ataxia usually affecting the legs initially. Extrapyramidal features of bradykinesia, facial masking, and postural instability may be observed. Tremor may occur, and frontal release signs such as grasp and snout reflexes may be found.

3. **Diagnosis.** Progressive cognitive impairment with clear sensorium and typical behavioral and motor features in an AIDS patient with low CD4 counts suggests the diagnosis. Opportunistic processes must be excluded by MRI and cerebrospinal fluid (CSF) analysis. MRI may show atrophy or symmetric leukoencephalopathy. CSF usually shows only protein elevation or is normal.

4. **Therapy.** See Figure 44-1.

   a. **Zidovudine (AZT)** inhibits HIV reverse transcriptase and is the only antiretroviral agent to date shown to have efficacy in HIVE, having been shown to produce improvement in cognitive function on serial neuropsychometric testing. There is some suggestive evidence that higher doses of AZT may be more effective, and we use 1200–2000 mg/day in five or six divided doses if tolerated. Myelosuppression is anticipated at these dosages and is counteracted by erythropoietin to maintain hemoglobin

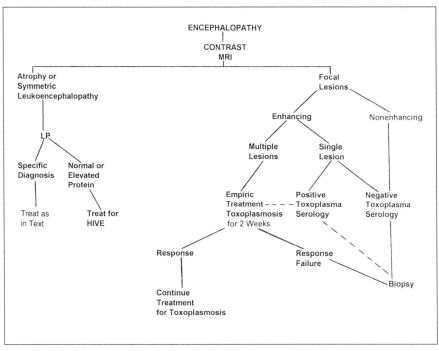

ENCEPHALOPATHY
|
CONTRAST
MRI

Atrophy or
Symmetric
Leukoencephalopathy

Focal
Lesions

Enhancing   Nonenhancing

LP

Specific   Normal or
Diagnosis   Elevated
                Protein

Multiple   Single
Lesions   Lesion

Treat as   Treat for
in Text   HIVE

Empiric   Positive   Negative
Treatment – – – – Toxoplasma   Toxoplasma
Toxoplasmosis   Serology   Serology
for 2 Weeks

Response   Response
                                      Failure

                                                            Biopsy

Continue
Treatment
for Toxoplasmosis

Figure 44-1. Approach to the AIDS patient with encephalopathy (HIVE = HIV encephalopathy; LP = lumbar puncture; MRI = magnetic resonance imaging).

levels above 10 g/dl and granulocyte colony stimulating factor to maintain absolute neutrophil counts above 1000/mm^3. In some instances, transfusions may be required. AZT also may cause headaches, myalgias, and a myopathy with increased creatine kinase levels, hepatotoxicity, nausea and emesis, and malaise. Because AZT, like other currently available antiretroviral agents, is virustatic, HIV resistance may develop, and some evidence suggests a limited duration of efficacy in HIVE.

  b. Other antiretroviral agents. Several other HIV reverse transcriptase inhibitors are currently available. The dideoxynucleosides (DDI, DDC, D4T) may have efficacy against strains of HIV resistant to AZT, but have not yet been shown to benefit patients with HIVE. Combination therapy with these agents is more effective. Adverse reactions to dideoxynucleosides include peripheral neuropathy, pancreatitis, hepatic toxicity, and gastrointestinal intolerance. A new class of antiretroviral agents called protease inhibitors are now available and appear to show synergistic effects when combined with reverse transcriptase inhibitors. The impact of such combination therapy on HIVE has not yet been established.

  c. Adjunctive therapy. Clinical trials are currently evaluating a number of agents proposed to counteract HIV-induced damage on the basis of in vitro effects on cytokine levels or HIV toxicity in cell cultures. Such agents, combined with antiretroviral therapy, might influence intermediate steps to achieve favorable modification of HIV neuropathogenesis.

  d. Supportive therapy

    (1) Apathy and withdrawal can be treated with methylphenidate at 5–10 mg bid-tid. Side effects include hepatotoxicity and gastrointestinal intolerance, delirium, seizures, anxiety, and sleep disturbances.

    (2) Depression can be treated with tricyclic antidepressants such as amitriptyline at dosages starting at 25 mg at bedtime, and increasing as tolerated in 25-mg increments every 1–2 weeks, or with serotonin reuptake inhibitors such as fluoxetine starting at 10–20 mg/day and increasing in 10-mg increments. Adverse reactions to amitriptyline and other tricyclic agents include anticholinergic effects (such as urinary retention, constipation, dry mouth, and ileus), cardiac conduction abnormalities and arrhythmias, hypotension, sedation that may be transient, toxic delirium, seizures, tremors, paresthesias, sleep disturbances, gastrointestinal intolerance, changes in appetite and increased weight, and alteration of taste, as well as uncommon effects such as myelosuppression, hepatic toxicity, and movement disorders. Adverse reactions to fluoxetine include chills, fevers, nausea, headache, cardiac conduction abnormalities and arrhythmias, angina, blood pressure elevation or depression, arthralgias, gastrointestinal intolerance, hepatotoxicity, tremors, ataxia, hypomania, agitation and restlessness, respiratory tract irritation, menstrual irregularities, and seizures. Uncommonly, movement disorders, syncope, and myelosuppression may occur.

(3) Seizures may occur in HIVE and can be treated with any of the anticonvulsants; however, because of frequent hypersensitivity and myelosuppressive reactions with other agents, phenobarbital may be best tolerated. Sedation is the most common adverse effect.

(4) Supervision. Progression of HIVE results in loss of ability to manage personal business and financial affairs. Provisions for legal transfer of decision-making powers for both financial and health-care decisions, and advance healthcare directives, should be made. Assistance in the home is eventually required for maintenance, provision of meals, and assistance with personal care. Residence in a sheltered facility may be considered when the need for assistance precludes independent living. Hospice programs may provide valuable support as the disease progresses.

5. **Outcome.** Limited studies suggest that AZT treatment extends survival and may decrease occurrence or delay progression of HIV-related dementias. Whether other antiretroviral agents or combinations of agents offer significant benefit is presently unknown. Monitoring of patients on high-dosage AZT should include monthly blood counts, liver function studies, and creatine kinase levels. Neurologic examinations should be performed serially. Abrupt changes in neurologic function should prompt evaluation for a superimposed opportunistic process.

B. **HIV myelopathy**

1. **Natural history.** Neuropathologic evidence of myelopathy is found in up to 40% of AIDS patients at autopsy and may affect 20% clinically, predominantly in the dorsal and lateral columns of the thoracic spinal cord. Concurrent encephalopathy is often present, and the condition typically is gradually progressive over months. The specific etiology is unknown, because active HIV infection is not usually found in the cord. An acute self-limited myelitis has rarely been reported as a seroconversion reaction.

2. **Clinical features.** Gradually progressive spastic paraparesis and sensory ataxia evolving over months in an AIDS patient with advanced immunosuppression are typical of vacuolar myelopathy. Disturbances of urinary bladder function commonly occur, and sensory deficits reflect dorsal column involvement with loss of vibration and position sensations. Up to 60% of patients may have associated HIV encephalopathy.

3. **Diagnosis** can be made on clinical grounds once other etiologies for chronic myelopathy have been excluded, particularly vitamin B_{12} deficiency, syphilis, human T-cell lymphotropic virus type I (HTLV-I) infection, and indolent opportunistic infections. MRI may be normal or show atrophic changes. CSF shows nonspecific protein elevation but is otherwise unremarkable.

4. **Therapy.** No direct therapy has been shown to prevent progression of myelopathy, and the best recommendation at present is to treat the associated encephalopathy in the manner described above. **Supportive therapy** is beneficial. Spasticity can be treated with baclofen at 5–20 mg tid-qid. Anticholinergic agents such as oxybutynin at 2.5–5.0 mg tid-qid may improve urinary frequency, urgency, and incontinence. External supports enhance safety and mobility in patients with sufficient leg strength, and motorized

wheelchairs can maintain mobility in weaker patients who are otherwise capable of independent activity. Adverse reactions to baclofen include gastrointestinal intolerance, hepatotoxicity, and, at higher dosages, lethargy or weakness. High dosages of baclofen cannot be stopped abruptly but should be gradually tapered to prevent withdrawal-related seizures and encephalopathy. Oxybutynin can produce anticholinergic side effects such as decreased gastrointestinal motility, dry mouth, abdominal cramping and nausea, urinary hesitation or retention, and decreased sweating. Lethargy or delirium may occur, and tachycardia or vasodilatation may be observed. Anticholinergics cause mydriasis and may increase intraocular pressure.

5. **Outcome.** Most patients with HIV myelopathy follow a progressive course marked by other HIV-related illnesses. Some, however, have extended survivals with retention of other faculties. Patients should be periodically reexamined neurologically to adjust supportive therapy. Abrupt changes should prompt evaluation for a superimposed opportunistic process.

C. **HIV distal sensory neuropathy (DSN).** See Figure 44-2.

1. **Natural history.** DSN is the most common neuropathy seen in AIDS patients, occurring clinically in about one-third of patients late in the disease course and demonstrable pathologically in up to 100% of small series. The etiology is unknown, but a progressive axonal degeneration with endoneurial and epineurial inflammation may be found on nerve biopsy.

2. **Clinical features.** DSN is characterized by a **distal symmetric sensory involvement** beginning in the feet and gradually ascending in the legs. Distal upper extremities are involved later and to a lesser degree. Patients complain of severe neuralgic pain described as burning or shooting in character. Feet are numb, and paresthesias in upper and lower limbs are usually present. Examination reveals impairment of vibration and pinprick perception distally, loss of or diminished ankle reflexes with variable depression of other reflexes, and sensory ataxia. Motor weakness in distal muscles may be present but is overshadowed by the sensory symptoms.

3. **Diagnosis.** The principal differential consideration is often toxic effects of dideoxynucleoside antiretroviral agents, which may mimic or exacerbate DSN. Other potentially neurotoxic agents are commonly used in HIV patients, including dapsone, INH, and vincristine. Vitamin B_{12} deficiency is common in this population. Lymphoma may produce neuralgia by direct invasion or by paraneoplastic effects. Alcohol, diabetes, and other conventional etiologies for neuropathy should be excluded. Electrophysiologic studies reveal diminished amplitudes and conduction in sural nerves and variable-amplitude decrements in other nerves with relatively preserved conduction. Symmetric denervation and reinnervation may be detected by electromyography (EMG).

4. **Therapy**

   a. Direct HIV therapy has variable benefit on DSN. Other treatment is directed at disabling sensory symptoms. Potential neurotoxic agents should be discontinued to the extent possible, particularly dideoxynucleosides. Toxic symptoms may persist for 6–8 weeks after discontinuation. Any metabolic deficiency should be corrected.

   b. Neuralgic pain may be treated with combinations of anticonvulsants such as carbamazepine (CBZ) or diphenylhydantoin (DPH) and tricyclic agents such as amitriptyline. CBZ can be initiated at dosages of 100 mg tid-qid and increased by 200 mg on a weekly basis to 800–1200 mg/day if tolerated. DPH is an alternative for patients unable to take CBZ and is given in dosages of 100 mg tid-qid. Gabapentin in dosages of 300–600 mg tid may also be tried. Amitriptyline is begun at 25 mg qhs and increased by 25 mg every 1–2 weeks as required up to 100 mg qhs. Patients who fail to respond may be given a trial of mexiletine at 150 mg bid, increased to 300 mg bid as required after anticonvulsants and tricyclics have been discontinued. Patients failing to obtain relief may require narcotic analgesia.

      (1) Adverse reactions to CBZ include drowsiness, ataxia, and gastrointestinal intolerance, which may be more likely when dosages are increased rapidly. Confusion, visual blurring, diplopia, headache, leukopenia, and thrombocytopenia may be observed, and aplastic anemia, cardiac arrhythmias, inappropriate antidiuretic hormone

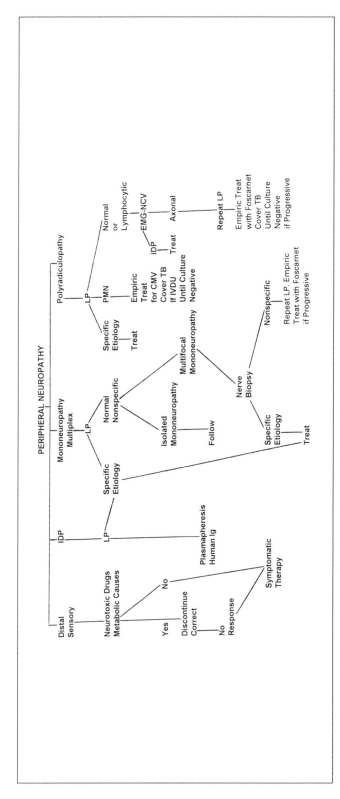

Figure 44-2. Approach to the AIDS patient with peripheral neuropathy (LP = lumbar puncture; CMV = cytomegalovirus; TB = tuberculosis; IVDU = intravenous drug user; IDP = inflammatory demyelinating polyneuropathy; Ig = pooled human immune globulin; PMN = polymorphonuclear leukocytes; EMG-NCV = electromyography-nerve conduction velocities).

secretion, hepatotoxicity, and Stevens-Johnson syndrome may occur in rare cases.

(2) DPH may produce thrombocytopenia, hepatotoxicity, hirsutism, gingival hyperplasia, nystagmus, and, at higher serum levels, ataxia, drowsiness, and confusion. A rash indicates common hypersensitivity and should prompt discontinuation to prevent progression to Stevens-Johnson syndrome. Less common side effects include fever, lymphadenopathy, lupoid or pseudolymphoma syndromes, and pulmonary infiltrates. Osteomalacia and peripheral neuropathy may occur after chronic use. Adverse reactions to amitriptyline are listed in sec. **II.A.4.d.** Mexiletine may produce cardiovascular toxicity with conduction block, arrhythmia, hypotension, or syncope; gastrointestinal intolerance including ulceration, hemorrhage, and dysphagia; hepatotoxicity; and, rarely, Stevens-Johnson syndrome.

5. Outcome. Symptomatic management may be helpful in alleviating discomfort, but reversal of DSN is unlikely. Abrupt changes in severity of DSN sometimes occur in association with active cytomegalovirus (CMV) infection, and screening for CMV may be indicated when compatible systemic symptoms are present.

D. Inflammatory demyelinating polyneuropathy (IDP). See Figure 44-2.

1. Natural history. Acute IDP usually occurs early in the course of HIV infection and may represent a reaction to seroconversion. Its natural history is similar to that of Guillain-Barré syndrome in the non-HIV-infected population and is presumed to result from an immune reaction that transiently causes peripheral demyelination. Chronic IDP may occur at any disease stage, also presumably a result of immune mediated demyelination. Neurologic symptoms of chronic IDP may be relapsing or progressive.

2. Clinical features. Acute IDP presents with progressive motor weakness, areflexia, and variable sensory and autonomic symptoms, evolving over days and usually beginning in the lower extremities and ascending. Some patients progress to respiratory insufficiency requiring mechanical ventilatory support. Chronic IDP may follow a progressive or relapsing course over months with similar motor weakness and areflexia but with more prominent sensory impairment.

3. Diagnosis. Typical clinical features are suggestive. Electrophysiologic studies reveal prominent slowing and motor nerve conduction blocks, prolonged or absent F-wave responses, and variable degrees of axonal damage and denervation. CSF typically shows prominent protein elevation. In contrast with the non-HIV-infected population, acute IDP may be associated with a moderate lymphocytic pleocytosis, and such a finding should lead to follow-up testing to exclude a seroconversion reaction when initial HIV serology is negative.

4. Therapy

a. Patients with IDP may recover spontaneously, but those with significant motor impairment should be treated with plasma exchange totaling 200–250 ml/kg divided into five exchanges over a 2-week period with 5% albumin replacement. An expensive but more convenient alternative is the use of pooled human immune globulin in dosages of 0.4 g/kg daily for 5 days given as an IV infusion at 0.05–4.0 ml/kg/hr as tolerated. Patients with chronic IDP require maintenance therapy with one treatment every 2–4 weeks. Intervals can be gradually extended as response occurs. Additional benefit may result from combining the two methods. Because of the potential for facilitating opportunistic infections, corticosteroid therapy for chronic IDP probably should not be used in the HIV-infected population. Patients with impending respiratory failure in acute IDP (vital capacity <1000 cc), should be electively intubated until adequate respiratory function returns.

b. Adjunctive therapy is important to prevent complications of immobility and maintain function in anticipation of neuromuscular recovery. Non-ambulatory patients should be given subcutaneous heparin at 5000 U q12h and intermittent calf compression to prevent deep-vein thrombophlebitis. Physical therapy should be initiated at the bedside for passive ranging to prevent contracture formation and should be advanced with improvement in strength. Occupational therapy should also be started early for individuals with upper-extremity weakness. Neuralgic pain may be treated in the same manner as in DSN (sec. **II.C.4.b**). As strength improves, mobilization may require support devices or orthotics, particularly in patients with chronic IDP.

   c. Adverse reactions to plasmapheresis include complications of hyper- or hypovolemia, hemolytic anemia, infection, allergic reactions, hypoglycemia, hemorrhage, and complications of catheter placement. Side effects of therapy with human immune globulin include risks of transmissible diseases, myalgias, arthralgias, headaches, lightheadedness, chills, tremors, gastrointestinal intolerance, and, in patients with IgA deficiency, hypotension and dyspnea. Many of these adverse reactions may be ameliorated by slowing the infusion rate.

   5. **Outcome.** Acute IDP usually resolves with complete recovery in most patients. Chronic IDP has a more variable outcome, and residual neurologic impairment often persists.

E. **HIV myopathy**
   1. **Natural history.** Myopathy may develop in HIV-infected patients as a result of AZT toxicity, an HIV-related polymyositis, or, rarely, opportunistic pathogens. AZT myopathy usually appears after at least 6 months of treatment and is thought to result from mitochondrial toxicity. The pathogenesis of HIV myopathy is unknown, and the disorder may occur at any stage of infection.
   2. **Clinical features.** A symmetric progressive proximal weakness with elevation of serum creatine kinase levels is typical of both HIV and AZT myopathies. Myalgias are variable.
   3. **Diagnosis.** The clinical pattern and elevated creatine kinase levels are suggestive. EMG demonstrates myopathic motor unit potentials with increased recruitment. Concurrent neuropathy is not uncommon. Muscle biopsy demonstrates scattered muscle fiber degeneration. Mitochondrial abnormalities and inclusions such as nemaline rod bodies may be observed. Scattered inflammatory infiltrates are typical.
   4. **Therapy.** Patients taking AZT who develop myopathy should discontinue the therapy. If no improvement occurs after 1–2 months, muscle biopsy should be considered. For patients with acute severe myalgia, biopsy should be pursued earlier to exclude opportunistic myositis. When inflammatory changes are demonstrated in a patient not taking antiretroviral agents, institution of AZT or other antiretroviral therapy may produce clinical improvement at conventional dosages. Progressive myositis in spite of these measures can be treated with corticosteroids. Prednisone may be started at 40–60 mg/day and tapered to lower, alternate-day dosages as response allows, but the risk of facilitating opportunistic infections must be recognized. Human immune globulin may be considered in accordance with the regimens described for IDP (sec. **II.D.4.a**). In addition to opportunistic infections, adverse effects from corticosteroid therapy include hyperglycemia, hypertension, hyperlipidemia, weight gain, osteoporosis, gastrointestinal ulceration and hemorrhage, myopathy, psychosis, mood changes, cataracts, and impaired healing of wounds.
   5. **Outcome.** Most patients respond to either withdrawal of AZT or institution of antiretroviral or steroid therapy. Failure to respond to empiric measures should prompt muscle biopsy to establish inflammation and exclude opportunistic myositis before starting corticosteroids.

F. **Aseptic meningitis** may appear with HIV seroconversion, typically presenting with headache, fever, neck stiffness, and occasionally cranial neuropathies and confusion or lethargy. This condition is self-limited and requires no therapy other than analgesia. Chronic, subclinical, aseptic meningitis is observed in many HIV-infected patients with moderate protein elevation, modest lymphocytic pleocytosis, elevated gamma globulin index, and occasionally oligoclonal banding. The importance of this condition lies primarily in its potential for causing diagnostic confusion during evaluation for possible neurosyphilis or opportunistic disease. As immunosuppression progresses, the pleocytosis tends to disappear. In patients with significant immunosuppression, aseptic meningitis should prompt investigation for opportunistic infection.

III. **Opportunistic diseases**
   A. *Cryptococcus*
      1. **Natural history.** *Cryptococcus neoformans* is the most common oppor-

tunistic meningitis in AIDS patients, affecting up to 10%. Extraneurologic cryptococcal infection may be found in lung, bone marrow, liver, and skin. Localized cryptococcomas may be found in brain parenchyma. The fungus is acquired by inhalation and spreads to the CNS hematogenously, becoming symptomatic with immune suppression.

2. **Clinical features.** The most common presentation is meningitis, and symptoms may be subtle with only headache and fever. Meningismus is present in no more than half the cases. Cranial neuropathies may be observed, and some patients have gastrointestinal symptoms. Seizures and focal neurologic signs may be observed with parenchymal involvement, which may occur in the absence of meningitis.

3. **Diagnosis.** Imaging studies may be normal or reveal meningeal enhancement in patients with meningitis. Cryptococcomas may or may not enhance with contrast. Cystic lesions caused by invasion of Virchow-Robin spaces in basal ganglia and other sites do not enhance. CSF pleocytosis may be present or absent. Depressed glucose levels and modest protein elevations may be observed but are nonspecific. Cryptococcal antigen titers are generally positive, and cultures always yield *cryptococcus* in patients with meningitis, but both may be negative when isolated parenchymal disease is present. Cryptococcal antigen can be measured in serum. Definitive diagnosis of isolated parenchymal lesions may require biopsy.

4. **Therapy**

   a. **Initial therapy** for cryptococcal meningitis may be undertaken with amphotericin B at 0.6–1.0 mg/kg/day with or without flucytosine at 25.0–37.5 mg/kg qid in patients with normal renal function. Alternatively, fluconazole at a dosage of 200 mg bid has been shown to produce similar response rates but less rapid CSF sterilization, and can be used in patients with less severe infections who have normal mentation and CSF cryptococcal antigen titers of less than 1:1000. Amphotericin B should be continued to a total dosage of about 1 g and followed by fluconazole at 200 mg PO bid for 10 weeks. Patients with sterile CSF can then be treated with a maintenance regimen.

   b. **Adjunctive therapy.** Patients with significant elevations of intracranial pressure can be treated with acetazolamide at 250 mg qid and/or mechanical drainage by serial lumbar puncture (LP) or CSF shunt.

   c. Successful sterilization of CSF with induction therapy should be followed by **lifetime maintenance therapy** with fluconazole at 200 mg/day.

   d. Adverse effects of amphotericin B are common. Fever and chills occur with administration and may be suppressed by ibuprofen, aspirin, or small doses of hydrocortisone. Nausea, emesis, headache, tachypnea, and hypotension also occur following infusion. Renal toxicity is significant, and hydration and dosage reduction for signs of renal insufficiency may prevent more serious impairment. Pain at the infusion site; arthralgias; myalgias; phlebitis; and electrolyte disturbances with hypocalcemia, hypo- or hyperkalemia, and hypomagnesemia are observed. Hepatotoxicity, thrombocytopenia, leukopenia and granulocytopenia, coagulopathy, seizures, ototoxicity, encephalopathy, neuropathy, and anaphylactoid reactions may occur. Cardiac arrest, arrhythmia or congestive heart failure, dyspnea, pulmonary edema, and hypersensitivity pneumonitis have been reported. Flucytosine commonly causes gastrointestinal intolerance and myelosuppression. Nephrotoxicity, delirium or confusion, ataxia, ototoxicity, headache, paresthesias, neuropathy, hypoglycemia, hypokalemia, hepatotoxicity, and colitis may occur. Fluconazole may produce gastrointestinal intolerance, headache, hepatotoxicity, anaphylactic reactions, seizures, and leukopenia. Stevens-Johnson syndrome, hypokalemia, hypercholesterolemia, and hypertriglyceridemia have been reported. In patients on concurrent therapy with warfarin or diphenylhydantoin, these latter agents may be potentiated, requiring dosage adjustments.

5. **Outcome.** Acute mortality for cryptococcal meningitis in AIDS is 10–25%. The most important factor affecting prognosis is the clarity of mentation and sensorium at presentation. Other factors thought to affect prognosis negatively are CSF cryptococcal antigen titers greater than 1:1024, extraneuro-

logic cryptococcal infection, elevated intracranial pressure, and hyponatremia. CSF should be sampled following completion of induction therapy. Persistently positive cryptococcal cultures should be treated with continued higher dosages of fluconazole. Serum cryptococcal antigen cannot be used to monitor responders.

6. **Prevention.** Retrospective studies suggest a decreased frequency of cryptococcal meningitis in AIDS patients taking fluconazole at dosages of 100–200 mg/day.

B. **CNS toxoplasmosis**

1. **Natural history.** *Toxoplasma gondii* is an intracellular parasite that typically is acquired by ingestion and that usually remains dormant unless immunosuppression permits reactivation. It is uncertain whether CNS toxoplasmosis in AIDS results from local reactivation or from hematogenous spread following reactivation. CNS toxoplasmosis is the most common opportunistic encephalitis in AIDS patients.

2. **Clinical features.** The most common presentation is a subacute illness beginning with headache and fever followed by progressive focal or diffuse neurologic deficits appearing over days to 1–2 weeks. Some patients present acutely with seizures.

3. **Diagnosis.** Imaging studies show multiple enhancing lesions in 80–85% of patients. MRI is more sensitive than CT. Most lesions appear as masses, but nonenhancing infarction-like patterns may be observed. Approximately 15–20% of patients may have single lesions, and the appearance of the lesions is not specific. Serologic studies for IgG antibodies to *Toxoplasma* are positive in 85% of cases, but IgM antibodies or convalescent rises in IgG titers are not often observed. Antibodies to toxoplasmosis and *Toxoplasma* DNA amplified by polymerase chain reaction (PCR) techniques can be detected in CSF when it can be obtained safely. Definitive diagnosis requires pathologic demonstration of organisms.

4. **Therapy**

   a. Because of the rapidity of the response to therapy, empiric treatment of HIV patients with multiple lesions typical of toxoplasmosis and positive serologies is warranted for a 2-week period before brain biopsy is considered. Single lesions with negative serology for toxoplasmosis should be biopsied. Optimal therapy combines sulfadiazine at 1.5 g PO q6h and pyrimethamine PO in an initial dose of 100 mg followed by 75 mg/day. Folinic acid at 10 mg/day PO is added to counteract myelosuppression from the pyrimethamine. Patients unable to take sulfa can substitute clindamycin at 600–900 mg qid with similar efficacy for acute infection. Corticosteroids should be avoided to prevent diagnostic confusion when treating empirically. Seizures should be treated with anticonvulsants.

   b. Successful initial therapy is continued for 6 weeks and is followed by **lifetime maintenance therapy** with sulfadiazine at 500 mg qid or clindamycin at 300 mg qid and pyrimethamine at 50 mg/day with continuation of folinic acid. Patients unable to take either sulfa or clindamycin can be treated with atovaquone at 750 mg PO qid, but efficacy may not be equivalent.

   c. Adverse effects of sulfa include allergy, nephrotoxicity, gastrointestinal intolerance, pancreatic and hepatic toxicity, and, less frequently, hemolytic anemia resulting from G6PD deficiency, toxic encephalopathy, neuritis, and dizziness. Adverse effects of clindamycin include gastrointestinal intolerance with diarrhea, pain, nausea, and emesis; hepatotoxicity; polyarthritis; and allergic reactions. Hypotension may occur after rapid IV infusion. Pyrimethamine produces thrombocytopenia, anemia, and leukopenia by causing folate deficiency, and rare CNS toxicity with headache, confusion, seizures, tremor, ataxia, depression, or insomnia. Atovaquone can cause gastrointestinal intolerance, fever, insomnia, headache, dizziness, and allergic reactions. Rare CNS toxicity, nephrotoxicity, and myelosuppression are also reported with quinones.

5. **Outcome.** Therapeutic monitoring is particularly important for patients treated empirically for CNS toxoplasmosis. Imaging should be repeated 2 weeks after initiation of antibiotic therapy. Failure of lesions to respond should prompt brain biopsy. If any lesion enlarges despite therapy, it should be biopsied to exclude a concurrent process irrespective of the behavior of

other lesions. Most patients who respond can maintain control of the infection by taking suppressive antibiotic therapy. About 10% of patients relapse, usually because of discontinuation of maintenance therapy. Recurrence despite adequate maintenance therapy should prompt biopsy to exclude an alternate process.

6. **Prevention.** Evidence from studies of patients taking sulfa to prevent pneumocystis pneumonia suggests that toxoplasmosis can also be prevented by daily trimethoprim-sulfamethoxazole DS or dapsone at 50 mg/day and pyrimethamine 50 mg/week.

C. CNS lymphoma

1. **Natural history.** Primary CNS lymphoma (PCNSL) affects 2–4% of AIDS patients. Prognosis is poor even with therapy, and most patients succumb to the tumor or to another AIDS-related illness within 3–6 months of diagnosis.

2. **Clinical features.** Subacutely progressive headache, lethargy, cognitive impairment, and focal neurologic deficits related to tumor location, such as hemiparesis, aphasia, ataxia, or visual field deficits, are common presentations. Cranial nerve palsies may be observed. Other patients present with seizures, which may produce symptoms resembling transient ischemic attacks (TIAs). AIDS patients may also have leptomeningeal lymphoma attributable to either seeding from a cerebral tumor or metastasis of a systemic lymphoma. Presentations include features of meningitis, meningoencephalitis, or meningoradiculitis.

3. **Diagnosis.** PCNSL typically produces enhancing mass lesions on cerebral imaging studies following contrast infusion. Single or multiple lesions may be present, and the lesions cannot be differentiated from CNS toxoplasmosis or other cerebral abscesses. Patients with leptomeningeal lymphoma may show meningeal enhancement on gadolinium-infused MRI scans. CSF may yield lymphoma cells in patients with leptomeningeal seeding, but diagnosis is generally made by brain biopsy in patients with mass lesions.

4. **Therapy.** PCNSL is radiosensitive, and referral for radiation therapy is appropriate for improvements in function and quality of life. Unfortunately, the therapy is palliative, with survival seldom exceeding 6 months. Currently, clinical trials are evaluating the impact of combined chemotherapy and radiation on duration and quality of survival. Patients who have access to participating centers should be considered for referral. AIDS patients with leptomeningeal lymphoma have a poor prognosis. They can be treated with intrathecal cytosine arabinoside (ara-C) at a dosage of 50 mg/m^2/week. Adverse effects of intrathecal ara-C include headache; nausea; myelosuppression that may require support with erythropoietin, granulocyte colony-stimulating factor (G-CSF), or transfusions; encephalopathy; and hepatotoxicity.

5. **Outcome.** Prognosis for AIDS patients with PCNSL is currently poor. Untreated individuals usually die from their tumors within 3 months. Patients treated with radiation therapy alone generally survive for 3–6 months, usually succumbing to opportunistic infection. Longer survivals following therapy occur on occasion, which stimulates interest in developing better treatment protocols. For patients who are treated, imaging studies are obtained monthly during therapy to evaluate tumor response. Patients with leptomeningeal lymphoma have a poor prognosis also and are monitored with serial CSF cytologic studies on samples obtained prior to each intrathecal treatment. Patients on chemotherapy require serial blood counts and liver function studies on a weekly basis during therapy.

D. Progressive multifocal leukoencephalopathy (PML)

1. **Natural history.** PML may affect up to 5% of AIDS patients and, of these, represent the initial presenting illness in up to 25%. This disease results from reactivation of a polyoma virus, called JC virus (JCV), acquired earlier in life but suppressed by normal immune function. Once symptoms appear, progression is usually inexorable, leading to death within 6 months. In some instances, however, the disease follows a more protracted course, with arrested or slowed progression and, rarely, spontaneous improvement.

2. **Clinical features.** Subacute progressive cognitive impairment, visual field defects, hemiparesis, ataxia, and speech or language disturbances evolving over weeks to months are typical presentations. Some patients present with seizures or strokelike acute onset of neurologic impairment.

3. **Diagnosis.** MRI scans typically reveal multiple asymmetric lesions in cere-

bral white matter that are best seen on T2-weighted images. The lesions generally do not enhance and rarely exhibit any mass effect. CT scans are less sensitive but may show areas of attenuation resembling infarctions. Single lesions are not uncommon when patients are seen early in the course. Definitive diagnosis requires pathologic confirmation of JC virus infection of oligodendrocytes. Studies utilizing PCR amplification techniques can detect JC virus DNA in tissue and CSF, but specificity and sensitivity of CSF assays have yet to be determined.

4. **Therapy.** No therapy has been proven effective in treatment of PML. Anecdotal reports have described cases appearing to respond to both high-dosage antiretroviral therapy and cytosine arabinoside (ara-C). A recent clinical trial conducted by the AIDS Clinical Trials Group (ACTG) comparing high-dosage combination antiretroviral therapy with ara-C given intravenously or intrathecally failed to show prolonged survival for any of these treatment regimens compared to the others.

5. **Outcome.** Untreated individuals with PML usually survive less than 6 months. Occasional longer spontaneous survivals rarely with disease regression hinder interpretation of anecdotal reports attributing responses to therapy. New clinical trials will provide treatment options in the future.

E. **Cytomegalovirus (CMV)**

1. **Natural history.** CMV is commonly acquired early in life, and serologic evidence of infection is present in the majority of American adults. Although a transient systemic illness may occur on acquisition, normal immune function prevents further manifestations. CMW is transmitted in body fluids, and virtually all HIV-infected people have serologic evidence of exposure. The most common symptomatic CMV infections in AIDS patients occur in the retina and gastrointestinal tract. Autopsy studies have demonstrated CMV in the brains of 10–40% of AIDS patients.

2. **Clinical features.** CMV affects all levels of the neuraxis in AIDS patients, but most commonly causes three syndromes. **CMV encephalitis (CMVE)** is characterized by subacute confusion, disorientation, or delirium; impaired attention, memory, and cognitive processing; and varying focal signs including cranial neuropathies, nystagmus, weakness, spasticity, and ataxia. Focal encephalitis with mass lesions and features of meningitis may occur. Clinical symptoms evolve over weeks. **CMV polyradiculomyelitis (CMV-PRAM)** presents as a subacute hypotonic motor weakness with areflexia and sphincter dysfunction (usually urinary retention), evolving over 1–3 weeks. Variable sensory features including painful paresthesias in perineal and lower-extremity regions, and signs of myelopathy such as sensory levels and Babinski's signs, may be found on examination. Symptoms involve the lower extremities and may ascend, superficially resembling Guillain-Barré syndrome. **CMV multifocal neuropathy** is a subacute process evolving over weeks to months and characterized by motor weakness, depressed reflexes, and sensory deficits involving nerves of both upper and lower extremities in an asymmetric pattern. Motor features generally overshadow the sensory findings, although paresthesias may be the initial symptoms. Less commonly, CMV may cause meningomyelitis or myositis.

3. **Diagnosis.** The clinical syndromes are suggestive but not pathognomonic for the diagnosis of CMV infection of the nervous system in AIDS. MRI scans with gadolinium contrast may reveal enhancement of ventricular ependyma in about 10% of patients with CMVE, of meninges in some patients with meningoencephalitis or meningomyelitis, and of lumbar nerve roots and conus medullaris in some patients with CMV-PRAM. Imaging studies are often normal or show nonspecific atrophic changes. CSF studies characteristically reveal a polymorphonuclear pleocytosis, hypoglycorrhachia, elevated protein, and, about half the time, positive cultures for CMV in patients with CMV-PRAM. With CMVE, pleocytosis is uncommon and CMV cultures are almost never positive. CSF is normal or reveals nonspecific protein elevation in patients with multifocal mononeuropathy. Recently, application of PCR amplification techniques have allowed detection of CMV DNA in CSF, and retrospective studies suggest that this is both a sensitive and a specific indicator of active CMV infection, although prospective studies of sensitivity have yet to be performed. Virtually all

AIDS patients with CMV infection of the nervous system have **systemic infection** as well, and ophthalmologic screening or evaluation of gastrointestinal symptoms may be revealing. CMV infection is also frequently found in the lung and adrenal glands.

4. **Therapy.** Two agents are currently available for treatment of active CMV infections in AIDS. Both are virustatic. Some authors recommend combination therapy in patients with CMV disease of the CNS.

   a. **Foscarnet** has better CSF penetration than ganciclovir and modest antiretroviral activity in addition to its efficacy against CMV. An induction dosage of 90 mg/kg IV bid in patients with normal renal function is given for 14–21 days followed by reduction to a maintenance dosage of 90–120 mg/day. An indwelling catheter suitable for long-term use is placed to provide access. Dosages must be reduced for patients with renal insufficiency. In addition to nephrotoxicity, adverse effects include fevers, gastrointestinal intolerance, electrolyte imbalances, headaches, paresthesias, seizures, and toxic encephalopathy. At times it may be difficult to distinguish adverse effects of foscarnet from CMV infection.

   b. **Ganciclovir** has also been shown to have efficacy against CMV infections of the nervous system in AIDS patients, with responses reported for both CMV-PRAM and multifocal neuropathy. Ganciclovir is given in an induction dosage of 5 mg/kg IV bid for 14–21 days followed by a maintenance dosage of 5 mg/kg/day. Myelosuppression, particularly neutropenia, is common with ganciclovir, especially when it is given concurrently with antiretroviral agents; dosages of antiretroviral agents usually must be reduced. Other potential adverse effects of ganciclovir include hepatotoxicity, gastrointestinal intolerance, headaches, seizures, lethargy, paresthesias, toxic encephalopathy, and nephrotoxicity. As with foscarnet, it may be difficult to distinguish adverse effects of ganciclovir from disease manifestations of CMV.

   c. **Viral resistance** may develop to either foscarnet or ganciclovir during prolonged therapy, and neurologic symptoms emerging during maintenance therapy for CMV retinitis or enteritis should be treated with the induction dosage of the alternate agent. Even when both drugs have failed individually, patients may respond to combined therapy, and this should be pursued.

5. **Outcome.** No prospective studies are available to guide therapy of CMV neurologic disease in AIDS, partly because of difficulties in premortem diagnosis. Responses to therapy for CMV-PRAM and multifocal neuropathy are reported anecdotally. Few data are available regarding responses in CMVE. Treated patients should be continued on maintenance therapy, although the optimal regimen is yet to be devised. CSF studies appear to be the best markers of disease activity and should be obtained on completion of induction therapy and for any progressive neurologic symptoms that occur during maintenance therapy. Recurrent inflammation and possibly persistent evidence of CMV DNA by PCR amplification may suggest active viral replication and imply resistance to the regimen employed.

F. **Herpes simplex virus (HSV)**
   1. **Natural history.** HSV is ubiquitous in the general population, and HIV-infected patients have a high frequency of HSV-2 genital-rectal infection. Many episodes of HSV-2 aseptic meningitis are self-limited, but symptomatic meningoradiculitis, encephalitis, or myelitis may be severe enough to require therapy. HSV-1 encephalitis has been reported in HIV-infected patients and may produce subtle and atypical pathologies in immunosuppressed patients.

   2. **Clinical features.** HSV-1 produces a focal encephalitis with a predilection for the deep frontal and temporal lobes. Seizures, headaches, personality changes, and focal language disturbances may progress to confusion, obtundation, and coma over days. Some HIV patients demonstrate less clinical progression. HSV-2 produces aseptic meningitis with fever and headache; meningoradiculitis, which may involve sacral roots producing urinary retention; and meningoencephalitis. Patients with meningomyelitis develop progressive weakness, spasticity, sensory impairment, and ataxia, typically affecting lower extremities, associated with variable sphincter disturbances. Patients with HSV-2 meningoencephalitis present with confusion, seizures, headaches, and fever, with variable motor impairment. Neurologic manifes-

tations of HSV-2 may be observed concurrently with or following genital-rectal eruptions, or may occur independently.

3. **Diagnosis.** HSV-1 encephalitis may be suspected when focal enhancing lesions are detected in the inferior frontal or temporal lobes on MRI with gadolinium contrast infusion. EEGs may show characteristic periodic spike discharges. Patients with focal encephalitis caused by HSV-1 in other locations have no characteristic features. CSF studies typically show a mixed pleocytosis, erythrocytes in some cases, modestly depressed or normal glucose levels, and elevated protein. Viral culture may yield HSV-1 on occasion. PCR amplification of HSV DNA in CSF is now available. When such confirmation to support diagnosis is lacking, HIV patients with isolated temporal or frontal lesions should be biopsied because of the range of possible pathologies. Patients with HSV-2 meningitis, meningomyelitis, or meningoencephalitis may show meningeal enhancement or have normal MRI studies. CSF reveals lymphocytic pleocytosis or normal cell counts, normal or modestly depressed glucose, and variable protein levels. Viral culture may be positive, and PCR amplification of HSV-2 DNA can support CSF diagnosis.

4. **Therapy**
   a. Acyclovir is a virustatic agent with efficacy against herpes viruses possessing thymidine kinase activity that initiates formation of acyclovir triphosphate, which inhibits viral replication. Acyclovir in a dosage of 10 mg/kg IV tid should be started immediately on suspicion of HSV CNS disease while other diagnostic studies are pending. Confirmed cases are treated for 10–14 days. Maintenance therapy is sometimes given for recurrent genital-rectal infections at a dosage of 200 mg PO 5 times daily. Resistant strains of HSV-2 are starting to appear, and patients with persistent or progressive neurologic manifestations of HSV should be treated with foscarnet at 60 mg/kg bid for 14–21 days.
   b. Adverse effects of acyclovir include nephrotoxicity, hepatotoxicity, gastrointestinal intolerance, and infusion-site irritation. Dosage must be reduced for patients with renal insufficiency. Patients may have headaches and dizziness, and rarely a toxic delirium with confusion, disorientation, hallucinations or delusions, and seizures may occur, usually with elevated serum acyclovir levels. Hypotension and myelosuppression have been reported.

5. **Outcome.** Few studies are available on the course of HSV meningitis or related CNS disease in AIDS. Many patients respond to therapy with acyclovir, but others do not because of either HSV resistance or inadequate immune function. Serial CSF studies are currently the best means of detecting resistance and should be obtained following completion of antiviral therapy and for recurrent neurologic symptoms.

G. **Varicella-zoster virus (VZV)**
   1. **Natural history.** VZV commonly occurs in HIV-infected patients at multiple stages of the disease and may produce encephalitis or myelitis in addition to radiculitis. The virus, which causes chicken pox, is acquired early in life and resides latently in sensory ganglia, where it can intermittently produce recurrent radiculitis. Retrograde extension to the CNS along contiguous sensory roots and fiber tracts has been shown to occur. Patients with radiculitis often have self-limited dermatologic eruptions, which may be accompanied by prolonged neuralgia. CNS extension may be marked by vasculitis, particularly after ophthalmic zoster, resulting in cerebral infarction. CNS extension may result in necrotizing myelitis and brainstem encephalitis. Focal or diffuse cerebral encephalitis may also occur.
   2. **Clinical features.** VZV radiculitis is usually heralded by painful paresthesias in a restricted dermatomal distribution of a thoracic or trigeminal root. A vesicular rash usually follows, but cases of VZV occur in the absence of dermatomal eruptions. The rash typically heals over weeks, with the vesicles crusting and then fading. Pain may persist. VZV myelitis is usually marked by weakness referable to the region of eruption, and sometimes by associated myoclonus. Myelitis may be limited or may be progressive, resulting in spastic weakness, sensory impairment, and sphincter dysfunction. A meningitis marked by lymphocytic pleocytosis, increased protein, and depressed or normal glucose levels is often associated. VZV myelitis may occur in the ab-

sence of dermatomal eruption. VZV encephalitis may be focal or diffuse in AIDS patients, presenting with seizures, confusion, progressive language and cognitive impairments, and sensory or motor abnormalities. Progression may be gradual and the level of immunosuppression modest. CSF profile is similar to that of myelitis. VZV vasculitis may result in acute focal features resulting from cerebral or spinal infarction.

3. **Diagnosis.** When the characteristic dermatologic eruption occurs, diagnosis is not difficult. For patients with isolated encephalitis or myelitis, however, the diagnosis may be elusive. CSF is nonspecific and rarely yields virus on culture. PCR amplification for identification of VZV DNA is now available and important in diagnosis of CNS VZV infection. Immunohistochemistry of pathologic specimens obtained by biopsy of progressive cerebral lesions may be required, but even histochemical techniques lack sensitivity. Imaged lesions may initially appear as focal areas of attenuation on CT or high signal on T2 MRI. More diffuse leukoencephalopathy or enhancing focal lesions may be observed.

4. **Therapy.** HIV-infected patients with VZV radiculitis should be treated with acyclovir at 800 mg PO 5 times daily until all lesions have crusted, despite limited evidence for efficacy of antiviral therapy in the nonimmunosuppressed population. If new lesions appear despite oral therapy, IV acyclovir at a dosage of 10 mg/kg tid should be used. IV therapy may also be considered for patients with recurrent eruptions occurring at different segmental levels. Neuralgia is best treated with carbamazepine at dosages of 100–200 mg qid-q4h or with diphenylhydantoin at 100 mg tid-qid. Amitriptyline at 25 mg qhs may be added and increased by 25 mg/day at weekly intervals to 100 mg qhs. Some patients who fail to respond to these agents may benefit from the addition of baclofen at 5–10 mg tid-qid or topical application of capsaicin to the involved cutaneous area tid-qid. Patients with encephalitis or myelitis should be treated with IV acyclovir for 14–21 days at 10 mg/kg tid. The role of maintenance therapy to prevent recurrent eruptions is unclear, because resistance of VZV to acyclovir has begun to emerge. VZV CNS disease refractory to acyclovir should be assumed to reflect resistance and should be treated with foscarnet at 60–90 mg IV bid for 10–21 days. Supportive therapy for myelitis is similar to that described for HIV myelopathy, including antispasticity agents, physical therapy, and orthotics as required, and anticholinergic agents for hypertonic neurogenic bladder. Anticonvulsants are used for patients with seizures. Adverse effects of these medications are covered in sec. **II.B.4.**

5. **Outcome.** Most patients with VZV radiculitis achieve resolution of their acute symptoms, although recurrences are common and may not involve the same distribution each time. Prognosis for progressive myelitis and encephalitis is variable, although only limited anecdotal data are available. The extent to which this reflects VZV resistance to acyclovir is unknown.

H. Tuberculosis

1. **Natural history.** *Mycobacterium tuberculosis* (MTB) in the HIV-infected patient appears to have a more aggressive course, with increased frequency of dissemination and cerebral mass lesions. MTB occurs more often in AIDS patients who use IV drugs. Response to therapy as measured by inpatient mortality, however, appears similar in HIV- and non-HIV-infected populations. Untreated MTB in HIV is progressive and often fatal.

2. **Clinical features.** AIDS patients with MTB may present with meningitis or meningoencephalitis marked by headaches, fever, confusion, lethargy, cranial neuropathies, ataxia, seizures, or hemiparesis. Contiguous extension of basal meningitis to blood vessels of the circle of Willis may result in cerebral infarction. Cerebral abscess formation results in focal symptoms, seizures, headaches, and signs of increased intracranial pressure.

3. **Diagnosis.** Imaging studies may reveal focal abscesses indistinguishable from toxoplasmosis or CNS lymphoma. Areas of attenuation typical of infarction, meningeal enhancement, exudate in basilar cisterns, or hydrocephalus in patients with MTB meningitis may be seen. CSF reveals mixed or lymphocytic pleocytosis, depressed glucose, and elevated protein levels. Smears for acid-fast bacteria are rarely positive, and cultures require weeks. PCR amplification of MTB DNA and MTB antigen assays may provide more rapid detection in CSF. Diagnosis of patients with mass lesions is generally

made by histopathologic examination of biopsy material. HIV patients with MTB are often anergic. Most have concurrent pulmonary disease.

   4. Therapy

   a. Combined therapies with combinations of isoniazid (INH) at 300 mg PO, rifampin at 600 mg PO, and ethambutol at 15–25 mg/kg/day PO, with pyrazinamide at 15–25 mg/kg PO daily added for the first 2 months, are commonly used. Pyridoxine (50 mg/day) is added for patients on INH. MTB resistance to these agents is now observed in up to 20% of isolates in urban areas, and failure to respond should prompt infectious disease consultation to modify therapy. Therapy should be continued for at least 6 months.

   b. Adverse effects of INH include hepatotoxicity, which is more likely after 35 years of age; gastrointestinal intolerance; hypersensitivity; and peripheral neuropathy resulting from vitamin B_6 deficiency. Other, uncommon effects are optic neuropathy; toxic encephalopathy with seizures, delirium, obtundation, and myoclonus; myelosuppression; lupoid reactions; and hyperglycemia. Rifampin imparts an orange color to urine and secretions. Adverse effects of rifampin include headaches, hepatotoxicity, gastrointestinal intolerance, fatigue, lethargy, and myalgias, as well as the uncommon effects of myelosuppression, hemolytic anemia, nephrotoxicity, myopathy, delirium or confusion, and hypersensitivity reactions. Ethambutol may produce optic neuropathy, gastrointestinal intolerance, peripheral neuropathy with paresthesias, headaches, toxic encephalopathy, thrombocytopenia, hyperuricemia, and hypersensitivity reactions. Pyrazinamide may cause polyarthralgia, myalgia, hyperuricemia, hepatotoxicity, gastrointestinal intolerance, anemia, and coagulopathy.

   5. Outcome. Hospital mortality is low in treated patients, but noncompliance with outpatient therapy may lead to therapeutic failure and emergence of resistant MTB after multiple short courses of therapy. Patients with MTB meningitis should have follow-up CSF studies at 1–2 months and on completion of primary therapy to detect persistent infection from resistant organisms. Mass lesions can be followed by serial imaging studies. Mass lesions that become enlarged despite therapy should be biopsied to detect resistant organisms or concurrent opportunistic processes. Potential drug toxicity should be monitored with serial CBC and chemistry profiles and ophthalmologic exams at 6-month intervals. Use of alcohol while on INH should be avoided.

I. Neurosyphilis

   1. Natural history. Although not an opportunistic infection, overlapping risk factors and atypical response to therapy make *Treponema pallidum* a frequent concern in HIV-infected patients. Failure of conventional therapy, particularly benzathine penicillin, to prevent neurosyphilis and recurrence of neurosyphilis despite IV penicillin has been reported.

   2. Clinical features. Meningitis, meningoradiculitis, meningovasculitis with infarctions of small vessels, meningomyelitis, and encephalitis may occur in AIDS patients. Mass lesions resulting from gumma formation may present with seizures, focal signs, and increased intracranial pressure. Cranial neuropathies, headache, and fever may mark syphilitic meningitis, and polyradiculitis may result in a cauda equina syndrome similar to CMV-PRAM. Luetic encephalitis and myelitis may be gradually or subacutely progressive.

   3. Diagnosis. Meningitis is nonspecific with variable lymphocytic pleocytosis and elevated protein. The Venereal Disease Research Laboratory (VDRL) test is often but not always positive in CSF, and specific treponemal antibody assays such as the *T. pallidum* hemagglutination assay (TPHA) and fluorescent treponemal antibody (FTA) indexes are more sensitive, and exclusionary when negative. Imaging studies may reveal infarctions or enhancing masses in patients with gummas, but such studies are not diagnostic, and mass lesions must be biopsied. Serum FTA should be obtained in all HIV-infected patients with neurologic disease, and CSF should be evaluated in all such FTA-positive patients.

   4. Therapy. Neurosyphilis should be treated with IV aqueous penicillin at a dosage of 2–4 million U q4h for 10–14 days. Patients with asymptomatic CNS syphilis may be offered 2.4 million U/day of procaine penicillin IM plus probenecid at 500 mg PO bid for a similar duration. No other therapy has proven efficacy, although ceftriaxone at 2 g/day IV for 10–14 days may be tried in penicillin-allergic patients who do not exhibit cross-sensitivity to cephalosporins. Patients with neurosyphilis who are allergic to both agents should be evaluated by an allergist and infectious disease specialist for desensitization therapy to allow treatment with penicillin.

5. **Outcome.** Although initial response is often good, recurrent neurosyphilis is common enough to warrant vigilance. Patients with luetic meningitis should have CSF studies after completion of therapy and at 6-month intervals until CSF VDRL stabilizes or becomes nonreactive. Subsequent neurologic symptoms should prompt evaluation for recurrence.

J. *Nocardia asteroides*

1. **Natural history.** *Nocardia asteroides* is a gram-positive intracellular bacterium found in soil and decaying organic matter and acquired by inhalation. In patients with immunosuppression, hematogenous spread to the CNS may result in meningitis or abscess formation.

2. **Clinical features.** In AIDS patients, *Nocardia* abscesses present as subacutely progressive mass lesions with headaches, fever, focal signs related to localization, obtundation, confusion, and lethargy.

3. **Diagnosis.** Imaging studies typically show contrast-enhancing mass lesions that often are multiloculated in appearance. CSF, when obtainable, shows depressed glucose and elevated protein levels with variable polymorphonuclear pleocytosis. Diagnosis is usually made from smears or cultures of abscess fluid.

4. **Therapy.** Optimal therapy combines abscess excision and antibiotics. Sulfadiazine at a dosage of 1.5 g PO qid or trimethoprim/sulfamethoxazole at 320–400/600–2400 mg qid may produce clinical response, but recurrences are observed despite maintenance therapy. Treatment should be continued indefinitely. Recurrences despite therapy can be treated with minocycline at 100–200 mg PO bid, which is an alternative for patients allergic to sulfa. Ceftriaxone at 2 g IV bid may be used with minocycline. Adverse effects of sulfa are listed in sec. **III.B.4.c.** Minocycline may produce gastrointestinal intolerance, pancreatic and hepatotoxicity, nephrotoxicity, photosensitivity, pseudotumor cerebri, hemolytic anemia, thrombocytopenia, neutropenia, eosinophilia, and hypersensitivity reactions including Stevens-Johnson syndrome.

5. **Outcome.** Relapses occur despite maintenance therapy, and vigilance is required for concurrent opportunistic infections. Lesion size should be followed by means of serial imaging studies. New lesions that fail to respond to brief trials of therapy directed at *Nocardia* should be biopsied.

K. **Other fungal opportunistic infections**

1. **Natural history.** Several other CNS fungal infections, including aspergillus, blastomycosis, coccidioidomycosis, histoplasmosis, and mucormycosis, are reported in small numbers of AIDS patients, usually in association with disseminated infection. Prognosis is generally poor despite therapy, although patients may respond occasionally.

2. **Clinical features.** Aspergillus may present with multiple cerebral infarctions resulting from colonization of blood vessels, abscess formation, or meningitis. The presence of sinus or airway disease should prompt consideration of the diagnosis. Mucormycosis also invades blood vessels and may occur in IV drug users or diabetics. Blastomycosis, coccidioidomycosis, and histoplasmosis may present with meningitis or cerebral abscesses. Meningomyelitis may also occur.

3. **Diagnosis.** CNS imaging is nonspecific. Diagnosis of these infections usually rests on examination of abscess fluid or culture of CSF when positive. Patients with meningitis and sinusitis or bronchitis may yield a diagnosis on culture of biopsied respiratory tract material.

4. **Therapy.** Amphotericin B at dosages of 0.5–1.0 mg/kg/day for at least 8 weeks is used initially. Maintenance therapy with itraconazole at 200 mg PO bid may be used for responders with aspergillus, coccidiomycosis, or histoplasmosis. Fluconazole at 200 mg PO bid may also be used for coccidiomycosis. Ketoconazole at 400 mg PO/day may be started with amphotericin B and continued as maintenance therapy for patients with blastomycosis. Adverse effects of amphotericin B and fluconazole are described in sec.

III.A.4.d. Itraconazole and ketoconazole may produce gastrointestinal intolerance, hepatotoxicity, hypertension, lethargy, headaches, dizziness, and pruritus. Ketoconazole also may result in impotence, gynecomastia, and menstrual irregularities. Thrombocytopenia, leukopenia, hemolytic anemia, and depression occur uncommonly.

  5. **Outcome.** Response is generally poor because of disseminated infection at the time of CNS presentation, immunosuppression, and delays and difficulties in diagnosis. Occasional responders should be continued on maintenance therapy indefinitely. New lesions should prompt aggressive evaluation to differentiate recurrence from alternative CNS opportunistic pathogens.

Recommended Readings

Bartlett JG. *The Johns Hopkins Hospital Guide to Medical Care of Patients with HIV Infection* (4th ed). Baltimore: Williams & Wilkins, 1994.

Baumgartner JE, et al. Primary central nervous system lymphomas: Natural history and response to radiation therapy in 55 patients with acquired immunodeficiency syndrome. *J Neurosurg* 73:206–211, 1990.

Berger JR, Levy RM. The neurologic complications of human immunodeficiency virus infection. *Med Clin NA* 77:1–23, 1993.

Berger JR, et al. Progressive multifocal leukoencephalopathy associated with human immunodeficiency virus infection. *Ann Int Med* 107:78–87, 1987.

Cohen BA, et al. Neurologic prognosis of cytomegalovirus polyradiculopathy in AIDS. *Neurology* 43:493–499, 1993.

Devinsky O, et al. Herpes zoster myelitis. *Brain* 114:1181–1196, 1991.

Drugs for AIDS and associated infections. *Med Letter* 35:79–86, 1993.

Goldstein JD, et al. Primary central nervous system lymphoma in acquired immunodeficiency syndrome. *Cancer* 67:2756–2765, 1991.

Gordon SM, et al. The response of symptomatic neurosyphilis to high-dose intravenous penicillin G in patients with human immunodeficiency virus infection. *N Engl J Med* 331:1469–1473, 1994.

Gray F, et al. Varicella-zoster virus encephalitis in acquired immunodeficiency syndrome: Report of four cases. *Neuropathol Appl Neurobiol* 18:502–514, 1992.

Holland NR, et al. Cytomegalovirus encephalitis in acquired immunodeficiency syndrome (AIDS). *Neurology* 44:507–514, 1994.

Kieburtz K (ed). Neurology of HIV infection. *Semin Neurol* 12:1–50, 1992.

Luft BJ, Remington JS. Toxoplasmic encephalitis in AIDS. *Clin Inf Dis* 15:211–222, 1992.

McArthur JC. Neurologic diseases associated with human immunodeficiency virus type 1 infection. In RT Johnson, JW Griffin (eds), *Current Therapy in Neurologic Disease* (4th ed). St. Louis: Mosby, 1993. Pp 146–152.

National Institutes of Health Symposium. Retroviruses in the nervous system. *Ann Neurol* 23(suppl):54–594, 1988.

Petito CK, et al. Vacuolar myelopathy pathologically resembling subacute combined degeneration in patients with the acquired immunodeficiency syndrome. *N Engl J Med* 312:874–879, 1985.

Porter SB, Sande MA. Toxoplasmosis of the central nervous system in the acquired immunodeficiency syndrome. *N Engl J Med* 327:1643–1648, 1992.

Powderly WG. Cryptococcal meningitis and AIDS. *Clin Inf Dis* 17:837–842, 1993.

Price RW, et al. The brain in AIDS: Central nervous system HIV-1 infection and AIDS dementia complex. *Science* 239:586–592, 1988.

Roullet E, et al. Cytomegalovirus multifocal neuropathy in AIDS: Analysis of 15 consecutive cases. *Neurology* 44:2174–2182, 1994.

Rovira MJ, Post MJD, Bowen BC. Central nervous system infections in HIV-positive persons. *Neuroimag Clin N Am* 1:179–200, 1991.

Saag MS, et al. Comparison of amphotericin B with fluconazole in the treatment of acute AIDS-associated cryptococcal meningitis. *N Engl J Med* 326:83–89, 1992.

Sidtis JJ, et al. Zidovudine treatment of the AIDS dementia complex: Results of a placebo controlled trial. *Ann Neurol* 33:343–349, 1993.

Simpson DM, Olney RK. Peripheral neuropathies associated with human immunodeficiency virus. *Neurol Clin N Am* 10:685–711, 1992.

Simpson DM, Tagliati M. Neurologic manifestations of HIV infection. *Ann Int Med* 121:769–785, 1994.

Spinal Cord Disorders
Edward C. Daly

I. **Developmental disorders** occasionally can cause pain or progressive neurologic dysfunction in adults. Others are found incidentally. Recent studies have suggested that maternal folate supplementation during pregnancy prevents neural tube defects in offspring.

  A. **Chiari malformations** are characterized by extension of the cerebellum through the foramen magnum with downward displacement of the medulla and kinking of the cervical spinal cord. Hydrocephalus, bony abnormalities of the skull base, and syringomyelia in the cervical cord are frequently found. Chiari I malformations (not associated with meningomyelocele) frequently do not manifest themselves until adulthood.

  1. No treatment is warranted if the patient is asymptomatic. Cranial nerve signs and a history of sleep apnea should be sought. Baseline pulmonary functions should be considered.

  2. If the patient is symptomatic, decompressive suboccipital craniectomy and upper cervical laminectomy with or without ventricular shunting are required.

  a. Respiratory depression is the most common postoperative complication requiring close monitoring.

  b. Approximately 50% of patients benefit, 25% show no change, and 25% deteriorate.

  B. **Spina bifida occulta** is the anomalous development of the posterior neural arch without an extraspinal cyst and is found in 5% of the population. Cutaneous anomalies often overlie the bony defect, and other lumbosacral anomalies may be found. Dermal sinus tracts can cause recurrent meningitis. Lipomas and dermoids may impinge on the cord or the cauda equina.

  1. Dermal sinus tracts are closed to prevent meningitis.

  2. Biopsy is indicated for tissue diagnosis of mass lesions.

  3. Surgery is indicated for progressive deficits.

  C. **Tethering of the cord** by adhesions, lipomas, or a tight filum terminale is the most common finding associated with spina bifida occulta. The syndrome often manifests itself after growth spurts. Pain can be predominant in adults.

  1. Surgery is controversial in asymptomatic children.

  2. Surgical release stabilizes progression without a marked effect on bladder dysfunction. Results are mixed for the relief of pain.

  D. **Diastematomyelia** is the splitting of the spinal cord by a bony or fibrous septum. The anomaly may become evident during growth spurts or minor traumas. Spina bifida occulta is often present. Pain is prominent in adults but not in children.

  1. The septum is removed in children in response to expected progression.

  2. Surgery in adults is reserved for those with severe pain or progression.

  E. **Platybasia** (an upward displacement of the floor of the posterior fossa) and **basilar invagination** (protrusion of the odontoid through the foramen magnum) result in a reduction in the diameter of the foramen magnum. They present in adults as spastic quadriparesis or lower cranial nerve dysfunction.

  1. Surgical options include decompressive suboccipital craniectomy with upper cervical laminectomy.

  2. Counseling is indicated for the apparent genetic basis of skull base disorders.

  F. **Syringomyelia** is a congenital pericentral cavity of the cervical spinal cord that may extend into the thoracic cord or upward into the medulla (syringobulbia). Chiari I malformation, arachnoiditis, or kyphoscoliosis may be present.

1. Syringomyelia usually presents in adolescence or adulthood. The classic syndrome of upper-extremity weakness and atrophy (often asymmetric) with dissociated sensation in a "cape distribution" is found in 75% of cases. Enlargement of the syrinx can result in Horner's syndrome and myelopathy.
2. Although this disorder is often slowly progressive, long periods of stabilization, as well as acute deterioration, may occur. Neck or arm pain is often a prominent complaint.
   a. Surgery may not be indicated if symptoms are minimal or very severe, if symptoms persist longer than 5 years, or if the cord is of normal size on MRI.
   b. Surgery may be indicated in the presence of mild deficits of short duration, enlargement of the cord on MRI, and predominant symptoms of pain or spasticity.
3. Surgery is indicated in progressive cases.
   a. Results of surgery: approximately one-third improve, less than one-half stabilize, and approximately one-quarter deteriorate.
      (1) Pain and paraparesis show the best responses.
      (2) Sensory loss, lower motor neuron signs, and brainstem findings are the symptoms least likely to improve.
   b. Success is less likely in the presence of arachnoiditis.
   c. If no Chiari malformation is found, draining and shunting of the cavity are less satisfactory. Secondary cavitation into a tumor should be considered.

II. Vitamin deficiencies

A. **Vitamin B$_{12}$ (cobalamin) deficiency** is the most common disorder of the spinal cord for which a specific medical therapy exists.

1. **Pernicious anemia (PA)** is the most common cause of vitamin B$_{12}$ deficiency and is thought to be an autoimmune disorder affecting all races and both sexes. Antibodies to parietal cells are found in almost 90% of patients, and antibodies to intrinsic factor are found in somewhat more than 60%. Increased clinical suspicion, automated RBC indices, and insidious onset (it takes 5–10 years to deplete normal body stores of cobalamin) make the fully developed classic hematologic and neurologic presentations clinical rarities today.

2. **Other causes** of vitamin B$_{12}$ deficiency include **gastrectomy, diseases of the terminal ileum** (Crohn's disease and diverticulosis), and a less severe **gastric atrophy** (causing a food-bound malabsorption). Dietary causes are thought to be uncommon except in vegans and their breast-fed infants. **Nitrous oxide exposure** during anesthesia can result in precipitous neurologic presentations in patients with "silent" deficiencies or marginal body stores. Nitrous oxide can also be the cause of an insidious myelopathy if abused.

3. **Clinical features**
   a. **Hematologic features.** The classic severe megaloblastic anemia of insidious onset is relatively rare. Approximately 25% of patients have normal hemoglobin, 25% have normal RBC indices, and 10–20% have completely normal CBC.
   b. **Neurologic features.** About 25–50% of patients with vitamin B$_{12}$ deficiency have neurologic symptoms or signs at diagnosis. One study found 27% of patients to be without neurologic complaints but to have abnormal signs. Most patients experience leg dysesthesias as the first symptom. Neurologic presentations include:
      (1) **Polyneuropathy,** orthostasis, and decreased visual acuity
      (2) **Subacute combined degeneration of the spinal cord** affecting the posterior and lateral columns
      (3) **Personality changes, dementia, and psychiatric illness,** including psychosis.

4. **Diagnosis.** In large-scale screening of elderly asymptomatic individuals, between 10–20% may be cobalamin-deficient.
   a. **Serum vitamin B$_{12}$ (cobalamin).** Sensitivity, specificity, and accuracy of this commonly used assay are controversial. Patients can have normal levels and cobalamin-responsive neurologic disorders; low levels and nonresponsive deficits; or low levels but no other evidence of deficiency. Despite these severe shortcomings, determination of serum cobalamin is

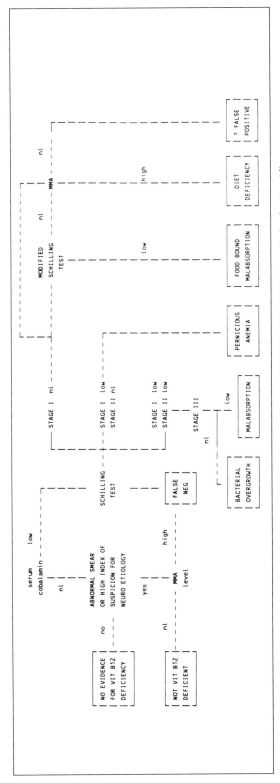

Figure 45-1. Diagnosis and evaluation of a suspected cobalamin deficiency in neurologic disorders (MMA = methylmalonic acid).

the screening test that is the most widely available. For most patients, serum folate should be determined at the same time.

b. The **peripheral blood smear** should be examined for macro-ovalocytes and hypersegmentation of neutrophils. It may be abnormal in the absence of clinically significant anemia.

c. Methylmalonic acid (MMA) (urine and serum) and **homocysteine** (serum) accumulate in vitamin B_{12} deficiency. Homocysteine is also elevated in folate deficiency. Assays for these metabolites can be helpful in selected cases. In comparison to serum cobalamin determination, these assays are characterized by the following:

(1) Advantages include possibly better sensitivity and specificity.

(a) These assays reflect the cellular status of cobalamin-dependent pathways.

(b) Urine MMA assay is comparable in cost to serum cobalamin; it may be used as a substitute when it becomes more widely available.

(2) Disadvantages are expense and limited availability.

(a) MMA levels are affected by dehydration and renal failure.

(b) The implicit assumption is that all tissues have identical cobalamin requirements for optimal function.

5. Once a deficiency is suspected, a variety of tests can help determine the etiology and appropriate treatment (Fig. 45-1).

a. The **Schilling test** measures absorption of radiolabeled crystalline vitamin B_{12} in the absence of exogenous intrinsic factor (stage I) and in its presence (stage II). The radioisotope in a 24-hour urine sample measures absorption. An abnormal stage I with a normal stage II indicates deficiency of intrinsic factor; if both stages are abnormal, malabsorption is suggested. A persistently low test after a 7–10-day course of antibiotics (stage III) suggests bacterial overgrowth as the etiology of malabsorption. Potential pitfalls are as follows.

(1) Incomplete urine collection and renal insufficiency are significant problems in the elderly. Placement of an indwelling catheter for 24 hours is often considered.

(2) Ileal mucosal injury in severe cobalamin or folate deficiency may prevent absorption of the cobalamin–intrinsic factor complex. Appropriate treatment for 1–3 months and repetition of the test clarifies the results.

(3) A normal test is found in patients who absorb crystalline cobalamin but not the dietary vitamin.

(4) Bone marrow examination and MMA level, if ordered, should be done beforehand. The flushing dose (1 mg) of cobalamin given during the Schilling test may normalize these tests within 24–48 hours.

b. The **food-bound Schilling test** measures absorption of cobalamin bound to protein (by mixing with egg yolks). Determination of administered dose is more difficult, and the test is not yet widely available.

c. Anti-intrinsic factor antibody testing is specific but suffers from low sensitivity (<60%). However, its low cost and simplicity make this test useful as an alternative first step in the confirmation of PA.

d. Antiparietal cell antibody testing is sensitive (>90%) but suffers from low specificity. A negative result makes PA unlikely.

6. Treatment

a. For patients with **PA, severe deficits,** or **poor compliance,** the usual treatment is cyanocobalamin in the following dosages: 1 mg/day IM for 7–12 days, then 1 mg/week IM for 3 weeks, and then 1 mg q1–3mo IM **for life.** Monthly injection is the standard **maintenance regimen** and provides the greatest ease of compliance. If longer intervals are used, MMA levels should document adequate treatment and compliance.

b. The patient or caregiver should be taught to give the shots to avoid the costs of office visits. If **self-injection** is not feasible, a visiting nurse can be very helpful with injections and compliance.

c. The unusual patient with PA and a strong aversion to injections may be offered **oral therapy** after initial cobalamin repletion. Large doses are needed, since only 1–3% of cobalamin is absorbed independently of intrinsic factor (IF). Checks of cobalamin levels are needed until compliance is assured. The dosage is 1 mg/day PO for life.

    d. For patients who are compliant, absorb oral vitamin B_{12} (i.e., the standard Schilling test is normal and the serum cobalamin normalizes), have mild deficits, and wish to avoid monthly injections, cyanocobalamin can be given at 50 μg/day PO for life.

  7. Prognosis. Degree of recovery is dependent on the severity and duration of deficits at diagnosis. Severe deficits or symptoms that have existed for more than one year often respond incompletely. Most improvement occurs within 6–12 months. If a patient has not shown some improvement after 3 months, a response is unlikely. Either the diagnosis was in error or a vitamin B_{12} deficiency was coexistent but not causal (commonly observed in dementia).

  8. Therapeutic strategy. Predicting which neurologic deficits will respond to vitamin B_{12} is imprecise. It is this author's belief that patients should be given a 6-month trial of vitamin B_{12} if other treatable disorders (including folic acid deficiency) have been eliminated and if there is a suggestion of a deficiency and a neurologic deficit compatible with that deficiency. A less rigorous strategy, with no attempt to confirm the diagnosis or determine etiology, will miss treatable disorders. A more rigorous strategy, withholding treatment unless deficiency is "proven," may be based on an overestimation of our knowledge of cobalamin and one-carbon metabolism.

B. Folic acid deficiency is not generally appreciated as a cause of neurologic dysfunction very similar to that found in vitamin B_{12} deficiency. As in vitamin B_{12} deficiency, the neurologic deficits can develop with normal or mildly abnormal hematologic parameters. The incidence of severe neurologic deficits may be lower in folate deficiency than in cobalamin deficiency.

  1. Dietary inadequacy is the most common cause of folate deficiency, especially in the elderly. Pregnancy, alcoholism, generalized malabsorption, antiepileptic medication, chemotherapy, and congenital defects in absorption or one-carbon enzymes are other potential etiologies.

  2. Clinical features

    a. Instances of dementia, depression, psychosis, polyneuropathy, and subacute combined degeneration of the spinal cord have all been shown to be responsive to folate supplementation. Changes in mental status and higher cortical functions may be the most common presentations in adults.

    b. An association between maternal folate supplementation and prevention of neural tube defects in the offspring has been found. Folate appears to correct a subtle block in one-carbon metabolism rather than replenish a deficiency.

  3. Diagnosis. See Figure 45-2.

    a. Low **serum folate** indicates a negative balance and predicts the likelihood of folate deficiency if uncorrected. The serum level is a poor predictor of total body stores.

    b. Red blood cell (RBC) folate indicates body stores during the lifetime of the red blood cell. If both the serum and RBC folate levels are low, an ongoing folate deficiency exists.

    c. Elevated **serum homocysteine** with a normal serum MMA is also a marker of folate deficiency. Although expensive and not widely available, such testing is helpful in equivocal cases. Because cobalamin deficiency also elevates homocysteine, MMA needs to be measured at the same time to distinguish the two deficiencies.

    d. A search for a GI disorder should be undertaken when signs of malabsorption exist or no etiology is clear. Radiologic examination of the small bowel is the usual first step. GI referral and jejunal biopsy should be considered.

  4. Treatment with folic acid at a dosage of 2.5–10.0 mg/day PO is sufficient in dietary deficiency. Parenteral (IM) doses are given in malabsorption syndromes. Treatment is for life or until body stores are repleted and etiologic factors corrected. A multivitamin should also be given. Compliance and adequacy of treatment can be monitored with a homocysteine level.

  5. There is uncertainty concerning the possible **epileptogenic properties** of folic acid. Folate deficiency should be confirmed by a serum homocysteine in patients with seizures. Unless severe hematologic or neurologic deficits are present, less aggressive dosing (1–2 mg/day) may be best. Normalization

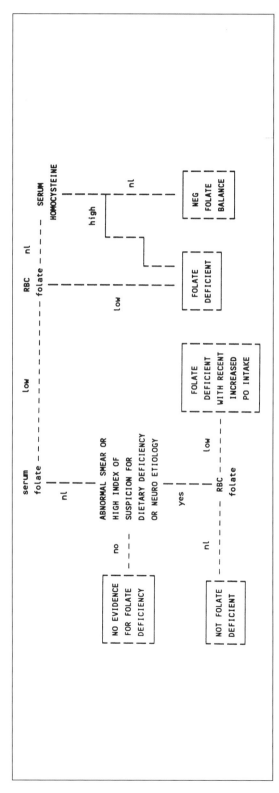

Figure 45-2. Diagnosis and evaluation of a suspected folic acid deficiency in neurologic disorders.

of serum homocysteine is necessary to document compliance and verify adequate treatment.
6. **Prognosis** is generally good if treatment is started early. Poor responses in cases of dementia or depression with folate deficiency probably represent the concurrence of two common disorders in the elderly.
C. **Vitamin E deficiency** can cause polyneuropathy, myopathy, and demyelination within the posterior columns and spinocerebellar tracts of the spinal cord. The ataxia and posterior column manifestations of **abetalipoproteinemia,** a rare autosomal recessive disorder of lipoprotein metabolism, are responsive to vitamin E supplementation. Rare adults with vitamin E deficiency usually present with long-standing **steatorrhea.** An isolated defect in absorption also exists. Reversal of neurologic deficits with vitamin E supplementation is variable but can be dramatic. Large oral dosages of vitamin E up to 3600 U/day or semi-weekly injections of alpha-tocopherol have been used.

III. **Acute spinal cord injury**
A. **Etiology.** The major causes of acute spinal cord injury are motor vehicle accidents, falls, recreational injuries, and acts of violence. Fracture and compromise of the spinal cord (or cauda equina) occur most often at cervical and thoracolumbar levels. Although thoracic fractures are less common, neurologic injury is more common because of the narrowness of the spinal canal.
B. **Natural history.** Spinal cord injury occurs most often in young males. Neurologic impairment is approximately evenly divided among complete quadriplegia, complete paraplegia, incomplete quadriplegia, and incomplete paraplegia.
C. **Prevention.** Proper use of passive and active restraints in automobiles and use of helmets by motorcyclists and bicyclists prevent head and spinal injuries. The "THINK FIRST" program, addressing educational issues for youth in grades K–12 and actively supported by the neurosurgical community, should be embraced by healthcare providers.
D. **Prognosis.** Improvement of even one level may make a dramatic impact on function, especially in cervical cord injuries (Table 45-1). Final neurologic function depends on severity of initial injury, prevention of secondary damage, and successful management of the complications and sequelae of the acute injury and intensive rehabilitation.
1. Features suggesting a possibility of neurologic improvement:
   a. Motor or sensory function below neurologic level
   b. Residual anal sphincter tone
   c. Preserved bulbocavernosus reflex
2. Features suggesting a poor prognosis:
   a. Absence of residual function after 72 hours
   b. Hemorrhage or multilevel edema on MRI
E. **Principles of treatment**
1. **Immobilization of the spine** at the scene, in transport, and in ER is critical in preventing further damage.
2. ABCs of **trauma care**
3. **Primary survey** of associated damage
   a. Alteration of sensorium requires investigation for accompanying head injury.
   b. Neurologic level may mask the usual symptoms and signs of thoracic, abdominal, pelvic, or extremity injury. More reliance is placed on objective tests.
4. **Radiologic evaluation** of skeletal injury level
5. **Skeletal traction** for stabilization and closed reduction
6. Assessment of **neurologic level of injury**
   a. The neurologic level of injury is the most caudal segment at which key motor groups retain full range of movement against gravity (grade 3 on the usual five-point scale) and at which key sensory areas retain reproducible sensation (Table 45-2).
   b. The completeness of the injury is defined by modified Frankel grades A through E, which describe function at least three levels below the neurologic level of injury. Grade A indicates a complete level, grade E indicates recovery, and grades B–D describe incomplete levels.
7. **Secondary survey** and stabilization of patient
8. **Transport** to spinal cord injury center
9. **Medications** to prevent secondary (i.e., oxidative) damage

Table 45-1. Functional potential for complete spinal cord lesions.

Neurologic level	Functional potential
C1-C4	Most patients require tracheotomy and ventilator; totally assisted cough Patient controls electric wheelchair with breath controls Microprocessor adaptations for environmental control Attendant needs to be available 24 hours
C5	Assisted cough Can eat with set-up and assistive devices Electric wheelchair with joystick Attendant full time; may assist with some activities of daily living
C6	Assisted cough supine, independent sitting Can eat with assistive devices Manual wheelchair indoors only, independent pressure relief Clean intermittent catheterization (CIC) requires attendant; most require indwelling or suprapubic May drive van with adaptations and lift Attendant for assistance; rarely able to live alone
C7	Assisted cough supine, independent sitting Independent in most self-care with assistive devices Manual wheelchair indoors, ramps, and simple transfers CIC very difficult, usually needs external collection system Can drive car or van with hand controls and adaptations Attendant for assistance; few can live alone
C8-T1	Assisted cough supine, independent sitting Independent with all self-care skills Independent in wheelchair, including transfers CIC possible Can drive car with hand controls Frequently can live alone; may need help with bowel care
T2-T10	Higher levels have less effective cough Stand with braces for exercises only Assistance not necessary but helpful
T11-L2	Potential for walking with long leg braces and forearm crutches, indoors only
L3-S3	Stair climbing with forearm crutches May ambulate outdoors with braces and crutches or canes Impotence Credé's maneuver if low pressure, double stress incontinence, dribbling

Adapted from Sipski ML, Hendler S, DeLisa JA, Rehabilitation of patients with spinal cord disease, *Neurol Clin* 9:705–725, 1991; Frost FS, Role of rehabilitation after spinal cord injury, *Urol Clin N Am* 20:549–559, 1993; and Donovan WH, Spinal cord injury, in RW Evans, DS Baskin, FM Yatsu (eds), *Prognosis of Neurological Disorders*, New York: Oxford University Press, 1992.

       a. The National Acute Spinal Cord Injury Study 2 (NASCIS 2) demonstrated a modest but significant benefit compared with placebo for high-dosage methylprednisolone if started within 8 hours of injury. The initial dose of 30 mg/kg IV bolus is followed by 5.4 mg/kg/hr infusion for 23 hours.

       b. Further NASCIS research protocols are in progress.

    10. Restoration and maintenance of spinal alignment

IV. Sequelae of spinal cord injuries

    A. Pressure sores are the most preventable complication of spinal cord injury. They are classified according to depth:

       Stage I: nonblanchable erythema of intact skin
       Stage II: partial-thickness skin loss
       Stage III: full-thickness skin loss
       Stage IV: extension into muscle and bone

       1. Prevention. Patient and family education are important. Pressure is relieved by turning in bed every 2 hours and "wheelchair" lifts for 5–10 sec-

Table 45-2. Key muscles and sensory areas for determination of neurologic level of injury.

Level	Muscle action	Key muscle	Key sensory area
C2	—	—	Occipital protuberance
C3	—	—	Supraclavicular fossa
C3-C5	Diaphragm	—	—
C4	Shoulder shrug	—	Top anterior shoulder
C5	Shoulder abduction	Deltoid	Lateral antecubital fossa
	Elbow flexion	Biceps	—
C6	Wrist extension	E. carpi radialis	Thumb
C7	Elbow extension	Triceps	Ventral middle finger
C8	Finger extension	E. digitorum	Ventral little finger
	Finger flexion	F. digitorum profundus	—
T1	Finger abduction	Abductor digiti minimi	Medial antecubital fossa
	Finger adduction	First dorsal interosseous	—
T2	—	—	Apex of axilla
T4	—	—	Nipple line
T6	—	—	Xiphisternum
T10	—	—	Umbilicus
T12	—	—	Inguinal ligament
L5	Great toe dorsiflexion	E. hallucis longus	Dorsum of foot at third meta-carpophalangeal joint
	Knee flexion	Hamstrings	
S1-S2	Ankle plantarflexion	Gastrocnemius	—
	Toe flexion	Peroneus longus/brevis	—
S1	—	—	Lateral heel
S2	—	—	Midpopliteal fossa
S3	—	—	Ischial tuberosity
S4-S5	—	—	Perianal area

Adapted from Gutierrez PA, Young RR, Vulpe M, Spinal cord injury. An overview, *Urol Clin N Am* 20:373–382, 1993.

onds every 15–30 minutes. Special mattresses and wheelchair cushions do not obviate the need for proper positioning and frequent repositioning. The skin is kept clean and dry.

2. **Pressure relief.** A repositioning schedule ensuring that the sore is always pressure-free needs to be rigidly followed, since the reduced number of possible weight-bearing positions make another sore more likely. Simultaneous treatment of more than one pressure sore requires special frames or flotation beds.

3. **Debridement.** Saline wet-to-dry gauze and whirlpool therapy are standard, but commercial enzyme preps are less labor-intensive. If the eschar is hard and blackened, necrotic tissue is removed surgically.

4. **Dressings.** Shallow ulcers are covered with sterile gauze. Occlusive dressings may promote more rapid healing and have to be changed less often, but are much more expensive. Deeper, pear-shaped ulcers are packed with saline-soaked gauze to prevent abscess formation and to promote "bottom-up" healing.

5. **Surgical excision** with a myocutaneous flap to fill the cavity is usually required for deeper ulcers. Reduction of bony prominences may be necessary.

B. **Deep venous thrombosis** is a serious concern in spinal cord injury. Pain may not be felt below a sensory level, and swelling may be masked by edema and vasomotor changes.

1. **Prophylaxis** is needed for at least 3 months or until the return of ambulation. Intermittent pneumatic compression stockings together with low-dosage heparin (5000 U q12h SC) or warfarin (5–10 mg/day PO, International Normalized Ratio [INR] of 2–3) are effective during the first 10–14 days. When the stockings are removed, heparin is increased (10,000–15,000 U q12h SC) to maintain the partial thromboplastin time (PTT) in the high normal range if warfarin is not being used.

2. **Treatment.** A loading dose of heparin (5000–7000 U IV) is followed by con-

tinuous infusion adjusted to maintain a PTT at 1.5–2.0 times control. Warfarin (5 mg/day) is started within 24 hours and adjusted to maintain the prothrombin time (PT) at an INR of 2–3. Heparin is then discontinued. The patient may sit in a chair at 5 days, resume therapy at 7 days, and resume range of motion (ROM) exercises in the affected limb at 14 days after initiation of treatment. Warfarin is continued for 3 to 6 months.

3. Vena cava filters are avoided in quadriplegics because of the risk of dislodgement by abdominal compression for cough.

C. Autonomic hyperreflexia. From 30–85% of quadriplegics and high paraplegics develop paroxysmal episodes of severe hypertension, sweating, flushing, and piloerection accompanied by headache, chest pain, and bradycardia or tachycardia in response to relatively benign stimuli below the level of injury. Pulmonary edema, intracranial hemorrhage, cerebral infarction, seizures, or death can result. Bladder and bowel distension, instrumentation, or irritation are the most common precipitating stimuli.

1. Etiology. In the setting of a spinal lesion above the major splanchic outflow tract (T6-L2), reflex activation of sympathetic discharge occurs below the lesion unchecked by descending inhibitory pathways from supraspinal centers.

2. Management. Initial treatment entails removal of the precipitating stimulus and medication for the hypertensive crisis.

  a. Removal of precipitating stimulus

    (1) Stop procedure.

    (2) Check for urinary catheter blockage.

    (3) Remove tight clothing, shoes, straps, etc.

    (4) Catheterize carefully with 2% xylocaine jelly.

    (5) Do kidney, ureter, and bladder (KUB) and rectal exam with xylocaine jelly to check for impaction.

    (6) Check for sores, infections, trauma, and fractures.

    (7) Consider acute abdomen and deep venous thrombosis.

  b. Treatment of hypertension

    (1) Elevate head of bed or place patient in sitting position to induce postural changes in blood pressure.

    (2) Administer **nifedipine** at 10–20 mg sublingual (SL); may be repeated after 15 minutes.

    (3) If blood pressure remains critical, IV protocols (hydralazine, diazoxide, sodium nitroprusside, etc.) for hypertensive crisis must be initiated.

  c. Treatment of profuse sweating without hypertension. Give probantheline at 15 mg PO (may be repeated after 10 minutes) or oxybutynin at 5 mg PO (may be repeated after 10 minutes)

3. Prophylactic medications

  a. Nifedipine 10 mg PO 30 minutes before procedure

  b. Phenoxybenzamine 10–20 mg PO tid

  c. Scopolamine patch may help with reflex sweating.

D. Central pain syndrome. Development of chronic dysesthesia or central pain at or distal to the level of injury poses a therapeutic challenge.

1. Predisposing factors include arachnoiditis; tethering of cord; posttraumatic syringomyelia; decubiti; and bowel, urologic, and musculoskeletal etiologies. Development of pain above the level of the lesion is suggestive of a posttraumatic syrinx.

2. Pharmacologic approach is by trial and error.

  a. Tricyclics

    (1) Amitriptyline (Elavil) 25 mg PO qhs; increase by 25 mg every 5–7 days as tolerated to 50 mg tid

    (2) Nortriptyline (Pamelor) 25–100 mg/day PO

    (3) Desipramine (Norpramin) 25–150 mg/day PO

    (4) Side effects include sedation, anticholinergic effects, orthostatic hypotension, and cardiac arrhythmias.

    (5) If side effects are not tolerable, a chemically unrelated compound—e.g., fluoxetine (Prozac) at 20–40 mg/day PO—may be tried.

  b. Anticonvulsants (usually in combination with tricyclics)

    (1) Carbamazepine (Tegretol) 100 mg PO bid; increase by 100 mg every 3 days as tolerated to serum level of 8–10 μg/ml, in 3–4 doses per day

        (a) Side effects include sedation, diplopia, GI upset, ataxia, weakness, rash, and blood dyscrasia.

        (b) Monitor CBC with platelets every 2 weeks for 3 months, then CBC, platelets, and liver function every 3–6 months.

    (2) Phenytoin or divalproex sodium

  c. Neuroleptics (with tricyclic; stop anticonvulsant)

    (1) Must warn of the risk of tardive dyskinesia with the use of neuroleptics.

    (2) Fluphenazine (Prolixin): start at 1 mg/day, then slowly increase to 10 mg/day as tolerated.

        (a) Periodically attempt to wean or discontinue.

        (b) If no relief is obtained, discontinue.

3. Physical methods may provide some temporary relief.

  a. TENS (transcutaneous electrical nerve stimulation)

  b. Warm or cool packs, and ultrasound

4. Surgical treatment should be considered only after conservative therapy has failed.

  a. Dorsal root entry zone (DREZ) surgery

    (1) Laminectomy and radiofrequency ablation of DREZ is performed two levels above and one level below site of injury.

    (2) Improvement is realized in 60–90% of patients. Best results are achieved in patients with pain at or just below the site of injury.

    (3) Complications include loss of one or two sensory levels, CSF leakage, hematomas, and bowel, bladder, and sexual dysfunctions.

  b. Avoid sympathectomies, rhizotomies, and cordotomies.

5. Narcotic therapy is indicated only after both conservative and surgical therapies have failed.

  a. Combination with tricyclics may be synergistic.

  b. The patient must be carefully selected and carefully supervised.

  c. Methadone (Dolophine) 5 mg PO bid at least 8 hours apart; may be increased slowly to 20 mg q8h.

    (1) A formal contract detailing expectations and criteria for termination of treatment is made with the patient.

    (2) Periodic attempts should be made to wean the medication.

    (3) Iatrogenic addiction rate is 5%.

    (4) Abuse rate is 17%.

    (5) Side effects include sedation, respiratory depression, constipation, and reduced sexual function.

E. Post-traumatic syringomyelia is recognized in 1–5% of spinal cord injury patients, but MRI and autopsy studies suggest an incidence closer to 20%. Symptoms present months to years after the original injury.

  1. Clinical symptoms are similar to those of autonomic hyperreflexia.

    a. Onset or exacerbation of **pain,** especially if perceived above the level of original injury

    b. Change in level or completeness of neurologic deficits

    c. Increased spasticity

  2. Treatment

    a. Untethering the spinal cord at site of injury

    b. Surgical shunting of cavity

    c. Pain, spasticity, and autonomic hyperreflexia respond best.

V. Spinal cord injury without radiologic abnormality

  A. More common in children: laxity of spinal ligaments

  B. Subtle or transient deficits may go unnoticed. There is a high risk of delayed neurologic dysfunction if the syndrome is not recognized and managed appropriately.

  C. Treatment

    1. Rigid immobilization

    2. Avoidance of precipitating activities, especially sports

VI. Central cord syndrome

  A. Etiology. Hyperextension injuries (frequently falls in the elderly with cervical spondylosis or athletic injuries in younger patients with congenital stenosis) without acute radiologic changes may produce spinal cord contusion primarily affecting the central gray matter. Lamination of tracts in the cervical cord (sacral fibers, lateral; cervical fibers, medial) explains the clinical picture.

B. Clinical features. Patients present with a picture of "inverted quadriparesis," in which upper-extremity weakness exceeds lower-extremity weakness. Transient burning dysesthesias in the hands with little weakness or urinary dysfunction can also occur. With recovery, the leg, bladder, and upper-extremity weaknesses improve. The fingers are last to recover.

C. Prognosis. Almost all patients show improvement, but often to an incomplete degree in the elderly. A delayed progressive myelopathy can develop in approximately 25% of cases.

D. Treatment

1. Conservative therapy consists of rigid immobilization of the neck, physical therapy, and consideration of a course of corticosteroids.

2. Surgical therapy. Guided by neuroimaging, patients who have not improved, have plateaued, or demonstrate instability of the spine are considered for surgical decompression.

VII. Hyperextension-flexion injury (whiplash injury)

A. Etiology. Automobile accidents account for approximately 85% of whiplash injuries. The roles of mild CNS injury and psychosocial factors are controversial.

B. Prevention. Automobile head restraints reduce flexion-hyperextension motion of the head in automobile accidents, especially during rear-end collisions. However, surveys have shown that they are frequently adjusted incorrectly.

C. Natural history. Rear-end collisions are involved in most whiplash injuries. Cynicism and controversy exist over the etiology of a chronic whiplash syndrome.

D. Prognosis. Although figures vary widely, approximately 25% of patients are still symptomatic after 6 months, and 5–10% sustain permanent medical disabilities.

E. Treatment

1. Positive attitude and encouragement

2. Ice for first 24 hours

3. Conservative therapy as detailed in Chap. 22

4. Trigger-point injections (0.1–0.6 ml sterile water) often make patients more comfortable but remain unproven.

VIII. Spasticity is one of the cardinal manifestations of chronic spinal cord disease. In acute spinal lesions, spasticity develops after a variable period of spinal shock, whereas in disorders with insidious onset it may be the first symptom noticed.

A. The decision to treat must be made on an individual basis. Treatment is indicated when the advantages of spasticity outweigh the disadvantages. Specific treatment goals need to be formulated.

1. Advantages

a. Bowel training maintains sphincter tone.

b. "Internal crutches" for ambulation

c. Enables weight bearing in transfers

d. Reduced osteopenia

e. Increased muscle bulk

f. Increased venous tone and possibly decreased deep venous thrombosis

2. Disadvantages

a. Pain and falls resulting from paroxysmal spasms

b. Impaired hygiene owing to hip adductor spasticity

c. Joint contractures

d. Formation of pressure sores

e. Renal damage as a result of external sphincter spasticity

f. Impairment or interruption of movements required for activities of daily living

B. Assessment of severity can be made using the modified Ashworth scale (Table 45-3).

C. A **changing pattern in a previously stable degree of spasticity** should alert the clinician to varying etiologies.

1. Medication: fluoxetine, sertraline, or trazodone

2. Anxiety

3. Tight clothing or shoes

4. Inadequate or prolonged postures

5. Formation of pressure sores

6. Development of deep venous thrombosis

7. Ingrown toenails

Table 45-3. Modified Ashworth scale for measuring spasticity.

Grade 0: Normal muscle tone
Grade 1: Slight increase in muscle tone; "catch" or minimal resistance at end of range of
motion (ROM)
Grade 2: Slight increase; "catch" followed by minimal resistance for remainder of ROM
Grade 3: More marked increase in tone through most of ROM; parts moved easily
Grade 4: Considerable increase in tone; passive movement difficult
Grade 5: Affected part(s) rigid in flexion or extension

Total score is the average of hip flexion and abduction, knee flexion, and ankle dorsiflexion
bilaterally.

Adapted from McLean BN, Intrathecal baclofen in severe spasticity, *Brit J Hosp Med* 49:262–267, 1993.

      8. Spinal instability
      9. Fractures
    10. Post-traumatic syringomyelia
    11. GI dysfunctions: impaction, hemorrhoids, and acute abdomen
    12. GU dysfunctions: infections; stones; blocked catheters; and disorders of testicle, prostate, vagina, uterus, or ovary.
  D. Management is based on a multidisciplinary approach with a rigorous program of both passive and active stretching.
    1. Physical modalities
      a. ROM and stretching exercises
      b. Heat or cold
      c. Vibration (increases presynaptic spinal inhibition)
      d. Splints, casts, and orthotics to prevent contractures and increase mobility
    2. Useful medications are summarized in Table 45-4.
    3. Nerve blocks
      a. Alcohol or **phenol** damages nerves nonselectively.
        (1) Useful for relieving spasticity in a specific muscle—e.g., obturator nerve and hip adduction
        (2) Test injections with a local anesthetic help determine whether or not this is a reasonable approach.
        (3) EMG-guided injection increases selectivity.
        (4) Parallel reductions in spasticity and strength
        (5) Not fully reversible; pain, scarring, and fibrosis at site are potential complications.
      b. EMG-guided botulinum toxin (Botox) injection is investigational for lower-extremity spasticity.
        (1) The time and effort required for multiple injections limit this technique to one or two key muscles.
        (2) Advantages are reversible block (6–12 weeks) and selectivity toward motor fibers.
        (3) The **disadvantage** is the expense.
    4. Neurosurgical procedures
      a. An **intrathecal baclofen pump** is a safe alternative to ablative surgery for intractable spasticity at experienced centers.
        (1) Patients with stable neurologic disorders and whose spasticity is both resistant to oral antispastic agents and severely interfering with the quality of life should be considered for referral to an experienced center.
        (2) Improvements are observed in muscle tone, spasms, musculoskeletal pain, mobility, and bladder function.
        (3) There is no improvement in central pain.
        (4) Although life-threatening, all instances of drug overdose have been completely reversible.
        (5) Experience and better pump design have decreased the complication rate to less than 5%.
        (6) In early series of patients, surgical revision was required in 20% for catheter-related problems.
      b. Selective posterior rhizotomy with interoperative EMG selection of

Table 45-4. Drug treatment of spasticity.

Drug	Daily dosage[a] (starting dosage)	Side effects/comments
baclofen (Lioresal)	10–160 mg (5 mg bid)	Drowsiness, weakness, tremor, ataxia, abrupt withdrawal with seizures, confusion/hallucinations
diazepam (Valium)	4–60 mg (2 mg at bed-time)	Sedation, cognitive changes, depression, weakness, dependence, abuse, with-drawal syndrome
clonidine (Catapres)	0.2–1.0 mg (0.1 mg at bed-time)	Dry mouth, hypotension, nausea, sedation, confusion, weakness
clonidine (Catapres-TTS)	0.1–1.0 mg	Same as above—find effective and toler-ated dose with tablets; patch permits once-a-week dose
dantrolene[b] (Dantrium)	25–400 mg (25 mg once a day)	Weakness, hepatotoxicity, confusion, sedation, nausea, diarrhea; monitor liver function closely
phenytoin (Dilantin)	200–400 mg (100 mg bid)	Drug interactions, rare hepatotoxicity, serious skin rash, dosage-dependent ataxia, mental confusion, rarely effec-tive; monitor CBC and liver function
carbamazepine (Tegretol)	400–1200 mg (100 mg bid)	Skin rash, dosage-dependent drowsiness, diplopia, rare hematotoxicity, hepato-toxicity, hyponatremia, rarely effective; monitor CBC and liver function

[a]It is important to start with a low dosage and gradually build to a target dosage as tolerance to the sedation and most other side effects of the medication develop.
[b]The potentially fatal hepatotoxicity of dantrolene is more common in adults and those taking estrogens. This drug probably should be avoided in those with preexisting liver disease.

rootlets for sectioning is useful in the management of cerebral palsy. Two-thirds of patients are improved with minimal sensory loss and few side effects.

   c. Percutaneous posterior rhizotomy is technically more difficult, and re-currence may be more of a problem.

   d. Efficacy of spinal cord stimulators is controversial.

   e. Peripheral neurectomies are occasionally used to relieve specific joint contractures.

   f. Longitudinal myelotomy, unselective posterior rhizotomy, and anterior rhizotomy are rarely done.

  5. Orthopedic procedures are used most often in a supportive role to relieve pain, increase mobility, and decrease deformity in cerebral palsy.

   a. Tendon release, lengthening, and transfer

   b. Osteotomy and arthrodesis

IX. Amyotrophic lateral sclerosis is a chronic degenerative disease involving **mo-toneurons** in the spinal cord and brain. Sensation and cognition are left intact. Eye movements and sphincters are affected very late, if at all. The etiology remains unknown, and approximately 5–10% of the cases appear to be familial. A **gene de-fect** recently found in familial cases is absent in sporadic cases.

  A. Prognosis. The course of the disorder is relentlessly progressive, leading to respiratory insufficiency secondary to weakness and death within an average of 3.5 years after the onset of symptoms. Approximately 20% of patients have a more benign course and survive for more than 5 years, but prognosis for an in-dividual patient is generally not possible at the onset. Patients who have promi-nent involvement of the bulbar muscles at onset have a more rapid course, with death occurring within 2.2 years on average.

  B. Most physicians refer the patient to a neurologist for a second opinion when the diagnosis is suspected. Presentation of the diagnosis to the patient and fam-ily is always difficult. A prompt (2–3 weeks) and extended follow-up visit gives the patient and family an opportunity to ask questions and allows the physician to present a positive therapeutic strategy. This strategy should not be so detailed at this time as to overwhelm the patient. Patients must be given time before they can be expected to be active participants in such plans.

C. **Treatment.** There is no specific treatment. The clinician offers **supportive care** for both the patient and family.

1. Addresses of **support groups** should be offered to the patient and family. These associations coordinate local groups, provide patient and family education, and can notify patients of current research protocols that are open. In addition, active electronic communities are beginning to form on the Internet. Two support groups are:

The ALS Association
21021 Ventura Blvd.
Suite 321
Woodland Hills, CA 91364
(818)340-7500

Muscular Dystrophy Association
3300 East Sunrise Dr.
Tucson, AZ 85718
(520)529-2000

2. A **multidisciplinary team,** with a leader readily identified by the patient and other team members, should consist of speech, dietary, respiratory therapy, neurologic nursing, social service, rehabilitation medicine, pulmonary, ENT, and neurology professionals.

3. The diagnosis and treatment of **dysphagia** and **dysarthria** are discussed in Chaps. 18 and 19.

   a. A speech pathologist experienced in neurologic problems as well as communication aids should be utilized early to maintain **socialization** of the patient.

   b. **Pseudobulbar palsy** is suggested by emotional lability and a brisk jaw jerk. It can frequently be helped with amitriptyline (Elavil) at 25 mg PO tid or amantadine at 100 mg PO bid.

   c. A **feeding tube** often frees the patient and family from the burden that meals become. Tube feeding allows adequate nutrition, as well as hydration to loosen secretions. Because of the dangers of general anesthesia, percutaneous placement is generally preferred.

4. **Salivation**

   a. **Drooling** can be helped with a portable suction machine and one of the following agents.

      (1) Amitriptyline (Elavil) 25–100 mg/day PO

      (2) Scopolamine (Transderm-Scōp) patch every 3 days

      (3) Glycopyrrolate (Robinul) 1–2 mg PO tid

   b. **Thickened secretions** are treated with hydration and expectorants.

      (1) Ensure adequate hydration.

      (2) Avoid caffeine beverages; stop diuretics if possible.

      (3) Dilute potassium iodide (SSKI) at 300–600 mg PO tid-qid, or

      (4) Guaifenesin (syrup or tablet) at 200–400 mg PO q4h

      (5) Dried secretions within the oropharynx can be loosened with a cotton swab dipped in meat tenderizer.

D. **Respiratory care**

1. **Pulmonary functions** are evaluated on a regular basis. Rate of decline in vital capacity correlates with prognosis.

2. **Orthopnea** (resulting from diaphragmatic weakness) and **sleep apnea** (possibly a result of bulbar weakness) are frequent problems that can be helped by sleep posture and nocturnal CPAP. Some physicians use theophylline for its possible stimulant effect on the diaphragm.

3. **Respiratory infections** should be treated aggressively.

4. **Influenza and pneumonia vaccines** should be kept up to date.

5. The possibility of **home ventilation** should be discussed with the patient and family. Social service, psychological, and pulmonary consultation should be available.

E. **Assistive devices** can help with activities of daily living.

1. The patient can refer to a catalog of self-help aids, such as:

Sammons Catalogue
145 Tower Drive, Dept. #423
Burr Ridge, IL 60521
(708)325-1700

2. The home should be inspected for modifications that will improve mobility and quality of life.
3. Microprocessor-controlled adaptive devices permit nearly complete control of the environment.
4. **Respite care** should be available to the caregiver.

F. **Hospice care** should be discussed in advance with the patient and family.

Recommended Readings

Balazy TE. Clinical management of chronic pain in spinal cord injury. *Clin J Pain* 8:102–110, 1992.

Colachis SC III. Autonomic hyperreflexia with spinal cord injury. *J Am Paraplegia Soc* 15:171–186, 1992.

Critchley E, Eisen A (eds). *Diseases of the Spinal Cord.* New York: Springer-Verlag, 1992.

Ditunno JF Jr, Formal CS. Chronic spinal cord injury. *N Engl J Med* 330:550–556, 1994.

Evans RW. Some observations on whiplash injuries. *Neurol Clin N Am* 10:975–997, 1992.

Evans RW, Baskin DS, Yatsu RM (eds). *Prognosis of Neurological Disorders.* New York: Oxford University Press, 1992.

Frost FS. Role of rehabilitation after spinal cord injury. *Urol Clin N Am* 20:549–559, 1993.

Green D, et al. Deep vein thrombosis in spinal cord injury. Summary and recommendations. *Chest* 102(suppl):633S–635S, 1992.

Gutierrez PA, et al. Spinal cord injury. An overview. *Urol Clin N Am* 20:373–382, 1993.

Johnson RT, Griffin JW (eds). *Current Therapy in Neurologic Disease* (4th ed). St. Louis: Decker, 1993.

Krendel DA, et al. Isolated deficiency of vitamin E with progressive neurologic deterioration. *Neurology* 37:538–540, 1987.

Leigh PN, Ray-Chaudhuri K. Motor neuron disease. *J Neurol Neurosurg Psychiat* 57: 886–896, 1994.

Mariani C, et al. The natural history and results of surgery in 50 cases of syringomyelia. *J Neurol* 238:433–438, 1991.

Maroon JC, et al. Central cord syndrome. *Clin Neurosurg* 37:612–621, 1991.

McLean BN. Intrathecal baclofen in severe spasticity. *Brit J Hosp Med* 49:262–267, 1993.

Pang D, Wilberger JE Jr. Tethered cord syndrome in adults. *J Neurosurg* 57:32–47, 1982.

Parry TE. Folate responsive neuropathy. *Presse Med* 23:131–137, 1994.

Parziale JR, Akelman E, Herz DA. Spasticity: Pathophysiology and management. *Orthopedics* 16:801–811, 1993.

Pruthi RK, Tefferi A. Pernicious anemia revisited. *Mayo Clin Proc* 69:144–150, 1994.

Schmitt J, Midha M, McKenzie N. Medical complications of spinal cord disease. *Neurol Clin* 9:779–795, 1991.

Smith RA, Gillie E, Licht J. Palliative treatment of motor neuron disease. In de Jong (ed), *Handbook of Clinical Neurology,* vol 15(59): *Diseases of the Motor System.* Amsterdam: Elsevier, 1991.

Trop CS, Bennett CJ. Autonomic dysreflexia and its urological implications: A review. *J Urol* 146:1461–1469, 1991.

Woolsey RM, McGarry JD. The cause, prevention, and treatment of pressure sores. *Neurol Clin* 9:797–808, 1991.

Young W. Medical treatments of acute spinal cord injury. *J Neurol Neurosurg Psychiat* 55:636–639, 1992.

46

Neuropathy
John Collins Kincaid

Peripheral neuropathy is a general term for abnormalities that affect the peripheral nervous system (PNS). The site of abnormality may be at the nerve cell bodies, the nerve roots, the nerve trunks, or the terminal branches. Abnormality of the axon or myelin sheath may be the pathologic substrate, as can abnormality of the connective and vascular tissue that invests the nerves. A primary step in devising therapy for peripheral neuropathy is determining whether there is a specific etiology that may be treated directly or whether a less specific plan to manage the symptomatic results of the neuropathy indirectly must be used. Some terms used in characterizing the site of lesion are as follows.

neuronopathy: abnormality of the nerve cell body, usually producing motor or sensory dysfunction separately
radiculopathy: abnormality at the level of the nerve root, usually affecting a single spinal level only and often the result of compression by a disk or osteophyte
polyradiculopathy: abnormality involving many if not most spinal root levels and often of inflammatory etiology
polyradiculoneuropathy: same as polyradiculopathy, but affecting the nerve trunks as well as the nerve roots
plexopathy/plexitis: abnormality at the level of the brachial plexus in the shoulder or lumbosacral plexus in the pelvis
mononeuropathy: abnormality of a single peripheral nerve, often resulting from entrapment or local trauma
polyneuropathy: abnormality of multiple peripheral nerves, usually in a symmetric fashion and affecting feet and legs before hands and arms
mononeuritis multiplex: abnormality of multiple peripheral nerves independently, often spreading in a patchy fashion such that one nerve is affected but an adjacent one of similar length is spared, and often observed with vasculitis
axonal neuropathy: neuropathy in which the pathology affects the axon
demyelinating neuropathy: neuropathy in which the myelin sheath is the primary site of pathology
entrapment neuropathy: neuropathy in which the nerve is compressed by the anatomic structure through which it is passing

I. **Management based on symptoms.** Despite known etiologies of some neuropathies and some specific treatments, the clinician, as either the generalist or the specialist, is presented with a group of symptoms that are often similar from one neuropathy to another. Management of the symptoms is also similar, and a general approach is presented. Neuropathic symptoms consist of:

Pain
Paresthesias
Sensory loss
Weakness
Unstable balance

A. **Pain** is often the most bothersome of the symptoms and is the most difficult to manage satisfactorily. The pain takes several different forms.
1. **Fiery, burning, constant pain,** which is often localized to the toes, bottoms of the feet, and fingertips, is very bothersome. This type of pain responds only partially to analgesics, which can be mild agents such as aspirin and acetaminophen or combinations such as acetaminophen-propoxyphene napsylate. There is no compelling evidence that nonsteroidal anti-inflammatory

drugs (NSAIDs) offer much relief for this type of pain, but they can be tried. If the pain is more severe, stronger analgesics—such as codeine, hydrocodone, or oxycodone, all in combination with acetaminophen—may be required. It is important that the patient understand that these medications may not provide complete relief of pain, which may help limit the tendency toward overuse in search of complete relief. This type of pain is often worse when the patient retires for sleep, and, if possible, the stronger analgesics should be reserved for these times.

This type of pain may also be significantly lessened by tricyclic antidepressants, which probably act through brainstem pain-modulating pathways. Pain is reduced in intensity but not fully relieved. Medications such as desipramine, amitriptyline, nortriptyline, and doxepin are the preferred agents. Antidepressants of the specific serotonin reuptake inhibitor (SSRI) class do not seem to provide any direct pain-modulating benefit in these conditions.

When starting these drugs, inform the patient that the medication can help relieve but will not eliminate the pain, that it can help improve the quality of sleep and leave the patient better equipped to handle the pain during the day, and that there may be some early side effects such as morning sedation, dry mouth, and blurred vision. These effects usually lessen within a few days. Start these medications at a low dosage such as 25 mg given 1 hour or so before bedtime. Pain benefit may begin within a few days but may take several weeks to become evident. Increase the dosage by 25 mg every 2–3 weeks if there has been no benefit at the initial dosage. A dosage of 50–75 mg is usually sufficient, but higher doses can be used within the bounds of the particular drug. Drug level monitoring does not help. If a medication is beneficial, it should be continued for at least 6 months. At that point, a taper of 10–25 mg every 2 weeks will reveal by worsening symptoms whether the agents are still effective. Long-term use may be needed.

Topical capsaicin creams are also potentially helpful for this type of pain. Neurotransmitter depletion in pain-sensing neurons is the proposed mechanism of action. These preparations are applied to the painful areas three or four times daily. Several weeks are required for benefit to appear, and a short-term increase in the pain may occur before the benefit begins. These drugs are moderately expensive and somewhat cumbersome to use. Like the other pain treatments, they may lessen but will not eliminate the pain.

2. **Short jabs of pain** are another form of neuropathic pain. These jabs are often felt in the feet, lower legs, or fingers. They last a second or two and move about from one occurrence to the next. These pains often respond to anticonvulsant drugs such as phenytoin at 100 mg bid-tid or carbamazepine at 100 mg bid up to 200 mg tid. The benefit often appears within a few days and is obvious to the patient. Monitoring of drug levels is probably not helpful in maximizing benefit but may be needed if higher dosages are used, so as to avoid toxicity. The CBC should be monitored in patients on carbamazepine.

3. **Tight or bandlike pressure pain** often felt in the feet or lower parts of the legs is relatively resistant to treatment. This pain usually occurs in combination with other types of pain that are often more bothersome. Encourage patients not to rely on their analgesics to provide full relief from this type of pain.

4. **Cold, frostbite-type painful sensations** may be felt in the feet and fingers. This type of pain is also poorly responsive to medications of any class.

5. **Painful hypersensitivity to touch** is often an accompaniment to spontaneous pain. The patient perceives light touch in the involved area as exquisitely uncomfortable during and a few seconds after the touch. Wearing light cotton socks or gloves can mollify these sensations, as can tents in the bed linens to keep the toes free of touch at night. Tricyclic antidepressants may relieve this type of pain to some degree.

B. **Paresthesias** are another form of sensory abnormality. These phenomena take the form of feelings of repetitive prickles, or "pins and needles" sensations. These sensations are felt in larger areas than the discrete jabs of pain discussed in sec. **I.A.2** above and may, for example, be felt in the toes, the feet, or the hands. They occur spontaneously or may be produced by touching of the body part. These sensations may respond to some degree to antiepileptic medications such as phenytoin and carbamazepine in the dosages mentioned for jabs of pain. Analgesics do not help these symptoms, but transcutaneous electrical nerve stimulation (TENS) may partly relieve them.

C. **Sensory losses** that produce feelings of the affected areas being "dead," or "like blocks of wood," or "leathery," do not respond to symptomatic treatment, and reliance on medications such as analgesics for relief should be discouraged. Because of the sensory loss, it is important that body parts in these areas be visually inspected at least daily for local trauma such as blisters or cuts. The tips of the toes and bottoms of the feet are particularly important areas for such inspection. Unrecognized lesions may lead to more serious problems such as ulcers and infections. Properly fitting shoes are important also.

D. **Weakness** in polyneuropathy is usually more notable distally and tends to be symmetric. It may be minor in degree, but if the condition worsens, foot drop and hand weakness can appear. Significant proximal weakness such as the weakness that makes it difficult to get up from chairs or the arm weakness that produces lifting difficulties is more often a feature of inflammatory demyelinating neuropathy, motor neuron disease, or myopathy. In radiculopathy or mononeuropathy, weakness is localized.

Foot drop or a slapping foot indicates ankle extensor weakness, as do complaints of unsteady walking or difficulty standing still without holding onto something. Imbalance in this setting may be markedly improved by bracing the foot with an ankle-foot orthosis. A cane may also be helpful.

Knee weakness may predispose patients to falling. Patients compensate for such weakness by keeping the knee locked in extension. A minor dislodgment from that position, caused by a shift in body position or a bump, may cause a fall. Compensation by bracing is more difficult for knee weakness than for weakness at the ankle. Bilateral knee weakness makes it difficult to arise from chairs or to climb stairs. An arm chair or lift chair may assist in getting up from sitting. Hand weakness can be aided by large-handle eating and personal hygiene utensils.

Physical and occupational therapy and evaluation by a physical medicine and rehabilitation physician can be very helpful in all of these conditions.

E. **Unstable balance** may cause problems ranging from mild inconvenience in walking or standing still to significant danger to the patient in terms of potential falls. This problem may result from sensory loss, cerebellar dysfunction, or weakness in the legs at the ankles and knees. In mild forms of this condition, no management other than caution by the patient may be required. More pronounced deficits require progressive aids such as another person to hold onto, a series of strategically placed pieces of furniture, a cane, a walker, a motorized scooter, or a wheelchair. Patients may have increased difficulty in darkness or in situations in which their eyes are closed, such as showering. The patient who has had several falls and who has an unmanageable condition should be encouraged to use a wheelchair to avoid further injury.

II. **Management of specific conditions**

A. **Acute inflammatory demyelinating neuropathy** (Guillain-Barré syndrome) presents as sensory loss and weakness usually beginning in the feet. The onset may follow a viral or other infectious-type illness by a week or two and may also appear spontaneously. The condition worsens over days to a few weeks. The motor and sensory deficits migrate proximally and appear in the upper extremities also. The deficits may remain mild or become severe. Weakness often brings the patient to medical attention.

The diagnosis is supported by findings of a progressive loss of muscle stretch reflexes along with weakness and sensory loss that are usually more pronounced distally. Laboratory findings of raised spinal fluid protein concentration along with normal or minimally abnormal WBC count support the diagnosis, as do electromyography (EMG) and nerve conduction studies (NCS) that show the major slowing of conduction velocity that is characteristic of a demyelinating neuropathy. Arsenic intoxication, porphyria, and tick bite paralysis can mimic this condition.

Patients suspected of having acute inflammatory demyelinating neuropathy should be hospitalized. Mild cases may not require direct intervention other than close observation for progression of the weakness. Weakness of a degree that causes significant impairment of walking or use of the arms benefits from treatment. The duration or severity of the attack can be lessened.

Two treatments—plasmapheresis and intravenous gamma globulin infusion—have shown benefits. Both probably work by reregulating the immune system. **Plasmapheresis,** also termed **plasma exchange,** is done by exchanging a portion of the plasma to filter off as yet undefined fractions that are the presumed mediators of the attack. The sequence usually involves an exchange every other day for four or five sessions. Access by means of peripheral veins is possible, but a central line is usually required. Treatments are generally well tolerated. Hypotension can occur, and therefore this mode may not be optimal for older patients with fragile cardiovascular systems. **Intravenous gamma globulin infusion** in a regimen of 0.4 g/kg/day for 5 days has been shown to be equally as effective as plasmapheresis. This treatment is logistically easier, because only peripheral vein access is required. Complications of this mode of treatment have been infrequent but have included vascular incidents presumably resulting from hyperviscosity from the large protein infusion and aseptic meningitis.

In both treatments, improvement may begin within a day or two of starting but may also appear only weeks later in the form of a shortening of the natural time course. A small percentage of the patients who show improvement with either of these treatments may relapse within a few weeks of the initial improvement. In such instances, another one or two plasma exchanges or gamma globulin infusions will reestablish the improvement. Near or full improvement occurs in a high percentage of patients, but even with these treatments some patients have a prolonged, severe course requiring weeks if not months of hospitalization including respiratory support. In the more severe cases, deficits of distal weakness, sensory loss, and paresthesias may show prolonged recovery over months to years or may persist.

Corticosteroids do not benefit this acute form of inflammatory neuropathy.

B. **Chronic inflammatory demyelinating neuropathy** is similar to the acute form but continues to worsen over a longer period, such as months. This form may not improve without treatment. Monoclonal gammopathy of the IgM type can mimic this condition. The laboratory and nerve conduction results are also similar to those of the acute form. The treatment options are the same also, with the exception that corticosteroids may benefit this type of neuropathy.

Prednisone at a dosage of 1 mg/kg/day for 1 month may produce dramatic improvement over a month or so. If a benefit occurs within 1 month, the dosage should be slowly tapered off to 10–20 mg/day over the next 2 months. If improvement is sustained at these low dosages, complete withdrawal should be attempted over another month or two. The need for prolonged low-dosage maintenance is signified by recurrence of the deficits as the dosage is reduced. This type of treatment can be significantly less expensive than plasmapheresis or gamma globulin infusion. Potential steroid side effects and the relative benignity of the other treatments merit consideration in choosing the type of management.

In some patients, one form of treatment may fail but another provide good benefit. Patients who are managed with either gamma globulin infusion or plasmapheresis and who show good initial response may require repeated treatments at about monthly intervals for an extended period of time. If symptoms recur, often within 3–8 weeks, a single session of treatment should be repeated and the patient observed for another month. Further treatment is then dictated by the continued remission or recurrence.

C. **Vasculitic neuropathy** occurs in the setting of inflammatory involvement of the vasa nervorum. This usually happens as part of a more generalized systemic disease but in rare cases may be limited to the vessels of the peripheral nerve alone. The presentation and evolution of this type of neuropathy tends to be unique. Progression occurs in a very patchy fashion such that a single nerve in a limb malfunctions and then a nerve in another location does the same. The deficits often appear rather suddenly and then accumulate over days to weeks. This pattern is referred to as **mononeuritis multiplex.** If unchecked, it evolves into what looks like a generalized symmetric polyneuropathy. Careful history-taking identifies the patchy pattern of onset.

Vasculitic neuropathy is potentially very serious and continues to progress if untreated. It may occur in association with polyarteritis nodosa, rheumatoid arthritis, systemic lupus erythematosus (SLE), or Wegener's granulomatosis and may be the presenting feature of these conditions.

The diagnosis is supported by laboratory studies that identify any of the abovementioned systemic illnesses. EMG may also help by showing a patchy pattern of involvement suggestive of mononeuritis multiplex. Biopsy of a peripheral nerve in an area of clinical involvement, such as the sural nerve in the leg or a superficial radial nerve in the arm, can provide strong support also.

Treatment requires immunosuppressive therapy. Prednisone at 1 mg/kg/day provides some improvement, but addition of cyclophosphamide is usually required for sustained benefit. Cyclophosphamide should be given by physicians familiar with its use. It can be administered by daily oral dosage or monthly IV pulse therapy. Recovery takes place over an extended period and appears first as a cessation of further worsening. Actual improvement appears over months, but severely affected areas may show persistent deficits.

D. **Alcoholic neuropathy** is a sensorimotor neuropathy that affects the legs initially and may progress into the arms if the excess exposure continues. The onset is insidious, and progression takes place over months or longer. Sensory symptoms include numbness, tingling paresthesias, and fiery pain. Motor abnormalities in the form of foot drop, hand weakness, and even proximal leg weakness can occur in more advanced cases. The neuropathy shows a pattern of axonal damage on EMG. Supporting laboratory findings include liver enzyme abnormalities and macrocytosis.

Therapy consists of discontinuance of alcohol and supplementation of the diet with thiamine at 100 mg/day. Improvement takes place over months. Unstable walking as a result of alcoholic cerebellar disease shows a poorer recovery than the neuropathy and may limit overall improvement.

Mononeuropathies also result from local compression of nerves during periods of obtundation. Radial neuropathy at the spiral groove of the humerus, causing wrist drop, is the classic lesion. The deficit clears spontaneously over days to a few weeks as the pressure-injured axons remyelinate. Foot drop from peroneal compression at the head of the fibula or ulnar neuropathy from compression in the retroepicondylar area of the medial epicondyle is also observed. Spontaneous improvement over the same time course as that of the radial lesion should be expected.

E. **Diabetic neuropathies** take several forms. There is still no specific regimen of management for diabetic neuropathies, but knowledge of these several conditions can help provide guidance for the patient. The principles of general symptom management outlined above should be followed.

1. **Sensorimotor polyneuropathy** causing bilateral foot and hand numbness with or without a painful component is the most common type of diabetic neuropathy. Good blood sugar control is the foundation of management, but neuropathic symptoms may occur regardless.

2. **Femoral neuropathy** or so-called "diabetic amyotrophy" is a distinctive syndrome observed with some frequency in diabetics (see Chap. 25, sec. **II.A**). It often occurs when blood sugar control goes from loose to better as in a change from an oral agent to insulin. The condition presents with spontaneous onset of unilateral pain in the low back, hip, groin, or thigh that can become quite severe over the next few days. Days to a few weeks after onset of the pain, paresthesias and sensory loss appear in the thigh and medial lower leg areas. Weakness of the quadriceps and hip flexor muscles appears about the same time. The weakness may present as a sudden fall as the leg gives out under the patient. Notable atrophy of the quadriceps muscles can occur after the weakness has appeared. The pain is often poorly responsive to analgesics but begins to improve spontaneously within a month or so after onset. The long-term prognosis is good. Occasionally, as the initially involved side is improving the opposite side becomes involved.

3. **Thoracic radiculopathy** is somewhat similar to femoral neuropathy in its time course and circumstances of onset. Unilateral pain begins spontaneously in the chest or upper lumbar region and is bandlike in nature. The pain is persistent and can be severe. There may also be cutaneous hypersensitivity such that clothing produces a very uncomfortable sensation when in contact with the involved area. Localized weakness of the lateral or anterior abdominal muscles may produce localized bulging of the abdominal wall, particularly in the standing position. Analgesics provide mild relief at best. Tricyclic antidepressants may also help ease the intensity of the pain and help the patient sleep. Local anesthetic nerve blocks of the involved der-

matome may help to some degree, as can use of a TENS unit. The pain persists for some months but eventually resolves.

4. **Diabetic polyradiculoneuropathy** is a distinctive syndrome but shares some features with femoral neuropathy and thoracic radiculopathy. This condition often presents at a time of change in the quality of blood sugar control. This change may be from loose to tight or may appear when previous good control becomes loose. Patients may report that they "just got sick." Symptoms appear over weeks to a few months. Patients often complain of loss of appetite and may lose notable amounts of weight. Neuropathic features can include back and flank pain, which can be bilateral, and leg weakness, which is usually proximal. The hip flexors, knee extensors, and adductors can be involved, at times severely, and leave the patient wheelchair-bound. This syndrome has a good long-term prognosis and tends to clear over months. The management regimen is similar to those described for thoracic radiculopathy in sec. **II.E.3** and for weakness in sec. **II.D.**

F. **Lyme disease** can have several types of peripheral neuropathy as manifestations. The bites of certain ticks of the *Ixodes* genus (e.g., *I. ricinus*) transmit the infectious agent *Borrelia burgdorferi*. The characteristic skin lesion erythema chronic migrans develops, as does a general "flulike" syndrome comprised of fever, malaise, and myalgias. The peripheral nerve lesions appear a few weeks to about 2 months later and are present in about one-third of infected patients.

Several different types of neuropathy are observed. The diagnosis of any of these syndromes as being related to Lyme disease depends on the history of the tick bite, the occurrence of the typical skin lesion, and positive serologic testing for antibodies to the infectious agent.

Antibiotic treatment appears to improve all of these manifestations either by shortening the durations of episodes—such as facial palsies—that might have eventually resolved spontaneously or by producing improvement in more persistent symptoms such as polyneuropathies. Oral antibiotics can be used to treat the skin rash and "flulike" phase of the initial stage of the infection, but IV penicillin or ceftriaxone is more appropriate when there is peripheral nerve involvement. Treatment for 10–21 days is the current norm.

1. **Facial neuropathy** produces a typical Bell's palsy syndrome including pain in the ear region. Bilateral involvement occurs more frequently in focal neuropathy than in idiopathic forms.

2. **Thoracic radiculitis** produces a syndrome similar to that described for diabetic neuropathies and consists of dermatomal pain that can reach a significant level of intensity. Sensory loss may occur in the affected dermatomes.

3. **Brachial plexitis** produces clinical features similar to those described in sec. **II.H.**

4. **Mononeuritis multiplex** produces a clinical picture similar to that described in sec. **II.C.**

5. A **symmetric polyneuropathy** that produces only mild distal paresthesias and minor abnormalities on examination can also occur. Patients may show somewhat more impressive NCS abnormalities than the mild clinical picture would suggest.

G. **Human immunodeficiency virus (HIV)** can have several types of peripheral neuropathies within its clinical spectrum.

1. Typical **acute inflammatory demyelinating neuropathy**, or Gullain-Barré syndrome, can occur early in the course of the infection. Cerebrospinal fluid (CSF) pleocytosis is the only feature that usually differentiates this condition from the typical idiopathic variety. Management is the same as for the idiopathic form of the disorder.

2. More bothersome to both the patient and the managing physician is the **generalized neuropathy** with predominant painful sensory symptoms that occurs when AIDS is clinically full-blown. Patients complain of painful paresthesias consisting of pressure- or burning-type sensations. The hands are involved to a lesser extent or spared. Weakness is minimal. CSF tends to be normal to minimally abnormal. Nerve conduction studies show a pattern of axonal damage. Treatment of this type of neuropathy is symptomatic only and not particularly satisfactory. The general guidelines for painful neuropathy presented in sec. **II.A** should be followed.

3. **Polyradiculitis** resulting from infection by **cytomegalovirus (CMV)** is an-

other distinctive neuropathy that affects AIDS patients in the advanced stage of the illness. This is a recognizable neuropathy. Patients complain of unilateral pain and weakness in lower extremities and the back. Within days to weeks, the opposite leg is also involved. Sensory loss develops in the perineal area, as do bladder and bowel incontinence. Progression to arm involvement is infrequent. Spinal fluid shows pleocytosis and elevated protein level. Pathologic specimens show inflammation of the nerve roots of the lumbar and sacral areas.

Treatment with ganciclovir may produce stabilization of the condition, but in general this lesion is a very poor prognostic indicator for survival.

H. **Brachial plexitis,** which is also known as **Parsonage-Turner syndrome** or neuralgic amyotrophy, is easily recognizable retrospectively but can be difficult to differentiate securely from cervical nerve-root compression or intrinsic shoulder disease at presentation or in the early stages of evolution. The upper trunk of the brachial plexus tends to be involved. Brachial plexitis may be idiopathic or may follow infections, immunizations, surgery, or childbirth.

The pain begins unprovoked in the neck, shoulder, or upper arm. It is constant and felt "deep in the bone" and is usually unilateral. The pain intensifies over hours to a few days and is often excruciating. Neck movements do not particularly worsen the pain, but arm or shoulder motions may do so. The patient often chooses to hold the arm quietly adducted to the side and flexed at the elbow. A week or longer after onset, symptoms of sensory loss and weakness appear. The sensory deficits occur in the radial forearm, thumb, and index and middle fingers whereas the weakness tends to be manifested in the deltoid, serratus anterior, biceps, and other shoulder muscles.

Significant atrophy can occur in affected muscles. The pain is poorly responsive to even major analgesics. The pain usually lessens within 3–6 weeks. The sensory loss and weakness improve over months, but long-term deficits may persist. Maintaining range of motion of the shoulder and, if affected, the elbow joint during the period of pain can help ensure a better substrate for recovery. Intrinsic shoulder disease should be evaluated for by joint examination and radiography. Differentiation from a cervical disk syndrome may require imaging studies of the spine. Even though the lesion is presumably inflammatory in nature, drugs such as corticosteroids have shown no definite benefits.

Recommended Readings

Brown MR, et al. Central and peripheral nervous system complications. *Diabetes* 31(suppl 1):65–70, 1982.

Dyck PJ (ed). *Peripheral Neuropathy* (3rd ed). Philadelphia: Saunders, 1993.

Halperin JJ, et al. Lyme disease: Cause of a treatable peripheral neuropathy. *Neurology* 37:1700–1706, 1987.

McKahnn GM. Guillain-Barré syndrome: Clinical and therapeutic observations. *Ann Neurol* 27(suppl):S13–S16, 1990.

Miller RG, et al. The spectrum of peripheral neuropathy with ARC and AIDS. *Muscle Nerve* 11:857–863, 1988.

Van Doorn PA, et al. Intravenous gamma globulin in treatment of patients with chronic inflammatory demyelinating polyneuropathy. *Arch Neurol* 48:217–220, 1991.

47 Myopathies
Raúl N. Mandler

Myopathies are diverse diseases of the skeletal muscles in which striated muscle cells or connective tissue elements may be affected. Myopathies can result from abnormalities of skeletal muscle proteins (Duchenne's muscular dystrophy), alterations of the sarcolemmal Na+ channels (hyperkalemic periodic paralysis), mitochondrial alterations (mitochondrial myopathies), or cell-mediated autoimmune mechanisms (polymyositis), just to name a few examples. Because of the myriad of abnormal mechanisms, treatments vary from one condition to the next. Progress in molecular biology, genetics, and immunology has considerably expanded our understanding of these complicated diseases. This chapter emphasizes current therapeutic approaches to patients with relatively common myopathies.

I. **Idiopathic inflammatory myopathies** are autoimmune diseases characterized by muscle weakness, pain, and fatigue, with inflammatory infiltrates on muscle biopsy. **Polymyositis,** the prototype of inflammatory myopathies, may occur in isolation, accompanying other connective tissue disorders or systemic autoimmune disorders (Crohn's disease, primary biliary cirrhosis, ankylosing spondylitis, Hashimoto's disease, psoriasis, etc.). **Dermatomyositis, inclusion body myositis,** and **polymyalgia rheumatica** comprise the other three major categories of idiopathic inflammatory myopathies. The incidence of these diseases is approximately 1 in 100,000.

A. **Natural history and prognosis**

1. **Polymyositis** usually affects upper and lower girdle muscles in a rather symmetric fashion after the second decade of life. Often, pharyngeal muscles and myocardium are affected. Patients with no family history of muscle weakness suffer from subacute (weeks to months), progressive weakness of deltoid, trapezii, neck flexors and extensors, biceps, triceps, iliopsoas, glutei, quadriceps, and other muscles, in contrast with muscular dystrophy patients, who have family histories and whose progression of weakness is usually measured in years.

Patients characteristically have problems arising from a sitting position, shampooing their hair, or walking up or down stairs. Muscle pain often accompanies the weakness, especially early in the course. Fatigue, weight loss, and malaise are common. Often the syndrome is preceded by an upper respiratory infection. In some cases the disease follows an acute course that can be complicated by myoglobinuria resulting from acute muscle necrosis. Pharyngeal muscle compromise may lead to dysphagia without dysarthria. The tongue is usually spared. Extraocular and facial muscles should not be impaired. Sensation is not affected. Cardiac involvement can occur in up to 40% of cases and can lead to heart failure or arrhythmias. Pulmonary involvement can result from primary weakness of respiratory muscles or from pulmonary interstitial fibrosis.

Polymyositis also occurs in association with connective tissue and systemic autoimmune disorders. Against popular belief, polymyositis does not carry an increased incidence of malignancy, and thus an extensive malignancy work-up is not justified simply because of a diagnosis of polymyositis. Inasmuch as tumors in polymyositis patients have been diagnosed by abnormal findings in medical histories and physical exams, a complete annual physical with pelvic and rectal examinations, urinalysis, CBC, blood chemistry, and chest x-ray should suffice. On the other hand, it appears that dermatomyositis has a higher risk of being accompanied by malignancy.

2. **Dermatomyositis** is characterized by a rash that accompanies or precedes the muscle weakness. The characteristic skin abnormality is the heliotrope rash (purple discoloration of the eyelids) with a red rash on the rest of the face and upper trunk and erythema of the knuckles, in contrast with the erythema of systemic lupus, in which the phalanges are involved and the knuckles are spared. The erythematous rash may also affect elbows, knees, neck, upper chest (V shape), or back and shoulders (shawl sign) and may be photosensitive. Subcutaneous nodular calcifications and dilated capillaries at the bases of the fingernails are rather characteristic. In children the extramuscular manifestations are more frequent. Dermatomyositis usually occurs alone but may be associated with systemic sclerosis, mixed connective tissue disease, other autoimmune conditions, or malignancies. Fascitis and skin changes similar to those found in dermatomyositis may also occur in patients with the eosinophilia-myalgia syndrome secondary to ingestion of contaminated tryptophan.

3. **Inclusion body myositis** characteristically involves distal muscles such as foot extensors and finger flexors. Weakness and atrophy can be asymmetric and selectively involve the quadriceps, simulating the femoral neuropathy or plexopathy observed in patients with diabetes. Often the diagnosis of inclusion body myositis is retrospectively made in patients who had presumptively been diagnosed with polymyositis and who did not benefit from therapy. Inclusion body myositis may also be associated with autoimmune or connective tissue disorders. Familial forms have also been described.

4. **Polymyalgia rheumatica** affects elderly men and women with a peak incidence at 74 years of age. Patients complain of diffuse muscle aching with neck and shoulder stiffness. Pain predominates over weakness or atrophy. Low-grade fever and anemia are found. Approximately 15% of the patients also suffer from temporal arteritis. The incidence of rheumatoid arthritis is also increased. The erythrocyte sedimentation rate (ESR) is elevated to more than 40 mm/h. Despite the severity of the symptoms, muscle biopsy is usually noncontributory.

5. Noninfectious inflammatory myositis also occurs in the contexts of systemic lupus erythematosus, progressive systemic sclerosis, Sjögren's syndrome, rheumatoid arthritis, mixed connective tissue disease, sarcoidosis, hypereosino-philic syndromes, and other disorders.

B. **Diagnosis.** In addition to the clinical features, the diagnosis of inflammatory myopathies is supported by **muscle enzymes, electromyography,** and **muscle biopsy.**

1. **Muscle enzymes.** Creatine kinase is released from the sarcoplasm into the serum following muscle destruction and may be elevated as much as 50-fold in polymyositis. Other muscle enzymes such as lactate dehydrogenase, aldolase, and aminotransferases are commonly elevated. Whereas creatine kinase levels often parallel disease activity, they can be normal in active polymyositis. In inclusion body myositis, creatine kinase may be elevated as much as 10-fold or remain normal. In some patients with active childhood dermatomyositis and in patients with associated connective tissue diseases, creatine kinase levels may be normal.

2. The main value of **electromyography (EMG)** resides in its ability to determine that peripheral neuromuscular weakness originates from the muscle itself and not from denervation or from a defect in neuromuscular transmission. It can also help determine disease activity. The classic EMG findings include short-duration, small-amplitude motor unit potentials (MUPs) and increased membrane irritability signaled by increased insertional activity, fibrillations, and complex-repetitive potentials. These findings should not be considered specific for inflammatory myopathies, because they also can be found in acute toxic/metabolic myopathies and in dystrophies.

3. **Muscle biopsy** helps establish the diagnosis. Light microscopy of paraffin-embedded sections displays inflammatory infiltrates, necrosis, atrophy and regeneration of muscle fibers, and increased amounts of connective tissue in polymyositis.

   In dermatomyositis, the inflammatory infiltrates are present around the vessels or in the interfascicular septa. In polymyositis and inclusion body myositis, the infiltrates are inside the fascicles. In dermatomyositis, blood vessels have hyperplastic endothelia and might be occluded. Group atrophy predominates in dermatomyositis whereas scattered atrophy prevails in polymyositis.

Inclusion body myositis is characterized by basophilic granular inclusions around the edges of vacuoles (rimmed vacuoles). Tissue should be prepared frozen and for electron microscopy, because paraffin processing may dissolve the granules. Muscle biopsy has limitations. Certain drugs (penicillamine and zidovudine) and parasites (toxoplasma, trypanosoma, cysticerci, etc.) may also produce focal or generalized myopathy, which requires differentiation from the idiopathic-autoimmune inflammatory myopathies depicted here. Sometimes biopsies fail to disclose abnormalities expected from the clinical presentation because of sampling errors.

C. Therapy

1. High-dosage prednisone is the initial line of treatment for polymyositis and dermatomyositis. The recommended dosage is 1.0–1.5 mg/kg/day given in a single daily dose before breakfast for 3–4 weeks. The total dosage should not exceed 100 mg. Daily administration should be used until unquestionable muscle strength improvement with recovery of ambulation occurs. In severely ill patients, initial, very high dosages of IV methylprednisolone (250 mg bid for 3–5 days, slowly over 2 hours with monitoring of ECG and potassium) may be required. Then the dosage can be slowly reduced over 10 weeks to 1 mg/kg every other day. If no deterioration occurs, the dosage is further reduced by 5–10 mg every 3–4 weeks until the lowest dosage that controls the disease is reached. The dosage should not be reduced if strength decreases. If treatment is effective, the strength should improve within 3 months. However, most patients may require prednisone for at least 1 year, if not longer. A feeling of well-being and a reduction of enzymes without increase in muscle strength are not sufficient parameters to decide that disease improvement has occurred. If after 3 months of therapy no improvement has been achieved, prednisone should be tapered off and another immunosuppressant medication begun.

   It is imperative that patients become acquainted with the numerous side effects of long-term prednisone treatment in order to better prevent them. Sodium chloride and fluid retention are prevented by a low sodium chloride diet. A low free sugar diet is also important to minimize weight gain. Potassium depletion might require careful monitoring and sometimes replacement. Possible development of hypertension requires systematic monitoring. Aseptic necrosis of the hip, osteoporosis, and bone fractures are major complications. Prevention of osteoporosis requires supplemental calcium gluconate or carbonate (500–1000 mg/day) and calcitriol (0.2–0.5 µg/day) as well as exercise and adequate passive range of motion maneuvers. Calcemia needs to be monitored. Flatulence, abdominal distention, and weight gain are common. Antacids and histamine-2 blockers should be used to prevent peptic ulcers. Periodic eye exams are required for diagnosis of incipient cataracts or glaucoma. Impaired wound healing, hirsutism, acne, moon face, propensity to infections, insomnia, personality changes, headache, dizziness, and diabetes are other important side effects.

   The use of prednisone might produce a steroid myopathy—namely, increased muscle weakness with normal creatine kinase. Distinguishing between worsening of polymyositis and development of steroid myopathy might be difficult. The decision to raise or lower the prednisone dosage needs to be made after careful consideration of the patient's history of muscle strength, mobility, creatine kinase levels, and changes in medications in the preceding months.

2. **Azathioprine** is considered when serious complications preclude the use of steroids, when the disease is not responding to adequate dosages of prednisone, or when it progresses rapidly and is accompanied by respiratory failure. A therapeutic response may take 3–6 months. Azathioprine is usually used in combination with prednisone at lower dosages than those used in prednisone monotherapy. This approach might reduce prednisone-related side effects. Azathioprine can be administered at 2 (up to 3) mg/kg/day for 4–6 months. The initial dosage should be about 50 mg/day with subsequent gradual increase. The total daily dosage should be divided bid or tid and given with meals. Dosage-independent side effects are fever, nausea, rash, and pancreatitis. Dosage-dependent side effects are bone marrow suppres-

sion and liver toxicity. CBC with differential and platelets, as well as liver function tests, should be monitored weekly for the first month and monthly thereafter. Other side effects include anorexia, hair loss, possible development of cancer, and teratogenicity. Concomitant administration of allopurinol is *contraindicated*. Azathioprine should not be used for children.

3. **Methotrexate** (0.5–0.8 mg/kg/week IM or up to 15–25 mg/week PO) is used when azathioprine is ineffective.

4. **High-dosage intravenous gamma globulin** is effective in inflammatory myopathies, including some cases of inclusion body myositis. The recommended dosage is 0.4 g/kg/day given daily for 5 days. The initial rate of treatment should be slow, at 0.01–0.02 ml/kg/min, and then be increased to 0.04 ml/kg/min. Several preparations are available, not all of them biologically equal. Improvement after this therapy might be followed by relapses. Repeated infusions might be required on a monthly basis. In some patients, high-dosage immunoglobulin produces worsening of the syndrome. Side effects include headaches, hypertension, and risk of acute renal failure and myocardial infarction owing to hyperviscosity. Aseptic meningitis as a result of high-dosage gamma globulin might respond to prednisone treatment. IgA-depleted preparations reduce the risk of reactions related to anti-IgA antibodies. Solvent detergent-treated, hepatitis B- and C-free, and HIV-free preparations are a must. Treatments are expensive. In spite of these reservations, high-dosage IV gamma globulin might benefit patients who have been unresponsive to other medications. High-dosage gamma globulin can be administered in outpatient settings such as day treatment units.

5. In refractory cases, especially when interstitial lung disease occurs, cyclophosphamide (1–2 g/square meter monthly, IV) might be required. Side effects include nausea, vomiting, alopecia, hemorrhagic cystitis, teratogenicity, bone marrow suppression, cancerogenesis, and pulmonary fibrosis. Responses to cyclosporine or plasmapheresis have been, in general, disappointing.

6. **Physical therapy** and **adequate diet** should be underscored.

7. In polymyalgia rheumatica, **prednisone** rapidly provides benefits, sometimes within hours. Duration of treatment and dosage need to be individualized and, because patients are elderly, monitored very carefully. In general, a starting dosage of 1 mg/kg/day should be appropriate. In mild cases, nonsteroidal anti-inflammatory agents can be used. In patients suffering from temporal arteritis, corticosteroid treatment may prevent blindness.

D. **Prognosis.** Dermatomyositis and, to a lesser degree, polymyositis are responsive to treatment, whereas inclusion body myositis is usually resistant. Patients with interstitial lung disease may have a high mortality and require treatment with cyclophosphamide. When the treatment of polymyositis is unsuccessful, the patient should be reevaluated and the muscle biopsy reexamined in order to exclude inclusion body myositis or muscular dystrophy of the limb-girdle type. Finally, it is important to underscore the need to evaluate the patient's strength and activities of daily living as measures of improvement, rather than simply adjust treatment on the basis of creatine kinase levels alone.

II. **Viral inflammatory myopathies.** Viruses and retroviruses may produce acute or subacute inflammatory myopathies. Acute viral myosites related to the influenzaviruses and coxsackieviruses are the most common. Viruses can also trigger a subacute polymyositis as in Reye's syndrome. Myopathies can also be associated with the human immunodeficiency virus (HIV) and its treatment with zidovudine (AZT).

A. **Natural history, prognosis, and treatment**

1. **Influenza myositis** presents in children and adults. Children suffer from a brief, febrile illness characterized by myalgias with prodromic fever, malaise, sore throat, and rhinorrhea. Occasionally there is vomiting or myoglobinuria. Strength, which is usually normal, may be difficult to assess because of the pain. A similar syndrome may be related to parainfluenza, respiratory syncytial virus, herpes simplex, or mycoplasma pneumonia. Most laboratory studies are normal, but creatine kinase may be elevated. The prognosis is usually favorable. Treatment consists of bed rest, fluids, and antipyretic agents other than aspirin. In adults the syndrome may be more severe. Cardiopulmonary complications, myoglobinuria, and renal failure may develop. In patients with myoglobinuria, intravenous hydration may be required to prevent acute renal failure.

2. **Coxsackievirus B** produces pleurodynia—epidemic myalgia of Born-holm—accompanied by an inflammatory myopathy. The disease occurs during the summer and fall, and it is contagious through the feces. The hallmark is the abrupt onset of excruciating pain in the lower thorax or abdomen, exacerbated by deep inspirations or coughing. The acute phase improves in a week, but fatigue and muscle pains may persist. Relapses may occur. Laboratory tests are negative and treatment is symptomatic.

3. **Reye's syndrome** is an acute encephalopathy with fatty degeneration of the liver that develops after varicella or influenza infections. This rare condition of children and adolescents begins with repeated vomiting and continues with personality changes, confusion, lethargy, and coma. Mortality is still high. Laboratory metabolic abnormalities relate to acute liver dysfunction. The creatine kinase MM isoenzyme derived from skeletal muscle may be increased 300-fold. The level of creatine kinase correlates with prognosis. Salicylates might precipitate the syndrome. Treatment is supportive.

4. **HIV** may produce a subacute or chronic myopathy early or late in relation to the infection. It has been reported in adults but not in children with HIV. Proximal, symmetric involvement of lower or upper limbs is manifested by weakness with or without atrophy. A concomitant myelopathy or peripheral neuropathy may occur. Serum creatine kinase levels may be elevated 10–15 times. The syndrome is practically identical to polymyositis. Thus, in the work-ups of patients with polymyositis, determination of HIV titers is now recommended. The electrophysiologic and biopsy findings may also be indistinguishable from those of polymyositis.

   a. In advanced AIDS, **HIV wasting syndrome** is characterized by marked disproportion between severe muscle mass loss and weakness, which might be mild or even absent. Creatine kinase is normal. Biopsy shows atrophy of type II fibers—a common, nonspecific finding in cachexia, immobilization, and malnutrition.

   b. **Pyomyositis** is a muscle abscess produced by *Staphylococcus aureus*. It should be suspected in AIDS patients with localized pain and swelling in a muscle, with or without fever or creatine kinase elevation. By examining the muscle with ultrasound, MRI, or contrasted CT, an enhancing lesion, often with fluid density, may be appreciated. Systemic antibiotics and local drainage are used. Predisposing factors may include muscle trauma and hematogenous spread of a bacterial infection, even with negative blood cultures.

   c. **Prognosis and treatment.** Because of the AIDS epidemic and the better management of AIDS patients, the number of individuals affected with AIDS myopathy has increased. Treatment remains empirical. If the myopathy is mild, a nonsteroidal anti-inflammatory agent can be used. Antiretroviral (AZT) therapy might be started if the myopathy progresses.

   d. **Zidovudine (AZT) myopathy** occurs with long-term use of this medication and results from mitochondrial toxicity in skeletal muscle. Patients complain of lower-extremity myalgias and proximal weakness. Creatine kinase elevation further increases after exercise. Symptoms are related to the dosage and duration of AZT treatment, often occurring after 1 year of therapy. The myopathy improves once treatment is discontinued. Differentiation from AIDS myopathy might be difficult solely on a clinical basis. Muscle biopsy demonstrates numerous "ragged red fibers," a sign of mitochondrial disease, and its presence supports the diagnosis of zidovudine myopathy. Electron microscopic examination of the biopsy specimen is very useful in determining mitochondrial damage. Treatment consists of stopping the medication. Nonsteroidal anti-inflammatory agents can be used. Whereas myalgias usually improve within weeks of discontinuing AZT, muscle weakness may persist for months.

III. **Parasitic inflammatory myopathies.** In North America, **trichinosis, cysticercosis,** and **toxoplasmosis** can produce myopathies. The incidence of these diseases has been raised by the AIDS epidemic and by various immunosuppressive treatments and conditions. *Trypanosoma cruzi*, the agent of Chagas' disease, predominates in South America, but a few cases have been detected in the United States, mainly attributable to contaminated blood transfusions.

   A. **Natural history, prognosis, and treatment**

   1. **Toxoplasmosis** is a protozoan infection produced by *Toxoplasma gondii*.

It is contracted by consuming parasited meats or by contact with cat feces. It can also be acquired transplacentally or by blood transfusions. Infections are more severe in patients with AIDS. Myopathy is just one of the manifestations of a systemic infection. The course is progressive, subacute, and clinically indistinguishable from that of idiopathic inflammatory myopathies. Fever, myalgias, lymphadenopathy, and neck pain sometimes occur. Serum creatine kinase is elevated. EMG demonstrates those changes observed in polymyositis. The diagnosis of toxoplasmosis is determined by serologic methods. Muscle biopsy is the definitive test for diagnosing toxoplasma myopathy when tachyzoites or cysts can be identified.

Diagnosing toxoplasma myositis as opposed to other myopathies has significant treatment implications. The treatment of choice is a combination of pyrimethamine and sulfadiazine or trisulfapyrimidines. Pyrimethamine is a folate antagonist, and thus folate should be given to lower the risk of bone marrow suppression.

2. **Cysticercosis** is contracted by eating uncooked pork or as a result of fecal contamination of food and water. This disease is produced by the larva of the intestinal tapeworm *Taenia solium.* It is found in Mexico and the southwestern United States. The disease may occur many years after primary infection. The embryos of the taenia invade many tissues, especially skeletal muscle, CNS, and eye. Involved muscle may present enlarged and painful nodules. Eosinophilia and eosinorrachia are common. Stools for ova and parasites, and serum and cerebrospinal fluid (CSF) antigen detection, assist in the diagnosis. Only muscle biopsy can provide the final diagnosis, when encysted larvae are detected by gross and microscopic inspection and by antigen detection techniques. The muscle pseudohypertrophy is related to the number of larvae present. Calcification of the degenerated cyst is common.

Niclosamide and antibiotic paromomycin have been effective in removing the adult worm. Praziquantel, commonly used in CNS cysticercosis, appears ineffective. Prednisone is used concomitantly to suppress the inflammation. The larvae can also be removed by surgery.

3. **Trichinosis** is caused by the nematode *Trichinella spiralis.* The larvae infiltrate many tissues, often muscle. The incubation period is 2–12 days following ingestion of uncooked pork containing encysted larvae. Often, a prodrome characterized by abdominal pain and diarrhea occurs, followed by fever, myalgias, and proximal muscle tenderness. Examination is remarkable for weakness that can also involve extraocular muscles, intercostal muscles, and the diaphragm. Periorbital swelling and ptosis may be observed. Myalgias reach their peak at the third week of illness. Myocarditis may also occur. EMG shows changes supporting an acute myopathy. Prominent eosinophilia may reach up to 60%. Antibodies against *T. spiralis* by flocculation assay can be detected 3 weeks after the infection. Definite diagnosis is made by identifying the larva in muscle biopsy. An inflammatory, calcified pseudocyst forms in affected muscle.

Albendazole (400 mg tid for 2 weeks) is the drug of choice against the larva and the adult worm. This medication should not be used for children or pregnant women. For patients with weakness, prednisone (1.0–1.5 mg/kg/day) should be used. Prognosis is grave for patients with severe cardiac myositis or encephalitis and those who are immunocompromised.

IV. **Periodic paralyses** are rare disorders characterized by episodes of flaccid muscle weakness that may evolve into paralysis. Attacks usually last for hours. Periodic paralyses are either primary autosomal-dominant disorders or secondary disorders.

A. **Natural history and prognosis**

1. **Primary hypokalemic periodic paralysis** predominates in men. The genetic abnormality is located in chromosome 1, at a gene that codes for the dihydropyridine receptor. This disease affects young and middle-aged people. Attacks usually occur at night. On awakening, patients may be paralyzed and unable to get out of bed. The flaccid paralysis usually spares the respiratory and cranial muscles, but in very severe cases respiration may be compromised. Often, precipitating factors include high carbohydrate consumption and strenuous physical activity. During attacks, the serum potassium decreases. If serum potassium is persistently low, the paralysis may be secondary. Electrocardiography (ECG) may reveal hypokalemic changes, in-

cluding progressive flattening of T waves, depression of ST segment, and appearance of U waves. In some families there is a tendency for the attacks to become more numerous with time. A few patients later develop a chronic myopathy, independent of the severity and frequency of the attacks. EMG does not record normal insertional activity during attacks. The presence of myotonia virtually rules out the diagnosis of hypokalemic periodic paralysis.

2. **Secondary hypokalemic periodic paralysis**
   a. **Thyrotoxic periodic paralysis** occurs 70 times more often in males than in females 20–40 years of age, in spite of the increased prevalence of hyperthyroidism in women. In nearly all cases, the condition is sporadic and the attacks cease when thyroid function is normalized.
   b. **Periodic paralyses secondary to urinary or gastrointestinal potassium loss** may result from primary hyperaldosteronism, excessive thiazide therapy, excessive mineralocorticoid therapy for Addison's disease, renal tubular acidosis, the recovery phase of diabetic coma, sprue, laxative abuse, villous adenoma of the rectum, or prolonged gastrointestinal intubation or vomiting.

3. **Primary hyperkalemic periodic paralysis** produces episodic attacks of weakness accompanied by elevations in serum potassium (up to 5–6 mM/l). It is often associated with myotonia (inability to relax the muscle) or paramyotonia (muscle stiffness worsened by exercise or cold that gives way to flaccid paralysis) and is inherited in an autosomal-dominant fashion. The genetic abnormality has been mapped to chromosome 17, linked to the sodium channel gene, which encodes for the alpha-subunit of the tetrodotoxin-sensitive (adult) sodium channel.

   Attacks occur in the first decade of life, usually in the morning before breakfast, and last 20 to 60 minutes. Rest, potassium salts, cold, and stress provoke attacks. Sustained mild exercise may prevent attacks. Ventricular and supraventricular cardiac arrhythmias are dangerous accompanying conditions and require careful monitoring and therapy.

   Pathogenically, the abnormal sodium channel of the sarcolemma fails to inactivate. Incomplete inactivation caused by abnormalities of the inactivation gate leads to a sustained influx of sodium, which results in sustained membrane depolarization. Simultaneously, the potassium leaves the sarcoplasma and increases in the serum.

B. **Prevention and therapeutic approach**
   1. **Primary hypokalemic periodic paralysis.** Low carbohydrate ingestion and avoidance of strenuous exercise prevent attacks. Mild attacks may not require treatment. For attacks of general paralysis, 0.25 mEq/kg of potassium chloride by mouth in an unsweetened 10–25% solution is the preferable therapy. The dose should be repeated every 30 minutes until the weakness improves. Muscle strength usually recovers within ½–1 hour. Patients are encouraged to exercise mildly. Carbohydrate-containing foods and IV fluids should be avoided. IV potassium *is not* recommended because of the danger of producing uncontrollable hyperkalemia and should be avoided as much as possible. However, if repeated vomiting precludes the administration of oral salts, IV potassium can be used carefully with serial ECG monitoring and serum potassium determinations. Potassium dosage should be adjusted in patients with renal disease. Intravenous KCl can be administered in a 5% mannitol solution (20–40 mEq/L) or by bolus (0.05–0.10 mEq/kg). Glucose and saline diluents should be avoided. Gastrointestinal irritation may occur with oral administration, and phlebitis may accompany IV administration.

      For prevention of attacks, acetazolamide is the drug of choice at a low starting dosage of 125 mg every other day, which can be raised to 250 mg tid. Side effects include increased incidence of nephrolithiasis, paresthesia, anorexia, and metallic taste. Dichlorphenamide, another carbonic anhydrase inhibitor, may be used when acetazolamide fails. The dosage is 25 mg tid. In severe cases, patients should be put on a low-salt diet and be given the aldosterone antagonist spironolactone (100 mg bid) or triamterene (150 mg/day). Both drugs promote renal potassium retention, sodium depletion, and mild acidosis. Supplemental potassium treatment is *contraindicated* with the latter two medications. Diazoxide and verapamil have also been used in refractory cases.

   2. **Thyrotoxic periodic paralysis.** Control of euthyroid status is imperative.

Potassium chloride by mouth can be used for the treatment of acute attacks, and a low-carbohydrate, low-sodium diet may prevent attacks until the patient becomes euthyroid. Acetazolamide is ineffective, sometimes making the disease worse. Propranolol (40 mg qid) and other beta-adrenergic blocking agents may prevent attacks, possibly by suppressing the adrenergic overactivity induced by hyperthyroidism.

3. **Primary hyperkalemic periodic paralysis.** Preventive measures consist of frequent meals rich in carbohydrates, low-potassium diet, avoidance of fasting, strenuous work, or exposure to cold. Slight exercise or the ingestion of carbohydrates at the onset of weakness may prevent or abort attacks. Staying in bed longer may precipitate attacks. Patients are advised to rise early and have a full breakfast.

   Thiazide diuretic, acetazolamide, or inhalation of a beta-adrenergic agent (metaproterenol or salbutamol) may abort the attack.

   For chronic preventive therapy, a thiazide diuretic or acetazolamide is recommended at the lowest possible dosage (hydrochlorothiazide, 25 mg every other day).

V. **Muscular dystrophies** are chronic, hereditary myopathies characterized by a progressive course and characteristic histologic abnormalities. Recent developments in the field of molecular genetics have widened our understanding of the pathophysiologies of many dystrophies. The most important dystrophies are **X-linked dystrophinopathies,** which include **Duchenne's** and **Becker's muscular dystrophies,** and **autosomal-dominant facioscapulohumeral, myotonic, limbgirdle, oculopharyngeal,** and **progressive ophthalmoplegic muscular dystrophies.**

A. **Natural history and prognosis**

1. **Dystrophinopathies** are recessive disorders caused by a mutation in the short arm, locus 21, of the X chromosome, in the enormous gene that codes for the protein **dystrophin.** Dystrophin is a filamentous protein present in striated and cardiac muscle and other tissues. Although the role of dystrophin has not yet been firmly established, anchoring and structural functions have been proposed for this protein. In the most severe dystrophinopathy— **Duchenne's muscular dystrophy**—practically no dystrophin is detected in skeletal muscle by immunohistochemistry. In milder allelic forms, phenotypically denominated **Becker's muscular dystrophy,** some muscle fibers express dystrophin, which might be structurally abnormal. Practically all patients with dystrophinopathies are male. Often the disease is caused by spontaneous mutations, which are more common than in other genetic disorders, probably because of the large size of the gene.

   a. **Duchenne's muscular dystrophy** affects children who have noticeable difficulties in walking early in life. Motor developmental delay may be noticeable after the first year, but disease is already present, because muscle necrosis and serum enzyme elevation can be found in neonates. Onset of walking may be delayed past 15 months of age. Signs might usually be recognized before the age of 5 years, including difficulties in running and climbing stairs. Lower-extremity, lower trunk, and pelvic muscles are affected first. Children develop hyperlordosis with prominent abdomen and calf pseudohypertrophy. Tiptoe walking is common. Progression is fast. In order to stand up from the floor, patients employ their hands (Gowers' sign). Joint contractures of the iliotibial bands, hip flexors, and heel cords develop in most patients 6–9 years of age. By the age of 10, many of these patients lose the ability to walk or stand, and become dependent on a wheelchair. By the midteens they lose upper-extremity function. Mental retardation occurs in 10% of cases. The disease is usually fatal by the end of the second decade. Death is usually related to pulmonary infections, respiratory failure, gastrointestinal complications, or cardiomyopathy. About 8% of female carriers have myopathies of the limb-girdle type. A small number of carriers may also suffer from isolated cardiomyopathy.

      Diagnosis of Duchenne's muscular dystrophy can be confirmed by an *absence* of dystrophin immunostaining in the muscle biopsy. DNA analysis in blood leukocytes using the polymerase chain reaction (PCR) technique is abnormal in more than two-thirds of Duchenne's patients. Prenatal diagnosis from chorionic villi is also feasible. Fast screening is done by measuring serum creatine kinase, which is markedly elevated in patients (up to the thousands or tens of thousands of units) and is also elevated in female carriers. With the advent of molecular diagnosis and in cases with documented family histories, muscle biopsy might not be required as much as in the past. In less-documented cases, muscle biopsy might be very useful in distinguishing this severe disease from others presenting similarly but carrying favorable prognoses (congenital myopathies of the nemaline and central core types, for example). Muscle biopsies in Duchenne's patients display abnormal variations in fiber size, fiber splitting, central nuclei, and replacement by fat and fibrous tissues. Dystrophin immunostaining in muscle biopsy is now commonly used to differentiate benign from malignant myopathies. Because of worsening caused by immobilization, it might be preferable to obtain the biopsy from mildly involved rectus abdominis rather than from the gastrocnemius or deltoid muscles. An EMG done early in the course of the disease shows findings compatible with a myopathy. Later, the number of motor units that are activated decreases and tissue may even become unexcitable.

   b. **Becker's muscular dystrophy** is a milder variety of dystrophinopathy, in terms of severity and molecular abnormalities. Patients may live up to many decades with mild to moderate symptoms, which can be indistinguishable from those of limb-girdle dystrophies. Onset is usually after 12 years of age. Calf pain during exercise, myoglobinuria, and creatine kinase elevation are common findings.

2. **Emery-Dreifuss muscular dystrophy** is an X-linked disease mapping at band Xq28 and characterized by early onset of elbow and ankle contractures followed by weakness and atrophy of humeroperoneal muscles. This disease has a longer course than the dystrophinopathies. Cardiac involvement is common. Patients suffer from conduction defects, bradycardias, and heart blocks, which can lead to syncope or sudden death. Early recognition of this disease might be lifesaving because timed insertion of a pacemaker may prevent a fatal conduction defect. The defective gene, when normal, codes for a protein named **emerin,** which is expressed in skeletal muscle and myocardium. The function of this protein is still unknown.

3. **Facioscapulohumeral (FSH) muscular dystrophy** is an autosomal-dominant disease that has high penetrance and usually better prognosis than Duchenne's and that affects both males and females starting before the age of 30. The gene for FSH maps to the telomere of chromosome 4. Neither the gene nor its product has yet been defined. Clinically, facial muscles, including the orbicularis oculi, orbicularis oris, and zygomaticus, are affected early, but the disease onset is often hard to establish, so that abnormal features may be taken to be nothing more than family traits. Masseter, temporalis, and extraocular muscles are not involved. Bell's phenomenon and drooping of the lower lip are noticeable. Patients may be unable to whistle. FSH also involves the trapezii, rhomboids, and serratus anterior scapular musculature. Scapular winging is maximized with forward movement because of serratus anterior weakness. Deltoid function and rotator cuff muscles are better preserved, whereas the pectoralis is very atrophic. Patients seek medical attention because of the involvement of the shoulder rather than of the facial muscles. If patients are not disrobed, the diagnosis can be easily missed. Lower-extremity weakness, especially of the anterolateral leg compartment, is found later in the disease. This disorder has wide phenotypic variability, even within the same family. Some patients remain ambulatory all their lives, whereas others become wheelchair-dependent, suffer from marked kyphoscoliosis, and die from respiratory insufficiency or infections. The heart is usually spared. Not uncommonly, atrophy and weakness are asymmetric. Truncal weakness may also occur.

4. **Oculopharyngeal muscular dystrophy** is an autosomal-dominant disease of late onset that occurs in certain ethnic groups including Jewish Americans, French Canadians, and Hispanic Americans from New Mexico and Colorado. This syndrome is manifested by ptosis, progressive dysphagia, rimmed vacuoles in muscle biopsy, and tubulofilamentous inclusions within the striated muscle cell nucleus. Differential diagnosis includes myasthenia gravis and oculocraniosomatic diseases with ragged red fibers (Kearns-

Sayre syndrome), which are mitochondrial myopathies characterized by slowly progressive involvement of extraocular musculature, proximal myopathy, peripheral neuropathy, and cardiomyopathy.

5. **Limb-girdle muscular dystrophies** comprise a heterogeneous collection of both autosomal-recessive and autosomal-dominant disorders that affect pelvic and upper girdle muscles and spare the face, with onset between the first and fourth decades. Molecular genetics and diagnostic techniques have confirmed the heterogeneity of these disorders, with mutations having been found in at least two different loci (chromosomes 5q and 15q). These diseases progress more slowly than Duchenne's.

6. **Myotonic dystrophy** is the most common muscular dystrophy in adults. Rather than being restricted to the skeletal muscle, it usually represents a multisystemic, autosomal-dominant disorder with varied expression, which may also involve the pancreas, gonads, thyroid, myocardium, and brain. Autosomal-dominant myotonic dystrophy is produced by a defective gene in chromosome 19 (19q13.2–13.3) that codes for myotonin protein-kinase, a ubiquitous enzyme related to protein phosphorylation. The generalized disorder may be explained by the wide distribution of the enzyme. The molecular gene defect is characterized by excessive triple repeats (triplet repeat amplification) of guanine-cytosine-thymine. The length of the repeat is directly correlated with the severity of the disease and inversely correlated with the date of onset.

   a. **Muscle features.** Weakness of facial muscles is typical. The face is hatched and thin, with early frontal balding. Ptosis is present but is not as severe as in myasthenia gravis or Kearns-Sayre syndrome. Temporalis and masseter atrophy is characteristic. Sternocleidomastoid weakness is out of proportion with shoulder and posterior neck muscles. Limb involvement is predominantly distal and late in appearing. Proximal limb muscles are usually preserved until the late stages. Thus, unlike patients with other dystrophies, myotonic dystrophy patients usually remain ambulatory. Myotonia is the delay of muscle relaxation after contraction. Often, myotonia is simply a sign that does not elicit complaints. Seldom do patients complain of stiffness. Myotonia can be elicited by percussion on the thenar eminence or tongue. Patients often demonstrate inability to release the grip after a handshake. Repetitive muscle contractions diminish the myotonia (true myotonia). Clinical diagnosis is supported by the presence of myotonic discharges on the EMG. Molecular diagnosis by the PCR technique can detect the triple repeat expansion.

   b. **Generalized features.** Many patients have predominant systemic symptoms rather than neuromuscular symptoms. These patients may never be diagnosed with myotonic dystrophy. Failure to diagnose the disease may jeopardize patients' good medical and preventive care. Common abnormalities include cataracts, tubular testicular atrophy, heart block, and arrhythmias, which can cause sudden death. Whereas severe cardiac arrhythmias may occur in phenotypically mild cases, cardiomyopathy is rare. Constipation and cholelithiasis are related to smooth muscle involvement. Diaphragmatic involvement produces hypoventilation. Hypersomnia is common. Because of the cardiorespiratory compromise, patients are susceptible to complications during surgery and anesthesia. Myotonia can increase with depolarizing relaxants. Opiates and barbiturates may induce respiratory failure. Unfortunately, the diagnosis of myotonic dystrophy is sometimes established only after cardiopulmonary complications secondary to general anesthesia have occurred. Mild mental retardation, apathy, and lethargy are not uncommon.

   Congenital myotonic dystrophy is the more severe form that is present since birth. These neonates display bilateral facial weakness, hypotonia, mental retardation, respiratory distress, hydramnios, and reduced fetal movements. The abnormal gene is transmitted exclusively through maternal inheritance.

B. **Prevention.** For the **dystrophinopathies** (Duchenne's and Becker's), preventive measures comprise prenatal diagnosis, carrier detection, and genetic counseling. Pedigree analysis, serum creatine kinase determination, and clinical, routine histologic and electromyographic studies are now complemented by dystrophin analysis in muscle biopsy, PCR analysis of heterozygotes, and restriction fragment length polymorphism analysis. Fetal abnormalities can be detected using molecular techniques in samples of chorionic villi during early pregnancy (after 8 weeks) or by amniocentesis. Muscle biopsy from fetus for dystrophin immunostaining can be obtained after 19 weeks of gestation with ultrasound guidance. A known carrier has one chance in two of giving birth to a Duchenne's boy or to a carrier female. About one-third of patients, however, do not have family histories.

For **myotonic dystrophy,** slit-lamp examination, insulin levels, ECG, prenatal care, and thorough cardiopulmonary assessment before surgical procedures can diminish the rate of complications.

C. **Therapeutic approach**

1. **Duchenne's muscular dystrophy**

   a. **Family and patient education** is of utmost relevance. The disease creates major distress in all aspects of family life. Not only the emotional stress but also the physical and financial limitations imposed by needing to transport and take care of the patient may become insurmountable. The goal is to keep the child ambulatory and functioning at home and at school. If no mental retardation is present, the child can start attending normal school. Physical adjustments will be needed to compensate for lack of ambulation and for upper-extremity weakness.

   b. **Physical therapy** is used to preserve mobility and to prevent early contractures, which are common in flexor muscles of hips, knees, and ankles. Passive range of motion exercises and adequate orthotics may prolong ambulation, but do not stop disease progression. Exercises may be useful in diminishing the risk of obesity, which further impairs ambulation and respiratory function. If patients can no longer walk, they are asked to stand at least 3 hours/day in divided periods. Bed rest is avoided, because weakness may become permanent. Excessive exercise, however, may be detrimental. Once patients can no longer ambulate without assistance, braces, crutches, or surgical procedures are used. Splints can keep the joints in neutral position and are used at night. When the patient becomes chair-bound, contractures and scoliosis worsen. Benefits of scoliosis surgery should be thoroughly counterbalanced against the potential risks of the procedure and anesthesia. The technique of segmental spinal stabilization of Luque is the method of choice. In general, surgery is used when the scoliosis evolves rapidly in combination with restrictive ventilatory failure, and when the scoliosis has not yet reached 40 degrees. Patients with Duchenne's muscular dystrophy are at high risk for side effects of general anesthesia. Succinylcholine or halothane should not be used, because patients may develop episodes that resemble malignant hyperthermia. Adverse effects may be reduced by using nondepolarizing muscle relaxants.

   c. **Respiratory therapy.** Breathing exercises or playing wind instruments may improve the quality of life. In the late stages, intermittent positive pressure ventilation is useful, especially when very advanced patients retain CO_2 and start suffering from nightmares. Good pulmonary exercises may reduce the propensity for pulmonary infections.

   d. **Medications.** Prednisone (0.75 mg/kg/day) is recommended only for special situations, such as very acute deterioration. Prednisone can improve neuromuscular strength after 1 month of treatment. The maximum effect is reached by 3 months. Benefits should outweigh possible side effects, which include insomnia, difficult behavior, and gastrointestinal symptoms. In controlled studies, benefits lasted for 3 years. A low-sodium, low-fat diet should be administered to prevent weight gain. Zoster immunoglobulin should be given if the child becomes exposed to chicken pox.

   e. **Gene therapy** is still experimental. Myoblast transplant therapy has succeeded in the *mdx* mouse model but so far has failed in patients. Gene therapy administered through viral vectors or liposomes is presently being tested in animal models.

   f. **Becker's muscular dystrophy** follows similar principles, as in Duchenne's. In mild cases, thorough follow-up with prevention of complications may suffice.

2. **Emery-Dreifuss muscular dystrophy** requires careful evaluation of the

heart and timely implantation of a pacemaker in many cases in order to prevent fatal arrhythmias.

3. **Facioscapulohumeral muscular dystrophy.** Physical therapy is empirically recommended. Posterior plastic ankle orthotics can correct foot drop. A motorized wheelchair with adjustable height control is invaluable for nonambulatory patients. In such patients, a brace may provide help for the excessive lumbar lordosis and prominent abdomen.

4. In **oculopharyngeal muscular dystrophy,** mild ptosis can be easily treated by the use of special glasses with props. In more severe cases, blepharoplasty with resection of the levator palpebrae may be required. The dysphagia may improve with cricopharyngeal myotomy.

5. In **limb-girdle dystrophies,** the main therapeutic objectives are the general premises described in sec. **V.C.1.**

6. In **myotonic dystrophy,** only when myotonia is disabling or bothersome, phenytoin (100 mg PO tid) can alleviate the myotonia with reasonable efficacy and relatively low risk. Quinine sulfate and procainamide can impair cardiac conduction, because they prolong the PR interval. In general, myotonic dystrophy patients do not complain much about the myotonia. The main goals are prevention and treatment of the systemic disease.

VI. **Metabolic myopathies** constitute a large, heterogeneous group of acquired and inherited disorders whose common denominator is a metabolic alteration. **Endocrine myopathies, malignant hyperthermia, acid maltase deficiency, McArdle's disease,** and **carnitine-O-palmitoyltransferase deficiency** will be reviewed.

A. **Natural history, prognosis, and treatment**
1. **Endocrine myopathies**
   a. **Thyrotoxic myopathy** presents with weakness and little muscle wasting. Fatigue and heat intolerance are also present. Bulbar and respiratory involvement may occur. Hypokalemic periodic paralysis (see sec. **IV.A.2.a**) and myasthenia gravis are associated with hyperthyroidism and should be included in the differential diagnosis. Treatment relies on correcting the hyperthyroid state. Beta-adrenergic blocking agents may be of help. Glucocorticoids should be used in the thyroid storm to block the peripheral conversion of T4 in T3.

   b. **Hypothyroid myopathy** presents with enlarged muscles, weakness, painful cramps, myoedema, and slow-recovery reflexes. This disease is more common in women. Rhabdomyolysis or respiratory muscle involvement may be present. Serum creatine kinase may be elevated. The diagnosis is supported by abnormal thyroid function tests. Treatment is to restore the euthyroid state.

   c. **Steroid myopathy** is characterized by proximal weakness and wasting that are worse in the lower extremities, difficulties in climbing stairs, and normal creatine kinase. If iatrogenic, the weakness reverses on discontinuation of steroid treatment. Fluorinated corticosteroids, such as dexamethasone and triamcinolone, have more myopathic potential. EMG reveals normal insertional activity and no spontaneous activity. Treatment includes dosage reduction to the lowest possible therapeutic level, conversion to a nonfluorinated steroid, and alternate-dose therapy. However, improvement may take weeks to months. Adequate diet and exercise should help the recovery.

2. **Malignant hyperthermia** is a severe syndrome observed during general anesthesia and characterized by rapid elevation in body temperature resulting from a fast, uncontrolled increase in skeletal muscle metabolism associated with rhabdomyolysis, and high mortality. This syndrome is a result of an autosomal-dominant susceptibility to general anesthesia, especially to halothane or succinylcholine. Body temperature may climb to 43°C with marked metabolic acidosis, tachycardia, muscle rigidity, disseminated intravascular coagulation, coma, areflexia, and death. Creatine kinase rises precipitously, sometimes to 10,000 times the normal values. Myoglobinuria, elevation of various muscle enzymes, and release of muscle potassium are observed also.

   a. **Prognosis** is guarded. Recognition of the syndrome is important in instrumenting rapid treatment, which can diminish the mortality. The pathogenesis is related to the malfunction of the calcium channel of the sarcoplasmic reticulum (the **ryanodine** receptor). The abnormal ryanodine receptor may accentuate calcium release. The gene for the ryanodine receptor maps to chromosome 19 (13-1). Malignant hyperthermia can occur in association with dystrophinopathies and central core-congenital myopathy.

b. **Neuroleptic malignant syndrome (NMS)** also presents with high fever, rigidity, tachycardia, and rhabdomyolysis. However, it has a slower onset, over days to weeks, it is not familial, and it usually is triggered by drugs that block central dopaminergic pathways, such as phenothiazines, lithium, and haldol, or can occur after discontinuation of L-dopa for Parkinson's disease.

c. **Prevention** includes early diagnosis of impending malignant hyperthermia when symptoms are still few, such as isolated trismus. Greater recognition of the syndrome by anesthesiologists and the availability of dantrolene have reduced morbidity and mortality. The use of barbiturate, nitrous oxide, and opiate–nondepolarizing relaxant anesthesias should not induce malignant hyperthermia.

d. **Treatment** of malignant hyperthermia depends on the severity, which is often related to the dosage and duration of the anesthesia. For mild cases, discontinuation of anesthesia may suffice. In more severe cases, correction of acid-base disturbance should be rapidly implemented in order to save the patient's life. Ventilation should be increased and IV sodium bicarbonate (2–4 mg/kg) given. Cooling blankets and cold IV fluids should be used until the temperature reaches 38°C. Volume loading and diuretics are necessary in the presence of myoglobinuria. Steroids are given for the acute stress reaction. Dantrolene is the specific therapy because it inhibits the calcium release from the sarcoplasmic reticulum. It should be used at 2 mg/kg IV q5min, up to 10 mg/kg, and should correct the associated hyperkalemia. The administration of calcium to correct the hyperkalemia should *not* be undertaken.

3. **Acid maltase deficiency** is an autosomal-recessive glycogen storage disease caused by a deficiency in lysosomal alpha-glucosidase, which normally participates in the metabolism of glycogen into glucose. The infantile form is called Pompe's disease, a generalized glycogenesis with severe cardiomyopathy. Milder cases with little or no heart disease may occur in adults. The genetic abnormality maps to chromosome 17. Infants with Pompe's disease suffer from hypotonia, macroglossia, cardiomegaly, and hepatomegaly. Usually the disease is rapidly fatal. Adults suffer from a slowly progressive myopathy with respiratory failure. Diaphragm, biceps, shoulder, and thigh adductor muscles are preferentially affected. Myotonic discharges can be found electrically, but patients usually do not have myotonia. Vacuolar myopathy with high glycogen content is conspicuous. The diagnosis is confirmed by leukocyte or urine acid maltase determination. Prenatal diagnosis can be established by chorionic villi biopsy. At the present, no specific therapy is available. Inspiratory exercises can be of use.

4. **McArdle's disease,** or myophosphorylase deficiency, affects children and adults who complain of exercise intolerance with myalgia, fatigue and muscle stiffness, myoglobinuria, renal failure, wasting, and seizures. Some patients can tolerate their deficits and learn to avoid the brief, strong exercises that precipitate attacks. Usually cramps and myoglobinuria develop during adulthood. Creatine kinase is increased. EMG shows changes supportive of a myopathy. The forearm ischemic exercise causes no increase in venous lactate. The disease is autosomal-recessive. The gene for muscle phosphorylase maps to chromosome 11. Prognosis is rather benign. Muscle biopsy discloses subsarcolemmal deposits of glycogen at the periphery. The histochemical reaction of the phosphorylase can confirm the diagnosis by being undetectable in patients with McArdle's disease. Experimental therapies with diets and branched-chain amino acids have been tried, but no definite treatment is yet available.

5. **Carnitine-*O*-palmitoyltransferase deficiency** also presents intermittently with cramps, myalgias, and myoglobinuria. Renal failure resulting from myoglobinuria, and respiratory failure, may ensue. During attacks, muscle strength is normal. The symptoms are precipitated by exertion. The capacity to perform short, demanding exercise is not impaired. Patients have no

warnings of the attacks, which usually follow prolonged exercise. Fasting, exposure to cold, high fat intake, viral infections, and general anesthesia can precipitate rhabdomyolysis. The disease is autosomal-recessive. The abnormal gene maps to chromosome 1. Creatine kinase is normal. No specific therapy is available.

Recommended Readings

Askari AD, Huettner TL. Cardiac abnormalities in polymyositis/dermatomyositis. *Semin Arthritis Rheum* 12:208–219, 1982.

Banker BQ, Victor M. Dermatomyositis (systemic angiopathy) of childhood. *Medicine* 45:261–289, 1966.

Brooke MH. *A Clinician's View of Neuromuscular Diseases.* Baltimore: Williams & Wilkins, 1986.

Brooke MH, et al. Duchenne muscular dystrophy: Patterns of clinical progression and effects of supportive therapy. *Neurology* 39:475–481, 1989.

Dalakas MC (ed). *Polymyositis and Dermatomyositis.* Boston: Butterworths, 1988.

Dalakas MC. Polymyositis, dermatomyositis, and inclusion-body myositis. *N Engl J Med* 325:1487–1498, 1991.

Dalakas MC, et al. Mitochondrial myopathy caused by long-term zidovudine therapy. *N Engl J Med* 322:1098–1105, 1990.

Dubowitz V, Brooke MH. *Muscle Biopsy: A Modern Approach.* Philadelphia: Saunders, 1973.

Ebers GC, et al. Paramyotonia congenita and hyperkalemic periodic paralysis are linked to the adult muscle sodium channel gene. *Ann Neurol* 30:810–816, 1991.

Emery AEH. *Duchenne Muscular Dystrophy* (2nd ed). New York: Oxford University Press, 1993.

Emery AEH, Dreifuss FE. Unusual type of benign X-linked muscular dystrophy. *J Neurol Neurosurg Psychiat* 29:338–342, 1966.

Engel AG. Acid maltase deficiency in adults. Studies in four cases of a syndrome which may mimic muscular dystrophy or other myopathies. *Brain* 93:599–616, 1970.

Engel AG, Emslie-Smith AM. Inflammatory myopathies. *Curr Opin Neurol Neurosurg* 2:695–710, 1989.

Engel AG, Franzini-Armstrong C (eds). *Myology* (2nd ed). New York: McGraw-Hill, 1994.

Fischbeck KH. The mechanism of myotonic dystrophy. *Ann Neurol* 35:255–256, 1994.

Greenlee JE, et al. Adult toxoplasmosis presenting as polymyositis and cerebellar ataxia. *Ann Intern Med* 82:367–371, 1975.

Griggs RC. Periodic paralysis. In JD Wilson, et al (eds), *Harrison's Principles of Internal Medicine* (12th ed). New York: McGraw-Hill, 1991. P 2121.

Griggs RC, Mendell JR, Miller RG. *Evaluation and Treatment of Myopathies.* Philadelphia: Davis, 1995.

Griggs RC, et al. Cardiac conduction in myotonic dystrophy. *Am J Med* 59:37–42, 1975.

Griggs RC, et al. Prednisone in Duchenne dystrophy. A randomized, controlled trial defining the time course and dose response. *Arch Neurol* 48:383–388, 1991.

Griggs RC, et al. Genetics of facioscapulohumeral muscular dystrophy: New mutations in sporadic cases. *Neurology* 43:2369–2372, 1993.

Hoffman EP, Brown RH, Kunkel LM. Dystrophin: The protein product of the Duchenne muscular dystrophy locus. *Cell* 51:919–928, 1987.

Hoffman EP, Fischbeck KH, Brown RH. Characterization of dystrophin in muscle-biopsy specimens from patients with Duchenne's muscular dystrophy. *N Engl J Med* 318:1363–1368, 1988.

Jablecki CK. Myopathies. In WF Brown, CF Bolton (eds), *Clinical Electromyography* (2nd ed). Boston: Butterworth-Heinemann, 1993. Pp 653–689.

Karpati G, Carpenter S. Idiopathic inflammatory myopathies. *Curr Opin Neurol Neurosurg* 1:806–818, 1988.

Kearns TP, Sayre GP. Retinitis pigmentosa, external ophthalmoplegia, and complete heart block. *Arch Ophthal* 60:280–287, 1958.

Lange DJ. Neuromuscular diseases associated with HIV-1 infection. *Muscle Nerve* 17:16–30, 1994.

Lotz BP, et al. Inclusion body myositis. Observations in 40 patients. *Brain* 112:727–747, 1989.

Rowland LP, Layzer RB, DiMauro S. Pathophysiology of metabolic muscle disorders. In AK Asbury, GM McKhann, WI McDonald (eds), *Disease of the Nervous System.* Philadelphia: Saunders, 1986. Pp 197–207.

Srinivasan AV, et al. Neuroleptic malignant syndrome. *J Neurol Neurosurg Psychiat* 53:514–516, 1990.

Victor M, Hayes R, Adams RD. Oculopharyngeal muscular dystrophy: A familial disease of late life characterized by dysphagia and progressive ptosis of the eyelids. *N Engl J Med* 267:1267–1272, 1962.

Walton JN (ed). *Disorders of Voluntary Muscle.* New York: Churchill-Livingstone, 1981.

48

Neuromuscular Junction Abnormalities

Robert M. Pascuzzi

I. Myasthenia gravis (MG) is an autoimmune disorder of neuromuscular transmission involving the production of autoantibodies directed against the nicotinic acetylcholine receptors. Acetylcholine receptor antibodies are detectable in the serum of 80–90% of patients with MG. The prevalence of MG is about 1 in 10,000–20,000. Women are affected about twice as often as men. Symptoms may begin at virtually any age, with a peak for women in the second and third decades and a peak for men in the fifth and sixth decades. Associated autoimmune diseases such as rheumatoid arthritis, lupus, and pernicious anemia are present in about 5% of patients. Thyroid disease occurs in about 10%, often in association with antithyroid antibodies. About 10–15% of MG patients have thymomas, and thymic lymphoid hyperplasia with proliferation of germinal centers occurs in 50–70% of cases.

A. Clinical manifestations

1. The hallmark of MG is **fluctuating or fatigable weakness.**
2. **Presenting symptoms.** Ocular symptoms are common, with 25% of patients initially presenting with diplopia, 25% presenting with ptosis, and, by 1 month into the course of the illness, 80% having some degree of ocular involvement. Other presenting symptoms are bulbar disorders (dysarthria or dysphagia) in 10% of patients, leg weakness (impaired walking) in 10%, and generalized weakness in 10%. Respiratory failure is the presenting symptom in 1% of cases.
3. Patients usually complain of symptoms resulting from focal muscle dysfunctions, such as diplopia, ptosis, dysarthria, dysphagia, inability to work with the arms raised over the head, and disturbance of gait. In contrast, patients with MG tend *not* to complain of "generalized weakness," "generalized fatigue," "sleepiness," or muscle pain.
4. In the classic case, fluctuating weakness worsens with exercise and improves with rest. Symptoms tend to progress later in the day. Many different factors can precipitate or aggravate weakness, such as physical stress, emotional stress, infection, or exposure to medications that impair neuromuscular transmission (perioperative succinylcholine and aminoglycoside antibiotics).

B. Diagnosis

1. A history of **fluctuating weakness** with corroborating findings on examination remains the basis for clinical diagnosis.
2. **Edrophonium (Tensilon) test.** The most immediate and readily accessible confirmatory study is the edrophonium test.
   a. To perform the test, choose one or two weak muscles to judge. Ptosis, dysconjugate gaze, and other cranial deficits provide the most reliable endpoints.
   b. Use a setting in which hypotension, syncope, or respiratory failure can be managed, because patients occasionally decompensate during the test. If the patient has severe dyspnea, do not perform the test until the airway is secure. Start an IV.
   c. Have IV atropine (0.4 mg) readily available in the event of bradycardia or extreme GI side effects.
   d. Edrophonium (10 mg, or 1 ml) is drawn up into a syringe, and 1 mg (0.1 ml) is given as a test dose while checking the patient's heart rate (to ensure the patient is not supersensitive to the drug). If no untoward side effects occur after 1 minute, another 3 mg is given. Many MG patients show improved power within 30–60 seconds of administration of the initial

4 mg, at which point the test can be stopped. If after 1 minute there has been no improvement, give an additional 3 mg, and if there is still no response, give the final 3 mg 1 minute later.

e. If the patient develops muscarinic symptoms or signs at any time during the test (sweating, salivation, or GI symptoms), one can assume that enough edrophonium has been given to effect an improvement in strength, and the test can be stopped.

f. When a placebo effect or examiner bias is of concern, the test is performed in a double-blind placebo control fashion. The 1-ml control syringe contains either saline, 0.4 mg of atropine, or 10 mg of nicotinic acid.

g. **Improvement** lasts for just a few minutes. When improvement is clear-cut, the test is positive. If the improvement is borderline, it is best to consider the test to be negative. The test can be repeated several times.

h. **Sensitivity** of the edrophonium test is about 90%.

i. **Specificity** is difficult to determine, because improvement following IV edrophonium has been reported in other neuromuscular diseases, including Lambert-Eaton syndrome, botulism, Guillain-Barré syndrome, motor neuron disease, and lesions of the brainstem and cavernous sinus.

3. Acetylcholine receptor antibodies

a. The standard assay for receptor-binding antibodies is an immunoprecipitation assay using human limb muscle for acetylcholine receptor antigen. In addition, assays for receptor modulating and blocking antibodies are available.

b. **Sensitivity.** Binding antibodies are present in about 80% of all myasthenic patients (50% of patients with pure ocular MG, 80% of those with mild generalized MG, 90% of patients with moderate to severe generalized MG, and 70% of those in clinical remission). By also testing for modulating and blocking antibodies, one can improve the sensitivity to 90% overall.

c. **Specificity** is outstanding, with false-positives being exceedingly rare in reliable labs. If blood is sent to a reference lab, the test results are usually available within a week.

4. EMG (electrophysiologic testing)

a. **Repetitive stimulation testing** is widely available and has variable sensitivity depending on the number and selection of muscles studied and various provocative maneuvers. In most labs, however, this technique has a sensitivity of about 50% in all patients with MG (lower in patients with mild or pure ocular disease).

b. **Single fiber electromyography (SFEMG)** is a highly specialized technique, usually available in major academic centers, with a sensitivity of about 90%. Abnormal single fiber results are common in other neuromuscular diseases, and therefore the test must be used in the correct clinical context. The specificity of single fiber EMG is an important issue in that mild abnormalities can clearly accompany a variety of other diseases of the motor unit, including motor neuron disease, peripheral neuropathy, and myopathy. Certainly, disorders of neuromuscular transmission other than MG can have substantial abnormalities on SFEMG. In contrast, receptor antibodies are not present in non-MG patients. In summary, the two highly sensitive laboratory studies are SFEMG and receptor antibodies; nonetheless, neither test is 100% sensitive.

C. Natural course. Appropriate management of the patient with autoimmune MG requires understanding of the natural course of the disease. The long-term natural course of MG is not clearly established other than being highly variable. Several generalizations can be made.

1. About half of MG patients present with ocular symptoms, and 80% exhibit such symptoms within 1 month. The presenting symptom is bulbar weakness in 10% of patients, limb weakness in 10%, generalized weakness in 10%, and respiratory weakness in 1%. By 1 month, symptoms remain purely ocular in 40%, generalized in 40%, limited to the limbs in 10%, and limited to bulbar muscles in 10%. Weakness remains restricted to the ocular muscles on a long-term basis in about 15–20% of cases (pure ocular MG).

2. Most patients with initial ocular involvement tend to develop generalized weakness within the first year of the disease (90% of those who generalize

do so within the initial 12 months). Maximal weakness occurs within the initial 3 years in 70% of patients. In the modern era, death from MG is rare.

3. Spontaneous long-lasting remission occurs in about 10–15% of cases, usually in the first year or two of the disease.

4. Most MG patients develop progression of clinical symptoms during the initial 2–3 years. However, progression is not uniform, as illustrated by patients (15–20%) whose symptoms remain purely ocular and those who have spontaneous remission.

D. Treatment options

1. Cholinesterase inhibitors (CEIs) are safe and effective, and are the first-line therapy for all patients.

a. Inhibition of acetylcholinesterase (AChE) reduces the hydrolysis of acetylcholine (ACh), increasing the accumulation of ACh at the nicotinic postsynaptic membrane. The CEIs used in MG bind reversibly (as opposed to organophosphate CEIs, which bind irreversibly) to AChE. These drugs cross the blood-brain barrier poorly and tend not to cause CNS side effects. Absorption from the gastrointestinal tract tends to be inefficient and variable, with oral bioavailability of about 10%.

b. Muscarinic autonomic side effects of gastrointestinal cramping, diarrhea, salivation, lacrimation diaphoresis, and, when severe, bradycardia may occur with any of the CEI preparations.

c. Cholinergic weakness. A feared potential complication of excessive CEI use is skeletal muscle weakness (cholinergic weakness). Patients receiving parenteral CEI are at the greatest risk of developing cholinergic weakness. It is uncommon (although not unheard of) for patients receiving oral CEI to develop significant cholinergic weakness even while experiencing muscarinic cholinergic side effects.

d. Commonly available CEIs are summarized in Table 48-1.

(1) Pyridostigmine (Mestinon) is the most widely used CEI for long-term oral therapy. Onset of effect is within 15–30 minutes of an oral dose, with peak effect within 1–2 hours, and wearing off gradually at 3–4 hours postdose. The starting dosage is 30–60 mg tid-qid depending on symptoms. Optimal benefit usually occurs with a dosage of 60 mg q4h. Muscarinic cholinergic side effects are common with larger dosages. Occasional patients require and tolerate more than 1000 mg/day, dosing as frequently as every 2–3 hours. Patients with significant bulbar weakness often time their doses about 1 hour before meals in order to maximize chewing and swallowing. Of all the CEI preparations, pyridostigmine has the least muscarinic side effects.

(2) Pyridostigmine may be used in several forms alternative to the 60-mg tablet. The syrup may be necessary for children or for patients who have difficulty swallowing pills. Sustained-release 180-mg pyridostigmine (Mestinon Timespan) is sometimes preferred for nighttime use. Unpredictable release and absorption limit its use.

(3) Patients with severe dysphagia or undergoing surgical procedures

Table 48-1. Cholinesterase inhibitors (CEIs).

Inhibitor	Unit dose	Average dosage
Pyridostigmine bromide tablet (Mestinon)	60-mg tablet	30–60 mg q4–6h
Pyridostigmine bromide syrup	12 mg/ml	30–60 mg q4–6h
Pyridostigmine bromide timespan (Mestinon Timespan)	180-mg tablet	1 tablet bid
Pyridostigmine bromide (parenteral)	5 mg/ml ampules	1–2 mg q3–4h ($\frac{1}{30}$ of oral dose)
Neostigmine bromide (Prostigmin)	15-mg tablet	7.5–15 mg q3–4h
Neostigmine methylsulfate (parenteral)	0.25–1.0 mg/ml ampules	0.05 mg q3–4h
Ambenonium chloride (Mytelase)	10-mg and 25-mg tablets	2.5–5.0 mg q4–6h

may need parenteral CEIs. Intravenous pyridostigmine should be given at about ⅟₃₀ of the oral dosage.

(4) Neostigmine (Prostigmin) has a slightly shorter duration of action and slightly greater muscarinic side effects.

(5) Ambenonium (Mytelase) has shown no significant advantages over the other CEIs but has been suggested to be of greatest use in treating appendicular weakness. Headache is an additional occasional side effect.

(6) For patients with intolerable muscarinic side effects at CEI dosages required for optimal power, a concomitant anticholinergic drug such as atropine sulfate (0.4–0.5 mg PO) or glycopyrrolate (Robinul) (1 mg PO) on a prn basis or with each dose of CEI may be helpful.

(7) Patients with mild disease can often be managed adequately with CEIs. However, patients with moderate, severe, or progressive disease usually require more effective therapy.

2. **Thymectomy.** Association of the thymus gland with MG was first noted at the beginning of the twentieth century, and thymectomy has become standard therapy over the past 50 years. Prospective controlled trials have not been performed for thymectomy. Nonetheless, thymectomy is generally recommended for patients with moderate to severe MG—especially those inadequately controlled on CEIs and those under age 55 years. All patients with suspected thymoma undergo surgery.

a. **Clinical response.** About 75% of MG patients appear to benefit from thymectomy. Patients may improve or simply stabilize. For unclear reasons, the onset of improvement tends to be delayed by a year or two in most patients (some patients seem to improve 5–10 years after surgery).

b. **Method.** The majority of centers use the transsternal approach for thymectomy, with the goal of complete removal of the gland. The limited transcervical approach has been largely abandoned because of the likelihood of incomplete gland removal. Some centers perform a "maximal thymectomy" in order to ensure complete removal. The procedure involves a combined transsternal-transcervical exposure with en bloc removal of the thymus.

c. **Patients who do not undergo thymectomy.** Patients with very mild or trivial symptoms do not have surgery. Most patients with pure ocular MG do not undergo thymectomy, although there has been some reported benefit in selected patients. Thymectomy is often avoided in children because of the theoretical possibility of impairing the developing immune system. However, reports of thymectomy in children as young as 2–3 years of age have shown favorable results without adverse effects on the immune system. Thymectomy has been largely discouraged in patients over age 55 because of expected increased morbidity, latency of clinical benefit, and frequent observation of an atrophic, involuted gland. Nonetheless, there are older patients who are reported to have benefited from thymectomy.

d. **Major complications** of thymectomy are uncommon as long as the surgery is performed at an experienced center with anesthesiologists and neurologists familiar with the disease and perioperative management of MG patients. Common, less serious side effects of thymectomy include postoperative chest pain (which may last several weeks), a convalescence period of 4–6 weeks, and incisional scarring.

3. **Corticosteroids.** There are no controlled trials documenting the benefits of corticosteroids in MG. However, nearly all authorities have personal experience attesting to the virtues (and complications) of corticosteroid use for MG patients.

a. In general, corticosteroids are used for patients with moderate to severe, disabling symptoms that are refractory to CEIs. Patients are commonly hospitalized for initiation of therapy to avoid the risk of early exacerbation. Opinions differ regarding the best method of administration.

b. For patients with severe MG it is best to begin with high-dosage daily therapy of 60–80 mg/day PO. Early exacerbation occurs in about half of patients, usually within the first few days of therapy and typically lasting 3 or 4 days. In 10% of cases the exacerbation is severe, requiring mechanical ventilation or a feeding tube (thus the need to initiate therapy in the hospital). Overall, about 80% of patients show favorable responses to steroids (with 30% attaining remission and 50% enjoying marked improvement). Mild to moderate improvement occurs in 15%, and 5% have no response. Improvement begins as early as 12 hours and as late as 60 days after initiation of prednisone, but most patients begin to improve within the first week or two. Improvement is gradual, with marked improvement occurring at a mean of 3 months and maximal improvement at a mean of 9 months. Of those patients having favorable responses, most maintain their improvement with gradual dosage reduction at a rate of 10 mg every 1–2 months. More rapid reduction is usually associated with a flareup of the disease. Although many patients can eventually be weaned from steroids and maintain their responses, the majority cannot. They require a minimum dosage (5–30 mg every other day) in order to maintain their improvement. Complications of long-term high-dosage prednisone therapy are substantial, including cushingoid appearance, hypertension, osteoporosis, cataracts, aseptic necrosis, and the other well-known complications of chronic steroid therapy. Older patients tend to respond more favorably to prednisone.

   c. An alternative prednisone treatment involves a low-dosage, alternate-day regimen on a gradually increasing schedule in an attempt to avoid early exacerbation. Patients receive prednisone at 25 mg alternate day (AD) with an increase of 12.5 mg every third dose (about every fifth day) to a maximum dosage of 100 mg AD or until sufficient improvement occurs. Clinical improvement usually begins within 1 month. The frequency and severity of early exacerbation are less than those associated with high-dosage daily regimens.

   d. High-dosage intravenous methylprednisolone (1 g/day for 3–5 days) can provide improvement within 1–2 weeks, but the clinical improvement is temporary.

4. **Nonsteroidal immunosuppressive drug therapy**

   a. **Azathioprine (Imuran)** is a cytotoxic purine analog frequently used for immunosuppressive treatment of MG. Experience in azathioprine treatment of MG is extensive but largely uncontrolled and retrospective.

      (1) **Dosage.** The starting dosage is 50 mg/day PO, with CBC and liver function tests weekly in the beginning. If the drug is tolerated and the bloodwork is stable, the dosage is increased by 50 mg every 1–2 weeks, aiming for a maximum dosage of about 2–3 mg/kg/day (about 150 mg/day in the average size adult).

      (2) **Side effects.** When azathioprine is first started, about 15% of patients have intolerable GI side effects (nausea, anorexia, and abdominal discomfort), sometimes associated with fever, leading to discontinuation. Bone marrow suppression with relative leukopenia (WBC 2500–4000) occurs in 25% of patients but is usually not significant. If the WBC drops below 2500 or the absolute granulocyte count goes below 1000, the drug is stopped (and the abnormalities usually resolve). Macrocytosis is common and of unclear clinical significance. Liver enzymes are elevated in 5–10% of patients, but this effect is usually reversible, and severe hepatic toxicity occurs in only about 1% of cases. Infection occurs in about 5%. There is a theoretical risk of malignancy (based on observations in organ transplant patients), but this increased risk has not been clearly established in the MG patient population.

      (3) **Clinical response.** About half of MG patients improve on azathioprine with onset about 4–8 months into treatment. Maximal improvement takes about 12 months. Relapse after discontinuation of azathioprine occurs in more than half of patients, usually within 1 year.

   b. **Cyclosporine** is used for patients with severe MG who cannot be adequately managed with corticosteroids or azathioprine.

      (1) **Dosage.** The starting dosage is 3–5 mg/kg/day given in two divided doses. Cyclosporine blood levels should be measured monthly (aiming for a level of 200–300) along with electrolytes, magnesium, and renal function (in general, serum creatinine should not exceed 1½ times the pretreatment level). Blood should be sampled before the morning dose is taken.

(2) **Clinical response.** Over half of patients improve on cyclosporine. The onset of clinical improvement occurs about 1–2 months after therapy is initiated, and maximal improvement occurs at about 3–4 months.

(3) **Side effects** include renal toxicity and hypertension. Nonsteroidal anti-inflammatory drugs and potassium-sparing diuretics are among the drugs that should be avoided while on cyclosporine. In patients on corticosteroids, the addition of cyclosporine can lead to a reduction in steroid dosage (although it is usually not possible to discontinue prednisone).

c. **Cyclophosphamide (Cytoxan)** is a nitrogen mustard antimetabolite occasionally used in severe refractory MG. A dosage of 150–200 mg (3–5 mg/kg/day) PO or 250 mg/day for 5 days IV therapy (followed by long-term oral therapy) is generally used. About half of patients improve beginning at about 1–2 months. Maximum improvement occurs by 6 months. The drug is discontinued if significant leukopenia or other major side effects occur. Alopecia, nausea, vomiting, anorexia, and infection are additional complications.

5. **Plasma exchange (plasmapheresis)** removes acetylcholine receptor antibodies and results in rapid clinical improvement.

a. **Protocol.** The standard course involves removal of 2–3 liters of plasma every other day or three times per week until the patient improves (usually a total of five or six exchanges).

b. **Clinical response.** Improvement begins after the first few exchanges and reaches a maximum within 2–3 weeks. The improvement is moderate to marked in nearly all patients but usually wears off after 4–8 weeks as a result of reaccumulation of pathogenic antibodies.

c. **Vascular access** may require placement of a central line.

d. **Complications** include hypotension, bradycardia, electrolyte imbalance, hemolysis, infection, and access problems (such as pneumothorax from placement of a central line).

e. **Indications** for plasma exchange include any patient in whom a rapid temporary clinical improvement is needed.

6. **High-dosage intravenous immunoglobulin (IVIG).** IVIG administration is associated with improvement in MG symptoms. The mechanism is unclear but may relate to downregulation of acetylcholine receptor antibody production or to the effect of anti-idiotype antibodies.

a. **Protocol.** The usual protocol is 2 g/kg spread out over 5 consecutive days (0.4 g/kg/day). Different IVIG preparations are administered at different rates (contact the pharmacy for guidelines).

b. **Clinical response.** The majority of MG patients improve, usually within 1 week of starting IVIG. The degree of response is variable. The duration of response, like that of plasma exchange, is limited to about 4–8 weeks.

c. **Complications** include fever, chills, and headache, which respond to slowing of the rate of the infusion and to antihistamines (diphenhydramine). Occasional cases of aseptic meningitis, renal failure, nephrotic syndrome, and stroke have been reported. Also, patients with selective IgA deficiency can develop anaphylaxis, which is best avoided by screening for IgA deficiency ahead of time. The cost of the treatment is high, comparable to that of plasma exchange.

E. **General guidelines for management**

1. **Be certain of the diagnosis.**

2. **Patient education.** Provide the patient with information about the natural course of the disease (including its variable and somewhat unpredictable nature). Briefly review the treatment options outlined in sec. **I.D,** pointing out their effectiveness, time course of improvement, duration of response, and complications. Provide the patient with educational pamphlets prepared by the Myasthenia Gravis Foundation or the Muscular Dystrophy Association.

3. **When to hospitalize the patient.** Patients with severe MG can deteriorate rapidly over a period of hours. Therefore, those having dyspnea should be hospitalized immediately in a constant observation or intensive care setting. Patients with moderate to severe dysphagia, weight loss, or rapidly progressive or severe weakness should be admitted urgently. This allows close monitoring and early intervention in the case of respiratory failure, and also ex-

pedites the diagnostic work-up and initiation of therapy.
4. **Myasthenic crisis** (Table 48-2) is a medical emergency characterized by respiratory failure from diaphragm weakness or severe oropharyngeal weakness leading to aspiration. Crisis can occur in the setting of surgery (post-op), in association with acute infection, or following rapid withdrawal of corticosteroids (although some patients have no precipitating factors). Patients should be placed in an ICU setting and have forced vital capacity (FVC) and forced expiratory volume one second (FEV-1) checked every 2 hours. Changes in arterial blood gases occur relatively late in neuromuscular respiratory failure. There should be a low threshold for intubation and mechanical ventilation. Criteria for intubation include a drop in the FVC below 15 ml/kg (or below 1 liter in an average-sized adult), severe aspiration from oropharyngeal weakness, or labored breathing regardless of the measurements. If the diagnosis is not clear-cut, it is advisable to secure the airway with intubation, stabilize ventilation, and only then address the question of the underlying diagnosis. If the patient has been taking a CEI, the drug should be temporarily discontinued in order to rule out the possibility of cholinergic crisis (see Table 48-2).
5. **Correct any underlying medical problems,** such as thyroid disease (hypo- or hyperthyroidism can exacerbate MG).
6. **Drugs to avoid in MG.** Avoid using d-penicillamine, chloroquine, quinine, quinidine, or procainamide. Aminoglycoside antibiotics should be avoided unless required for life-threatening infections. Neuromuscular blocking drugs such as pancuronium and d-tubocurarine can produce marked and prolonged paralysis in MG patients. Depolarizing drugs such as succinylcholine can also have prolonged effects and should be used only by a skilled anesthesiologist who is well aware of the patient's MG.
F. **Indications for specific therapies** (Table 48-3). Treatment must be individualized. Mild diplopia and ptosis may not be disabling for some patients, but for an airline pilot or a neurosurgeon, mild intermittent diplopia may be critical. In a similar fashion, some patients may tolerate side effects better than others.
1. **Mild or trivial weakness,** either localized or generalized, should be managed with a CEI (pyridostigmine).
2. **Moderate to marked weakness,** either localized or generalized, should initially be managed with a CEI. Even if symptoms are adequately controlled, patients under age 55 undergo thymectomy early in the course of the disease (within the first year). In older patients, thymectomy is usually not performed unless the patient is thought to have a thymoma. Thymectomy is performed at an experienced center with the clear intent of complete removal of the gland (by either a transsternal or "maximal" technique). All patients with suspected thymoma (by chest scan) should have

Table 48-2. The acutely deteriorating myasthenic patient.

Myasthenic Crisis
Respiratory distress
Respiratory arrest
Cyanosis
Increased pulse and BP
Diaphoresis
Poor cough
Inability to handle oral secretions
Dysphagia
Weakness
Improves with edrophonium

Cholinergic Crisis
Abdominal cramps
Diarrhea
Nausea and vomiting, excessive secretions, miosis
Fasciculations, diaphoresis
Weakness
Worsens with edrophonium

Table 48-3. Treatment of myasthenia gravis.

Mild, trivial weakness: cholinesterase inhibitors (CEIs)
Moderate to marked localized or generalized weakness:
  CEIs
  Thymectomy for patients under age 55 (complete removal)
If symptoms are not controlled by cholinesterase inhibitors, use immunosuppression:
  Prednisone if severe or urgent
  Azathioprine if:
    Prednisone is contraindicated
    Prednisone fails
    Prednisone causes side effects
Plasma exchange:
  Impending crisis, crisis
  Preoperative
  Refractory chronic disease
If the abovementioned treatments fail:
  Search for residual thymus tissue
  Cyclosporine
  Cyclophosphamide
  High-dosage IVIG
  Referral to neuromuscular specialty group

thymectomy, even if their myasthenic symptoms are mild. Unless a thymoma is suspected, patients with pure ocular disease are usually not treated with thymectomy.

3. If symptoms are inadequately controlled on a CEI, immunosuppression is used. High-dosage corticosteroid therapy is the most predictable and effective long-term option. If patients have severe, rapidly progressive, or life-threatening symptoms, the decision to start corticosteroids is clear-cut. Patients with disabling but stable symptoms may instead receive azathioprine, especially if there are particular concerns about using corticosteroids (i.e., the patient is already overweight, is diabetic, or has cosmetic concerns). Those patients who respond poorly or have unacceptable complications on steroids are started on azathioprine.

4. **Plasma exchange** is indicated in:
   a. Rapidly progressive, life-threatening, impending myasthenic crisis or actual crisis, particularly if prolonged intubation with mechanical ventilation is judged hazardous.
   b. Preoperative stabilization of MG (such as prior to thymectomy or other elective surgery) in poorly controlled patients.
   c. Disabling MG refractory to other therapies.

5. **IVIG** should be considered an alternative to plasma exchange with the same indications, especially if plasma exchange is not available or vascular access cannot be obtained.

6. If these options fail, use cyclosporine.

7. If the patient remains poorly controlled despite appropriate treatment, perform a repeat chest CT scan to look for residual thymus. Some patients improve after "repeat thymectomy." Check for other medical problems (diabetes, thyroid disease, infection, and coexisting autoimmune diseases).

8. **Referral** to a neurologist or center specializing in neuromuscular disease is advised for all patients with suspected MG and can be particularly important in complicated or refractory cases.

G. **Miscellaneous forms of MG**
   1. **Transient neonatal myasthenia** occurs in 10–15% of babies born to mothers with autoimmune MG. Within the first few days after delivery, the baby has a weak cry or suck, appears floppy, and occasionally requires mechanical ventilation. This condition is caused by maternal antibodies that cross the placenta late in pregnancy. As these maternal antibodies are replaced by the baby's own antibodies, the symptoms gradually disappear, usually within a few weeks, and the baby is normal thereafter. Infants with severe weakness are treated with oral pyridostigmine at 1–2 mg/kg q4h.

2. **Congenital myasthenia** represents a group of rare hereditary disorders of the neuromuscular junction. The patients tend to have lifelong, relatively stable symptoms of generalized fatigable weakness. These disorders are nonimmunologic, without acetylcholine receptor antibodies, and therefore patients do not respond to immune therapy (steroids, thymectomy, or plasma exchange). Most patients improve on CEIs.

II. **Lambert-Eaton Syndrome (the myasthenic syndrome)**

A. **Clinical features** (Table 48-4). The Lambert-Eaton myasthenic syndrome (LES) is a presynaptic disease characterized by chronic fluctuating weakness of proximal limb muscles. Symptoms include difficulties in walking, climbing stairs, and rising from a chair. In LES there may be some improvement in power with sustained or repeated exercise. In contrast, the ptosis, diplopia, dysphagia, and respiratory failure of MG are far less common. In addition, LES patients often complain of myalgias, muscle stiffness of the back and legs, distal paresthesias, metallic taste, dry mouth, impotence, and other autonomic symptoms of muscarinic cholinergic insufficiency. LES is rare compared with MG, which is about 100 times more common. About half of LES patients have underlying malignancies that are usually small cell carcinomas of the lung. In patients without malignancy, LES is an autoimmune disease and can be associated with other autoimmune phenomena. In general, patients over age 40 are more likely to be men and to have associated malignancies, whereas younger patients are more likely to be women and to have no neoplasm malignancy. LES symptoms can precede detection of the malignancy by 1–2 years.

B. **Diagnosis.** The diagnosis is confirmed with EMG studies, which typically show low amplitude of the compound muscle action potentials and a decrement to slow rates or repetitive stimulation. Following brief exercise, there is marked facilitation of the compound muscle action potential (CMAP) amplitude. At high rates of repetitive stimulation, there may be an incremental response. Single fiber EMG is markedly abnormal in virtually all patients with LES. The pathogenesis involves autoantibodies directed against voltage-gated calcium channels at cholinergic nerve terminals. These IgG antibodies also inhibit cholinergic synapses of the autonomic nervous system (ANS). Over half of LES patients demonstrate these antibodies to voltage-gated calcium channels in serum, providing another useful diagnostic test.

C. **Therapy** (Table 48-5)

1. In patients with associated malignancy, successful treatment of the tumor can lead to improvement in the LES symptoms.

2. Symptomatic improvement in neuromuscular transmission may occur with the use of cholinesterase inhibitors such as pyridostigmine.

3. **Guanidine** has shown some benefit, but its use has been limited by bone marrow, renal, and hepatic toxicity. Guanidine increases the release of ACh by increasing the duration of the action potential at the motor nerve terminal.

4. **DAP.** The quaternary ammonium compound 4-aminopyridine increases ACh release by blocking voltage-dependent potassium conductance and thereby prolonging depolarization at the nerve terminal and enhancing the voltage-dependent calcium influx. CNS toxicity may result in seizures, agitation, and confusion. However, a less toxic derivative, **3,4-diaminopyridine (DAP)**,

Table 48-4. Lambert-Eaton syndrome: Symptoms and signs.

Symptoms
Proximal limb weakness
Fatigue or fluctuation of symptoms
Difficulty rising from a sitting position
Difficulty walking, climbing stairs
Dry mouth, metallic taste
Anticholinergic symptoms

Clinical Signs
Proximal limb weakness (legs more than arms)
Hypoactive muscle stretch reflexes
Transient improvement in muscle power following exercise

Table 48-5. Treatment of Lambert-Eaton syndrome.

Treat the associated neoplasm
Symptomatic improvement in neuromuscular transmission:
   Cholinesterase inhibitors (pyridostigmine)
   Guanidine (hepatic, bone marrow, and renal toxicity)
   3,4-diaminopyridine (limited availability)
Immunosuppressive therapy:
   Corticosteroids
   Azathioprine
   Plasma exchange

appears to have more limited access to the CNS and therefore to be less toxic. DAP has been shown clearly to improve most LES patients with relatively mild toxicity. However, this compound is largely unavailable (except through a research center).

   5. **Immunosuppressive therapy** is used for patients with disabling symptoms. Long-term high-dosage corticosteroids, azathioprine, plasma exchange, and IVIG have all been used with moderate success. In general, the use of these therapies should be tailored to the severity of the patient's symptoms.

III. Botulism

  A. Classic botulism occurs after ingestion of food contaminated by botulinum toxin. Eight different toxins have been identified, but disease in humans is caused by types A, B, and E. Type E is associated with contaminated seafood. All types produce similar clinical pictures, although type A may cause more severe and enduring symptoms. In all three types, the condition can be fatal.

    1. **Clinical features** begin 12–48 hours after ingestion of contaminated food. Bulbar symptoms, including diplopia, ptosis, blurred vision, and speech and swallowing difficulties, occur initially and are followed by weakness in the upper limbs and then in the lower limbs. Severe cases produce respiratory failure requiring mechanical ventilation. The tendency for paralysis to start in the cranial muscles and then descend down the body distinguishes the presentation from that of Guillain-Barré syndrome (which more often causes an ascending paralysis). Botulism produces autonomic dysfunctions, including constipation, ileus, dry mouth, and abnormal pupils.

    2. **Management**

      a. The patient should be placed in an intensive care setting, and pulmonary functions with FVC should be monitored every 2–4 hours. If FVC goes below 1 liter or 15 ml/kg or if the patient appears to be having respiratory difficulty, intubation and mechanical ventilation are necessary.

      b. Use of trivalent botulinum antitoxin is controversial, because adverse side effects occur in about 20% of patients. There is some evidence that antitoxin shortens the duration of clinical illness, especially for type E.

    3. **Course.** Even with aggressive support, the overall mortality remains about 5–10%, usually from respiratory or septic complications. The other patients tend to improve over a period of several weeks to several months. In patients who survive, recovery is nearly complete. Several years after the illness, some patients still have subjective fatigue and ANS abnormalities including constipation, impotence, and dry mouth. Clinical recovery results from the formation of new nerve terminals.

  B. Infant botulism is the most frequently reported form of botulism in recent years. The infant ingests spores of *Clostridium botulinum*, which lodge in the intestinal tract, germinate there, and produce botulinum toxin in the gut. The typical presentation is an infant between the ages of 6 weeks and 6 months who exhibits generalized weakness and constipation. The weakness may start in the cranial muscles and then descend, causing a weak suck, a poor cry, and reduced spontaneous movement. The cranial muscles are weak, with poor extraocular movements, reduced gag reflex, and drooling. The diagnosis is validated by finding *C. botulinum* in feces. The toxin is usually not detectable in the serum. EMG studies can point to this diagnosis in 80–90% of cases. Infantile botulism can range from mild to severe. Management centers around observation and general support (including respiratory stability). The recovery tends to be excellent over the course of weeks to months.

C. **Wound botulism** occurs when toxin produced from *C. botulinum* infects a wound. The symptoms are similar to those of classic botulism except that the onset may be delayed for up to 2 weeks after contamination of the wound. The diagnosis is supported by EMG studies, demonstration of toxin in the patient's blood, or finding the organism in the patient's wound. Wounds that lead to botulism include direct traumas, surgical wounds, and wounds associated with drug use (e.g., intravenous and intranasal cocaine).

Recommended Readings

Buckingham JM, et al. The value of thymectomy in myasthenia gravis: Computer assisted matched study. *Ann Surg* 184:453–458, 1976.

Cherington M. Botulism. *Sem Neurol* 1(1):27–31, 1990.

DeBaets MH, Oosterhuis HJGH (eds). *Myasthenia Gravis*. Boca Raton, FL: CRC, 1993.

Finley JC, Pascuzzi RM. Rational therapy of myasthenia gravis. *Sem Neurol* 10(1):70–82, 1990.

Grob D, et al. The course of myasthenia gravis and therapies affecting outcome. *Ann NY Acad Sci* 505:472–499, 1987.

Howard JF Jr. Adverse drug effects on neuromuscular transmission. *Sem Neurol* 10:89–102, 1990.

Lanska DJ. Indications for thymectomy in myasthenia gravis. *Neurology* 40:1828–1829, 1990.

McEvoy KM. Diagnosis and treatment of Lambert-Eaton myasthenic syndrome. *Neurol Clin N Amer* 12(2):387–399, 1994.

McEvoy KM, et al. 3,4-diaminopyridine in the treatment of Lambert-Eaton myasthenic syndrome. *N Engl J Med* 321:1567–1571, 1989.

O'Neill JH, et al. The Lambert-Eaton myasthenic syndrome. *Brain* 11(1):577–596, 1988.

Pascuzzi RM, Coslett B, Johns TR. Long-term corticosteroid treatment of myasthenia gravis: Report of 116 patients. *Ann Neurol* 15:291–298, 1984.

Phillips LH. The epidemiology of myasthenia gravis. *Neurol Clin N Amer* 12(2):263–271, 1994.

Rivner MH, Swift TR. Thymoma: Diagnosis and management. *Sem Neurol* 10:83–88, 1990.

Sanders DB, Scoppeta C. The treatment of patients with myasthenia gravis. *Neurol Clin N Amer* 12(2):343–368, 1994.

Seybold ME, Drachman DB. Gradually increasing doses of prednisone in myasthenia gravis. *N Engl J Med* 290:81–84, 1974.

Tindall RSA, et al. A clinical therapeutic trial of cyclosporine in myasthenia gravis. *Ann NY Acad Sci* 681:539–551, 1993.

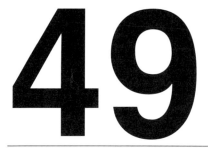

Migraine, Cluster, and Tension Headaches

James R. Couch, Jr.

I. Migraine therapy and management

A. Algorithm for approach to the migraine patient.
Figure 49-1 provides an algorithm for diagnosing the headache patient. Migraine is essentially a clinical diagnosis and not one that is associated with specific laboratory or radiologic tests at this time. It is a diagnosis of exclusion in which the physician must rule out other possible etiologies for the headache process.

Table 49-1 outlines the process of developing a headache profile. This profile, by enabling the physician to compare the patient's headaches with established headache profiles, can be very useful in establishing the diagnosis and developing an approach to the headache patient.

B. Migraine therapy

1. Therapies for migraine can be divided into symptomatic and prophylactic or preventive therapies. Symptomatic therapy can be further subdivided into nonspecific therapies and specific abortive therapy. An algorithm for migraine therapy is presented in Figure 49-2.

Symptomatic therapies for migraine are oriented primarily toward relief of pain. Pain is the symptom that brings the majority of patients to seek medical help. Nausea and vomiting are the next most common symptoms that lead patients to seek medical help, and antinauseants may often be part of a successful migraine treatment regimen.

It is of note that successful treatment of the pain and nausea of migraine usually produces remission of the entire migraine syndrome. Typically, the various symptoms of the migraine syndrome tend to occur together. In some cases, migrainous neurologic or gastrointestinal (GI) symptoms may occur in the absence of pain, a syndrome known as migraine-sans-migraine. There are, however, occasional examples of prolonged migrainous aura that do not respond to antimigrainous therapy.

2. Nonspecific symptomatic therapy

a. Analgesics. The simplest treatment for migraine is nonsteroidal anti-inflammatory drug (NSAID) such as aspirin, ibuprofen, or naproxen, all of which are now available in over-the-counter preparations and may be effective for a large number of patients many of whom are never seen by physicians. At times, larger dosages of NSAIDs, such as 800 mg of ibuprofen, 600 mg of fenoprofen, or 500 mg of naproxen, may be effective in relieving migraine. Addition of an antinauseant such as promethazine or hydroxyzine (25–50 mg) may be helpful in relieving the GI symptoms of migraine as well as extending the effect of the analgesic medication.

Acetaminophen is an analgesic but has no anti-inflammatory action. Some patients find 500–1000 mg of acetaminophen an effective treatment for migraine.

b. Minor narcotics. The next step is to use minor narcotics such as codeine (30–60 mg), hydrocodone (5–7.5 mg), oxycodone (5 mg), or propoxyphene (65 mg) to relieve pain. As with the NSAIDs, use of 25 mg of promethazine or hydroxyzine with the minor narcotic extends the effect of the narcotic and helps relieve the GI symptoms of migraine.

c. Narcotic agonist/antagonist. A narcotic agonist/antagonist medication such as butorphanol (Stadol) at 2–4 mg IM or nalbuphine (Nubain) at 10 mg IM is the next step in nonspecific pain relief. These narcotic agonist/antagonist medications stimulate opiate receptors at low dosages

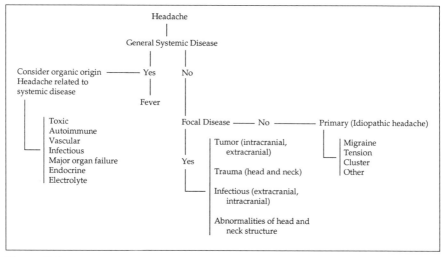

Figure 49-1. Approach to the diagnosis of headache.

but become narcotic antagonists and can elucidate withdrawal syndromes at higher dosages.

    d. Major narcotics. If these medications are ineffective, use of a stronger narcotic, such as meperidine (25–100 mg) or morphine (5–15 mg), may be indicated. These agents are usually given intramuscularly but can be given intravenously at lower dosages. Use of an antinauseant often extends the effect of the narcotic and allows it to be effective at a lower dose. Promethazine or hydroxyzine at 25–75 mg usually is quite effective when given with a narcotic. By and large, the use of narcotics should be limited to patients who have only occasional severe headaches that are refractory to other nonspecific analgesic approaches or to the specific abortive therapies discussed in sec. **I.B.3,** below.

    e. Adjuvant pain medications. Occasionally an antinauseant such as metoclopramide (10 mg) or prochlorperazine (10 mg) given intravenously is very helpful by itself. This approach should be considered before using narcotics.

Table 49-1. Key features of a headache profile (complete a profile for each type of headache).

Frequency of headache in terms of number per week, month, year, or even day
Duration of headache in terms of hours or days
Intensity of headache
    Mild: does not interfere with activity
    Moderate: interferes with activity to some extent but more than 50% of usual activity is possible
    Severe: some activity is possible but less than 50% of activity is carried out
    Disabling: patient must go to bed with the headache
Symptoms associated with headache
    General symptoms: photophobia, phonophobia, osmophobia
    Gastrointestinal and other autonomic symptoms
    Neurologic symptoms
    Mood changes
    Other symptoms
Precipitating factors for headache
    Exogenous: exposure to fumes, solvents, foods, weather changes, etc.
    Endogenous: relation to menstrual cycle
    Psychological
Age of onset of headache

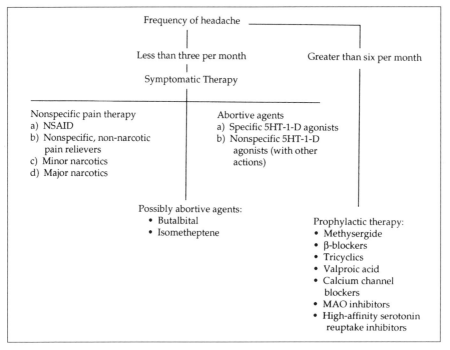

Figure 49-2. Approach to migraine therapy.

3. **Specific symptomatic (abortive) therapies for migraine** generally are not analgesics or narcotics—that is, they do not stimulate the opiate receptors and are not reversible by naloxone. These medications appear to provide specific antimigrainous effects but to have no effect on other types of pain. A possible exception is sumatriptan, discussed in sec. **I.B.3.b** below, which has been reported to produce relief in patients with headaches of inflammatory origin related to subarachnoid hemorrhage.

Current theory suggests that abortive medications work by stimulation of the serotonin 1-D (5HT-1-D) receptor, a presynaptic receptor on trigeminal nerve endings. Stimulation of presynaptic receptors depolarizes the synapse and reduces transmitter release. Thus, stimulation of presynaptic 5HT-1-D receptors or trigeminal nerve endings decreases release of substance P, calcitonin gene–related peptide, and neuropeptide Y, in turn decreasing neurovascular inflammation.

a. **Ergotamine,** which was isolated from the rye fungus in 1925, was the first abortive medication. The pharmacology of ergotamine is very complex. Ergotamine stimulates most of the aminergic receptors, and as a result has many pharmacologic actions. Table 49-2 outlines the use of ergotamine.

Ergotamine has a strong arterial vasoconstrictive effect as well as a venoconstrictive effect. The vasoconstrictive action has long been thought to be the basis for the antimigraine action of ergotamine, but this antimigraine effect is likely to be related to stimulation of the 5HT-1-D or 5HT-1-B receptor. In pharmacodynamic experiments, ergotamine does not appear to cross the blood-brain barrier. Nevertheless, a significant number of individuals who take ergotamine report anxiety, difficulty with concentration, or "loosening of thoughts." Frank hallucinations rarely occur. Occasionally, however, ergotamine has been used as a substitute for LSD in the street drug culture. Patients occasionally complain that the side effects of ergotamine, which may last for up to 24 hours and may persist after the headache pain has remitted, are as bad as the migraine headache itself.

Table 49-2. Use of ergotamine.

Principles
  Use ergotamine early in the headache to achieve maximal effect; later use may be
    ineffective.
  Do not exceed recommended dosage.
  May be given as a pill, sublingual preparation, or suppository
Oral therapy
  1 mg at onset of headache
  1 mg at 30 minutes if needed
  1 mg hourly up to 6 mg/day
  Maximum of 6 mg/day or 10 mg/wk
Therapy by suppository (usual suppository is 2 mg)
  2 mg at onset
  May repeat in 1 hour if needed; may repeat again in 6–12 hours
  Maximum of three suppositories (6 mg) per day, or five suppositories (10 mg) per week
  Suppositories can be cut into halves or quarters. Some patients may respond to as little as
    0.5 mg of ergotamine given by suppository.
Precaution: Ergotamine is potentially habituating and can precipitate rebound-withdrawal
  headache in the habituated patient. Because of a long life at tissue receptors, as little as 1 mg
  every other day may produce a habituation-withdrawal cycle.

Ergotamine may also cause coronary vasoconstriction, and there have been several reports of myocardial infarction associated with ergotamine use.

Ergotamine can cause vasoconstriction in the digits. This is usually a relatively insignificant finding. With chronic use of ergotamine, however, peripheral cyanosis, acroparesthesia, and peripheral neuropathy all may result. It is unclear whether these findings are related to microvascular constriction, including constriction of vasa nervorum, or whether there is a separate direct neurotoxic effect of ergotamine.

Between 50 and 80% of patients who take ergotamine respond to this medication. For some patients with intermittent migraine, the ergotamine may be all that is necessary to treat the headache. In other patients, the response is relatively inadequate or the extent of side effects is great enough that different or additional medications are required.

Ergotamine provides a degree of psychic stimulation along with its other effects and thus can be abused. Ergotamine abuse can cause a habituation-withdrawal headache. This type of headache cannot be brought under control without discontinuing the ergotamine.

The pharmacodynamics of ergotamine are deceiving. The serum half-life of the medication is only 2 hours. If, however, the digital vasoconstrictive effect is used to assay ergotamine activity, a single dose of ergotamine in a naive subject may produce digital vasoconstriction for up to 7 days. Even if a patient is taking ergotamine as seldom as every other day, there still is a potential that the drug will lead to habituation-withdrawal headaches.

  b. **Sumatriptan** is a specific 5HT-1-D and 5HT-1-B receptor agonist. Table 49-3 outlines the effects of sumatriptan and dihydroergotamine (DHE) on aminergic receptors. Sumatriptan and DHE both have very strong effects on the 5HT-1-D and 1-B receptors. Sumatriptan has very little effect on any other aminergic receptors, whereas DHE affects several other receptors.

The demonstration that specific 5HT-1-D receptor agonism produced relief of migraine headache stimulated a great deal of research into the pharmacology of these receptors. This research has resulted in the development of sumatriptan, which is a highly specific migraine-abortive medication.

Sumatriptan is a water-soluble medication that can be given either intramuscularly or subcutaneously, and an oral form is also available. This medication has a half-life of approximately 2–4 hours when given as a subcutaneous injection or taken orally.

Table 49-3. Use of sumatriptan, dihydroergotamine (DHE), and isometheptene (Midrin).

Sumatriptan
Use: 6 mg SC
Repeat: may repeat in 4–6 hours to a maximum of 12 mg the first day and 6 mg/day thereafter
Side effects: chest pressure, anxiety, and (rarely) dissociation or speeding of thoughts
Rare myocardial infarctions have been reported in patients at risk for coronary disease.
Evaluate for coronary disease before use. Obtain ECG for all patients more than 50 years old.
  Do not use for patients at risk for myocardial infarction.

Dihydroergotamine (DHE)
IV use (Raskin protocol):
  Metoclopramide or prochloperazine 10 mg IV over 60 seconds
  Wait 5 minutes to allow distribution.
  DHE 0.5 mg IV over 60 seconds
  Wait 3–5 minutes.
  May repeat 0.5 mg IV if no relief
Repeat: may repeat every 8 hours for up to 4–6 days
Side effects: chest pressure, anxiety, speeding or dissociation of thoughts, and nausea
SC or IM use: 1 mg; may be used without antinauseant
Repeat: may repeat every 8 hours, but for longer-term use, suggest once a day.
Side effects: similar to sumatriptan
Evaluate for coronary disease before use. Obtain ECG for all patients more than 50 years old.
  Do not use for patients at risk for myocardial infarction.

Isometheptene (Midrin)
Use: capsules at onset; repeat hourly if needed up to 6 capsules/day.
Repeat: maximum of 6 capsules/day or 10 capsules/week
Side effects: drowsiness, bad taste, and (rarely) elevated blood pressure

Pharmacologically, sumatriptan has a fairly highly specific effect on cerebral vasculature, causing constriction of the cerebral vessels. It has a much lower potency for constriction of arteries in other locations but can cause some constriction of the coronary arteries.

At the cellular level, sumatriptan has a highly specific effect on the serotonin 1-D (5HT-1-D) receptor. Stimulation of this receptor appears to decrease pain and headache. Side effects of sumatriptan include a generalized feeling of warmth, a sensation of pressure over the body, and a sensation of chest pressure. The sensation of pressure over the chest is thought to relate to esophageal constriction. In the experimental work on sumatriptan, patients who had this side effect during ECG monitoring did not show ECG changes. In rare cases, however, myocardial infarctions have been reported in association with sumatriptan. Rare patients have also reported frank hallucinations and severe anxiety. Overall, the spectrum of side effects may be similar to that for ergotamine, but the side effects of sumatriptan are of lower intensity and shorter duration.

Sumatriptan has a remarkable effect on migraine headache when given as a subcutaneous injection. The onset of action with reported relief usually occurs within 20–120 minutes, and some patients report relief within 9–10 minutes. In studies of sumatriptan that employed a 6-mg dose, 70–80% of patients reported mild pain or no pain, and 80% reported mild disability or no disability, within 2 hours. In the comparable placebo group, only 28% of the patients had responses of this degree.

A dose of 8 mg of sumatriptan elicited slightly better responses with regard to headache but also produced greater side effects.

The recommended dosage of sumatriptan is 6 mg SC at the time the headache becomes moderate in severity. Studies on sumatriptan given during the aura have indicated that it is not effective if given before the headache reaches "moderate" intensity.

A dose of 6 mg may be repeated in 6–12 hours, not to exceed 12 mg in a 24-hour period.

For oral treatment, 25–50 mg may be given and can be repeated in

1 hour. This may be repeated in 8–12 hours, with a maximum dosage of 200 mg in 24 hours.

Sumatriptan has a relatively short half-life, and recurrence of headache following an initial good response to the medication occurs in 40–50% of patients. There is debate as to whether the recurrence is related to the short half-life and therefore relatively brief antiheadache effect afforded by sumatriptan or whether it is a rebound-type phenomenon precipitated by the short half-life of sumatriptan and relative withdrawal of the medication and the circulation.

Occasionally, patients continue to have recurrent headaches following several repeated shots of sumatriptan and have to allow the headache to "run its course" by not taking any more sumatriptan.

c. **DHE.** Dihydroergotamine mesylate (DHE, or DHE 45) is an agonist for most aminergic receptors, including the 5HT-1, 5HT-2, catecholamine, and dopamine receptors. It is equipotent to sumatriptan as a 5HT-1-D agonist.

Given intravenously, 1 mg of DHE is as potent as subcutaneous sumatriptan in migraine relief. Table 49-3 outlines the protocol employed by Raskin. Given IV, DHE can produce relief in 15–30 minutes. DHE has not been found to produce habituation-withdrawal or rebound-withdrawal headache.

DHE has a half-life of 10 hours. There is accumulation of metabolites over time with repeated dosing. The uncontrolled study of Belgrade et al. suggested that 70–80% of patients had good relief with IV DHE and that 50% of those were headache-free. Raskin's group, and later Silberstein, have used DHE in treatment of intractable migraine on status migrainous with good results. The protocol in Table 49-3 is repeated every 8 hours for 2–4 days or until the patient is headache-free. If, however, the patient does not respond to the first two or three doses, other approaches should be taken.

DHE is primarily a venoconstrictor whereas ergotamine has a greater effect on arterioles. The side effects of DHE are similar to those of ergotamine but are less intense. The incidence of peripheral and coronary vasospasm is much lower with DHE than with ergotamine.

DHE can also be used as a 1-mg IM or SC injection. Studies have shown a slower onset of action but 60–70% good headache relief. Patients may be trained to give their own injections and thus use the medication at home.

d. **Isometheptene (Midrin)** is a combination of 65 mg of isometheptene mucate, a weak catecholamine agonist; 100 mg of dichloralphenazone, an antihistamine; and 325 mg of acetaminophen. Receptor pharmacology has not been studied, but this medication appears to have an abortive antimigraine action. The dosage schedule is listed in Table 49-3. Side effects are very few, and tolerance has not been reported. Some patients respond to isometheptene very well.

e. **Cost.** Table 49-4 presents the costs of drugs used for symptomatic therapy of headache. Average wholesale and retail prices are given. Note the wide variation in cost. The patient's resources must be taken into account when prescribing.

4. **Preventive antimigraine therapy.** The concept of prevention of migraine rather than symptomatic therapy for individual headaches dates from the late 1950s. Although earlier attempts at preventive therapy had been made with various medications, the first successful preventive medication was methysergide. The concept of preventive medication is to provide the patient who is having frequent headaches with a medication that will prevent the headaches from occurring. For this type of medication to work, the assumption of "critical factors" must be made. This could be theoretically envisioned as follows. Migraine is a state that is dependent on some type of trigger precipitating an event. This event leads to a cascade of physiologic changes, which develop into the migraine headache. If this cascade can be interrupted, the migraine headache can be prevented.

The mechanism of migraine prophylaxis remains speculative. It has been suggested that stimulation of the 5HT-2 receptor is related to the migraine-preventive effect. Because the exact mechanism of migraine is unknown, the

Table 49-4. Costs of medications for acute migraine treatment (all treatments per headache).

Medication	Dosage	AWP[a]
Isometheptene (Midrin)	1 capsule, then 1/h (max 5 q12h)	$1.94
APAP/isometheptene/ dichloralphenazone		.94
Fiorinal tabs, Fiorinal caps	1–2 q4h (max 6/h)	2.98
		2.98
ASA/caffeine/butalbital tabs		.27
Stadol NS spray	1 spray/nostril; repeat once in 3–5 h	60.28
Dihydroergotamine (DHE 45)	1 mg IM; repeat up to twice at 1-h intervals (3 mg)	10.68
Cafergot	1 rectal suppository; can repeat once at 1 h	8.20
Ergotamine 2 mg/caffeine 100 mg		5.48
Ergotamine 1 mg/caffeine 100 mg	2 tabs, then 1 q30min 4 times prn (max 6)	3.39
Sumatriptan (Imitrex)	6 mg IM; repeat once at 4 h if needed	77.77 (kit)[b]
50-mg tablets	50–100 mg; repeat at 1 h (max 300 mg)	12.18
25-mg tablets	25–50 mg; repeat at 1 h (max 300 mg)	10.74

[a]Average wholesale price.
[b]The kit contains two doses of 6 mg.

mechanism by which the 5HT-2 receptor stimulation might prevent migraine is also unknown.

a. General principles of preventive therapy. The decision whether or not to use preventive medication is based on the following factors (see Table 49-1): (1) frequency of migraine, (2) intensity of migraine, (3) duration of headache, (4) the patient's willingness or desire to try the prophylactic approach, and (5) extent and tolerability of side effects of the medication. Typically three or four headaches per month or 6–8 days per month with headache are reasonable guidelines. Two severe headaches lasting 4 days each per month would prompt many patients to consider prophylactic therapy. On the other hand, four headaches of 4 hours each per month would likely result in a request for symptomatic therapy.

It is not uncommon for patients to have significant side effects. Weight gain, sedation, and impaired thinking can occur as side effects with most of these agents. In each patient, the therapeutic benefit must be balanced against the extent of side effects to maximize the overall therapeutic result.

The drugs that have been most successful in migraine prevention are the antiserotonin drug methysergide, beta-adrenergic blocking agents, and tricyclic antidepressant agents. Other drugs for this purpose include cyproheptadine (an antihistamine with a tricyclic structure), calcium channel blocking agents, and, more recently, valproic acid.

The preventive medications have multiple side effects and are not well tolerated by all patients. The usual procedure is to start with a small dosage and build up the dosage gradually until either a therapeutic effect or limiting side effects are observed.

The effective prophylactic antimigraine agents are outlined in Table 49-5. These agents will be considered by classes.

b. Beta-blocking agents. The beta-adrenergic blocking agent propranolol was approved for migraine prophylaxis in 1974. The beta-adrenergic blocking agents without intrinsic sympathomimetic activity (ISA) appear to have a preventive antimigraine effect. Those with ISA appear to have a minimal effect on migraine prophylaxis. Propranolol will be discussed as the representative of this group.

The pharmacology of propranolol is complex. As a nonspecific beta-adrenergic blocking agent it has many pharmacologic effects, including decreases in blood pressure, heart rate, and cardiac contraction; inhibition of bronchodilation, and diminishment of the gluconeogenic response in diabetics or insulin. Propranolol also has an antianxiety effect in small doses and has been used to diminish panic attacks and to control stage fright.

Table 49-5. Prophylactic antimigraine agents.

Beta-adrenergic blocking agents	Agent	Range of effective dosage (mg/day)	Usual effective dosage (mg/day)
Nonspecific beta-blockers	Propranolol	20–360	80–240
	Nadolol	40–160	40–80
	Timolol	10–40	20–30
Specific beta 1 blocking agents	Atenolol	25–150	50–100
	Metoprolol	25–150	50–100
Tricyclic antidepressants	Amitriptyline	25–300	75–150
	Doxepin	25–300	75–150
	Nortriptyline	10–150	50–100
	Imipramine	25–250	75–150
	Protriptyline	10–60	20–40
Tricyclic antihistamine	Cyproheptadine	4–40	12–24
Calcium channel blocking agents	Verapamil	80–480	120–240
Nonsteroidal anti-inflammatory agents	Naproxen	500–1000	500–1000
Monoamine oxidase inhibitor	Phenelzine	15–90	30–60
Antiserotonin agent	Methysergide	2–8	4–6
Gamma-aminobutyric acid agonist	Divalproex	500–2000	500–1000

Propranolol has been found to be most effective in patients with intermittent migraine. In propranolol studies that were controlled and blinded, approximately 50–55% of patients were improved by more than 50%.

The side effects of propranolol include fatigue or a lack of energy as well as sedation. Orthostatic hypotension and syncope can result if the hypotensive effect is too great. The slowing of heart rate is occasionally significant enough that the patient develops a heart rate below 50 beats per minute. At this rate, the patient may have great difficulty carrying on usual activities.

Because of the negative chronotropic and inotropic effects of propranolol, patients may find their responses to exercise diminished. Usually this is a problem only when maximum exercise tolerance is tested. Some patients, however, find that just carrying out activities of daily living causes dyspnea. In patients with limited cardiac reserve, propranolol can induce cardiac failure or worsen existing failure.

The dosage of propranolol may vary from as little as 20 to 30 mg/day to as much as 480 mg/day. In most patients who respond to propranolol, dosages of 80–240 mg/day provide good headache prophylaxis. There is not a dose-response relationship but rather an apparently idiosyncratic relationship between dosage and headache relief. The usual method of initiating propranolol therapy is to start with a relatively low dosage and then build up the dosage gradually to a point at which the patient has either relief from the headaches or significant side effects, whichever comes first. Typically a dose of 20 mg bid is tolerated initially. The dosage can be advanced by 20 mg every third day to a maximum of 40 mg tid. The dosage usually can then be increased by 40 mg every week or every month until maximum dosage is reached.

Two contraindications should be mentioned: (1) propranolol should not be given to diabetics, because it masks the response to hypoglycemia; and (2) propranolol may precipitate asthmatic reactions in patients with actual or latent asthma.

Other beta-blocking agents without ISA appear to be equivalent to propranolol in their potency and range of effectiveness (see Table 49-5). Although some of these agents may have desirable properties such as longer half-life, there has been very little evidence that use of one beta-blocking agent without ISA is better than any other. Typically, if one beta-blocking agent fails, better results are seldom obtained with trials of other beta-blockers.

c. **Tricyclic antidepressants (TCAs)** have been generally favored for chronic tension headache and chronic daily headache whereas the beta-adrenergic blocking agents have typically been more effective in the patient with pure intermittent migraine, but TCAs may be effective for intermittent migraine as well. In this author's experience, amitriptyline and doxepin are the two most effective preventive antimigraine agents, and the other agents listed in Table 49-5 are relatively less effective. Some patients, however, are found to respond to other tricyclic agents when amitriptyline and doxepin have failed. Although there are no studies on this subject, anecdotal experience suggests that some patients may respond better to doxepin than to amitriptyline, or vice versa. If only a modest response is obtained to one of the agents, it is usually worthwhile to give the other a try to see if it has better therapeutic efficacy.

The pharmacology of TCAs is complex. These agents inhibit reuptake of 5HT and norepinephrine at nerve endings and also have anticholinergic, beta-adrenergic blocking, and sedative effects.

For amitriptyline, a starting dosage of 25–50 mg at bedtime is usually tolerated. The dosage may be increased by 25 mg every 1–2 weeks to a maximum of 300 mg/day. The dosage is determined by either (1) good headache relief or (2) occurrence of unacceptable side effects. The response to TCAs, like that to propranolol, is more idiosyncratic and not closely related to blood levels. If the patient has no side effects and no relief, continue to increase the dosage. At dosages above 200 mg/day, an amitriptyline level should be obtained. If the tricyclic level amitriptyline plus nortriptyline exceeds 300 mg/ml, the dosage should be decreased. Typically, the dosage should be divided, with 50% at bedtime and the remainder in divided doses during the day.

The typical side effects of the tricyclics are drowsiness along with the anticholinergic effects of a dry mouth, constipation, difficult or slowed urination, and blurred vision. Anxiety and paradoxical stimulation with difficulty sleeping occur in 2–5% of patients. Tardive dyskinesia has been reported rarely, and TCAs may lower seizure threshold. Amitriptyline and imipramine have been associated with sudden death in rare cases. These drugs have rarely been associated with fatal arrhythmias. To date, doxepin has not been reported to have cardiac side effects. For patients over age 50 or who have significant risk factors for cardiac disease, an ECG is recommended before these agents are administered. This precaution is also recommended for most of the preventive antimigraine agents listed in Table 49-5.

Combinations of amitriptyline in dosages of 75–150 mg/day and propranolol at 80–160 mg/day have been used by headache experts for several years in treating migraine. In some patients, a significant additive effect is observed.

d. **Cyproheptadine.** Pharmacologically, cyproheptadine has a tricyclic structure, but its major effect is that of an antihistamine. Cyproheptadine produced more than 50% improvement in 45–50% of subjects in two trials. The potential side effects and potential toxic problems of cyproheptadine are the same as those of amitriptyline, although cyproheptadine usually has fewer side effects than amitriptyline. Dosages of 12–24 mg/day are the usual effect dose in those who respond. Doses of up to 40 mg/day may be tried if not limited by side effect.

e. **Valproic acid (VPA)** was first reported to be effective in treating migraine in 1987. Other anecdotal trials that confirmed the original report ensued, which led to several controlled trials in which approximately 50% of subjects treated with VPA were improved more than 50%.

Valproic acid formulated as divalproex sodium (Depakote) has a higher tolerability. The earlier formulation had a higher incidence of nausea and gastric irritation. The major side effects of VPA as divalproex sodium are weight gain, tremor, and hair loss. These symptoms remit when VPA is discontinued.

Alterations of liver function by changes in carnitine metabolism occur and may result in elevated blood ammonia. Hepatoxicity may occur and is a greater risk in the setting of polytherapy. Children are at greater risk than adults, and the extent of potential hepatoxicity in adults is unknown. VPA may also be associated with bone marrow suppression, but this occurs rarely if at all.

The dosage for divalproex sodium is 250 mg bid-tid initially and then is increased to 500 mg tid if needed. It is unclear if higher dosages are effective when these doses are not.

f. **Methysergide** is a serotonin receptor blocking agent, although it also has significant potency for blocking norepinephrine receptors. Methysergide is effective for migraine prophylaxis, with 55–60% of subjects reporting more than 50% relief. Methysergide, however, has a very high side-effect profile. The most common side effects are nausea and abdominal cramping, which may occur in 10–20% of patients. Other acute side effects include coolness of the digits as a result of vasoconstriction, acroparesthesia, neuropathy, limb edema, rashes, and psychiatric side effects consisting of dissociation of thoughts, anxiety, nervousness, and, rarely, hallucinations.

In patients who have taken methysergide for prolonged periods of time (greater than 2 years), inflammatory fibrosis may develop in the retroperitoneal area, in the lungs, or in the myocardium. Typically, patients so affected are those who have taken methysergide uninterruptedly for more than 2 years and often for as much as 5 years.

It is recommended that methysergide be given for no more than 6 months at a time without at least a 1-month drug holiday. Usually the patient receives the medication for 5 months, takes a 1-month holiday, and then resumes treatment for another 5 months.

Methysergide should be started at 2 mg/day and increased by 2 mg/day to a level of 2 mg tid.

Patients should be monitored periodically for serum creatinine. Some authorities recommend that periodic intravenous pyelograms or CT scans of the kidney with contrast be taken as part of the monitoring process.

Comment: The five medications listed above (propranolol, amitriptyline, cyproheptadine, valproic acid, and methysergide) have typically been the most effective in a compilation of studies carried out to determine the extent to which patients were improved by at least 50%. The results showed that 58% of a group of 1500 patients taking methysergide, 55% of a group of 100 patients on amitriptyline, 51% of a group of 210 patients on propranolol, and 48% of a group of 50 patients on cyproheptadine reached this criterion in various double-blind studies in a comparison of medication versus placebo. No definite dosage-response relationship has been found for any prophylactic antimigraine medication. The prophylactic antimigraine response is idiosyncratic as far as we now know.

g. **Calcium channel blocking agents** generally have been disappointing in their effects on migraine prophylaxis. Initial expectations for these agents were high, but the calcium channel blocking agents have shown very poor effectiveness in double-blind studies against placebos. There appears, however, to be a smaller group of patients who respond very well to calcium channel blocking agents. These patients often develop tachyphylaxis after 2 or 3 months on the medication and require a period of 1 month off the medication to restore responsiveness.

The representative of this group is verapamil. When it is effective, it is usually at dosages of 80–240 mg/day. Verapamil is typically more effective when used as the regular formulation and less effective as a slow-release agent or long-acting agent. Usually 80 mg tid is a reasonably effective dosage. The dosage may be increased to 120 mg qid if tolerated.

h. **Clonidine,** an alpha agonist, was also once thought to be an agent with a bright future in migraine prophylaxis. Several trials of clonidine have been carried out, but none has shown significant potential. In this author's experience, rare patients who have been refractory to other medications have responded to clonidine.

i. **Monoamine oxidase inhibitors (MAOIs)** have been studied primarily in an anecdotal fashion. Phenelzine has been used most commonly. Because of the risk of paradoxical hypertension and the need for a special diet low in tyramine, MAOIs are used only when other drugs have failed. Occasionally, patients may respond to phenelzine at 15–30 mg tid. The reader is referred to drug compendia for pharmacology and side effects.

j. **Cost of therapy.** The preventive or prophylactic antimigraine medications vary widely in cost. Table 49-6 reviews the costs of 1-month supplies of these medications at their usual daily dosages. The average wholesale price is presented.

II. **Cluster headache therapy and management**

A. **Symptomatic therapy.** The therapies for cluster headache can be divided into symptomatic and prophylactic approaches (Fig. 49-3). The symptomatic treatment can be further subdivided into nonspecific analgesic medications and specific abortive medications.

1. **Analgesic or narcotic nonspecific medications** generally represent a very ineffective way of treating cluster headache. Because of the usual brief duration of the cluster headache and gastroparesis during the headache, analgesic medications usually do not have time to be fully absorbed and become effective by the time the headache terminates. Even for more prolonged headaches, where the medications have time to be effective, the results are usually poor with oral or injected medications. Typically, analgesic and narcotic medications provide relatively little relief for cluster headache patients.

2. **Abortive medications** include ergotamine, dihydroergotamine, and sumatriptan as well as oxygen.

Ergotamine, as a therapy for cluster headache, can be given by pill or suppository. Cluster headache is associated with a relative gastroparesis that slows absorption of ergotamine. Nevertheless, studies by Kudrow showed that ergotamine by mouth can be effective in producing pain relief in approximately 10 minutes. The dosage guidelines for ergotamine in cluster headache are similar to those employed for migraine.

Dihydroergotamine given as a subcutaneous (SC) or intramuscular (IM) injection can produce good relief for cluster headache patients. Onset of action is within 5–10 minutes with a dosage of 1 mg IM.

Sumatriptan at a dosage of 6 mg SC usually produces rapid relief from cluster headache. Studies on oral sumatriptan have also shown good effectiveness.

Oxygen delivered with a mask at a rate of 2–3 l/min can produce good relief from cluster headache with onset of effect in a few minutes. Typically

Table 49-6. Cost of medication: Migraine prophylaxis, one-month supply.

Medication	Daily dosage (mg)	Tablet size (mg)	No. tablets/m	AWP*
Methysergide (Sansert)	4	2	60	$102.60
Propranolol (Inderal)	240	80	90	90.32
Propranolol (generic)	240	80	90	20.69
Amitriptyline (Elavil)	50	50	30	20.67
	100	50	60	41.55
Amitriptyline (generic)	50	50	30	2.32
	100	50	60	4.70
Doxepin (Sinequan)	50	50	30	19.09
	100	50	60	36.18
Doxepin (generic)	50	50	30	5.99
	100	50	60	12.10
Divalproex (Depakote)	750	250	90	67.29
Verapamil (Calan)	240	80	90	44.64
	240 (sustained release)		30	40.78
Verapamil (generic)	240	80	90	5.07
	240 (sustained release)		30	34.86

*Average wholesale price.

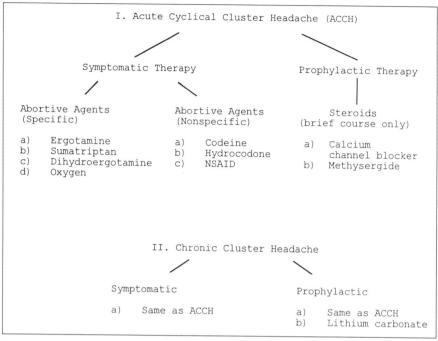

Figure 49-3. Approach to cluster headache therapy.

the patient must continue oxygen administration for 15–30 minutes. In a significant number of patients, the headache recurs shortly after oxygen administration is discontinued.

B. Prophylactic therapy of cluster headache is often preferable. Because of the stereotyped nature of the headache, its tendency to occur in cycles, and the frequency of headaches during the cycles, patients usually prefer a preventive approach if possible.

1. Steroids. Corticosteroids are highly effective in temporary prophylaxis of cluster headache. The most commonly employed steroid preparation is prednisone, although equipotent dosages of other corticosteroid preparations show the same degree of activity. For this reason, the recommendations noted will be given in terms of dosage of prednisone.

The dosages of prednisone that have been reported to be effective in cluster headache vary from 10–100 mg/day. Typically, a higher dosage is needed to initiate steroid therapy. As steroid dosage is tapered, it is common for the cluster headaches to recur at dosages of or equivalent to 20 mg of prednisone per day. As a result, steroids are usually best employed for temporary prophylaxis and for gaining control of the cluster headache, with either verapamil or methysergide being employed for longer-term prophylaxis.

Steroids may not be used for prolonged periods without risk of significant side effects. The side effects, well known to physicians, include increased fragility of blood vessels and skin, osteoporosis, aseptic necrosis of the head of the femur, obesity, myopathy, and psychosis.

2. Methysergide was the first medication to demonstrate a prophylactic effect in cluster headache patients. Loughlin, when reporting on this treatment in 1952, noted that 70% of patients responded well in the first cycle or cluster that was treated, 48% of the group responded the second time, and 25% responded the third time. Although there have been few formal studies, this author's experience has been similar to that of Kunkel. The dosages of methysergide vary from 4–8 mg/day. Side effects of methysergide are outlined in sec. **I.B.4.f.**

3. Calcium channel blocking agents. Verapamil, a calcium channel blocking agent, has been shown to have a prophylactic effect in cluster headache patients. Because of the lower incidence of side effects, it has become the preferred agent for prophylaxis. Dosages of verapamil may vary from 120–480 mg/day depending on the patient and whether the patient has side effects of bradycardia, hypotension, or constipation. The results with verapamil are generally similar to those of methysergide, with a tendency for subsequent cycles of therapy to diminish in effectiveness. Verapamil should not be used in sick sinus syndrome, A-V block, and Wolff-Parkinson-White syndrome if there is left ventricular failure.

4. **Combined therapy.** A therapeutic approach combining steroids and either verapamil or methysergide has provided good results in this author's experience. Typically the patient is treated with prednisone at 60–100 mg/day for 3 days with a rapid taper of 20 mg every 2 days until the prednisone is discontinued. At the same time that prednisone is started, the patient is started on verapamil at a dosage of 80 mg tid or methysergide at 2 mg bid or tid. The verapamil or methysergide is then continued for 60–90 days. This combined therapy has achieved good results in 70–80% of first-time trials. In treatment of subsequent cycles, however, the effectiveness of verapamil and methysergide may diminish, as indicated in secs. **II.B.2** and **3.**

The routine medications for prevention of migraine headache are relatively ineffective for cluster headache. Relatively poor results are obtained with beta-adrenergic blocking agents, tricyclic antidepressants, cyproheptadine, or clonidine.

III. Chronic cluster headache

A. Prescribing therapy for chronic cluster headache is very difficult. Lithium has been reported to be effective in several studies. The typical dosages are 600–1200 mg/day, controlling the blood level at 0.6–1.2 mEq/L. The usual signs of lithium toxicity include confusion, disorientation, drowsiness, seizures, thirst, and rashes. Patients should be warned about, and observed for development of, these side effects. Blood levels should be monitored if lithium is to be used. In patients for whom lithium is successful, tachyphylaxis often develops over time. When this occurs it is necessary to discontinue the lithium and restart it after 4–6 weeks to restore responsiveness.

Combinations of steroids with either verapamil or methysergide, and occasionally tricyclic antidepressants or MAOIs, may be beneficial in treating chronic cluster headache.

B. For patients who have chronic cluster headaches that do not respond to any medical therapy, surgery on the trigeminal nerve has been somewhat effective. Two procedures have been prescribed: a trigeminal gangliotomy by radiofrequency lesioning and a preganglionic nerve-root section. Both of these procedures produce numbness and diminished sensation in the distribution of the trigeminal nerve. Patients who have had these procedures often note that they still have sensations as if they were having cluster headaches but no longer have the pain. To date, there have been no serious complications noted in the small series that have been recorded. Longer-term follow-up is still inadequate to determine if these procedures will produce long-term relief.

IV. Tension headache therapy is based on chronicity of occurrence for the acute tension headache. Use of nonsteroidal anti-inflammatory agents or a combination of butalbitol (50 mg) and an analgesic such as aspirin (Fiorinal) or acetaminophen (Fioricet) may be very helpful. At times, addition of a muscle relaxant in a low dosage, such as 2 mg of diazepam or 50 mg of orphenadrine, may be helpful. Very often, however, the patient with pure tension headache does not worry about medication unless the tension headache develops into a migraine.

For chronic tension headache, a different situation exists. Chronic tension headaches typically have combined symptoms of tension and migraine headaches and fit into the category of chronic daily headache. Typically, the first-approach therapy is to use tricyclic antidepressant agents. Any of the other preventive antimigraine agents can also be used. Not infrequently, combination therapies combining a tricyclic with one of the other medications may be attempted, although there are relatively few standard data on response to these combination regimens. For this type of patient, it is necessary to limit access to habituating medication. Because of the chronicity of the pain problem, patients are very likely to overuse medications that are potentially habituating. This overuse may lead to a rebound-withdrawal (habituation-withdrawal) type of headache. In these situations, the medication becomes part of the problem instead of part of the solution.

V. Referral. Many headache patients are treated very capably by primary care physicians, but additional opinions and specialized care are sometimes required. One of the questions often asked is when a patient should be referred to a headache specialist. Situations that may require referral include:

1. a new, unexplained headache
2. development of new, unexplained neurologic findings
3. poor response to the treatments with which the physician is comfortable
4. a situation in which the referring physician is uncomfortable with the patient for medical or psychological reasons

The first area of consideration is a new, unexplained headache. If the patient has a headache that is severe enough to cause continual complaints and the treating physician is unable to find an adequate etiology, the patient probably should be referred to a specialist with greater knowledge of headaches.

If the patient develops new and progressive neurologic findings that cannot be explained on the basis of available testing and insight, the patient should be seen by a headache specialist.

The third situation deals with treatment of the headache. If the primary physician is unable to provide the patient with adequate relief, referral should be considered. If the pain can be relieved only by increasing the dosage of an analgesic/narcotic medication and the possibility looms that the patient may develop a habituation-withdrawal headache in response to that medication, the patient should be referred.

Finally, if the physician simply feels uncomfortable with the situation and believes that his or her skills may be inadequate to help the patient, referral is advised. The difficult headache patient usually has a very chronic pain problem, which may be exacerbated by psychological factors. If the patient is manifesting a significant degree of chronicity and if communication and trust between the patient and the physician begin to break down, referral is indicated.

Patients with chronic diseases often "doctor shop" to see if some other physician can provide a better level of treatment. If a patient asks for a referral, it is best to proceed with the referral. The patient will respect the physician for assisting the patient to continue searching for pain relief. The physician's ready agreement to refer the patient demonstrates to the patient that the doctor's first concern is the patient's well-being.

There are several specialized headache centers throughout the country. The American Association for the Study of Headache and the American Council of Headache Education can provide patients with information about these centers. The address for both organizations is 875 Kings Highway, Suite 200, Woodbury, New Jersey 08096-3172.

Recommended Readings

Belgrade MJ, et al. Comparison of single-dose meperidine, butorphanol, and dihydroergotamine in the treatment of vascular headache. *Neurology* 39:590–592, 1989.

Callahan M, Raskin N. A controlled study of dihydroergotamine in the treatment of acute migraine headache. *Headache* 26:168–171, 1986.

Couch J. Cluster headache: Characteristics and treatment. *Semin Neurol* 2(1):30–40, 1982.

Couch J. Medical management of recurrent tension-type headache. In CD Tollison, RS Kunkel (eds), *Headache Diagnosis and Treatment*. Baltimore: Williams & Wilkins, 1993. Pp 151–162.

Couch J. Complexities of presentation and pathogenesis of migraine headache. In RK Cady, AW Fox (eds), *Treating the Headache Patient*. New York: Marcel Dekker, 1995. Pp 15–40.

Couch J, Hassanein RS. Amitriptyline in migraine prophylaxis. *Arch Neurol* 36:695–699, 1979.

Couch J, Micieli G. Prophylactic pharmacotherapy. In J Olesen, P Tfelt-Hansen, KMA Welch (eds), *The Headaches*. New York: Raven, 1993. Pp 537–542.

Ferrari MD, Saxena PR. Clinical and experimental effects of sumatriptan in humans. *Trends Pharmacol Sci* 14:129–133, 1993.

Hoffert MJ, et al. Transnasal butorphanol in the treatment of acute migraine. *Headache* 35:65–69, 1994.

Humphrey PPA, Feniuk W. Mode of action of the anti-migraine drug sumatriptan. *Trends Pharmacol Sci* 12:444–445, 1991.

Kudrow L. Plasma testosterone levels in cluster headache: Preliminary results. *Headache* 16:28–31, 1976.

Loushin L. Treatment of histaminic cephalgia with methysergide (UML-491). *Dis Nerv System* 24:3–7, 1963.

Mathew N. Clinical subtypes of cluster headache and response to lithium therapy. *Headache* 18:26–30, 1978.

Mathew NI, et al. Migraine prophylaxis with divalproex. *Arch Neurol* 52:281–286, 1995.

Moskowitz MA. Neurogenic versus vascular mechanisms of sumatriptan and ergot alkaloids in migraine. *Trends Pharmacol Sci* 13:307–311, 1992.

Silberstein SD, Young WB. Safety and efficacy of ergotamine tartrate and dihydroergotamine in the treatment of migraine and status migrainosus. *Neurology* 45:577–584, 1995.

The Subcutaneous Sumatriptan International Study Group. Treatment of migraine attacks with sumatriptan. *N Engl J Med* 325:316–321, 1991.

Tfelt-Hansen P, Johnson ES. Ergotamine. In J Olesen, P Tfelt-Hansen, KMA Welch (eds), *The Headaches*. New York: Raven, 1993. Pp 313–322.

Tfelt-Hansen P, Johnson ES. Nonsteroidal anti-inflammatory drugs in the treatment of the acute migraine attack. In J Olesen, P Tfelt-Hansen, KMA Welch (eds), *The Headaches*. New York: Raven, 1993. Pp 305–311.

Tfelt-Hansen P, Saxena PR. Antiserotonin drugs. In J Olesen, P Tfelt-Hansen, KMA Welch (eds), *The Headaches*. New York: Raven, 1993. Pp 373–382.

Tfelt-Hansen P, Shanks RG. B-adrenoceptor blocking drugs. In J Olesen, P Tfelt-Hansen, KMA Welch (eds), *The Headaches*. New York: Raven, 1993. Pp 363–372.

Toda N, Tfelt-Hansen P. Calcium antagonists. In J Olesen, P Tfelt-Hansen, KMA Welch (eds), *The Headaches*. New York: Raven, 1993. Pp 383–390.

50

Chronic Pain
Bette G. Maybury

Chronic pain has been described by various pain authorities as pain lasting longer than 1, 3, or 6 months or pain that persists past the "usual" time for a given disorder to heal. Obviously certain chronic and degenerative diseases by their very nature include chronic pain as part of the illness. The International Association for the Study of Pain (IASP) defines chronic pain as pain that is present for 3 months.

Chronic pain is a significant health problem contributing to physical, psychological, and psychosocial impairment at great cost to patients, their families, and society. This chapter discusses treatment of the various types of chronic pain in general terms.

I. Types of chronic pain
A. Neuropathic pain
1. **Symptomatology.** Neuropathic pain may have more than one aspect in a given patient. Characteristics frequently described include burning, ripping, throbbing, aching, prickling, lancinating, shocklike sensations, and jabbing. The painful symptoms may be associated with numbness, weakness and atrophy, fasciculations, and muscle cramps. Restless legs are observed with some types of neuropathic pain.
2. **Etiologies**
   a. **Polyneuropathies.** (The reader is referred to a more detailed description in Chap. 46, sec. **II.**)
      (1) Metabolic: e.g., diabetes mellitus, uremia
      (2) Nutritional: e.g., vitamin deficiency and alcoholism
      (3) Toxic: e.g., heavy metals, organic compounds, and medications
      (4) Vasculitic/inflammatory: e.g., rheumatoid arthritis, systemic lupus erythematosus, Guillain-Barré syndrome, and chronic inflammatory demyelinating polyradiculopathy
      (5) Infectious: e.g., HIV
      (6) Malignancy: e.g., paraneoplastic
      (7) Inherited: e.g., hereditary sensory motor neuropathies and Fabry's disease
      (8) Ischemic: e.g., peripheral vascular disease
      (9) Idiopathic
   b. **Mononeuropathies/mononeuropathy multiplex**
      (1) Metabolic: e.g., diabetic amyotrophy
      (2) Vasculitic/inflammatory: e.g., collagen vascular diseases, periarteritis nodosum, and sarcoidosis
      (3) Infectious: e.g., herpes zoster, infectious mononucleosis, and leprosy
      (4) Malignant: e.g., direct or metastatic invasion
      (5) Traumatic/surgical
      (6) Idiopathic
B. Musculoskeletal pain
1. **Symptomatology.** Musculoskeletal pain may include deep or superficial aching, throbbing, burning, or tenderness, which may be diffuse or local. The pain is frequently associated with muscle spasms, stiffness, and decreased range of motion.
2. **Etiologies**
   a. Arthritides
   b. Fibromyalgia and myofascial pain
   c. Myopathies
   d. Trauma/postoperative

e. Metabolic bone and muscle diseases

C. Psychological/psychosocial pain. Depression, anxiety, and insomnia frequently accompany chronic pain. Patients may markedly decrease physical activity, withdraw socially, or both. Treatment to reverse or diminish these symptoms and behaviors is imperative to prevent a vicious cycle of increasing pain, dysfunction, and impairment.

In some patients, psychological or psychosocial dysfunction may be the primary cause of the chronic pain rather than secondary to it. In either situation, a formal psychological/psychiatric evaluation and ongoing treatment can be helpful. The majority of patients are amenable to this recommendation if approached in a positive manner. An acknowledgment by the primary physician that psychological and emotional stress are to be expected with chronic pain allows patients to accept intervention to aid them in coping with their illnesses.

II. Treatment of chronic pain

A. Remove the causative agent or treat the underlying disease process.

B. Medications

1. **Opioids** (Table 50-1). If possible, opioids should be avoided in chronic benign pain management. In reality, however, they are sometimes necessary. Guidelines are as follows.

   a. Use preparations with the least abuse potential and the fewest or mildest side effects. Prescribe oral medications if possible.

   b. Use the lowest dosages needed for analgesia. (Concomitant use of NSAIDs often greatly potentiates efficacy.)

   c. Prescribe fixed dosages with monitoring for abuse—i.e., multiple pharmacies or physicians.

   d. Treat side effects—e.g., constipation and nausea. The opioid medications exert their effects by interacting with several types of opioid receptors in both the PNS and CNS. They not only produce analgesia, but may also have side effects of sedation, respiratory depression, nausea, cognitive impairment, pruritis, dizziness, hypotension, constipation, and urinary retention.

   Avoid concomitant use of pure agonist and agonist-antagonist medications or use of agonist-antagonist agents following chronic use of pure agonists.

2. **Nonsteroidal anti-inflammatory drugs (NSAIDs)** (Table 50-2) are thought to produce their analgesic and anti-inflammatory effects by inhibiting prostaglandin production. Other nonprostaglandin effects are likely, and central effects have been postulated as well.

   Use of a given NSAID should be dictated by patient response in regard to efficacy and side effects. Sequential trials of different medications are warranted, because effectiveness varies from one patient to another. Medication trials should last about 4 weeks unless side effects intervene.

Table 50-1. Equivalent opioid dosages.

Medication	Dosage (mg)	
	IM	Oral
Pure Agonists		
Morphine	10	30
Hydromorphone	1.5	7.5
Hydrocodone	—	5–10
Oxycodone	15	30
Meperidine	100	300
Codeine	130	200
Propoxyphene napsylate	—	400
Propoxyphene hydrochloride	—	300
Agonist-Antagonists		
Butorphanol	2	2 (nasal spray)
Pentazocine	60	180*

*Oral analgesia is weak and unpredictable.

Table 50-2. NSAID daily dosages.

Medication	Maximum daily dosage (mg)	Dosing schedule
Acetylsalicylic acid	6000	qid
Choline magnesium trisalicylate	6000	Daily or bid
Diflunisal	1500	bid
Ibuprofen	3200	qid
Ketoprofen	300	tid
Fenoprofen	3200	qid
Flurbiprofen	300	tid
Diclofenac	200	tid
Naproxen/naproxen sodium	1500/1375	bid
Etodolac	1200[a]	tid
Nabumetone	2000	Daily or bid
Indomethacin	200	tid
Sulindac	400	bid
Tolmetin	2000	qid
Piroxicam	20	Daily
Meclofenamate	400	bid
Ketorolac[b]	10	qid
Oxaprozin	1200	Daily

[a]For patients weighing 60 kg or less, maximum dosage is 20 mg/kg.
[b]Not recommended for continuous chronic use.

NSAIDs should be taken with food. Side effects include heartburn, bloating, flatulence, diarrhea, gastric ulceration and bleeding, hepatic and renal dysfunction, and inhibition of platelet aggregation.

3. **Antidepressants** (Table 50-3). Use of antidepressants as pain medications should be explained to the patient to avert suspicion that "the doctor just thinks I'm depressed." The mechanism of action as pain medication is unknown but is likely to be multifactorial—i.e., decreased synaptic transmission, potentiation of endogenous opioids, improved sleep, and an antidepressant effect. In general, lower dosages are required for treatment of pain

Table 50-3. Antidepressant daily dosages.

Medication	Dosage (mg)	
	As a pain reliever	As an antidepressant
More Sedating		
Amitriptyline	10–75 at bedtime	150–250 at bedtime
Doxepin	10–75 at bedtime	150–250 at bedtime
Trazodone*	50–150 at bedtime	200–400 tid
Less Sedating		
Nortriptyline	10–50 at bedtime	75–100 at bedtime
Desipramine*	10–75 at bedtime	100–250 at bedtime
Imipramine	10–75 at bedtime	150–250 at bedtime
Newer Agents		
Fluoxetine	Insufficient data	20–60 daily
Fluvoxamine	Insufficient data	150 bid
Nefazodone	Insufficient data	100–300 daily
Paroxetine	Insufficient data	20–40 daily
Sertraline	Insufficient data	50–200 daily
Venlafaxine	Insufficient data	25–75 tid

*Less anticholinergic.

than for treatment of depression. Begin with a low dosage (10–25 mg) and titrate upward as needed and tolerated.

Side effects include sedation, dry mouth, constipation, orthostatic hypotension, urinary retention, dizziness, confusion, and weight gain. Amitriptyline sometimes paradoxically causes agitation rather than sedation. Substituting doxepin usually circumvents this problem. Concomitant use of monoamine oxidase inhibitors (MAOIs) with antidepressants should be avoided.

4. **Anticonvulsants** (Table 50-4). The mechanism of action of anticonvulsants is probably decreased synaptic transmission. Anticonvulsants are the most useful medications for lancinating or jabbing pain. Side effects include sedation, nausea, dizziness, ataxia, and diplopia. Bone marrow suppression and hepatic dysfunction occur rarely. Development of a generalized rash requires immediate discontinuation. CBC, differential, platelet count, and liver enzymes should be monitored at intervals. A modest but stable elevation of gamma-glutamyltransferase (GGT) is common and is no cause for concern.

   a. **Phenytoin (Dilantin).** Start with 300 mg/day, and increase as needed and tolerated. Steady-state blood levels may take as long as 2 weeks to be reached. Loading may be accomplished by giving 1000 mg orally in divided doses over 12–24 hours. Unique side effects include gingival hyperplasia, hirsutism, and acne. Lymphadenopathy, fever, and arthralgias occur rarely. Late complications are uncommon but can include peripheral neuropathy, osteoporosis, and cerebellar atrophy. Calcium and vitamin B supplementation are recommended for long-term use.

   b. **Carbamazepine (Tegretol).** Start with 100 mg bid, and increase the daily dosage by 100 mg every 3 days up to 200 mg tid or until symptoms are relieved or side effects occur. Leukopenia is common, but WBC counts as low as 2500/mm^3 with absolute granulocyte counts greater than 1000/mm^3 are acceptable. Hyponatremia may develop and limit use. Concomitant use of propoxyphene, erythromycin, and cimetidine markedly increases carbamazepine levels.

   c. **Sodium valproate (Depakote).** Start with 125 mg bid, and increase the daily dosage by 125 mg every 3–4 days until symptoms are relieved or side effects occur. If GI side effects are problematic at the lowest dosage, use 125-mg sprinkles. Addition of baclofen may augment effectiveness. Weight gain and peripheral edema are relatively common side effects. At higher dosages, tremor and/or hair loss may develop. Thrombocytopenia is not uncommon and is dosage-related, usually resolving with decreases in dosage.

   d. **Gabapentin.** Start with 300 mg/day, and increase to 300 mg bid-tid as needed and tolerated. Side effects are uncommon but include sedation, dizziness, and ataxia. These effects can be minimized by using smaller increases in dosage or, if necessary, by using 100-mg capsules to start at a lower dosage. Because gabapentin has low protein binding and renal clearance, it has fewer drug interactions than other anticonvulsants.

5. **Neuroleptics** (Table 50-5). In addition to central effects, neuroleptics are believed to decrease peripheral sensory transmission.

   Many practitioners prefer to avoid neuroleptics because of the danger that tardive dyskinesia (TD) will develop with long-term use. The lower dosages used for pain treatment make TD less likely but do not guarantee that it will not develop. Elderly patients are at higher risk. Long-term use over years is

Table 50-4. Anticonvulsant daily dosages.

Medication	Dosage for pain treatment (mg)	Dosing schedule
Phenytoin	300–400	bid
Carbamazepine	200–600	tid
Sodium valproate	250–1000	bid-tid
Gabapentin	Insufficient data	

Table 50-5. Neuroleptic daily dosages.

Medication	Oral dosage for pain treatment (mg)
Chlorpromazine	10–50
Thioridazine	10–75
Perphenazine	1–5
Trifluoperazine	1–5
Fluphenazine	1–3
Haloperidol	1–3

to be avoided. Other side effects include parkinsonian symptoms, dystonia, cognitive impairment, sedation, and orthostatic hypotension. Neuroleptics may cause myocardial depression and potentiate cardiac arrhythmias in susceptible patients. Less common are bone marrow suppression, hepatic toxicity, and neuroleptic malignant syndrome.

Medications for extrapyramidal side effects should be used only if the symptoms actually occur. Diphenhydramine (Benadryl) at 10–25 mg tid has a milder anticholinergic side effect than that of either benztropine (Cogentin) at 1–6 mg/day or trihexyphenidyl (Artane) at 2–10 mg/day.

6. **Anxiolytics** (Table 50-6). In general, antianxiety medications should be avoided in chronic pain syndromes. Buspirone may be an exception. If anxiety is judged to be a major problem, guidelines for benzodiazepine use are as follows.
   a. First try nonpharmacologic methods such as exercise, biofeedback, and relaxation training.
   b. Use briefly and intermittently.
   c. Practice gradual upward titration and weaning.
   d. Be aware of additive effects with other psychoactive medications.
   e. Assess the patient frequently.
   f. Avoid use in patients with known histories of drug overuse or abuse.
7. **Muscle relaxers** (Table 50-7). Muscle relaxant medications are most suited for short-term use. They may be more effective for chronic pain if used intermittently. Patients taking baclofen or diazepam must be weaned slowly from high dosages. Sedation is a common side effect and may limit use. A bedtime dose only is sometimes helpful, particularly for patients having primarily nocturnal muscle spasms or morning muscle stiffness and difficulty in sleeping.
8. **Other agents**
   a. Quinine sulfate 300 mg daily at bedtime for cramps and restless legs
   b. Clonazepam (Klonopin) 0.5 mg at bedtime for cramps and restless legs
   c. Carbidopa/levodopa (Sinemet) 12.5 mg/50 mg–25 mg/100 mg for cramps and restless legs

Table 50-6. Antianxiety daily dosages.

Medication	Oral dosage (mg)
Benzodiazepines	
Clorazepate	3–15
Chlordiazepoxide	15–30
Diazepam	2.5–10
Alprazolam	0.5–3.0
Lorazepam	2–5
Oxazepam	10–15
Nonbenzodiazepines	
Hydroxyzine	100–400
Buspirone*	15–60

*Avoid concomitant use of monoamine oxidase inhibitors (MAOIs).

Table 50-7. Muscle relaxant daily dosages.

Medication	Oral dosage (mg)	Dosing schedule
Baclofen	60–80*	tid
Carisoprodol	1050–1400	tid-qid
Cyclobenzaprine	20–40	bid-tid
Diazepam	6–40	tid-qid
Methocarbamol	4000–4500	tid-qid

*Start with 5 mg bid and titrate upward.

> **d.** Clonidine (Catapres) at 0.1 mg/day has an intrinsic analgesic effect and potentiates opioids both endogenous and exogenous.
> **e.** Capsaicin 0.025–0.075% topical cream applied to the affected area tid or qid. The mechanism is thought to be depletion of substance P. Expect initial increase in pain (for 2–4 weeks) as substance P is released. If discontinued, substance P reaccumulates and pain recurs.
> **f.** Calcium channel blockers may be effective for metabolic myopathies and sympathetic mediated pain.
>> **(1)** Verapamil (Calan, Verelan, or Isoptin) 40–160 mg tid
>> **(2)** Nifedipine (Procardia) 10–30 mg tid
> **g.** Mexiletine (Mexitil) 100–300 mg tid
> **9. Nerve or trigger-point anesthetic blockade**

C. Nonpharmacologic modalities. A key aspect of the treatment of chronic pain is prevention, if possible. This includes thorough evaluation, avoidance of unnecessary surgery, and aggressive treatment of acute pain. Once chronic pain is established, multiple strategies should be employed, if needed, to promote the best patient outcome.

> **1. Physical and occupational therapy,** including massage, heat/cold, ultrasound, exercise, and bracing
> **2. Electrical stimulation,** including transcutaneous electrical nerve stimulation (TENS), dorsal column stimulators, or thalamic stimulators. The classical proposed mechanism of action of TENS is that large-fiber stimulation closes a sensory "gate" opened by excessive firing of small, pain-carrying fibers.
>
> TENS is a noninvasive but relatively expensive treatment modality. Application of electrodes by an experienced technician for optimum effect will increase the likelihood of success. Contraindications include cardiac pacemakers, pregnancy, and patient inability to use the device properly.
> **3. Psychological interventions**
>> **a. Personal and/or family counseling**
>> **b. Behavior modification**
>> **c. Biofeedback and/or relaxation training**

III. Referral. Consider referral to an anesthesiologist experienced in pain management for trigger-point injection or for peripheral nerve, epidural, or sympathetic blockade. Referral to a psychiatrist or psychologist experienced in pain management is indicated for patients with prominent symptoms in this area that require more counseling or support than can be provided in a general practice setting and for patients who do not respond well to psychotropic medications. A physiatrist can be helpful in management of musculoskeletal pain (which can accompany neurologic disease or injury resulting in weakness with resultant strain on compensating muscles). If the patient remains disabled and dysfunctional, referral to a multidisciplinary pain center should be considered.

Recommended Readings

Bonica JJ, et al. (eds). *The Management of Pain.* Philadelphia-London: Lea & Febiger, 1990.

Cailliet R. *Pain: Mechanisms and Management.* Philadelphia: Davis, 1993.

Tollison CD, Satterthwaite JR, Tollison JW (eds). *Handbook of Pain Management.* Baltimore: Williams & Wilkins, 1994.

Warfield CA (ed). *Manual of Pain Management.* Philadelphia: Lippincott, 1991.

Warfield CA (ed). *Principles and Practice of Pain Management.* New York: McGraw-Hill, 1993.

51

Reflex Sympathetic Dystrophy

R. Venkata Reddy
Kevin Edward Macadaeg

Reflex sympathetic dystrophy (RSD) is a chronic pain syndrome characterized by varying degrees of pain, autonomic dysfunction, sensory changes, and loss of voluntary function. The International Association for the Study of Pain (IASP) in 1986 defined RSD as "continuous pain in a portion of an extremity after trauma, which may include fracture but does not involve a major nerve, associated with sympathetic hyperactivity." Causalgia is defined similarly except that incomplete injury to a major nerve is involved. RSD is associated with a wide variety of precipitating factors (Table 51-1). Trauma is the most common precipitating event in the development of RSD, with an estimated 5% of traumatic cases resulting in RSD.

I. **Pathophysiology.** Various hypotheses put forth over the years have generally favored either a peripheral or a central mechanism.
   A. **Peripheral mechanisms** do not address the issues of spread of pain beyond a dermatomal territory and pain occurring in patients without nerve injury. They are of four types.
      1. C-nociceptive afferent sensitization as a result of high-frequency firing-induced biochemical changes in the involved peripheral nerves
      2. Abnormal activation of peripheral nociceptors by sympathetic efferents
      3. Generation of aberrant nerve sprouts at the site of injury, developing into neuroma
      4. Artificial synapses formed at the site of nerve injury, allowing "ephaptic" transmission between sympathetic efferent and sensory afferent fibers
   B. **Central mechanisms** are of two types.
      1. Self-sustaining loops of abnormal interneuronal firing in the dorsal horn, after being propagated by a peripheral irritative focus, giving rise to ascending projections of pain and descending sympathetic hyperactivity
      2. Long-term sensitization or "wind-up" of wide-dynamic-range (WDR) neurons in the spinal cord resulting from ongoing nociceptive stimulation from the periphery. Continuous stimulation of C fibers causes a progressive increase in response of WDR neurons. Subsequent non-noxious stimulation of the same peripheral area results in stimulation of these spinal neurons to the same degree as that of a painful stimulation. The signs commonly observed in RSD are thought to result from disuse atrophy and extreme guarding behavior secondary to the pain, and not from abnormal sympathetic activity.

II. **Diagnosis and course**
   A. **Diagnosis** of RSD is generally made on the basis of history and clinical findings. The patient reveals varying degrees of clinical features (Table 51-2). The most useful test for confirming the diagnosis of RSD is sympathetic neural blockade with a local anesthetic.

   Methods used in aiding difficult cases of diagnosis and various severities of RSD include radiography and scintigraphy.
      1. **Radiography.** Plain x-rays may show patchy osteopenia in half of all patients. Plain radiography remains useful in detecting or excluding other bony abnormalities.
      2. **Scintigraphy.** The three-phase technetium bone scan (TPBS) is helpful in confirming the diagnosis and staging of RSD. It detects physiologic changes rather than anatomical details, with a sensitivity of 60% and a specificity of 86%. TPBS may also be positive in other patients with osteomyelitis; stress fractures; degenerative arthritis; bone infarctions, malignancies, osteomas; Reiter's disease; and thoracic outlet syndrome. A TPBS is used in three ways.

Table 51-1. Precipitating factors in the development of RSD.

Soft-tissue injury	Malignancy
Fracture	Arthritis
Sprain	Bursitis
Joint dislocation	Peripheral nerve injury
Operative procedures	Carpal tunnel release
Immobilization with a cast or splint	Venipuncture
Arthroscopic surgery	Myocardial infarction
Brachial plexopathy	Polymyalgia rheumatica
Radiculopathy	Myelopathy
Stroke	Dental extraction
Spinal cord injury	Prolonged bed rest
Drugs (isoniazid, phenobarbital, ergotamine, cyclosporine)	

   a. **"Blood flow" phase.** Rapid sequence images of the involved extremity are obtained on IV injection of a radionuclide tracer to evaluate the vascularity of a region.
   b. **"Blood pool" phase.** Images are obtained immediately after the blood flow phase to evaluate regional perfusion including that of soft tissue.
   c. **"Bone scan" phase.** Static images are obtained 2–3 hours after initial injection that detects abnormal osteoblastic activity, reflected locally as increased periarticular uptake in the affected extremity.
 B. **Course.** RSD is a dynamic process that may progress through three stages.
   1. **Stage 1 (acute).** The pain is described as aching or burning aggravated by physical contact or emotional upset and typically restricted to a vascular or peripheral nerve or root territory. Some patients complain of abnormal sensations, whether spontaneous or evoked (paresthesias). Light touch can induce pain (allodynia). Tissue swelling and local vascular, bony, and trophic changes occur in the affected part. Roentgenography may show diffuse bony changes. TPBS may reveal increased radionuclide uptake in all phases. Stage 1 is usually observed 1–3 months following injury.
   2. **Stage 2 (dystrophic).** This stage is characterized by spontaneous burning pain radiating proximally or distally from the site of injury, associated with pronounced hyperpathia (prolonged painful sensation to touch), decreased hair growth, brittle nails, and indurated edematous tissue. Roentgenography may show patchy osteoporosis. TPBS demonstrates normalization in blood flow and blood pool phases with the bone scan phase remaining intense. Stage 2 is usually observed 3–6 months following injury.
   3. **Stage 3 (atrophic).** Pain tends to subside or diminish in intensity. The skin is cool, thin, and shiny. Irreversible trophic changes occur with subcutaneous atrophy and wasted fingertips. Roentgenograms may show severe patchy osteopenia. TPBS demonstrates reduced blood flow and blood pool phases and bone scan phase normalization. Stage 3 is usually observed 6 months to years following injury.

Table 51-2. Clinical features of RSD.

Feature	Examples
Autonomic deregulation	Temperature, vasomotor, and sudomotor instability
Blood flow alterations	Hyperhydrosis, hypohydrosis, edema, and discoloration
Sensory abnormalities	Burning pain, hyperpathia (prolonged painful sensation to touch), allodynia (pain resulting from a stimulus that is normally painless—e.g., touch), and dysesthesia (an unpleasant abnormal sensation)
Motor dysfunction	Weakness, tremor, and joint stiffness
Trophic changes	Skin thinning, hair loss, and brittle nails
Psychological disturbances	Anxiety, depression, and suicidal ideation
Radiologic changes	Patchy osteoporosis, soft-tissue edema, and articular erosion

III. **Prevention** is best accomplished through early recognition and treatment. The unnecessary use of braces, casts, splints, and immobilization should be avoided. If RSD is suspected, heat should be applied rather than cold. Alcohol is better avoided because it affects temperature regulation and may aggravate soft-tissue damage by increasing hyperoxide activity in the area of damage.

IV. **Management.** RSD remains one of the most perplexing chronic pain syndromes to treat. The treatment goals early in the course of the disease are cessation of aberrant sympathetic hyper- or hypoactivity, desensitization of normal sensory pathways transmitting pain, and maintenance of normal musculoskeletal function. Reasonable approaches for the treatment of upper- and lower-extremity RSD are presented in the form of algorithms in Figures 51-1 and 51-2.

A. **Pharmacologic therapy**

1. **Anti-inflammatory agents.** Proposed mechanisms of the actions of non-

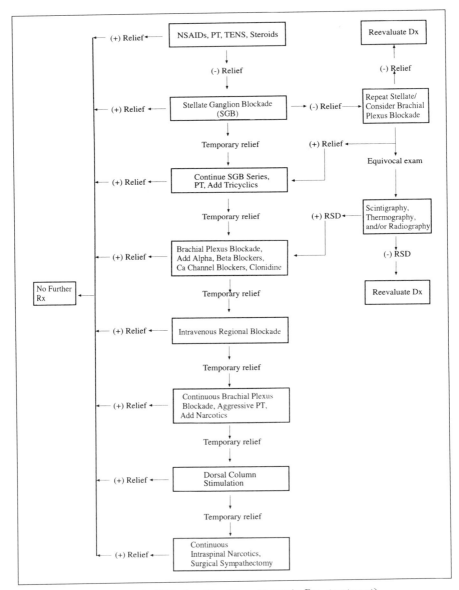

Figure 51-1. Upper-extremity RSD algorithm (Dx = diagnosis; Rx = treatment).

steroidal anti-inflammatory drugs (NSAIDs) in the prevention of RSD include reduced swelling with increased mobility of muscles and joints, inhibition of prostaglandin synthesis causing reduced sensitivity of pain receptors; and thromboxane inhibition causing interference with vasoconstriction.

NSAIDs are usually started in patients with early, mild symptoms—particularly when an inflammatory process (e.g., arthritis) is a component of the painful condition. Regardless of the agent chosen, the dosage should be maximized for optimal control of pain. NSAIDs are of minimal beneficial value, however, in the treatment of longstanding RSD.

An IV regional blockade technique with **ketorolac** at a dosage of 60 mg, in saline or 0.5% lidocaine, to volumes of 40 ml in the upper extremity and 50 ml in the lower extremity, has produced prolonged pain relief with no serious side effects in some patients.

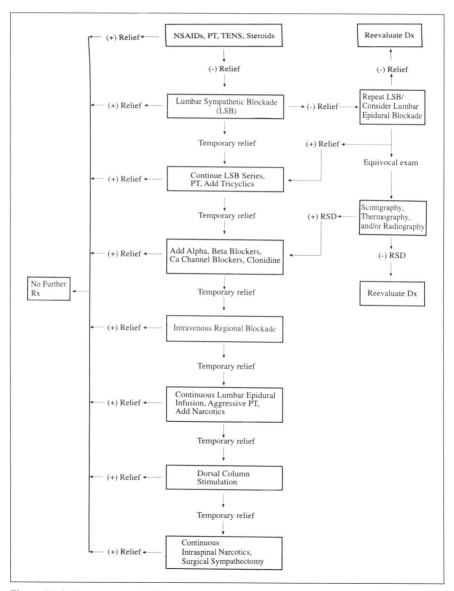

Figure 51-2. Lower-extremity RSD algorithm (Dx = diagnosis; Rx = treatment).

2. **Antidepressants** are effective adjuvants and are commonly used in RSD. They have direct analgesic effects, and proposed mechanisms include (1) potentiation of descending inhibitory pain-modulating pathways by blockade of presynaptic reuptake of the neurotransmitters serotonin and norepinephrine; (2) a neuronal membrane–stabilizing effect; (3) alterations in adrenergic, anticholinergic, and adenosinergic effects; and (4) a synergistic effect with opioid analgesics through bioavailability enhancement. Their direct antidepressant and sedative effects are beneficial in treating the depressive and anxious states that patients with chronic pain are likely to exhibit. There are no clear-cut studies demonstrating a significantly higher quality of analgesia for any one antidepressant, and hence the choice of drug depends on the patient's medical profile and previous response to antidepressants.

   Amitriptyline is the prototype tricyclic antidepressant and is the most widely used. Its propensity for norepinephrine reuptake blockade is greater than that for serotonin. Two weeks of treatment may be required before its analgesic effect is observed. Treatment should begin with small dosages of 10–25 mg at bedtime, which should be increased by 10–25 mg every 1–2 weeks, while assessing for side effects, until a beneficial effect is achieved or a maximum of 150 mg is reached.

   Antidepressants may interfere with the reuptake mechanism of bretylium, an agent commonly used in an IV regional sympathetic blockade technique. Antidepressant therapy should be discontinued for at least 2 weeks prior to initiation of IV bretylium blocks.

   Complications of antidepressant use include sedation, orthostatic hypotension, dry mouth, blurred vision, and urinary retention.

3. **Systemic corticosteroids.** In addition to having anti-inflammatory effects, steroids may have inhibitory effects on spontaneous neural discharge. Their effects are only temporary and they do not inhibit the sympathetic reflex mechanism in RSD.

   A standardized regimen of high initial dosage and subsequent tapering of dosage consists of prednisone (or an equivalent) at 15 mg qid, 10 mg qid, 10 mg tid, 10 mg bid, 15 mg every morning, 10 mg every morning, and 5 mg every morning for 4 days each.

   Injections of depot steroids directly into inflamed muscles and joints may significantly reduce pain in an affected extremity and serve adjunctively as a treatment for RSD.

   Potential harmful effects of steroids include osteoporosis, hyperglycemia, adrenal suppression, glucose intolerance, and sodium and water retention.

4. **Narcotic analgesics** are rarely required in the treatment of RSD. Intermittent use of narcotic analgesics as a prophylactic measure may be beneficial prior to exercise therapy.

   In severe, dystrophic stages associated with longstanding pain not controlled by other medical therapy or nerve block procedures, narcotic analgesics may become a necessary adjunct to long-term care. In such cases, administration by means of an intrathecal morphine pump, as discussed in sec. **IV.F.2,** may be appropriate.

   The risks of tolerance and dependence that attend long-term narcotic use must be carefully weighed against the benefits.

5. **Calcium channel blockers** are utilized in RSD for their peripheral vasodilatory effects as well as their antagonistic effects with norepinephrine on arterial and venous smooth muscles.

   Nifedipine has the most vasodilatory effect of all the calcium channel blockers. A hypothermic extremity, as typically observed in RSD, is an appropriate indication.

   Side effects of calcium channel blockers include an increase in pain, hypotension, myocardial depression, and cold intolerance as a result of peripheral vasodilatation.

6. **Alpha-2 agonists** have been studied in recent years to determine their analgesic effects on chronic pain states.

   Clonidine, a centrally acting alpha-2 agonist, causes decreased sympathetic outflow and vasodilatation. Clonidine administered transdermally by application of a patch causes inhibition of norepinephrine release from peripheral presynaptic adrenergic terminals. Clinically, it produces a substantial reduction in hyperalgesia in response to mechanical stimuli confined primarily to the skin beneath the patch. Reports of systemic analgesic effects of clonidine are conflicting. Therefore, this agent may be most useful for patients with RSD limited to only small areas. The recommended method of application is to place a patch over an area of allodynia, starting with 0.1 mg placed every 3 days and increasing the dosage by 0.1-mg increments every 12 days, to a dosage of 0.3 mg. The skin should be checked for desensitization underneath the patch on replacement, and tolerance of side effects should be noted before the dosage is increased. The localized analgesia effect is typically seen within 36–48 hours and subsides within a week of discontinuance.

Clonidine administered in a 300-μg dose within the epidural space produces effective analgesia in patients with refractory RSD, but long-term relief has not been fully addressed.

Significant side effects of clonidine include hypotension, bradycardia, and sedation.

7. **Alpha-1 antagonists** have been shown to be of some help to patients with RSD.

Terazosin, an oral alpha-1 antagonist, appears to be effective for some patients and can be used on a once daily dosing regimen. It can be started at 1 mg at bedtime and titrated slowly upward to 3 mg at bedtime.

Use of alpha-blockers is limited by their prominent side effects of hypotension, reflex tachycardia, fatigue, and dizziness.

8. **Anticonvulsants** stabilize abnormal hyperexcitability in both peripheral and central neurons and are thus hypothesized to inhibit excessive discharge of regional sympathetic nerves. Phenytoin at a dosage of 100 mg qid or carbamazepine at 200 mg tid may be used for management of dysesthesia.

9. **Calcitonin,** given parenterally or intranasally, is widely employed for RSD pain in the United Kingdom. It has analgesic activity and inhibits bone resorption activity.

B. **Physical therapy** is a very useful adjunct in the management of RSD. It is used to treat and minimize dystrophic changes in muscles and joints. Compliance is increased if adequate pain relief can be achieved prior to initiation of physical therapy.

1. **Range of motion (ROM) and stretching exercises** are used for progressive stretching of restrictive tissue for maintenance of flexibility.

2. **Strengthening exercises** employ progressive resistance to the musculoskeletal system to maintain strength and coordination of the musculature. These exercises include isotonic, isometric, isokinetic, and aerobic exercises. If a lower extremity is involved, the therapy should focus on gradual increase in the weight-bearing capability of the limb.

3. **Deep friction massage** is useful as a desensitization technique in those patients who can tolerate such manipulation.

C. **Psychotherapy.** Patients with RSD exhibit a wide range of behavioral changes, including depression, anxiety, suicidal ideation, and drug addiction. Patients who develop these traits at or before the time of injury are considered at higher risk of developing and maintaining symptoms of RSD. Therefore, all such patients should be considered for psychological consultation.

Psychotherapeutic management of RSD includes counseling and cognitive-behavioral techniques.

1. **Counseling** is a means whereby the patient is helped to cope with the pain, irrespective of how well it may be controlled by pharmacologic and/or physical treatments. The services of a psychiatrist, psychologist, or social worker are used when appropriate.

2. **Cognitive-behavioral techniques** include biofeedback, relaxation, and hypnosis.

D. **Transcutaneous electrical nerve stimulation (TENS).** According to the gate theory put forth by Melzack and Wall in 1965, painful transmission from the periphery carried by afferent C fibers causes a loss of interneuronal large-diameter A-fiber inhibition in the dorsal horns of the spinal cord. Both sets of fibers synapse on interneurons in the substantia gelatinosa of laminae II and III before secondary fibers transmit across the midline to ascending tracts and eventually synapse in the thalamus and higher cortical centers. Thus, TENS is thought to provide pain relief by closing this gating mechanism through preferential stimulation of large-diameter A fibers and inhibition of the smaller fibers within the substantia gelatinosa or by causing the release of endorphins and enkephalins, or both. Overall, TENS relieves symptoms of RSD in the majority of children but in only about 25% of adults.

E. **Sympathetic blockade.** The mechanism of continued pain relief from sympathetic blockade is not completely understood. The improvement of symptoms of early RSD through the inhibition of sympathetic activity seems to be a paradoxical effect considering that this stage is typically characterized by a picture of sympathetic hypoactivity consisting of vasodilation, redness, warmth, and sweating. Possible explanations for this effect include blockade of afferent nerve fibers transmitting pain, blockade of efferent fibers eliminating sensitization of nociceptors, and inhibition of localized vasospasm.

Sympathetic blockade may be performed on the cervical sympathetic chain, primarily the stellate ganglion, for head, neck and upper-extremity dystrophy and on the lumbar sympathetic chain for lower-extremity dystrophy. For a sympathetic blockade to be used as a therapeutic intervention, several criteria should be met. First, the blockade should demonstrate a desired effect. Efficacy is assessed subjectively by the degree of pain relief and objectively by the degree of functional improvement of the extremity. Second, the effect should last longer than the known duration of the local anesthetic. Third, the patient must be willing to continue a series of sympathetic blockades in order for the therapy to be effective.

Once a sympathetic blockade has been shown to be effective, a series of frequent blocks is performed. Initially, the time interval between procedures should roughly equal the time it takes for the pain to return and limit rehabilitation. This typically equates to intervals ranging from daily to no more than weekly. After the first three to five blockades, the time interval is extended to approximately 1.5 times the period of pain relief and improved function. Medical therapy, physical therapy, and desensitization techniques are used in conjunction. As long as the patient's condition continues to improve, this therapy is continued. Resolution of symptoms is typically seen within four to eight blocks. If pain remains after sympathetic blockade, the diagnosis of RSD should be reconsidered.

The patient's condition is considered refractory if the pain relief is incomplete or if the painful condition returns after a series of sympathetic blockades has been performed.

1. **Stellate ganglion block.** The stellate ganglion is the irregularly shaped ganglionic mass derived from the fusion of the inferior cervical and first thoracic sympathetic ganglia. Preganglionic fibers destined for the upper extremity originate from upper thoracic segments to approximately T8.

   The stellate ganglion block involves instillation of local anesthetic at the anterior tubercle of C6. These blockades are repeated one to three times per week, up to 10 in a series, until a long-term effect is achieved. If pain relief remains inadequate, a brachial plexus block or IV regional bretylium block is attempted.

   a. **Indications.** RSD and causalgia of the upper extremity are the two most common indications for stellate ganglion block.

   b. **Complications.** Most injections result in Horner's syndrome and temporary hoarseness. Performance of stellate ganglion blocks bilaterally is not recommended because of the possibility of bilateral recurrent laryngeal nerve paralysis and loss of cardioaccelerator activity. Block of the phrenic nerve results in temporary paralysis of a hemidiaphragm. Injections into the vertebral artery may result in seizures or cerebral embolisms. Intradural injections can result in unconsciousness, respiratory paralysis, seizures, and sometimes cardiovascular collapse. Other complications include brachial plexus block, pneumothorax, and osteitis of the transverse process.

2. **Lumbar sympathetic block.** The abdominal portion of the sympathetic trunk that supplies the lower extremities is situated anterolateral to the bodies of the lumbar vertebrae L1-L3 along the medial margin of the psoas major muscle. Blockade of the lumbar sympathetic nerves can be performed with a spinal, epidural, or peripheral nerve block, but relief after lumbar sympathetic blockade most clearly delineates the etiology of the pain as sympathetically mediated.

  a. **Indications** include sympathetically mediated pain, postherpetic neuralgia, phantom limb pain, and stump pain.

  b. **Complications** of lumbar sympathetic blockade include back pain, somatic nerve block, intraspinal anesthesia, intravascular injection, kidney trauma, and bowel perforation.

3. **Intravenous regional sympathetic blockade.** Bretylium, like guanethidine, selectively inhibits peripheral sympathetic nerve transmission by entering the preganglionic nerve endings by means of active transport and displacing norepinephrine from its storage sites. Its concentration builds up at these sites and prevents reuptake of norepinephrine and release of any remaining norepinephrine in response to neuronal stimulation. The norepinephrine depletion results in impairment and eventual loss of sympathetic adrenergic nerve function. This blockade lasts for many hours, for days, and sometimes for weeks because of the drug's strong binding and slow elimination. In sufficient concentration, guanethidine can cause permanent damage to the norepinephrine reuptake pump.

  a. **Indications.** Intravenous regional sympathetic blockade with bretylium or guanethidine remains a viable alternative for those patients who fail to respond to block procedures. This procedure is less invasive and can be carried out by physicians who are unfamiliar with the use of regional anesthesia. It is also useful for patients for whom regional anesthesia is contraindicated.

  b. **Complications.** Placement of an Esmarch bandage and tourniquet on an extremity may be intolerable to a patient with painful RSD. Agent not taken up by the tissue on release of the tourniquet may enter the systemic circulation and cause hypertension and tachycardia. Orthostatic hypotension may result from the chemical sympathetic blockade. Bretylium in high concentrations has local anesthetic and neuromuscular blocking properties. These drugs should not be administered to patients taking monoamine oxidase inhibitors (MAOIs) or to patients with known pheochromocytoma. Other side effects include dysrhythmias, dizziness, diarrhea, edema, and nausea.

F. **Other treatments for RSD**

1. **Dorsal column stimulation (DCS)** has recently become a more widely accepted mode of therapy for refractory RSD. The mechanisms of DCS are explained by the gate-control theory of pain and/or an increase in production of endogenous endorphins.

  a. **Indications.** DCS is indicated for patients suffering from chronic intractable pain. Patient-selection criteria include failure of conservative therapies, absence of drug abuse or psychological history, absence of contraindication to spinal implantation, and a successful trial of DCS using temporary electrodes.

  b. **Complications.** Complications include infection, arachnoiditis, a high long-term failure rate, and mechanical failure.

2. **Intraspinal opioid programmable pump.** Preganglionic sympathetic intermediolateral columns of the spinal cord are modulated by projection from multiple supraspinal nuclei, including the nucleus raphae magnus (NRM). Intrathecal morphine may be effective in relieving refractory RSD by increasing NRM inhibition of sympathetic outflow, in addition to its inhibitory effects on nociceptive neurons. Moreover, intrathecal morphine administered continuously through a programmable pump permits stable cerebrospinal fluid (CSF) concentrations, resulting in fewer episodes of pain breakthrough or drug overdose. It may also reduce the overall dosage requirements and delay the development of tolerance.

  a. **Indications.** The intraspinal opioid programmable pump is reserved for RSD patients who are unresponsive to all other forms of less invasive measures. A successful trial of intrathecal morphine placed percutaneously is required.

  b. **Complications.** A significant disadvantage of an intraspinal opioid infusion pump is the high cost of implanting and maintaining the device. In addition, physical tolerance and dependence complicate therapy for many patients. Other problems of intraspinal opioid programmable pump therapy include infection, arachnoiditis, mechanical failure, unremitting breakthrough pain, and opioid tolerance and dependence.

G. Surgical sympathectomy. For upper-extremity RSD, surgical sympathectomy involves extensive ablation of the thoracic sympathetic ganglia from T1 to T6 or T7 by means of a transthoracic approach. Surgical sympathectomy for lower-extremity RSD involves ablation of the lumbar sympathetic chain from L1 to L4. The pain relief derived from surgery may be inadequate or transient owing either to incomplete sympathetic denervation or to subsequent nerve regeneration.

    1. Indications. Surgical sympathectomy is usually reserved for RSD patients who have been able to obtain definite but only temporary relief from repeated sympathetic nerve blocks and remain incapacitated by the disease.

    2. Complications. Potential morbidity, including wound complications, permanent Horner's syndrome, and painful neuralgia, warrants exhaustive physical, pharmacologic, and psychological therapy prior to consideration of surgical sympathectomy.

V. Referral. Cases of RSD should be referred to a chronic pain specialist or neurologist if (1) signs and symptoms remain persistent despite a 6-week trial of conservative measures, (2) pain is severe and intractable at any time after the inciting event, (3) a new-onset neurologic deficit is noted, or (4) signs and symptoms have spread to other parts of the body.

Recommended Readings

Besson JM, et al. Peripheral and spinal mechanisms of nociception. *Physiol Rev* 67:67–186, 1987.

Bonica JJ. Causalgia and other reflex sympathetic dystrophies. In JJ Bonica (ed), *The Management of Pain*. Philadelphia: Lea & Febiger, 1990. Pp 220–243.

Chaturvedi SK. Phenytoin in reflex sympathetic dystrophy. *Pain* 36:379–380, 1989.

Cline MA, et al. Chronic hyperalgesia and skin warming caused by sensitized C-nociceptors. *Brain* 112:621–647, 1989.

Davis KD, et al. Topical application of clonidine relieves hyperalgesia in patients with sympathetically maintained pain. *Pain* 47:309–317, 1991.

Demangeat JL, et al. Three-phase bone scanning in reflex sympathetic dystrophy of the hand. *J Nucl Med* 29:26–32, 1988.

Doupe J, et al. Post-traumatic pain and the causalgic syndromes. *J Neurol Neurosurg Psychiat* 7:33–48, 1944.

Geertzen JHB, et al. Reflex sympathetic dystrophy: Early treatment and psychological aspects. *Arch Phys Med Rehabil* 75:442–446, 1994.

Gobelet C, et al. The effect of adding calcitonin to physical treatment on reflex sympathetic dystrophy. *Pain* 48:171–175, 1992.

Hord AH, et al. Intravenous regional bretylium and lidocaine for treatment of reflex sympathetic dystrophy: A randomized, double-blind study. *Anesth Analg* 74:818–821, 1992.

International Association for the Study of Pain, Subcommittee on Taxonomy. Classification of chronic pain: Descriptions of chronic pain syndromes and definitions of pain terms. *Pain* 3(Suppl):S1–S226, 1986.

Kanoff RB. Intraspinal delivery of opiates by an implantable, programmable pump in patients with chronic, intractable pain of nonmalignant origin. *JAOA* 94(6):487–493, 1994.

Lynch ME. Psychological aspect of reflex sympathetic dystrophy: A review of the adult and pediatric literature. *Pain* 49:337–347, 1992.

Melzack R, Wall PD. Pain mechanisms: A new theory. *Science* 150:971–975, 1965.

Payne R. Neuropathic pain syndromes, with special reference to causalgia and reflex sympathetic dystrophy. *Clin J Pain* 2:59–73, 1986.

Prough DS, et al. Efficacy of oral nifedipine in the treatment of reflex sympathetic dystrophy. *Anesthesiology* 62:796–799, 1985.

Raja SN. Reflex sympathetic dystrophy: Pathophysiological basis for therapy. *Pain Digest* 2:274–280, 1992.

Rauck RL, et al. Epidural clonidine treatment for reflex sympathetic dystrophy. *Anesthesiology* 79:1163–1169, 1993.

Roberts WJ. A hypothesis on the physiological basis for causalgia and related pains. *Pain* 24:297–311, 1986.

52

Primary Central Nervous System Tumors
Bertrand C. Liang
Diane M. Liang

There are approximately 20,000 **primary central nervous system tumors** diagnosed each year in the United States. These tumors tend to affect younger patients and comprise the second most frequent cause of cancer-related death in children, the third most frequent cause of cancer-related death in patients aged 15–35 years, and the fourth most frequent cause of cancer-related death in patients aged 36–45 years. However, the incidence of the histologically more malignant tumors seems to be rising, especially in the elderly.

Primary CNS tumors are thought to arise from precursor cells to nervous system elements. In tumor cells, there is an accumulation of genetic events that allows dysregulation of differentiation and growth, resulting in neoplastic proliferation. This proliferation results in the development of a mass, which becomes clinically apparent with neurologic symptoms. This chapter discusses some of the more frequent tumors, including **gliomas** (astrocytoma, anaplastic astrocytoma, glioblastoma, and oligodendroglioma), **primitive neuroectodermal tumors** (medulloblastoma), **ependymomas,** and **meningiomas.** Also discussed are **primary CNS lymphomas,** which are being seen with increasing frequency in the immunocompromised population.

I. **Gliomas** are the most common intracranial tumors, comprising about 60% of all primary CNS neoplasms. Although there are several grading systems currently in use, the three-tiered classification system has become the most popular, with the astrocytoma representing the most well-differentiated and lowest-grade tumor, the anaplastic astrocytoma being an intermediate-grade tumor, and the glioblastoma being the most malignant and poorly differentiated glioma. The most malignant form, the glioblastoma, is the most common, representing 50–60% of gliomas diagnosed. Most studies in all grades of glioma show either no sex preponderance or a slight male bias. These tumors do not tend to be inherited, except in a few rare syndromes (e.g., neurofibromatosis, Li-Fraumeni syndrome, tuberous sclerosis, and ataxia-telangiectasia). No definite environmental association of these tumors has been noted in comparisons of urban and rural populations.

A. **Astrocytoma**

1. **Natural history.** About 30% of diagnosed gliomas are astrocytomas. These low-grade neoplasms tend to occur in younger patients, typically in the fourth decade or earlier. There is a paucity of prospective information regarding the natural history of astrocytoma; retrospective analysis has shown age to be an important predictive factor, with younger patients (especially those less than 20 years old) having the highest 5-year survival rate. The incidence of malignant transformation and response to therapy are not well known. Total surgical resection and good postoperative performance status have been associated retrospectively with prolonged survival. One exception to the lack of information on low-grade tumors is the **pilocytic astrocytoma,** which occurs most often in children and occasionally in adults. With only surgical intervention, these tumors have an excellent prognosis and only rarely transform to malignant neoplasms. Other tumors that fit into the rubric of low-grade astrocytomas include **ganglioglioma** and **neurocytoma;** these tumors also tend to behave in a benign fashion and to require only surgical intervention.

2. **Therapy.** Except as noted, there are no prospective studies that evaluate the efficacy of therapeutic intervention in low-grade astrocytomas. It is accepted that surgical excision is a reasonable initial approach to these tumors, although any further therapy is based only on anecdotal or retrospective analyses. Currently there are no generally accepted guidelines for

radiation therapy in low-grade astrocytomas, although many clinicians feel that, for the occasional older patient, treatment with high-dosage radiation (~6000 cGy) is appropriate. At least initially, chemotherapy is not felt to play a part in management of these patients because of the slow growth of these tumors. However, many astrocytomas progress to higher-grade neoplasms, in which case therapy is referable to the more malignant tumor (see secs. **B** and **C**). Typically, follow-up CT or MRI scans are done at 6-month intervals and when the patient presents with clinical changes.

3. **Prognosis.** Astrocytoma patients with the best prognoses are young, have had gross total tumor resections, and have minimal or no postoperative neurologic or other deficits. In these patients, the 5-year survival rate is greater than 80%. Further specific prognostic assessment in other patient subgroups is difficult, but at least a fraction of astrocytomas in such patients progress to higher-grade neoplasms requiring other types of therapy. In any patient with a diagnosis of astrocytoma (with the exception of pilocytic astrocytoma, ganglioglioma, and neurocytoma), continuous follow-up is necessary, because malignant transformation can occur at any time.

B. **Anaplastic astrocytoma**

1. **Natural history.** Anaplastic astrocytoma is diagnosed much less frequently than its lower- and higher-grade counterparts. Part of the reason for this revolves around the pathologic criteria for anaplastic astrocytoma compared with those for glioblastoma (i.e., anaplasia without necrosis in the specimen). Even with these criteria, there may still be an overestimation of the incidence of anaplastic astrocytoma because of sampling errors that occur when subtotal resections or stereotactic biopsies are sent to pathologists for review. It has been estimated that up to 30% of tumors diagnosed as anaplastic astrocytomas by stereotactic biopsy are of higher grade (glioblastoma). Apart from difficulties with histologic grading, few prospective analyses of these tumors have been performed. Retrospective studies have shown anaplastic astrocytoma to occur typically in the fifth decade, usually with a long (greater than 1 year) history of neurologic symptoms. The most important favorable prognostic factors include younger age and good performance status. Surgery has not been found to influence survival, perhaps because anaplastic tumors tend to be diffusely infiltrating. A high percentage of these tumors recur at higher pathologic grades.

2. **Therapy.** Patients with anaplastic astrocytoma require a multidisciplinary approach similar to that used for glioblastoma.

a. **Surgery and corticosteroids.** Surgery should be considered if the diagnosis is in question, if there would be benefit of cytoreduction (i.e., reduction of mass effect), or if surgery is indicated because of clinically emergent conditions. As noted, surgery does not seem to affect survival per se. Corticosteroids may be necessary to decrease symptoms of increased intracranial pressure. Dexamethasone is often given at a starting dosage of 4 mg qid, titrated to relief of symptomatology. Dosages greater than 32 mg/day are rarely useful. Minimizing dosages of corticosteroids because of known side effects should be an important goal after radiation treatment.

b. **Radiation therapy** is an important aspect of treatment of anaplastic astrocytoma, with a current recommended dosage of about 6000 cGy. The fractionation schedule of the radiotherapy usually ranges from 180–200 cGy/day. Focal radiation of 4500 cGy within a 3-cm margin, with a boost of 1500 cGy for the 1.5-cm margin surrounding the area of enhancement of the tumor, has been found to be as effective as whole-brain irradiation.

c. **Chemotherapy.** Anaplastic astrocytoma is treated with both adjuvant and recurrent chemotherapy. Adjuvant chemotherapy (given within 2 weeks after the completion of radiation) usually consists of a combined regimen of procarbazine (60 mg/m^2 PO, days 8–21), CCNU (lomustine) (110 mg/m^2 PO, day 1), and vincristine (1.4 mg/m^2 IV, days 8 and 29) (PCV) every 6–8 weeks for 1 year or until tumor recurrence. At recurrence, high-dosage IV BCNU (carmustine) (250 mg/m^2) is administered every 6–8 weeks until further tumor progression. The administration of these drugs requires that specific laboratory values and clinical cautions be assessed periodically (see sec. **VI.B** and Tables 52-1 and 52-2). Further

Table 52-1. Chemotherapy dosages and monitoring laboratory tests.

Drug	Dosage	Laboratory tests
BCNU	200–250 mg/m^2	CBC, electrolytes, BUN, creatinine, liver function tests, pulmonary function tests
Procarbazine	PCV: 50–100 mg/m^2 Alone: 150 mg/m^2	CBC, electrolytes, liver function tests
CCNU	100–150 mg/m^2	CBC, electrolytes, BUN, creatinine, liver function tests, pulmonary function tests
Vincristine	1.0–1.4 mg/m^2	CBC, electrolytes, BUN, creatinine, urinalysis
Cyclophosphamide	15 mg/kg	CBC, electrolytes, BUN, creatinine, urinalysis
Methotrexate (with leucovorin)	IA: 2.5 g IV: 1 g/m^2 IT: 12 mg	CBC, electrolytes, BUN, creatinine, liver function tests, urinalysis
Ara-C	3 g/m^2	CBC, electrolytes, BUN, creatinine, liver function tests

CBC = complete blood count; BUN = blood urea nitrogen; liver function tests include AST, ALT, and bilirubin; pulmonary function tests should include diffusion coefficient; IA = intraarterial; IV = intravenous; IT = intrathecal.

therapy at this point usually revolves around phase I/II drugs or other experimental therapies. Consultation with a neuro-oncologist is often necessary. Follow-up CT or MRI evaluation should be performed 6 weeks subsequent to completion of radiation therapy and prior to each cycle of chemotherapy.

3. **Prognosis.** With implementation of surgery, radiation, and chemotherapy, patients with anaplastic astrocytoma have a median survival of more than 3 years. Typical time to first tumor recurrence is about 2.5 years, with time to death after progression of 8 months. Patients less than 40 years old have the highest chances for response to treatment and prolonged survival. Few patients more than 60 years old respond to this multimodal approach to therapy, and patients in this age group have the most frequent incidence of significant side effects resulting from treatment. Clinical judgment and careful consideration of the patient's wishes are necessary prior to any decision regarding therapeutic intervention—especially chemotherapy.

C. **Glioblastoma**
  1. **Natural history.** Glioblastoma is the most frequently diagnosed primary CNS neoplasm. Its natural history, in contrast to those of astrocytoma and anaplastic astrocytoma, is well defined. This tumor is the most malignant of the gliomas and has a poor prognosis with inexorable progression to death. Glioblastoma patients usually present in the sixth decade, with a short history (less than 6 months) of neurologic symptoms. The best predictors of survival and response to chemotherapy are the same as those for anaplastic astrocytoma—patient age and performance status. A shorter duration of symptoms prior to diagnosis has also been associated with longer survival. Currently it is unclear whether extent of surgery is an important prognostic factor.
  2. **Therapy.** Treatment of glioblastoma is similar to that of anaplastic astrocytoma. Maximal surgical debulking is usually suggested for patients who can undergo the procedure safely, with subsequent administration of radiation therapy of high dosage (~6000 cGy or higher) as noted for the anaplastic tumors. Adjuvant chemotherapy with BCNU is usually initiated within 2 weeks after completion of radiation treatments and is given every 6–8 weeks. Recurrence is then treated with PCV, high-dosage oral procarbazine alone (each cycle consisting of 150 mg/m^2/day for 28 days, followed by a 28-day rest), or either phase I/II agents or other experimental therapy. As

Table 52-2. Treatment toxicity.

Treatment	Toxicity
Radiation Therapy	
Acute	Worsening of neurologic symptoms, symptoms of increased intracranial pressure
Early delayed	Somnolence, fatigue, worsening of neurologic symptoms
Late delayed	Worsening of neurologic symptoms, radiation necrosis
Chemotherapy[a]	
BCNU/CCNU	Pulmonary fibrosis, hepatic necrosis, encephalomyelopathy
Procarbazine	Malignant hypertension (sensitivity to amines)
Vincristine	Sensorimotor neuropathy, SIADH,[b] diminished levels of phenytoin
Cyclophosphamide	Hemorrhagic cystitis, water retention, alopecia
Methotrexate	Hepatic dysfunction, renal failure, stomatitis, motor neuropathy
Ara-C	Cholestasis, mucositis

[a]Hematologic/infection (all).
[b]Syndrome of inappropriate antidiuretic hormone.

noted previously, consultation with a neuro-oncologist is necessary at this point. CT or MRI scanning should be performed prior to each cycle of chemotherapy.

3. **Prognosis** for patients with glioblastoma is poor. Patients who are treated with surgery alone have a median survival of 14–26 weeks; the addition of radiation therapy increases survival to 40 weeks. Administration of chemotherapy with nitrosureas such as procarbazine and BCNU further increases median survival to 50 weeks and the proportion of patients surviving 18 months. Nevertheless, with multimodality therapy, median survival is less than 1 year, and less than 15% of patients survive for 2 years.

D. **Oligodendroglioma**

1. **Natural history.** Oligodendrogliomas arise from presumed oligodendroglial precursors and usually present in the fourth or fifth decade. These tumors occur in proportion to the volume of white matter, and hence the frontal lobes are the areas most frequently affected. There is an inconsistent relationship between histologic grade and malignant behavior. Few data are available regarding the frequency of malignant degeneration, although it is well known that some oligodendrogliomas transform into glioblastomas. Better prognostic factors include more benign histology, postoperative radiation therapy, complete surgical resection, and good pre- and postoperative performance status. Close follow-up is necessary in the management of these patients, especially given the long-term survival of particular subsets.

2. **Therapy.** Management of the different types of oligodendroglioma is evolving. Maximal surgical excision is considered the initial step in management of these tumors. Radiation therapy can follow surgery in a manner similar to that of anaplastic astrocytoma or glioblastoma. Although there is no strict relationship between histologic anaplasia and malignant potential, most neuro-oncologists suggest that patients with anaplastic oligodendrogliomas be treated with multiagent chemotherapy—i.e., PCV. Patients with nonanaplastic oligodendrogliomas typically are followed without further therapy after radiation, and are given PCV chemotherapy only at recurrence. Radiographic imaging with MRI or CT should be performed prior to administration of chemotherapy and every 6–8 weeks for anaplastic tumors or every 3 months for nonanaplastic oligodendroglioma for the first year and, if there is no evidence of recurrence, every 6 months thereafter.

3. **Prognosis** for oligodendroglioma is more favorable than that of either anaplastic astrocytoma or glioblastoma. Overall, the median survival is more than 5 years, and the 10-year survival rate is 24%. Selected patients with particularly good prognostic factors, as noted above, will survive even longer.

II. **Primitive neuroectodermal tumors**

A. **Natural history.** Primitive neuroectodermal tumors (PNETs) are primarily neoplasms of children. These tumors constitute the most frequently diagnosed soft-tissue malignancies in the pediatric ages but account for less than 1% of all adult tumors. In adults, the median age of diagnosis is 24 years. The most often diagnosed PNET is the medulloblastoma, which typically occurs in the posterior fossa. There is a male-to-female ratio of 2:1. These tumors are graded according to the Chang criteria (T-M system), although there is no influence per se on prognosis. Medulloblastoma is a malignancy that can metastasize throughout the craniospinal axis, as well as outside the nervous system, up to 10 years after initial diagnosis. Bone, lymph nodes, lung, pleura, liver, and breast are the most frequent sites of seeding outside the nervous system. Prolonged survival is associated with high-dosage posterior fossa radiation accompanied by additional radiation therapy of the whole brain, spinal cord, and coverings, as well as with early treatment. The extent of surgery is important in relapse-free, but not overall, survival.

B. Therapy. Maximal surgical resection and radiation are the mainstays of treatment for medulloblastoma. Radiation dosages of 5200–5500 cGy for the posterior fossa and 2500–3500 cGy for the remaining neuraxis are considered appropriate. Treatment of recurrent disease typically revolves around chemotherapy, although the most beneficial regimen has not yet been defined. However, most neuro-oncologists recommend a multidrug protocol with drugs such as the nitrosureas, a platinum-based compound, and steroids. Consultation is required to determine the most current regimen. Imaging studies should be obtained after radiation therapy and before each cycle of chemotherapy. Because recurrences are not uncommon, follow-up for these patients (including periodic radiographic evaluations) should be performed for at least 10 years after the completion of therapy.

C. Prognosis. With maximal treatment (with radiation being paramount in importance), the 5-year survival rate is 50–76%, and the 10-year survival rate is 33–60%. Recurrence, when it is observed, is typically in the posterior fossa. Some patients with more extensive tumors may benefit from chemotherapy in either an adjuvant or a recurrence setting. Those patients who metastasize, especially outside the nervous system, have worse prognoses than those who have solitary recurrences in the posterior fossa.

III. Ependymomas

A. Natural history. Ependymomas, like PNETs, are tumors of the young and are uncommon in adults. These tumors arise most frequently in the central canal of the spinal cord or the filum terminale, as well as in white matter adjacent to a ventricular surface. Like the medulloblastomas, ependymomas tend to seed throughout the nervous system, although the likelihood of such seeding is defined by the grade of the tumor. Ependymomas are graded in a variety of different ways, but can be most conveniently divided into differentiated (low-grade, myxopapillary) and anaplastic (high-grade) ependymomas. The anaplastic tumors are most often associated with neuraxial spread. A particular subtype of ependymoma, the ependymoblastoma, has an especially high frequency of seeding. However, the usual area of recurrence for all ependymomas is the primary site, although seeding can accompany local treatment failure in the higher grades. Better prognostic factors include low grade, treatment with surgery, and high-dosage radiation therapy.

B. Therapy. Evaluations of the entire nervous system and cerebrospinal fluid (CSF) for malignant cells are often recommended in the treatment of ependymoma. Maximal surgical resection and radiation therapy are the necessary initial treatments. In low-grade tumors, a dosage of 5400 cGy applied to the primary tumor is considered standard, with no additional therapy of the remainder of the nervous system. In anaplastic tumors, 5400 cGy is applied to the primary tumor site and 3500–4000 cGy to the neuraxis. Chemotherapy is given at recurrence, although only anecdotal data on the most beneficial regimen are available. Hence, the chemotherapeutic protocol to be followed as recurrence therapy should be determined by consultation with a neuro-oncologist to determine the most current regimen. Imaging should be performed subsequent to radiation therapy and prior to each chemotherapeutic intervention. Continuous follow-up is necessary because of the possibility of late recurrence.

C. Prognosis. Patients with ependymomas of low grade treated maximally with surgery, radiation, and chemotherapy have a 5-year survival rate of 60–80%. Higher-grade disease has a significantly worse prognosis: 10–47% of patients survive for 5 years. As with medulloblastomas, seeding carries a worse prognosis.

IV. Meningiomas
   A. **Natural history.** Meningiomas are common nervous system tumors, constituting about 15% of all CNS neoplasms. There is a slight female preponderance. Although the peak age of diagnosis is 45 years, asymptomatic tumors are common in older adults as well. These neoplasms grow slowly, and typically are benign in behavior. However, the recurrence rate for totally resected tumors is still 10%, with 15% of meningiomas recurring if a dural attachment remains after surgery, and 39% recurring if only a subtotal resection can be accomplished. These tumors occur most frequently in the parasagittal and falx regions, and can be associated with inherited syndromes (e.g., neurofibromatosis). Malignant meningiomas, which are rare, display anaplastic pathology and behavior and require continuous monitoring and treatment.
   B. **Therapy.** Surgical removal is the treatment of choice for meningiomas. Cauterization or embolization have been performed on particularly vascular tumors to ease removal. Radiation and chemotherapy play no role in the typical meningioma, although malignant tumors may require these additional interventions. Imaging studies should be obtained on a yearly basis for at least 3 years and if symptoms develop.
   C. **Prognosis** for meningioma is good. Tumors can recur, however, and recurrence necessitates additional surgery or, for malignant meningiomas, radiation and chemotherapy.

V. Primary CNS lymphomas
   A. **Natural history.** Primary CNS lymphoma (PCNSL) is a rare tumor in the immunocompetent population, comprising less than 2% of all brain tumors and extranodal lymphomas. Pathologically, these tumors are typically non-Hodgkin's B-cell tumors, although T-cell tumors are occasionally observed. The incidence of PCNSL has been rising, primarily because of the increasing population of acquired immunodeficiency syndrome (AIDS) patients; moreover, other immunocompromised patients such as renal transplant patients are also developing PCNSL with increasing frequency. Other immunodeficiency diseases that have been reported in association with PCNSL include Wiskott-Aldrich syndrome, agammaglobulinemia, and ataxia-telangiectasia. Although concurrent non-Hodgkin's lymphomas at other extranodal sites are very uncommon in these patients, staging evaluation of a patient found to have PCNSL should include radiographic imaging (CT or MRI) of the chest, abdomen, and pelvis as well as a bone marrow aspirate. Because PCNSL can occur in ocular and meningeal tissues, slit-lamp and CSF examinations should be performed. Finally, human immunodeficiency virus (HIV) testing should be performed on all patients with diagnoses of PCNSL. Combination chemotherapy and radiation therapy has been found to prolong survival significantly in comparison with surgery and radiation alone.
   B. **Therapy.** Use of biopsy alone to establish the diagnosis of PCNSL is the sole surgical intervention required; no additional benefit is derived from subtotal or total resection of any visualized mass. Radiation therapy can be given either initially after biopsy or at recurrence after adjuvant chemotherapy. The optimal regimen has yet to be defined, but combination therapy with both radiation and chemotherapy has been successful in prolonging median survival to more than 40 months, although in some regimens leukoencephalopathy and cognitive changes have been noted. Unfortunately, although treatment of AIDS patients with PCNSL has shown tumor regression, ultimately there has been no increase in overall survival rate for these patients.

   In the treatment of PCNSL, the two most successful regimens have used significant dosages of chemotherapy. In the first, blood-brain barrier disruption with mannitol has been used with efficacy. Intravenous cyclophosphamide (15 mg/kg) and intra-arterial methotrexate (2.5 g) are administered with the disruption, oral leucovorin (20 mg q6h) is given 36 hours after the completion of the infusion of methotrexate and continued for 5 days, and procarbazine (100 mg/day PO) and dexamethasone (24 mg/day PO) are given for 14 days after the disruption. This cycle is repeated every 28 days for 1 year. Radiation therapy is given at relapse. In the second regimen, chemotherapy is combined with radiation therapy as adjuvant treatment. Dexamethasone (16 mg/kg PO) is given until an Ommaya reservoir has been placed, and then IV methotrexate (1 g/m^2) is begun, given on days 1 and 8. Intrathecal methotrexate (12 mg through the Ommaya reservoir) is administered on days 1, 4, 8, 11, 15, and 18, with a dexamethasone taper. Whole-brain radiation (4000 cGy) with a cone down boost (1440 cGy) is then given; three weeks later, ara-C (3 g/m^2) is given intravenously for 2 days and repeated 3 weeks later. Both regimens show high response rates, with median survival of more than 40 months. Imaging (preferably MRI) should be performed prior to each intervention and every 6–8 weeks thereafter.

C. **Prognosis** for PCNSL is better than that for the malignant glial tumors. With radiation and chemotherapy, median survival of patients with PCNSL can be expected to be greater than 3.5 years. Although each of the regimens described in sec. **V.B** have been associated with limited side effects, some studies using high-dosage chemotherapy with radiation for PCNSL have noted both leukoencephalopathy and cognitive changes with treatment. Thus, careful assessment and follow-up of neurologic status is very important. Patients with AIDS respond to such regimens; however, prognosis in that patient population is related to the underlying disease process.

VI. **Treatment toxicity**

A. **Radiation toxicity** can be conveniently classified according to the time of presentation into **acute reactions, early delayed reactions,** and **late delayed reactions.**

1. **Acute reactions** occur during the course of treatment, and consist of symptoms of increased intracranial pressure or worsening of existing neurologic symptoms. These symptoms are usually mild and transient, and are thought to result from radiation-induced edema. Occasionally it is temporarily necessary to administer or increase the dosage of a corticosteroid.

2. **Early delayed reactions** occur several weeks to months after completion of radiation treatment. These reactions also may present with worsening symptoms, or be manifested by increasing somnolence and fatigue. It is felt that these symptoms are caused by a temporary inhibition of myelin synthesis. Although this syndrome is typically temporary and mild, there have been reports of severe reactions requiring intensive medical support. Careful consideration is necessary to avoid interpreting an early delayed reaction as a treatment failure without enlargement of tumor mass on radiographic imaging.

3. **Late delayed reactions** may occur months to years after completion of radiation therapy. The major type of late delayed reaction is radiation necrosis, which can mimic tumor recurrence in that it can be progressive, irreversible, and fatal. This effect may be a result of damage to small and medium-sized arterioles or a direct effect on glial cells. Radiation necrosis is difficult to diagnose without biopsy; use of a variety of anatomic (MRI and CT) and functional (positron emission tomography and single-photon emission CT) imaging modalities has not reliably differentiated necrosis from tumor recurrence. Treatment of suspected or confirmed radiation necrosis usually consists of surgery; however, only total resection (cf. biopsy) is clinically beneficial. There is anecdotal evidence that anticoagulants (heparin and warfarin) may be useful in treatment of radiation necrosis at dosages used in stroke management.

B. **Chemotherapy toxicity.** All drugs used in the treatment of gliomas can result in myelosuppression, which is typically delayed and cumulative. As a result, weekly blood counts, electrolytes including calcium and magnesium, and liver function tests should be performed on a weekly basis during each cycle. Procarbazine inhibits monoamine oxidase and thus predisposes patients to autonomic sensitivity; avoidance of foods containing high amounts of tyramine (e.g., red wine, cheese, and tomatoes) as well as any sympathomimetic drugs (tricyclic antidepressants, hypnotics, antihistamines, narcotics, and phenothiazines) is necessary during therapy. The nitrosoureas (BCNU and CCNU) can also cause hepatic necrosis and pulmonary fibrosis, which are related to cumulative dosing (above 1500 mg/m^2). Current recommendations include avoiding nitrosourea therapy for patients with significant pulmonary disease and monitoring pulmonary function tests every few cycles. Nitrosoureas should be discontinued when a cumulative dosage of 1500 mg/m^2 is attained. Vincristine causes a sensorimotor neuropathy and can produce mental status changes, result in syndrome of inappropriate antidiuretic hormone (SIADH), and diminish levels of phenytoin. Methotrexate/leucovorin may be associated with stomatitis. Ara-C has been shown to cause cholestasis and mucositis in some patients. Cyclophosphamide can cause a hemorrhagic cystitis, water retention, and alopecia. Table 52-1 lists the chemotherapeutic interventions, dosages, and lab values that need to be monitored, usually weekly, while these drugs are being given. Table 52-2 gives the possible side effects of therapy in patients with glial tumors.

VII. Ancillary support

    A. Diagnosis and recurrence. With the exception of the more benign tumors (e.g., meningioma, pilocytic astrocytoma, ganglioglioma, and neurocytoma), the vast majority of primary CNS tumors recur and require terminal care. Because cancer, especially cancer of the brain, is such a devastating diagnosis, it is important to realize and understand the anxieties of the patient and family. As a result, most neuro-oncologists are members of teams of physicians, nurses, and social workers who specialize in the care of brain tumor patients and their families. Each member of the healthcare team should speak with the patient and concerned family members and provide both practical and emotional support. A mutual understanding of the disease process and long-term expectations provides a better overall working relationship and maximizes the quality of life for the patient and family. At recurrence, the patient and family may need additional support.

    These issues can be addressed by either the nursing or social work staff in addition to the treating physician. Patient care concerns need to be especially identified during this aspect of the treatment course. Hence, education is a particularly important aspect of patient care, and includes teaching of patient and family about chemotherapeutic intervention(s), daily medications, and specific nutritional or equipment requirements. Support staff can also act as facilitators in identification and accessing of community resources and services such as home care nursing and cancer support groups.

    B. Terminal care. In the United States, once terminal care is required, it is appropriate to contact local hospice services. Hospice provides the patient and family with emotional support, respite care, equipment and supply services during the period when death is imminent. The importance of hospice care, in conjunction with frequent contact with the healthcare team, cannot be overemphasized because of the emotional consequences of such an impending loss. This combination of care can be helpful in making the patient as comfortable as possible and can aid in the later transition of the family after death has occurred.

Recommended Readings

Bloom HJG, Bessell EM. Medulloblastoma in adults: A review of 47 patients treated between 1952 and 1981. *Int J Rad Onc Biol Phys* 18:761–772, 1990.

Burger PC, et al. Glioblastoma multiforme and anaplastic astrocytoma: Pathologic criteria and prognostic implications. *Cancer* 56:1106–1111, 1985.

DeAngelis LM, et al. Primary CNS lymphoma: Combined treatment with chemotherapy and radiotherapy. *Neurology* 40:80–86, 1990.

DeAngelis LM, et al. Combined modality therapy for primary CNS lymphoma. *J Clin Onc* 10:635–643, 1992.

Devita VT, Hellman S, Rosenberg SA (eds). *Cancer: Principles and Practice of Oncology* (4th ed). Philadelphia: Lippincott, 1993.

Garton GR, et al. Medulloblastoma: Prognostic factors and outcome of treatment: Review of Mayo Clinic experience. *Mayo Clin Proc* 65:1077–1086, 1990.

Glantz MJ, et al. Influence of the type of surgery on the histologic diagnosis in patients with anaplastic gliomas. *Neurology* 41:1741–1744, 1991.

Grant R, et al. Age influences chemotherapy response in astrocytomas. *Neurology* 45:929–933, 1995.

Hubbard JL, et al. Adult cerebellar medulloblastomas: The pathological, radiographic, and clinical disease spectrum. *J Neurosurg* 70:536–544, 1989.

Kornblith PL, Walker MD, Cassady JR. *Neurologic Oncology.* Philadelphia: Lippincott, 1987.

Levin VA, et al. Superiority of post-radiotherapy adjuvant chemotherapy with CCNU, procarbazine, and vincristine (PCV) over BCNU for anaplastic gliomas: NCOG 6G61 final report. *Int J Rad Onc Biol Phys* 18:321–324, 1990.

Liang BC, et al. Malignant astrocytomas: Focal tumor recurrence after focal external beam radiation therapy. *J Neurosurg* 75:559–563, 1991.

Liang BC, et al. Primary central nervous system lymphoma: Treatment outcome with multiagent systemic and intrathecal chemotherapy with radiation therapy. *Int J Onc* 3:1001–1004, 1993.

Neuwelt EA, et al. Primary CNS lymphoma treated with osmotic blood-brain barrier dysruption: Prolonged survival and preservation of cognitive function. *J Clin Onc* 9:1580–1590, 1991.

Newton HB, et al. Procarbazine chemotherapy in the treatment of recurrent malignant astrocytomas after radiation and nitrosourea failure. *Neurology* 40:1743–1746, 1990.

Packer RJ. Chemotherapy for medulloblastoma/primitive neuroectodermal tumors of the posterior fossa. *Ann Neurol* 28:823–828, 1990.

Shaw EG, et al. Radiation therapy in the management of low grade supratentorial astrocytomas. *J Neurosurg* 70:853–861, 1989.

Soffietti R, et al. Prognostic factors in well-differentiated cerebral astrocytomas in the adult. *Neurosurgery* 24:686–692, 1989.

Sonneland PRL, Scheithauer BW, Onofrio BM. Myxopapillary ependymoma: A clinical and immunocytochemical study of 77 cases. *Cancer* 56:883–893, 1985.

Thomas DGT (ed). *Neuro-oncology: Primary Malignant Brain Tumors.* Baltimore: Johns Hopkins University Press, 1990.

Vick NA, Bigner DD (eds). *Neurologic Clinics: Neuro-oncology.* Vol 3(3). New York: Saunders, 1985.

Whitaker SJ, et al. Postoperative radiotherapy in the management of spinal cord ependymoma. *J Neurosurg* 74:720–728, 1991.

53

Nervous System Complications in Cancer

Jack M. Rozental

Nervous system complications in cancer can be metastatic, treatment-related, or remote (paraneoplastic). They can cause significant cognitive and/or motor disability or death even when systemic disease seems to be under control. Timely recognition and aggressive management of some complications can be beneficial to the patient's quality and length of life. In most instances, the treatment of nervous system complications is only palliative, and so quality-of-life factors may be more significant than longevity in making therapeutic decisions.

I. Metastases to the brain parenchyma

A. Approximately 20% of cancer patients develop metastatic disease of the central nervous system (CNS), but only one-half of these patients are symptomatic.

   1. The tumors that cause 75% of brain metastases are lung (50%), breast (15%), and melanoma (10%); gastrointestinal (GI) and other pelvic malignancies such as prostate and ovary tumors cause another 10%.

   2. About 50% of metastases are single.

   3. About 20% of patients have just two metastases.

   4. Patients with breast, GI, and pelvic tumors tend to develop single brain lesions.

   5. Patients with lung cancer, melanoma, and tumors of unidentified origin usually develop multiple metastases.

   6. CNS structures are colonized in rough proportion to their relative masses.

      a. Most metastases localize to the frontal and parietal lobes, and few (1%) localize to the brainstem.

      b. Metastases prefer the arterial border zones of the major vessels (anterior-middle and middle-posterior cerebral arteries), presumably as a result of decreased vascular caliber and flow.

B. Among metastases from pelvic (prostate, ovary, or uterus) or GI tumors, about 50% are to the posterior fossa; only 10% of other primary tumors metastasize to the posterior fossa.

C. Management

   1. The brain has no lymphatics nor can it expand within the skull, and therefore edema contributes to the mass effect and increased intracranial pressure (ICP) produced by tumors.

   2. Increased ICP from an intracranial mass is managed with dexamethasone at a dosage of 10 mg IV followed by 4 mg IV or PO qid for maintenance.

   3. In a patient with minimal deficit, treatment can begin with dexamethasone at 4 mg PO qid.

   4. If the initial steroid dosage is inadequate, dexamethasone may be increased to 6, 8, or more mg IV or PO qid.

   5. Clinical improvement should become apparent within 24–48 hours of treatment, continue for several days, and then plateau.

   6. Dexamethasone should be tapered as tolerated after the patient has become stable and has begun more definitive therapy.

D. Steroids should be used carefully.

   1. An antacid regimen should be started with the steroid as prophylaxis against gastric bleeding, ulceration, or perforation.

   2. A Stevens-Johnson syndrome may occur in a patient on steroid and anticonvulsant therapy who is receiving brain irradiation.

E. Patients in extremis from increased ICP may require an osmotic diuretic such as mannitol (1 g/kg IV), which acts within minutes.

1. Smaller doses of mannitol (0.25–0.50 g/kg) can be repeated, but ICP must be monitored.
2. Only short-term hyperosmolar therapy is useful, for the following reasons.
    a. When serum sodium rises to more than 160 mEq/L, the treatment stops being useful.
    b. Dehydration may lead to cardiovascular collapse.
    c. Rebound increase in ICP occurs despite continued treatment, especially on rehydration.
3. Patients on diuretics should have bladder catheters.

F. **Hyperventilation** also causes ICP to drop rapidly. Hyperventilation and osmotics should be used only if precisely indicated and if a definitive end point is first established.

G. **Seizures**
1. Approximately 15–30% of patients with brain metastases develop seizures.
2. Status epilepticus is treated in the standard manner with intubation and IV anticonvulsants.
3. The drug of choice for patients who present with seizures is phenytoin (Dilantin).
    a. It is easily administered PO or IV.
    b. It is well tolerated.
    c. Its long half-life allows once-daily administration.
    d. Most patients can start at the usual maintenance dosage of 300 mg/day PO.
    e. If a patient has had several seizures in the preceding hours, load with 15–20 mg/kg (1000–1200 mg) IV or divided into three or four oral doses over 12–24 hours.
    f. **Therapeutic levels**
        (1) If the loading dose is administered intravenously, a therapeutic level (10–20 mg/dl) is reached at the end of the infusion.
        (2) If the load is administered orally all at once, a therapeutic level is reached in 4–6 hours.
        (3) If the oral dosage is divided, attaining a therapeutic level takes 24 hours.
        (4) If only a maintenance schedule is initiated, it takes 4–7 days to reach a therapeutic level.
    g. If seizures continue, the phenytoin dosage and blood level can be increased beyond the customary therapeutic range until dosage-related toxicity occurs.
    h. Patients who suffer subsequent seizures almost invariably have subtherapeutic drug levels.
4. If seizures cannot be controlled, use carbamazepine (Tegretol) (titrated up to 200 mg PO tid-qid), phenobarbital (90–150 mg/day), or valproic acid. One of several newly approved anticonvulsants (e.g., Neurontin or Lamictal) may also be considered. When seizures are controlled, the phenytoin is withdrawn slowly and the dosage of the second anticonvulsant is adjusted to keep the patient seizure-free.
5. Except for patients with melanoma (50% of whom develop seizures), there is no consensus regarding the use of prophylactic anticonvulsants in patients with brain metastases.
6. Posterior fossa metastases are not epileptogenic.
7. Dexamethasone and phenytoin have complex interactions.
    a. Each may increase the required dosage of the other.
    b. When phenytoin, dexamethasone, and whole-brain irradiation are used concurrently, the risks of erythema multiforme and erythema multiforme bullosa (Stevens-Johnson syndrome) are increased.

H. **Surgical management**
1. The patient with minimal disability, a single circumscribed accessible lesion, inactive systemic disease, and a long interval between diagnosis of the primary tumor and the brain metastasis is the ideal candidate for surgery.
2. A shunt is indicated for obstructive hydrocephalus.
3. In up to 10% of cases, an intracranial mass in a cancer patient is not a metastasis; the differential diagnosis includes primary CNS tumor, abscess, and arteriovenous malformation (AVM). Therefore, a biopsy is advisable if it can be done safely.

4. Current areas of controversy
  a. Reoperation may be indicated for metastases that recur in the original tumor bed with minimal further parenchymal invasion.
  b. Excision of multiple metastatic masses. If one or two of several metastases are symptomatic or life-threatening, a palliative resection should be considered. When resection is indicated, the result is as gratifying as that of surgical removal of a single lesion.
I. Radiation therapy
  1. Radiation is the primary treatment for brain metastases.
    a. Dosages range from 30–40 gray (Gy) in 180–200 cGy fractions to the whole brain over 2–4 weeks.
    b. Patients with radiosensitive tumors may benefit from a boost to the tumor bed.
    c. Complications from radiation are few (mild headache, hair loss, and asthenia) if dexamethasone is administered concurrently. Without dexamethasone, edema can lead to severe headaches, nausea, vomiting, papilledema, and death.
    d. Long-term toxic effects from radiotherapy include leukoencephalopathy, radiation necrosis, accelerated atherosclerosis, mineralizing microangiopathy, and impaired cognition.
    e. If high dosages of methotrexate are used concurrently with radiation, a necrotizing encephalopathy may occur within several months.
    f. CNS tolerance to radiation is inversely proportional to the volume irradiated.
  2. Prophylactic cranial irradiation is controversial because, although it lowers the incidence of subsequent brain metastases from small cell lung cancer, it does not impact significantly on patient survival.
  3. Stereotactic radiosurgery (either linear accelerator–based or "gamma knife") is a noninvasive technique that delivers a single large fraction or several smaller fractions of ionizing radiation to a well-defined, limited intracranial target with sharp peripheral dosage fall-off, resulting in minimal exposure to normal surrounding brain.
    a. A 10–25-Gy fraction can be administered as a boost either before or after conventionally fractionated radiation to tumor volumes of up to 30 cm^3 (maximum tumor diameter of about 4 cm).
    b. To remain within brain tolerance parameters, the dosage varies inversely with collimator size and number of isocenters.
    c. Initial clinical data suggest that tumor control rates higher than 80% can be achieved, with complete response rates of about 40%.
    d. Tumors with volumes less than 2 cm^3 may respond better than those with volumes greater than 10 cm^3.
    e. Metastases invade surrounding brain to varying degrees, and thus peripheral recurrences may emerge.
  4. Brachytherapy
    a. Brachytherapy uses a series of catheters stereotactically implanted directly into the tumor bed and afterloaded with high-activity iodine 125 (^{125}I) or iridium 192 (^{192}Ir).
    b. The target includes the contrast-enhancing tumor plus a 1-cm margin.
      (1) The target receives 45–60 Gy of radiation at a dosage rate of 40–50 cGy/hour.
      (2) The dosage delivered to surrounding normal tissue is minimal; it decreases by the square of the distance from the source.
      (3) The therapeutic ratio improves at continuous low dosage rates because tumors are less able to repair sublethal damage and the radiosensitivity of hypoxic cells depends less on oxygen.
  5. The patient with radiation necrosis presents with acute or subacute neurologic deterioration and signs and symptoms of a mass lesion.
    a. Neither computed tomography (CT) nor magnetic resonance imaging (MRI) scans can differentiate a necrotic mass from a recurrent tumor.
    b. Necrosis can be managed conservatively with steroids.
    c. Resection is indicated if neurologic deterioration continues, escalating steroid dosages become necessary, or intolerable steroid toxicity develops.
J. Chemotherapy

     1. Chemotherapy is not routinely indicated for treatment of CNS metastases.
       a. Most tumors are relatively drug-resistant.
       b. CNS metastases most frequently occur in patients with advanced cancer who have not responded to chemotherapy.
     2. Chemotherapy may be considered in some cases.
       a. The patient with a chemosensitive tumor, a good performance status, and inactive systemic disease whose CNS metastasis recurs following radiation with or without surgery is the ideal candidate for chemotherapy.
       b. CNS metastases from small cell lung cancer, breast cancer, lymphoma, and germ cell tumors may respond to chemotherapy with response rates comparable to those of the concurrent systemic tumor.
       c. The precise indications remain to be resolved.

K. Cerebellar metastases
     1. The signs are gait or limb ataxia with or without nystagmus and papilledema.
     2. The symptoms are instability of gait, headache, dizziness, vomiting, and double vision.
     3. Initial treatment considerations are the same as for supratentorial metastases—i.e., dexamethasone and irradiation.
     4. Acute complications from irradiation are more common with cerebellar than with supratentorial metastases, and therefore dexamethasone should be started at least 48 hours before radiotherapy is initiated.
     5. The risk of brain herniation following lumbar puncture (LP) is greater in patients with posterior fossa masses.
     6. The indications for resection are the same as for supratentorial metastases, but any sign of clinical instability or deterioration, an expanding mass, hydrocephalus, or nonresponse to dexamethasone should prompt consideration of immediate neurosurgical intervention.

II. Pituitary apoplexy
  A. Acute panhypopituitarism may occur from a metastasis to the sella turcica or to the pituitary, which causes necrosis or hemorrhage of the gland.
  B. This syndrome is characterized by headache, ophthalmoplegia, bitemporal hemianopsia or amaurosis, encephalopathy, or coma.
  C. This disorder is life-threatening when the patient becomes unable to maintain blood pressure despite fluids and pressors.
  D. Pituitary apoplexy is an emergency, and its treatment consists of high-dosage intravenous corticosteroids—e.g., dexamethasone at 6–12 mg IV q6h.

III. Metastases to the skull base
  A. The hallmark of metastases to the skull base is involvement of the cranial nerves as they exit through the basal foramina.
  B. Five major syndromes are recognized.
     1. Orbital syndrome presents as dull, continuous, and progressive pain over the affected eye with proptosis and ophthalmoplegia. There is decreased sensation over the distribution of the first division of the trigeminal nerve (CNV).
     2. Parasellar syndrome (cavernous sinus metastasis) is manifested as unilateral frontal headache and ophthalmoplegia. There may be decreased sensation over the distribution of the first division of CNV. If sinus thrombosis occurs, there are chemosis, edema of the eyelid and forehead, proptosis, and papilledema with retinal hemorrhages. This disorder is a cause of Tolosa-Hunt syndrome.
     3. Middle fossa syndrome (gasserian ganglion) is signaled by pain, numbness, or paresthesias over the distribution of the second or third division of CNV. The initial presentation may be a numb chin (or lip) syndrome; 65% result from breast cancer and 15% from lymphoproliferative tumors. About 50% of patients have mandibular metastases, 15% have skull base lesions, and 20% have carcinomatous meningitis.
     4. Jugular foramen syndrome manifests as hoarseness and dysphagia (CNX), with or without pain (CN IX or X). Examination may reveal asymmetric palatal elevation (CN IX), weakness of the ipsilateral sternocleidomastoid and trapezius muscles (CN XI), and a Horner's syndrome (sympathetic). Weakness and atrophy of the tongue may be found if CN XII is compromised by extension of the tumor to the adjacent hypoglossal canal.
     5. Occipital condyle syndrome presents as stiff neck and severe occipital

pain that increases with neck flexion. There is dysarthria and dysphagia from unilateral involvement of CN XII.

IV. Spinal epidural metastases

A. Metastatic epidural spinal cord compression occurs in 5–10% of patients with cancer; it is a neuro-oncologic emergency.

B. Prognosis. The most important determinant is neurologic performance status at presentation.

1. Of ambulatory patients, 90% remain so after treatment and have a 75% probability of surviving 1 year.
2. Only 50% of paraparetic and 13% of paraplegic patients with "radiosensitive" tumors become ambulatory after treatment.
3. Fewer than 10% of nonambulatory patients survive 1 year.
4. Once sphincter control is lost, it is unlikely to be regained.
5. Once neurologic dysfunction begins, paraplegia and loss of sphincter control follow within hours. Once established, the neurologic deficit usually is irreversible.
6. "Metastatic epidural spinal cord compression" is not an adequate term, because the challenge is the timely diagnosis of metastatic epidural tumor, prior to compromise of the spinal cord, rather than established spinal cord compression.

C. Epidural tumor must be suspected on clinical grounds and must prompt timely confirmation and treatment.

1. Approximately 60% of epidural metastases arise from prostate, lung, breast, and kidney cancers.
2. About 50% of adults with acute transverse myelopathies have spinal cord compression from epidural metastasis. In half of those patients it is the initial manifestation of cancer, and in half of those the primary tumor is in the lung.

D. Presentation

1. About 95% of patients with epidural tumors have progressive axial pain with or without a radicular or referred component.
2. Some weakness and sensory disturbance are present in 80%.
3. Almost 60% have sphincter dysfunction—a poor prognostic sign that implies bilateral cord or root damage.

E. Site of involvement

1. In about 85% of epidural tumors from solid cancers, the bony vertebral column is the site of metastasis.
   a. The vertebral body is involved in 45%.
   b. The posterior arch and pedicle are involved in 40%.
   c. The entire vertebra is involved in 15%.
2. From 50–70% involve the thoracic spine.
3. From 20–30% involve the lumbosacral spine.
4. From 10–20% involve the cervical spine.
5. At least one-third of patients with breast and prostate cancer have metastases at multiple levels.
6. Most patients with lung cancer have metastases at only one level.

F. Tumor may also reach the epidural space by direct invasion of a paravertebral mass through the intervertebral foramen; this is the mechanism in 75% of cord compressions resulting from lymphoma.

G. Diagnosis

1. A neuroimaging study should be performed in all cases of suspected epidural tumor to establish the diagnosis, the upper and lower limits of tumor invasion, and whether tumor exists at discontinuous levels.
   a. MRI is the imaging modality of choice for confirmation, visualization of extent of disease, and treatment planning. The best approach, however, is to obtain whatever study is available (and safe) in a timely fashion.
   b. If a myelogram is to be performed on a patient with signs or symptoms of increased ICP, a focal examination, or widespread metastases, safety dictates that intracranial metastases be ruled out first.
2. Plain spinal x-rays are inexpensive, readily available, and the most important diagnostic procedure for evaluation for epidural tumor.
   a. Plain x-rays correlate with vertebral metastases in 85–95% of patients with epidural compression from solid tumors, but in only one-third of patients with lymphoma.

b. Patients with back pain or with focal examinations and abnormal spinal films have a probability of cord compression of 90%.
c. If spinal films are normal, the probability of cord compression drops to 10%.
3. **Initial management**
   a. If cord compression is suspected, or on confirmation, a 10-mg IV bolus of dexamethasone is administered.
   b. A maintenance dosage of dexamethasone (4 mg IV or PO q6h) is instituted and then tapered as tolerated.
   c. The contribution of steroids to patient outcome is unknown.
   d. Steroids rarely produce dramatic reversal of established neurologic disability, but prognosis is better when they do.
   e. The bladder should be catheterized to determine postvoiding residual volume, and an indwelling catheter should be inserted if necessary.
   f. Prophylaxis against deep-vein thrombosis and a stool-softening regimen also should be started.
H. Although the intent of therapy remains palliative, several treatment options are available.
   1. **Decompressive laminectomy** works only temporarily and fails because the metastatic tumor generally is located in the vertebral body (that is, anterior to the spinal cord) and not in the neural arch, and because the procedure may contribute to spinal instability.
   2. **Anterior vertebral body resection**
      a. This is the only technique that debulks the tumor.
      b. It must be coupled with surgical stabilization of the spine.
      c. Debilitated patients are ineligible.
      d. Operative morbidity (10%) centers around nonhealing, breakdown, or infection of the wound and failure to stabilize the spine.
I. Radiation
   1. A total of 20–40 Gy is the usual dosage.
   2. The port should encompass two vertebral bodies above and two below the epidural defect and any discontinuous lesions.
   3. Radiation is indicated promptly after the diagnosis is made and should follow the administration of dexamethasone.
   4. If the surgery is performed first, radiation should follow after the wound heals.
   5. The tumors that most commonly produce epidural metastases—lung, breast, prostate, and lymphoma—are likely to respond to radiation.
   6. If neurologic deterioration continues, surgical intervention should be considered.
   7. **Complications** of radiation are as follows.
      a. Bone marrow depression
      b. Radiation myelopathy and/or a syrinx (from 6–18 months after therapy)
      c. A subacute syndrome characterized by Lhermitte's sign (a shocklike sensation down the back to the legs when the neck is flexed) may appear several weeks after radiation.
   8. **Laminectomy plus radiation.** There is no evidence that combining laminectomy with radiation results in an outcome better than that of radiation alone.
   9. **Recurrent spinal epidural metastases**
      a. Local metastases develop within two vertebral bodies of a previous lesion and within 3 months of the original diagnosis; they represent failure of tumor control at the margin of the radiation port.
      b. Distant metastases develop three or more vertebral bodies from a previous lesion and 15 months or longer after the original diagnosis.
      c. Patients who previously responded to radiation may be considered for reirradiation. They may benefit while not surviving to suffer the consequences of exceeding the spinal cord tolerance for radiation.
V. Leptomeningeal metastases
   A. Leptomeningeal carcinomatosis is most often caused by advanced or rapidly progressive lung and breast cancer, lymphoma, or melanoma.
   B. Presentation
      1. Hydrocephalus with no intracranial mass lesion
      2. Neurologic dysfunction at different levels of the neuraxis

3. Chronic, worsening, unremitting headache or somatic pain without apparent cause

C. The diagnostic hallmarks in the CSF are as follows.
1. Malignant cells
   a. Occasionally, multiple specimens must be taken.
   b. Cytology should be based on cytospin samples, not on stained smears.
   c. Cytology is more likely to be positive if taken near the symptomatic site, and thus cervical or cisternal punctures should be done if lumbar CSF is negative and suspicion is high.
2. Low glucose
3. Elevated protein
4. Myelography may reveal nodular masses or a block.

D. The major **differential diagnosis** comprises bacterial or fungal meningitis.

E. **Initial treatment**
1. In deciding whether or not to treat, the systemic disease status and likelihood of successful palliation should be considered.
2. Dexamethasone rarely provides symptomatic improvement. It may protect the CNS during radiation and/or chemotherapy, and it should be tapered after more definitive treatment has been initiated.

F. **Craniospinal radiation**
1. Either 30 Gy to the entire neuraxis, or 24 Gy to the most symptomatic areas, is usually administered.
2. Irradiating the entire neuraxis rarely controls leptomeningeal disease.
3. Craniospinal radiation aggravates or produces severe bone marrow depression, and most patients are unable to tolerate a complete course.

G. **Intrathecal chemotherapy**
1. Intrathecal chemotherapy is useful because tumor diffusely infiltrates the leptomeninges.
2. After systemic administration, most drugs reach CSF concentrations from 1–25% of the plasma concentration. Hence, the dosage intensity of treatment in the CSF is decreased, predisposing to CNS failure.
3. The volume of distribution in the CSF is small, and so high concentrations can be achieved with small drug dosages.
4. Drug clearance half-lives tend to be longer in the CSF than in plasma, maximizing exposure.
5. Intrathecal chemotherapy can be used alone or with neuraxis irradiation.
6. The first few doses may be administered by LP, but if this is continued it may lead to an epidural hematoma, CSF leaks, and virtual subdural or epidural compartments through which drug can be lost.
7. Other constraints to delivery by LP are related to the dynamics of CSF flow, which is craniocaudal, tends to bypass the ventricles, is affected by patient position, and may be severely disturbed in the presence of meningeal tumor with or without increased ICP.
8. A ventricular catheter with subcutaneous (Ommaya) reservoir should be implanted for drug delivery.
   a. The major, but uncommon, complication of Ommaya reservoirs is infection, and therefore proper sterile technique should be followed with each use.
   b. Fever, headache, lethargy, and CSF extravasation around the reservoir are signs of infection.
9. Except for lymphomas, the success rate in treatment of leptomeningeal cancer is poor.

VI. **Metastases to the spinal cord parenchyma**
A. Treatment is palliative.
B. Dexamethasone is the initial emergency treatment, and should be followed by irradiation of the whole cord.
C. Because approximately 75% of these cases are secondary to lung cancer, breast cancer, or lymphoma, some clinical improvement can be expected, especially if treatment is initiated before a myelopathy develops.
D. Surgical decompression accomplishes little, because the disease is intrinsic to the spinal cord and resection of the lesion itself generally is not feasible.

VII. **Metastases to the peripheral nervous system (PNS)**
A. **Presentation**
1. With pain, numbness, paresthesias, or weakness

2. Must be differentiated from radiation plexopathy
3. Pain, paresthesias, and weakness are more frequent with neoplastic involvement than with radiation plexopathy.
4. Horner's syndrome frequently occurs, with metastasis to the brachial plexus.

B. Treatment
1. Aggressive pain relief is imperative.
2. Non-narcotic drugs fail early, and adequate dosages of narcotics should be prescribed.
3. If narcotics fail, several procedures are available through anesthesia or neurosurgery.
4. Radiation or chemotherapy is instituted as appropriate.

VIII. Neurologic complications from chemotherapy
A. Most cytotoxic drugs are capable of nervous system toxicity.
B. Important reasons for recognizing iatrogenic toxicity are as follows.
1. Drug-induced complications may obscure or mimic the presentation of metastases, paraneoplastic syndromes, or primary neurologic disease.
2. Neurotoxicity may contribute to morbidity, disability, and death.
3. Neurotoxicity can result from a metabolic derangement of therapy or from cancer-induced end-organ failure.
4. Recognize and discontinue or modify the dose of the offending agent during treatment with a multidrug regimen.

C. Common complications attributable to chemotherapy
1. Peripheral neuropathy
a. Peripheral neuropathy is observed in almost all patients treated with vincristine, vinblastine, cisplatin, or paclitaxel (Taxol).
b. Peripheral neuropathy is dosage-limiting for vincristine, and is a function of the cumulative dosage.
   (1) Loss of the distal muscle stretch reflexes, although asymptomatic, is almost universal; foot and wrist drop may occur.
   (2) The most common complaints are paresthesias of the feet or hands with minor, if any, objective deficit.
   (3) Cranial nerve toxicity can present as a palsy of the recurrent laryngeal nerve, as bilateral facial nerve palsies, as diplopia resulting from an oculomotor nerve palsy, or as ptosis.
   (4) Occasionally, jaw or thigh pain occurs within a few hours of vincristine administration.
   (5) Complete or partial recovery of a vincristine-related deficit occurs several months after the drug is discontinued.
c. An **autonomic neuropathy** from vincristine manifests with orthostasis and constipation.

2. Transient, dosage-dependent myalgia may occur several days after administration of paclitaxel.

3. CNS complications
a. The prototype drug for CNS complications is methotrexate (MTX).
b. Route of administration, dosage, and simultaneous use of MTX with other neurotoxic therapy (particularly cranial irradiation) may cause additive or synergistic toxicity.
c. Intrathecal MTX produces aseptic meningitis within a few hours after administration (the meningitis lasts several days and subsides without sequelae) and transient or permanent myelopathy.
d. Leukoencephalopathy is a delayed effect of either intrathecal or high-dosage systemic administration; it may occur in up to 45% of patients if MTX is combined with cranial irradiation or other neurotoxic drugs.
e. High-dosage MTX can produce an acute, self-limited neurologic syndrome characterized by encephalopathy (seizures, delirium, and confusion) or, sometimes, a strokelike syndrome of unknown etiology.

4. Cerebellar toxicity
a. Purkinje cells are very sensitive to chemotherapy.
b. Cerebellar toxicity occurs in 8–50% of patients given high-dosage ara-C (dosages >48 g/m^2).
   (1) Symptoms occur within 24–48 hours with nystagmus and mild ataxia, followed by a florid encephalopathic and ataxic syndrome.

(2) Patients may improve within 1 week and recover completely within 2 weeks.

(3) The pathogenesis of this syndrome relates to the minimal amounts of cytidine deaminase (which inactivates ara-C) in the CNS.

c. 5-Fluorouracil causes abrupt cerebellar dysfunction in up to 7% of patients between a few days to months after the start of treatment; the dysfunction resolves after the drug is discontinued. Cerebellar dysfunction is likely with schedules that employ one or more weekly boluses of more than 15 mg/kg of 5-fluorouracil.

5. Some simple treatment strategies are of value.

a. Physical and/or occupational therapy could determine whether a patient is functional or disabled.

b. An ankle-foot orthosis for a foot drop may preserve the patient's ability to walk or help avoid tripping.

c. Neuropsychology may assist in the management of cognitive disability from leukoencephalopathy.

IX. Other complications

A. Encephalopathy

1. Seizures

a. Encephalopathic conditions can cause seizures, and seizures can cause encephalopathy.

b. A postictal state can mimic an encephalopathy; in debilitated, elderly patients, it may last 1 week.

2. If treatable causes are excluded, the management is supportive.

B. CNS infections

1. The most frequently encountered organisms are: *Listeria monocytogenes*, *Cryptococcus neoformans*, and *Aspergillus fumigatus*.

2. Next in frequency are gram-negative rods, *Candida albicans*, and herpes zoster.

3. Latent mycobacterial infections may reactivate.

4. Presentation

a. CNS infections present with fever, mental status changes, and seizures.

b. Headache and stiff neck may be subtle if the patient is unable to mount an adequate inflammatory response.

c. In severely leukopenic patients, the CSF may not be purulent and the infecting organism may not be readily detectable.

d. Gram or Ziehl-Neelsen staining of a cytospin sediment may reveal the pathogen before cultures turn positive.

5. Lumbar puncture (LP) should be approached with caution, because a patient with increased ICP may herniate or a thrombocytopenic patient may develop an epidural hematoma.

6. Treatment consists of antibiotics and support.

7. Progressive multifocal leukoencephalopathy (PML)

a. CNS infection with an opportunistic papovavirus, the JC virus.

b. Rarely, cases go into long-term remission.

c. PML presents with mental status changes, speech and visual deficits, and weakness.

d. Diagnosis is by biopsy of a focal (nonenhancing) white-matter brain lesion.

e. Treatment, with adenine arabinoside (ara-A) or cytosine arabinoside (ara-C), is of unproven benefit.

C. Cerebrovascular complications

1. At autopsy, about 15% of cancer patients have cerebrovascular disease (CVD), half of which are symptomatic.

2. Atherosclerosis remains the leading cause of infarction, but only about 15% of the infarcts are symptomatic.

3. Cancer patients may also develop CVD as a complication of the neoplastic process or its treatment.

4. Ischemic infarcts, rather than hemorrhages, predominate among patients with carcinoma. Nonbacterial thrombotic endocarditis and intravascular coagulation are frequent causes of symptomatic cerebral infarcts in this population.

5. The most frequent causes of intraparenchymal hemorrhage are coagulopathy and hemorrhage into metastases from melanoma and germ cell tumors.

6. Mucinous cancers may produce infarcts from widespread occlusions (by mucin) of any cerebral artery.

7. A large proportion of symptomatic patients with CVD and leukemia develop hemorrhagic infarcts.

8. There is no specific treatment for these complications.

9. Chemotherapy, especially cisplatin, may cause both acute and late vasculo-occlusive complications.

   a. Acute vascular occlusions may be related to endothelial injury.

   b. Late occlusions relate to vasospasm from hypomagnesemia.

10. Late effects of radiotherapy include a noninflammatory arteriopathy that causes large- and small-vessel occlusion, mineralizing microangiopathy, and accelerated atherosclerosis.

11. Dural sinus thrombosis, particularly of the superior sagittal sinus, is under-diagnosed.

   a. It is frequently asymptomatic and eventually recanalizes.

   b. It is most frequent in leukemic patients receiving chemotherapy and in patients with coagulopathy or widespread cancer.

   c. It presents with headache, seizures, papilledema, focal motor signs, and encephalopathy.

   d. The diagnosis is made by angiography, contrast CT, MRI, or MRI angiography.

   e. Treatment is supportive. Limited-term anticoagulation may be initiated if there is no hemorrhage, but its indication is controversial.

12. Neoplastic angioendotheliosis or intravascular lymphomatosis is the intravascular occlusion of small blood vessels by malignant mononuclear cells.

   a. This disorder is a rare complication of lymphoma.

   b. When the occluded vessels are in the CNS, patients develop multifocal deficits and encephalopathy with short-term or subacute progression to death.

   c. This disorder is difficult to differentiate from PML, vasculitis, or multiple emboli.

D. Syncope in patients with head and neck cancer

1. This syndrome presents in advanced or recurrent disease with syncope accompanied by paroxysmal head and face pain.

2. An abnormally strong carotid sinus reflex mediates the syncopal attacks.

3. A relationship between the syncope and sudden death exists and should prompt a search for recurrent carcinoma.

4. Pain is treated with carbamazepine.

5. Syncope is managed with anticholinergic drugs such as propantheline at a dosage of 15–30 mg PO qid. Ephedrine, at 25 mg PO qid, may be added if there is a vasodepressor component.

X. Paraneoplastic syndromes

A. The remote or paraneoplastic effects of cancer are thought to originate from production of an antibody to antigens shared by the tumor and the CNS.

1. Paraneoplastic syndromes must be differentiated from treatment-related toxicity and from metastasis.

2. Individual syndromes might distinguish patients whose prognoses differ from those of others with the same tumors.

B. Paraneoplastic cerebellar degeneration (PCD)

1. Presentation

   a. Acute onset of diplopia, vertigo, and vomiting

   b. Rapid progression to severe ataxia, coarse tremor, dysarthria, and nystagmus

   c. Stabilization with severe disability within several weeks to months

   d. Follows a course independent of that of the primary tumor, but individual patients may improve with control of the primary disease, after plasmapheresis, or with IV IgG

2. PCD occurs in fewer than 1% of patients with cancer.

3. PCD is described most frequently in patients with carcinomas of the ovary, lung, and breast, and with lymphomas.

4. This disorder is characterized by loss of Purkinje and granule cells from the cerebellum.

5. PCD is associated with high titers of antibodies to Purkinje cells, such as the anti-Yo antibody, in the sera and CSF.

C. Myasthenic syndrome (Eaton-Lambert syndrome)
  1. Presentation
     a. This syndrome presents with proximal muscle weakness with depressed muscle stretch reflexes, pain in the large muscle groups, dry mouth, and impotence.
     b. Weakness of the respiratory and extraocular muscles (diplopia) is less common but may occur.
     c. Strength improves transiently after repeated muscle contractions.
  2. In 75% of patients, myasthenic syndrome is associated with small cell carcinoma of the lung, and its diagnosis in an otherwise healthy person should prompt a search for this tumor.
  3. This syndrome is an autoimmune disorder in which an antibody to the voltage-gated calcium channel (VGCC) on small cell lung cancer is produced. This antibody cross-reacts with the VGCC on presynaptic cholinergic nerve terminals, resulting in reduced calcium entry into the nerve during depolarization and a consequent decrease in the number of transmitter quanta released.
  4. Treatment
     a. Eaton-Lambert syndrome may regress after successful antitumor treatment.
     b. The drugs most used for treatment are guanidine (starting at 5–10 mg/kg and increasing up to 35–45 mg/kg) and 3,4-diaminopyridine, both of which increase the number of quanta released by nerve impulses.
     c. Plasmapheresis is effective because it removes circulating antibodies.
     d. Intravenous immunoglobulins shut down production of endogenous immunoglobulins.
D. Paraneoplastic sensory neuronopathy and/or encephalomyelitis (PSN/E)
  1. Presentation
     a. PSN/E presents as rapidly or subacutely progressive pure sensory neuropathy affecting all modalities and complaints of distal numbness and paresthesias, areflexia, and sensory ataxia.
     b. Patients may develop limbic encephalitis (dementia), brainstem encephalitis (cranial nerve dysfunction), PCD (similar to the anti-Yo syndrome), transverse myelitis, motor neuron disease (similar to amyotrophic lateral sclerosis, or ALS), and autonomic dysfunction (orthostatic hypotension, neurogenic bladder, and constipation).
     c. PSN/E follows a course independent of the tumor.
  2. PSN/E occurs in fewer than 1% of patients with small cell lung cancer.
     a. There is inflammation and loss of neurons in the dorsal root ganglion in association with high titers of the anti-Hu antibody.
     b. Carcinomatous meningitis should be ruled out.

Recommended Readings

Byrne TN. Spinal cord compression from epidural metastases. *N Engl J Med* 327: 614–619, 1992.

Cybulski GR. Methods of surgical stabilization for metastatic disease of the spine. *Neurosurgery* 25:240–252, 1989.

Delatrre JY, et al. Distribution of brain metastases. *Arch Neurol* 45:741–744, 1988.

Graus F, Rogers LR, Posner JB. Cerebrovascular complications in patients with cancer. *Medicine* 64:16–35, 1985.

Greenberg HS, et al. Metastasis to the base of the skull: Clinical findings in 43 patients. *Neurology* 31:530–537, 1981.

Mehta MP, et al. Defining the role of radiosurgery in the management of brain metastases. *Int J Rad Onc Biol Phys* 24:619–625, 1992.

Posner JB. *Neurologic Complications of Cancer.* Philadelphia: Davis, 1995.

Rottenberg DA (ed). *Neurological Complications of Cancer Treatment.* Boston: Butterworth-Heinemann, 1991.

Rozental JM. Neurologic complications of cancer. In MC Brain, PP Carbone (eds), *Current Therapy in Hematology-Oncology* (5th ed). St. Louis: Mosby-Year Book, 1995.

Willson JKV, Masaryk TJ. Neurologic emergencies in the cancer patient. *Semin Oncology* 16:490–503, 1989.

54

Neurotoxicology and Iatrogenic Neurology
Margaret A. Laycock

Neurotoxins may be characterized by the source of the exposure, the mode of the exposure, and the signs and symptoms of the neurotoxicity. The signs and symptoms of neurotoxicity are common to many agents, and seemingly minor historical details may prove to be of invaluable significance. Signs and symptoms of neurotoxicity may be characterized as follows:

1. *Constitutional:* anorexia, weight loss, malaise, fatigue, nausea, vomiting, and insomnia
2. *CNS:* headache, dizziness, mental status changes, changes in behavior and personality, seizures, stroke, ataxia, movement disorders, encephalopathy, aseptic meningitis, benign intracranial hypertension, psychosis, and myelopathy
3. *PNS:* paresthesias, dysesthesias, visual changes, hearing loss, vertigo, and autonomic disorders including hypotension, bladder dysfunction, diaphoresis, piloerection, and sexual dysfunction
4. *Neuromuscular junction and muscle:* weakness, myalgias, myotonia, muscle cramps, myopathy, and myasthenic syndromes

The following overview of common neurotoxins includes toxins from industrial, commercial, environmental, medicinal, and recreational exposure sources. Detailed information and extensive lists of agents capable of causing similar clinical scenarios can be found in textbooks of neurotoxins and pharmaceuticals.

I. Industrial/commercial/environmental neurotoxins
    A. Metals (e.g., lead, arsenic, mercury, thallium, gold, and bismuth)
        1. Lead
            a. Common exposure sources. Lead-based paint (especially prior to 1972); ceramic glazes; automotive industry; lead smelters; petroleum refineries; shooting galleries; paper, rubber, and plastics industries; and battery manufacturing
            b. Modes of exposure. Inhalation and ingestion
            c. Systemic symptoms. Gastrointestinal (GI) symptoms
            d. Clinical signs of significance. Gingival lead lines may be seen in those with poor oral hygiene.
            e. Neurologic disorders
                (1) Children. The most common disorder among children is encephalopathy, with symptoms ranging from poor school performance and headaches to seizures and coma. Peripheral neuropathy may occur infrequently.
                (2) Adults. The most frequent disorder among adults is an asymmetric axonal peripheral neuropathy with motor fibers affected more severely than sensory fibers. The neuropathy commonly presents with wrist drop or foot drop. Encephalopathy occurs less commonly than in children.
            f. Diagnosis
                (1) Clinical picture and history of exposure
                (2) Laboratory
                    (a) CSF. Mild pleocytosis and elevated protein
                    (b) Blood. Elevated lead level and microcytic anemia with basophilic stippling and increased delta-aminolevulinic acid
                    (c) Urine. Increased lead level, increased total urinary delta-aminolevulinic acid, and increased coproporphyrin level
                (3) Radiographic. Lead lines in growth plates of long bones, ra-

601

diopaque lead in GI tract in cases of ingestion, and cerebral edema in severe intoxication

g. **Treatment**
(1) Identify the source and remove the patient from exposure.
(2) Refer for outpatient neurologic evaluation on a semiurgent basis (less than 1 week) if the patient is asymptomatic and the source is easily removed; inpatient evaluation is necessary if the patient is symptomatic, the exposure source is unidentified, or the blood lead level in an asymptomatic patient is higher than 70.
(3) Provide supportive therapy for seizures, cerebral edema, and coma, if necessary. Avoid steroids, concomitant iron supplementation, and overhydration.
(4) Administer chelation therapy with edetate ethylenediaminetetraacetic acid (EDTA) for lead levels of 20–70; EDTA and dimercaprol (BAL) for levels above 70. Hydration, renal function, and electrolyte status must be carefully assessed prior to treatment. Only the mildest cases can be treated on an outpatient basis. Most require inpatient treatment by neurologists, nephrologists, and intensivists.
(5) Penicillamine has been given orally after chelation with EDTA and BAL, although it is not FDA approved for this use.
(6) Additional courses of treatment may be necessary as stores are mobilized. Follow-up blood levels must be performed.
(7) Careful monitoring for BAL toxicity (headache, hypertension, and seizures) and EDTA toxicity (headache, myalgias, and tetany) is necessary.

2. **Arsenic**
a. **Common exposure sources.** Attempted homicide/suicide, insecticides, taxidermy, battery manufacturing, etching, printing/bookbinding, and adulterants in alcohol
b. **Modes of exposure.** Ingestion, inhalation, and skin contact
c. **Systemic signs and symptoms.** Gastrointestinal symptoms, dermatitis, fever, hemolysis, jaundice, diaphoresis, and nephropathy
d. **Clinical signs of significance.** Mees' lines (transverse white lines in the nailbeds, observed approximately 1 month after exposure), dermatitis and hyperkeratosis prominent in palmar and plantar surfaces and skin folds, and garlic odor on breath
e. **Neurologic disorders** range from acute to latent signs and symptoms, with onset usually within 2 weeks but occasionally after months.
(1) **CNS.** Headache, vertigo, changes in mental status, encephalopathy (may be hemorrhagic or acute/subacute/chronic), seizures, coma, and myelopathy
(2) **PNS.** Painful sensorimotor peripheral neuropathy with axonal features, occasionally pure sensory neuropathy; optic neuropathy with loss of vision
(3) **Muscle.** Cramps and myalgias
f. **Diagnosis**
(1) Clinical picture and history of exposure may or may not be available (e.g., homicide/suicide attempt)
(2) **Laboratory**
(a) **Hair and nail samples** are most reliable for chronic or remote exposure. Abnormal arsenic levels are greater than 0.1 mg/100g hair.
(b) **Urine and blood** may be negative despite significant arsenic intoxication. High arsenic levels in urine following seafood ingestion may occur. Urine and blood may be negative for arsenic if greater than 14 days has elapsed since exposure. Abnormal arsenic levels are greater than 0.1 mg/l.
(c) **CSF.** Mild increase in protein, increased number of red cells in cases with hemorrhagic encephalopathy, and possibly increased opening pressure
(d) **Radiographs** may show radiopaque arsenic in gut after ingestion.
g. **Treatment**

(1) Identify the source and remove the patient from exposure.
(2) Refer for inpatient evaluation by neurologists, intensivists, and nephrologists.
(3) Provide supportive treatment for seizures, coma, and concomitant systemic dysfunction.
(4) Perform aggressive GI lavage, administer cathartics, and forced emesis for ingestion. Gastric wash with protein solution or milk may reduce toxin absorption from the GI tract.
(5) Begin chelation therapy with BAL (dimercaprol).
  (a) Administer by IM route in initial dosages ranging from 2.5 mg/kg q6h to 3 mg/kg q4h and gradually taper over 10–14 days.
  (b) Avoid concomitant iron preparations.
  (c) Precautions regarding renal function, hydration, and electrolyte status are the same as in treatment for lead intoxication.

3. Mercury
a. Common exposure sources
(1) **Organic mercury.** Contaminated seafood and grain treated with antifungal agents containing mercury
(2) **Inorganic mercury.** Paints; insecticides; industries involving production of electrical equipment, paper, chlorine, plastics, and felt; and amalgam for dental fillings

b. Modes of exposure. Ingestion, inhalation, skin contact, and in utero (organic mercury)
c. Systemic signs and symptoms. GI symptoms (may have hemorrhagic diarrhea), hypersalivation, stomatitis, renal failure, and shock. Metallic taste in mouth. Chronic intoxication in children may include symptoms of hypertension and erythematous skin (pink disease).
d. Clinical signs of significance. Gingival hypertrophy with bluish line along gingival margin
e. Neurologic disorders
(1) **Acute intoxication.** Mental status changes ranging from irritability to psychosis with coma, tremor, and myoclonus in inorganic mercury intoxication; ataxia, cortical blindness, and peripheral neuropathy in organic mercury poisoning
(2) **Chronic intoxication.** CNS changes as above; seizures; visual changes (cortical and cranial nerve); hearing loss; painful, axonal peripheral neuropathy or ALS-like motor neuronopathy; ataxia
(3) **In children.** Painful neuropathy with autonomic nervous system (ANS) dysfunction
(4) **In utero exposure** may lead to mental retardation or cerebral palsy.

f. Diagnosis. Clinical presentation/history of exposure. Blood, hair, and urine tests for elevated mercury levels. Urine and blood may be negative if more than 2 weeks have elapsed since exposure.
g. Treatment
(1) Identify the source and remove the patient from exposure.
(2) Refer for inpatient consultation with neurologists, intensive care specialists, and nephrologists.
(3) Provide supportive treatment for seizures, coma, and concomitant systemic disorders (e.g., renal failure and oliguria).
(4) Initiate gastric lavage and forced emesis, followed by charcoal or gastric wash with albumin or protein solution (may also use 5% solution sodium formaldehyde sulfoxalate to slow absorption).
(5) Begin chelation therapy with BAL works best for acute intoxication and less so for chronic intoxication. Penicillamine may be more useful in chronic mercurialism.
(6) EDTA is contraindicated in all forms of mercurialism.
(7) Cholestyramine and osmotic agents (such as sorbitol) may be given to prevent constipation and reabsorption of mercury from the GI tract

4. Costs and availability of agents for treatment of heavy metal intoxication
a. EDTA injectable (1 g ampule) is widely available and has an estimated hospital cost of $26.00/g.

      b. BAL is not readily available and has an estimated hospital cost, before processing for use, of $35.00/g.

      c. Penicillamine (250 mg capsules) is widely available and has an estimated hospital cost of $0.65/capsule.

B. Solvents (e.g., toluene, benzene, ethylene glycol, acetone, isopropyl alcohol, and formaldehyde)

  1. Most cases of solvent intoxication involve mixtures of solvents rather than single agents.

  2. Exposure sources

    a. Recreational ("sniffing"). Substances commonly used are aerosols, model cements, and glues.

    b. Occupational. Paint thinners and lacquers, furniture polish, dyes and paints, model cements and glues, aerosols, gasoline and explosives, dry cleaning agents, perfumes, and plastics

  3. Modes of exposure. Inhalation, ingestion, and skin contact

  4. Systemic signs and symptoms. Severe metabolic acidosis and renal failure

  5. Neurologic disorders. Alterations in behavior, personality, and mental status; hallucinations; movement disorders; ataxia; visual changes; and peripheral neuropathy often affecting motor nerves to a greater extent than sensory nerves

  6. Clinical signs of significance. Odor of solvent on breath or clothing

  7. Diagnosis. Clinical picture and history of exposure

  8. Treatment

    a. Identify the source and remove the patient from exposure.

    b. Initiate inpatient evaluation for acute intoxication. Seek consultation with neurologists, intensive care specialists, and nephrologists.

    c. Provide supportive therapy for poor mental status, concomitant renal failure or acidosis, and electrolyte disturbances.

    d. Give activated charcoal or laxatives for ingestion.

    e. Dialysis may be necessary (hemodialysis and peritoneal).

    f. Specific therapies may be useful if the particular solvent is known (e.g., ethyl alcohol for ingestion of antifreeze).

C. Gases

  1. Carbon monoxide

    a. Sources of exposure. Automotive industry, fire fighting, furnaces and hot water heaters, cigarette smoke, suicide/homicide attempts

    b. Neurologic disorders

      (1) Acute. Mental status changes, dizziness, headaches, seizures, and coma

      (2) Chronic. Headache, memory and concentration disturbances, visual and hearing losses, polyneuropathy, pyramidal and extrapyramidal signs, tremor, ataxia, and encephalopathy

      (3) Fulminant CNS demyelination may follow 1–3 weeks after acute intoxication.

    c. Systemic signs and symptoms. Related to ischemia with end-organ damage

    d. Clinical signs of significance. Anoxia without cyanosis; "cherry red" appearance of skin

    e. Diagnosis. Clinical picture and history of exposure may or may not be available (e.g., suicide/homicide attempt). Elevated carboxyhemoglobin levels are found on blood sampling.

    f. Treatment

      (1) Remove the patient from the source.

      (2) Provide supportive therapy.

        (a) Maintain airway and circulation.

        (b) Administer 100% O_2.

        (c) Transfer patients with mental status changes to hospital. Severe cases require ICU care. Hyperbaric oxygen and exchange transfusion may help if available.

        (d) Seek consultation with internists and neurologists for all hospitalized patients and psychiatric consultation for all suicide attempts.

        (e) Treatment of cerebral edema should be managed by neurologists.

        (f) Decrease the metabolic needs for oxygen (helps limit the degree of damage) by:
            (i) Bed rest and mild sedation for severe agitation
            (ii) Aggressive treatment of fevers
            (iii) Use of cooling blanket to lower body temperature (but avoid shivering)
            (iv) Aggressive treatment of seizures

2. Nitrous oxide
    a. Sources of exposure. Occupational exposure in dentistry and health-care and abuse by those with access to inhaled anesthetics
    b. Neurologic disorders. Paresthesias, ataxia, and axonal sensorimotor polyneuropathy; may have upper motor neuron involvement similar to subacute combined degeneration
    c. Treatment
        (1) Remove the patient from the source.
        (2) Administer 100% O_2.
        (3) Provide drug abuse and addiction counseling if appropriate.

D. Pesticides (e.g., organophosphates and other acetylcholinesterase inhibitors)
    1. Sources of exposure. Occupations in agriculture, gardening, crop dusting, and manufacture of pesticides
    2. Modes of exposure. Ingestion, inhalation, and skin contact
    3. Systemic symptoms. Nausea, vomiting, diarrhea, abdominal pain, diaphoresis, pupillary constriction, excessive salivation, bronchospasm (inhalation), increased lacrimation and respiratory secretions, and local skin swelling (skin contact)
    4. Neurologic disorders. Paresthesias, tremor, fasciculations, dysphagia, decreased mental status, miosis, diffuse weakness and respiratory failure, late-onset progressive peripheral neuropathy, myopathy, and upper motor neuron signs
    5. Diagnosis
        a. Clinical picture and history of exposure
        b. Urine and gastric fluid tests for identification of organophosphate by gas chromatography
    6. Treatment
        a. Identify the source and remove the patient from exposure, which may necessitate flushing contaminated skin with large amounts of water or use of aggressive gastric lavage (for ingestion).
        b. Provide supportive treatment for respiratory and circulatory failure. Secure airway and IV access, then transfer to emergency treatment facility. Consult with emergency medical team and with neurologists.
            (1) Pralidoxine at a dosage of 0.5–1.0 g IV immediately. Repeat if no change in status; may need to repeat periodically after initial response.
                (a) Pralidoxine (1-g ampule) may be limited in availability at smaller hospitals.
                (b) Estimated hospital cost: $23.00/g
            (2) Atropine at 1–2 mg IV. Repeat every 3–5 minutes if needed initially and then repeat as needed for control of bradycardia. May also administer atropine subcutaneously if no IV access is present. May give atropine orally if the patient is awake and able to swallow.

II. Medicinal neurotoxins. Many patients who enter a general practitioner's office have experienced adverse effects from medicinal agents. Maintaining a high index of suspicion of medication-induced nervous system dysfunction is crucial in diagnosis.
    A. Treatment of medication-induced neurotoxicity is multifaceted and hinges on establishing the diagnosis.
        1. Identify potential medicinal neurotoxins available to the patient.
            a. Obtain a complete medication history from the patient and family.
            b. Ask the patient to bring all medications and over-the-counter preparations to the office.
            c. Obtain a list of prescribed medications from the patient's pharmacy and specialty physicians.
        2. Identify patient risk factors for toxicity.
            a. Usage of multiple drugs or access to other persons' drugs

b. History of noncompliance with medications, incorrect dosing, or intentional overdose

c. Tendency toward self-treatment, or history of alcohol or substance abuse

d. Coexistent systemic, neurologic, or psychiatric disease

3. Exclude other possible etiologies of observed neurologic symptoms such as infection, metabolic disturbances, trauma, cardiovascular disease, and psychiatric illness.

4. Identify the agent most likely to be responsible for the neurologic disorder.

   a. Assess historical factors.

   (1) Recent changes in drug dosages may lead to toxicity or drug interactions.

   (2) Correlation of symptom onset with initiation or withdrawal from a medication is frequently found.

   (3) The patient's concurrent medical, social, and psychiatric history may suggest possible etiologic agents.

   b. Be aware of side-effect profiles of common medications.

   c. Observe changes in neurologic signs and symptoms after discontinuing or changing the dosage of a suspicious agent. Reinstituting a drug in suspected withdrawal may be of diagnostic benefit.

   d. Withdraw several suspected medications (if possible) with reintroduction of single agents if the patient is on several medications that could be responsible for the neurologic signs and symptoms.

5. Identify patients who potentially require advanced support, monitored observation, and invasive intervention.

   a. Acute overdose or intoxication (accidental or intentional)

   b. Alteration or rapid deterioration of neurologic function, or significant changes in cardiovascular or respiratory status that could threaten independent functioning

   (1) Intensive care specialists and neurologists may assist in identifying which patients need transfer to acute care facilities.

   (2) Poison control centers and emergency room staff may be valuable in providing information on simple and possibly critical interventions that can be undertaken prior to transfer.

B. Diagnosis is dependent on the practitioner's recognition of the spectrum of neurotoxicity associated with common medications.

1. Headaches

   a. Drugs may induce headaches in a variety of ways:

   (1) By aggravating a preexisting headache disorder or unmasking an underlying tendency for headaches (e.g., birth-control pills, hormone preparations, steroids, and sympathomimetics)

   (2) By vasoactive effects (e.g., caffeine, ergots, nitrates, nifedipine, hydralazine, pseudoephedrine, and bronchodilators)

   (3) By resulting in withdrawal syndromes or "rebound" headaches (e.g., analgesics, NSAIDs, ergots, caffeine, and narcotics)

   (4) By inducing aseptic or chemical meningitis (e.g., ibuprofen, intrathecal methotrexate, and inadvertent intradural injection of epidural anesthetic agents)

   (5) By precipitation of benign intracranial hypertension (e.g., several antibiotics, steroids, birth-control pills, and anesthetics)

   b. Treatment is initiated by discontinuing or weaning the appropriate agent and may require additional intervention in instances of aseptic meningitis and benign intracranial hypertension. Neurologic consultation should be considered in instances of diagnostic dilemmas, additional neurologic symptoms, abnormal neurologic exam, or failure of improvement after discontinuation of the suspected agent.

   c. When discontinuation of a given agent is not possible, symptomatic treatment may be necessary and patient support and counseling may be beneficial in continuing compliance with the responsible medication. Altering the dosing schedule may improve the patient's ability to function despite symptoms.

2. Changes in mental status, behavior, and personality

   a. Most medications can cause alterations in mentation and behavior either by direct nervous system action or by indirect mechanisms (e.g., by hepatic or renal toxicity). Symptoms are frequently functions of dosage.

b. Drugs commonly associated with alterations in mentation and behavior include analgesics, benzodiazepines, sleeping agents, and strongly anticholinergic medicines such as antihistamines and tricyclic antidepressants.

c. Less obvious agents include medications for treatment of Parkinson's disease (bromocriptine, L-dopa, and amantadine), cardiovascular disease (beta-blockers, clonidine, digitalis, and calcium channel blockers), epilepsy, peptic ulcer disease (cimetidine and ranitidine), diabetes (oral hypoglycemic agents), glaucoma (eye drops), and infections (isoniazid and sulfonamides).

d. Some chemotherapeutic drugs (methotrexate and cytosine arabinoside) may induce severe toxic brain damage known as leukoencephalopathy, which commonly presents as changes in mentation and may progress to coma and death. Concomitant radiation and intrathecal administration appear to increase the risk of this complication.

e. Withdrawal syndromes must be considered for patients taking medications with known addictive potentials.

3. Hallucinations

a. Hallucinations, which are usually visual in nature, may occur as toxic reactions to treatment with barbiturates, sleeping agents, anticholinergic drugs (tricyclic antidepressants, atropine, antihistamines, and eye drops for glaucoma), anti-Parkinson's agents (L-dopa and bromocriptine), cimetidine, and sulfonamides, as well as others.

b. Hallucinations may also be symptoms of withdrawal from barbiturates and benzodiazepines.

4. Gait disturbances

a. Toxin-induced gait disturbances may result from sedation or from direct effects on the cerebellum, spinal cord, or peripheral nerves, and may be either transient or irreversible.

b. Any medication with sedative properties may cause instability of gait. The concomitant alteration in mental functioning helps to identify these agents as potential causes of walking difficulties. Elderly patients and young children are particularly vulnerable to these effects.

c. Cerebellar ataxia may be observed in patients treated with chemotherapeutic agents (5-FU and cytosine arabinoside), anticonvulsants (phenobarbital, phenytoin, carbamazepine, and mysoline), lithium, and neuroleptics.

(1) Chemotherapy-induced ataxia must be differentiated from ataxia observed in paraneoplastic syndromes. The presence of serum and CSF antibodies to Purkinje cells, such as the anti-Yo antibody, and the progression of the dystaxia despite drug withdrawal favor the diagnosis of a paraneoplastic syndrome (see Ch. 53, sec. **X.B**).

(2) Ataxia associated with anticonvulsant use (phenytoin, phenobarbital, and carbamazepine) is most often observed when serum levels exceed the therapeutic range, although some patients may become toxic at levels within this range. Some evidence suggests that long-term phenytoin use may lead to cerebellar atrophy and associated irreversible cerebellar ataxia.

d. Toxic myelopathy can occur in patients treated with intrathecal methotrexate or cytosine arabinoside, and is occasionally observed after exposure to nitrous oxide. Compressive myelopathy may result from corticosteroid-induced epidural lipomatosis. Myelopathy presents as lower-extremity weakness and may have associated symptoms of bowel and bladder dysfunction.

5. Movement disorders

a. The spectrum of involuntary movements associated with medication use is astounding and is part of the differential diagnosis of all patients with movement disorders.

b. These involuntary movements include tremor, myoclonus, dystonias, akathisia, tardive dyskinesia, chorea, athetosis, and parkinsonism.

c. Medications frequently responsible for causing movement disorders include sympathomimetics, neuroleptics, tricyclic antidepressants, antiemetics, anti-Parkinson's agents, lithium, and valproic acid.

6. Seizures

a. Medications may precipitate seizures in a variety of ways:
   (1) By lowering the seizure threshold in susceptible patients (e.g., those with prior histories or family histories of seizures)
   (2) As a result of excessively high drug levels (e.g., secondary to overdose, failure of drug metabolism, or drug interactions)
   (3) As part of a withdrawal syndrome
   (4) Indirectly by toxicity on other organ systems and resultant metabolic disturbances
b. Most medication-associated seizures are generalized, and some have initial focal features.
c. Drugs commonly implicated in precipitating seizures include analgesics (cocaine and meperidine), anesthetics (lidocaine and ketamine), high-dosage antibiotics (penicillin, ampicillin, imipenem, and cephalosporins), anticonvulsants (with toxic dosages), bronchodilators, immunosuppressants and chemotherapeutic agents (cyclosporine A, methotrexate, and vincristine), sympathomimetics (ephedrine, pseudoephedrine, and phenylpropanolamine), baclofen, benzodiazepines (e.g., clonazepam), and barbiturates.

7. Autonomic dysfunctions
a. Hypotension is a problem commonly associated with antidepressants, diuretics, nitrates, and medications with anticholinergic properties.
b. Bladder and bowel dysfunctions in the forms of urinary hesitancy, incomplete voiding, urinary incontinence, and constipation are frequently caused by use of medications with anticholinergic properties (e.g., antihistamines and antidepressants). Underlying diseases, such as diabetes, multiple sclerosis, and benign prostatic hypertrophy, can increase the risk of bladder and bowel dysfunctions.
c. Sexual dysfunction may also occur and is caused by the same classes of drugs that may lead to hypotension and bladder dysfunction.

8. Neuromuscular junction disorders
a. Many drugs may interfere with neuromuscular junction activity, and patients with underlying diseases localized to the neuromuscular junction are at increased risk for such adverse effects. Aminoglycoside antibodies, muscle relaxants, and neuromuscular blocking agents may exacerbate weakness in susceptible people; and muscle relaxants and neuromuscular blocking agents may cause transient weakness in normal people. Drugs with potential neuromuscular junction effects should be avoided if possible in patients with myasthenia gravis and Eaton-Lambert syndrome.
b. Penicillamine may cause a neuromuscular junction disorder that is clinically indistinguishable from myasthenia gravis.
c. Combinations of sedatives and neuromuscular blocking agents are commonly used during management of patients requiring mechanical ventilation and may lead to prolonged neuromuscular blockade. This entity should be considered in the event of ventilator dependence despite absence of medical illness sufficient to prolong the need for artificial support. Prolonged blockade can be diagnosed by electromyography (EMG). Treatment entails withdrawal from sedatives and neuromuscular blockers while continuing respiratory support until adequate neuromuscular junction recovery occurs.

9. Peripheral neuropathies
a. Drug-induced peripheral neuropathies are usually symmetric, and are characterized by a stocking-and-glove distribution. They may present as a gradually progressive or fulminant process, and may cause permanent damage. Some may resolve completely after withdrawal of the responsible drug. Pure sensory forms and mixed sensorimotor neuropathies are common.
b. Medications commonly associated with complication of peripheral neuropathies include antimicrobials (e.g., nitrofurantoin, some aminoglycosides, isoniazid, and metronidazole), anti-inflammatories (gold and colchicine), chemotherapeutic agents (cis-platinum, vincristine, and procarbazine), pyridoxine, lithium, and amiodarone.
c. Prevention of peripheral neuropathy is the best means of treatment and includes:

(1) Discontinuing medications with potential peripheral nerve toxicity at first indication of toxicity (e.g., complaints of numbness, tingling, or tinnitus)

(2) Following drug levels of known potential neurotoxins (aminoglycosides) and avoiding levels that exceed recommendations

(3) Adjusting medication dosages in patients with impaired renal or hepatic function, or using alternative drugs that can be more easily metabolized (e.g., avoiding nitrofurantoin in patients with renal impairment or dehydration)

d. Ototoxicity may or may not present concurrently with a generalized neuropathy and is most commonly associated with the use of aminoglycoside antibiotics (e.g., streptomycin, gentamycin, and tobramycin) but may also occur as a complication of treatment with cis-platinum, salicylates, quinine, furosemide, and ethacrynic acid.

10. Myopathies

a. Atrophic, inflammatory, or necrotizing myopathies may be observed as complications of medication use.

b. Steroid myopathy is the most common drug-induced myopathy and is characterized by painless, proximal muscle weakness. Diagnosis can be difficult in patients taking steroids for polymyositis and may require serial clinical observations during dosage reduction, weaning from steroids, or changing to alternative immunosuppressants. EMG is normal in isolated steroid myopathy, and muscle biopsy shows type IIB muscle fiber atrophy.

III. Recreational neurotoxins (illicit drug use). Recreational drug use permeates every level of society, and most physicians are involved in treating patients involved in these practices and the associated complications. Identifying and treating these patients can be extremely difficult, even in the best of circumstances, because of patients' typical reluctance to admit to their recreational habits or believe that they are the sources of medical sequelae. Substances commonly abused include solvents, cannabis, cocaine, and opiates, among others.

A. Solvents

1. The most popular agents are those with high concentrations of toluene, such as spray paints and lacquers, model cements, and glues.

2. See sec. **I** for clinical syndrome, diagnosis, and treatment.

B. Cannabis (marijuana, "grass," "hash")

1. Modes of abuse. Ingestion and inhalation (by smoking)

2. Neurologic signs and symptoms. Cognitive impairment, confusion, and incoordination

3. Diagnosis. Clinical picture and history, odor of burnt leaves on clothing, and urine screen positive for tetrahydrocannabinol (THC)

4. Treatment. Counseling for substance abuse

C. Cocaine ("coke," "snow," "crack")

1. Modes of exposure. Powdered form is used intranasally ("snorting") and intravenously. Crystalline forms ("crack" or "rock") are inhaled by smoking.

2. Neurologic signs and symptoms. Headaches; changes in mentation; psychosis; vascular events such as transient ischemic attacks (TIAs), ischemic or hemorrhagic infarctions, and subarachnoid hemorrhages; and focal and generalized seizures

3. Diagnosis. Clinical picture and history; accompanying systemic disorders such as cardiac arrhythmias, hypertension, and respiratory suppression; positive drug screen for cocaine; and needle "tracks"

4. Treatment

a. Transfer suspected overdose patients to acute care facilities and consultation with appropriate specialists.

b. Provide supportive treatment for respiratory failure, arrhythmias, and severe hypertension. Appropriate therapy for seizures and intracranial events should be guided by neurologists.

c. Administer haloperidol for severe agitation and psychosis.

d. Initiate drug abuse and addiction counseling.

D. Amphetamines ("uppers," "speed," "crank")

1. Modes of abuse. Ingestion and IV injection

2. Neurologic signs and symptoms are similar to those observed with cocaine use: hypervigilance, anxiety, tremulousness, seizures, cerebral vascular events, vasculitis, and psychosis (usually paranoid).

   3. Diagnosis. Clinical picture and history; accompanying systemic signs such as hypertension, tachycardia, and other arrhythmias; and drug screen positive for amphetamines or derivatives
   4. Treatment
      a. Transfer suspected overdose patients to acute care facilities and consult with appropriate specialists.
      b. Provide supportive therapy for arrhythmias, respiratory failure, severe hyperthermia, and hypertension.
      c. Appropriate therapy for seizures and intracranial events should be guided by neurologists.
      d. Administer haloperidol and benzodiazepines for agitation and psychosis.
      e. Initiate forced emesis, gastric suctioning, and cathartics for ingestion.
      f. Acidification of urine may increase excretion of amphetamines.
      g. Refer patient for drug abuse counseling.
   E. Opiates (e.g., morphine and heroin)
      1. Modes of abuse. Ingestion, inhalation by smoking, intranasal, intradermal, intramuscular, and intravenous
      2. Neurologic signs and symptoms. Altered mental status, hypoxic encephalopathy, coma, cerebral edema, seizures, movement disorders, polyneuropathy, rhabdomyolysis, cerebrovascular events, cerebral abscess, and meningitis
      3. Diagnosis. Clinical picture and history; accompanying systemic signs of respiratory depression, pupillary constriction (may be dilated in hypoxia), and endocarditis; evidence of needle tracks and skin popping (round, shallow scars); and withdrawal symptoms including rhinorrhea, diaphoresis, chills, anxiety, abdominal cramps, nausea, vomiting, and diarrhea
      4. Treatment
         a. Transfer suspected overdose patients to acute care facilities and consult with appropriate specialists.
         b. Provide supportive therapy for respiratory and cardiovascular compromise and for withdrawal symptoms.
         c. Initiate treatment of associated infections (e.g., endocarditis and abscess) and seizures under specialists' guidance.
         d. Administer naloxone for overdose (0.4 mg IV q4–5min as needed).
         e. Refer patient to detoxification programs, methadone centers, and drug abuse and addiction counseling.

Recommended Readings

Alldredge BK, et al. Seizures associated with recreational drug abuse. *Neurology* 39:1037–1039, 1989.

Aminoff M (ed). *Neurology and General Medicine.* New York: Churchill-Livingstone, 1989.

Argov Z, Mostagliz F. Disorders of neuromuscular transmission caused by drugs. *N Engl J Med* 301(8):409–413, 1979.

Bleecker M (ed). *Occupational and Clinical Neurotoxicology.* Baltimore: Williams & Wilkins, 1994.

Blum K, Manzo L (eds). *Neurotoxicology.* New York: Marcel Dekker, 1985.

Goetz CG. *Neurotoxins in Clinical Practice.* New York: Spectrum, 1985.

Harmes JC, Filley C, Rosenberg N. Neurologic sequelae of chronic solvent vapor abuse. *Neurology* 36:698–702, 1986.

Hensen-Flaschen J, Cowen J, Raps E. Neuromuscular blockade in the intensive care unit. *Am Rev Resp Dis* 147:234–236, 1993.

Kaplan RS, Wiernik P. Neurotoxicity of antineoplastic drugs. *Semin Oncology* 9(1): 103–130, 1982.

Pascual-Leone A, et al. Cocaine-induced seizures. *Neurology* 40:404–407, 1990.

Patchell RA. Neurologic complications of organ transplantation. *Ann Neurology* 36:688–703, 1994.

Rowland L (ed). *Merritt's Textbook of Neurology* (8th ed). Philadelphia: Lea & Febiger, 1989.

Singer R. *Neurotoxicity Guidebook.* New York: Van Nostrand Reinhold, 1990.

Spencer P, Schaumberg H (eds). *Experimental and Clinical Neurotoxicology.* Baltimore: Williams & Wilkins, 1980.

Towfighi J, et al. Glue sniffer's neuropathy. *Neurology* 26:238–243, 1976.

55

Sleep Disorders
Phyllis C. Zee

Sleep disorders are prevalent in the general population, and it is estimated that approximately 10 million Americans consult physicians for sleep problems. Patients who complain of disturbed sleep generally describe one or more of three types of problems: insomnia, excessive daytime sleepiness; and abnormal motor activities, complex behaviors, or sensations during sleep.

The International Classification of Sleep Disorders (ICSD) lists 84 sleep disorders. The ICSD has four major categories: dyssomnias—that is, disorders of initiating and maintaining sleep and disorders of excessive sleepiness, the parasomnias, disorders associated with medical or psychiatric disorders, and proposed sleep disorders. In order to assist the clinician in diagnosing sleep disorders, a differential-diagnosis-based classification that was adapted from the ICSD is used in this chapter.

I. **Insomnia** is the inability to fall asleep, the inability to maintain sleep, or the perception of inadequate sleep. The three main categories of insomnia are psychophysiologic insomnia, idiopathic insomnia, and sleep state misperception.

A. **Psychophysiologic insomnia**

1. **Natural history.** To be diagnosed as suffering from psychophysiologic insomnia, a patient needs to demonstrate sleep difficulties that significantly affect daytime functioning and a learning or conditioning component that typically involves one or more of the following: daily worries about not being able to fall asleep or stay asleep accompanied by intense efforts to fall asleep each night; paradoxical improvement in sleep when the patient is away from the usual sleep environment (i.e., in another room of the house or away from home); and somatized tension associated with bedtime and the subject of sleep.

   The most difficult differential diagnosis is with generalized anxiety disorder, in which anxiety is pervasive and involves most aspects of daily life rather than exclusively the inability to sleep. Differentiation from affective disorders is also important.

2. **Treatment and outcome.** A multivaried individualized approach is indicated for most patients. Treatment involves teaching of good sleep hygiene, behavioral therapy, and hypnotic medications. Although pharmacologic intervention has an important role in the treatment of insomnia, it is not the basic, long-term approach. A 4–6-week trial of sleep hygiene counseling, behavior modification, and judicious use of hypnotics is recommended. If insomnia does not improve after this period of treatment, referral to a sleep specialist should be considered and nocturnal polysomnography performed.

   a. **Behavioral therapy.** There are four important factors in sleep hygiene. The first factor includes circadian rhythm and the structuring of sleep-wake cycles; the second factor involves changes in sleep physiology that accompany aging; the third factor is the important effects on sleep exerted by social and recreational drugs such as nicotine, caffeine, and alcohol; and the fourth factor concerns conditions and activities that promote arousal during sleep time. Sleep hygiene instructions that address these four areas are listed in Table 55-1.

   The most widely used behavioral therapy program in the treatment of insomnia includes relaxation techniques, stimulus-control therapy, and sleep-restriction therapy. Relaxation techniques may include progressive muscle relaxation, biofeedback, deep breathing, meditation, guided imagery, and other techniques to control cognitive arousal. These techniques are first taught during training sessions and then practiced daily

Table 55-1. Sleep hygiene instructions.

Homeostatic Drive for Sleep

Avoid naps, except for a brief 10–15-minute nap 8 hours after arising; but check with your physician first, because in some sleep disorders naps can be beneficial.

Restrict sleep period to average number of hours you have actually slept per night in the preceding week. Quality of sleep is important. Too much time in bed can decrease quality on the subsequent night.

Get regular exercise every day, preferably 40 minutes of an activity that causes sweating. It is best to finish exercise at least 3 hours before bedtime.

A warm non-caffeine-containing drink may help you relax as well as warm you.

Circadian Factors

Keep a regular out-of-bed time 7 days a week.

Do not expose yourself to bright light if you have to get up at night.

Get at least a half-hour of sunlight within 30 minutes of your out-of-bed time.

Drug Effects

Do not smoke to get yourself back to sleep.

Do not smoke after 7:00 P.M., or give up smoking entirely.

Avoid caffeine entirely for a 4-week trial period; limit caffeine use to no more than three cups no later than 10:00 A.M.

Avoid alcoholic beverages after 7 P.M. Alcohol can fragment sleep over the second half of the sleep period.

Arousal in Sleep Setting

Keep clock face turned away, and do not find out what time it is when you wake up at night.

Avoid strenuous exercise after 6:00 P.M.

Do not eat or drink heavily for 3 hours before bedtime. A light bedtime snack may help.

If you have trouble with regurgitation, be especially careful to avoid heavy meals and spices in the evening. Do not retire too hungry or too full. Head of bed may need to be raised.

Keep your room dark, quiet, well ventilated, and at a comfortable temperature throughout the night.

Use a bedtime ritual. Reading before lights-out may be helpful if it is not occupationally related.

Learn to use simple self-hypnosis when you wake up at night. Do not try too hard to sleep; instead, concentrate on the pleasant feeling of relaxation.

Use stress management and relaxation techniques in the daytime.

Be sure your mattress is not too soft or too firm and your pillow is of the right height and firmness.

An occasional sleeping pill is probably acceptable.

Use bedroom only for sleep; do not work or do other activities that lead to prolonged arousal.

---

for a period of 20–30 minutes by the patient at home, usually around bedtime. Stimulus-control therapy is very useful in the treatment of conditioned insomnia. This technique attempts to break the conditioning by teaching the patient to associate the bedroom with sleep behavior. The instructions for stimulus-control behavioral therapy are listed in Table 55-2. Sleep-restriction therapy involves curtailment of bedtime to a few hours per night until the patient learns to use the time in bed for sleeping.

b. **Hypnotics.** The most widely used prescription hypnotics are the benzodiazepines. More recently, a new class of hypnotics called imidazopyridines (e.g., zolpidem) were introduced for the treatment of insomnia. These medications are indicated for occasional sleepless nights to break the vicious cycle of patients needing sleep so desperately that they become tense, which perpetuates their insomnia. The choice of hypnotic may depend on the nature of the sleep complaints. For example, if the predominant problem is falling asleep, a fast-acting, short-half-life hypnotic may be preferable, whereas if the problem is frequent awakenings and sleep maintenance insomnia, a longer-acting hypnotic may be more effective. Hypnotics that are long-acting as well as those that contain active metabolites may cause "hangover" side effects in the morning. Con-

Table 55-2. Stimulus-control behavioral therapy.

Go to bed only when sleepy. Stay up until you are really sleepy, then return to bed. If sleep still
  does not come easily, get out of bed again. The goal is to associate bed with falling asleep
  quickly.
Use the bed only for sleeping: do not read, watch television or eat in bed.
If unable to sleep, get up and move to another room.
Repeat the preceding step as often as necessary throughout the night.
Set the alarm and get up at the same time every morning, regardless of how much you slept
  during the night. This helps the body acquire a constant sleep-wake rhythm.
Do not nap during the day.

tinued use of hypnotics on a daily basis should be avoided, because they
can be addictive, usually lose their effects (requiring escalation of dosage), and may produce rebound insomnia when withdrawn. Rebound insomnia and development of tolerance occur less frequently with zolpidem than with benzodiazepines. However, zolpidem lacks anxiolytic
properties and therefore is not useful in the treatment of insomniacs
who may benefit from the anxiolytic effects of hypnotics. The most
widely used prescription hypnotics and their properties are listed in
Table 55-3. Although patients with chronic insomnia rarely become
"great" sleepers after treatment, most can manage their predisposition
for insomnia by using the combination of sleep hygiene, behavioral treatment, and occasional hypnotics.

B. Idiopathic insomnia
  1. Natural history. Idiopathic insomnia is a lifelong inability to sleep, presum-
     ably associated with a neurologic predisposition for insomnia resulting from
     an abnormality of the sleep-wake cycle. Patients with this condition consti-
     tute a heterogeneous group. Most have been poor sleepers since childhood,
     and the insomnia, although it persists over the entire life span, can be aggra-
     vated by stress and tension. It is also interesting to note that patients with id-
     iopathic insomnia may show atypical reactions to stimulants and sedatives.
         Idiopathic insomnia is often accompanied by other factors, such as poor
     sleep hygiene or psychiatric disorders. Therefore, there tends to be a contin-
     uum from idiopathic insomnia to psychophysiologic insomnia to insomnia
     associated with psychiatric problems.
  2. Diagnosis. A diagnosis of idiopathic insomnia is made when there is no
     clear emotional or other trauma that is believed to have initiated the insom-
     nia. Psychiatric and medical causes must be ruled out. The severity of the in-
     somnia is such that waking function is impaired.
  3. Treatment and outcome. There is no consistent approach to treatment of
     idiopathic insomnia, because each case is different and a highly empirical
     approach may be necessary. Some patients respond to treatment with hetero-
     cyclic antidepressants such as amitriptyline or trazodone at bedtime. Effec-
     tive dosages vary greatly, ranging from low (i.e., 25 mg) to high (i.e., 200 mg).
     In addition to medication, referral for supportive psychological treatment is
     often necessary, as is good sleep hygiene.
C. Sleep state misperception
  1. Natural history. It is not uncommon for patients to overestimate sleep la-

Table 55-3. Benzodiazepine hypnotics pharmacology.

Drug	Onset of action	Duration of action	Active metabolites	Recommendation dosage
Estazolam	15–30 min	6–8 hr	Yes	1–2 mg
Flurazepam	15–30 min	8–10 hr	Yes	15–30 mg
Quazepam	15–30 min	8–10 hr	Yes	7.5–15 mg
Temazepam	40–60 min	6–8 hr	No	15–30 mg
Triazolam	15–30 min	3–4 hr	No	.125–.25 mg
Zolpidem	15–30 min	2–3 hr	No	5–10 mg

tency and underestimate total sleep time. In sleep state misperception, this tendency is extreme. Patients who claim not to sleep at all typically sleep several hours when studied in the laboratory.

2. **Diagnosis.** Sleep state misperception is indicated when the patient complains of persistent insomnia, although sleep duration and quality are normal. This condition can be diagnosed only in the laboratory, because one needs to document that sleep is normal.

3. **Treatment and outcome.** Confronting patients with the fact that their sleep is normal and that they sleep longer than they think they do, and behavioral treatments as discussed above, are effective.

D. **Insomnia associated with psychiatric disorders**

1. **Natural history.** Psychiatric conditions are major causes of insomnia. Epidemiologic studies suggest that as many as 57% of those with insomnia have a psychiatric condition or will develop one within 1 year. The underlying conditions are usually mood disorder, anxiety disorder, somatoform disorder, personality disorder, and schizophrenia. It is rare to encounter a patient with a mood disorder who does not also have sleep-wake problems. Sleep in major depression is characterized by early morning awakening (2–4 hours after sleep onset) and frequent nocturnal awakening with inability to reinitiate sleep. The incidence of insomnia among patients with anxiety disorders is also high. The typical complaints are sleep initiation difficulty and, to a lesser degree, nocturnal awakenings. Tiredness is common, but napping is unusual. Patients with anxiety disorders are very susceptible to conditioning factors that produce psychophysiologic insomnia.

2. **Treatment and outcome.** Treatment should first address the underlying psychiatric disorder. For major depressive disorders this involves use of antidepressants or serotonin-specific reuptake inhibitors (SSRIs). A compound with potent sedative properties is favored over a less sedating one for patients with insomnia complaints. Administration 30 minutes before bedtime also promotes sleep. Amitriptyline, trimipramine, doxepin, and trazodone are the most sedating, whereas protriptyline and SSRIs such as fluoxetine may even have stimulating effects. Benzodiazepines may also be useful in the anxious depressed patient and facilitate psychotherapeutic or pharmacologic treatment. Anticholinergic side effects of the tricyclic antidepressants (cardiotoxicity, urinary retention, erectile dysfunction, and dry mouth) can be a problem, particularly in the elderly.

The treatment of intense anxiety may require supportive psychotherapy with pharmacotherapy. The benzodiazepines are the medications of choice for an anxiolytic effect, and they have the added advantage of being hypnotics as well. The choice of the type of benzodiazepine is individualized on the basis of the patient's predominant symptoms. For example, if the main problem is difficulty initiating sleep, a single bedtime dose of a drug with an intermediate duration, such as alprazolam, lorazepam, or oxazepam, may be preferred over longer-acting ones such as flurazepam and chlordiazepoxide, which may be more useful in providing anxiolytic and hypnotic relief for patients with sleep maintenance insomnia. If this condition is suspected, referral to a sleep specialist or psychiatrist is recommended for evaluation of the underlying psychiatric disorder.

II. **Insomnia associated with circadian rhythm disorders**

A. **Natural history.** Circadian rhythms are generated by a neural clock located in the suprachiasmatic nucleus of the hypothalamus. Disruption of biological timing results in circadian rhythm disorders that are most often associated with the complaint of insomnia. Circadian rhythm disorders are characterized by essentially normal sleep that is not synchronized with conventional environmental light-dark cycles and periods of sleep. Diagnosis requires specialized assessment, including use of sleep logs, and careful history-taking to elicit the appropriate major diagnostic criteria.

The most common sleep disturbances that have been associated with disruption of circadian rhythmicity are the **sleep phase syndromes.** Delayed sleep phase syndrome (DSPS) is the persistent inability to fall asleep until the early morning hours (1 to 3 A.M., and sometimes later), and, if allowed, the patient will sleep until the late morning or early afternoon (10 A.M. to 2 P.M.). When the patient is forced to rise at 7 or 8 A.M., sleep is curtailed and daytime sleepiness develops. Despite the daytime sleepiness, patients find that in the evening they become more alert, and remain unable to fall asleep until the early morning hours. The advanced sleep phase syndrome (ASPS) is characterized by early evening sleep onset (8 to 9 P.M.) and early morning awakening (3 to 5 A.M.). Although DSPS predominates at younger ages and ASPS at older ages, both syndromes may be chronic and result in sleep complaints throughout the patient's life. Because many features of the sleep of patients with depression (early morning awakening) resemble those of ASPS, depression needs to be considered in the differential diagnosis.

Another type of circadian rhythm disorder encountered in practice is the **irregular sleep-wake pattern.** This condition differs from the phase disorders in that there is loss of circadian rhythmicity, which results in the lack of a long, consolidated sleep period. Sleep usually is broken into short sleep periods or naps during the course of the 24 hours. Irregular sleep-wake patterns are observed in patients with Alzheimer's disease and in other institutionalized nursing home elderly.

B. **Treatment and outcome.** The traditional treatment approach is chronotherapy, which is a behavioral technique in which bedtime is systematically delayed (for DSPS) or advanced (for ASPS) by 3-hour increments each day until the desired sleep phase is achieved. The patient is then instructed to maintain the newly established bedtime rigidly. Although this approach works, it is an arduous procedure, and maintenance of its effect has been difficult.

A new approach in the treatment of sleep phase disorders is bright light therapy. Light intensity greater than 2500 lux is considered to be bright. Appropriately timed bright light exposure can alleviate DSPS and ASPS. Exposure to bright light in the early morning results in an advancement of circadian phase, whereas exposure to light in the evening delays circadian rhythms. Therefore, for treatment of DSPS, exposure to light is usually scheduled for a period of 1–2 hours in the morning (6–8 A.M.). For ASPS, light exposure is recommended in the evening, approximately 2–4 hours before scheduled bedtime. Despite high rates of success in achieving the desired sleep phase under acute treatment, many patients fail to continue to comply with the light regimen and relapse. Some patients are able to maintain a normalized phase without maintenance of light exposure for up to several months, whereas others drift back toward the pretreatment phase within a few days.

Treatment of irregular sleep-wake patterns and associated behavioral problems in this group of patients provides a significant challenge. Treatment with sedative-hypnotics is prevalent in nursing homes. These medications have side effects that may not be well tolerated in older patients. Some promising studies have indicated that structured activity programs and timed bright light exposure may alleviate these sleep-wake and behavioral disorders. An initial evaluation by a sleep specialist and ophthalmologic consultation are recommended before treatment with bright light therapy is initiated. The costs of these light units range from $150–300.

III. **Disorders of excessive sleepiness.** Survey studies have found that approximately 4–5% of the general population complain of excessive daytime sleepiness (EDS). Sleepiness is excessive and an indication of a sleep disorder when it occurs at undesirable times, such as while driving and during social activities. Excessive daytime sleepiness may be divided into two types: extrinsic and intrinsic. Some extrinsic etiologies include environmental factors, drug dependency, sleep-disordered breathing, and movement disorders during sleep. The more common intrinsic hypersomnias are usually associated with primary CNS disorders such as narcolepsy and idiopathic hypersomnia.

A. **Narcolepsy**

1. **Natural history.** Narcolepsy is a manifestation of a dissociation between wakefulness and sleep, particularly rapid eye movement (REM) sleep. The onset usually occurs in adolescence or young adulthood, and males are affected more often than females. Studies have demonstrated a strong genetic association of narcolepsy with the DR2 DQw1 (DR15 Dqw6 under the new nomenclature) human leukocyte antigen (HLA).

2. **Clinical features.** Narcolepsy is a syndrome characterized by excessive daytime sleepiness, irresistible sleep attacks, cataplexy, and, less often, sleep paralysis and hypnagogic hallucinations. The presence of cataplexy is pathognomonic for narcolepsy. Moreover, nocturnal sleep is often disrupted

in patients with narcolepsy. Decreased quality and quantity of nocturnal sleep exacerbate the EDS even further.

3. **Diagnosis.** It is generally accepted that, in addition to history-taking, nocturnal polysomnography and multiple sleep latency testing (MSLT) are performed to establish a diagnosis of narcolepsy REM sleep in naps. If the results of the sleep studies are inconclusive, results of HLA typing may provide additional aid in establishing the diagnosis.

4. **Treatment and outcome.** Treatment approaches in narcolepsy emphasize control of narcoleptic symptoms in order to allow optimal social and professional productivity by maintaining the patient's alertness throughout the day. Choice of treatment must take into account that narcolepsy is a lifelong disorder and that patients will have to take medications for many years.

   Clinicians are not unanimous in their approach to treatment of narcolepsy. The drug treatments recommended in this chapter form a reasonable guideline for the treatment of most patients with narcolepsy. The drugs that are commonly used to treat the symptoms of EDS and sleep attacks are the CNS stimulants methylphenidate, dextroamphetamine, and pemoline. Because of frequent side effects, such as irritability, tachycardia, elevated blood pressure, and nocturnal sleep disturbance, amphetamines are no longer the first-line treatment. The use of methylphenidate is preferable because of its lower incidence and severity of these side effects. Pemoline, another stimulant with a long half-life and slower onset of action, is less effective than methylphenidate but well tolerated. Modafinil, a stimulant medication currently under investigation in the United States, has been reported to be effective in alleviating excessive sleepiness in patients with narcolepsy. Medications used in the treatment of EDS and their dosages are listed in Table 55-4. Drugs with norepinephrine-releasing properties have the greatest impact on sleepiness. However, even at the highest recommended dosages, no drug brings narcoleptics to a normal level of alertness.

   The treatment of cataplexy, sleep paralysis, and hypnagogic hallucinations involves tricyclic antidepressant medications. Protriptyline and clomipramine have been used widely, often with good results. Other tricyclic medications, such as imipramine, desipramine, and amitriptyline, are

Table 55-4. Narcolepsy drugs currently available.

Drug	Usual dosage[a]
Stimulants:	
Dextroamphetamine	5–60 mg/day
Methamphetamine	20–25 mg/day
Methylphenidate	10–60 mg/day
Mazindol	4–8 mg/day (divided dosage)
Pemoline	37.5 mg/day
Adjunct-effect drug[b]:	
Protriptyline	2.5–10 mg/day
Drugs for Treatment of Auxiliary Effects	
Tricyclic antidepressants with atropinic side effects:	
Protriptyline	2.5–20 mg/day
Imipramine	25–200 mg/day
Clomipramine	25–200 mg/day
Desipramine	25–200 mg/day
Antidepressant without atropinic side effects:	
Fluoxetine	20–60 mg/day
Experimental Drugs or Drugs Available in Few Countries	
Modafinil	—
Gamma-hydroxybutyrate	—

[a]Occasionally, depending on clinical response, the dosage may be outside the usual dosage range. All drugs administered orally.
[b]Adjunct-effect drugs improve excessive daytime sleepiness (EDS) if associated with a stimulant.

also effective; however, anticholinergic side effects (particularly impotence in men) limit the ability of many patients to tolerate these medications, particularly if high dosages are needed to treat the cataplexy. Fluoxetine is somewhat less effective for cataplexy, but it has the added advantage of being a mild stimulant. An example of an initial treatment regimen for narcolepsy in adults is provided in Table 55-5.

A third approach to the treatment of narcolepsy is to improve the nocturnal sleep of narcoleptics. Improvement of nocturnal sleep not only decreases EDS but may also help cataplexy. Nocturnal sleep disturbances may be related to periodic leg movements of sleep, which are frequently observed in patients with narcolepsy, but may also be complications of treatment with stimulants and tricyclic medications. Treatment of periodic leg movements with dopamine agonist drugs such as carbidopa/levodopa (Sinemet, 10–100 mg) or benzodiazepines such as clonazepam (0.5 mg) may be helpful.

The nonpharmacologic treatment approaches—scheduled short naps and support therapy—must also be emphasized. Short naps of 15–20 minutes taken three times during the day help maintain alertness. Narcolepsy patients often experience social and professional difficulties as a result of their sleepiness and cataplexy. Narcolepsy can result in unemployment, rejection by friends, and depression. For these reasons, it is important to encourage patients with narcolepsy to join support groups and to provide referral for psychotherapy when required.

5. **Side effects of stimulant medications.** Hypertension, abnormal liver function, alterations in mood, and psychosis are the most commonly reported complications of stimulant therapy for narcolepsy. Moreover, tolerance and, less frequently, addiction may be observed with drugs such as amphetamines. Interestingly, with high dosages of amphetamines (100 mg/day), a paradoxical effect of increased sleepiness may result. This paradoxical effect disappears with reduction of the daily dosage. Other common side effects include increased jitteriness, verbal aggressiveness, "racing thoughts," increased heart rate, tremor, and involuntary movements.

B. **Idiopathic CNS hypersomnia**

1. **Natural history.** Idiopathic CNS hypersomnia is a very disabling illness, characterized by excessive daytime sleepiness but without clearly defined

---

Table 55-5. Example of an initial treatment plan for narcolepsy in adults.

Avoid shifts in sleep schedule.
Avoid heavy meals and alcohol intake.
Regular timing of nocturnal sleep: 10:30 P.M. to 7:00 A.M.
Naps. Strategically timed naps, if possible (e.g., 15 minutes at lunchtime and 15 minutes at 5:30 P.M.)
Medication. The effects of stimulant medications may vary widely among patients. The dosing and timing of medications should be individualized to optimize performance. Additional doses, as needed, may be suggested for periods of anticipated sleepiness.

    Methylphenidate: 5 mg (three or four tablets) or 20 mg SR* in morning (on empty stomach)
    If difficulties persist:
        Methylphenidate (SR*): 20 mg in morning
                    5 mg after noon nap
                    5 mg at 4 P.M.
    If no response:
        Dexedrine spansule (SR*): 15 mg at awakening
                    5 mg after noon nap
                    5 mg at 3:30 or 4 P.M.
        (or 15 mg at awakening and 15 mg after noon nap)
    For cataplexy:
        Clomipramine at 75–125 mg, or
        Protriptyline at 10–20 mg, or
        Imipramine at 75–125 mg

---

*SR = sustained-release tablet.

sleep attacks and other features associated with narcolepsy. The age of on-set varies greatly, usually from adolescence to middle age. The symptoms are lifelong, with some worsening in old age.

2. **Clinical features.** Patients complain of sleepiness throughout the day, asso-ciated with prolonged naps that are nonrefreshing. In addition, automatic behaviors may occur during periods of drowsiness. These behaviors are of-ten inappropriate, and patients usually do not have any recollection of these events. Patients also have severe difficulty awakening in the morning.

3. **Diagnosis.** It is important to differentiate CNS hypersomnia from nar-colepsy and nocturnal sleep disorders such as sleep-disordered breathing or periodic movements of sleep, which are associated with daytime sleepiness. Therefore, the diagnosis is made by elimination of other causes of daytime sleepiness. Polysomnography should be performed to rule out these possi-bilities, and MSLT should be performed to document the level of objective daytime sleepiness.

4. **Treatment and outcome.** Because multiple etiologic factors may be re-sponsible for CNS hypersomnia and because of the relative lack of under-standing regarding its pathophysiology, treatment is symptomatic and not very effective. Behavioral therapies and sleep hygiene instructions should be recommended but have only modest positive impacts. The only medica-tions that provide partial relief of excessive sleepiness are stimulant drugs. The most commonly recommended medications are pemoline, methylpheni-date, and dextroamphetamine. Tricyclic antidepressants, selective serotonin agonists, clonidine, bromocriptine, amantadine, and methysergide have been used with varying success. Sometimes combinations of the abovemen-tioned drugs yield better control of sleepiness. Even with the highest recom-mended dosage, complete control of daytime sleepiness is seldom achieved in this group of patients. Therefore, prescribing more than 60 mg of methylphenidate or 40 mg of dextroamphetamine does not provide signifi-cant additional symptomatic relief. The patient should be advised not to drive or engage in potentially dangerous activities that require high levels of alertness.

IV. **Parasomnias** are conditions that occur during sleep or are associated with arousal from sleep. These conditions include enuresis, sleepwalking, night terrors, dream anxiety attacks, nocturnal complex seizures, and REM behavior disorder. The ones that are most often observed in adult clinical practice will be discussed here.

A. **Non–rapid eye movement (non-REM) parasomnias.** Sleepwalking and sleep terrors are a group of episodic behaviors that occur during non-REM stages of sleep, usually when the patient is coming out of slow wave sleep. Be-cause sleepwalking (somnambulism) and sleep terrors (pavor nocturnus) in adults are most often associated with each other, their key features are dis-cussed together.

1. **Natural history.** The prevalence of sleepwalking and sleep terrors is esti-mated at approximately 6% of the population. These parasomnias are most frequent in children and often disappear by adolescence. These behaviors may be considered to be normal in children, but in a significant number of people they persist into adulthood. Patients often report family histories of parasomnias.

2. **Clinical features.** During these episodes, patients exhibit stereotyped be-haviors, such as talking, sitting up, and getting up to walk. These episodes are potentially dangerous, because patients may bump into walls and win-dows or fall down stairs. With sleep terrors, extreme autonomic discharge and screaming are present. Patients usually have only vague recollections of these events and are confused if awakened.

3. **Diagnosis.** In the elderly, a thorough evaluation of abnormal nocturnal be-havior should be performed to differentiate non-REM parasomnias from other pathologic entities and from side effects of medications.

4. **Treatment and outcome.** Therapy for non-REM parasomnias includes sev-eral approaches consisting of preventive measures, psychological interven-tions, and medications.

a. **Preventive measures and psychological interventions.** Preventive measures are taken to avoid serious injuries during episodes of sleep-walking. The patient should be advised to locate the bedroom on the first floor, lock windows and doors, cover windows and glass doors with heavy draperies, and remove hazardous objects from the house.

Hypnosis and psychotherapy have also been used in the treatment of parasomnias. Hypnosis has been shown to be helpful, at least for a short time, in young adults. The need for psychotherapy depends on the association of psychological factors with the parasomnia. Psychotherapy has been used most widely in young adults for the treatment of sleep terrors. Most parasomnias increase in severity and frequency with psychological stress. Therefore, in addition to psychotherapy, progressive muscle relaxation and biofeedback may be beneficial.

   b. **Medications.** The benzodiazepines—most commonly alprazolam, clonazepam, and diazepam—have been used. In the treatment of sleep terrors, tricyclic antidepressants (particularly imipramine) have been used either alone or in combination with benzodiazepines to provide control of symptoms. In addition, several studies have shown that treatment with carbamazepine (Tegretol) may also be beneficial. An example of an initial therapeutic approach is to start with clonazepam (0.5–1.0 mg) approximately 30 minutes before bedtime. If the response is inadequate, the dosage should be increased by balancing the side effects, which may include confusion and daytime drowsiness, particularly in the elderly. A secondary line of treatment may include initiation of low dosages of tricyclic antidepressant drugs or carbamazepine at bedtime.

   Results of treatment of non-REM parasomnias are poorly documented. However, the little information in the literature indicates that response to combinations of pharmacologic and nonpharmacologic therapies is excellent, with up to 70% of adult patients reporting disappearance of their symptoms after various lengths of time.

B. REM sleep behavior disorder (RBD)

   1. **Natural history.** REM sleep is normally accompanied by muscle atonia. There are, however, pathologic conditions, such as REM sleep behavior disorder (RBD), in which there is a loss of REM atonia or excessive motor activation during sleep. Patients with this disorder most commonly complain of vigorous sleep behaviors that are accompanied by vivid dreams. These behaviors may be quite violent and result in serious injuries. RBD occurs in both acute and chronic forms. The acute form is usually associated with toxic metabolic etiologies—most commonly, drug withdrawal states (particularly delirium tremens). Loss of REM atonia may also be observed in patients taking medications that suppress REM sleep, such as tricyclic antidepressants and fluoxetine. The chronic form usually is associated with neurologic illness (stroke, space-occupying lesions, demyelinating disease, and degenerative disease) or is idiopathic. Chronic RBD is more common in older adults, in patients with CNS diseases, or in patients taking psychoactive medications.

   The differential diagnosis of RBD includes non-REM parasomnias, sleep apnea, periodic movements of sleep, nocturnal seizures, and nocturnal rhythmic movements. It is important to recognize this condition and differentiate it from other nocturnal behaviors, because RBD can be treated effectively.

   2. **Treatment and outcome.** Treatment of RBD involves pharmacologic therapy and interventions that address issues concerning environmental safety. The most effective drug therapy is clonazepam at a dosage of 0.5–1.0 mg at bedtime. Clonazepam may be taken earlier (1–2 hours prior to bedtime) by patients who complain of sleep-onset insomnia or morning drowsiness as a result of the medication. It is effective in 90% of cases, with little evidence of abuse and infrequent tolerance in this group of patients. Beneficial effects are observed within the first week of treatment. Typically, treatment with clonazepam results in control of vigorous, violent sleep behaviors, but mild to moderate limb movement, sleeptalking, and other complex behaviors may persist. Discontinuation of treatment usually results in recurrence of symptoms. Tricyclic antidepressant medications and other serotonergic and dopaminergic drugs are sometimes effective in the treatment of RBD. There have been few reported cases of successful treatment with desipramine, carbidopa/L-dopa, or clonidine.

   Environmental safety is also a very important issue in the treatment of

RBD. Patients should be advised to remove potentially dangerous objects from the house, to pad hard and sharp surfaces around the bed, to cover windows with heavy draperies, and even to place the mattress on the floor to avoid falling out of bed. The combination of drug therapy and implementation of safety precautions offers safe and effective treatment for RBD.

Nocturnal seizures should be considered in the differential diagnoses of many of these parasomnias. Therefore if the history is suggestive of possible seizure disorder or if symptoms are not controlled, referral to a neurologist or sleep specialist for further evaluation is recommended.

C. Restless legs syndrome (RLS) and periodic leg movements of sleep (PLMS)

1. Natural history. The restless legs syndrome (RLS) is characterized by creeping, crawling, and disagreeable sensations of the legs and occasionally of the arms that are associated with irresistible movements of the extremities. The symptoms are present at rest and are relieved by movements such as stretching, rubbing, and walking. Lying down in bed and falling asleep is a major problem for patients with RLS. Dysesthesias and the need to move the legs are the most severe at bedtime and often are associated with sleep-onset insomnia. Many patients also report severe dysesthesias and leg jerks in the middle of the night with difficulty returning to sleep. The severity of symptoms varies greatly. Patients may experience sudden remissions or relapses without clear cause.

The majority of patients with RLS also experience periodic leg movements of sleep (PLMS). However, PLMS can occur without RLS and has its own diagnostic category. It is characterized by stereotyped repetitive rhythmic movements (lasting 0.5–5.0 seconds with an intermovement interval of 20–40 seconds) of the legs (commonly, dorsiflexion of the foot) and occasionally may also involve the arms. PLMS is usually more frequent during the first half of the night, but can be present throughout sleep. Movements may be associated with sleep disruption and, if numerous, result in nocturnal awakenings and excessive daytime sleepiness. The prevalence of PLMS increases with age, from 5% of those under age 50 to 44% of those 65 years of age or older.

In most patients with RLS or PLMS, the etiology is unknown and therefore termed idiopathic. In many cases, RLS is familial. However, both RLS and PLMS may be associated with anemia resulting from iron, folic acid, or vitamin B_{12} deficiency; neuropathies; myelopathies; rheumatoid arthritis; thyroid dysfunction; and uremia. Furthermore, PLMS may be induced or exacerbated by tricyclic antidepressants, as well as by withdrawal from a variety of hypnotics. Therefore, these conditions should be entertained in the differential diagnosis of these periodic movement disorders so that patients receive the appropriate therapies. If these conditions are suspected, referral to the appropriate specialist is recommended.

2. Treatment. The three major classes of drugs that have been shown to be effective in the treatment of RLS and PLMS are benzodiazepines, dopaminergic drugs, and the opioids. Several benzodiazepines, including clonazepam, nitrazepam, lorazepam, and temazepam, have been found to improve nocturnal sleep in patients with RLS and PLMS. Of these, clonazepam is the most widely used. Clonazepam's therapeutic action most likely results from its ability to reduce the number of arousals caused by leg movements. The usual starting dosage of clonazepam is 0.5–1.0 mg taken at bedtime for treatment of PLMS. Treatment of RLS may require additional doses to control symptoms during the day. Because benzodiazepines are CNS depressants, they may aggravate sleep apnea, particularly in older persons.

Several studies have shown that L-dopa is an effective treatment for RLS and PLMS. At the onset, carbidopa/L-dopa (25 mg/100 mg) is given at bedtime, and the dosage is increased progressively until a therapeutic effect is obtained. Usually a dose of carbidopa/L-dopa (50 mg/200 mg) is sufficient to control RLS and PLMS. A second administration during the day may be necessary if patients complain of an increase in leg movements in the morning. Treatment with controlled-release carbidopa/L-dopa (Sinemet CR) may also alleviate the rebound effect. The side effects of L-dopa treatment are generally minimal. The major side effects are rebound symptoms of dysesthesias or leg movements during the day. The use of longer-acting carbidopa/L-dopa and addition of benzodiazepine during the day may be beneficial. Dyskinesias associated with long-term L-dopa treatment, as observed in patients with Parkinson's disease, are uncommon in this group of patients. Finally, bromocriptine and other dopaminergic drugs are also effective in treating RLS and PLMS.

The opioids are very effective in the treatment of RLS and PLMS. However, the risks of abuse, addiction, and tolerance limit their clinical use. In severe cases that are refractory to other treatments, intermittent therapy with opioids provides some relief. Other proposed treatments include carbamazepine, clonidine, and baclofen.

V. Sleep-disordered breathing. The most commonly encountered types of abnormal nocturnal breathing are the sleep apneas and hypopneas. Sleep apneas are cessations of breathing for at least 10 seconds caused by obstruction of the upper airway (obstructive sleep apnea), loss of respiratory effort or rhythmicity (central apnea), or a combination of the two (mixed apnea). Hypopneas are decreases in airflow, which may be obstructive or central in origin. Most patients with sleep apnea have combinations of the central and obstructive types, which suggests that the mechanisms of the different types of sleep apnea overlap.

A. Central sleep apnea

    1. Natural history. Patients with central sleep apnea constitute less than 10% of the total sleep apnea population who are studied in sleep laboratories. Therefore, only a few studies have been reported, which limits our knowledge of this disorder. Very little information is available regarding the cardiovascular sequelae of central sleep apnea. The most common finding is sinus arrhythmia with bradycardia. Oxygen desaturation in patients with central sleep apnea tends to be generally mild to moderate when compared with that in patients with obstructive sleep apnea. Although the etiology of central sleep apnea in most cases is unknown, it has been associated with certain disease processes that should be considered in the differential diagnosis and treatment of this disorder. These diseases include central alveolar hypoventilation (Ondine's curse), obesity-hypoventilation (pickwickian) syndrome, congestive heart failure (Cheyne-Stokes breathing pattern), autonomic dysfunctions (Shy-Drager syndrome, familial dysautonomia, and diabetes mellitus), neuromuscular disorders (muscular dystrophy, myasthenia gravis, and motor neuron disease), and brainstem lesions.

    2. Treatment of central sleep apnea is limited and not very satisfactory. Studies regarding treatment have usually involved small numbers of patients, and very few have addressed the long-term efficacy of the proposed treatments. One approach is noninvasive nocturnal ventilation delivered by means of a nasal mask with a volume- or pressure-cycled ventilator. This approach is used only in the most severe cases of central alveolar hypoventilation or in patients with neuromuscular disorders.

In patients with medical or neurologic conditions known to be associated with central sleep apnea, the condition should be treated specifically and the central apnea reassessed. However, if the problem persists or if an etiology is not found, several pharmacologic agents can be used. Acetazolamide, a carbonic anhydrase inhibitor, has been shown to treat central sleep apnea. In a small number of patients, acetazolamide has been shown to reduce substantially the number of central apneas. The recommended dosage is 250 mg qid. There are even fewer studies that address the long-term efficacy of this treatment. The side effects associated with mild metabolic acidosis are usually well tolerated in this group of patients.

Other medications, such as theophylline, naloxone, and medroxyprogesterone acetate, have been used with varying degrees of success. Tricyclic antidepressants—particularly clomipramine—have also been used successfully in a small number of patients. Because none of these medications has been studied systematically, more precise recommendations regarding their use is currently not available.

Some patients with central sleep apnea have been shown to benefit from therapy with nasal continuous positive airway pressure (CPAP). This type of therapy is most beneficial in obese patients who also have signs of upper-airway obstruction with predominantly central apneas. Nasal CPAP has also been shown to be effective in some patients with congestive heart failure in whom central apneas and periodic breathing are observed during sleep. Finally, oxygen therapy has also been useful in treating central apneas.

B. Obstructive sleep apnea (OSA)

1. **Natural history.** The presenting symptoms of obstructive sleep apnea (OSA) syndrome are loud snoring, excessive sleepiness, fatigue, morning headaches, memory problems, alterations in mood, and apneas witnessed by the bed partner. OSA is associated with significant morbidity, including sleep fragmentation, daytime sleepiness that may lead to vehicular and industrial accidents, nocturnal hypoxemia, and cardiovascular as well as cerebrovascular sequelae (e.g., stroke, right heart failure, and hypertension). OSA is generally caused by upper-airway obstruction resulting from obesity and skeletal and soft-tissue abnormalities. Examination of the nose and throat may indicate a possible cause. However, some patients with obstructive sleep apneas may have normal physical examinations. If OSA is suspected, polysomnography should be performed to ascertain the severity of the breathing disorder, which will determine the appropriate therapy. Some patients who have symptoms indistinguishable from those of OSA may have predominantly sleep hypopneas. The sleep hypopneas syndrome should be treated in the same manner as the sleep apnea syndromes. The apnea-hypopnea (AH) index (number of respiratory events per hour of sleep) is used to measure sleep-disordered breathing. An index of 5 is generally accepted as the upper limit of the normal range. An AH index greater than 20 has been shown to result in increased mortality. Therefore, all patients with indexes greater than 20 should be treated. In addition, patients who have milder indexes but whose respiratory events are accompanied by moderate to severe oxygen desaturation and who have additional risk factors such as hypertension, history of heart disease, high cholesterol, and cigarette smoking should be treated also.

2. **Therapy.** The approach for treatment of obstructive sleep apnea and hypopnea syndromes involves both general measures and interventions that address specific abnormalities. In the majority of patients, nasal CPAP is the most effective treatment for control of sleep apnea.

   a. **General measures** for identifying and addressing coexistent lifestyle issues that exacerbate OSA should be part of therapy for all patients. Although difficult to achieve, weight loss is a very important factor in the treatment of obese apneics. Sleep apnea generally improves with weight loss and may even be abolished with significant weight loss of 40–50 pounds. In addition to dietary control, this approach requires an exercise program and psychological counseling for long-lasting results. Unfortunately, results indicate that most patients regain the weight within 2 years.

   Alcohol, hypnotics, and other CNS depressant drugs interfere with the arousal response that terminates apneic episodes. Therefore, patients should avoid alcohol use and should not receive hypnotics or sedatives.

   If a specific cause for upper-airway obstruction is found, an ENT or maxillofacial evaluation is recommended for possible surgical interventions and trials of orthodontic devices, including tonsillectomy or adenoidectomy for enlarged tonsils or adenoids and correction of retrognathia or micrognathia. Recent results indicate that dental devices may be useful in patients with mild to moderate sleep apnea who have some degree of retrognathia. If chronic rhinitis is found, an inhaled nasal steroid such as beclomethasone may be beneficial.

   b. **Nasal continuous positive airway pressure (CPAP).** If no specific cause of upper-airway obstruction is found, nasal CPAP is the treatment of choice. In fact, this treatment is effective in the majority of patients with obstructive apneas and hypopneas. The level of CPAP should be determined by titration of the therapeutic pressure in a sleep laboratory, with respiratory data being obtained in all sleep stages. Nasal CPAP requires patency of the nasal airway, and therefore this procedure may not be effective for patients with severe nasal obstruction. The most common causes of intolerance to nasal CPAP are nasal symptoms, discomfort from the mask, and social/psychological factors of having to use this appliance during sleep. With higher pressures, bilevel positive airway pressure (BiPAP) may be a more comfortable alternative to CPAP. Most home care companies provide both nasal CPAP and BiPAP services.

Although improvement of symptoms including daytime sleepiness may be observed within 1 or 2 days of treatment with nasal CPAP, maximal improvement may not occur for several weeks. Follow-up studies indicate that long-term compliance with nasal CPAP is a significant problem, with many patients not using CPAP throughout the night and on a daily basis. Compliance is increased with closer follow-up. A follow-up visit should be scheduled 1 month after starting CPAP and every 6 months thereafter.

If the patient with sleep apnea also demonstrates a low baseline oxygen saturation during the day or during sleep, referral to an internist or pulmonologist is recommended.

c. **Uvulopalatopharyngoplasty (UPPP)** is a surgical procedure in which excess soft tissues of the soft palate, uvula, and sometimes tonsils and adenoids are removed. A recent advance in this type of approach is laser-assisted uvuloplasty (LAUP). The advantages are that LAUP is an office-based procedure and that the amount of tissue removed can be titrated to effect. However, the efficacy of these procedures as treatments for sleep apnea is variable. It is estimated that UPPP is effective only 40–50% of the time, and there is very little information on the efficacy of LAUP. Both of these treatments are quite effective for snoring, and thus patients may continue to have silent obstructive apneas following surgery.

d. **Drug therapy.** When nasal CPAP is not an option, patients with mild to moderate OSA may benefit from drug therapy. Protriptyline at a dosage of 10 mg at bedtime with upward adjustment depending on response and side effects may be an alternative treatment. Drug therapy is generally unsatisfactory for treatment of OSA.

Recommended Readings

ASDC Case Series Committee (RM Coleman, Chairman). Diagnosis, treatment and follow-up of about 8,000 sleep-wake disorder patients. In C Guilleminault, E Lugaresi (eds), *Sleep/Wake Disorders: Natural History, Epidemiology and Long-Term Evolution.* New York: Raven, 1983. Pp 87–97.

Bootzin RR, Epstein D, Wood JM. Stimulus control instructions. In P Hauri, *Case Studies in Insomnia.* New York: Plenum, 1991.

Coccagna G. Restless legs syndrome/periodic movements in sleep. In MJ Thorpy (ed), *Handbook of Sleep Disorders.* New York: Dekker, 1990. Pp 457–478.

Coleman RM, et al. Epidemiology of periodic movements during sleep. In C Guilleminault, E Lugaresi (eds), *Sleep/Wake Disorders: Natural History, Epidemiology and Long-Term Evolution.* New York: Raven, 1983. Pp 217–229.

Czeisler CA, et al. Chronotherapy: Resetting the circadian clocks of patients with delayed sleep phase insomnia. *Sleep* 4:1–21, 1981.

Diagnostic Classification Steering Committee (MJ Thorpy, Chairman). *International Classification of Sleep Disorders: Diagnostic and Coding Manual.* Rochester, MN: American Sleep Disorders Association, 1990.

Ekbom KA. Restless legs syndrome. *Neurology* 10:868–873, 1960.

Guilleminault C. Sleep disorders. In JAM Frederiks (ed), *Handbook of Clinical Neurology: Clinical Neuropsychology.* New York: Elsevier, 1985. Pp 129–145.

Guilleminault C. Amphetamines and narcolepsy: Use of Stanford database. *Sleep* 16:199–201, 1993.

Guilleminault C, Faull KF. Sleepiness in non-narcoleptic, nonsleep apneic EDS patients: The idiopathic CNS hypersomnolence. *Sleep* 5:S175–S181, 1982.

Hauri P, Fisher J. Persistent psychophysiologic (learned) insomnia. *Sleep* 9:38–53, 1986.

Issa F, Sullivan C. Reversal of central sleep apnea using nasal CPAP. *Chest* 90:163–171, 1986.

Kavey NB, et al. Somnambulism in adults. *Neurology* 40:749–752, 1990.

Kryger MH, Roth T, Dement WC. *Principles and Practice of Sleep Medicine.* Philadelphia: Saunders, 1994.

Langdon N, et al. Fluoxetine in the treatment of cataplexy. *Sleep* 9:371–372, 1986.

Mahowald MW, Ettinger MG. Things that go bump in the night: The parasomnias revisited. *J Clin Neurophysiol* 7:119–143, 1990.

Mitler M, Erman M, Hajdukovic R. The treatment of excessive somnolence with stimulant drugs. *Sleep* 16:203–206, 1993.

Moldofsky H, Musisi S, Phillipson EA. Treatment of case of advanced sleep phase syndrome by phase advance chronotherapy. *Sleep* 9:61–65, 1986.

National Institute of Mental Health, Consensus Development Conference. Drugs and insomnia: The use of medications to promote sleep. *JAMA* 251:2410–2414, 1984.

Reynolds CF III, Shipley JE. Sleep in depressive disorders. In RE Hales, AJ Frances (eds), *Psychiatry Update: The American Psychiatric Association Annual Review* (vol 4). Washington: American Psychiatric Press, 1985. Pp 341–351.

Sanders MH, Kern N. Obstructive sleep apnea treated by independently adjusted inspiratory and expiratory positive airway pressures by nasal mask. *Chest* 98:317–324, 1990.

Schenck CH, Mahowald MW. Motor dyscontrol in narcolepsy: Rapid eye movement (REM) sleep without atonia and REM sleep behavior disorder. *Ann Neurol* 32:3–10, 1992.

Schenck CH, et al. Chronic behavioral disorders of human REM sleep: A new category of parasomnia. *Sleep* 9:293–308, 1986.

White D, et al. Central sleep apnea: Improvement with acetazolamide therapy. *Arch Intern Med* 142:1816–1819, 1982.

Zorick F, et al. Effects of uvulopalatopharyngoplasty on the daytime sleepiness associated with sleep apnea syndrome. *Bull Eur Physiopathol Respir* 19:600–603, 1983.

Zorick FJ, et al. Evaluation and diagnosis of persistent insomnia. *Am J Psychiatry* 138:769–773, 1981.

56

Dizziness and Vertigo

Bradley Todd Troost
Melissa A. Waller

Dizziness and **vertigo**, particularly dizziness, represent one of the most common complaints presenting to the primary care physician. Although dizziness is usually benign and readily treatable, some forms are life-threatening and require immediate attention and action. Isolated rotary vertigo is usually a manifestation of peripheral vestibular or inner ear dysfunction. For example, in the setting of an upper respiratory infection, acute rotary vertigo without associated complaints of double vision, perioral numbness, limb weakness, or ataxia is usually a benign, self-limited condition that should be managed conservatively.

On the other hand, for patients with complaints of diplopia or other brainstem signs, immediate attention should be given to the possibility of brainstem or cerebellar infarction. An immediate CT or, preferably, MRI scan should be performed to rule out a developing cerebellar stroke, which may require immediate surgical intervention. Cardinal features suggesting CNS abnormalities are history, associated complaints, and posterior fossa signs of (1) direction-changing nystagmus, (2) ataxia, (3) weakness, and (4) falling in the direction of the most prominent nystagmus.

Dizziness may be very vaguely described, including complaints such as unsteadiness, lightheadedness, and instability. It may be produced by a variety of conditions including peripheral vestibulopathy (inner ear), systemic disorders such as postural hypotension or the nonspecific effects of drugs or cardiac arrhythmia, and CNS disorders.

The major causes of dizziness and vertigo are otologic or peripheral vestibular, central neurologic, and systemic or medical (Table 56-1). Vertigo is the illusion or hallucination of movement. If the sensation is of rotary vertigo, the etiology is almost always the peripheral vestibular apparatus—i.e., the inner ear or labyrinth. Because the inner ear is anatomically juxtaposed to the cochlea or hearing apparatus, auditory symptoms are often present, as in Ménière's disease.

The sensation of balance and the ability to maintain posture are dependent on input from three major sensory systems: the inner ear, the eyes, and proprioceptive input from the peripheral nerves. Hearing is also important, because auditory cues may aid postural stability. All the sensory information must be integrated by the brain and coordinated by the cerebellum and motor pathways of the CNS to maintain posture and ambulation.

I. Otologic or peripheral vestibular causes of vertigo
A. Benign paroxysmal positional vertigo (BPPV)

1. **Natural history and prognosis.** BPPV is characterized by brief attacks of vertigo produced by changes in head position. BPPV may follow previous attacks of labyrinthitis or head trauma. This disorder is caused by loose particles in the posterior semicircular canal of the inner ear. BPPV is responsible for at least 50% of all cases of vertigo. Its frequency increases with age, and it is estimated to be present, at one time or another, in 40% of patients aged 70 years or older. It is usually benign and self-limiting, disappearing spontaneously. There are, however, many patients who have recurrent attacks of BPPV over months or even many years, which can be disabling. Specific intervention in the form of exercise therapy is needed to reposition the particles so that attacks no longer occur.

2. **Prevention.** There is no specific method for preventing BPPV. Individual attacks are prevented by avoiding specific provocative head positions.

3. **Therapeutic approach.** The primary therapeutic option is one form or another of exercise therapy. The severity of individual attacks and the accompanying nausea may be lessened by medical therapy, but such therapy does not prevent future attacks.

   Exercise therapy is indicated for all patients with BPPV. There are two

Table 56-1. Major causes of vertigo.

Otologic or Peripheral Vestibular Causes of Vertigo
Benign paroxysmal positional vertigo (BPPV)
Labyrinthitis or vestibular neuronitis
Ménière's disease
Ototoxicity
Perilymph fistula (PLF)
Tumors involving the eighth nerve
Central Neurologic Causes of Vertigo
Brainstem ischemia and infarction
Basilar artery migraine
Seizures
Multiple sclerosis
Chiari malformations
Medical or Systemic Causes of Vertigo
Postural hypotension
Cardiac arrhythmia
Metabolic causes: hypoglycemia and hypothyroidism
Drug effects
Multiple afferent sensory loss

general approaches to therapy: a single treatment session in an outpatient office setting, and a series of exercises performed by the patient at home. Each will be described briefly.

a. Office single treatment approach. Among the single treatment approaches are the canalith repositioning maneuver (CRP) and its modifications. One standard protocol is described below. This technique works best for patients in whom a specific head position, such as with the left ear down, produces attacks of vertigo. Often the examiner notices a characteristic rotary vertical nystagmus accompanying the vertigo when the head is placed in the offending position (Figs. 56-1 and 56-2).

Treatment protocol for the left ear

(1) The patient is moved quickly from a seated position back over the end of the examination table with the head extended and turned approximately 45 degrees with the left ear down. (In each position in this protocol, nystagmus may be induced as a result of the change from the prior head position.) The patient is kept in this position until the nystagmus or symptoms subside—typically for 10–15 seconds.

(2) The head is slowly rotated so that the right ear is turned 45 degrees down, keeping the head extended.

(3) The head and body are rotated to the right until the patient is facing downward. This position is maintained for approximately 15 seconds.

(4) The patient is then brought gradually up to a seated position with the head turned to the right.

(5) The head is turned forward with the chin slightly depressed.

Over the next 24–48 hours, some recommend that the patient remain upright as much as possible. Another variation is to apply a hand-held mechanical oscillator to the head in each position. The overall success rate of this single treatment is reported to be 50–75%.

b. Home exercise therapy. The patient is first instructed carefully about the type of exercise to be performed (Fig. 56-3).

Treatment protocol for either ear

(1) In a seated position, on the edge of a couch or bed, the patient is asked to lie quickly on one side, placing the worst ear (if this can be determined) down first (Fig. 56-4). The patient is asked to move rapidly from the sitting position and to rest the head on a pillow or other support. The patient should not move so forcefully as to produce a neck injury.

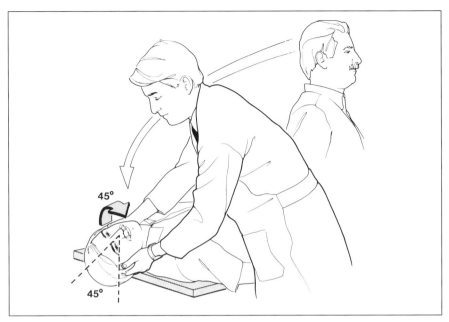

Figure 56-1. Provocative maneuvers for positional vertigo and nystagmus. The patient is abruptly moved from a seated position to one with the head hanging 45 degrees below the horizontal and rotated 45 degrees to one side, and is then observed for benign paroxysmal positional nystagmus (BPPN). The maneuvers are repeated with the head straight back and turned to the other side. (Reprinted with permission from Troost BT, Patton JM. Exercise therapy for positional vertigo. *Neurology* 42:1442, 1992.)

    (2) The patient then returns rapidly to an upright seated position and remains there for 30 seconds or until the symptoms subside.

    (3) The patient rapidly lies down on the other side and remains there for approximately 30 seconds or until the symptoms subside.

    (4) The patient then returns to the upright seated position. This constitutes a single repetition.

        Twenty repetitions should be performed two times each day. Each session lasts approximately 30 minutes. Some patients have intense symptoms at the onset of the BPPV, including vomiting. These patients may need hospital admission or hydration in an outpatient setting, with the concurrent administration of vestibular suppressant medications. It is clear that patients who experience extreme discomfort during these maneuvers will not be likely to pursue them on their own outside of the office or hospital setting. Most patients are willing to perform exercises at home. This protocol is particularly useful for BPPV patients who have (1) bilateral BPPV, (2) uncertainty as to which ear is involved, or (3) failure of single office treatment protocols.

        Recovery can be quite rapid, occurring during the first few days of exercise therapy. Others progressively improve over weeks or months, which suggests that the vestibular system may adapt to whatever abnormal perturbation is causing the symptoms.

4. Expected outcome. Approximately 50% of patients who have well-defined vertigo and nystagmus in certain head positions show improvement following the single treatment maneuver. Variations include the use of a hand-held oscillator or longer durations at each single position. The home set of maneuvers, known as the Brandt-Daroff maneuvers, may take weeks or even months to produce a cure, but progressive improvement of symptoms should be noticed by the patient within the first few weeks. It is estimated

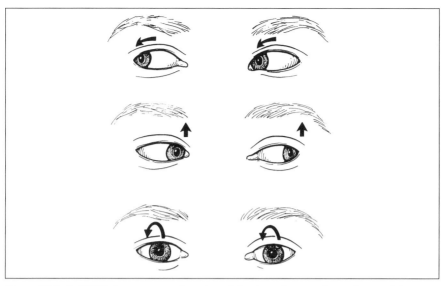

Figure 56-2. In BPPN, the nystagmus fast phase is horizontal-rotary directed toward the undermost ear when gaze is directed toward the undermost ear (upper panel). The nystagmus fast phase is upward toward the forehead when gaze is directed to the uppermost ear (middle panel). With the eyes in the central orbital position, the nystagmus fast phase is vertical upward and rotary toward the down ear (bottom panel). (Reprinted with permission from Troost BT, Patton JM. Exercise therapy for positional vertigo. *Neurology* 42:1443, 1992.)

that approximately 20% of patients have recurrences within the first year, and either of the maneuvers described above may be repeated with a high expectation of further improvement. The overall success rate of exercise therapy approaches 90%, even among patients who have been symptomatic for years.

5. **Referral.** Persistence of BPPV, after repeated exercise therapy of either general type has failed, indicates the need for referral to an otolaryngologist or neuro-otologist. Rare instances of persistent disabling positional vertigo, unresponsive to exercise therapy, may require a surgical approach—either sec-

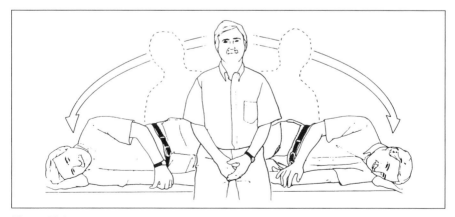

Figure 56-3. Exercise therapy. The patient begins in the seated position and then leans rapidly to the side, placing the head on the bed or table. The patient remains there until the vertigo subsides and then returns to the seated upright position, remaining there until all symptoms subside. The maneuver is repeated to the opposite side, completing one full repetition. Ten to 20 repetitions should be performed three times a day. (Reprinted with permission from Troost BT, Patton JM. Exercise therapy for positional vertigo. *Neurology* 42:1443, 1992.)

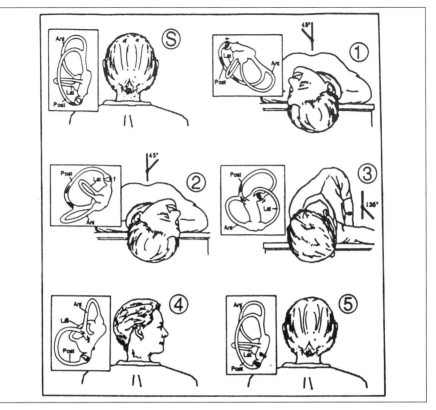

Figure 56-4. Positioning sequence for left posterior semicircular canal (PSC) shows orientation of left labyrinth and gravitating canaliths. S (start). Patient is seated with operator behind patient. Oscillation is started. 1. Head is placed over end of table, 45 degrees to left, with head extended. (Canaliths gravitate to center of posterior semicircular canal.) 2. Head is rotated 45 degrees to right; head is kept well extended in process of coming from position 1. (Canaliths reach common crus.) 3. Head and body are rotated until facing downward 135 degrees from supine. (Canaliths traverse common crus.) 4. Patient is brought to sitting position; head is kept turned to right in process of coming from position 3. (Canaliths enter utricle.) 5. Head is turned forward with chin down about 20 degrees. (Reprinted with permission from Epley JM. Fine points of canalith repositioning procedure for treatment of BPPV. *Insights Otolaryngol* 9:7, 1994.)

tioning of the nerve to the posterior semicircular canal or a surgical canal plugging operation. The vast majority of patients who have BPPV are readily diagnosed. Most of these patients do not need expensive work-ups that include MRI scanning. If the diagnosis is unclear, it is less expensive to refer the patient to specialists in the area, who may make the diagnosis on the basis of history and careful physical examination without the need for neuroimaging procedures.

B. Labyrinthitis. Peripheral vestibulopathy encompasses disorders such as vestibular neuronitis, labyrinthitis, and viral neurolabyrinthitis. **Vestibular neuronitis,** strictly speaking, is characterized by a single episode or recurrent episodes of true vertigo lasting from hours to days and often associated initially with vomiting. When the condition is associated with hearing loss, the entire labyrinth is assumed to be involved and the term **labyrinthitis** is used. Despite this technical distinction, many neuro-otologists, otologists, and neurologists use the terms "vestibular neuronitis" and "labyrinthitis" interchangeably, whether or not auditory symptoms are present. In such patients, the vertiginous sensation may be worsened by head movement, but not necessarily by a particular head position. Whether or not isolated viral involvement of the vestibular nerves is the cause of acute or episodic vertigo is controversial. Many prefer the terms "acute peripheral vestibulopathy" and "recurrent peripheral vestibulopathy." In the acute phase, most patients present with sudden and severe vertigo, nausea, and vomiting without any hearing disturbance or facial weakness.

1. **Natural history and prognosis.** In general, the prognosis is good. At least 90% of patients have only a single attack with no apparent residual deficit.
2. **Prevention.** There is no specific preventive therapy for acute inner ear inflammation. However, patients with middle ear infections or otitis media should be treated with appropriate antibiotic therapy to prevent spread to the inner ear.
3. **Therapeutic approach.** Therapy is outlined for symptomatic treatment of acute dizziness presumed to be caused by labyrinthitis. Classes of drugs are listed in Table 56-2.

   Although most of the drugs used for dizziness are loosely referred to as vestibular suppressants, it is often unclear which agent will be effective in a given patient and what its true mechanism of action is likely to be. The primary vestibular afferent system could be suppressed directly or indirectly through the inhibitory portion of the major vestibular efferent system. An important function of some agents may be to act on other sensory systems such as proprioceptive or visual inputs to the vestibular nuclei of the brainstem.

   Many of the agents commonly used are empirical. Few controlled studies have investigated the response of patients with presumed peripheral vestibular dysfunction. Many of the drugs used by physicians for treating such patients are based on studies of the prevention of motion sickness in normal subjects or of the various regimens employed by otologists in the management of patients diagnosed as having Ménière's disease. Each class of drugs is discussed separately.

Table 56-2. Medical therapy for vertigo.

Antihistamines
Meclizine (Antivert, Bonine)
Cyclizine (Marezine)
Dimenhydrinate (Dramamine)
Promethazine (Phenergan)

Anticholinergics
Scopolamine (hyoscine)
Atropine

Sympathomimetic
Ephedrine

Antiemetics
Trimethobenzamide (Tigan)
Prochlorperazine (Compazine)

"Tranquilizers"
Diazepam (Valium)
Prazepam (Vestran)
Haloperidol (Haldol)
Chlorpromazine (Thorazine)

Combination Preparations and Others
Scopolamine with ephedrine
Scopolamine with promethazine
Ephedrine with promethazine
Buclizine hydrochloride (Bucladin)
Cyclandelate (Cyclospasmol)
Diuretics
Diet

a. **Antihistamines** (Table 56-3) are among the agents most commonly employed in the treatment of dizziness. The drug usually employed initially is meclizine hydrochloride in dosages up to 50 mg tid. Because the main side effect of antihistamines is drowsiness, the smallest dosage should be used initially, even as low as 12.5 mg bid-tid.

For dizziness, the antihistamines in the H_1 antagonist group are used. Possibly the H_1 blockers, effective in motion sickness, act by central antagonism of acetylcholine (ACh), as does scopolamine. An excellent drug as a second choice is promethazine, a phenothiazine with the strongest ACh-blocking action. The usual starting dosage is 25 mg tid, but if this produces drowsiness and still has a positive effect, the dosage can be reduced to 12.5 mg tid.

b. **Anticholinergics** (Table 56-4) that block the muscarinic effect of ACh have been widely used and studied for the prevention of motion sickness. Atropine acts centrally to stimulate the medulla and cerebrum, but the closely related alkaloid scopolamine is more widely used.

Transdermal delivery of scopolamine may prevent or mitigate the nausea and vomiting associated with motion sickness, but not the dizziness. In general, transdermal scopolamine is not useful for patients with acquired vestibulopathy. Frequent side effects are blurred vision and dry mouth, in addition to occasional confusion. Some patients have significant difficulty when they try to discontinue the use of scopolamine patches. A side effect of low-dosage scopolamine or atropine is transient bradycardia (four to eight fewer beats per minute) associated with the peak action of oral scopolamine at 90 minutes and diminishing thereafter.

c. **Sympathomimetics** have been used in the treatment of motion sickness, particularly in combination with anticholinergics. The sole agent in this class that may have an application in combination with other drugs is ephedrine. Tolerance may develop after a few weeks of treatment.

d. **Antiemetics** (Table 56-5) may be used when prominent nausea is an accompanying feature of the patient's complaint. Many of the antihistaminic and anticholinergic drugs listed in Tables 56-3 and 56-4 are also used for their antiemetic actions. Prochlorperazine (Compazine) should be used with caution, particularly by the intramuscular route, because of the high incidence of dystonic reactions. Because promethazine (Phenergan) has a significant antiemetic effect, it is particularly useful when there is prominent nausea.

e. **Tranquilizers** (Table 56-6) is the general name given to drugs from different classes having central and probably peripheral effects. Such drugs include benzodiazepines, butyrophenones, and phenothiazines. Diazepam is one of the most widely prescribed drugs for the treatment of dizziness. Many believe it should not be the first choice, primarily because of the significant potential for habituation and depression, and because it can be the actual cause of dizziness. Nonetheless, it does remain the first choice of many otoneurologists and otologists. Other longer-

Table 56-3. Antihistamines for dizziness.

Generic name	Trade name	Dosage*
Ethanolamines		
Diphenhydramine hydrochloride	Benadryl	50 mg qd-bid
Dimenhydrinate	Dramamine	50 mg qd-bid
Piperazines		
Cyclizine hydrochloride	Marezine	50 mg qd-bid
Meclizine hydrochloride	Antivert, Bonine	25–50 mg tid
Phenothiazine		
Promethazine hydrochloride	Phenergan	25–50 mg/day

*Usual adult starting dosage can be increased by a factor of 2–3 with drowsiness as the most common side effect.

Table 56-4. Anticholinergics for dizziness.

Generic name	Trade name	Dosage*
Scopolamine	Donphen*	1 tablet tid
Scopolamine	Donnatal*	1 tablet tid
Scopolamine hydrobromide tablets	—	0.45–0.50 mg qd-bid
Scopolamine	Transderm-V	1 0.5-mg patch, change every 3 days

*The combination preparations Donphen and Donnatal each contain a mixture of atropine alkaloids with approximately ¼ gr (15.0–16.2 mg) of phenobarbital.

acting benzodiazepines may be helpful for certain patients, but no study has substantiated their effectiveness.

Haloperidol in low oral dosages (0.5 mg tid) is effective for many patients with peripheral vestibular dysfunction who are not helped by other antidizziness medications.

f. **Combination preparations,** including agents listed in Table 56-2, are frequently useful, particularly the combination of ephedrine and promethazine. Some other agents and regimens used primarily in the medical management of Ménière's disease are listed in the same table. Low-sodium diets and diuretics have been helpful for some patients. In the belief that in some cases an effect on blood supply to the peripheral end organ might be a factor, agents such as cyclandelate have been used. The general approach to the patient with an acute or chronic vestibulopathy is first to employ an antihistamine such as meclizine hydrochloride. If this is not helpful, the next step is to use promethazine (Phenergan), and if this is ineffective, low-dosage diazepam can be tried, always keeping in mind the habituation potential of benzodiazepines. The majority of these medications are relatively inexpensive. Single drugs such as antihistamines are less expensive than the combination preparations.

4. **Expected outcome.** It should be expected that some patients with peripheral vestibular dysfunction will respond to medical therapy with significant lessening of symptoms. Medication may need to be taken daily by patients with chronic peripheral vestibulopathy.

5. **Referral.** Patients who do not respond to medical therapy should be referred to a neuro-otologist or a neurologist.

C. **Ménière's disease**

1. **Natural history and prognosis.** Ménière's disease is characterized by attacks of severe vertigo and vomiting, tinnitus (often described as roaring), fluctuating hearing loss, ill-described aural sensations of fullness and pressure, and spontaneous recovery in hours to days. Most often the patient develops a sensation of fullness and pressure along with decreased hearing and tinnitus in a single ear. These symptoms are followed by severe vertigo attacks that reach peak intensity within minutes and slowly subside over hours, with a persistent sense of disequilibration for days after an acute episode. On some occasions, patients with Ménière's disease experience

Table 56-5. Antiemetics.

Generic name	Trade name	Dosage*
Trimethobenzamide	Tigan	250 mg qd-bid PO
		200 mg qd-bid PR
Phenothiazines:		
Promethazine	Phenergan	12.5–25.0 mg tid-qid PO
		12.5–25.0 mg suppository
Prochlorperazine	Compazine	5–10 mg tid-qid PO
		25-mg suppository

*Interactions with other drugs and extrapyramidal side effects, especially with Compazine, should promote caution.

Table 56-6. "Tranquilizers" for dizziness.

Generic name	Trade name	Dosage
Benzodiazepines		
Diazepam	Valium	5–10 mg qd-tid
Prazepam	Verstran	10 mg/day
Butyrophenone		
Haloperidol	Haldol	0.5–1.0 mg qd-bid[a]
Phenothiazines		
Promethazine hydrochloride	Phenergan	25–50 mg/day
Chlorpromazine	Thorazine	10–50 mg/day[b]

[a]Note very low dosage compared with usual antipsychotic levels. Still, patients should be observed for dystonias.
[b]Usual precautions for phenothiazines. We have not used chlorpromazine for dizziness, but it is used as an adjunct by some.

such severe attacks that they suddenly fall to the ground. Consciousness is not lost in such episodes, although awareness of surroundings may be altered by the intensity of the accompanying sensation.

Ménière's disease usually develops between the ages of 30 and 50 and is slightly more common in women than in men. The prognosis is for progressive reduction in hearing along with increasing frequency of attacks. Although some patients' stabilizers "burn out," they are left with residual hearing loss, but no subsequent attacks of severe vertigo. Approximately 50% of Ménière's patients become bilateral. The hearing loss often progresses to a moderated deficit and then stabilizes.

2. **Prevention.** There is no specific intervention or therapy that prevents the development of Ménière's disease.

3. **Therapeutic approach.** The usual first-line treatment for patients with Ménière's disease is vestibular medications such as those described in sec. **I.B.** All these forms of therapy have, in certain patients, lessened the severity of attacks, and have provided successful management of many patients. However, there is a subset of patients who are unresponsive to standard medical therapy and for whom surgical intervention must be considered. Labyrinthectomy or vestibular nerve section is a main mode of therapy. A medical labyrinthectomy may be performed by the use of aminoglycoside drugs—those particularly destructive to the peripheral vestibular hair cells in the inner ear. In this procedure, a drug such as gentamicin is injected through the tympanic membrane with the idea that there will be selective destruction of vestibular hair cells but relative sparing of hearing. Surgical or medical labyrinthectomy is usually a last resort for patients who have clearly defined severe attacks of Ménière's disease that are unresponsive to medical therapy.

Various shunting procedures have been used in the treatment of Ménière's disease, such as an endolymphatic shunt from the inner ear to the mastoid.

The indication for surgical therapy is complete failure of medical treatment. There are no specific contraindications to labyrinthectomy depending on the general state of the patient's health, but the procedure has certain limitations and pitfalls. Labyrinthectomy should generally be limited to patients who have severe reduction or complete loss of hearing, because patients lose hearing following labyrinthectomy. Selective posterior fossa sectioning of the vestibular nerve may spare hearing. Complications of the procedure are the standard ones for any surgical procedure, such as postoperative infection and leakage of cerebrospinal fluid (CSF) with subsequent meningitis.

4. **Expected outcome.** It is expected that many patients will respond favorably to medical treatment with less severe attacks of vertigo. The therapy will not prevent the progressive hearing loss. Surgical therapy in unilateral Ménière's patients is expected to be curative. The patient is subsequently free of attacks following an initial period of days to a few weeks, then experiences increased disequilibration resulting from loss of vestibular input on

one side. Bilateral surgical patients, although they may be free of future attacks of severe vertigo, have a persistent state of some disequilibrium and have difficulty making rapid turns. There is also a sensation of movement of the visual environment with rapid head movement, known as oscillopsia.

5. **Referral.** Patients with suspected Ménière's disease should be referred to an otologist.

D. **Ototoxicity**
1. **Natural history and prognosis.** The usual cause of bilaterally reduced vestibular function is treatment with ototoxic antibiotics, particularly gentamicin. The patient experiences severe ataxia and oscillopsia.

Prognosis for complete recovery is only fair. It is very unusual to have complete loss of vestibular hair cells bilaterally, and therefore some recovery is to be expected; however, it usually takes months or even years.

2. **Intervention.** Diligent monitoring of aminoglycoside levels during therapy is extremely useful in avoiding ototoxicity. Some patients are unusually sensitive, and treatment should be stopped, except for a life-threatening illness, at any sign of imbalance or vertigo during therapy. Extreme caution should be used in treating patients with renal dysfunctions, because aminoglycosides are exputed through the kidneys. A major reduction in aminoglycoside dosage should be made in patients with concomitant renal insufficiency. It is, therefore, important that any patient considered for aminoglycoside therapy have a careful assessment of renal function before the treatment is begun.

3. **Therapeutic approach.** The primary therapeutic option is to avoid the occurrence of ototoxicity. No specific therapy is available once ototoxicity has occurred. Further reduction of vestibular function with medications such as those used to treat labyrinthitis are generally not helpful, although an occasional patient with bilateral, but asymmetric, aminoglycoside ototoxicity may experience modest improvement.

4. **Expected outcome.** As mentioned in sec. **B.3,** some patients experience modest relief from the use of vestibular suppressant medication, but significant improvement is unusual.

5. **Referral.** Patients with bilaterally reduced vestibular function should be referred to an otologist or a neurologist specializing in balance disorders.

E. **Perilymph fistula (PLF)** usually follows barotrauma (such as in scuba diving) or a blow to the ear resulting in a rupture between the fluid in the semicircular canals and the middle ear.
1. **Natural history and prognosis.** Patients experience extreme pressure sensitivity with attacks of vertigo or imbalance and ataxia associated with increased pressure in the ear. On occasion, symptoms are exacerbated by certain head positions. Small perilymph fistulas may close spontaneously.

2. **Prevention.** During deep-sea diving, careful monitoring of pressure is mandatory to protect the inner ear from barotrauma. Ear protection should be worn in any situation where there may be aural trauma.

3. **Therapeutic approach.** When PLF is diagnosed, the initial treatment should be prolonged bed rest with the avoidance of sudden increases in pressure, such as from a Valsalva's maneuver. The rest promotes spontaneous sealing of the fistula. Persistent symptomatology after 2 weeks of bed rest, however, should lead to surgical exploration of the inner ear with an attempt to localize and seal the fistula. The surgical technique includes occlusion of the fistula, usually with biological material such as muscle. Most surgical patients are kept at bed rest for 2 weeks with strict avoidance of activities that might reopen the fistula, such as coughing or straining at stool. A significant limitation is an inability to find the exact location of the fistula during surgical exploration lest an inadvertent new rupture be caused by the procedure itself.

4. **Expected outcome.** Most patients experience relief, either with bed rest or with surgical therapy. Reexploration may be necessary.

5. **Referral.** Patients suspected of having perilymph fistulas should be immediately referred to an otolaryngologist.

F. **Tumors involving the eighth nerve**
1. **Natural history and prognosis.** Tumors of the cerebellopontine angle rarely present solely with episodic vertigo. The most common tumor in this location results from a proliferation of Schwann cells, hence the name schwannoma. Most of these tumors arise under the vestibular portion of the

eighth nerve within the internal auditory canal. They progressively enlarge, deforming the internal auditory canal and compressing adjacent neurostructures, such as the acoustic portion of the eighth nerve, the facial nerve, the trigeminal nerve, and eventually the brainstem and cerebellum. The most common symptoms associated with eighth nerve tumors are progressive unilateral sensorineural hearing loss and tinnitus. Intermittent vertigo occurs in approximately 20% of patients, but a symptom of imbalance or disequilibration is more common, approaching 50%. The prognosis for untreated tumors of the cerebellopontine angle is determined by the type of tumor and the rate of growth. Ultimately, untreated tumors affect hearing and vestibular functions and, as they enlarge, involve nerves such as the seventh nerve and compress the brainstem. Surgical intervention is required.

2. **Prevention.** There is no specific means of preventing tumors of the cerebellopontine angle, but prevention of subsequent neurologic damage can be accomplished by early diagnosis. Any patient with progressive unexplained unilateral hearing loss, with or without vertigo, should have neuroimaging studies to detect or rule out the presence of a tumor.

3. **Therapeutic approach.** The primary therapeutic option is surgery. Small tumors may be approached through the ear by an otolaryngologist or through the posterior fossa by a neurosurgeon. Monitoring of seventh and eighth nerve function during surgery may permit preservation of function. Once a tumor is suspected, the patient should have high-resolution MRI with contrast of the posterior fossa. It is less expensive to proceed immediately to a focused neuroimaging test and referral to an appropriate specialist than to delay until the tumor has grown significantly.

4. **Expected outcome.** Tumors involving the eighth nerve inevitably progress, causing losses of hearing, balance, and other cranial nerve functions, as discussed earlier. Prognosis for benign tumors detected early and operated on is excellent.

5. **Referral.** Patients suspected of having eighth nerve tumors should be referred to neurosurgeons or otolaryngologists specializing in neuro-otology.

II. **Central neurologic causes of vertigo**

A. **Brainstem ischemia and infarction**

1. **Natural history and prognosis.** Vertigo, including brief episodes of isolated vertigo, may be caused by posterior circulation disturbance. The posterior circulation supplies blood to the brainstem, the cerebellum, and the peripheral vestibular apparatus. It is not surprising that vertebrobasilar ischemia may be accompanied by vertigo. In general, brainstem transient ischemic attacks (TIAs) should be accompanied by neurologic symptoms or signs in addition to vertigo, before a clear-cut diagnosis is entertained. Symptoms include transient clumsiness, weakness, loss of vision, diplopia, perioral numbness, ataxia, drop attacks, and dysarthria.

The prognosis following a definite posterior circulation TIA is uncertain. It is estimated that at least one-third of patients have strokes within 3 years. Therefore, prevention and therapy are paramount.

2. **Prevention.** All risk factors for ischemic stroke should be evaluated, including hypertension, hyperlipidemia, diabetes, and smoking. The patient should also be evaluated for possible cardiac sources of emboli. It is clear that the best treatment of stroke is its prevention.

3. **Therapeutic approach.** Once an actual infarction has occurred, the therapy is primarily supportive. Therapeutic approaches are directed toward preventing future incidence of TIAs and preventing actual infarction. The first-line therapy is antiplatelet drugs, including aspirin and ticlopidine. In situations in which there is increasing frequency of TIAs or a suspected source of emboli, the patient should be hospitalized, and intravenous heparin may be given. Patients with suspected cardiac sources of emboli are candidates for long-term warfarin therapy.

A history of gastric ulcers or bleeding is a significant contraindication to anticoagulation. Therapy for ischemic cerebrovascular disease is discussed in Ch. 36, sec. **II.**

4. **Expected outcome.** The appropriate therapy for diminishing risk factors may significantly reduce the likelihood of permanent defects resulting from infarction. Some patients may have strokes despite therapy.

5. Referral. Any patient suspected of having brainstem ischemia and infarction should be referred for a complete neurologic and neurovascular evaluation.

B. Basilar artery migraine

1. Natural history and prognosis. This condition is usually diagnosed in young women who have episodic events such as diplopia, dysarthria, vertigo, ataxia, and bilateral visual loss followed by diffuse throbbing headache. There may be a significant family history of sick headaches. When vertigo is followed by diffuse headache, this condition should be considered. Prognosis is variable, with some episodes disappearing spontaneously. Rare patients, however, may have brainstem infarctions so that intervention is paramount.

2. Prevention. Prophylactic therapy for migraine may eliminate attacks, but overall is less successful than for migraine without aura (common migraine).

3. Therapeutic approach. There are two general approaches to therapy of migraine. One is acute abortive treatment with agents such as ergotamines or sumatriptan. However, when there are significant neurologic symptoms, prophylactic therapy with calcium channel blockers, beta-blockers, amitriptyline, or methysergide should be considered. Migraine therapy is presented in Ch. 49, sec. **II.**

4. Expected outcome. Ideally, patients with basilar artery migraine should be controlled with prophylactic therapy so that they have no attacks with accompanying neurologic symptoms such as vertigo.

5. Referral. Patients with neurologic symptoms precipitating or accompanying migraine attacks should be referred to a neurologist for management.

C. Seizures

1. Natural history and prognosis. Seizures are a rare cause of isolated vertigo. There is alteration of consciousness or accompanying features with complex partial seizures (such as lip smacking, drooling, or even associated motor activity). Even if there are some episodes of isolated vertigo, sooner or later most patients have episodes of clear alteration of consciousness. The prognosis at that point depends on the cause of the seizure. The prognosis is worse if there is a tumor and is generally much better if there is a small cortical scar that can be removed surgically.

2. Prevention. There is no specific prevention for the onset of seizures, but individual patients may find certain precipitants that can be avoided such as alcohol or sleeplessness.

3. Therapeutic approach. Primary therapy for recurrent seizures is properly selected antiepileptic drugs. Therapy for seizure disorders is covered in sec. **II** of Chs. 38 and 39.

4. Expected outcome. Ideally, patients are completely managed with anticonvulsant therapy. Complex partial seizures can be refractory and even require surgical intervention.

5. Referral. Once a diagnosis of seizure disorder has been made, the patient is often referred to a neurologist.

D. Multiple sclerosis

1. Natural history and prognosis. Multiple sclerosis is diagnosed primarily on the basis of a history of different neurologic signs or symptoms in the CNS that are separated in time—e.g., a patient may have an episode of vertigo at one time and an attack of optic neuritis at another time. Clinical diagnosis is usually confirmed by MRI. Multiple sclerosis tends to progress, with new neurologic signs and symptoms occurring over many years. Prognosis depends on the extent of the neurologic involvement.

2. Prevention. There is no known specific preventive therapy for multiple sclerosis, but severity of individual attacks may be lessened by therapy.

3. Therapeutic approach. Therapy for multiple sclerosis includes acute treatment with intravenous solumedrol and a variety of interventions designed to prevent future attacks and progression. Therapy for multiple sclerosis is discussed in Ch. 40, sec. **II.**

4. Expected outcome. It is believed that with appropriate therapy, individual attacks can be lessened in severity and future attacks lessened by regimens discussed in Ch. 40, sec. **II.**

5. Referral. Patients with suspected or known multiple sclerosis are often referred to neurologists.

E. Arnold-Chiari malformation
1. **Natural history and prognosis.** The adult type of Arnold-Chiari malformation is a brainstem or cerebellar herniation through the foramen magnum. The condition usually presents with unsteadiness or vertigo and a downbeating nystagmus, particularly on sideward gaze. Ocular oscillation may produce a sense of tumbling when the patient looks to the side. The natural history is one of progression of all symptoms. The patient may begin to experience sudden headache with coughing as the brainstem compression progresses over years.
2. **Prevention.** There is no remedial action that can slow the progression of the illness.
3. **Therapeutic approach.** Once a symptomatic condition has been identified, there should be surgical intervention with decompression of the posterior fossa.
4. **Expected outcome.** Surgical intervention usually halts the progression of the brainstem signs and symptoms and may improve them.
5. **Referral.** Once the symptomatic Arnold-Chiari malformation has been identified through the use of MRI, the patient is often referred to a neurologist, who may then refer the patient for neurosurgical intervention.

III. Medical or systemic causes of vertigo and dizziness

A. Postural hypotension
1. **Natural history and prognosis.** Patients usually describe the symptom complex of postural hypotension as lightheadedness rather than a sensation of spinning. Episodes are usually associated with changes in posture such as from lying to standing, but may take several minutes to develop. There may be an accompanying graying-out of vision or even actual fainting. The natural history and prognosis depend on the specific cause if the postural hypotension is the result of an autonomic neuropathy, because in diabetes it tends to worsen progressively with time. If it is the result of a medication such as an antihypertensive medication, major improvements can be achieved by changing the drug regimen.
2. **Prevention.** There is no known specific preventive treatment for autonomic neuropathy. Careful monitoring of blood pressure can usually prevent postural hypotension caused by an antihypertensive medication.
3. **Therapeutic approach.** The therapy for postural hypotension resulting from autonomic neuropathy is difficult. Some episodes may be prevented by the use of elastic stockings or pantyhose. Sodium-retaining steroids such as fludrocortisone (Florinef) may be helpful, but care must be taken not to produce congestive heart failure.
4. **Expected outcome.** The outcome depends on the specific cause, but when the disorder is a medication side effect the expectation is that it can be ameliorated.
5. **Referral.** Patients with postural hypotension resulting from autonomic system failure are often referred to neurologists specializing in autonomic neuropathy. Difficult-to-manage hypertensive patients should be referred to internists or primary care physicians.

B. Cardiac arrhythmia
1. **Natural history and prognosis.** Once presyncope or syncope with lightheadedness has been diagnosed, secondary to cardiac arrhythmia through monitoring, the usual history is of worsening attacks. The prognosis is for further attacks and even life-threatening periods of asystole.
2. **Prevention.** Medications that can interfere with cardiac arrhythmia, such as beta-blockers, should be avoided.
3. **Therapeutic approach.** Patients with cardiac arrhythmia as the cause of dizziness may be treated with antiarrhythmics or pacemakers under the direction of a cardiologist.
4. **Expected outcome.** With proper identification and management, most cardiac arrhythmias can be treated.
5. **Referral.** Patients with cardiac arrhythmias are referred to cardiologists.

C. Metabolic causes of dizziness and vertigo including hypoglycemia and hypothyroidism
1. **Natural history and prognosis.** Metabolic causes of dizziness are unusual and often difficult to diagnose. The symptom complex is not usually one of spinning vertigo, but rather vague episodes of disequilibration. This specific prognosis depends on the exact etiology and correction of the metabolic condition.
2. **Prevention.** Episodic hypoglycemia may be prevented by frequent small

meals or regulation of oral hypoglycemic or insulin therapy when it occurs in diabetics.

3. **Therapeutic approach.** Therapy for endocrine disorders producing disequilibration depends on the specific metabolic abnormality identified. The therapy is directed at correcting the metabolic anomaly.

4. **Expected outcome.** Correction of the metabolic abnormality is usually beneficial with lessening of dizziness or disequilibration.

5. **Referral.** Patients with identified metabolic abnormalities suspected of causing disorders of equilibrium should be referred to internists or endocrinologists.

D. **Drug effects**

1. **Natural history and prognosis.** Disorders of balance may be produced by a wide variety of medications—particularly anticonvulsants, hypnotics, and some tranquilizers. Unless medication specifically affects blood pressure so as to produce lightheadedness, the symptom complex is described as unsteadiness or incoordination. Patients have persistent symptoms as long as they remain on the drugs.

2. **Prevention** depends on the awareness that certain medications, including those used to treat dizziness (such as benzodiazepines), may have medication side effects.

3. **Therapeutic approach.** The general approach is gradual withdrawal, whenever possible, of the medication believed to be producing the side effects. In the case of antiepileptic drugs (AEDs), which are required to control seizure disorders, alternative AEDs may be employed. Very gradual reductions in benzodiazepines may be required if there is a problem of habituation.

4. **Expected outcome.** There is usually significant improvement in symptoms of dizziness and disequilibration once offending medications have been replaced or withdrawn.

5. **Referral.** Patients on AEDs experiencing ataxia or disequilibration should be referred to a neurologist. When other medications such as hypnotics, sedatives, or tranquilizers are suspected to be possible causes of disequilibration, they may be selectively decreased or eliminated by the primary care provider.

E. **Multiple afferent sensory loss**

1. **Natural history and prognosis.** In the elderly, a constellation of sensory deficits, such as combined hearing loss, visual loss, age-related vestibular change, and peripheral neuropathy, as well as a significant sense of disequilibration, unsteadiness, and falls, may ensue. All of these sensory systems work together to produce a sense of stability and balance. The ultimate prognosis depends on factors that are correctable. For example, cataract removal may significantly enhance balance.

2. **Prevention.** Awareness that multiple sensory deficits may produce unsteadiness in the elderly should promote specific endeavors to correct the remedial problems and improve function.

3. **Therapeutic approach.** Specific interventions such as cataract removal or proper refractive correction can improve vision, and hearing aids may improve auditory sensitivity. A specific therapeutic maneuver that may improve balance is the use of a "dragging cane." The proprioceptive input from the cane being moved across the ground may significantly improve postural stability. Depending on the degree of disequilibration, some patients may be forced to use other assistive devices such as walkers.

4. **Expected outcome.** When specific sensory deficits are improved, there may be a significant improvement in balance.

5. **Referral.** Patients with significant visual problems should be referred to ophthalmologists and those with auditory disorders to otolaryngologists.

Recommended Readings

Amarenco P. The spectrum of cerebellar infarctions. *Neurology* 41:973–979, 1991.

Baloh RW, Honrubia V. *Clinical Neurophysiology of the Vestibular System* (2nd ed). Philadelphia: Davis, 1990.

Brandt T. *Vertigo: Its Multisensory Syndromes.* London: Springer-Verlag, 1991.

Caplan LR. *Stroke: A Clinical Approach* (2nd ed). Boston: Butterworth-Heinemann, 1993.

Epley JM. The canalith repositioning procedure: For treatment of benign paroxysmal positional vertigo. *Otolaryngol Head Neck Surg* 107:399–404, 1992.

Froehling DA, et al. Does this dizzy patient have a serious form of vertigo? *JAMA* 271:385–388, 1994.

Grad A, Baloh RW. Vertigo of vascular origin: Clinical and electronystagmographic features in 84 patients. *Arch Neurol* 46:281–284, 1989.

Oas JG, Baloh RW. Vertigo and the anterior inferior cerebellar artery syndrome. *Neurology* 42:2274–2279, 1992.

Sharpe JA, Barber HO. *The Vestibulo-Ocular Reflex and Vertigo.* New York: Raven, 1993.

Troost BT. Dizziness and vertigo. In WG Bradley, et al. (eds), *Neurology in Clinical Practice* (2nd ed). Stoneham, MA: Butterworth (in press).

Troost BT, Patton JM. Exercise therapy for positional vertigo. *Neurology* 42:1441–1444, 1992.

Troost BT, Waller M. Hearing loss and tinnitus without dizziness/vertigo. In WG Bradley, et al. (eds), *Neurology in Clinical Practice* (2nd ed). Stoneham, MA: Butterworth (in press).

Troost BT, Waller M. Neuro-otology. In WG Bradley, et al. (eds), *Neurology in Clinical Practice* (2nd ed). Stoneham, MA: Butterworth (in press).

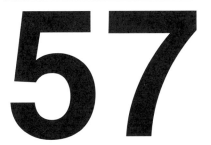

Neurologic Diseases in Pregnancy
Kathleen B. Digre
Michael W. Varner

Pregnancy is common. In the United States there are 4,000,000 live births per year. At any given time, 10% of all women of reproductive age are pregnant. It is therefore not unusual or rare to see neurologic conditions occur in association with pregnancy. Furthermore, physiologic changes in pregnancy contribute in part to neurologic symptoms. Not only can neurologic conditions be affected by pregnancy, but treatment frequently must be altered to accommodate a developing fetus. Finally, pregnancy-specific conditions can present with neurologic symptoms and signs.

I. Normal physiologic changes in pregnancy
A. Cardiovascular
1. Increase (30–50%) in cardiac output
2. Increase (30–50%) in blood volume
3. Midpregnancy decrease in blood pressure
B. Pulmonary
1. Increase (20–30%) in minute volume
2. Increase in respiratory rate
C. Renal
1. Increase (30–50%) in renal blood flow
2. Decreased serum BUN and creatinine
D. Gastrointestinal
1. Decreased motility
2. Elevated alkaline phosphatase (placental). Other liver function tests are normal.
E. Hematologic
1. Decreased hematocrit
2. Increased WBC
3. Decreased platelets
F. Coagulation factors
1. Increased plasminogen, fibrinogen, and factors VII, VIII, IX, and X
2. No change in factor V, antithrombin III, or platelet adhesion
G. Connective tissue. Thickening and fragmentation of reticular fibers with mild hyperplasia of smooth muscle cells
H. Evaluating neurologic conditions in pregnancy. See Table 57-1.
I. FDA risk factor classification of drugs in pregnancy
1. **Class A.** Controlled studies show no risk to fetus in first trimester; fetal harm is remote.
2. **Class B.** There are no controlled studies, but no known risks.
3. **Class C.** Studies on animals may show effects on fetuses, but no controlled studies are available. The drug can be used if the risk is justified.
4. **Class D.** There are positive risks, but the drug may be used if serious disease or life-threatening conditions exist.
5. **Class X.** Human and animal studies show risk. The risk of use outweighs any benefit.

II. Seizure disorders in pregnancy
A. Frequency. 1.0% of the population
1. 2.8 million in the United States, including 1.1 million women of reproductive age
2. In an unselected population, frequency should be 7–8 per 1000 deliveries ($1000 \times 0.01\% \times \frac{9}{12}$).
B. Heredity
1. 2–5% if parent is affected with "idiopathic" epilepsy

Table 57-1. Evaluating neurologic conditions in pregnancy.

Test	Risk to mother	Risk to fetus	Contraindications
MRI	None	None known	Metal, cardiac pacemaker, otologic implant
MRI with gadolinium	None	None known	Same as above
CT	None	Minimal*	None
CT with contrast	None	Minimal*	Dye allergy
Angiography	Minimal in most centers	Minimal*	Dye allergy
Lumbar puncture	None	None	Incipient herniation or mass lesion
Ultrasound	None	None	None
EEG	None	None	None
NCV/EMG	None	None	None
Tensilon test	Minimal	Minimal	Heart failure
Visual fields	None	None	None
Dilated eye examination	None	None with punctal occlusion	Incipient glaucoma
Fluorescein angiogram	None	Minimal	Allergies

*Abdominal shielding.

      a. Relatively higher if mother
      b. Relatively lower if father
   2. No significant transmission if disease is acquired
C. Natural history in pregnancy
   1. Best figures for disease activity during pregnancy are:
      a. Improved, 22%
      b. Exacerbated, 24% (most likely to occur in the first trimester)
      c. No change, 54%
   2. Postulated mechanisms for changes in frequency during pregnancy include:
      a. Physiologic
         (1) Hormonal
         (2) Metabolic
      b. Sleep deprivation
      c. Noncompliance
      d. Pharmacokinetic decreases in drug levels
      e. Folate supplementation
      f. Stress/anxiety
      g. Alcohol or other drug use
   3. Seizure frequency during pregnancy does not correlate with:
      a. Maternal age
      b. Seizure type(s)
      c. Drug regimen
      d. Seizure frequency in previous pregnancies
D. Therapeutic options
   1. Pharmacologic
      a. Be certain of the diagnosis.
      b. Be familiar with and use the few drugs that are the most effective for the various types of seizures.
   2. Surgery, in general, should be addressed before or after pregnancy.
   3. General
      a. Maintain daily habits (meals, sleep, minimize stress)
      b. Avoid alcohol and sedatives
      c. Avoid hazardous situations
E. Drug dosages, plasma levels, and clinical management
   1. Anticonvulsant drug levels decline during pregnancy in almost all women. This does *not* equate with a need to increase dosage.

    a. Free drug. Equates with clinical status (seizure control and side effects)

    b. Total drug. Usual result

    c. With the exception of valproic acid, the average decline in free levels is less than that for total levels. In difficult cases, there is no substitute for obtaining free levels.

2. Frequency of levels

    a. Ideally, preconceptional total and free levels should be obtained.

    b. Obtain total levels every 2–3 months when:

        (1) Seizure types do not interfere with activities of daily life.

        (2) There are other, well-controlled forms of epilepsy.

    c. Obtain monthly free levels when:

        (1) Uncontrolled seizures interfere with activities of daily life during the year prior to conception.

        (2) Previously controlled seizures recur during pregnancy.

        (3) Seizures are controlled but total drug levels decrease by more than 50% on routine screens.

3. Changing drug dosage

    a. Reasons not to change dosage

        (1) Declining total drug levels in a woman with well-controlled seizures (unless >30% decline in free levels and a history of poor control)

        (2) A woman taking two or more drugs discovers that she is pregnant (the time to change to monotherapy is preconceptional).

    b. Reasons to change dosage

        (1) Increased tonic-clonic seizures

        (2) Complex partial or other seizure types that interfere with activities of daily life and the patient wants better control

        (3) A decline of more than 60% in total level (75% for valproate) or a decline of more than 30% in free levels in a seizure-free patient who has had seizures within the year before becoming pregnant

        (4) Troublesome or disabling side effects

    c. It is reasonable to stop medications if a patient has been seizure-free for more than 2 years.

4. Antiepileptic drugs used in pregnancy

    a. Phenobarbital (risk factor D)

        (1) Dosage. 1–2 mg/kg/day; 90–120 mg/day

        (2) Indications. Generalized seizures

        (3) Problems. Sedation

    b. Phenytoin (risk factor D)

        (1) Dosage. 4–5 mg/kg/day; 300–400 mg/day

        (2) Indications. Generalized seizures

        (3) Problems. Levels need to be followed; may be low in early pregnancy and frequently high in the immediate puerperium

    c. Primidone (risk factor D)

        (1) Dosage. 250 mg tid

        (2) Indications. Generalized and partial complex seizures

        (3) Problems. Folate deficiency

    d. Carbamazepine (risk factor C)

        (1) Dosage. 10–30 mg/kg/day

        (2) Indications. Partial complex and generalized seizures

        (3) Problems. Possible 0.5% risk of fetal neural tube defects; otherwise, few

    e. Valproic acid (risk factor D)

        (1) Dosage. 15–60 mg/kg/day

        (2) Indications. Generalized seizures

        (3) Problems. Approximately 1% risk of fetal neural tube defects

    f. Lamotrigine (risk factor C)

        (1) Dosage

        (2) Indications. Adjunctive therapy for partial seizures

        (3) Problems. Decreased folate in fetal rats; thus may have a risk of neural tube defects equivalent to those of other anticonvulsants.

    g. Felbamate (risk factor C)

        (1) Dosage. 300–400 mg tid

        (2) Indications. Partial onset with secondary generalized seizures or Lennox-Gastaut syndrome

(3) Problems. Aplastic anemia
h. Gabapentin (risk factor C)
  (1) Dosage. 300–600 mg tid
  (2) Indications. Adjunctive for generalized seizures
  (3) Problems. Renal clearance
5. Other drugs to add or consider for patients with epilepsy
  a. Folic acid
    (1) Requirements are further increased because of malabsorption, competitive metabolism, and increased hepatic metabolism.
    (2) Increased supplementation may precipitate seizures by lowering anticonvulsant levels.
    (3) Best advice is to maintain usual supplementation.
  b. Vitamin K should be administered (10 mg IM) to all pregnant women receiving antiepileptic drugs beginning 1–3 weeks before expected delivery until birth to minimize the risk of neonatal hemorrhage.
  c. Vitamin D
    (1) Anticonvulsants can induce clinical osteomalacia and rickets or, more commonly, asymptomatic hypocalcemia.
    (2) Unlikely to be of clinical significance in well-nourished women
    (3) Not routinely supplemented
6. Anticonvulsant teratogenesis
  a. Fetal hydantoin syndrome occurs in 3–5% of epileptic women, and can be observed in association with any anticonvulsant medication.
    (1) Craniofacial and digital dysmorphic changes
    (2) Growth deficiency
    (3) Microcephaly
    (4) Cardiac defects
    (5) Mental retardation
  b. Other factors that may explain the increased incidence of anomalies in infants of epileptic mothers are as follows.
    (1) Increased incidence of anomalies in infants of epileptic mothers not taking medication. The only anomalies that are more common in phenytoin-exposed fetuses are hypertelorism and digital hypoplasia.
    (2) Increased incidence of characteristic malformations in infants of epileptic fathers, described as being intermediate between treated and untreated epileptic mothers
    (3) A specific metabolic defect may predispose to damage:
      (a) Epoxide hydrolase deficiency—teratogenic in animals
      (b) Inherited as autosomal codominant
      (c) Correlates highly with the incidence of fetal anomalies
    (4) Epilepsy may represent an underlying genetic disease.
    (5) The defects may result from a relative folate deficiency. (Folate antagonists are known abortifacients/teratogens.)
  c. Valproic acid and neural tube defects
    (1) Risk is 1–2%.
    (2) The relative risk is dosage-related.
    (3) If the drug is absolutely necessary for seizure control, the patient should be offered maternal serum alphafetoprotein (MSAFP) and ultrasound (US) screening.
    (4) Women of reproductive age who are taking valproic acid should receive folate supplementation.
    (5) Carbamazepine may be associated with an intermediate increased risk (~0.5%).
  d. Trimethadione is clearly teratogenic and is contraindicated in pregnancy.
7. Breast-feeding
  a. Most anticonvulsants cross into breast milk, although in low levels. Ratios between concentrations in breast milk and serum include:
    (1) Phenytoin, 0.10
    (2) Carbamazepine, 0.41
    (3) Phenobarbital, 0.39
  b. Contraindications to breast-feeding include:
    (1) Poorly controlled maternal seizures

(2) An initially hungry infant who rapidly becomes somnolent, suggesting a drug effect

F. Onset of seizures during pregnancy—differential diagnosis

1. Tumor

a. Especially likely to present in the first trimester

b. Meningiomas tend to expand during pregnancy.

2. Arteriovenous malformation

3. Cortical venous thrombosis—especially late in pregnancy and in the immediate puerperium

4. Gestational epilepsy

a. A diagnosis of exclusion

b. Represents only a small fraction of all women who have their initial seizures while pregnant

5. Rule out eclampsia.

G. Status epilepticus during pregnancy

1. Less than 1% of all epileptics during pregnancy

2. Not an indication for termination of pregnancy

3. Management should include:

a. Hospitalization

b. Secure the airway.

c. IV access with normal saline and B vitamins

d. Baseline lab studies including electrolytes, CBC, glucose, calcium, and arterial blood gases

e. Maternal and fetal vital signs (VS), including ECG and fetal heart rate monitoring

f. Glucose bolus (50 ml of D50)

g. Thiamine (100 mg IM or IV)

h. Begin IV diazepam (5–15 mg IV in 5-mg boluses) or lorazepam (0.1 mg/kg IV, not to exceed 2 mg/min) and phenytoin (18 mg/kg, not to exceed 50 mg/min, with ECG and BP monitoring, administered in non-glucose-containing fluids).

i. If seizures persist, intubate and begin either IV phenobarbital (15 mg/kg, not to exceed 100 mg/min) or diazepam.

j. If seizures still persist, institute general anesthesia with halothane and neuromuscular junction (NMJ) blockade.

III. Headache

A. The **most common diagnoses** in headache clinics are:

1. Migraine

a. Unilateral or bilateral throbbing headaches associated with photophobia, phonophobia, nausea, and/or vomiting

b. Particularly prominent in women of reproductive age

2. Tension

a. All day, worse in the evening, local soreness, frequently commences in the neck and/or back of the head

b. Not associated with nausea or vomiting

3. Depression is often worse in the morning, and often accompanied by other symptoms of depression.

B. Most patients with headaches do *not* have underlying structural disease, but remember:

1. Signs and symptoms may be helpful in identifying the patient with evolving structural disease:

a. Sleep disturbances

b. Exertional headaches

c. Adult-onset paroxysmal headaches

2. Brain tumor (intermittent, dull, nonthrobbing, exacerbated by exercise, associated with nausea or vomiting)

3. Subarachnoid hemorrhage. Sudden onset of the worst headache of one's life

C. Migraine in pregnancy

1. The majority of women with migraine improve when pregnant. This is especially true of:

a. Menstrual migraine

b. Migraine onset at menarche

2. Approximately 10–20% get worse or have the initial onset during pregnancy, usually in the first trimester.
3. Migraineurs have no increased risk of complications during pregnancy, but headaches usually recur in the puerperium.
4. **Differential diagnosis** of migraine occurring for the first time in pregnancy includes:
   a. Intracranial hemorrhage
   b. Cerebral venous thrombosis
   c. Intracranial hypertension
   d. Severe preeclampsia
5. **Treatments**
   a. **Nonmedication treatments**
      (1) Avoidance of dietary/environmental trigger factors
      (2) Biofeedback, relaxation therapy, massage
      (3) Physical therapy
      (4) Heat/ice packs
   b. **Acute medication treatment principles**
      (1) Prevent nausea (Table 57-2).
      (2) Treat pain (Table 57-3).
      (3) Sedation (Table 57-4)
   c. **Prophylactic treatment.** In general, avoid daily medications, but if headaches are too severe or interfere excessively with life, daily treatment may be required. In general, monotherapy should be attempted. The lowest dosage should be encouraged. See Table 57-5.

IV. Tumors
   A. Incidence
      1. Probably less than 100 per year nationwide
      2. Pregnancy does not increase the risk of brain tumors but does increase the likelihood of symptomatology.
      3. The types of tumors are identical to those observed in nonpregnant women of the same age—primarily gliomas (32%), meningiomas (29%), acoustic neuromas (15%), and others (24%).
   B. Clinical features
      1. Headache
      2. Nausea and vomiting
      3. Focal deficits and/or seizures
   C. Diagnosis
      1. MR with contrast (gadolinium)
      2. CT with contrast
   D. Treatment
      1. **Dexamethasone (risk factor C)**
         a. **Dosage.** 6 mg q6h or 4 mg q4h
         b. **Problems.** Gastrointestinal; cushingoid changes with prolonged use
      2. **Mannitol** for acute swelling
   E. Pituitary tumors
      1. **Natural history**
         a. Microadenomas are rarely symptomatic (5%).
         b. Macroadenomas are symptomatic in 15–35% of cases.
      2. **Visual field evaluation** must be performed for macroadenomas.
      3. **Treatment**

Table 57-2. Acute migraine treatment in pregnancy: Nausea prevention.

Drug	Dosage	FDA schedule	Side effects
Promethazine (PO, PR, IM)	25–75 mg	C: trimester 1	—
		B: trimester 2–3	—
Hydroxyzine (PO, IM)	25–75 mg	C	Fatigue
Prochlorperazine (PO, PR, IM, IV)	10–25 mg	C	Dystonic reaction
Trimethobenzamide (PO, PR)	—	C	—
Chlorpromazine	25 mg	C	Dystonic reaction
Metoclopramide	5–10 mg	B	Dystonic reaction

Table 57-3. Acute migraine treatment in pregnancy: Pain treatment.

Drug	Dosage	FDA schedule	Side effects
Acetaminophen	350–500 mg	B	—
Aspirin	325–650 mg	C	Bleeding diathesis, in utero closure of ductus arteriosus, oligohydramnios
Caffeinated compounds	—	B	—
Butalbital-acetaminophen	—	C	Possible neonatal withdrawal with heavy use
Isometheptene (Midrin)	Two at onset, then one/hour to maximum of five/24 hours	Not established	—
NSAIDs*:			
Ibuprofen	200–800 mg	B	—
Naproxen	200–500 mg	B	—
Sumatriptan	—	C	—
Butorphanol	—	B	—
Narcotic (use with antiemetic):			
Meperidine	50–100 mg	B	Nausea
Ergotamine (DHE or ergotamine)	Avoid	X	Possible abortifacient

*NSAIDs = nonsteroidal anti-inflammatory drugs.

    a. Bromocriptine may be taken throughout pregnancy if tumor enlarges.
    b. If vision is threatened, surgical treatment is appropriate.
  4. Sheehan's syndrome involves pituitary infarction, frequently associated with tumor.
    a. Presents as failure to lactate, hypopituitarism, hypothyroidism
    b. Treatment involves steroid and thyroid replacement.
V. Pseudotumor cerebri (benign intracranial hypertension) is characterized by increased intracranial pressure not caused by an intracranial space-occupying lesion demonstrable by MRI or CT. Pregnancy does not cause pseudotumor cerebri. However, it can present during pregnancy. Pregnancy does not by itself cause visual loss. Pseudotumor cerebri does not cause miscarriage.
  A. Symptoms and signs
    1. Headache is the most common symptom (>90%). Patients are otherwise alert and healthy.
    2. Papilledema
    3. VI nerve palsy, and possibly VII nerve palsy
    4. Obesity
  B. Differential diagnosis of papilledema and no mass lesion in pregnancy
    1. Venous thrombosis

Table 57-4. Acute migraine treatment in pregnancy: Sedation.

Drug	Dosage	FDA schedule	Side effects
Chloral hydrate	500–1500 mg	C	—
Pentobarbital	—	D	Withdrawal
Hydroxyzine/promethazine	25–75 mg	C	—
Meperidine (plus antiemetic)	—	B	—
Diazepam	5–10 mg	D	—
Lorazepam	—	D	—
Clonazepam	0.5–1.0 mg	C	—
Chlorpromazine	25–50 mg	C	—

Table 57-5. Migraine prophylaxis in pregnancy.

Drug	Dosage	FDA schedule	Side effects/comments
Beta-blockers:			
Propranolol	20–80 mg	C	Intrauterine growth retardation (IUGR),* prematurity, hypotension
Nadolol	10–40 mg	C	—
Timolol	10–30 mg	C	—
Tricyclic antidepressants:			
Amitriptyline	10–75 mg	C-D	Limb deformities
Nortriptyline	10–75 mg	D	—
Imipramine	10–75 mg	D	—
Desipramine	—	C	—
Cyproheptadine	4 mg tid	B	Weight gain; occasionally effective
Calcium channel blockers:			
Verapamil	—	C	—
Nifedipine	—	C	—

*Contraindicated drugs: methysergide, valproic acid.

    2. Venous hypertension
    3. Meningitis
    4. Syphilis
  C. Evaluation must include an imaging procedure (MRI or CT), cerebrospinal fluid (CSF) with opening pressure, and CSF constituents. Because the greatest threat to the patient is visual loss, visual acuity and visual field examinations must be followed frequently.
  D. Treatment options
    1. Medical treatment
      a. Weight loss
      b. Frequent lumbar puncture (LP)
        (1) Safe
        (2) Painful, often difficult
      c. Acetazolamide (500–2000 mg) after the first trimester
      d. Steroids (prednisone, methylprednisolone)
    2. Surgical treatment
      a. Optic nerve sheath decompression is the preferred procedure to save vision.
      b. Lumbar peritoneal shunt can be problematic in a pregnant patient.
VI. Cerebrovascular disease
  A. Stroke or vascular occlusion. The causes of stroke during pregnancy are listed in Table 57-6.
    1. Arterial
      a. Characteristically presents with paresis but without altered consciousness or seizures
      b. Represents 90% of strokes during pregnancy
    2. Venous
      a. Characteristically presents with headache, seizures, increased intracranial pressure, and alteration of consciousness
      b. Represents 80% of strokes during puerperium
    3. Intracranial hemorrhage characteristically presents with sudden onset of headache, loss of consciousness, and accompanying signs of neck stiffness and altered blood pressure.
    4. Diagnosis
      a. CT scan
      b. Angiography
      c. Cardiac evaluation
      d. Appropriate laboratory studies
    5. Treatment is directed at the underlying cause.
      a. Heparin does not cross the placenta and can therefore be used safely

Table 57-6. Causes of stroke in pregnancy.

   I. Arterial occlusive disease
     A. Thrombotic cause
       1. Atherosclerotic
       2. Fibromuscular dysplasia
     B. Embolic source
       1. Cardiac
         a. Peripartum cardiomyopathy
         b. Mitral valve prolapse
         c. Rheumatic heart disease
         d. Endocarditis (bacterial and nonbacterial)
         e. Paradoxical embolus
       2. Amniotic/air embolism
  II. Venous occlusive disease
     A. Hypercoagulable state
     B. Infection
 III. Drug abuse
 IV. Hypotensive disorders
     A. Watershed infarction
     B. Sheehan's pituitary necrosis
  V. Hematologic disorders
     A. Lupus anticoagulant
     B. Thrombocytopenic purpura
     C. Sickle cell disease
     D. Protein C, antithrombin III, protein S deficiencies
 VI. Arteritis
     A. Systemic lupus erythematosus
     B. Infectious arteritis (syphilis, tuberculosis, meningococcal)
     C. Cerebral angiitis
     D. Takayasu's arteritis
 VII. Intracerebral hemorrhage
     A. Eclampsia and hypertensive disorders
     B. Venous thrombosis
     C. Choriocarcinoma
     D. Arteriovenous malformation
     E. Vasculitis
VIII. Subarachnoid hemorrhage
     A. Aneurysm (saccular, mycotic)
     B. Arteriovenous malformation (cerebral, spinal cord)
     C. Eclampsia
     D. Vasculitis
     E. Choriocarcinoma
     F. Venous thrombosis
 IX. Other
     A. Carotid cavernous fistula
     B. Dural vascular malformation

---

        during pregnancy.
     b. Warfarin crosses the placenta and is contraindicated during pregnancy. However, it can be used when breast-feeding.
     c. Low-dosage aspirin (<80 mg/day) can be used safely in pregnancy when clinically indicated.
  B. Cerebral venous thrombosis
     1. Occurs primarily postpartum, with signs and symptoms including:
       a. Headache
       b. Seizures
       c. Hemiplegia

     d. Papilledema
     e. Obtundation/coma
    2. Diagnosis is now optimum by means of MRI.
    3. Treatment
     a. Correction of predisposing factors
     b. Control of seizures
     c. Use of antiedema agents
     d. Anticoagulation (see secs. **VI.A.5.a–c,** above)
   C. Drug abuse
   D. Hematologic disorders
    1. Anticardiolipin antibody syndrome is associated most frequently with recurrent miscarriage and severe preeclampsia/eclampsia.
    2. Sickle cell disease
    3. Deficiencies of antithrombin III, or protein C or S
   E. Subarachnoid hemorrhage. (See Table 57-7 for differentiating causes.)
    1. Intracranial aneurysm
     a. Thought to be present in 1% of all women of reproductive age
     b. A significant contributor to maternal mortality
     c. Rupture is probably equally likely throughout pregnancy.
     d. More likely to occur in older, parous women
     e. Diagnosis requires CT scan (and LP) and angiography.
     f. Optimum outcomes occur with surgical correction.
     g. Avoid nitroprusside because of its cyanide effect on the fetus. Hypertension may be controlled with verapamil or nimodipine.
     h. Vaginal delivery should be anticipated after successful clipping unless obstetric contraindications exist. If delivery occurs before clipping, cesarean section or forceps delivery with epidural anesthesia is indicated.

Table 57-7. Differentiating causes of subarachnoid hemorrhage.

Clinical features	Aneurysm	Arteriovenous malformation	Eclampsia
Age	25–37 (increases with age)	15–20 (younger)	Any age
Headache	Severe	May be severe	60% frontal
Parity	Multiparous	Primiparous	Both
Epigastric pain	−	−	+
Nausea/vomiting	+/−	+/−	+
Trimester	3rd	3rd	2nd–3rd
Loss of consciousness	⅓–⅔	⅓–⅔	All
Nuchal rigidity	Prominent	May be present	Rare
Seizure	15–30%	Present	100%
Hypertension	30–50%	After bleed	90% >140/90
Proteinuria	30%	14%	All
Focal weakness	20%	Frequent	Rare
Cerebrospinal fluid	Blood	Blood	Clear/some blood
Recurrent hemorrhage	Less than 2 weeks	+	No
Subsequent pregnancy	Good if mother treated	+++	May recur, especially with predisposing causes
Prognosis	Mother treated: 11% maternal mortality and 5% fetal mortality. Mother untreated: 63% maternal mortality and 27% fetal mortality	Recurrence untreated = 32% maternal mortality	Good if mother delivered. Fetus— variable, depends on gestational age

    i. Vasospasm can be treated with nimodipine; volume expansion must be monitored.

  j. Outcome

    (1) Grades 1–3. With expedited surgery, expect 95% successful outcome.

    (2) Grade 4. 45–75% mortality

    (3) Fetal outcomes. 27% mortality rate without surgery

  k. Subsequent pregnancies after successful clipping have good prognoses.

  l. Asymptomatic aneurysm should be treated if greater than 7 mm in diameter.

2. Arteriovenous malformation

  a. Characteristically occurs in younger, less parous women

  b. Diagnosis requires CT scan (and LP) and angiography.

  c. Should be corrected, if possible, surgically and/or embolically

  d. Stereotactic radiotherapy is not indicated during pregnancy.

  e. Vaginal delivery epidural: low-outlet forceps

3. Eclampsia/severe preeclampsia

  a. Definition

    (1) 5–7% of pregnancies

    (2) Severe preeclampsia

    (3) Eclampsia

    (4) HELLP syndrome

  b. Symptomatology and physical findings

    (1) Headache, dizziness, scotomata, nausea, vomiting

    (2) Generalized edema

    (3) Fundoscopic findings: segmental vasospasm, serous retinal detachment

    (4) Neurologic finding: hyperreflexia

    (5) Bedside testing: Amsler grid for detection of scotomata

  c. CT and MRI findings

    (1) CT. Edema 75%, hemorrhage 9%

    (2) MRI. Severe preeclampsia: deep white matter T_2 signals; eclampsia: T_2 signals at gray-white matter junctions (particularly in the parietal/occipital areas), cortical edema, hemorrhage

  d. Treatment

    (1) Delivery

    (2) Magnesium sulfate

    (3) Antihypertensive medications: hydralazine

    (4) Anticonvulsants: diphenylhydantoin

    (5) Nimodipine

    (6) Treat cerebral edema or herniation with hyperventilation, steroids, or mannitol after delivery.

  e. Postpartum eclampsia

  f. Outcome

    (1) Recent maternal mortality rates: 1–5%

    (2) Recent perinatal mortality rates: 13–30%

  g. Complications

    (1) Intracranial hemorrhage

    (2) Congestive heart failure

    (3) Intrahepatic hemorrhage

VII. Multiple sclerosis (MS)

  A. MS does not affect pregnancy per se, or vice versa.

    1. Patients who have sphincter disturbances or are paraplegic may experience increased difficulties during pregnancy.

    2. There is no evidence of vertical transmission.

  B. There is an increased incidence of exacerbations in the first 3–6 months postpartum.

  C. Treatment of acute MS in pregnancy

    1. Steroids (see Ch. 40, sec. **V.B.1**)

    2. Betaseron is not yet established for use in pregnancy.

VIII. Paraplegia

  A. Pregnancy is associated with increased risks of:

    1. Urinary tract infections

    2. Pressure sores

B. Labor progresses normally. Maternal perception depends on the level of the block:

1. Above T10: painless
2. Below T10: painful

C. Autonomic hyperreflexia

1. Occurs only if the block is at or above T5-T6
2. Develops in association with excessive activity of any viscus (i.e., labor)
3. Characteristic signs and symptoms include:
   a. Throbbing headache
   b. Hypertension
   c. Reflex bradycardia
   d. Sweating
   e. Nasal congestion
   f. Cutaneous vasodilatation and piloerection above the level of the lesion
4. Symptoms are caused by the sudden release of catecholamines, so treatment may include reserpine, atropine, clonidine, glyceryl trinitrate, or hexamethonium.
5. May be misdiagnosed as preeclampsia

IX. Root lesions and peripheral neuropathies

A. Lumbar disk

1. Signs and symptoms are the same as in nonpregnant patients.
2. Generally treated nonoperatively. Consider surgery if:
   a. Bilateral symptoms
   b. Disturbance of sphincter function

B. Carpal tunnel syndrome

1. Pain and paresthesias commonly are worse at night and also tend to be worse in the dominant hand.
2. Tinel's sign
3. Symptoms usually respond to nocturnal wrist splinting and resolve within 3 months postpartum.

C. Bell's palsy

1. Facial paresis of lower motor neuron type when no other specific etiologic agent can be found. Signs and symptoms include:
   a. Abrupt onset, often with pain around the ear
   b. The face feels stiff and pulled to one side.
   c. Difficulty closing the eye on the affected side
   d. Taste disturbances
   e. Hyperacusis
2. About three times more likely to occur during pregnancy, primarily in the third trimester or immediately on initiation of puerperium
3. Steroids are probably effective if given within the first 5–7 days. Surgery is ineffective.

D. Other cranial nerve palsies

1. Nerve IV
2. Nerve VI

E. Meralgia paresthetica

1. Causes numbness in the lateral aspect of the thigh
2. Usually resolves within 3 months postpartum

F. Sciatica and back pain. Lumbosacral disk surgery should be reserved only for progressive atrophy or bowel/bladder dysfunction.

G. Guillain-Barré syndrome

1. Causes are not generally affected by pregnancy.
2. Labor and delivery are otherwise normal.

X. Myasthenia gravis (MG)

A. Variable weakness and fatigability of skeletal muscles, resulting from defective neuromuscular transmission (reduced acetylcholine receptors in the neuromuscular junction)

B. Does not affect labor progress, except for voluntary efforts in the second stage

C. Certain drugs should be avoided, including:

1. Ester anesthetics: tetracaine (Pontocaine), chloroprocaine (Nesacaine)
2. Curare (and other nondepolarizing muscle relaxants)
3. Halothane (Fluothane)
4. Aminoglycoside antibiotics
5. Quinine and quinidine

6. Magnesium sulfate. The antidote is edrophonium (Tensilon), not calcium.
D. Treatment
  1. Antepartum
    a. Pregnancy per se does not affect the severity of preexisting disease.
    b. Perinatal mortality is increased because of an increased risk of premature delivery as well as neonatal myasthenia.
    c. Pharmacologic treatment of MG is not altered by pregnancy.
  2. Intrapartum
    a. Oral medications should be discontinued at the onset of labor and their intramuscular equivalents continued until oral medications can again be ingested. Equipotent dosages are:
      (1) Neostigmine 0.5 mg IV
      (2) Neostigmine 0.7–1.5 mg IM
      (3) Neostigmine 15 mg PO
      (4) Pyridostigmine 60 mg PO
    b. Analgesia and anesthesia for labor require the utmost caution because of the risks of respiratory depression and/or aspiration.
    c. MG does not affect the progress of labor and is not an indication for cesarean section.
  3. Postpartum
    a. Exacerbations are more likely to occur postpartum and tend to be sudden and severe in their onset.
    b. Women with severe disease or whose babies become symptomatic after nursing should not breast-feed.
    c. Most women return to their preconceptional oral dosages, with modest increases in dosage to allow for the additional stresses of early parenthood.
E. Neonatal myasthenia
  1. Occurs in 10–15% of cases
  2. Results from transplacental transfer of maternal antibody against acetylcholine receptors
XI. Myotonic dystrophy
  A. Clinical characteristics
    1. Autosomal dominant
    2. Weakness and wasting in muscles of face, neck, and distal limb
    3. Myotonia of hands and tongue
    4. Variable age of onset. Mothers are sometimes diagnosed only after an affected child is born.
    5. Predisposed to cardiac arrhythmias
    6. Treatment
      a. Dystrophy: none
      b. Myotonia: phenytoin (Dilantin), quinine, procainamide
  B. Effects on pregnancy
    1. Increased spontaneous abortion
    2. Increased premature labor and polyhydramnios
    3. Normal first stage of labor
    4. Normal response to oxytocin
    5. Prolonged second stage of labor
  C. Labor management
    1. Outlet forceps
    2. Regional anesthesia
    3. Avoid succinylcholine.
      a. May cause hyperthermia
      b. Nonpolarizing agents are safe.

Recommended Readings

Berg G, et al. Low back pain during pregnancy. *Obstet Gynecol* 71:71–75, 1988.

Bernardi S, et al. The influence of pregnancy on relapses in multiple sclerosis: A cohort study. *Acta Neurol Scand* 84:403–406, 1991.

Birk K, et al. The clinical course of multiple sclerosis during pregnancy and the puerperium. *Arch Neurol* 47:738–742, 1990.

Branch DW. Antiphospholipid antibodies and pregnancy: Maternal implications. *Semin Perinatol* 14:139–146, 1990.

Briggs GG, Freeman RK, Yaffe SJ. *Drugs in Pregnancy and Lactation* (3rd ed). Baltimore: Williams & Wilkins, 1990.

Carr SC, et al. Antenatal treatment of myasthenia gravis. *Obstet Gynecol* 78:485–489, 1991.

Chanceller MD, Wroe SJ. Migraine occurring for the first time during pregnancy. *Headache* 30:224–227, 1990.

Cornelissen M, et al. Supplementation of vitamin K in pregnant women receiving anticonvulsant therapy prevents neonatal vitamin K deficiency. *Am J Obstet Gynecol* 168:884–888, 1993.

Davis RK, Maslow AS. Multiple sclerosis in pregnancy: A review. *Obstet Gynecol Surv* 47:290–296, 1992.

Dias MS, Sekhar LN. Intracranial hemorrhage from aneurysms and arteriovenous malformations during pregnancy and the puerperium. *Neurosurgery* 27:855–866, 1990.

Digre KB, Varner MW. Diagnosis and treatment of cerebrovascular disorders in pregnancy. In HP Adams (ed), *Handbook of Cerebrovascular Diseases*. New York: Marcel Dekker, 1993. Pp 258–286.

Digre KB, Varner MW, Corbett JJ. Pseudotumor cerebri and pregnancy. *Neurology* 34:721–729, 1984.

Digre KB, et al. Cranial MR imaging in severe preeclampsia versus eclampsia. *Arch Neurol* 50:399–406, 1993.

Donaldson JO. *Neurology of Pregnancy.* London: Saunders, 1989.

Goldstein PJ (ed). *Neurological Disorders of Pregnancy.* New York: Futura, 1986.

Holcomb W, Petrie R. Cerebrovascular emergencies in pregnancy. *Clin Obstet Gynecol* 33:467–472, 1990.

Jaffe R, et al. Myotonic dystrophy and pregnancy: A review. *Obstet Gynecol Surv* 41:272–278, 1986.

Maymon R, Fejgin M. Intracranial hemorrhage during pregnancy and puerperium. *Obstet Gynecol Surv* 45:157–179, 1990.

Nygaard I, Bartscht K, Cole S. Sexuality and reproduction in spinal cord injured women. *Obstet Gynecol Surv* 45:727–732, 1990.

O'Brien MD, Gilmour-White S. Epilepsy and pregnancy. *Br Med J* 307:492–495, 1993.

Omtzigt JCG, et al. The risk of spina bifida aperta after first-trimester exposure to valproate in a prenatal cohort. *Neurology* 42:119–125, 1992.

Perry K. The diagnosis and management of hemoglobinopathies during pregnancy. *Semin Perinatol* 14:90–102, 1990.

Peterson CM, Kelly JV. Pseudotumor cerebri in pregnancy. Case reports and review of literature. *Obstet Gynecol Surv* 40:323–329, 1985.

Plauche WC. Myasthenia gravis in mothers and their newborns. *Clin Obstet Gynecol* 34:82–99, 1991.

Ratinahirana H, Darbois Y, Bousser MG. Migraine and pregnancy: A prospective study in 703 women after delivery. *Neurology* 40(suppl 1):437, 1990.

Roelvink NCA, et al. Pregnancy-related primary brain and spinal tumors. *Arch Neurol* 44:209–215, 1987.

Rosa F. Spina bifida in infants of women treated with carbamazepine during pregnancy. *N Engl J Med* 324:674–677, 1991.

Simolke G, Cox S, Cunningham FG. Cerebrovascular accidents complicating pregnancy and the puerperium. *Obstet Gynecol* 78:37–42, 1991.

Simon RH. Brain tumors in pregnancy. *Semin Neurol* 8:214–221, 1988.

Uknis A, Silberstein SD. Review article: Migraine and pregnancy. *Headache* 31:372–374, 1991.

Varner MW, Digre KB. Myasthenia gravis. In CB Coulam, WP Faulk, JA McIntyre (eds), *Immunological Obstetrics*. London: Norton, 1992. Pp 666–676.

Wand JS. Carpal tunnel syndrome in pregnancy and lactation. *J Hand Surg* 15:93–95, 1990.

Yerby MS. Pregnancy and epilepsy. *Epilepsia* 32(suppl 6):51–59, 1991.

Yerby MS, Freil PN, McCormich K. Antiepileptic drug disposition during pregnancy. *Neurology* 42:12–16, 1992.

Appendixes

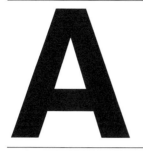

Clinical Signs and Ancillary Diagnostic Studies for Delirium

John C. Andrefsky
Jeffrey I. Frank

↓ LOC = decreased level of consciousness; ↑ = increased; ↓ = decreased; NR = nuchal rigidity; HA = headache; N/V = nausea and vomiting; FNF = focal neurologic findings.

Etiology	Clinical comments	Laboratory diagnosis	Neuroimaging and other diagnostics
Systemic infection (including sepsis, pneumonia, etc.)	Can cause ↓ LOC; fever; hypotension; tachycardia; symptoms and signs of local infection	*Laboratory*—↑ peripheral WBC; metabolic acidosis (sepsis); respiratory alkalosis and hypoxia (pneumonia); pyuria (urinary tract infections)	
Bacterial meningitis	Can cause ↓ LOC; HA; NR; seizures; rarely FNF; fever; hypotension; tachycardia	*Laboratory*—↑ peripheral WBC *Lumbar puncture*— ↑ WBC 100–100,000 cells/cm³; neutrophils 85–95%; protein usually >100 mg/dl; glucose <50% serum; (+) Gram stain and cultures; ↑ CSF pressure	*CT scan*—early: normal; later: with enlarged ventricles secondary to communicating hydrocephalus *MRI scan*—early: T1-weighted images (T1WI) with gadolinium with meningeal enhancement
Tuberculous meningitis	Can cause ↓ LOC; ocular palsies; HA; NR; FNF; evidence of systemic tuberculosis; cough; weight loss	*Laboratory*—↓ serum sodium (SIADH) *Lumbar puncture*— ↑ WBC 50–500 cells/cm³; early: neutrophils and lymphocytes; later: lymphocytes; protein 100–200 mg/dl; glucose <40 mg/dl; (+) culture (may take weeks to become positive); ↑ CSF pressure	*CT scan*—with plaquelike dural thickening or dural calcifications around basilar cisterns
Cryptococcal meningitis	Subacute onset of HA; NR may be lacking; ataxia; spastic paraparesis; usually without FNF; fever; cough if	*Laboratory*—↓ serum sodium (SIADH) *Lumbar puncture*— ↑ WBC <500 cells/cm³, usually lymphocytes;	*CT scan*—usually not useful, but can identify hydrocephalus when present *MRI scan*—T2-weighted images (T2WI) with multifocal basal ganglia

Etiology	Clinical comments	Laboratory diagnosis	Neuroimaging and other diagnostics
	respiratory involvement	↑ protein; glucose <50 mg/dl; (+) culture; (+) India ink prep and cryptococcal antigen; ↑ CSF pressure	and midbrain hyperintensities that represent cryptococcomas
Meningeal syphilis	Confusion may occur anytime within 2 years of inoculation; cranial nerve palsies; NR; N/V if hydrocephalus present; seizures; afebrile	*Laboratory*—(+) RPR suggests active syphilis, but high false negative and false positive rate; (+) MHA-TP or FTA-ABS implies prior syphilitic infection *Lumbar puncture*— ↑ WBC 200–300 cells/cm³, mostly lymphs; ↑ protein 40–200 mg/dl; glucose normal; (+) CSF VDRL, but high false negative rate	
Tertiary syphilis	Insidious onset of confusion 15–20 years after inoculation; dementia; Argyll-Robertson pupils; dysarthria; myoclonic jerks; action tremor; seizures	*Laboratory*—see meningeal syphilis *Lumbar puncture*— ↑ WBC 10–200 cells/cm³, mostly lymphs; ↑ protein 40–200 mg/dl; (+) CSF VDRL, but high false negative rate	
Herpes simplex encephalitis (HSE)	Confusion over days; ocular palsies; occasional NR; ataxia; seizures; hemiparesis; fever	*Lumbar puncture*— ↑ WBC 10–500 cells/cm³ (usually <200), mostly lymphocytes; ↑ RBC up to the thousands; ↑ protein; normal to slightly ↓ glucose; virus is rarely isolated from the CSF, but PCR can be helpful	*CT scan*—early: normal or with low attenuation in the temporal lobe with mass effect *MRI scan*—early: T1WI with gyral edema; T2WI with high signal in the temporal lobe *EEG*—with periodic (2–3/second) lateralizing epileptiform discharges (PLEDS) over the temporal regions
Progressive multifocal leukoencephalopathy (PML)	Confusion over days to weeks; dementia; aphasia; hemiparesis; quadriparesis	*Lumbar puncture*— usually normal but may have mildly ↑ protein	*CT scan*—with nonenhancing areas of low attenuation in white matter *MRI scan*—T2WI with multifocal oval or round supratentorial and infratentorial white matter hyperintensities
Human immunodeficiency virus	Subacute onset of confusion; slowly or rapidly progressing dementia; ataxia of	*Laboratory*—(+) HIV serology *Lumbar puncture*— normal or have mild lymphocyto-	*CT scan*—with atrophy and multiple areas of low attenuation in deep white matter *MRI scan*—T2WI with

	gait and limbs; seizures	sis and mildly ↑ protein	diffuse, patchy, or confluent increased signal lesions
Brain abscess	HA; signs of ↑ CSF pressure; focal or generalized seizures; fever during suppurative phase	*Laboratory*—↑ peripheral WBC *Lumbar puncture**—moderately ↑ WBC mostly neutrophils; moderately ↑ RBC; ↑ protein; normal glucose; (+) cultures (50% of patients)	*CT scan*—early: normal or with subcortical low attenuation that later is better defined; (+) ring enhancement with contrast *MRI scan*—early: T2WI with subcortical hypointensity; later: with central area becoming hyperintense; T1WI with gadolinium with intense rim enhancement
Epidural abscess	NR; fever; malaise	*Laboratory*—↑ peripheral WBC *Lumbar puncture**—mildly ↑ WBC; mildly ↑ protein; cultures usually normal	*CT scan*—with large volume of fluid between cranium and dura; contrast may enhance dura and detectability of more subtle epidural fluid collections
Subdural empyema	Confusion preceded by HA; can cause ↓ LOC; aphasia; NR; N/V; focal seizures; hemiplegia; hemianesthesia; fever; malaise	*Laboratory*—↑ peripheral WBC *Lumbar puncture*—↑ WBC 50–1000 cells/cm^3, mostly neutrophils; ↑ protein 75–300 mg/dl; normal glucose	*CT scan*—with low attenuation crescentic extraaxial fluid collections *MRI scan*—T2WI with a mildly hyperintense collection; gadolinium enhanced T1WI with a surrounding membrane
Toxoplasmosis	Acute onset of confusion; most asymptomatic; retinochoroiditis; NR; myoclonus; asterixis; seizures; neurologic manifestations very common in AIDS patients; can have fever; splenomegaly; if immunocompromised: myositis; fever; rash; myocarditis; pneumonitis; malaise; hepatomegaly	*Laboratory*—(+) serum antibody to toxoplasmosis *Lumbar puncture**—↑ WBC mostly lymphocytes; ↑ protein	*CT scan*—with solitary or multiple ring enhancing masses with contrast *MRI scan*—T1WI with multifocal hypointense lesions that are hyperintense on T2WI; T1WI with gadolinium usually with prominent rim enhancement of the lesions
Subacute spongiform encephalopathy (Creutzfeldt-Jakob disease)	Subacute delirium with rapid progression; behavioral changes; depression; myoclonic jerks lateralized at first then generalized; sleep disturbances; fatigue; weight loss	*Lumbar puncture*—normal	*EEG*—early: with diffuse and nonspecific slowing; later: with stereotyped high-voltage slow and sharp waves on a flat background *Brain biopsy*—with diffuse loss of neurons and vacuoles within glial cells and neurons
Whipple's disease	Subacute confusion; supra-	*Laboratory*—anemia; biopsy of je-	

Etiology	Clinical comments	Laboratory diagnosis	Neuroimaging and other diagnostics
	nuclear ophthal-moplegia; oculo-masticatory myo-rhythmia; myo-clonus; ataxia; seizures; hyper-somnia; fever; weight loss; ab-dominal pain; hyperpigmenta-tion; lymph-adenopathy	junal mucosa has macrophages filled with PAS-positive material *Lumbar puncture—* usually normal or ↑ WBC to 400 cells/cm^3, mostly monocytes; mod-erately ↑ protein; CSF histiocytes or macrophages laden with PAS-positive material are often present	
Acute dissemin-ated encephalo-myelitis (ADEM)	Acute onset of confusion; can cause ↓ LOC; HA; NR; myoclonic movements; choreoathetosis; ataxia; if spinal cord involve-ment then para-plegia; quadri-plegia; ↑ or ↓ deep tendon reflexes; variable degrees of bowel and bladder dysfunc-tion; fever; often postinfectious	*Lumbar puncture—* ↑ WBC 20–200 cells/cm^3, mostly lymphocytes; mildly ↑ protein <100 mg/dl; nor-mal glucose; ↑ CSF pressure (50% of patients)	*MRI scan—*T2WI with multifocal subcortical hyperintense foci; not all lesions enhance with gadolinium
Hypernatremia and hyperosmolality	Temporal profile of onset is vari-able; can cause ↓ LOC; hypoten-sion and tachy-cardia particu-larly when asso-ciated with vol-ume depleted state	*Laboratory—*con-fusion usually with serum osmo-lality ≥320 mOsm/kg of H$_2$O	
Hyponatremia and hypo-osmolality	Variable onset of confusion; can cause ↓ LOC; myo-clonus; seizures; generalized weakness	*Laboratory—*confu-sion usually with serum sodium <120 mEq/L	
Central pontine myelinolysis (CPM)	Confusion due to severe electro-lyte disturbance (hyponatremia); extreme hyper-osmolality or rapid correction of hyponatremia causes syndrome characterized by subacute quadri-plegia, variable	*Laboratory—*recent extreme hyperos-molality or rapid correction of hyponatremia of <130 mEq/L *Lumbar puncture—* normal (50% of patients) or mildly ↑ monocyte count; ↑ CSF pressure; ↑ protein	*CT scan—*normal or with low-attenuation white matter changes and cen-tral pontine cavitation *MRI scan—*T1WI with hypointense lesions and T2WI with hyperintense lesions; mostly nonen-hancing; the presence of pontine and basal gang-lia lesions is specific for CPM

	pseudobulbar palsy, and locked-in syndrome	
Hypokalemia	Areflexic paralysis; generalized weakness; cardiac arrhythmias; paralytic ileus; renal tubular damage; rhabdomyolysis; myoglobinuria	*Laboratory*—serum potassium <2.0 mEq/L
Hypercalcemia	Confusion; can cause ↓ LOC; depression; proximal weakness; restless leg syndrome; cardiac arrhythmias, asystole	*Laboratory*—confusion usually with calcium level >12 mg/dl; but variable symptomatic threshold
Hypophosphatemia	Can cause ↓ LOC; paresthesia; seizures; generalized weakness; myocardial; hepatic, erythrocyte, leukocyte, and platelet dysfunction	*Laboratory*—confusion usually with serum phosphate <0.1 mg/dl
Hypermagnesemia	Hypotension; bradyarrhythmias; asystole	*Laboratory*—curare-like effects if serum magnesium >10 mEq/L
Hypomagnesemia	Can cause ↓ LOC; N/V paresthesia; seizures; generalized weakness; paralytic ileus; fatigue	*Laboratory*—confusion usually with serum magnesium <0.1 mEq/L
Respiratory acidosis	See Hypercapnia	
Metabolic acidosis	Confusion caused by etiology of metabolic acidosis; can cause ↓ LOC; mild diffuse muscle hypertonus; cardiac depression	*Laboratory*—if uncomplicated metabolic acidosis then ABG will have pH <7.35 and HCO_3 <24 mEq/L; symptomatic usually when pH <7.24
Respiratory alkalosis	Light-headedness; paresthesia; circumoral numbness	*Laboratory*—if uncomplicated respiratory alkalosis then ABG will have pH >7.45 and P_{CO_2} <40 mm Hg
Metabolic alkalosis	Tetany; neuromuscular irritability; cardiac depression with severe alkalosis	*Laboratory*—if uncomplicated metabolic alkalosis then ABG will have pH >7.45 and HCO_3 >24 mEq/L

Etiology	Clinical comments	Laboratory diagnosis	Neuroimaging and other diagnostics
Diabetic keto-acidosis	Can cause ↓ LOC; hyperosmolar state contributes to symptom complex; HA; N/V; generalized weakness; abdominal pain	Laboratory—variable symptomatic threshold	
Hyperosmolar non-ketotic hyperglycemia	Can cause ↓ LOC; severe dehydration; similar to hypernatremia	*Laboratory*—confusion usually with serum osmolality >320 mOsm/kg of H_2O; but variable symptomatic threshold	
Hypoglycemia	Can cause ↓ LOC; HA; myoclonic twitching; seizures; nervousness; trembling; sweating; hunger	*Laboratory*—confusion usually with levels <30–40 mg/dl	
Hypercapnia	Can cause ↓ LOC; papilledema; HA asterixis; action tremor; course twitching of muscles; seizures	*Laboratory*—if uncomplicated respiratory acidosis then ABG will have pH <7.35 and P_{CO_2} >40 mm Hg	
Hypoxia	Can cause ↓ LOC; poor judgment; shortness of breath; cyanosis	*Laboratory*—confusion may be present with P_{O_2} <55 mm Hg	
Hypotension	Can cause rapid ↓ LOC; cyanosis	*Vital signs*—onset of confusion usually with systolic blood pressure (BP) <60 mm Hg; may be higher in hypertensive patients	
Uremia	Confusion may be episodic; can cause ↓ LOC; irritability; apathy; muscular twitching; asterixis; tetany; fatigue	*Laboratory*—confusion is usually related to the rapidity of renal failure and not to clear thresholds *Lumbar puncture*—mildly ↑ WBC; mildly ↑ protein	EEG—with triphasic waves or diffuse slowing
Hepatic encephalopathy	Early: confusion with agitation; later: ↓ LOC; signs of ↑ CSF pressure; myoclonus; asterixis; FNF are rare; icteric sclera; spider telangiectasia; caput medusae; ascites;	*Laboratory*—hypoglycemia; hyperammonemia; ↑ prothrombin time (PT); elevated liver enzymes *Lumbar puncture*—if protein is ↑ search for another cause; ↑ CSF glutamine	EEG—with triphasic waves or diffuse slowing

	splenomegaly; jaundice		
Reye's syndrome	Onset of confusion is rapid as is progression to ↓ LOC; confusion preceded by one week of vomiting, fevers, and upper respiratory infections	*Lumbar puncture*— usually acellular; normal protein; ↓ glucose; ↑ CSF pressure	
Pancreatic encephalopathy	Acute onset of confusion; can cause ↓ LOC; agitation; hallucinations; dysarthria; N/V quadriplegia; midabdominal pain; upper abdominal tenderness	*Laboratory*—serum amylase usually increases later and may remain elevated for several days	
Acute intermittent porphyria	Confusion resolves over days to weeks and precedes the severe cases of polyneuropathy; psychosis; ocular palsies; facial paralysis; hypertension; tachycardia; colicky pain	*Laboratory*—↑ urinary delta-aminolevulinic acid and porphobilinogen *Lumbar puncture*— normal or mildly ↑ protein	
Hyperthyroidism	Subacute onset of confusion; agitation; emotional lability; tremor; seizures; proximal weakness; heat intolerance; palpitations; tachycardia; atrial fibrillation; fatigue; weight loss	*Laboratory*—abnormal thyroid function tests *Lumbar puncture*— normal, occasionally ↓ protein	
Hypothyroidism	Confusion may be mild; can cause ↓ LOC; paranoia; confabulation; ataxia; peripheral neuropathy; delayed relaxation of deep tendon reflexes; cold intolerance; bradycardia; periorbital swelling; hair loss	*Laboratory*—abnormal thyroid function tests *Lumbar puncture*— normal, occasionally ↑ protein	
Cushing's syndrome	Psychosis; depression; hallucinations; proximal muscular weakness; hyperten-	*Laboratory*—abnormal dexamethasone suppression test	*CT scan*—with cerebral atrophy

Etiology	Clinical comments	Laboratory diagnosis	Neuroimaging and other diagnostics
	sion; obesity; hirsutism; incessant activity or immobility		
Adrenal cortical insufficiency	Irritability; seizures; generalized weakness; hypotension; fatigue; weight loss; skin hyperpigmentation	*Laboratory*—abnormal cortisol stimulation test	
Pituitary apoplexy	Acute onset of confusion; can cause ↓ LOC; acute HA; bilateral amaurosis; ophthalmoplegia	*Lumbar puncture*—can be consistent with subarachnoid hemorrhage or ↑ WBC and ↑ protein	*CT scan*—with an enlarged sella with infarction of pituitary tumor; hemorrhage noted in and above the sella; often misread as normal
Wernicke's encephalopathy	Signs of alcohol withdrawal; loss of long-term memory; anterograde amnesia; confabulation; ocular palsies; gaze palsies; nystagmus; gait ataxia; peripheral neuropathy; dyspnea; postural hypotension; precipitated or aggravated by glucose load in malnourished; prevented with thiamine supplement	*Laboratory*—low transketolase activity and elevated blood pyruvate *Lumbar puncture*—normal or mildly ↑ protein	*MRI scan*—T2WI with hyperintensities surrounding the third ventricle and aqueduct; T1WI with gadolinium with enhancement of the above areas and the mammillary bodies
Pellagra	Acute onset of confusion; depression; myelopathy involving posterior and lateral columns; fatigue; scaly dermatitis; diarrhea	*Laboratory*—decreased excretion of urinary N-methyl-nicotinamide	
Vitamin B_{12} deficiency	Confusion usually begins after spinal cord involvement; depression; paranoia; general weakness and paresthesia can progress to ataxic paraparesis; bowel and bladder dysfunction	*Laboratory*—megaloblastic anemia; low B_{12} level (usually <200 pg/ml); ↑ serum methylmalonic acid *Lumbar puncture*—usually normal or mildly ↑ WBC or mildly ↑ protein	
Acute alcohol intoxication	Can cause ↓ LOC; unrestrained behavior; incoordination; atrial	*Laboratory*—confusion usually with level >200 mg/dl but variable symp-	

	flutter; acute gas- tritis; diuresis	tomatic threshold
Acute alcohol with- drawal (delirium tremens)	Onset of delirium is usually 2–4 days after the cessation of alco- hol and is fairly acute; agitation; dilated pupils; seizures (7–48 hours after the cessation of alco- hol); fever; tachy- cardia; perspira- tion	*Laboratory*—alco- hol level does not need to be 0 mg/dl for withdrawal to occur
Opioid intoxica- tion	Constricted pupils; N/V; hypother- mia; bradycar- dia; respiratory depression; con- stipation	*Laboratory*—(+) drug screen
Cocaine intoxica- tion	Agitation; psy- chotic behavior; pupillary dilatation; N/V; seizure; tachycardia; car- diac arrhythmias; respiratory de- pression; nares may have ero- sions	*Laboratory*—(+) drug screen
Amphetamine intoxication	Same as cocaine; except no psycho- motor agitation, but maladaptive behavior or psy- chological change may be present	*Laboratory*—(+) drug screen
Phencyclidine (PCP)	Can cause ↓ LOC; nystagmus; dys- arthria; muscle rigidity; tremor; hyperacusis; ataxia; seizures; decreased respon- siveness to pain; ↑ BP; tachycardia	*Laboratory*—(+) drug screen
Sedative-hypnotic; barbiturate intoxication	Can cause ↓ LOC; slurred speech; nystagmus; in- coordination; unsteady gait; hypothermia; hy- potension; res- piratory depres- sion	*Laboratory*—(+) drug screen; if bar- biturate is sus- pected check level
Barbiturate with- withdrawal	Delirium develops following convul- sive phase; with- drawal begins about 12 hours after the last	*Laboratory*—check barbiturate level

Etiology	Clinical comments	Laboratory diagnosis	Neuroimaging and other diagnostics
	dose; if chronically intoxicated then withdrawal may take 48–72 hours; tremor; insomnia; generalized seizures occur 7 days from the last dose; fever; tachycardia		
Benzodiazepine intoxication	Onset of delirium is during or shortly after the ingestion of drugs; can cause ↓ LOC; hostile behavior; slurred speech; hypotension; syncope	*Laboratory*—(+) drug screen	
Benzodiazepine withdrawal	Onset of confusion is 2–3 days after last dose with short-acting drugs or 5–6 days with long-acting ones; anxiety; dysphoria; N/V; tremor muscle twitches; occasional seizures; intolerance for bright lights and loud noises; sweating	*Laboratory*—(+) drug screen	
Lithium intoxication	*Level 1.5–2.0:* onset of confusion; N/V; nystagmus; slurred speech; ataxia; dizziness; abdominal pain *Level >2.0:* can cause ↓ LOC; clonic limb movement; seizure; syncope; circulatory failure	*Laboratory*—↑ peripheral WBC, ↑ sodium, magnesium, calcium, and glucose levels; ↓ potassium and phosphorus levels	
Carbon monoxide poisoning	*10–30% carboxyhemoglobin:* HA; N/V *30–40% carboxyhemoglobin:* confusion; severe HA; dizziness *>50% carboxyhemoglobin:* can cause ↓ LOC; seizures; shock; tachypnea	Laboratory—elevated carboxyhemoglobin level	*CT scan*—with low attenuation in the watershed regions especially in the basal ganglia and parasagittal regions *MRI scan*—T2WI with hyperintensities in the watershed regions; T1WI with gadolinium with striking enhancement

Subarachnoid hemorrhage	Confusion may occur with the original hemorrhage, associated vasospasm, or hydrocephalus; acute onset HA; NR; N/V; ↑ BP; tachycardia	*Laboratory*—check PT, PTT, disseminated intravascular coagulation (DIC) profile and platelet count *Lumbar puncture*—↑ RBC; ↑ protein; ↓ glucose; ↑ CSF pressure (50% of patients)	*CT scan*—with high attenuation following the course of the gyri; may be localized but usually diffuse, especially within the cisterns; frequently misread as normal *Angiogram* is usually diagnostic of aneurysm or AVM
Acute subdural hematoma (<3 days)	Confusion may appear at the time of trauma or be delayed as hematoma enlarges; can cause ↓ LOC; aphasia; seizures; hemiparesis	*Laboratory*—check PT, PTT, and platelet count *Lumbar puncture*—unnecessary with modern imaging	*CT scan*—with high attenuation crescent-shaped fluid collection over the underlying hemisphere *MRI scan*—hyperacute: T1WI with isointense and T2WI with isointense to hyperintense hemorrhage; acute: T1WI with isointense to moderately hypointense hemorrhage; T2WI with very hypointense hemorrhage
Subacute (3 days to 3 weeks) and chronic (>3 weeks) subdural	Variable onset of confusion; may be intermittent; can cause ↓ LOC; dementia; HA; transient ischemic attack-like episodes; seizures	*Laboratory*—check PT, PTT, and platelet count *Lumbar puncture*—unnecessary with modern imaging	*CT scan*—subacute: with nearly same attenuation as underlying cortex; chronic: low attenuation when compared with enhancing membrane; may be loculated *MRI scan*—subacute with hyperintensity on both T1WI and T2WI; chronic: variable; T1WI usually isointense to hypointense; T2WI hyperintense
Epidural hematoma	Confusion may appear acutely after trauma or may appear after a lucid interval; can cause rapid ↓ LOC; HA; FNF	*Lumbar puncture*—unnecessary with modern imaging	*CT scan*—with high attenuation biconvex mass with mass effect *MRI scan*—acute: T1WI with isointense epidural mass; T2WI with hyperintense epidural mass
Concussion	Confusion occurs after head injury with subsequent resolution; HA; N/V	*Lumbar puncture*—normal	*CT scan*—normal
Contusion	Onset of confusion after injury; can have progressive brain swelling with ↓ LOC; FNF; fever; tachycardia	*Lumbar puncture*—unnecessary with modern imaging	*CT scan*—early: normal or with patchy ill-defined low-attenuation frontal or temporal lesions mixed with smaller high-attenuation foci of petechial hemorrhage; edema; contusions may enhance; common locations are inferior frontal and anterior temporal lobes

Etiology	Clinical comments	Laboratory diagnosis	Neuroimaging and other diagnostics
			MRI scan—acute: T1WI with some hyperintense signal abnormalities (hemorrhage); T2WI with multiple superficial hyperintense signal abnormalities on T2WI
Transient ischemic attack	Confusion begins with the onset of ischemia; FNF may be present depending on the areas of the brain affected with full resolution of deficits; see cerebral infarction for specific areas	*Lumbar puncture*—normal	Imaging studies are normal
Cerebral infarction	Confusion begins with the onset of the stroke; HA large vessel occlusions; visual field deficit if posterior cerebral arteries are involved Localizations that can be associated with confusion: 1. parahippo-campal-fusi-form-lingual gyri on either side of the brain 2. right posterior parietal 3. right prefrontal region 4. bilateral PCA territories 5. transient confusion if left PCA involved	*Lumbar puncture*—unnecessary with modern imaging	*CT scan*—early: normal or with sulcal effacement and loss of gray-white junction; later: with low attenuation in a specific vascular territory *MRI scan*—early: T1WI with brain swelling; T2WI with hyperintensity after 8 hours
Intracerebral hemorrhage (ICH)	Confusion begins with the onset of the hemorrhage; HA; see cerebral infarction for localizations that can be associated with confusion	*Laboratory*—check PT, PTT, and platelet count *Lumbar puncture*—unnecessary with modern imaging	*CT scan*—with an area of high attenuation representing the hematoma; degree of mass effect is related to size and location of hematoma *MRI scan*—see acute SDH for the intensities of the hematoma on T1WI and T2WI
Vasculitis	Usually subacute confusion; HA; aphasia; FNF	*Lumbar puncture*—normal or ↑ WBC; ↑ protein; glucose usually normal; CSF pressure can be normal, ↓, ↑	*CT scan*—with multiple areas of low attenuation

Cerebral venous sinus occlusion	Subacute onset of confusion; can cause ↓ LOC; aphasia; papilledema; signs of ↑ CSF pressure; HA; seizures; FNF	*Lumbar puncture*— if idiopathic: normal or ↑ protein; if septic thrombophlebitis: CSF is similar to cases of meningitis; if hemorrhagic infarction: then ↑ RBC; ↑ CSF pressure if thrombosis is acute	*CT scan*—without contrast: with high attenuation in sinus representing thrombus; with or without cortical or subcortical hemorrhage; with contrast: sinus with low attenuation with enhancement around thrombus (empty delta sign); possible focal area of low attenuation representing area of venous infarction *MRI scan*—acute: T1WI with isointense clot; subacute: T1WI or T2WI with hyperintense clot *MR venography*—with no flow noted in the occluded sinus
CNS tumors	Onset of confusion is subacute and progressive; irritability; abulia; aphasia; signs of ↑ CSF pressure; seizures	*Lumbar puncture*— all parameters are variable and depend on histologic type of tumor, location, presence of ↑ CSF pressure, and hemorrhage	*CT scan* and *MRI scan*— results are variable and depend on histologic tumor type, location, presence of ↑ CSF pressure, and hemorrhage
Limbic encephalitis	Onset of confusion is subacute; dementia; retentive memory defect; depression; agitation; anxiety; hallucinations; seizures	*Laboratory*—systemic evidence of carcinoma; usually oat-cell of the lung *Lumbar puncture*— ↑ WBC 10–50 cells/cm^3, mostly lymphocytes; mildly ↑ protein	*CT scan*—usually normal *MRI scan*—with high signal intensities in the medial temporal lobe; almost identical to herpes simplex encephalitis
Generalized seizure (absence)	Onset of confusion is with the seizure or postconvulsive; can cause ↓ LOC; automatisms; myoclonic jerks	*Laboratory*—if seizure remains focal; no lab abnormalities; if generalized tonic-clonic then ↑ peripheral WBC; metabolic acidosis *Lumbar puncture*— may have mildly ↑ WBC if done within 72 hours of a generalized tonic-clonic seizure; assuming no recent CNS injury, infection, or stroke	*CT scan* and *MRI scan*— results are variable and depend on the cause of the seizure *EEG*—interictal: may be normal; ictal: with generalized 3/second spike and wave
Partial seizure	Onset of confusion with onset of seizure; auras; illusions; hallucinations; anxiety; fear; automatism; persistence of com-	*Laboratory*—if seizure remains focal; no lab abnormalities; if generalized tonic-clonic then ↑ peripheral WBC; metabolic acidosis *Lumbar puncture*—	*CT scan* and *MRI scan*— results are variable and depend on the cause of the seizure *EEG*—interictal: may be normal or with intermittent spikes or sharp waves; ictal: may be

Etiology	Clinical comments	Laboratory diagnosis	Neuroimaging and other diagnostics
	plex acts; amnesia; may see secondary generalization; ↑ BP; tachycardia; ↓ respirations	may have mildly ↑ WBC if done within 72 hours of a generalized tonic-clonic seizure; assuming no recent CNS injury, infection, or stroke	normal or with repetitive focal spike discharges
Postconvulsive (after generalized or complex partial seizures)	Confusion occurs after a seizure; duration of confusion is variable; aphasia; postconvulsive paralysis	*Lumbar puncture*—see seizure for results	*CT scan* and *MRI scan*—results are variable and depend on the cause of the seizure *EEG*—with diffuse or focal slowing
Hypertensive encephalopathy	Rapid onset of confusion and ↑ BP; can cause ↓ LOC; papilledema; HA; N/V; seizures; visual disturbances	*Lumbar puncture*—↑ protein usually <100 mg/dl; ↑ CSF pressure in many cases	*CT scan*—with generalized cerebral edema as manifested by loss of gray-white junction, diffuse loss of sulci and cisternal spaces, and small ventricles
Beclouded dementia	Patients are demented and have ↑ confusion secondary to another etiological factor; signs of dementia	*Laboratory*—abnormal results depend on etiology	*CT scan* and *MRI scan*—results are variable and depend on the cause of the dementia; diffuse atrophy and ex vacuo hydrocephalus are usually observed
Postoperative delirium	Onset of confusion occurs after surgery; fever; hypothermia; BP changes; tachycardia	*Laboratory*—electrolyte abnormalities; anemia; hypoxemia; or multiple etiologies may be present	*CT scan* and *MRI scan*—results are variable and depend on the cause

*Only if indicated to make therapeutic decisions and no contraindications are present (see Chap. 1, sec. **III.D.1**).

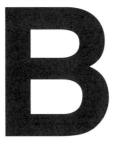

Imaging Choices and Alternatives for Patient Presentation Categories

Buckley terPenning

Clinical problem	Working diagnosis	Modality of choice	Advantages	Disadvantages	Protocol
Headache, chronic and complicated	Sinus disease	CT	Structural detail	Ionizing radiation	Thin coronal images
	Venous thrombosis	MRI/MRA	Sensitivity	Availability	Coronal images useful, contrast useful
	Tumor	MRI	High sensitivity	Availability	With and without contrast
	AV malfor-mation	MRI/MRA	Shows nidus and vessels	Availability	T1, T2 axial MRI plus TOF MRA
	Hydroceph-alus	CT	Availability	Availability	Routine, noncon-trast
	Infection, chronic	MRI	Sensitivity	Availability	Coronal images useful, contrast useful
	Pseudotumor cerebri	CT	Availability	Ionizing radiation	Routine, noncon-trast
	Vasculitis	See Headache, acute			
	Cranial neuralgia	MRI	Shows intra-cranial nerves	Availability	Tailored to the patient
Headache, acute	Subarachnoid hemorrhage	CT	High sensitivity	Ionizing radiation	Routine, noncon-trast
	Arterial dis-section	MRA	Very low risk	Artifacts	Time of flight
		Angiography	High sensitiv-ity	Invasive	Include ex-ternal car-otid
		CT angiog-raphy	Low risk	Bone foramina or canals interfere	Requires contrast and fast (helical) CT imager
	Intracerebral hemorrhage	CT	High sensitiv-ity	Somewhat limited in posterior fossa	Routine, noncon-trast

Clinical problem	Working diagnosis	Modality of choice	Advantages	Disadvantages	Protocol
		MRI	High sensitivity	May miss SAH	T1 and T2 axial images
	Intracerebral vasculitis	MRI	High sensitivity	Low specificity	T1 and T2 axial images
		Angiography	Moderately high sensitivity	Low yield, invasive	Cut film or high resolution digital subtraction
Facial pain	Neuralgia	MRI	Best visualization of vessels and nerves	Availability	Oblique sagittal planes may demonstrate cranial nerves
Neck pain, nontraumatic	Nonradicular	No imaging	Avoid radiation		
	Radicular or myelopathic: disk or joint disease, tumor	MRI	Best visualization of disks and spinal cord	May not examine bone and neural foramina well	Protocols vary
	See also Myelopathy	Plain films	Bone definition and foramina	Ionizing radiation	AP, lateral, obliques
		CT myelogram	Bone and thecal sac definition	Invasive	Cervical myelogram followed by CT
	Instability	Plain films	Alignment and bone definition	Cord not evaluated	AP, lateral, obliques, flexion and extension
		MRI	Poor bone visualization	Cord evaluated	Protocols vary
Low back pain	Disk or joint disease, infection, tumor	No imaging	90% of painful conditions resolve	2–3 week delay of surgery in 2%	Conservative management
		MRI	Best visualization of disks and spinal cord	May not examine bone and neural foramina well	Sagittal T1, spin-density, T2, or spin-echo, with axial T1
Myelopathy	Multiple sclerosis, tumor, spinal stenosis (DDD/DJD), syrinx	MRI	Best visualization of disks and spinal cord	Availability	Sagittal T1, spin-density, T2, or spin-echo, with axial T1
Failed back	Recurrent disk, post-	MRI	Best soft-tissue visuali-	Availability	Sagittal and axial T1,

	operative scar, infection		zation, best enhancement		each without and then with contrast
Alterations in consciousness and cognition (stupor, coma, dementia, amnesia)	Alzheimer's, toxic-metabolic	MRI	Best soft-tissue visualization	Poor specificity does not add to management	T1 and T2 axial images; coronal images occasionally illustrative
	Tumor, hydrocephalus, SAH, ICH	CT	Fast, available	Ionizing radiation	IV contrast for tumor
	Basilar artery thrombosis	Transcranial Doppler	Fast, portable	Availability	Operator-dependent
		Angiography	Accurate, permits possible therapy	Invasive; thrombolytic therapy requires prior CT	
	Stroke, trauma	See Chap. 32, sec. **XIV**			
Aphasia		See TIA and stroke			
Dysphagia	See Chap. 32	Videofluoroscopy	Evaluates anatomy and physiology	Ionizing radiation	Elaborate protocol
Seizure, neonate	Benign convulsions, errors of metabolism, drug-related	No imaging	Avoid unnecessary sedation		
	Hypoxic-ischemic, intracranial hemorrhage, CNS infection, migration abnormalities	MRI	Best soft-tissue visualization	Availability, sedation required	T1 and T2 axial images
Seizure, child	Febrile, absence, infantile spasm, Lennox-Gastaut	No imaging	Avoid unnecessary sedation		
	Benign partial seizure, generalized tonic-clonic, tumor, trauma, heterotopias, vascular abnormalities	MRI	Best soft-tissue visualization	Availability, sedation required	T1 and T2 axial images
Seizure, adult	Tumor, AVM, stroke, trauma,	MRI	Best soft-tissue visualization	Availability	T1, spin-density, and T2

Clinical problem	Working diagnosis	Modality of choice	Advantages	Disadvantages	Protocol
	alcohol-related, heterotopias, hippocampal sclerosis				axial images; T2 coronal images
Hearing loss	Dysmorphology, infection, tumor	CT (conductive hearing loss)	Very good resolution of fine bone structures	Ionizing radiation	Thin-section images, both axial and direct coronal
	Stroke, infection, tumor	MRI (sensorineural hearing loss)	Good soft-tissue visualization	Coarser spatial resolution than CT	T1, spin-density, and T2 axial images; coronals occasionally
Vertigo	Drugs, toxins	No imaging			
	Trauma	See Trauma			
	Stroke, labyrinthitis, tumor	MRI	Best soft-tissue visualization	Availability	
Vision	See Chap. 32	MRI	Good soft-tissue visualization	Availability	Axial T1, spin-density, and T2 images
		CT	Best bone imaging for trauma	Ionizing radiation to ocular lens	Axial and direct coronal
TIA and stroke	Large vessel disease, penetrating artery disease; cardiogenic, venoocclusive, vasculitic	MRI	Excellent brain visualization	Availability	T1, spin-density, and T2-weighted axial images
		CT	Good brain visualization	Not as sensitive for brain lesions as MRI	Noncontrast, contrast if equivocal
		Ultrasound	Low-cost screen for carotid disease	80–90% accurate	Tailored to patient
		MRA	Screen for carotid disease during MRI	80–90% accurate	Time of flight
		Angiography	Required for endarterectomy	Invasive	Aortic arch, both carotids, cerebral
Trauma	Penetrating	CT	Detects blood,	Metal may	Routine

head, fractures		bone, and metal for surgical planning	cause artifact	NCCT
Closed head trauma	CT	Fast assessment of intracerebral edema or hemorrhage	Patients usually require MRI after acute period	Routine NCCT
	MRI	Sensitive to small contusions and shear injuries	Insensitive to fractures	T1, spin-density, and T2-weighted axial images
	MRA	Sensitive for large artery dissections	More artifacts than angiography	Time of flight
	Cervical spine plain film series	Spine injury often unsuspected	Difficult to obtain good films in acute period	AP, lateral, odontoid, obliques
	Cervical spine CT	Spine injury often unsuspected	Availability	Spiral CT superior to incremental CT
	Angiography	Best evaluation of arterial injury	Invasive	Aortic arch, both carotids

Note: Patients cannot be exposed to the strong magnetic field of an MR imager if they bear the following: cardiac pacemaker; brain aneurysm clip; spinal, cardiac, or other implanted electrodes; metallic heart valve replacement; insulin pump; cochlear implant; or metal lodged in eyes. Uncertainty can be solved with a plain film to look for the metal or device.

Other patients may require plain film screening prior to exposure to MRI: patients with histories of sheet metal work, toolmakers, metal lathe operators.

The following items can interfere with the MR exam: spinal fusion rods, hearing aids, metal mesh, dentures, partial plates, metal plates, screws, shrapnel, bullets, BBs.

Index

Index

Basilar invagination, 498
BCNU. *See* Carmustine (BCNU)
Bechterew sign, 274*t*
Beck depression and anxieties inventories, 85
Becker's muscular dystrophy, 529, 530
  prevention of, 531–532
  therapy for, 532
Beclouded states, acute confusional, 4*t*, 5
  ancillary diagnostic studies for, 672
Bed spins, 164–165
Behavior disturbance(s)
  in child, 364–365
  in drug toxicity, 606–607
  in multiple sclerosis, 442–443
  in phenytoin side effects, 426
Behavioral therapy
  in Alzheimer's disease, 463–464
  in psychophysiologic insomnia, 613*t*, 613–614,
    614*t*
Bell's palsy
  diagnostic approach in, 153
  differential diagnosis in, 151
  facial weakness in, 148, 150*f*
  headaches in, 214
  paresthesias in, 284
  in pregnancy, 652
Benadryl (diphenhydramine)
  in dizziness and vertigo, 632*t*
  in Parkinson's disease, 451
Benedikt's syndrome, 124
Beneficence, 368
Benign focal epilepsy of childhood, 56
  with centrotemporal spikes (BFECTS),
    402–403
  not yet internationally accepted, 403
  with occipital spike waves (BEOSW), 403
  with somatosensory evoked spikes, 403
Benign intracranial hypertension (BIH)
  headaches in, 220–221, 226
  in pregnancy, 647–648
Benign myoclonic epilepsy in infancy, 403–404,
    406
Benign neonatal familial convulsion(s), 403
Benign paroxysmal positional vertigo (BPPV),
    155, 626–630, 628*f*–630*f*
  diagnosis of, 164–165
  exercise in, 627–628, 629*f*, 633*f*
  Frenzel's goggles and, 161
  variants of, 167
Benzodiazepine(s)
  in chronic pain, 567*t*
  dizziness from, 157
  dopaminergic neurotransmission suppression
    and, 455–456
  in essential tremor, 457–458
  intoxications from, 667–668
  in multiple sclerosis spasms, 441
  in non–rapid eye movement sleep disorders,
    620
  in parasomnias, 620
  in restless legs syndrome, 618
    in sleep disorders, 621
  in status epilepticus, 431–432
    in child, 415
  in West's syndrome, 405
  withdrawal from, 668
Benztropine (Cogentin), 450*t*
BEOSW (benign focal epilepsy of childhood
    with occipital spike waves), 403
Best interests standard, 369
Beta-adrenergic blocking agent(s) in migraine
    headaches, 554–556

in pregnancy, 648*t*
Betaseron, 447
BFECTS (benign focal epilepsy of childhood
    with centrotemporal spikes), 402–403
Bicarbonate in blood, syncope and, 68
Bicipital tendinitis, 258
BIH (benign intracranial hypertension)
  headaches in, 220–221, 226
  in pregnancy, 647–648
Bilateral visual loss from homonymous hemi-
    anopia, 104–105
Bilirubin, cerebrospinal fluid, 8
Binocular diplopia, 119. *See also* Diplopia
  cover test for, 125
  differential diagnosis in, 128
Binocular visual loss
  with abrupt onset, 102, 103*t*
  from chiasmal damage, 102–104
Binswanger's disease, 81*t*
Biopsy
  brain, 9
  in headache evaluation, 226–227
  muscle, 313
    in inflammatory myopathies, 523–524
  nerve, 313–314
  skin, in epilepsy of childhood, 410
Bladder, urinary
  dysfunction of
    atonic, with overflow incontinence, 322,
      323*t*
    in multiple sclerosis, 444–445
    in stroke, 382–383
  function assessment of, 273
  neuroanatomy of, 319
  training of, 322
Blastomycosis in AIDS, 495–496
Bleeding disorder(s)
  in hemorrhagic strokes, 393–394
  lumbar puncture contraindicated in, 348–349
Blepharospasm, 292*t*, 293
Blink reflex, facial numbness and, 139
Blockade
  nerve
    multiple sclerosis and, 437–438
    in reflex sympathetic dystrophy, 576–577
    in spinal cord injury spasms, 510
  neuromuscular, quadriplegic myopathy after,
    316
  receptor
    adrenergic. *See* Adrenergic blocker(s)
    calcium channel. *See* Calcium channel
      blocker(s)
Blood alcohol level in acute confusional state,
    8
Blood count(s)
  in headaches, 208, 226
  syncope and, 68
Blood dyscrasia(s) in phenytoin side effects,
    426
Blood flow, cerebral
  imaging of, 336, 673–674
  syncope and, 64
Blood gas(es)
  in headaches, 209
  in sleep-induced respiratory impairments,
    85–86
  syncope and, 68
Blood pressure
  coma and, 47–48
  in hypokinesia, 303
  strokes and, 383, 398
Blood vessel disorders

in chronic pain, 566, 566*t*
generic substitutions and, 423
in HIV distal sensory neuropathy, 483
in multiple sclerosis, 443
in myotonic dystrophy, 533
in partial seizures, 424–425
pharmacokinetics of, 422*t*, 426–427
praziquantel levels and, 478
in pregnancy, 643
in primary generalized epilepsies, 425
in secondary generalized epilepsies, 426
in seizures
  in bacterial meningitis, 472–473
  in herpes encephalitis, 475
  in status epilepticus, 473
in seizures from central nervous system
  metastases, 590
in spinal cord injury spasms, 511*t*
in status epilepticus, 432
teratogenicity of, 644
toxicity of, 426
in zoster infections in AIDS, 493
Pheochromocytoma, 221
PHN (postherpetic neuralgia), 143–144, 145
Phobia(s) in Alzheimer's disease, 464
Phonation, speech, 194
abnormal, 196–198, 200–201
testing for, 199
Phonophobia, 206
Photic stimulation, 338
Photophobia, 206
Phycomycosis, orbital, 122, 130
Physical activity
  risk factors for stroke and, 382
  upper extremity pain and paresthesias after,
    247
Physiologic tremor, 294
Pick's disease, 35, 467
Pickwickian syndrome, 86–87
Pigment changes in child, 364
Pilocarpine, 116–117
Pilocytic astrocytoma, 580
PIN (posterior interosseous nerve) compres-
  sion, 254
Piroxicam, 565*t*
Pituitary apoplexy, 103–104
  ancillary diagnostic studies for, 666
  in cancer complications, 592
  diplopia and, 123, 130
Pituitary tumor(s) in pregnancy, 646
Plantar neuropathies, 265–266
Plantar reflex(es), 273
Plaque in multiple sclerosis, 437
Plasma exchange. *See* Plasmapheresis
Plasmapheresis
  in inflammatory demyelinating neuropathy,
    485, 518
  in Lambert-Eaton syndrome, in cancer com-
    plications, 599
  in myasthenia gravis, 542, 544*t*
Platybasia, 498
PLEDs (periodic lateralized epileptiform discharges), 56, 296, 340
Pleocytosis, cerebrospinal fluid, 349
Plexitis
  brachial, 521
  defined, 515
Plexopathy(ies)
  acute, 282, 289, 314
  brachial, 256–257, 314
    with malignancy, 257
  defined, 515

electromyography and nerve conduction
  study of, 344
PLF (perilymph fistula), 155, 166, 635
PLMD (periodic limb movement disorder), 84*t*, 87
  in sleep disorders, 618, 621–622
PML (progressive multifocal leukoencephalopathy)
  in AIDS, 489–490
  ancillary diagnostic studies for, 660
  in cancer metastases, 597
PNETs (primitive neuroectodermal central nervous system tumors), 583–584
Poisoning. *See also* Neurotoxin(s). Toxin(s)
  carbon monoxide, 306, 604–605, 668
  memory impairment and, 38
  organophosphate, 315, 668
Poliomyelitis, 314
  dysphagia after, 190–191
Polymerase chain reaction(s) (PCR), cerebrospinal fluid, 9
Polymyalgia rheumatica, 522
  natural history of, 523
  prednisone in, 525
Polymyositis, 312–318, 522
  in HIV, 526
  natural history of, 522
  prognosis in, 525
Polymyositis/dermatomyositis (PM/DM), 316
Polyneuropathy(ies), 312–318
  acute
    in acute sensory loss, 282–290
    overlap, 314
  chronic pain in, 563
  defined, 515
  electromyography and nerve conduction
    study of, 344
  inflammatory demyelinating, 485–486, 520
  sensorimotor, in diabetes, 519
Polyradiculitis in AIDS or HIV, 520–521
Polyradiculomyelitis in AIDS, 491
Polyradiculoneuropathy
  defined, 515
  diabetic, 520
Polyradiculopathy
  acute, in acute sensory loss, 282, 314
  defined, 515
Polysomnography (PSG), 83, 84*t*, 347
  in advanced sleep-phase syndrome, 90
  in central sleep apnea, 86
  in circadian rhythm disorders, 90
  in cluster headaches, 93
  in delayed sleep-phase syndrome, 90
  in fibrositis syndrome, 93
  in insomnia, 84*t*, 85
  in irregular sleep-wake pattern, 91
  in movement disorders of sleep, 87, 88
  in narcolepsy, 91
  in nocturnal paroxysmal dystonia, 89
  in obstructive sleep apnea, 86
  in sleep-induced respiratory impairments, 84*t*,
    85–86
  in sleepwalking, 89
Pooled human immune globulin in inflammatory demyelinating polyneuropathy, 485.
    See also Immunoglobulin(s)
Porphyria, acute intermittent (AIP), 315, 665
Port-wine stain, 363–364
Position
  benign paroxysmal positional vertigo and,
    626–630, 628*f*, 629*f*, 630*f*
  testing for sensation of, 283
Positional tremor in parkinsonism, 303

Torticollis—*Continued*
paroxysmal, in nonepileptiform paroxysmal
events in child, 354
TOS (thoracic outlet syndrome), 256–257
Touch, sensation of, 283
Tourette's syndrome (TS), 295–296, 454–455
in child, 360
Toxin(s). *See also* Neurotoxin(s). Poisoning
in acute myopathy, 316
barium salt, 315
central nervous system tumor treatment and,
586–587
in dementia differential diagnosis, 16*t*
dystonia and, 293
exposure to, in acute confusional state, 7
in hypokinesia, 300, 301, 306–307
memory impairment and, 37–38
myoclonus from, 297
organophosphates as, 315, 605
in seizures, 55–56
Toxoplasmosis
in AIDS, 488–489
ancillary diagnostic studies for, 661
in myopathies, 526–527
t-PA (tissue plasminogen activator), 387, 388*t*
Tranquilizer(s), dizziness and vertigo and, 631*t*,
632–633, 634*t*
Transcortical mixed aphasia, 25*t*, 27–28
Transcortical motor aphasia, 25*t*, 27
Transcortical sensory aphasia, 25*t*, 27
Transcranial Doppler ultrasonography in basilar
artery thrombosis, 333
Transcutaneous electrical nerve stimulation
(TENS)
in chronic pain, 568
in reflex sympathetic dystrophy, 575–576
Transderm-V. *See* Scopolamine (Donphen, Don-
natal, Transderm-V)
Transection of spinal cord, complete, 287–288
Transient evoked otoacoustic emission
(TEOAE), 183, 184*f*
Transient global amnesia (TGA), 10, 39
Transient ischemic attack (TIA)
ancillary diagnostic studies for, 669–670
dizziness and vertigo in, 155–156, 167
facial numbness from, 286
headaches in, 212, 220
imaging in, 336, 676
stroke and, 380
syncope and, 66
Transient monocular visual loss (TMVL),
99–102, 100*t*
Transient neonatal myasthenia gravis, 544–545
Transient unresponsiveness in elderly, 52
Transient visual loss in childhood nonelepti-
form paroxysmal events, 354
Transient visual obscuration (TVO), 102, 107*t*
Transtentorial herniation, 123
Transverse myelitis, acute, 288
Tranxene (clorazepate)
in childhood epilepsies, 413
in chronic pain, 567*t*
Trauma
central nervous system. *See also* Head trauma
acute confusional state in, 3, 4*t*
in dementia differential diagnosis, 16*t*
cervicocephalic arterial dissection in, 212
craniocerebral
occult, 392
strokes versus, 395
dental, numbness from, 134
facial, numbness from, 134

head. *See* Head trauma
headaches after, 221–222
cluster, 144
in hypokinesia etiology, 300
imaging in, 336–337, 676–677
neck pain in, 229–230
parkinsonism from, 307
in seizures, 56
sensory loss in, 284
upper extremity pain and paresthesias after,
247
vertigo after, 157, 165, 166
Trazodone
in chronic pain, 565*t*
in idiopathic insomnia, 614
in multiple sclerosis, 443
Tremor, 294, 457–458
in acute confusional state, 6
in parkinsonism, 302–303, 449
referral for, 298
in valproic acid side effects, 428
Trendelenburg gait, 272
Triamterene, 528
Triazolam, 614*t*
Trichinosis, 526, 527
Trichloroethylene, 137
Tricyclic antidepressant(s)
in central pain syndrome in spinal cord injury,
507
in chronic pain, 565*t*, 565–566
in HIV distal sensory neuropathy, 483
in HIV encephalopathy, 481–482
in migraine headaches, 556
in pregnancy, 648*t*
myoclonus from, 297
in narcolepsy, 617*t*, 617–618
in non–rapid eye movement sleep disorders,
620
in parasomnias, 620
in reflex sympathetic dystrophy, 574
Trifluoperazine, 567*t*
Trigeminal nerve, 132–133, 133*f*
in cutaneous sensation from face, 282–283
gasserian ganglion and, 135*f*, 136*t*
neuralgia of. *See* Trigeminal neuralgia (TN)
sensory neuropathy of, 136, 137
tumors of, 136
Trigeminal neuralgia (TN), 142–143
headaches in, 214
in multiple sclerosis, 443
referral for, 145
Trigger zone
facial pain and, 142
in multiple sclerosis tonic spasms, 444
Trihexyphenidyl (Artane), 450, 450*t*
Trimethadione, teratogenicity of, 644
Trimethobenzamide (Tigan), 633*t*, 646*t*
Trimethoprim-sulfamethoxazole
in *Nocardia asteroides* infections in AIDS,
594
in toxoplasmosis in AIDS, 489
Trochlear nerve lesions, diplopia in, 124
Tropia, cover test for, 125
Trunk, sensory loss in, 286–288
TS (Tourette's syndrome), 295–296, 454–455
in child, 360
Tuberculosis
in AIDS, 493–494
in meningitis, 477, 659
Tuberous sclerosis in child, 363
Tumor(s). *See also* Neoplasm(s)
in ataxia in child, 359